DON'T GO SHOPPING FOR HAIR-CARE PRODUCTS WITHOUT ME

Over 4,000 products reviewed,
plus the latest hair-care information

PAULA BEGOUN

Contributing Author: Bryan Barron
Editors: Sigrid Asmus, John Hopper, Jennifer Forbes Provo,
   Stephanie Parsons
Art Direction, Cover Design, and Typography: Erin Smith Bloom,
   Beginning Press
Printing: Publishers Book Services, Inc.
Research Director: Kate Mee
Research Assistant: Lauren Graham

Copyright © 2004, Paula Begoun
Publisher:
   Beginning Press
   13075 Gateway Drive, Suite 160
   Seattle, Washington 98168

1st Edition Printing January 1995
2nd Edition Printing January 2000
3rd Edition Printing September 2004

ISBN   187798831-6
        10 9 8 7 6 5 4 3 2 1

This book is distributed to the United States book trade by:
Publishers Group West
1700 Fourth Street
Berkeley, California 94710
(510) 528-1444

And to the Canadian book trade by:
Raincoast Books Limited
9050 Shaughnessy Street
Vancouver, British Columbia, V6P 6E5 CANADA
(604) 633-5714

STAY UPDATED WITH PAULA'S WEB SITE
www.CosmeticsCop.com

Beauty Bulletin

Keep up with the latest new product reviews, Paula's Choice specials, and "Dear Paula" Q&As that cover everything from cosmetic surgery and wrinkles to the latest innovations in skin and hair care.

Specials
Find out about exclusive savings each month!

Learn
Check out product reviews, read "Dear Paula" letters, and learn how to best take care of your skin. You'll find pages and pages of free information, what's fact and what's fiction, beauty shortcuts, and much more.

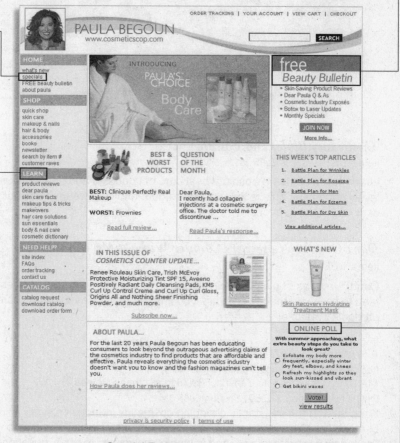

Special Features
Free reviews of monthly Best and Worst Products and intriguing "Dear Paula" questions.

Online Poll
Cast your vote in our fun and informative bi-weekly polls.

ALSO BY PAULA BEGOUN...

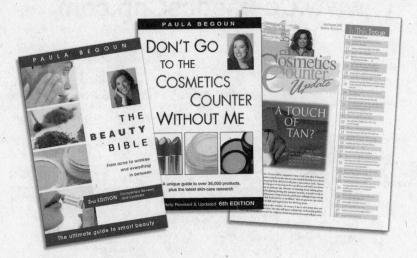

The Beauty Bible, 2nd Edition

Item # BB2 $18.95 US

Learn how to take the absolute best care of your skin and apply makeup flaw-
lessly and easily. This is the most up-to-date and comprehensive book on skin
care and makeup ever.

Don't Go to the Cosmetics Counter Without Me, 6th Edition

Item # DG6 $27.95 US

Candid reviews of over 30,000 specific products from almost 250 lines! Guaranteed to save you money and help you find the best skin-care and cosmetic
products available.

Cosmetics Counter Update Newsletter

Item # SUB, 1-year subscription (6 issues)
$18.75 to U.S., $26.25 to Canada, $33.75 to all other countries
Online subscription $12.50 (all countries)
Keep up with the constantly changing cosmetics industry. In every issue of Paula's
bi-monthly newsletter, read the latest evaluations of new cosmetics and hair-care
lines, new product reviews, and valuable answers to readers' questions.

---

(800) 831-4088 (U.S. and Canada) • **www.CosmeticsCop.com**

Beginning Press • 13075 Gateway Drive, Suite 160 • Seattle, WA 98168

PUBLISHER'S DISCLAIMER

The intent of this book is to present the author's ideas and perceptions about the marketing, selling, and use of hair-care products. The author's sole purpose is to present consumer information and advice regarding the purchase of hair-care products. The information and recommendations presented strictly reflect the author's opinions, perceptions, and knowledge about the subject and products mentioned. Some women may find success with a particular product that is not recommended or even mentioned in this book, or they may be partial to hair-care products the author has reviewed negatively. It is everyone's inalienable right to judge products by their own criteria and to disagree with the author.

More importantly, because everyone's hair, scalp, and skin can, and probably will, react to an external stimulus at some time, any product could cause a negative reaction on skin at one time or another. If you develop skin sensitivity or hair problems from using a hair-care product, stop using it immediately and consult your physician. If you need medical advice about your hair or scalp, it is best to consult a dermatologist.

ACKNOWLEDGMENTS

I have written the words that follow about Bryan Barron, my co-writer, and Kate Mee, my research director, before. They are more true than ever and I want to sing their praises once again with the same message: There are no words that can adequately express the challenge and commitment required to write a book of this scope and nature. The energy and resourcefulness needed to research, compile, review, write, and edit a book of this scope is an almost endless undertaking. If it were not for my co-writer Bryan Barron and research director Kate Mee, this book would not have been possible. Their perseverance and devotion to completing the project go beyond anything I could have hoped for. Not only did they meet deadline after deadline, they did it with an accuracy and exactness that exceeded my every expectation. Bryan and Kate bring new meaning to the concepts of proficiency and integrity. I am blessed to have these two people in my life. Without their feedback, patience, and contributions, this book would have been a very good idea, but an absolutely unconquerable task.

TABLE OF CONTENTS

CHAPTER FOUR—HAIR-CARE FORMULATIONS

CHAPTER FIVE—HAIR PROBLEMS VERSUS SCALP PROBLEMS

CHAPTER SIX—HAIR OF A DIFFERENT COLOR

CHAPTER SEVEN—PERMS AND RELAXERS

CHAPTER EIGHT—FOR WOMEN OF COLOR

CHAPTER NINE—STYLING HAIR

CHAPTER TEN—PRODUCT REVIEWS

CHAPTER 11—THE BEST PRODUCTS

APPENDIX

About the Author

Paula Begoun is the author of several best-selling books on the cosmetics industry. Her first book, *Blue Eyeshadow Should Be Illegal*, was published in 1985, and has had more than two dozen reprints and four separate revised editions. In 1992, Paula wrote the first edition of *Don't Go to the Cosmetics Counter Without Me*, now in its sixth edition. In 1995, she wrote the first edition of *Don't Go Shopping for Hair-Care Products Without Me*, and in 1997 she wrote *The Beauty Bible*, now in its second edition. Altogether, Ms. Begoun has sold more than 2.5 million copies of her books. She is also a syndicated columnist with Knight Ridder News Tribune Service and her newspaper column, Dear Paula, appears in newspapers across the country.

Over the years Paula has become a nationally recognized consumer expert on the topics of cosmetics and skin care, appearing on hundreds of national and local talk shows and news programs, including *The Today Show*, *20/20*, *Dateline NBC*, *The Early Show* on CBS, ABC's *Primetime*, *Oprah*, *The View*, and repeat appearances on CNN.

Using the information and knowledge she has gained from more than 20 years of experience working in the cosmetics industry and years of study; extensive research of medical journals and cosmetics industry magazines; and comprehensive personal interviews with dermatologists, oncologists, cosmetics chemists, and cosmetic ingredient manufacturers, Paula analyzes and evaluates the cosmetics industry and the products they sell. In an entertaining and compelling style, Paula reviews products, clarifies formulation similarities and differences, ascertains what skin or hair needs to function optimally, and explains how products can be harmful or helpful to skin and hair.

In 1995 Paula launched her Web site, www.cosmeticscop.com. Hundreds of articles and continuing product reviews are featured on this valuable, in-depth, and information-rich site. Paula also publishes a bimonthly subscription newsletter, *Cosmetics Counter Update*, and her free bi-weekly *Beauty Bulletin* is also available. These lively and informative news sources are enjoyed by hundreds of thousands of women the world over.

CHAPTER ONE

Don't Go Shopping for Hair-Care Products Without Me

GETTING BEYOND THE HYPE

Over the years, my books, newspaper columns, and newsletters have been based strictly on my earnest desire to get beyond the hype and chicanery of the cosmetics industry and to provide straightforward information that a consumer can really use to look and feel more beautiful.

Though I have studied many aspects of the cosmetics and hair-care industry over the past 20 years, I am not a cosmetics chemist, a doctor, or a scientist. My expertise is—just like the expertise of many other consumer reporters who cover a wide variety of topics, from food to cars to toys—based on extensive research in the area about which I am writing. What makes my situation unique is that I also have years of personal experience working as a professional makeup artist and aesthetician, along with extensive work with hairstylists and hair-care formulators.

Using my reporting background to continually and extensively research the cosmetics and hair-care industry, I base all my comments on comprehensive interviews with dermatologists, oncologists, chemists, and cosmetic and hair-care ingredient manufacturers and on information I've gleaned from industry magazines and medical journals. I constantly review scientific abstracts and studies. I do not capriciously or abruptly draw conclusions. Everything I report is supported by studies and information from experts in the field. Naturally, there are many who disagree with my assertions, and I do my best to present other points of view whenever I can. However, I assure you that a great number of people in the industry agree with my conclusions, even if they can't do so publicly.

In many ways, I am surprised that reviewing, researching, investigating, and questioning the beauty industry is what I do for a living. But a direct course of action and purpose has led me since 1978, when I started working in the beauty industry, as I've tried to uncover the truth inside the bottles and behind the sales pitches of the skin-care, makeup, and hair-care industry.

The demand from consumers to know what works and what doesn't has grown since I wrote my first book back in 1985, primarily because the industry itself has grown—to monstrous proportions. The number of new product lines emerging every day is sheer madness. Between the Internet, infomercials, multilevel direct-marketing lines, home shopping network lines, new lines at the department stores and drugstores, and the endless parade of new product launches from existing lines, it turns out that the first and second editions of this book were only the beginning.

SIMPLE BUT EFFECTIVE

The hair-care industry has gone through some major changes over the years. In many ways, it has gotten more complicated as the research into hair care has increased and become more technical and specific. But on the other hand, in many ways it has stayed the same, and remains truly far more mundane and repetitive than any part of the makeup or skin-care industry. It turns out that there are only so many ingredients that can clean hair, only so many that can cling to hair and condition it, and even fewer ingredients that can keep hair in place during and after styling. When it comes to skin-care or makeup formulations, a cosmetics chemist can choose from literally thousands of ingredients that can have a positive impact on the skin. In comparison, thanks to the differences between skin and hair, there are only a handful of effective ingredients available to a hair-care chemist. In some ways that makes the job of analyzing hair-care products far easier than analyzing skin-care or makeup products.

On the other hand, because hairstyling is such a core beauty issue for most women and the variables around hairstyles and preferences are so vast, it makes it that much more important—and difficult—to separate the hype and hyperbole from the honesty. We all want to have perfect hair and it must be that next product that will give us what we want!

My goal with this edition of *Don't Go Shopping for Hair-Care Products Without Me* is to examine, evaluate, and clarify all the new hair-care data and research in an effort to help each person choose the best products and services possible for his or her specific needs.

HOW I DO MY REVIEWS

If you've ever felt uncertain about a hair-care product, or didn't have the time, energy, or knowledge about ingredients to figure out which shampoos wouldn't build up on your hair, which conditioners would really make coarse, dry hair feel silky and soft, which hairsprays didn't create helmet hair, which gels didn't flake or leave a sticky residue, whether or not you can repair or restore hair, or wondered if any of the claims on the labels were true, I hope this book will answer those questions for you. I've also included a summary chapter of best finds and buys to create the best look for your hair type—but try not to jump to that section first. It is important to read the chapters about formulation and hair facts so you have a better understanding about what is genuinely possible for your hair and what are marketing fictions and deceptions. It is also important for you to read the individual product reviews so you understand *exactly* what you are buying. I might recommend 20 good shampoos for thin or fine hair, but each one might be good for a different reason.

In the product review chapter of this book (Chapter Ten, "Product Reviews"), each product is described in terms of its reliability, value, performance, effect, and feel. For every category of product—shampoos, conditioners, treatments, dandruff shampoos, hair serums, pomades, gels, mousses, hairsprays, and specialty products—I established specific criteria (I explain those criteria at length in Chapter Ten, "Product Reviews"), and I use those criteria to evaluate the products. For example, according to my criteria, a shampoo for someone with an oily scalp should be gentle but effective, and contain no conditioning agents (which can add emollients or oils to the scalp), minimal detangling agents (which can build up on the hair and make it feel limp and heavy because they add to the weight of the oil already on your scalp), and no irritants (which can cause an itchy, dry scalp). Conditioners for coarse, dry hair should leave a soft, smooth feel on the hair with no heavy or greasy after-feel. Hairsprays that claim they provide a firm hold should do just that, but not feel sticky, flake, or be hard to brush through. I relied on my 15 years of researching the hair-care industry, myriad interviews with hair-care chemists, and discussions with hundreds of hair-care professionals to establish guidelines for the quality of every product type.

Many elements of what a product would do for hair care were evaluated by analyzing the ingredient list and comparing it to the claims made about the product. If a shampoo claims it won't strip hair color or that it is good for sensitive skin, but it contains ingredients that break down the hair shaft or irritate the scalp, it would be rated poorly and not be recommended. If a conditioner claims it can hydrate hair, then it should contain ingredients that can keep moisture in the hair and not dehydrate it with drying ingredients. If a conditioner claims it can make hair feel silky, it should contain ingredients that create that effect. If a gel or mousse claims it can hold hair in place without feeling sticky, it shouldn't contain sticky ingredients. In addition, I have made a point of challenging the inflated claims made about such ingredients as herbal extracts, botanicals, seaweed extracts, placenta extracts, vitamins, minerals, and other overly hyped ingredients. Until a company provides substantiated or peer-reviewed research to support its claims, you should treat their claims as nothing more than snake oil and marketing artifice. I applied this standard of substantiation to all product types.

While ingredient evaluations played a large part in my assessments, I also purchased thousands of dollars' worth of hair-care products (all of the styling products) selected from each of the lines reviewed in this book. Each product was applied to hair and examined for texture and performance. If a product said it could make hair feel thicker and fuller but it didn't, then it was not recommended for that purpose. If a product said it wouldn't leave a film or sticky residue but it did, then it was not recommended, and so on.

HAIR-CARE CHEMISTS

Although I complain profusely about the way hair-care companies invent or twist the truth about their products and about some cosmetics companies not granting me interviews, I give my heartfelt thanks to the companies that actually do provide me with information and interviews. I know this might seem like a strange departure, given that I don't always agree with the information that I'm sent or told, but these resources are always welcomed and appreciated more than I can say. It is my intent to provide the best information possible, and whenever I can see the cosmetics and hair-care industry's point of view, my reporting is that much more accurate. Granted, it often fans the flames of my ire about false claims and misleading information, but it also helps me tell consumers when and where there are wonderful products.

And there are wonderful, exquisite products out there. I know I tend to emphasize the negative when it comes to crazy claims, exorbitant prices, and poor quality, but I also want to be sure to celebrate and extol the boundless parade of superlative products. I am hardly anti-hair care! Far from it. I am in awe of how well hair-care products work. Where would we be without the brilliant work of the hair-care chemists who make the exquisite products we use? It is because of their astonishing skill that we have shampoos that effortlessly clean hair, conditioners that make hair easy to comb and silky to touch, dyes that can change hair color in a matter of minutes, perms that can alter the very structure of hair, changing curly manes into straight tresses and vice versa—and of course, glorious styling products that keep hair exactly where you want it to be and looking beautiful.

I want to sincerely thank all the companies that have taken the time to provide me with so much information for this book, as well as for my newsletter and my other books. We often don't see eye to eye, yet despite our differences, more companies than ever have been generous and forthcoming with information and products.

The following hair-care companies were exceptionally helpful, either providing information about their products or actually sending us their entire line of products for review: African Pride, American Crew, Aussie, Avon, Back to Basics, bain de terre, Binge by (pH) Beauty Labs, Biosilk, Clairol, d:fi, Daily Defense, Folligen, Frederic Fekkai, Free & Clear, Giga Hold, Graham Webb, Hayashi, ICE, Inner Science, ION, ISO, j.f. lazartigue, Jheri Redding, John Freida, Joico, Kenra, Lange, Mop (Modern Organic Products), Neutrogena, Nexxus, Ouidad, Pantene Pro-V, Paul Mitchell, Philip B., Physique, Phyto, Proxiphen & Nano, Pureology, Quantum, Redken, Revlon Realistic, Rusk, Salon Grafix, Scruples, Sexy Hair Concepts, Sukesha, Terax, and TIGI.

I also want to thank all the hair-care chemists everywhere who strive to produce better and better products that continue to make the beauty industry so incredibly beautiful. I also want to ask those same chemists to do the best they can, whenever they can, to combat the insane marketing departments they have to work with. I know most of you don't believe even a fraction of what the advertisements, salespeople, infomercial hucksters, or editorials in fashion magazines say about the products you create. Your work is rooted in science, not hyperbole. I know this is a risky business. After all, creating products that no one buys is not going to get anyone a promotion, and the marketing department knows all too well what women love to hear, no matter how ridiculous it may be. But please try anyway, just to put a bit of fresh air into an otherwise very hazy and sometimes polluted business.

INDUSTRY STATISTICS

Collectively, United States consumers spend over $7 billion a year on our hair, whether it is on shampoos (about $1.5 billion) or conditioners (about $900 million). We also spend a lot of money getting our hair cut, styled, permed, or dyed at the salon—in 2002 we spent over $55 billion at salons for services and products combined (Sources: www.klinegroup.com; *The Green Book Directory*, 2003).

We also spent about $700 million on hairsprays, $600 million on gels and mousses, $2 billion on hair-coloring products, $150 million on men's hair products, and $400 million on permanents and hair straighteners. Perhaps the most astounding finding is that an estimated 48% of American women over the age of 25 color their hair. At least 85% of the technical work being done in salons concerns changing hair color or concealing gray, while only 15% is in the realm of providing permanent waves. Salons that cater to African-American clientele consistently perform permanent waves—for straightening hair—for approximately 85% of their customers, with an increasing number having braiding done. From any angle, it's obvious we have a lot invested in trying to make our hair look good (Sources: www.marketresource.com; www.packagedfacts.com; and www.klinegroup.com).

Statistics may not have much to do with your own personal hair-care needs, but they tell companies how to approach their marketing campaigns, and that affects how you spend money. It can cost millions of dollars to introduce a new product to consumers, and it's how a product is presented that determines its success or failure. Because we are coloring our hair more and more frequently, those of us who never had damaged hair are now battling frizzies, split ends, and "grow-out." These problems, in turn, require new products and new guarantees. Many current product innovations are aimed directly at the needs of the newly graying consumer. Aging baby boomers (I'm in this category, too) need to believe that the products they are buying will protect their hair, prevent fading, slow grow-out, and repair the damage of the chemical assaults.

The explosion of styling products filling shelf space in salons and drugstores is directly related to the diverse range of hairstyles adorning movie stars and models month after month in fashion and celebrity magazines. From flat-ironed straight hair to curly tresses, spiked ends, carefully arranged messy dos, or swept-up chignons, the novelties abound, and those who desire to reproduce those styles for themselves require very specific products.

To say that statistics drive product marketing is an understatement. Another clear example is the fact that approximately 40% of women in the United States complain that their hair is too fine, too limp, or too flat. Full, thick hair is the order of the day, and women feel it acutely when their hair won't behave accordingly. Cosmetics and hair-care companies are very aware of this huge number because it represents such a vast segment of the hair-care product–buying population. The result? Scads of lines and product types promising thicker, fuller hair.

No matter what the claim may be, promising some kind of miracle for your hair is what this industry is all about. Hair-care marketing is filled with just the right buzz words to convince women their hair will be repaired, rehydrated, strengthened, nourished, freed of split ends, energized, protected from rain and humidity, and even able to grow anew, along with everything else in between. Yet relying on marketing won't help your hair because most of the claims by hair-care companies just aren't possible.

DETANGLING AN INDUSTRY

Because there are many who will take issue with the information in this book, let me state from the very beginning: I have nothing against hairstylists. In fact, just the opposite is true. I unconditionally encourage women to put their trust, tresses, and money in the hands of a talented and skilled hairstylist. In comparison to buying hair-care products, it is almost impossible to waste money on a good stylist whose work you admire. Because I believe in the irrefutable value of a good stylist, I want to make it abundantly clear that this book does not in any way, shape, or form try to replace the expert service performed by an accomplished hairstylist.

I also want to state up front how wonderful I think many hair-care products really are. You will find a plethora of products that are nothing less than modern-day sensations. Shampoos that efficiently and gently clean hair, conditioners that make hair feel like new, dyes that change color in an instant and can actually make hair feel better, perms that alter the hair's very structure, and styling products that allow you to keep just about any shape you can coerce out of your clean, conditioned, dyed, and styled locks. Amazing! Simply amazing!

While I frequently find skin-care and makeup products that are actually harmful to skin, I (gladly) can't often say the same about hair-care products. There are far more great hair-care products than there are bad ones, and it's actually difficult to find really bad or harmful hair-care products. Yes, there are definitely some that can cause an itchy scalp; dry, flyaway hair; allergic reactions; and skin irritation; or that can't remotely live up to their claims. And (unfortunately) there are some, albeit very few, that can be exceedingly disappointing to the consumer. But more often than not, hair-care products perform well and live up to at least some aspect of the claim on the label.

After all this praise, you may be wondering why, if I have such deep respect for hairstylists and hair-care formulations, I would write a book suggesting that women should only go shopping for hair-care products with me instead of trusting the recommendations of their hairstylist or the companies that make hair-care products. The answer is simple. **You can't rely on the information you receive from your hairstylist or from the hair-care company that makes the products you are thinking of buying.**

The fundamental fact is that most hair-care companies don't tell you the truth about their products! The majority make bogus or misleading claims about what their products can and can't do, and that can hurt your hair as well as your pocketbook. Because of this industry-wide deceit, it is essential for every consumer to have objective information so we don't waste our money or damage our hair.

What about hairstylists? After conducting hundreds of interviews, I found that most hairstylists were not intentionally trying to be misleading or purposely giving out erroneous information about hair-care products. Quite the contrary; they seemed to earnestly believe what they were saying regarding what they knew about hair. Yet, more often than not, their information was wrong or ambiguous. (I untangle some of these myths at length throughout the book.) In fact, the only knowledge most hairstylists have about hair-care products comes directly from the hair-care companies whose products they are selling. Therein lies the problem, and I mean a really big problem. **Hairstylists are being trained by the very companies that make the false or misleading claims about their hair-care products.** Hairstylists don't perform complicated chemical analyses or peruse research findings; rather, they echo the falsehoods they've been taught by the companies who provide their training, namely, those designers or salon lines that come up with a wide variety of specious justifications to warrant their overinflated prices. Even the best hairstylists can be vulnerable to a hair-care company's marketing pitch, or fall for the numerous claims made for all manner of hair-care products.

Between the advertising and the guidance from hairstylists, there isn't much accurate information available to the consumer, and fashion magazines only make things worse. Consumers must be very skeptical about what they read in fashion magazines. When you think about it, how often do you see an article in a fashion magazine that doesn't have something nice to say about a hair-care product, or about a cosmetics line that happens to be one of the advertisers? About as often as you see an overweight model, right? If an article doesn't cast a critical eye on a particular company's claims or product selection or if it buries the cautionary words in the middle of the report, be suspicious. I always love it when fashion magazines offer their lists of the "Top 100 Products Our Readers Like Best." As long as the magazine was taking the time to find out what products their readers liked best, what about the products they didn't like? There isn't a woman anywhere in the world who hasn't purchased lots of hair-care products she hated! Why not provide that information as well? Because fashion magazines can't do that!

The majority of fashion reporters have their journalistic hands tied by the demands of the companies that advertise in the publications for which they write. And there is little impetus to change things. A magazine depends on advertisers, and it is simply counterproductive to tick off such a vital source of revenue. When cosmetics companies spend thousands or millions of dollars each year advertising in a magazine, a writer for that magazine cannot be expected to criticize that company's products and remain employed. **This commingling of editorial and advertising control results in gushing "news" stories that are little more than company publicity pieces and biased product recommendations. All the news that's fit to print—as long as it's what the cosmetics industry wants the consumer to know.**

Inasmuch as I find the technical or editorial information in fashion magazines to be swayed and prejudiced by the power of the magazines' advertisers (and therefore completely unreliable), the pictorial essays regarding the latest hairstyles or hair-color trends are nothing less than brilliant. Fashion magazines are the quintessential source for fashion news and lore and should be consulted whenever the need arises for a fashion update. It is when we go beyond the pictures to the product *advertorials* (not editorials, because they are hardly independent or autonomous) that the issue gets lost. By the time you finish reading this book you will have a better understanding of just how crazy much of the hair-care information you are receiving—from many different sources—really is.

WHY HAIR IS SO IMPORTANT

Feeling and looking beautiful is a wonderful, satisfying, joyous process as well as a state of mind in which women can revel with much pleasure and reward. Yet all the delightful and beautiful possibilities can get zapped by frustration caused by poor information and broken promises. It is more than vexing to spend $20 on a lavishly hyped conditioner or $50 on a whole new range of hair-care products, or to pay anywhere from $5 (for a drugstore product) to $300 (at a high-end salon) for a new hair color or perm, only to end up with more problems than you started with and none of the changes you were hoping for.

The truth is, hair care and hairstyling are not easy. No matter how much we would like to believe otherwise, and no matter how convincingly products claim they can do the impossible with no effort, nothing could be further from the truth. Hair-care needs, conditions, and problems, from both external and internal sources, are exceedingly technical and difficult to understand. Just to begin with, there are over 100,000 hairs on your head. That's a lot of hair to take care of! Also, hair isn't stagnant; it changes from day to day, depending on the weather (particularly the humidity), month to month (hormonal activity can affect its growth), season to season (drier versus wetter months), and year to year (because hair changes radically as we get older). And then there's the scalp's complex structure and function, which depend on a whole array of factors, from genetics, hormones, health, and the environment to the products you use. Taking all this into account makes it an understatement to say that hair care is a complex and multifaceted issue.

Hair biology and physiology are indeed fundamental issues, but beyond basic good health, it's the way they affect our appearance that is of vital concern. The hair on our head is one of the first things people notice about us and, whether we like it or not, it reveals to the world where we stand in terms of beauty, fashion, and age. In our culture, attentively coifed tresses are an obligatory component of beauty. For some, that means having smooth, silky, flowing tresses; for others it can mean a precisely cut Mohawk dyed a rainbow of colors; or it can mean a voluminous mane of tightly twisted curls; or perhaps a short, neatly trimmed haircut. Whatever direction you choose, the attention your hair receives makes your product choices important.

Two other aspects of our hair complicate matters even further. The first is that we often don't like the hair we are born with; it is either too thick, too thin, too straight, too curly, too coarse, too dry, or too *something* we don't like. Altering the structure of our hair (which results from genetics) is a struggle for many. The second aspect is that hair displays the effects of time by turning gray or becoming thinner well before any of us want to see that happen. Trying to prevent or hide those changes is a preoccupation for many of us. Preventing loss, hiding gray, or making hair go against its natural predisposition is technically more complicated than all the other needs of hair care combined. But overall, the best and most effective way to truly take care of any or all of these issues is to begin with factual information, and to ignore the half-truths and misleading claims that are so prevalent in the hair-care industry.

TRUE OR FALSE

Before you buy another hair-care product, the best place to start is with some basic facts so you can better differentiate between truth and fiction when it comes to your hair. Understanding these facts before you go shopping for hair-care products, before you see another infomercial promising flawless results, before a friend introduces you to a new multilevel company selling hair-care products, or before you read another fashion magazine will give you a better perspective on what you are really buying, what the products can and can't do, whether what you are using is worth the money, and, most important, whether any of the products can actually be damaging to your hair.

Following are some of the major myths I hope to dispel for you by the time you are done reading this book:

- Expensive hair-care products are better than inexpensive ones. (VERY FALSE)
- Inexpensive hair-care products are watered down, while expensive hair-care products are more concentrated. (FALSE)
- Salon products are better than drugstore products. (FALSE)
- Natural ingredients are better than synthetic ones. (COMPLETELY FALSE)
- Silicone is bad for hair. (1,000% FALSE)
- You can repair damaged hair. (FALSE—It's not possible)
- You can protect hair from heat damage caused by blow dryers, flat irons, or curling irons. (TRUE—Somewhat possible)

- Dyeing hair isn't damaging. (FALSE)

- You can perm and color hair without causing more damage if you wait a few weeks between treatments. (FALSE)

- Dyeing hair is dangerous and can cause cancer. (FALSE—Controversial, but definitely not substantiated)

- Inexpensive hair-care products can strip hair color, expensive products won't do this. (FALSE)

- Some hair-care products can protect hair from sun damage. (FALSE)

- Sodium lauryl sulfate and other hair-care ingredients cause cancer. (FALSE)

- Cosmetic hair-care products can grow hair. (ALMOST FALSE—Cosmetics company products can't, but products from pharmaceutical companies containing FDA-approved drugs can)

Here are the facts that I will explain at length in the chapters that follow:

1. **According to the United States Food and Drug Administration (FDA) (www.fda.gov), hair-care companies get to legally mislead or indirectly lie to you.** Hair-care companies do not have to substantiate claims or prove efficacy of any kind. The only part of a hair-care product firmly regulated by the FDA is the ingredient labeling, and that is impossible for most consumers to decipher.

2. **Expensive hair-care products are not better than inexpensive ones. Women who spend more money on hair-care products do not have better hair than those with a tighter budget.** Of course, women who can afford great stylists can have great haircuts—though all women who overprocess their hair have hair like straw— no matter who the stylist is.

3. **Believing that a particular hair-care line is the best one and has all the answers for your hair doesn't make sense.** In the world of hair care, the similarities between products from all price ranges is nothing less than startling, and there are no patented secrets or exclusive ingredients that are known or available to only one company. Not to mention that many expensive lines are produced by the same companies that produce the inexpensive lines.

4. **Start reading ingredient lists and you will notice there is little to no difference between products in inexpensive lines and expensive lines.** And the fancy ingredients are often irrelevant because they are either washed, brushed, or styled off the hair.

5. **Hair-care chemists are not chained to one company, so there is no reason to believe that one company has secrets another one isn't privy to.** Plus, if the research is legitimate, it is published and accessible to everyone. Beyond that,

what appears in an ingredient list is FDA-mandated information that is (or should be) on every hair-care product being sold.

6. **We have all bought products we disliked from expensive lines, so that should dispel the belief that expensive automatically means better.** Regardless of what we empirically know to be true, the pressure from advertisements, hairstylists, and infomercials often overpowers our own knowledge. The bottom line: There are good and bad products in a wide variety of price ranges. In the realm of hair-care products, price is not an indicator of quality.

7. **There is no such thing as an all-natural hair-care product.** Even ingredients derived from natural sources such as coconut, palm trees, silk, wheat, milk, or soy do not retain their "natural" composition once they are processed and altered to be a cleansing or conditioning agent. In the cosmetics industry, there are indeed wonderful "natural" ingredients that have remarkable benefits for skin—but that's not the case for hair. Natural ingredients, particularly vitamins, minerals, and plant extracts, in and of themselves, cannot clean hair, cling to hair, or perform any function of conditioning or styling. Plus, because hair is not alive these ingredients can't function the same as they can on skin. The very notion is ludicrous. And beyond that, plenty of natural ingredients turn out to be problematic for the hair and scalp, while there are lots of synthetic ingredients you do not want to do without.

   Most of the natural ingredients included in hair-care products are there for marketing purposes only, and more often than not actually get in the way of a product's performance. It only takes a quick glance at an ingredient list to notice that names like cetrimonium bromide, quaternium-16, cocamidopropyl betaine, cocamide DEA, disodium EDTA, PVP/DMAPA acrylates copolymer, and PEG-150 pentaerythrityl tetrastearate are not natural in the least, although they and hundreds of other "unnatural" ingredients are the backbone of every hair-care product you will ever use, even those products that assert their natural content.

   What is most insidious is the plethora of companies on the Internet making claims about "all-natural," extolling what their products don't contain, but then never providing a complete ingredient list. Do not buy a product unless you know every ingredient that's in it. If an ingredient list contains only plants, it's always a lie!

8. **There are no miracle ingredients that can cure your hair-care woes.** It's a great dream, but there are no patented or exclusive marvels that separate one product's performance from another.

9. **When a model's hair looks beautiful in an ad or on television, it is never simply because of the products being advertised.** Instead, what you see is due to the model's genetics, hours of diligent work by a hairstylist, great lighting, the

photographer's talent, and lots of digital touch-ups before the picture is ever shown to the public.

10. **What does make a great deal of difference to your hair is the kind of styling tools you use and how you use them.** Learning good styling techniques is a far better use of your time than spending endless hours shopping for hair-care products.

11. **There are no hair-care products that can repair, fix, correct, restructure, reform, change, reconstruct, restore, rebuild, or alter damaged hair.** Hair is dead (I will remind you of that fact frequently throughout this book), so it cannot be repaired or permanently reverted back to normal in any way. You can no more mend a hair strand than you can mend a dead leaf or soften a rock.

12. **There are no hair-care products that can completely protect hair from heat damage.** Hairstyling tools can get as hot as 350ºF, transferring about 200ºF to the hair. You cannot prevent that kind of heat from causing some harm to hair. Could you imagine protecting skin from that kind of heat with a hair-care product? If you can't do it for skin, you can't do it for hair.

13. **Advertising is a one-sided game of beautiful photography and overblown claims.** It is very easy to be seduced by new advertising, new products, or a new product line from the hair-care industry, but "new" does not automatically mean better, and the ads never make any product sound bad.

14. **Sun is damaging for hair.** There is no way around that. Sun causes hair color to fade, breaks down the hair shaft, and actually degrades the structure of hair.

15. **There are no products that can protect hair from sun damage.** The FDA does not allow hair-care products to have a Sun Protection Factor (SPF) rating because there is no reliable or consistent way to keep the necessary protective ingredients (which can be kept on and do protect skin) attached to the hair shaft (Source: www.fda.gov). Rinsing, styling, and brushing hair removes or degrades sunscreen ingredients so the protection is either nonexistent or short-lived. The only sure-fire way to protect your hair from sun damage is to wear a hat! Until there is a way to keep these ingredients on the hair and assign an SPF rating for hair-care products, the claims about sun protection are fraudulent and completely unreliable.

16. **There are no cosmetic hair-care products that can make hair grow.** None, period! However, this does not include Rogaine (minoxidil), which is not a cosmetic; it is a pharmaceutical that has met radically different FDA testing and substantiation requirements. Keep in mind, however, that hair-care products that do not contain pharmaceutical or over-the-counter regulated drug ingredients can wantonly make claims without meeting a requirement of proof, and they don't need to substantiate either their effectiveness or safety.

17. **Please think twice (or change channels) when buying products from an infomercial or from a home shopping network.** These are long, overextended ads, nothing more. No matter how wonderful they make their products sound, you are receiving a bizarrely one-sided point of view. Each "show" is more glorious and spectacular than the next, and what you choose to believe is based on how seduced you are by the claims and the enthusiastic responses of the participants. Clearly, the producers of the infomercial are not going to include people who have a contradictory or dissenting point of view.

18. **Terms and phrases like "hypoallergenic," "dermatologist tested," "exclusive formula," "all natural," and other such unsupported generalizations about a product are simply untrue.** There are no FDA guidelines or specifications for any of these marketing claims or terms. As I will remind you throughout this edition, according to the FDA, hair-care companies do not have to prove their claims.

MORE MYTH-BUSTING

Being misled or lied to can result in you not only wasting money but also choosing the wrong products for your hair type. I want to address a few hair-care myths that most women, maybe yourself included, have accepted without question. Let's separate fact from fiction.

MYTH: You need to change or alternate shampoos because your hair adapts to them. The hair and scalp can't "adapt to" shampoos. Hair is dead, so it cannot adapt or become used to something. What can happen is that the conditioners, emollients, and slip agents (such as silicones) found in many shampoos can build up on the hair shaft over time, making the hair limp, sticky, or dull. That buildup is easily washed away with a different shampoo that does not contain those specific ingredients. Then the cycle starts all over again when you switch back and the original shampoo's conditioning and styling agents start building up.

Shampoos containing conditioning agents, emollients, and slip agents are formulated in such a way that the detergent cleansers lift the dirt and oil away from the hair, allowing the water to rinse them away while leaving the conditioners behind. Cosmetics chemists do a great job devising shampoos that clean the hair but allow the conditioners to stay put despite the pressure of cascading water as you rinse. It is the nature of these shampoos that they do not remove the very conditioners they contain because the conditioners in them are designed to do just the opposite—stick to the hair. When you change to a new shampoo without conditioning agents, that new formulation can cut through the previous shampoo's conditioning agents, leaving the hair feeling new and full again. If the new shampoo contains different conditioning or styling agents, they will leave their traces, and the buildup cycle will begin again, though at first your hair may appear renewed and free of buildup. It is this subtle process that leads to the belief that hair adapts to shampoo.

Changing shampoos is a simple way to remove the buildup, especially if you choose a shampoo that contains no conditioning agents. I should mention that not all cosmetics chemists agree with this theory about changing shampoos. Some believe it is more a factor of perception or changes in weather conditions than a result of the products you are using. But given consumer feedback and the information I've received, I still favor the idea that changing shampoos makes sense.

MYTH: You need to change or alternate conditioners because your hair adapts to them. The truth about this one is pretty much the same as it is for the shampoos. Hair *can't* adapt to conditioners, but conditioners *can* build up on the hair. That's especially true for conditioners that are formulated specifically for damaged, chemically treated, or dry hair and are used in conjunction with shampoos that also contain conditioning agents. In that case, the shampoo with conditioners might not wash out the buildup every time you shampoo, and repeated use of the same conditioner and the same shampoo with conditioners can impart a sticky, heavy, or dull appearance to the hair. But you don't need to throw out the conditioner; you just need to alternate it with a shampoo that does not contain conditioning agents, and that will cut through the residue and thoroughly clean the hair.

The same is true for leave-in conditioners. Because they aren't rinsed off, the ingredients tend to cling better to hair and are somewhat more difficult to shampoo out, especially if you're also using a shampoo that contains conditioning and film-forming agents.

MYTH: I know a particular shampoo will be gentle enough for my dry, fine hair because it says on the label I can wash my face with it. Being able to use a product on your face doesn't say anything about how well it will clean your hair or whether it is really gentle. Some facial cleansers contain the exact same detergent cleansing agents as shampoos (facial cleansers just omit the ingredients that produce copious lather). But simply because a shampoo can be used on the face doesn't mean it should be used on your hair. Besides, facial cleansers that contain the same menu of ingredients as a shampoo are quite often drying for the face. And finally, a too gentle (meaning mild) shampoo might not be able to clean the buildup that can result from conditioners and styling products.

MYTH: You need to lather twice to make hair look and feel clean. Absolutely not! If anything, overwashing the hair can dry it out, and the more you handle your hair, the greater the chance of roughing up and damaging the cuticle. Shampooing the hair twice may be necessary for women who use a lot of styling products, who favor heavy or waxy conditioners, or who have extremely (and I mean *extremely*) oily hair, but that's it. In those situations, the ingredients and oils can be hard to break down, and a second lather may be just what it takes to get through the debris. But beyond that, the only reason hair-care companies suggest shampooing twice is to sell more shampoo!

MYTH: Shampooing oily hair can make it oilier. Oil production is a process affected by our hormones, which generate signals that trigger oil glands to be overproductive, and there is literally nothing you can do from the outside to stop or change that activity.

It would be great if you could use products for the face that absorb oil, but unfortunately, they cause the hair to feel heavy or limp.

MYTH: My hair is oily, so it is best if I wash with a shampoo designed for my hair type. Shampoos for oily hair often contain detergent agents that are stronger than is really necessary for an oily scalp or hair condition. These strong detergent agents can dry out the hair, and that can add to your problems. Of late, shampoos for oily hair have also been including ingredients such as peppermint, menthol, balm mint, eucalyptus, orange, grapefruit, and lemon, none of which has any effect on oil production or any real benefit for hair. However, these are all serious skin irritants and they can cause an itchy, flaky scalp or other skin irritation or allergic reactions.

MYTH: Everyone needs to use a conditioner. The only reason to use a conditioner is if your hair is dry, you have difficulty getting a comb through it, your scalp is dry, or you use styling tools, such as blow dryers and curling irons. If none of the above is true and your hair naturally feels soft and smooth, then there is very little reason for you to use a conditioner. Contrary to what advertisements would have you believe, conditioners are not automatically necessary for all heads of hair. In fact, using a conditioner when you don't need one can make your hair limp, heavy, and difficult to style.

PARTIAL MYTH: The longer you leave a conditioner on, the more effective it will be. Depending on the ingredients, this is entirely true. There is plenty of evidence that certain ingredients can penetrate the cuticle better when left on longer. However, that doesn't mean the ingredients will be better able to repair damage or restructure the hair shaft.

There is discussion in the world of hair care about the permeability of the hair shaft. Can ingredients penetrate beyond the cuticle into the hair shaft? Given that hair can absorb water, why not other compounds? If hair wasn't permeable, then humidity couldn't get in and change the hair's appearance, hair dyes couldn't get inside and become permanent, and perms wouldn't change the curl status of the hair. The question that leaves experts arguing is, how much benefit is derived from the absorption of such ingredients as amino acids, panthenols, biotin, and the like?

One thing we can be fairly certain of is that these microscopically tiny ingredients are absorbed to some degree. However, this absorption occurs in a laboratory setting, using high concentrations and pure forms of these ingredients. In contrast, given that the amount of these ingredients included in shampoos and conditioners is negligible and that the products are rinsed off or manipulated during the styling process, and then exposed to the elements, it is almost impossible for them to have any effect on hair whatsoever. Besides, what most of us already know from our own experience is that even the most expensive hair products in the world won't change damaged hair, and those lovely ingredients are gone the next time you wash your hair.

MYTH: I have oily hair, so it is best for me to avoid conditioners. If you have oily hair it is because your scalp is producing oil and the oil accumulation is making its way down the hair shaft. Other than that, hair itself is not oily, which means the hair farthest away from your scalp can be dry or damaged. In that case, you do need a conditioner, but you should use it on the ends only and be careful not to get it anywhere near the scalp.

MYTH: Hair needs to be squeaky in order to tell if it's really clean. All the experts I've interviewed said hair doesn't have to squeak to be clean. The reason hair squeaks is because of calcium deposits left on the hair by hard water, not because it's clean. It turns out that most households in the United States have hard water. We've come to associate squeaky hair with being clean because when the hair doesn't squeak it can mean detergent residue has been left on the hair. Most women feel it's important to hear their hair resonate through their fingers after washing for it to be really clean. I'm torn between what the experts tell me, what I personally feel, and what other women repeatedly tell me. When I can't hear my hair squeak after I wash and condition it, I almost always feel it doesn't style as well or look as full.

Because of the disparity between scientific evidence and what I've heard from women and hairstylists, I would say this is a personal decision, or at least one you have to experiment with for yourself. Nonetheless, because most people live in hard-water areas, and the expense of putting in a water softener system can be steep, your hair might squeak whether you like it or not.

MYTH: Lots of lather means the hair is getting thoroughly clean. I know this may be shocking—it still shocks me—but lather is unrelated to the cleaning ingredients in shampoo. Lather ingredients are added to shampoo for the emotional appeal they provide. They have no effect on cleaning. Why do we associate the amount of lather with clean hair? Because the amount of lather you get while shampooing is directly affected by the amount of oil and debris on the hair. The more oils, conditioning agents, or styling-product residue on the hair, the less lather will be produced when you shampoo. So the hair may be clean, but the lather ingredients were deactivated by the presence of the oil and other stuff you want to wash away. That is why hair generally lathers better the second time you wash it, because it was cleaned on the first go around, and now the lather agents can foam unimpeded.

MYTH: Baby shampoos are milder and gentler, so they are the best to use for my dry scalp and dried-out ends. No way! It's true that baby shampoos do omit ingredients that can sting the eyes (to some extent), which is nice, but because they are formulated with cleansing agents that are less drying and irritating they also have less cleaning ability. Obviously, it's rare for younger children to be using styling products, applying emollient conditioners, perming or coloring their hair, overusing blow dryers or curling irons, or doing any of a number of other problematic things that adults inflict on their hair. If you want to handle adult hair issues, adult shampoos and conditioners are the only way to go.

MYTH: Brushing the hair 100 times is good for the hair. Nothing could be further from the truth! Brushing the hair roughs up the cuticle, eventually chipping it away and exposing the cortex, leaving the hair porous and frayed.

MYTH: **Even though two hair-care products list the same ingredients, they are not the same product because the quality of the ingredients varies.** Most cosmetics companies would like you to believe that you can't tell anything from reading the ingredient list, and suggest that the quality of the ingredients is what counts. Having spoken with many raw-ingredient manufacturers and cosmetics chemists from most of the major hair-care companies and contract manufacturers, I assure you that the overall quality of the ingredients is fairly consistent. There are only a small number of raw-ingredient manufacturers, and they are not in the business of producing inferior materials for companies looking for a bargain. Every time I have asked an expensive hair-care line to show me proof that their ingredients are of a better grade or quality, I'm told they can't reveal their sources. Sources aren't a secret; if they were, the ingredient manufacturers couldn't earn a living. If a company can't substantiate a claim, then they have made it up, knowing that most consumers will fall for the line and won't press for details.

MYTH: **Products within a line are designed to work together, so it is best never to mix products from other lines.** Do not assume that hair-care products from the same line are all wonderful or that all of them will be compatible with your hair. Experiment with what works best for your hair's needs, not the needs of the hair-care line selling you products.

MYTH: **Cutting your hair makes it thicker.** Cutting hair does *not* make it thicker. However, because damaged ends can feel sparse, look thin, and may lie in a fuzzy layer, cutting them off can make your hair look newly thick. And it can stay looking and feeling healthy if you don't start re-torturing the ends. Also, depending on the talent of your hairstylist, a specific hairstyle can make the hair appear thicker through layering or stacking.

MYTH: **Hair can be double-processed without causing damage, or hair can be double-processed if you wait a few weeks between treatments.** In other words, you can perm *and* color your hair at the same time or a few weeks apart and not worry about excessive decomposition of the cuticle or hair shaft. Well, nothing could be further from the truth, even though some hairstylists would like us to believe otherwise. And why shouldn't they? A perm and a color job add up to a lot of technical work, plus the intensive hair treatments the hair will require if it is to endure your fashion indulgence. Hair coloring, as well as perms or relaxers, are treatments that require an alkaline base to make a permanent change in the color or shape of the hair. That process causes the hair shaft to swell, making it more porous and damaging the cuticle. Doing that to the hair twice is twice as damaging. And because hair isn't alive, waiting won't heal it. Damaged hair cannot be repaired. Nothing can restore the hair from the problematic effects of one chemical process, let alone two.

MYTH: **You can double-process the hair if the products being used are gentle and don't contain any harmful ingredients.** If it were possible to find gentle dyes and perms I would agree with this statement, but the basic characteristics of dyes and perms (those that create lasting change to the full length of hair—until the roots start showing) mean that these products are damaging to the hair. What you have to put the hair through to change its color, cover gray, and straighten or curl it is damaging to the hair. Doing both is doubly damaging. Products often claim they will be less damaging to the hair because they don't contain peroxide or ammonia. What they don't tell you, however, is that the ingredients they use instead, which don't sound like peroxide or ammonia, do exactly the same thing to the hair as peroxide and ammonia. You may not recognize the names, but they are just as damaging.

MYTH: You can protect your hair from chemical damage by using a good conditioner or conditioning treatment before you color or perm your hair. The ingredients in dyes and perms easily penetrate past conditioning ingredients (they have to or they wouldn't be able to change your hair color or shape), and that is where the damage takes place, inside the hair shaft.

PARTIAL MYTH: The best way to make limp, thin hair full is to perm it. To some extent that's true—perming can make hair look markedly fuller—but perming the entire head, especially on small rods and on a regular basis (to keep up with grow-out), is not a viable solution if you want full hair that looks good. When perming was all the rage in the 1980s, we saw plenty of evidence of what happens when thin, fine hair gets permed on a regular basis or when small rods are used to set in curl as opposed to fullness. Hair can't easily handle repeated perms without the risk of becoming a frizzy mess. Grow-out can look terrible, and re-perming only makes matters worse. A root perm is an option (only the root area is treated with perm solution, while the rest of the hair is protected with conditioner, creams, or oils), but it takes a very savvy hairstylist to do it well.

MYTH: Taking vitamins can make hair stronger and healthier. If you started taking special vitamin supplements for your hair, it would take months for the effect, if any, to show up. Hair has to grow to be affected by a new addition to your diet. So the promise of instant hair health with a vitamin supplement is sheer nonsense. This includes taking gelatin capsules or consuming gelatin with the hope of making your hair stronger.

Additionally, there are no definitive studies indicating that taking any vitamin changes the texture or appearance of the hair. Trace minerals and drugs can show up in hair analysis after the hair is chemically broken down and treated, but that doesn't mean you would be able to detect a difference in your hair between the months you took the vitamin supplements and the months you didn't.

DOES EXPENSIVE MEAN BETTER?

The number one myth you need to come to terms with is the notion that expensive or salon hair-care products are somehow superior to their drugstore counterparts. Before I can convince you of what you probably already suspect I'm building up to, I want to explain how to separate perceptions, emotional reactions, and opinions from fact.

Many consumers feel that if they buy salon products they will achieve a "salon look" for their hair. In many ways that's a logical conclusion. Most of us know that after a salon appointment we always look better. A good hairstylist can make hair defy gravity, smooth out frizzies as if they never existed, coax previously flat, limp hair into abundant voluminous waves, and transform perfectly straight hair into winsome, natural-looking curls. We know their talent plays a large part in what they can do, but when we see those products being strategically applied we assume there must be something special inside those bottles of conditioner, jars of gel, and cans of hairspray. And since most hairstylists wince every time a client confesses to using a drugstore product instead of a salon version, it creates an image and a powerful false impression, one that is repeated time and time again. On top of all that, hairstylists' explanations of what to use and how important it is for your hair to use the best products are so convincing it is hard to see through it all. Surely a stylist who can perform magic with your hair must know all there is to know about hair-care products! All this glamour, allure, and professionalism seem to provide more than enough evidence to persuade us that there must be something exceptional about salon products. But it isn't the truth.

Another reason many women become enamored with salon products is because drugstores are just so overwhelming. At the drugstore we are presented with literally hundreds of product choices. In our bewilderment, the only differences we see are the colors of the bottles, the names we are most familiar with from advertisements, and, if we are bargain-hunting, the price tags. There is no easy way to discern the actual differences, and no one to tell us which product will do what we want and need.

At the hair salon, there is none of this confusion. Not only is the selection much smaller (most salons carry only a handful of lines, versus the dozens and dozens at large drugstores and beauty supply houses), but eager stylists and the people behind the counter are there to gush over the effectiveness of each of the products they sell. It is important to recognize that your hairstylists' recommendations are most likely influenced more by the commission they receive for selling the products than they are by whether or not they truly like them. I have interviewed many hairstylists who confided that they prefer products purchased at the drugstore or lines their salon doesn't sell, but that they were required to promote (and use on their clients) the products sold by the salon.

Ultimately, there is also the issue of prestige. A stylist who charges $60 to $150 for a haircut and $80 to $200 for a hair color service, but recommends Citre Shine Shampoo at $5 for 12 ounces or L'Oreal's Vive Color-Care conditioner at $3.99 for 13 ounces seems to be doing something contradictory or bad for your hair. Whether or not the drugstore product is better is irrelevant because it just doesn't carry the distinction and élan of the salon lines. Forget the fact that most of the more expensive products are either made by the same companies that make the less expensive products, or that the same basic contract manufacturer uses the same ingredients to make many salon lines as well as many of the drugstore lines. Think about the fact that L'Oreal owns Redken, Matrix, Kerastase, Softsheen Carson, and Garnier Fructis; and that Proctor & Gamble owns Aussie, Clairol, Infusium 23, Pantene, Thermacare, Physique, Sebastian, and Wella? How does that figure into the equation?

With all this status pressure and the stylist's image at stake, it's a wonder that women ever deign or dare to buy hair-care products from the drugstore. How could drugstore products even begin to compete with the salon setting and its influence on us? Often, they can't—despite their quality—and that's where our emotions get in the way of reality.

It is true that good products can help generate a change in your hair and make it look better, but there are excellent products in all price ranges! I have yet to find a cosmetics chemist or an ingredient manufacturer who will state that expensive hair-care products are better than inexpensive ones, or that the inexpensive versions are somehow watered down or contain harsher ingredients. If ingredient manufacturers sold only to the pricey lines, they would go out of business. Expensive has nothing to do with quality! Salon products aren't what make your hair look so wonderful after leaving the salon. What creates the final results is the skill of the hairstylist, regardless of the products being used. The most wonderful products in the world can't make up for a lack of artistic ability or technique! A blow dryer held at the proper angle and used with the right brush can yield miracles. The perception that the products are controlling the effect is not reality. They may be good products, but the assumption that they are the only products that will work is sheer fantasy.

You may be shocked to learn that drugstore lines or lines we perceive as being "cheap" or a bargain (and therefore not very good) are often the very lines that spend the most money on research and development of their products. Companies like Revlon, Procter & Gamble, and L'Oreal spend millions of dollars a year on product research. Smaller companies cannot even begin to afford that kind of expenditure. L'Oreal has some of the most stunning, state-of-the-art laboratories you can imagine, and spends an average of $360 million a year for product development that is performed by a veritable brigade of cosmetics scientists and researchers.

Regardless of the price tag, the technology and the scientific capacity (meaning what it takes to create the products) don't change. The ingredients are the same and come from the same sources—only the color, shape, and design of the bottles and boxes are different. Let go of the illusion that salon lines spend more money on research and that the quality of their products is somehow superior; the facts tell us otherwise.

We have so many misconceptions and misunderstandings about salon versus drugstore products that the fallacies spiral around each other in a maze of propaganda. **I'm not suggesting there aren't reasons to shop for hair-care products at salons, because there are, but those reasons should be based on fact, not on advertising or media hype.**

Following are some of the myths and partial myths we believe about buying salon products rather than drugstore products.

- **Everyone needs pampering in a salon.** Absolutely! But buying products that might not be worth the money is not being pampered, it is wasting money.

- **Drugstore lines are weak and full of alcohol. Salon lines are more concentrated.** That is not what my research reveals, and I couldn't find any information, research, or sources (other than hair-care companies) showing that expensive products are formulated better. "Watery" products can be found both at salons and drugstores, and the same goes for products containing alcohol. Besides, alcohol is not necessarily a hair culprit—in a hairspray, for example, no other ingredient will dispense the holding ingredients in a way that doesn't wreck your hairstyle. All in all, there is nothing inherent in salon products that will make them last one hour longer or be any more effective than a drugstore product.

✂ **Salon products have fewer surfactants (cleansing agents) and wax-type ingredients than drugstore lines.** Nothing could be further from the truth. In fact, just the opposite can be true. It takes only a quick review of the ingredient list to determine the truth about this one. Surfactants are uniform throughout the industry. You will not find one shampoo ingredient in a salon line that can't also be found in a drugstore line. The same is true for conditioning and thickening agents. In the long run, what a product contains depends on the individual product.

✂ **Salon products use better grades of cosmetics than drugstore products.** I have heard this more times than I can count, although I have yet to find proof. I have called dozens and dozens of ingredient suppliers to ask if they sell different grades of ingredients, and the answer has always been a resounding "No." That's not to say that ingredient manufacturers don't have their selling angles to prove their quality and service is better, but these claims don't hold up when it comes to the ingredients' actual specifications and performance.

✂ **Drugstore products can damage hair or fade hair color.** Because the same shampoo and conditioning agents are used in virtually all hair-care products, with nothing but minor variations, that statement is completely unfounded. There are indeed ingredients that can cause hair problems, but they show up in both the inexpensive and the expensive stuff.

✂ **Hairstylists can pick the right product for your needs.** That definitely is true. However, that doesn't mean there aren't inexpensive options that are equally effective if not better. While most hairstylists are intimately familiar with the hair products they sell and with the results that can be achieved with those products, they are almost always unfamiliar with the brands found at drugstores. For that reason, using the products your stylist recommends is certainly one way to go. It's just that there are viable and often superior options available at the drugstore, too.

✂ **You can try hair-salon products first.** This is perhaps the best and only reason to buy the products your hairstylist recommends: you can evaluate a product's performance because your hairstylist used it on your hair first and you experience it personally. However, keep in mind that the way your hair feels and looks after you visit your stylist might not have anything to do with the products, but rather with the way your hair was styled. Remember, similar products could be available for less, but unless you can interpret the ingredient list, there is no way for you to know.

✂ **I am overwhelmed by the selection of products at the drugstore. It is just too large for me to make a comfortable decision.** Boy, is that the truth! A sea of products and a dearth of reliable information—it's enough to make anyone crazy. But that's why you're reading this book! It takes a good deal of the guesswork and worry out of your choices.

✂ **I would never feel confident dyeing my hair with drugstore products.** I understand the feeling. Yet all the evidence indicates that the risk of using drugstore products is the same as the risk of having a hairstylist do it for you. This is particularly true if the goal is only to lighten or darken the hair a shade or two or to cover gray. There are horror stories from both the salon and the drugstore sides of the color world (I've experienced a few myself). Hairstylists can custom-blend a color for you, but it still doesn't mean your hair will end up being the color you want. Nevertheless, I strongly suggest that if you want to make a drastic change in hair color (going three or more shades lighter or radically changing your hair color), it is probably best to start at the hair salon before you venture to the drugstore.

✂ **Salon products contain fewer potentially allergic ingredients than drugstore products.** Nothing could be farther off the mark than this. Hair-care products in all price ranges and from all types of companies have shockingly similar ingredients. Just read the labels: The evidence is plainly written in the ingredient list. From the cleansing agents to the preservatives and plant extracts, and everything else in between, salon and drugstore products have more similarities than differences. Moreover, hair-care products in all price ranges are often loaded with botanicals and fragrance, yet more often than not, those are the very plants and essential oils that cause allergic reactions and skin sensitivities.

✂ **Styling products available at the drugstore are just awful in comparison to those sold in hair salons.** My research just does not support this. Regardless of price, the crux of the matter is that almost all hair-care companies have good and bad products.

As you read the chapters on product formulation and the specific product reviews, you will discover that hair-care products sold by hair salons are not intrinsically better, more sophisticated, more appropriate, or superior to drugstore lines. In many cases, just the opposite is true, or, at the very least, there is no real difference between the expensive versus the inexpensive.

What is 100% true is that while there may be differences—both negative and positive—between any two products or product lines, they are not identifiable by the price or by the celebrity name on the package.

✄ **It must be good, because everyone's buying it.** Popularity is hardly a sign of value. Cigarettes are continually sold, slasher movies rake in huge dollars, overprocessed white bread is a staple in most households, and there are lots of popular hair-care products not everyone would rate as wonderful or effective. Length of time on the market or popularity doesn't prove anything except that uninformed consumers can, at the very least, waste their money or, at the very worst, cause themselves harm.

THE SALON GUARANTEE

Perhaps the most powerful draw for buying salon hair-care products is the "salon guarantee," although it is, for the most part, nothing more than a gimmick. The labels on the back of the container of products from companies such as Aveda, KMS, Paul Mitchell, Sebastian, Matrix, Scruples, Back to Basics, and dozens of other hair-care lines usually state something like this: "Retail sale of this product by anyone other than a professional styling salon is unauthorized by the manufacturer, and warranties do not apply."

So, what do these "guarantees" actually guarantee, and how is the consumer protected because the products are sold only at a hair salon instead of anywhere else? Good question, but the answer isn't clear.

For all the hoopla about product guarantees, none of the salon owners I interviewed agreed about what was guaranteed, or were even sure what the guarantees referred to. Comments ranged from assurances that you would be certain to get an authentic, salon-only product and not an imitation, to a belief that it meant the salon was getting the rights to an "exclusive" line, or that it was merely a return policy. According to the companies, the guarantee indeed refers to accepting returns and is a warranty that you are getting the right stuff *if* it is being sold in the right venue. In other words, if you buy a salon-only product at a drugstore or a discount store (and they are increasingly available outside of salons), the manufacturing company won't give you a refund if you're not happy with it. They will refund your money only if you purchased the product at a hair salon. However, if you check the drugstore's return policy (and most are flexible if you have the receipt), there is no need to worry about returning a product you don't like to the manufacturer, because you can simply return it to the store where you bought it.

The real problem with such guarantees is that they make the salon products sound more exclusive than they really are. Further, women rarely return hair-care products that don't work; women collect hair-care products much the same way they collect makeup. When they don't like a product they put it aside and buy another. The woman who asks for her money back is the exception.

So how does a salon-only product end up at a drugstore in the first place? No one is exactly clear or forthcoming about this, but unless the hair-care company sues (and a couple of them have), people are not arrested for selling salon-only products in a drugstore. More often than not, it isn't a distribution problem at all. Some hair-care companies simply sell their products wherever they can to improve their cash flow. Many hair-care companies even have a professional line and a drugstore line with, not surprisingly, identical ingredient lists.

Some salon-only companies told me the only way you can be sure you aren't getting a cheap imitation or a knockoff is to buy the product only at a hair salon. That is possibly a valid concern, but not a serious one—because even on the off chance that you aren't getting an authentic product, the level of risk to the consumer is nonexistent. Other companies do openly claim to reproduce popular formulas, and these imitations are clearly marked as such, so most consumers are not in any doubt about what they are buying.

Whether knockoffs of this nature are an ethical direction appropriate for cosmetics companies is debatable. I for one take offense at the practice. First of all, it suggests that there is something superior about the products being knocked off, and that isn't always the case. Paul Mitchell may indeed have some very good products, but there is nothing about awapuhi or The Conditioner that is necessarily worth knocking off. I also agree with the position of the salon-only hair-care companies about knockoffs, because these brands are capitalizing on another entrepreneur's efforts. I wouldn't want someone to do that to me! What if someone came out with a book called *Don't Go Shopping for Salon or Drugstore Hair Products Without This Book*? I would not be happy. Products should stand on their own, each with its own identity and marketing plan. While generics are probably a fine option for the consumer to try, putting the emphasis on one line's success and not on the value of an individual product is a misleading way to sell products.

What the professional or salon-only guarantee really turns out to be is a marketing device used to enhance value and add price points. Salons don't want to sell products the consumer can get from any drugstore shelf at a discount—where is the exclusivity in that? And where would the status and prestige be if the prices were so reasonable? Most women need to believe that their hair will be more beautiful if they spend more money on it, and hairstylists are more than willing to encourage that attitude.

NATURALLY ABSURD

The "natural" concept, as a marketing hook for hair-care products, is at the center of the fastest-growing and largest segment of the hair-care industry. Consumers are more likely to be swayed to purchase if some aspect of a shampoo, conditioner, or styling product appears to be formulated from natural ingredients. Although most cosmetics chemists cringe or laugh when you bring up the "natural" idea, they recognize that their products would be ignored without it. Almost all natural-sounding ingredients are nothing more than a game, but it is a charade in which the hair-care chemist, hair-care company, and hairstylist are all participating, either wittingly or unwittingly.

Each product celebrating this trend beckons to the consumer with a menu-like list of ingredients that sound good enough to eat. However, the drop of vitamins, dash of lavender, hint of rosemary or ginseng, or myriad other plant offerings is there almost solely for image and little else.

Most consumers are so enamored with the power of "natural" that there is no question in their minds whether any of this natural stuff is really good. Sadly, while some natural ingredients do indeed have beneficial properties for skin, most natural ingredients in hair-care products have little to no impact or influence on the health, cleanliness, strength, or smoothness of hair. If only I had a dime for every woman who has said to me, "Well, the products I'm using must be good—they're all natural and pure." And if only I had the opportunity to say in response, "The products you are using cannot be remotely or even partly all natural. You simply have bought into one of the biggest and most successful marketing scams of all time, because the functional ingredients in your products are not natural in the least."

In essence (and with the exception of nonvolatile plant oils in products for dry hair), you could take all of the natural-sounding ingredients out of a product and you would still have an effective shampoo, conditioner, or styling product that would leave hair clean, soft, and manageable. Take out all the so-called chemical-sounding ingredients and all you would have is tea (which is what plant extracts often are) and dirty, unconditioned, and unmanageable hair.

Consumers want to believe that natural ingredients such as plant extracts and vitamins can somehow nourish the hair and revitalize it, changing it into something better than it was before. Nothing could be further from the truth. All of the plants and vitamins in the world can't bring a dead leaf back to life, or put fallen petals back on a rose, and they can't change the very dead hair on your head. There is no trustworthy evidence that any of these ingredients provide any substantive benefit for hair. When you read the ingredient lists for these so-called natural products, you find that all the standard hair-care ingredients, used throughout the industry, are also listed there.

When pushed for evidence that natural ingredients make a difference, companies stoop to references to folklore or history for proof, but who knows what that means. Egyptians may well have used certain plants for their hair, but that doesn't mean they worked. Cleopatra might have used exotic plants to take care of her hair, but we have no proof she had great hair! Are we assuming she looked like Elizabeth Taylor in *Cleopatra*? We simply don't know if hair treatments from the past worked; we know only that they were used. When it comes to hair, I would, without question, choose the standard, far-from-exotic-sounding ingredients such as polyquaternium-16, dimethicone, cyclomethicone, or PVP (polyvinylpyrrolidone) to make my hair feel soft and stay in place over lavender extract or vitamin D, and so would hair-care chemists. Paying for the illusion of benefit from natural ingredients does absolutely nothing for your hair, but, because products boasting natural ingredients tend to cost more, it can surely hurt your pocketbook (Sources: *Cosmetics & Toiletries*, May 2003, pages 18 and 28–30, and May 2004, pages 64–68).

TRUTH IN ADVERTISING?

The United States Federal Trade Commission (FTC) and the Food and Drug Administration (FDA) have similarities and differences in their regulations concerning cosmetics. Neither the FDA nor the FTC have efficacy or safety requirements of any kind for hair-care products or cosmetics, they merely rely on the information provided by the cosmetics or hair-care company. What the FDA cares about is the content of a cosmetic, meaning that it should contain only cosmetic ingredients, and ruling that when a product does contain over-the-counter drug ingredients it must meet the (much more stringent) regulatory demands for that ingredient.

It is within the purview of the FTC to be concerned about deceptive or erroneous advertising claims. "When the substantiation claim is express (e.g., 'tests prove,' 'doctors recommend,' and 'studies show'), the Commission expects the firm to have at least the advertised level of substantiation" (Source: FTC *Policy Statement Regarding Advertising Substantiation*, www.ftc.gov). That means all the FTC cares about is that some kind of "study" for claims asserted in the ad does exist. But it doesn't have to be a published study and it doesn't have to meet any scientific standards or prove efficacy; it just needs to comply with some level of the statement "our studies show." For example, a study showing that a hair-care product "repairs" hair merely has to demonstrate the hair *looks* repaired, not that it *is* repaired. Or if a study states that hair looked 80% better, that only has to be the subjective opinion of the observer, who is someone hired by the company to conduct the study. That can pass the FTC standards for proof of claim, but it doesn't help the consumer know whether the product really works.

Further, an advertising claim (such as "repairs hair," "non-irritating," "reduces free-radical damage," "sun protection," "contains vitamins," "makes hair fuller," "is all natural," and other similar wording) is just that, a claim. And a claim is not the same thing as research showing whether a product is effective, worth the price, or safe to use. So if a hair-care product contains vitamins, that doesn't tell you if or how it is helpful for hair, how the product compares to other similar products, or even how much of the vitamins the product contains.

Another question has to do with exactly what *deceptive* means. As it stands, it's up for debate, which is why the FTC doesn't act on cosmetics advertising issues very often. For example, if a hair-care product claims to protect from sun damage, the FTC guidelines aren't concerned about whether the product does or does not have an SPF rating, or whether the product contains only enough active ingredients to warrant an SPF of 2. Similarly, when a hair-care product claims to repair hair, the FTC doesn't take issue with the fact that the "repair" claim is a temporary or aesthetic comment and that the actual structure of the hair hasn't really been changed. Claims that assert a product can make hair stronger, healthier, or more resilient are not enough to raise red flags for the FTC.

If major hair-care companies have legal and claim departments that accumulate evidence to substantiate their claims, I have yet to see any of that evidence. My team has called every cosmetics company whose products we've ever reviewed asking for proof of their claims, and over the years we have received almost none (I can count on one hand the number of studies cosmetics companies have sent to me).

One more point: It is interesting to note that there are definitely times when the FTC has made companies alter their advertising claims (I read about these all the time in the industry newsletter *The Rose Sheet*). However, by the time the ad is pulled or rewritten, the consumer has already been deluged with the frivolous claims, which are neatly planted in their thoughts before the retraction and correction take place, and by then the same company has launched another ad with a whole new bevy of claims.

PATENTED SECRETS

Are there really secret formulas in hair-care products? After all, if you're spending $15 to $25 for a conditioner with impressive claims, you want to believe you're purchasing an exclusive product that justifies the exorbitant price. Salespeople and marketing departments make much ado about patented or patent-pending formulas that are available only to their line. And when you look at the product label, there it is in black and white: a "patented" or "patent-pending" formula. It must be special, right? Well, yes and no.

The fact that a formula has an exclusive patented ingredient or group of ingredients doesn't tell you anything about how well the product works. It is not the patent office's responsibility to verify whether the patented formula or ingredient can do anything for the hair. There are millions of cosmetics patents, and not one has any meaning when it comes to effectiveness. This is because patents are granted for formulation procedures or for use claims, not because the products can really do something. Variations and potential uses are endless (which is why there are millions of patents), but the basic fact is that a patent doesn't have anything to do with effectiveness, only with the specifics of the formula.

Even when a patented product or formula actually does do something positive for the hair, as in the instance of two-in-one shampoos, it doesn't necessarily take much for another company to come up with a very similar (and equally patentable) formula. Next time your hairstylist or someone selling hair-care products carries on about an exclusive patented formula, remember that a patent doesn't tell you anything about how well the product works, and it definitely doesn't tell you whether or not there is a similar product on the market that does a better job.

SAFE SHOPPING RULES

Learning to abide by the shopping precepts below will help you save money, avoid endless disappointment, and become a savvy hair-care consumer.

1. **You must be willing to change some of your beliefs about hair care.** A hair-care company does not necessarily have your best interests at heart. If you are willing to keep buying a product that is overpriced or doesn't work, they will keep selling it, because there is no reason for them to change. It doesn't matter that hair can't be repaired or reconstructed by a conditioner or that hair can't be restored by a moisturizing pack or treatment. As long as people buy these products, why should the hair-care companies stop selling them?

2. **Almost every hair-care line has good and bad products.** Actually, most hair-care lines have fairly good products. It's the labels that give misleading information about which products are best for specific hair-care needs that cause the confusion. Many lines have their share of useless, overly perfumed, unreliable, and *overpriced* products that can't live up to the claims on the label. However, they also have products that work, even if these products are often overpriced. Also, just because a product works doesn't mean it's worth $20; there absolutely are $3 or $5 equivalents available elsewhere.

3. **Give up line loyalty.** It is great when you find a line you are comfortable with. For example, you might like Sebastian styling products and conditioners or Joico's treatment pack and shampoos. But that doesn't mean that every other product in those lines is also guaranteed to please you or be good for you, or that you need more of what the line offers. No matter how enthusiastic salespeople are about their terrific line, they are not unbiased bystanders; they have a vested interest in what you decide to buy.

4. **Do not buy impulsively or quickly.** That statement speaks for itself, but it isn't always easy! There you are at the salon, the stylist has just finished making you look stunning, and the premium products he or she used are staring you in the face. With just this small additional purchase of $35, $50, or $60, you think, you can get your hair to look the same between visits. Stop and breathe. Consider what you already have at home. Try to remember how I rated the products you're looking at. It would also be beneficial to remember the last time you bought the products recommended by a hairstylist and ask yourself whether those really made a difference, before you jump in and buy again.

5. **Hair-care advertisements may be alluring and interesting, but they are ads, not documentaries.** Just because the ads are sensual doesn't mean the products featured in the ads are, and it doesn't mean they'll make *you* more sensual. Accept seductive ads for what they are—seductive ads, not reliable sources of facts.

6. **Don't pretend you are above being affected by cosmetics advertising.** All advertising, especially cosmetics advertising, is a very, very powerful stimulus in our lives. Hair-care advertising, like any advertising, is designed to make us buy a specific product or be attracted to a specific company. Whether we like it or not,

advertising strongly affects how we make decisions. If advertising didn't influence us, companies wouldn't spend billions of dollars advertising their products to us. It is unwise to ignore the fact that advertising sells products, and sells them very well, because the hair-care companies wouldn't keep throwing money at something that produced no financial return. The next time you think you are not being affected by cosmetics and hair-care advertising, think again.

7. **Hair-care products are not a bargain just because they are less expensive than products offered by other areas of the cosmetics industry.** Because hair-care products are so much less expensive than products in the rest of the cosmetics industry (particularly skin-care products), and because you need fewer products to maintain your hair than your skin (at least for some women), it is easy to consider the price of a $15 hairspray or $20 shampoo a mere pittance in comparison to the $75 moisturizer or $100 antiwrinkle creams the skin-care industry sells. Still, it all adds up. A savvy hairstylist or salesperson can sell you a line of hair-care products for $40 before you know it. When you consider how often you make these purchases and realize that there are excellent products available in less expensive price ranges, it should give you pause.

8. **When it comes to hair-care products, there are no miracle ingredients, trade secrets, exotic ingredients, patented secrets, or salon-tested formulas that will permanently repair your hair.** If there were a magic potion for hair, it wouldn't stay under wraps. Every line would get their hands on it. Chemists are entirely capable of analyzing a product's ingredients and duplicating whatever they want. Sophisticated technologies make reproducing a product's components, even when they are patented, as easy as assembling a jigsaw puzzle when all of the pieces are included. And speaking of patented secrets, this is an oxymoron. U.S. patent law is very clear: In order for an ingredient or group of ingredients to be patented, the exact components and precise formulation details must be disclosed in full. It doesn't take much for a hair-care company to figure out an alternative to a patented formula; and if that's not feasible, they can buy the licensed right to use the formula. Realistically, if a product could repair hair, you should only have to use it a few times and then your hair would be repaired. That isn't what happens. You have to reapply these products every time you shampoo because their effect is only temporary, nothing more.

9. **Truly superior shampoos, conditioners, styling products, and special treatments can be found in inexpensive lines.** Formulations vary, and some products are better than others, but on the whole I find just as many great products at the drugstore as I do at the hair salon—and just as many bad ones. Marketing creates mystique, not reality.

10. **Shopping for hair-care products in a salon may feel more elegant than shopping at the drugstore, but that is a perception about the environment, not about the quality of the products.** The elegance lies in the pampered feeling you get from the earnest, helpful information and advice the salon stylist provides. If that environment is important to you and expense is not an issue, there are great products available at the salon. However, there is no research, evidence, or proof that salon products are formulated any better than drugstore products. In fact, after interviewing dozens of cosmetics chemists and cosmetic ingredient manufacturers, it is clear to me that nothing could be further from the truth.

CHAPTER TWO

To the Root of the Matter

HAIR BASICS 101

If you take no other information in this book to heart, the two following facts are the ones you must understand to take better care of your hair:

1. **Hair is dead (notice that when you cut hair, you don't say ouch), and once it has been damaged it cannot be repaired in any way, shape, or form.** Repeated blow drying, brushing, styling, chemical processing, and sun exposure degrades hair, and the damage cannot be mended or undone.

2. **Hair has a particular genetic or hormonally generated nature; you can work with it and spend time controlling it, and find products that simulate a different feel, but you cannot change how it grows.** Perms, straighteners, and dyes can make a drastic change in the appearance of your hair (and there are definite negative consequences to these processes), but the effects grow out, and that's an entirely different story from thinking that some quality of your hair can be altered for good.

The pursuit of products that will finally make your dream hair come true is endless. What most women desire and hope for is that they will find a product line (at any cost) that will make thick, heavy hair lighter and fuller; thin hair thicker and fuller; curly, frizzy hair straighter and smoother; straight hair curlier; coarse hair silkier; and on and on and on. Whatever it is you want to hear, the hair-care industry is willing to tell you. To name just a handful of claims: Overprocessed, completely destroyed hair can somehow be brought back to life. Split ends can be mended into a harmonious whole. Frizzy manes can be miraculously transformed into flowing, silky waves. Thin hair can be made thick. Dandruff can be cured. And dyeing hair won't cause damage. Is any of this possible? I know you want me to say "yes" unequivocally, but the truth is that the answer is both yes and no.

Primarily, what you can expect depends less on the products you use and far more on the actual texture and structure of your hair, how adept you are at wielding styling tools, and how much time and trouble you are willing to go through to achieve the desired results. And that all varies from hair type to hair type and from person to person.

For example, if you have thin, limp hair you can do only so much to change how thick it can really feel or how full it can really look. Most of the products that simulate (notice I said *simulate* and not create) a thick feel can also build up and make the hair appear limp and sticky. Likewise, products that help hold the hair aloft for an appearance of fullness can leave a film on the hair. If your hair is coarse and naturally frizzy, flat irons (with the right products) can work temporary miracles—but you can't change the nature of your hair over the long term without straightening it.

Now that you know what you can't expect, here's what you can expect. There are wonderful products on the market that can temporarily, washing to washing, do some fairly incredible things to hair. Several ingredients can produce amazing results, from filling in the holes and tears in damaged hair cuticles to imparting a silky-smooth texture to the rough sections of the hair shaft. Many ingredients can, to some extent, be absorbed by the hair shaft to help make the hair feel soft and manageable. Conditioners and shampoos can deposit temporary color on the hair to extend the life of your hair dye between touch-ups. Advances in sprays, gels, styling creams, and mousses allow deftly formed styles to be kept in place with a relative amount of softness and ease of brushing.

Does this have to be expensive? Absolutely not. As I get more into actual product formulations you will be shocked at how the same basic ingredients appear over and over again in hair-care products. In the world of skin care, cosmetics chemists have thousands of different ingredients at their disposal from which they can create a vast array of products with an almost limitless range of textures and performance traits. Hair-care formulations by comparison do not have that scope. **There is only a mere handful of ingredients that can clean hair or condition it.** Hair is very specific about what will cling to it and what you can use to clean it. The truly insane disparity in the prices of products from different lines in no way reflects differences in the products. Again, the information is all there on the ingredient list.

HAIR IS DEAD!

First and foremost, you need to know and remember that the hair you see on the top of your head, every inch of it, is dead as a doornail. The only portion of your hair that isn't dead is the hair you can't see, growing inside the hair follicle under your scalp. Because hair is dead, your options as to what you can do to take care of it are limited.

Hair-care companies want to convince you that, much like Frankenstein's monster, dead hair can be changed into ostensibly alive hair. How many products have you bought that said they would repair and reconstruct damaged hair, only to have your hair return to the original state of affairs after the next washing or when the weather changed? Yes, we all know that hair products, such as conditioners and gels, and hair implements, such as blow dryers and flat irons, can temporarily reshape hair. The trouble begins when we are led to believe it is possible to *permanently* alter or improve damaged hair structure with shampoos, conditioners, and treatments. The only way hair can truly be altered is with certain hair-coloring products and with perms. That's it—and even so you are not necessarily guaranteed long-term positive results. Everything else is a sort of Band-Aid remedy that is easily removed by washing.

Before you go shopping for hair-care products again, or before you venture into a hair salon to get your hair dyed or permed, you need to know some basic facts about your hair if you are to be a discerning, clear-eyed consumer. This isn't the most fascinating aspect of hair, but it is one more crucial step that will let you take better care of your hair.

THE THIN AND THICK OF HAIR

A single strand of hair is only 0.02 to 0.04 millimeters thick, but it is remarkably strong, with a tensile strength equivalent to a thin strand of wire. Why then does hair seem so fragile? Hair stretches easily (unlike wire) and is just fine even when extended by 30% of its original length. However, once it exceeds 30%, damage is certain, and at much past 80% of its original length the hair shaft fractures. Hair is even more vulnerable to breakage when the hair shaft is wet or damaged, but more about that later. For now, the percentage of stretch explains why the tension placed on hair from pulling it during blow drying with a round brush—or by tying the hair up tightly in a ponytail—can be so damaging.

Hair is composed primarily of a protein called keratin, which makes up about 70% to 90% of its structure. Keratin is a solid, resilient, strong, fibrous, and water-resistant form of protein. Getting a bit more technical, keratin is made up of amino acids linked together in a chain. As far as amino acids go, keratin contains mostly the amino acid called cysteine. Cysteine is important to hair because it contains sulfur, and sulfur can link together to create a disulfide bond, which is what gives hair its shape, strength, and flexibility.

Hair-care companies love to brag about the keratin and amino acids in their products, but they won't work to reinforce those elements in your hair. As conditioning agents, keratin and amino acids cling poorly to the hair and so are washed down the drain, which explains why you so rarely see them at the top of a product's ingredient list. And if keratin contains sulfur, why don't they brag about the sulfur in their products, when that's what is really responsible for the strength of your hair? Well, keratin is a much easier concept to sell to the consumer than smelly old sulfur. In the end, neither keratin nor amino acids end up being very good as hair-care ingredients.

The outer layer of the hair shaft is called the cuticle, where most of the keratin in hair is found. As far as hair is concerned the cuticle is all-important because it is the protective coating for the hair shaft. That's why this rather uninteresting structure is probably the most relevant one when it comes to the health of your hair. As the cuticle goes, so goes the hair! When the cuticle is intact you have healthy hair. When the cuticle is damaged you have problems that cannot be cured. Most of what you can do to keep your hair healthy involves taking care of the cuticle.

Under an electron microscope, magnified several thousand times, the cuticle resembles fish scales, layers of bark on a tree trunk, or shingles on the roof or side of a house. These overlapping layers form a tight barrier to the outside world's repeated attacks of washing, brushing, styling, and sun exposure. Sadly, the cuticle is not, shall we say, as tough as nails, and it can withstand our daily grooming rituals only up to a point before it starts to break down.

WHAT IS THE CUTICLE PROTECTING?

The cuticle protects a surprisingly elastic backbone of the hair called the cortex, as well as the sometimes-present medulla, which is the innermost part of the hair shaft. (Mentioning the medulla may be a bit confusing, because for some unknown reason this mysterious, innermost part of hair isn't present in all hair shafts. No one is sure what the medulla does or doesn't do, so for now there is little else to say about it.)

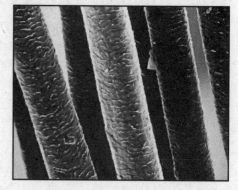

Hair damage of an extreme type can cause a change in hair texture or can create split ends. Under that same electron microscope, what you would really be looking at is a cuticle layer that has been chipped away and eliminated, exposing the fragile protein fibers of the cortex. Under the microscope these look much like the frayed strands of any worn material.

A healthy and intact cuticle and cortex work together to allow hair to look and perform the way it is supposed to (you may not like the way it performs, but at least it isn't damaged). When we change what the hair naturally wants to do, with perms, hair dyes, brushes, styling tools, or even simple things like shampooing and brushing, we start to break down the hair's outer coat of armor and its inner source of strength and elasticity. Regrettably, it doesn't take much to rip off pieces of cuticle and, given the demands of fashion, it is surprising we have any hair left on our heads! Yet what we do know about the cuticle can save our hair in more ways than one.

When the cuticle is healthy and intact, lying flat and tight against the hair shaft, the hair reflects light evenly, producing a wonderful luster and shine. When the cuticle is bruised, swollen, or eroded by chemical processes, heat, any kind of manipulation (even simple brushing or combing), or alkaline products, the edges of the cuticle scales begin to lift and separate from the hair shaft. Initially, that can have a positive effect on the appearance of your hair. A roughed-up cuticle causes the edges of the scales to stand up, spacing the hairs farther apart from one another and giving the hair a fuller appearance. One of the reasons permed or dyed hair can appear thicker (if the hair is not overly permed or dyed and is not multiprocessed) is because the chemicals from the dye and perms cause the cuticle to lift this way. The same is true for hair that is backcombed or "ratted." Backcombing the hair roughs up the cuticle, lifting the edges so the hairs grab each other at the overlapping, raised edges, creating a pretty tough matrix that keeps the hair aloft. That's why backcombed hair can stay in place for a fairly long period.

Up to a point, none of this is a serious problem—but only to a point. Hair can become overprocessed or overworked to the point of no return. When the cuticle is repeatedly mistreated, chips of cuticle are torn away from the hair shaft, literally peeling away like the layers of an onion until there is nothing left but the exposed core.

Bottom line: When the cuticle, the hair's first line of defense, is broken down and the cuticle's seven to ten layers are eroded away, there is little hope left for the cortex, the heart of the hair shaft.

THE SHAPE AND HEART OF THE HAIR

When you look at hair through an electron microscope, you can see that the cortex and the medulla, when it is present, have a porous, almost sponge-like appearance. The cortex is where vital factors such as the color, moisture content, elasticity, texture, and resilience of the hair reside.

One strand of hair all by itself appears to the naked eye to be nothing more than a wiry string with muted, dull color. Using an electron microscope to magnify that same ultra-thin hair a thousand times allows us to see the outer cuticle layer (made of protein), which resembles the scales on a fish or the overlapping shingles of a roof. Deeper inside, when you look at a tiny slice of hair cut in half under the same microscope, you can see rings that look like the rings in a tree trunk. These rings are more layers of cuticle, about seven layers, depending on the head of hair.

Inside these cuticle layers is the cortex, the heart and soul of the hair. Along with its open, sponge-like structure, the cortex has long protein filaments, called microfibrils and macrofibrils, that extend the length of the hair. These filaments are what determine the strength, resilience, and moisture content of the hair. If the medulla is present it is the innermost structure, but little is known about it. Strangely, the medulla is less likely to be present in hairs on your head than in hairs on other parts of your body.

Within these major structures, the form and shape of the hair are determined by even tinier components of the hair known as hydrogen and disulfide bonds. Disulfide bonds are created by the sulfur component of the amino acids that form the hair's protein, and they are incredibly strong and not easily broken. Hydrogen bonds, on the other hand, are quite weak and change easily with humidity and wetness. Hydrogen bonds affect the temporary day-to-day, shampoo-to-shampoo shape of your hair. The reason wet hair becomes longer and temporarily changes shape is because the hydrogen bonds have been broken. As the hair dries, the hydrogen bonds quickly reform and reestablish the hair's natural shape.

These hydrogen bonds explain why using rollers or blow dryers on wet hair can change its natural shape temporarily—because you've altered and then reformed or set the flexible hydrogen bonds with heat. Of course, once the hair becomes wet again (from water or humidity) the hydrogen bonds break and revert back to their original curl or lack thereof. **Hair's hydrogen bonds have a great memory, so unless you are there with** heat or formidable styling products in hand to convince those bonds to go in another direction, they will move the way they normally would.

Disulfide bonds, unlike hydrogen bonds, are not so easily persuaded to take on another form. Any permanent change in hair curl or straightness means you must break down these tenacious bonds. Because disulfide bonds are so strong, it takes potent chemicals to modify their shape. Permanent-wave or hair-straightening solutions (which actually use the same formulas—the hair is merely configured differently depending on what you want it to do) are highly alkaline solutions that actually fracture the disulfide bonds.

Once the disulfide bonds are broken, they are ready to be reformed, which is accomplished during the time the alkaline solution sits on the hair and the hair is molded to its new shape. If you curl your hair up in rollers (or comb your hair straight) and then soak it in an alkaline solution, the disulfide bonds will break and, with time, take on the shape of the roller (or be kept straight). As soon as the alkaline solution is neutralized, the reforming process stops and the new shape is set.

Remember, these disulfide bonds are stubborn. They want to go back to their original form. It takes a good deal of processing time and strong chemicals to get the disulfide bonds to do exactly what you want them to do, particularly if you have stick-straight or ultra-curly hair. And don't think for one second that the process of reforming disulfide bonds is anything less than damaging to your hair. Even breaking the weak hydrogen bonds and reforming them with heat is damaging to hair over time. But compared to that, breaking the disulfide bonds is a heavy burden to put on anyone's hair, and you can't expect it to come out anything but damaged. So-called "gentle" perms do exist, but they are gentle because they have a lower pH, not because they contain natural or special ingredients. Regrettably, the lower pH also makes these products not very effective on perfectly straight or extremely curly hair if the goal is to straighten out the curls or put in tighter ones. For more information on perms and straighteners, see Chapter Seven, "Perms and Relaxers" (Sources: *Chemical and Physical Behavior of Human Hair*, Clarence R. Robbins, Springer-Verlag, December 2001; and *Global Cosmetic Industry*, September 2001, pages 14–15).

UNDERSTANDING HAIR DAMAGE

Damaging the cuticle is the principal way we ruin all the things about hair that most of us want and envy, and, sadly, the hair is easily damaged. As the cuticle is chipped away, eliminating the hair's entire protective structure, it exposes the cortex and allows its protein fibers to get torn apart; eventually you end up with a stripped, weak, vulnerable hair shaft.

Split ends happen when most of the damage takes place on the ends of the hair. Since damage is almost always cumulative, it makes sense that split ends are a typical problem—those ends have been around the longest and have been subjected to repeated abuse.

Another typical problem occurs when hair breaks off in the middle rather than at the ends. This can result from concentrated damage at that specific site, overextending the hair shaft beyond its capacity (particularly during styling), or a genetic weak link in hair growth.

For those who repeatedly perm and/or color their hair, and especially if the hair is stripped (bleached) and then toned—by adding another color after the hair has been stripped—the result can be soft, mushy, dry, and brittle hair that breaks off in chunks. **This breakage happens when excessive overprocessing destroys most of the cuticle layer as well as the inner cortex.**

Unfortunately, it is all too easy to damage the hair shaft, yet we can hardly help ourselves. Many things can make the cuticle fall apart, yet most of the damage is not caused by the hair-care products we use. (Yes, that's ten points for the hair-care companies! On the whole, they are not making products that destroy hair, and the rare exceptions are thankfully few and far between.) Most of the abuse is caused by what we do to our hair in the name of fashion and simple hygiene, and the havoc we wreak in the name of style is often irreversible and irreparable. What causes the damage? The answers will amaze and disturb you. They certainly disturb me.

In essence, hair is damaged by almost everything we do to it. Common, everyday actions can cause breakage, splitting, frizzing, and dryness. **Friction and heat are the primary sources of cuticle damage. Friction occurs when you rub your hair against itself; for example, when you towel-dry your hair, or when your loved one runs his or her fingers tenderly through your hair. When you move the hair against itself, especially roughly, you start breaking apart the cuticle. Brushing hair also tears apart the cuticle.** Every time the brush smoothes through your locks, separating the shafts from one another, little bits of cuticle are being chipped away.

Stretching is particularly damaging to hair, such as when you are trying to undo a knot or untangle a mussed hairdo. Blow drying on the hottest setting, and using hot rollers, curling irons, and flat irons are all activities that fry off tiny, and sometimes large, parts of the cuticle every time, and the closer the heat, the greater the damage. Even shampooing causes damage when you massage the lather into the length of the hair by rubbing the hairs against each other.

It is interesting to note that, in studies, air-drying the hair causes no damage, blow drying the hair without brushing and simultaneous styling causes minor surface damage, and even brushing hair without heat causes moderate surface damage. The most damage occurs when hair is blow dried and brushed, meaning styled, at the same time. Blow dryers and flat irons accelerate the damage from brushing and combing (Source: *Global Cosmetic Industry*, January 2002, pages 30–32).

Towel-drying the hair in a tousling manner by rubbing the towel over the hair (instead of just gently squeezing) itself damages the cuticle, and hair is already more prone to damage when it is wet than when it is dry because the hydrogen bonds that in part give hair its shape are not intact when hair is wet. Yet, as many of us know, blow dryers work best on wet hair. That's why your hairstylist rewets your hair after it's been cut: to blow it dry in a better, longer-lasting shape. Braiding hair, tying it back into a bun or ponytail, and rolling it up on curlers (especially the relatively new Velcro rollers) all damage the hair. Environmental conditions also diminish the health of your hair, as sunlight, wind, pollution, salt water, and chlorine from pools can all cause damage.

By the way, chlorine can dry hair but it doesn't turn hair green. The green discoloration comes from swimming in pools with copper plumbing. Mineral deposits of copper from the plumbing are dissolved in the water and then cling to the hair shaft (Source: *Cutis*, July 1995, pages 37–40).

And don't forget that chemical processes such as perms and dyes are damaging. Doing these over and over again, or at the same time, is almost a guaranteed cuticle destroyer. Once hair has undergone a chemical process, the cuticle layer becomes more and more depleted, and eventually, when the cortex (the heart of the hair shaft) is exposed, hair loses its tensile strength and smoothness and becomes spongy and brittle.

Sounds hopeless, doesn't it? What are we supposed to do, never touch our hair again? Don't despair. It is neither hopeless nor impossible to change problematic habits once you are aware of them. A total hands-off ultimatum isn't the answer. You just need up-to-date information, a change of perspective, and a new relationship with your hair. **Once you become aware of what you can do and what it takes to have really healthy hair, you can start protecting your hair immediately.**

Keep in mind that the daily damage is cumulative and that it takes effort on your part to bring about change. Luckily, the cuticle is seven to ten layers thick, and there are a lot of hairs on your head, and your hair grows, replenishing itself with a new healthy base every month or two. You absolutely have some slack in the area between looking out for the welfare of the cuticle and styling your hair. Moreover, you don't have to buy products that promise to protect the hair (although some of them do help), because there are better, more reliable solutions that require action, not money.

Dear Paula,

My stylist recommended a product for me, and it's supposed to be geared toward long hair. The stylist told me it was specially formulated to keep the ends of hair from splitting since that is what makes most people have to get haircuts. Therefore, if your hair is long, you can keep it that way by using that product and not getting as many haircuts. This whole argument sounded silly and untrue to me. How does it know I have long, short, or medium length hair? After all, people with shorter hair than mine can have split ends if they overprocess their hair or damage it with styling tools, right?

Donna, via email

Dear Donna,

You are my kind of woman. When a sales pitch clearly sounds bogus, you don't let it get the better of you, assuming there may be something to it just because the stylist should know more than you. That's not necessarily the case, after all, at least not when it comes to product formulations and the physiology of hair.

First, you are right: There is no way for a shampoo to know how long or how damaged your hair is, it can only deposit the ingredients it contains on the hair it comes in contact with, regardless of the length.

The second issue is that there are no products that can prevent or repair split ends. Split ends result from hair being repeatedly damaged over a period of time. Ends of long hair have been subjected to months (sometimes years) of recurring insult—like high heat from styling tools, sun exposure, chemicals in pools, salt in oceans, hair dyes, perms, hairbrushes, and more. All of these things chip away at the cuticle, the protective outer layer of the hair. When the cuticle is finally worn down, it is irreplaceable. You can't mend it or put it back together, and there are no hair-care products that can undo the damage. However, what you *can* do, no matter the length of your hair, is reduce the amount of damage that takes place by doing the following:

Reducing how often you get your hair dyed or permed helps the most. Also, extreme color changes (going from brunette to light blonde) are the most damaging.

Avoiding using the high-heat setting on your blow dryer or flat iron (though be aware that high heat does help control hair better). Also, never let the heat stay in one place on the hair for more than a moment and keep it moving over the hair.

Styling products with conditioning agents (most of them have some), especially silicone, provide a small amount of protection from styling tools.

Keeping your hair covered when you are out in the sun makes a huge difference in the health of your hair.

Brushing your hair only when needed and never backcombing it.

Beyond that, the only way to deal with split ends when they appear is to cut them off.

STOPPING DAMAGE

In reality you really can't completely eliminate damage to your hair. That would mean never washing, brushing, styling, dyeing, or perming your hair again. Oh, and it would also mean never letting your hair see the light of day, at least not unless it was neatly tucked up under a hat. However, you can slow down or reduce the amount of damage that takes place. Not only will the techniques I list below improve the quality of your hair, they will also prevent breakage and hair loss, and that goes a long way toward improving the appearance of your hair.

For all intents and purposes, taking care of your hair is all about taking care of the hair cuticle. As I noted earlier, the cuticle is the microscopic layer of protection that surrounds each strand of hair, made up of tiny overlapping layers. Keeping the cuticle layer healthy—or as healthy as possible—will go a long way toward your having stronger, shinier, and smoother hair, and you'll have fewer bad hair days. You will need to change your ways, though, and that can take some getting used to. For many of us, the way we care for our hair, and I use the term *care* loosely, is actually just a daily assault of stresses that chip away at the structure of our hair until practically none is left. Our old hair-grooming rituals may have become second nature, but, with time, they will begin to seem strange, and the new habits will feel as natural as brushing your teeth.

Brush or comb your hair as infrequently and as gently as possible. Without question, brushing is one of the most damaging things you do to your hair, especially if you repeat it frequently during the day and use hard-bristled brushes. Every time you brush through your hair, the bristles or spikes chip away at the cuticle. Be good to your hair and leave it alone as often as you can. That doesn't mean never brushing, but rather brushing only when needed and using soft-bristled or soft-feeling brushes. The farther apart the bristles are, the better. If they are close together, make sure they have a soft, flexible feel. When you run the brush through your hair, take care to start at the base of your scalp, using as little force as possible. Avoid slamming the brush into your hair and driving it through to the ends. Brush your hair in sections starting at the top and working your way down, being the most gentle with the ends. Avoid backcombing, which chips pieces of cuticle away. If you want your hair to look its fullest, throw your head forward and brush from the nape of your neck toward your face, avoiding the ends. Then throw your head back and smooth the top and ends without digging into the hair. If you want to distribute the oil from your scalp throughout your hair, brushing it once in the morning, afternoon, and evening should take care of that. During the day you can also separate your hair with your fingertips, smoothing it with your hands.

Never use a brush on wet hair, and don't over-brush wet hair. Wet hair is more easily damaged than dry hair (when hair is wet its hydrogen bonds have been broken and the hair is therefore in a more vulnerable state). On wet hair, it's best to use either a wide-toothed comb or a wide-bristled brush with rounded tips.

Choose your brushes and combs carefully. Some brushes and combs are more damaging than others. As a general rule, the softer the brush or comb, the less it will damage the hair. If it tears and pulls at your hair as you brush or comb, it's hurting the cuticle. Combs with rough teeth and brushes with hard bristles (not to mention rubber bands!) can all tear and chip away at the cuticle, causing unnecessary damage.

When drying your hair, never tousle, twist, or wring it dry with a towel or with your hands; instead, squeeze it dry gently using either a towel or your hands. Friction erodes the cuticle. The less the hair is rubbed against itself or by or with anything else, the better off it will be.

Handle your hair as little as possible. Friction is the culprit here, too. Rubbing one strand against the surface of another, or across another surface, causes friction and fractures the cuticle. The less you interact with your hair, the better. If you have the habit of mindlessly running your hands through your hair (I know I do), try to develop another habit.

Use indirect heat (three to six inches away from the hair is best) to remove excess moisture from your hair before you style your hair with a blow dryer and brush. Hair is more vulnerable to damage when it is wet. However, hair is difficult to control and style with a blow dryer when it is completely dry, so the goal is to not dry the hair completely, but only to remove the excess moisture, leaving it damp, but not soaking wet. Then you can go through your hair and create the style you want with your blow dryer and brush. This step of removing excess moisture before styling will go a long way toward reducing damage.

It is interesting to note that mild heat is not a problem. In fact, low levels of heat can help conditioners penetrate the layers of the cuticle better, making hair feel soft and increasing flexibility.

When styling your hair with a blow dryer, avoid applying high, intense levels of heat directly to the hair. This rule is probably the hardest to comply with because high heat in direct contact with hair is what it takes to create most hairstyles, particularly if your goal is to change hair from curly to straight or straight to curly. If you are diligent about keeping the nozzle of the dryer moving over the hair so it doesn't rest in any one place for more than a moment, that helps a great deal in preserving the integrity of your hair. I recommended above that you keep the nozzle of the blow dryer at least three to six inches away from the hair. That indeed will prevent damage, but you've never seen a hairstylist do that because it won't help you style your hair. So do the best you can to get the style you want by keeping the heat moving over the hair.

Use your blow dryer, curling iron, hot rollers, or other heat implements as infrequently as possible, and try to use the least amount of heat you can and still achieve the style you want. Intense heat damages hair! There is no escape from this one either. The same way high heat can burn your skin, it can burn your hair. It's a dilemma, and this is where you may be tempted to ignore my warning. All you have to do is believe the claims that many styling products or conditioners make: that they can coat the hair and reduce damage caused by styling implements. Unfortunately, the claims don't add up to an accurate picture. These products do offer some protection, but how much is totally dependent on how thoroughly you saturate the hair and how hot your styling tool gets. High heat applied directly, along with brushing and pulling (a necessary element of using styling tools) for more than a few minutes will exhaust the product's ability to protect and will allow heat to easily get through to the cuticle.

Before using a flat iron or curling iron on your hair, be sure the hair is 100% dry. Any excess moisture left in the hair can literally boil when you use a flat iron or curling iron. Water boils at 212°F and most curling irons and flat irons get far hotter than that. What can happen when the curling iron or flat iron comes in contact with the hair, especially if you leave it in one place for too long, is that the water inside the hair shaft boils and turns to steam, which causes the hair to break or rupture in that area. Interestingly, there is research showing that there is minimal damage and even a slight improvement in the strength of hair when a flat iron or curling iron is used on completely dry hair using minimal tension and keeping the implement moving over the hair instead of resting in one spot (Source: *Journal of Cosmetic Science*, January–February 2004, pages 13–27).

When using a flat iron, move the implement smoothly over the hair to prevent concentrating the heat in one area. As mentioned above, flat irons can heat up well past the boiling point, and that can damage hair. Keep the implement moving over the hair to prevent too much heat from being concentrated in one area.

Perming and/or coloring hair causes damage. There is no way around this one! Even worse is perming and then coloring your hair, too (or vice versa), which causes terrible damage. Changing hair from dark brown to blonde is also extremely damaging. And once hair is damaged there is no way to repair it (Source: *Journal of Cosmetic Science*, September–October 2001, pages 329–333).

AVOID THE SUN

You are probably aware of how damaging any amount of unprotected sun exposure is for skin. What you may not realize is that unprotected sun exposure is also damaging to the hair. The sun's ultraviolet light energy impacts the cuticle almost the same way as bleaching the hair. Repeated or prolonged sun exposure literally wears away the hair's cuticle (the outer protective layer) by breaking down its keratin protein composition. Depending on the amount of exposure and how damaged or naturally porous your hair is, you end up with weakened, dry, brittle, and degraded hair.

Aside from the sun damaging the hair's structure, it can also affect hair color. Color pigment in the hair is held in a group of molecules that are relatively fragile and unstable. That's good news for those of us who want to change our hair color because it means the pigment can be altered or removed with the right chemical dyes or bleaches. The downside is that prolonged, unprotected sun exposure can have a similar effect by breaking down the pigment molecules inside the cortex, causing color loss. The destruction of hair color this way is another cause of damage to the cortex, the heart of the hair.

Protecting hair from the sun is a good idea, but it cannot be done reliably with hair-care products. Recognizing the limitations of sunscreen protection for hair, the FDA doesn't allow hair-care products to have an SPF rating because that would be deceptive.

Sunscreen ingredients just do not cling to hair very well, and they definitely do not hold up when hair is shampooed or when conditioner is rinsed out of hair. Leave-in conditioners or hair-styling products with sunscreens have a better chance of staying on your hair, yet after hair is styled with blow dryers, curling irons, or flat irons, those ingredients are diminished to the point of being nonexistent. Even if sunscreen ingredients could cling to hair and hold up under styling, when a product doesn't have an SPF rating there is no way to know how much protection you are getting. Let's say the product contained only enough sunscreen ingredient to rate an SPF 2 or SPF 4—that would provide only about 30 minutes to one hour of sun protection, hardly enough to adequately protect the hair throughout the day, and that's also assuming you don't do anything to manipulate the hair after the sunscreen ingredient is applied to it.

How can you best protect your hair? A hat and/or staying out of direct sunlight (which is best for your skin, too) are the only viable alternatives. Another possible option, though not necessarily aesthetically pleasing, would be to take whatever SPF product you apply to your skin and apply a generous amount evenly through your hair after it is dried. This works only if you use a sunscreen with an SPF 15 or higher rating that also contains a UVA-protecting ingredient—either titanium dioxide, zinc oxide, or avobenzone (which may also be listed as butyl methoxydibenzoylmethane or Parsol 1789). For more information about sun protection and the critical difference between UVA and UVB sun damage, refer to my Web site, www.cosmeticscop.com (Sources: *Journal of Photochemistry and Photobiology*, May 2004, pages 109–117; *Journal of Cosmetic Science*, January–February 2004, pages 95–113, and November–December 2001, pages 377–389; and *Skin Pharmacology*, July 1994, pages 73–77).

HAIR AND pH

Hair-care companies often proclaim their products are pH balanced and can return hair to its natural pH. But exactly what is hair being balanced to? It turns out that hair, when dry, actually has no pH. Only liquids or liquid solutions can have pH. So, when hair is dissolved in a liquid solution it has about the same pH as skin, about 4.5 to 5.5, which is acidic. Water has a neutral pH of 7. However, it's not the hair itself that has a pH. Rather, there is what's called an acid mantle covering the hair shaft, made up of oil and perspiration, and this is what creates the pH of hair. This invisible layer actually protects the hair. Applying a substance with a pH greater than 7 (more alkaline than hair) decomposes the hair's acid mantle and begins eating away at the hair's outer cuticle layer. A product with a pH less than 2 (more acidic than hair) also decomposes hair. Therefore, anything with a pH greater than 7 or less than 3 is bad for hair. And any product with a pH of 4.5 to 7 works great for hair, either by complementing the hair's natural acid mantle or just by leaving it alone and not disturbing it! The goal of any hair-care product should be to leave the pH of hair alone or to move it slightly in the acidic direction (to help the cuticle layer lie flat), and that's about it.

However, you don't have to run out and buy special pH paper to test your hair-care products. It turns out that almost every hair-care product being sold (except for hair dyes and perms) is formulated in a hair-friendly pH range. High-pH hair-care products that can damage your hair are largely a thing of the past and no longer a concern for your tresses.

Ms. Science: You can do your own hair-strand test to prove how hair reacts to acid versus alkaline solutions. Take a few strands of hair from your hairbrush (this works better if you have longer hair) and soak one strand in a tablespoon or so of lemon juice (this is the acid) and another in an equal amount of baking soda and water (one tablespoon baking soda to two tablespoons water; this is the alkaline). Then rinse both strands gently and allow them to dry. Run your fingers back and forth over the strands and notice how they feel and look. You should notice that the hair soaked in the lemon juice and water will feel smoother and look shinier than the strand soaked in baking soda and water.

SCALP FACTS

Your hair and your scalp are vastly different, yet intricately related. Oil production and dry scalp are probably two of the biggest headaches women have to deal with when deciding what shampoo and conditioner to use. Both oily and dry scalps can adversely affect the appearance of your hair on a daily basis. But even for someone with normal hair, a healthy scalp can play a significant role in the appearance of the hair over the long haul.

Like the skin on your face, your scalp goes through a shedding process. In both cases, the lowest layers of skin are where new cells are generated. Unlike other parts of your body that are not protected by a dense covering of hair, the scalp rarely, if ever, has any sun damage, and that makes it some of the healthiest skin on your body. But with overshampooing, buildup of styling products, and skin disorders such as dandruff and psoriasis, the scalp can have its problems, too.

As skin cells go through their life cycle, they transform, begin to die, and move toward the outside, changing shape and function along the way. By the time they get to the outer surface they are dead and ready to fall off. Meanwhile, emerging from the scalp via hair follicles embedded deep within it, are single strands of hair. Each hair follicle is connected to a sebaceous (oil-producing) gland, nerve endings, and blood vessels. Circulation at the base of the hair follicle feeds the developing hair cells, helping to make a strong, healthy strand of hair.

Your oil glands provide their own conditioning agent to the hair shafts. As oil makes its way along the hair shaft (which is aided by brushing), it adds shine, protection, flexibility, and smoothness by covering and filling in the spaces around and between the layers of cuticle.

Oil production is controlled almost entirely by hormonal activity. There is no way to stop oil production from the outside in. This means that so-called oil-control products are a bit of a joke, because while some of them can clean away oil or absorb excess oil, none can change the amount of oil that is being produced (Source: *Cosmetic Dermatology*, April 1999, pages 13–15).

For many reasons, oil production is both good and bad for hair. Oil is a problem when it makes hair look heavy, greasy, and limp, but oil from your oil glands is also good for hair because it protects the hair from drying out. Essentially, what a conditioner does is the same thing that your own oil provides naturally. The oil gland produces oil, the oil melts over the surface of the scalp and onto the hair shaft, and the oil then moves along the hair toward the ends. On straight hair, the oil follows the path of the hair and moves easily downward along the hair shaft toward the ends. On curly hair the oil also follows the exact path of the hair, moving along the twists and curves. That convoluted path makes it difficult for the oil to make its way to the ends of the hair. So, someone with straight hair and an oily scalp may experience far oilier conditions (meaning limp, greasy hair) than someone with curly hair and an oily scalp.

When you have an oily scalp, it is a never-ending struggle, because the oil you wash away is so rapidly replaced. Yet using stronger surfactant shampoos isn't the answer because you can only remove the oil that's already there—something that is relatively easy for even the most gentle shampoos. Using stronger products to try and stop the oil really can't do anything more, but it can definitely dry out the hair and scalp, making matters worse.

The most effective way to deal with almost all scalp types and to reduce damage to the hair shaft is to focus most of your shampooing attention on your scalp and not on your hair. That doesn't mean treating the scalp roughly or overscrubbing, it means gently massaging the scalp with your fingertips, and gently moving your nails along the scalp. This massaging action not only helps to remove dead skin cells, but also increases circulation as you shampoo. Gently increasing circulation is one of the only ways to help nourish the root of the hair follicle from the outside in to help maintain healthy growth. It won't produce miracles like helping to grow hair where there isn't any, but improving circulation can be subtly beneficial. Don't be concerned that you won't be getting the length of your hair clean; despite the way products can build up on the hair, it actually gets pretty clean without much manipulation. Moreover, the less you manipulate the hair shaft, the less you damage the cuticle.

There are also a couple other factors that come into play. Given how much oil is usually present at the roots of the hair, the roots require less conditioner. Similarly, less conditioner is needed thanks to the root's healthy state (it hasn't been around long enough to be damaged by styling tools, sun exposure, dyeing, or perming). So, just as it is important to clean the scalp more scrupulously than the length of hair, it is far more important to condition the length of hair than the scalp. Adding conditioner to the scalp is often like adding a moisturizer to oily skin on the face: It just makes matters worse.

So, regardless of the apparently close relationship between scalp and hair, it is essential to treat your scalp and your hair as if they were not at all related or even existing on the same head. Remember, the scalp is part of a living system, and the hair you see and need to maintain is dead. Scalp needs and hair needs are very different.

GENETIC DESTINY?

Many of us find that, regardless of how good we are to the cuticle or how diligent we are about taking care of our scalp, our hair still does not do exactly what we want it to, especially in the areas of thickness, fullness, and density. Alas, the strands that grow out of your head are genetically fated, and there isn't much any hair-care product can do to alter your inherited traits. How full your hair appears mainly has to do with two things: the number of hairs on your head and the size and curl of the hair shaft, both of which are predetermined at birth. The average head of hair has about 100,000 to 150,000 strands. Blonde and light brown hairs have very thin, narrow shafts, while black, dark brown, and red hairs have the thickest. This explains why, even though blondes tend to have more hair strands, their hair often appears less full—that's because the individual hairs themselves are not as thick.

Fine hair is twice as easy to break as medium-textured hair. Fine hair has fewer cuticle layers and thus is easier to damage, while medium- and coarse-textured hair is far more durable.

African hair is the thinnest and most fragile, for two reasons—because the hair shafts are very thin and because it has repeated twists and turns, with each twist being a potential break point. Asian hair, on the other hand, is rather thick and substantial, and most typically stick straight. You can change the hair you were born with, but big changes take time, energy, money, and skill (Sources: *Household and Personal Product Industry*, HAPPI, April 2004, pages 86–98; and *Cosmetics & Toiletries*, February 2004, pages 53–58).

Seeing the endless onslaught of seductive models with their long, flowing, diligently coifed manes causes angst in many of us. While the ads want us to believe the company's shampoo or conditioner created those results, it is not even vaguely possible. First, the models have great hair, which is why they're models and we're not! We also sometimes fail to recognize the energy and time it takes for a hairstylist to get hair to do what we see in ads and commercials. If you haven't seen a photo shoot or a commercial taping, you probably aren't aware of the contributions of the camera person, the lighting crew, or how any of a dozen details culminate in creating the enticing image. Fans are strategically placed to blow the hair into billowing fullness, and constant rebrushing and styling keep the do in place. **All the things we don't see are what really makes those models look so good, and yet the ads suggest that a simple product change can create those results. We want to believe it is really that simple, and the hair-care companies encourage us to do just that.**

I know I'm not telling you anything you don't already know, either from your own experience or your familiarity with ingredient lists. But with fashion magazines and hair-care companies incessantly telling you to expect the impossible, it is easy to fall prey to the advertising traps waiting to ensnare you.

HAIR COLOR AND GRAY HAIR

Hair color is created by pigment-producing cells called melanocytes, which make a pigment called melanin. For hair color, the two primary types of melanin are eumelanin and pheomelanin. Eumelanin generates shades of blonde, brown, and black hair color, while pheomelanin produces shades of red hair color (Source: www.medicine.net).

Whether we like it not, somewhere between the ages of 30 and 50 (and even as young as 12) gray hairs begin growing from the exact same hair follicle from which our previously blonde, brown, red, or black hair originated. Even more so than wrinkles, gray hair is associated with aging. Statistics show that for Caucasians, 50% of the hair you have will, to some degree, be gray by the age of 50.

Though rarely a health concern, gray hair is definitely a fashion concern for many men and women. Hair color changes to gray as a result of decreasing pigment production in the hair follicle. For unknown reasons, gray hair often starts being produced near the temple area and then spreads back through the crown. Others might experience a general diffuse graying all over the head, and less frequently swatches of gray can appear in just one section of the scalp (Sources: *Micron*, April 2004, pages 193–200; and *Experimental Gerontology*, January 2001, pages 29–54).

One of the pervasive myths about gray hair is that you can turn gray overnight as the result of some kind of emotional trauma. It isn't possible—well, not unless you dye your hair gray. Hair color over the entire length of the hair cannot change faster than the speed that hair grows, much less overnight. Hair color is produced deep in the scalp at the base of the hair follicle and it can take months or years before the change of color is visible in any appreciable length. Once the hair emerges from the scalp with a particular color, it cannot change itself to another color. Hair is dead, and the color does not alter or leach out unless influenced by hair dyes or prolonged sun exposure.

Equally persistent is the myth that if you pull out one gray hair two or more will grow back. If that were the case, why wouldn't pulling out a brown or blonde hair produce more hair from that follicle? What a way to make hair thicker! Of course, that's a myth, not fact; pulling out a hair does not generate the growth of another hair, or create a new follicle for hair to grow from. If anything, the number of hairs you have on your head is the number you had on the day you were born, and there's no way to create more follicles after that. What does happen is that the hair's texture, color, and growth pattern change as you get older; the number of hair follicles stays the same.

WHAT CAUSES BAD HAIR DAYS?

Bad hair days can happen overnight. Perfect hair one day, nightmare hair the next, and you did nothing different. The scenario goes something like this: You wake up on a Tuesday and your hair is perfect; it moves just the way you want it to and goes into just the style and shape you have in mind, and you don't even try very hard. The next day,

Wednesday morning, you wake up much as you did the day before, get dressed the same way you did the day before, everything is identical—except your hair now has a mind of its own and it has decided to be spiteful and bad-tempered. No matter how you blow it dry or what styling products you use, it goes this way instead of that and, to add insult to injury, it moves stiffly and seems to have cowlicks that were never there before. What happened?

We know the damage we inflict on our hair can cause styling problems. What we may not know is that conditioning agents and styling products can build up on the hair and eventually, although seemingly overnight, cause the hair to feel heavy and lifeless. This recurring phenomenon is often the cause of bad hair days. It is also why the myth about your hair adapting to hair-care products got started. It's not that your hair adapts, it's that the ingredients in conditioners and styling products that cling to hair are not easy to wash off, and tend to build up. That buildup can greatly affect the appearance and quality of hair.

Another thing that might be causing your hair's confusion are your hormones. Increased estrogen production the week before you get your period can trigger increased oil production, making hair limp and dull. Hormones also affect how you view yourself, and the premenstrual blues can make any feature that looked fine the day before seem like an eyesore the next. Everything probably looks the same, but with PMS eyes, you can't see it realistically. The significance of this should not be taken lightly. Women often waste more money on grooming products, fighting this time of month, when it has nothing to do with what really exists, but is a result of their own emotionally blurred vision. Depression and stress can cause the same misinterpretation of the facts. Realizing that you really haven't changed can help prevent your low spirits from getting even lower.

It's bad enough having your emotions and hormones play tricks on you, but the environment can also cause bad hair days. Humidity, dryness, or a change in the weather can alter your hair, whether it's due to the change of seasons or a weather pattern moving through your area. Hair takes on moisture from the air with relative ease, and it also releases its moisture content to the air when it is dry outside. If you've ever gotten on an airplane when the humidity was high or at least normal, with your curls bouncing neatly in place, you may have noticed that by the end of the trip they've gone flat and dry. The lack of humidity in the airplane virtually sucks the water out of the hair, causing it to go flat and look dry. During the winter, dry heat at home and in the office can have the same effect. Dry air can also cause static electricity, making hair go flyaway. On the other hand, increased relative humidity can cause naturally curly hair to swell and become more frizzy, more curly (where you don't want curls), and harder to control, while making thin or limp hair look even flatter and more limp.

Bad hair days are also affected by timing. **Hair behaves differently when it is dried at various degrees of wetness, and that behavior varies from person to person. Generally, if you start styling your hair when it is wet, you have a better chance of getting it**

to do what you want. Perhaps your bad hair experience occurred on a day when you got to your blow dryer a little later than usual and your hair had dried a bit more than it should in order for you to style it with ease. Hair is finicky, and finding your hair's personal nuances can sometimes let you come to the rescue on bad hair days. For example, if you rewet your hair to style it the next day, consider getting the roots wetter than the ends, because it's the way the roots slant that is predominantly responsible for determining the movement, lift, and shape of the hair. That's why the way you sleep on your hair can set it into a cowlick that all the heat in the world won't correct.

Finally, damaged hair is particularly susceptible to all the variations of humidity, dryness, hormonal activity, and styling nuances. When it's damaged, hair is so much more porous and its cuticle so much rougher that these hazards are twice as likely to cause problems.

WHY HUMIDITY IS WORSE THAN RAIN

It always baffled me why my hair held its style so much better day after day in the endless rainy weather months in the Pacific Northwest where I live (and, yes, it does seemingly rain here all the time) than it does on a sunny, hot, and humid day in Florida. How can it be that the water I *can't* see in the air makes my fastidiously and neatly flat-ironed hair frizz and curl despite all the styling lotions, hairsprays, silicone serums, and various forms of pomades I've used, while the water I *can* see, whether it is pouring or misting, tends to leave my hair intact as long as I keep the rain off it? The answer is simple: Because there is no way to keep the water you can't see off your hair.

It turns out that even healthy hair is exceptionally porous. Water is readily absorbed into hair, which is why hair changes so radically when it is wet. Even when hair is dry, it still holds about 20% water in the cortex. That's why anything more than 20% of water in the hair can destroy any hairstyle. Ironically, the lack of water in the hair can do the same thing, by making hair dry and lifeless.

Think of humidity as the amount of water in the air between the raindrops. That's the water you can't see and that's why high humidity (moisture in the air) can be present on a sunny day in Florida but not on a rainy day in Seattle. Relative humidity is a measure of the amount of moisture in the air. It is expressed in a percentage of how much moisture the air can possibly hold. The "wetter or damper" the air feels, the higher the relative humidity. Conversely, the drier the air feels the lower the relative humidity. So, while you can keep the rain off your hair with an umbrella or hood, which keeps it from penetrating into the hair shaft and altering your coif, there is no way to keep high humidity in the air out of your hair. Humidity in air is everywhere, omnipresent and invasive, even under umbrellas and in the space between your hat and hair. On days with higher relative humidity there is more water in the air, and that increases the likelihood it will be absorbed into your hair, wrecking your hairstyle the same way sprinkling water on your hair would.

STATIC ELECTRICITY

Dry conditions in your home, office, or environment can cause static electricity to build up whenever two surfaces are rubbed against each other. That explains why static electricity is more prevalent in the winter than in the summer: hot dry air in homes and offices sets the stage for static electricity, even just from shoes moving over a carpet or from your hand running through your hair. When dry hair is brushed, combed, or rubbed with material such as a hat or scarf, static electricity builds up on the hairs. When this electrical charge builds up, each strand of hair is repelled by the others, causing the hairs to fly away from each other. Humidity and moisture reduce the chances of a static electricity buildup. However, it wouldn't make sense to add water to your hair because that would ruin your hairstyle, but well-conditioned hair can help a great deal to control the flyaway effect. During the winter you may want to change the conditioner you use to one designed more for dry hair; adding a silicone serum to your hair before styling can help as well. And yes, rubbing a sheet of Bounce over your hair or spraying your brush or hat with Static Guard Anti-Static is also helpful.

CHAPTER THREE

Hair Growth—Hair Loss

HOW DOES HAIR GROW?

Depending on the individual, approximately 5 million hair follicles cover the surface of the body at any given time. Of that total, about 100,000 to 150,000 strands are growing on the head. Surprisingly, blondes usually have more hair on their heads than those with red or darker hair colors. All those millions of hair follicles are developed and in place before a person is born. Biologically, it is impossible to grow more hair after birth—all the hair you are ever going to have is already there when you arrive in this world (Source: *Structure and Function of Hair Follicles*, http://www.aad.org/education/hairfollicles.htm).

Inside the hair follicle, deep below the skin, hair is going through a life cycle all its own. At any given time, each hair on your body is going through one of three phases—growing, resting (or dormant), or shedding. The first phase is the **anagen (growth) phase.** At this point, the hair is very busy developing in the hair follicle, the pocket-like structure that houses the bulb-shaped root of the hair. At the very base of this root is an intricate network of capillaries and nerves that feed the developing hair. During the growth stage, each individual hair is formed by rapidly dividing cells that push forward and up through the follicle. As they multiply and expand, the cells reach the surface, where they die and harden into what we know (and see) as hair. The growth stage can last anywhere from two to six years. During this phase, hair grows an average of about half an inch per month, or six inches per year (but that is only an average and it varies drastically from very active hair growth to very slow growth for different people).

Over the entire growth phase, the hair can reach a length of approximately three feet, about the middle of the back for most women, before it stops growing and proceeds to the **catagen (resting) phase.** Naturally, there are variations in length potential, and women with tresses six feet long have been reported, but there are also women who can't grow hair much past their shoulders. The reason for these variations is that length of hair is genetically predetermined, and that explains why some women feel they can never get their hair to grow past a certain point, while other women can't seem to get to a hairdresser often enough to keep up with the grow-out.

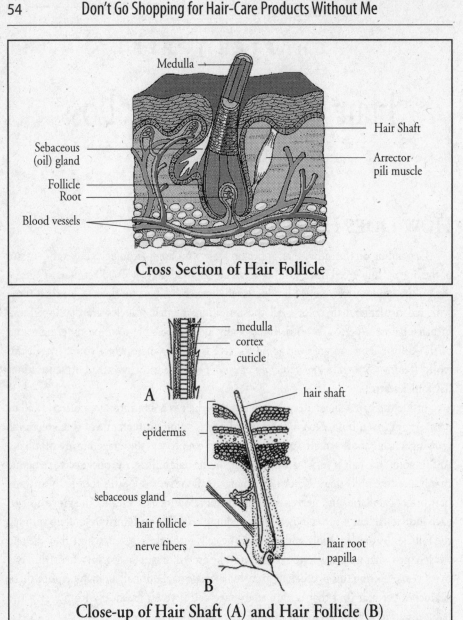

Cross Section of Hair Follicle

Close-up of Hair Shaft (A) and Hair Follicle (B)

The **catagen phase** also includes a **transition (intermediate) phase.** After about three to six years of growth, the hair cells stop reproducing and the growth process is over. For about two to six weeks, the hair just lies around taking it easy while the root slowly moves up to the skin's surface.

Entering its last phase of life, the hair is ready to literally jump ship and shed. The **telogen (final) phase** is short-lived. At this point the hair root has moved almost to the surface (near the opening of the oil gland), where it is completely separated from the base of the follicle. In a matter of weeks the anagen (growth) stage will begin again at the base of the hair follicle. Hair cells again start dividing and multiplying, generating a new shaft. When the new hair sprouts to the surface, it simply pushes the old hair out of its way. **So all that hair collecting on your brush, in the bottom of your drain, or on your clothing—about 25 to 100 hairs a day—is usually hair that has passed from the growth phase through the transition plateau and into the final period of shedding.**

At any given time, approximately 88% of scalp hair is in the anagen phase, 1% in the catagen phase, and 11% in the telogen phase. Thankfully, hair is predominantly in the growing phase (at least if male pattern baldness or some other form of hair loss has not started to occur), which explains why we end up having more hair than less, despite the strands we lose daily.

Although everyone's hair goes through the same life cycle, not all hair is the same; hair has very distinct inherited differences. African hair grows mostly in an alternating curved/flat sequence that imparts a coiled, corkscrew-like shape to the hair, a form that produces weak spots at every turn. Asian, Native American, and Hispanic hair is straight to slightly wavy, coarse, thick, and almost always black. European and Hindu hair textures vary greatly, from straight to curly, thick to thin, fine to coarse, and they have a wide range of colors. Generally, what distinguishes African hair from European or Asian hair is the tight, spiral growth pattern. The fragile nature of this corkscrew structure causes endless problems for African-American hair (see Chapter Eight, "For Women of Color") (Sources: www.aad.org; *Hair Loss: Principles of Diagnosis and Management Alopecia*, Jerry Shapiro, Taylor & Francis Group, December 2001; *Disorders of Hair Growth: Diagnosis and Treatment*, McGraw-Hill, Inc., 1994; *Dermatology Clinics*, October 1996, pages 573–583; *The Molecular and Structural Biology of Hair*, Annals of the New York Academy of Science, 1991).

WHY DOES HAIR STOP GROWING?

Alopecia is the technical name for hair loss, but that's just the beginning. There are so many complicated and multifaceted factors that affect hair growth the subject is too vast and complex for this book to tackle in detail. For example, reasons for hair loss can include **scarring alopecia** (also referred to as pseudopelade, a condition where for no known reason the hair follicle is destroyed, resulting in permanent hair loss); **nonscarring alopecia** (also referred to as **alopecia areata**, which results in hair loss that can grow back); **androgenetic alopecia** (more commonly known as male pattern baldness); **scleroderma** (a chronic connective-tissue disease believed to be an autoimmune rheumatic disease); **some tick bites; lichen planopilaris** (an inflammatory disease of unknown origin that usually affects the skin but can also affect hair and can result in permanent hair loss); **psoriasis; lupus** (an autoimmune disorder causing chronic inflammation, especially of the skin, but can also affect hair growth); **seborrheic dermatitis; trichotillomania** (an impulse-control disorder that causes people to pull out their own hair); **traction alopecia** (resulting from inadvertent pulling on hair from styling hair too tightly); **physical injury** (particularly burns that destroy hair follicles); **hemochromatosis** (an inherited disorder that causes the body to absorb and store too much iron, damaging the organs in the body); **surgery; cancer; rapid weight loss;** and **thyroid abnormalities**.

There is also a long list of **medications** that can cause hair loss, and there are no cosmetic products that can reverse their effect, though hair growth is almost always restored once the drug is not being taken. These include the cholesterol-lowering drugs clofibrate (Atromis-S) and gemfibrozil (Lopid); Parkinson's medication levodopa (Dopar, Larodopa); ulcer drugs cimetidine (Tagamet), ranitidine (Zantac), and famotidine (Pepcid); anticoagulants coumarin and heparin; drugs for gout treatment, including allopurinol (Loporin, Zyloprim); anti-arthritics penicillamine, auranofin (Ridaura), indomethacin (Indocin), naproxen (Naprosyn), sulindac (Clinoril), and methotrexate (Folex); drugs derived from vitamin-A isotretinoin (Accutane) and etretinate (Tegison); anticonvulsants for treating epilepsy trimethadione (Tridione); beta-blocker drugs for high blood pressure such as atenolol (Tenormin), metoprolol (Lopressor), nadolol (Corgard), propranolol (Inderal), and timolol (Blocadren); and anti-thyroid medications carbimazole, iodine, thiocyanate, and thiouracil.

Before you even begin to think about what products to use for hair growth, you must know the source of your hair loss. Each of these causes requires medical evaluation and a determination of treatment. Hair loss is not merely an aesthetic issue, it can also be a health issue (Sources: *Cosmetic Dermatology*, December 2003, pages 48–51; *Anagen Effluvium*, August 14, 2000, www.emedicine.com; *American Academy of Dermatology*, www.aad.org; American Hair Loss Council, www.ahlc.org; and *Journal of the American Academy of Dermatology*, October 2003, pages 667–671, and April 2000, pages 549–566).

MALE PATTERN BALDNESS

Although there are many forms of alopecia, the most prevalent by far is androgenetic alopecia, better known as male pattern baldness. About 95% of all cases of hair loss are the result of male pattern baldness, but this number also includes women, who can have a version of hair loss referred to as female androgenetic alopecia or female pattern baldness. Approximately 25% of men begin balding by age 30; two-thirds begin balding by age 60. For women, androgenetic alopecia was found in 3% of women ages 20 to 29 years, 16 to 17% of women ages 30 to 49, 23 to 25% of women ages 50 to 69, 28% of women ages 70 to 79, and 32% of women ages 80 to 89. In some research, statistics indicate that 40% of women are affected by androgenetic alopecia. As you can tell by these numbers, female pattern baldness increases dramatically just before and after menopause.

For men, male pattern baldness develops in a horseshoe pattern, with the hair receding from the forehead back toward the neck. Male pattern baldness can also take place from the center of the scalp out toward the sides. For women, the location is more diffuse, with hair loss taking place all over the scalp (Sources: *Male Pattern Baldness*, American

Medical Association Medical Library, www.medem.com; *Hair Loss & Restoration in Women*, International Society of Hair Restoration Surgery, www.ishrs.org; and *Dermatologic Surgery*, January 2001, pages 53–54).

The key element you need to be aware of to understand whether the products being sold to improve or restore hair growth will work is how hormones affect hair growth. This is because, for both male pattern baldness and female pattern baldness, hormones are the primary cause of hair loss. First, let's start with some basic information about the hair growing on your head.

Hair growth basically has a lot to do with hormonal activity, and is especially related to the male sex hormone group called androgens. (Androgens are male hormones such as testosterone and dihydrotestosterone.) Many different types of hormones influence hair growth, but androgens are believed to have the largest impact on the process. Testosterone and dihydrotestosterone (DHT, a hormonal by-product of testosterone) are produced in large quantities by the testes in men, and in smaller quantities by the ovaries in women. These hormones are responsible for the development of secondary male sex characteristics for both genders. They are also responsible for increasing the size of hair follicles early in life, and, ironically, for decreasing and shrinking the hair follicles later in life.

Technically, what is in part believed to be taking place in the hair follicle is that over time testosterone is changed to dihydrotestosterone (DHT) by the enzyme 5-alpha reductase (5AR). When DHT becomes concentrated in the hair follicle it eventually slows, and ultimately stops, hair growth. It is also believed that the effect of DHT is compounded or enhanced by an individual's genetic hair-follicle traits (Sources: *Androgenetic Alopecia*, October 2, 2003, www.emedicine.com; *Journal of Alternative and Complementary Medicine*, April 2002, pages 143–152; *British Journal of Dermatology*, April 2004, pages 750–752; *Journal of the American Academy of Dermatology*, May 2004, pages 777–779; *Journal of Investigative Dermatology*, December 2003, pages 1561–1564; and *American Journal of Clinical Dermatology*, 2003, volume 4, issue 6, pages 371–378).

For women, it appears that their increased levels of estrogen (the primary female sex hormone) act against the effects of male androgens on hair growth. This explains why, when estrogen levels decrease as women approach menopause, androgen-related balding can begin to appear. There is some research indicating that topical application of estrogen can induce hair growth in women (Source: *Journal of Investigative Dermatology*, January 2004, pages 7–13).

BLOOD FLOW AND HAIR LOSS

While research concerning hair loss has focused primarily on the involvement of hormones, there is a good deal of discussion about another concept, especially on Web sites selling products claiming to regrow hair. According to these sources, the status of the hair involves the issue of blood supply to the hair follicle. Some hair-care companies want you to believe that reduced or impeded blood flow is the primary factor affecting hair growth. Improve the blood flow, they say, and you should be able to improve hair growth. As logical as that sounds, it doesn't work that way in reality.

Although an adequate oxygenated blood supply is necessary for any and all of the tissues of the body to function properly, not all disorders of the body (including hair loss) are related to decreased blood flow. Consider this: When hair follicles are transplanted from the back of the head to the front they do not become thin and they do not fall out. There seems to be plenty of blood flow in the same bald areas where the newly trans-planted hair thrives. If the areas that became bald were damaged as a result of poor blood flow, then the transplanted hair follicles should suffer the same fate—yet they don't. If anything, the new hair becomes beautifully thick and healthy (Source: *British Journal of Dermatology*, February 2004, pages 186–194). Needless to say, this is one example of a hair-loss solution that sounds plausible, but the facts paint a different picture.

BALD-BUSTING

The myths surrounding baldness have been around a long time, and most are a mixed tangle of fabrications wound around a kernel of fact.

Only men experience male pattern baldness. Yes, the term does say "male"—but as the research discussed above clearly shows, "male pattern baldness" absolutely affects women, and is the most prevalent form of hair loss they experience.

Male pattern baldness skips a generation on your father's side; it is inherited from your mother's side of the family. We've all heard at least one of these, but it's time to stop blaming your relatives. Hair loss does have a genetic component, but no one is quite sure what it is. It is also probably related to several genes, not just one, and most likely a combination of genetic inheritance from both parents (Source: *Journal of Investigative Dermatology*, December 2003, pages 1561–1564).

Male pattern baldness or thinning hair is caused by hair mites. This theory is pro-moted mainly by the hair-care company Nioxin, which sells a product called Semodex designed specifically to kill the *Demodex folliculorum* mite. The problem with this theory is that lots of people have the *Demodex folliculorum* mite present in the sebaceous glands that are attached to the hair follicles. Up to 75% of the United States population—men, women, and children—have it, and not all of them are balding (especially not kids), or have thin hair. The other significant proof is similar to the blood-flow myth explained below: If the *Demodex folliculorum* mite was the factor in male pattern baldness then hair transplants wouldn't work, but work they do, and very well. There has never been a case where transplanted hair follicles fell out or became thinner, and male pattern baldness does not return, even though the *Demodex folliculorum* mite may still be present (Source: www.keratin.com).

Vitamin deficiency is responsible for hair loss. This myth is close to actually being true. There are definitely vitamin deficiencies that can result in hair loss. However, watch out for the notion that it takes some miraculous combination or secret blend of vitamins to restore hair, because that's where the myths abound, especially on Web sites selling supposedly special hair-growing pills. In reality, the vitamins believed to be responsible for hair growth are the B vitamins, with biotin arguably the most important. Vitamin C and vitamin A can both affect hair growth, but it's interesting to point out that excessive intake of vitamin A can cause a toxic reaction that can trigger hair loss (Source: www.keratin.com).

Mineral deficiency is responsible for hair loss. This is another myth that has some truth to it—but again, there is no magic mineral supplement that will regrow hair. There is research showing that iron deficiency in women can be a factor in female hair loss. Low levels of the essential amino acid L-lysine, or of magnesium and copper in the diet also seem to play a part in hair loss. Research on zinc supplements shows little evidence that it has any effect on hair growth, but there is controversy and the research is not in agreement about this (Sources: *Clinical & Experimental Dermatology*, July 2002, pages 396–404; *Obesity Surgery*, February 1996, pages 63–65; and *Acta Dermato-Venereologica*, May 1995, pages 248–249).

Poor blood flow causes pattern baldness. This isn't true in the least. As any hair transplant doctor will tell you, the scalp's healthy blood flow, even in areas where balding has taken place, is one of the reasons hair transplants work so well—there is thriving blood flow to supply the newly implanted hair. Not to mention that when you cut the scalp it bleeds profusely—hardly something indicating constricted or depleted blood flow.

Stress causes hair loss. There is some truth to this. However, because there are myriad reasons why hair can fall out and not grow back, it is important to have your concerns checked out by a dermatologist. Stress can be a factor in hair loss, but it is extremely low on the list of reasons for hair loss, especially in comparison to male pattern baldness, health issues (particularly taking certain medications and rapid weight loss), hair breakage caused by problematic styling techniques, and physical trauma or injury (Sources: *Cosmetic Dermatology*, February 2004, pages 123–126; and *The Journal of Dermatology*, December 2003, pages 871–888).

Wearing your hair in a ponytail can cause hair loss. This isn't quite a myth because it all depends on how tightly hair is pulled back and how often. Just because you wear a ponytail doesn't mean that it's going to affect hair growth. Yet in extreme cases, some hair loss can be attributed to frequent, intense, and constant pressure on the hair follicle. There is actually a name for this: **traction alopecia**. Women who wear extremely tight ponytails, especially those with fine or thin hair, can experience bald spots, particularly around the hairline. African-American women who weave heavy hair extensions or braids into their own hair, plait beadwork into cornrows, or wear tightly patterned braids are very susceptible to this kind of hair loss. Thankfully, traction alopecia is almost immediately rectified when the pressure is relieved. And less pressure is what's needed, because there are no vitamins, shampoos, or special products to handle this predicament.

Pregnancy can make hair grow. As wonderful as pregnancy can be it's not automatically guaranteed that it will make hair grow in thicker or healthier. In many cases pregnancy causes hair loss. Pregnancy focuses a large amount of the body's energy on taking care of the developing fetus and that priority can reduce or stop the hair's anagen or growth phase. When a hair falls out during the telogen or shedding phase of hair growth (it is natural to lose as many as 100 hairs a day), there is no new hair preparing to emerge and start the growth phase. On the other hand, some pregnant women whose female hormones are flourishing have an extended anagen phase of hair growth and their hair just keeps growing! At some point after the baby is born, the telogen/shedding phase finally kicks in and noticeable, sudden hair loss can be scary. Either way, don't be concerned: These are both temporary conditions that almost always return to normal sometime during the first few months after the baby's birth or, in some cases, after the breast-feeding stage is over. Just be patient. Don't rush out and buy products in an effort to change what is happening; they won't work (Sources: *Journal of the American Academy of Dermatology,* October 2003, pages 774–775; *American Journal of Dermatopathology,* April 1998, pages 160–163; *Journal of Cutaneous Medicine and Surgery,* May–June 2002, pages 236–240; and *Archives of Family Medicine,* March 1993, pages 277–283).

Clogged pores on the scalp cause hair loss. This one is complicated because the fundamental process of how hair actually grows is so intricate and so involved with chemistry and biology that it is difficult to understand the complexities unless you happen to be a scientist. Suffice it to say, there is a kernel of truth in this myth, but it isn't so much about pores being clogged as it is about the presence of sebum (oil) in the pores. All sebaceous glands produce some amount of oil, which contains testosterone and DHT, the by-product of testosterone that causes hair to stop growing. The sebaceous gland is also an area where 5AR, the enzyme that converts testosterone to DHT, is active. Therefore, as the theory goes, if you reduce oil production, you reduce the ability of 5AR to turn testosterone into DHT. Just keep in mind that this relationship between oil production and hair loss is a theory, and there is little research supporting it.

Some hair-care companies are capitalizing on this theory that clogged pores are the problem, claiming they can undo that blockage and thereby stimulate hair growth. Yet that is far from what is taking place. Oil production is regulated by hormones, and there is no way to turn that off by applying something topically (Sources: *Dermatology Clinics,* July 1999, pages 561–568; and *Endocrine Reviews,* August 2000, pages 363–392).

CAN THEY REALLY STOP HAIR LOSS?

I'm sure you've seen the ads: Grow Hair in 12 Weeks! Stop Hair Loss Today! Stop Baldness Without Costly Drugs, Chemicals, or Surgery! Turn Fallout into Grow-out with Only One Hour of Your Time a Week! Wouldn't that be nice? Then all you'd have to do is send in your three easy payments of $29.95 and receive a combination of vitamins, a special shampoo or conditioner, several scalp masks, a battery-operated scalp massager, and who knows what else, and you, too, would look like the before-and-after pictures in the advertisements. Bald spot one day, waves of bushy hair a few weeks later. If any of this were possible, why would anyone be bald? There wouldn't be a naked scalp in the house!

Some popular ingredients such as emu oil, zinc, superoxide dismutase, and green tea have some minor studies showing they have some ability to generate hair growth, but the research is not enough to warrant much attention. Nonetheless, these ingredients are promoted and glorified to the point of absurdity by companies selling products that contain them. The information enthusiastically states that there is abundant definitive research proving efficacy, when in reality the research is at best questionable, not done double-blind, and there are no additional, follow-up studies to verify the results of earlier studies. One study alone cannot by anyone's definition generate conclusive evidence. That means the evidence is more like guessing than anything, and something you shouldn't bank on with your hair follicles.

Regrettably, almost all of the concoctions being sold for hair growth are nothing more than snake-oil treatments, here today and gone tomorrow. You would be better off throwing your money out the window, at least then you wouldn't be funding the unscrupulous businesses that lure other hopeful but soon-to-be-deceived consumers into wasting their money.

HAIR GROWING POSSIBILITIES

Minoxidil is still the only over-the-counter, topical pharmaceutical whose claims regarding hair regrowth have been approved by the FDA. Minoxidil, at one time available only under the trade name Rogaine, is now available under different names from several different companies and can increase hair growth by a statistically significant percentage in both men and women. Extensive research and statistics suggest that this fairly inexpensive treatment works incredibly well for some people.

According to the Mayo Clinic's *Women's Health Report* (May 1998), minoxidil is successful for 44% to 63% of women who try it. It is actually far less effective for men, working in only about 20% of men who use it. Dermatologist Arthur P. Bertolino, M.D., Ph.D., director of the hair consultation unit at New York University, in an article published in the December 1991 FDA *Consumer* magazine, said that minoxidil ". . . approximately 90 percent of the time at least slows down hair loss."

Using minoxidil (the active ingredient in Rogaine) at any available strength is extremely safe (Source: *Journal of Cutaneous Medicine and Surgery*, July–August 2003, pages 322–329). Two strengths are available, 2% and 5% concentrations, and for women it seems that the 5% strength works better than the 2%. A study reported in the *Journal of the American Academy of Dermatology* (April 2004, pages 541–553) looked at 381 women who used either the 5% or 2% minoxidil solution for hair loss. Both the 5% and 2% solutions were superior to using nothing, which means both helped hair grow back, but the group that used 5% minoxidil demonstrated better hair growth than the 2% minoxidil group.

Despite this success, there is concern for women that both the 2% and 5% strengths can cause hair growth where you don't want it, namely on the face and other parts of the body.

A study published in the *Journal of the European Academy of Dermatology and Venereology* (May 2003, pages 271–275) found that in a review of 1,333 women who were using either 2% or 5% minoxidil, 4% experienced unwanted hair growth, and that there was a higher incidence of unwanted hair growth in the group using the 5% strength. The study also pointed out, however, that a large percentage of the women in a part of this study (27%) reported that they experienced facial hair growth *before* they began using minoxidil, so it's possible that the women who reported the unwanted hair growth before applying minoxidil were more prone to the potential for that growth when using minoxidil. It is important to note that the unwanted hair growth is not permanent and reverses itself once you stop treatment.

The question is: Would you fall into the 4% group who experienced hair growth in annoying places, and is that worth the risk to you? If you already have a problem with too much hair growth in unwanted places, perhaps minoxidil isn't right for you. I should mention that personally I use the 5% strength. I had been using the 2% strength and didn't see the improvement I was hoping for. I changed to the 5% strength and the receding areas at my hairline grew back in just under four months. I also found that I was allergic to Rogaine (it made me itch and flake terribly), so I changed to the generic version of minoxidil and it worked just fine with no problem in the several months I've been using it. And it's definitely less expensive.

No one is certain yet just how topical minoxidil works, though work it does. The most common side effects with this medication are itching and skin irritation, and once you stop using it, any hair that grew as a result of the drug will fall out.

Propecia (technical name **finasteride**) is an oral medication that was approved by the FDA in 1998 to treat men with male pattern baldness. It works by inhibiting the 5 alpha-reductase enzyme, the enzyme that converts testosterone into DHT (the hormone that causes male pattern baldness). An article in *Cosmetic Dermatology* (January 1998) reported that "The FDA's Dermatologic and Ophthalmic Drugs Advisory Committee agreed in discussions that Propecia is efficacious in treating male pattern baldness." The article cited three studies "involving 1,879 men, ages 18 to 41, who had mild to moderate but not complete hair loss…. These studies, which lasted 24 months demonstrated that treatment with Propecia prevented further hair thinning, and significantly increased hair growth in the majority of men (86%)." However, as an article in *Newsweek* (November 17, 1997) pointed out, 42% of the men in the placebo group also showed improvement. Still, 86% is an impressive number.

But don't get too excited—there are negatives to taking this drug. Propecia can cause birth defects for pregnant women and may decrease men's libido. However, as several doctors pointed out to me, the research showed the libido decrease was minor and that it was not significantly different from that of the placebo group. What the study warnings didn't point out was that in some people finasteride raised the levels of testosterone and increased the libido! For some that's a great side effect, and you may get some of your hairline back at the same time (Sources: *Journal of the American Academy of Dermatology*, June 1999, pages 930–937; *European Journal of Dermatology*, January–February 2002, pages 38–49; and *Archives of Dermatology*, August 1999, page 990).

There is also research showing that a combination of applying minoxidil topically while taking the oral medication Propecia has the most impressive and long-lasting results (Sources: *Dermatologic Surgery*, November 2003, pages 1130–1134; and *Journal of Dermatology*, August 2002, pages 489–498).

I should point out that one study, published in *Dermatologic Surgery* (May 2004, pages 761–763) and conducted at the University of California Los Angeles, showed significantly fewer desirable results than every other study published about finasteride (Propecia). A total of 1,261 patients were monitored every three months with telephone calls after finasteride was initially prescribed. After 12 months, a detailed questionnaire was sent to all patients. The study noted that 32% (414 men) continued to take finasteride daily for one to three years, that 24% (297 men) discontinued the drug between 3 and 15 months because of poor results, and that the remaining 44% (549 men) dropped out of the study for unknown reasons. Of the 414 men who continued to take the medication, less than half returned their detailed questionnaires; a small percentage of this group felt that they grew hair and the others noted poor results.

Saw palmetto is a popular herbal supplement sometimes recommended for hair growth. However, there are absolutely no reliable studies that have investigated saw palmetto in relation to hair growth (the only one that does exist was performed by the company that sells a saw palmetto supplement, and it studied only ten people; given the special interest and the small sample number this is a bogus study). There are abundant studies for saw palmetto in relation to its ability to improve benign prostatic hyperplasia (BPH). Saw palmetto got its reputation for hair growth inadvertently due to the relationship between BPH and male pattern baldness, both of which are affected by the production of DHT. If saw palmetto could affect DHT, it was only a short stretch to assume that it might be effective in treating male pattern baldness, too. But theory isn't always good medicine. There is also research suggesting that saw palmetto does not affect DHT and that it exerts some other action that may be the reason for the improvement in BPH symptoms. Further, there is no reason to assume that saw palmetto is safer than Propecia (active drug ingredient finasteride). In fact, there are reports of similar side effects (Sources: www.naturaldatabase.com; *Journal of the American Medical Association*, November 1998, pages 1604–1609; *American Family Physician*, March 2003, pages 1281–1283; *Urological Research*, June 2000, pages 201–209; *Cochrane Database of Systematic Reviews*, 2002, volume 3; and www.hairlosstalk.com).

Tretinoin (trade name Retin-A or Renova) is a topical cream or gel that may influence improvement in cell development, making it beneficial for many skin-care problems, ranging from acne to wrinkles. Surprisingly, no one is actually sure why tretinoin can do that, but there are lots of studies indicating that it does. Some dermatologists have begun formulating their own treatments for male pattern balding by mixing tretinoin with minoxidil for topical application. It is thought that tretinoin can increase the absorption of minoxidil into the scalp (Source: *Archives of Dermatology*, June 1996, pages 714–715).

Azelaic acid is typically prescribed for rosacea and some acne conditions. Recently, the potential for using azelaic acid to treat androgenetic alopecia has been discussed. According to Kevin J. McElwee, an immunologist/dermatologist involved in research on hair loss and regrowth, "Studies carried out in France in the late 80's were to assess the effects of zinc sulfate and azelaic acid on the human skin. The result of these studies demonstrated that at high concentrations, zinc could completely inhibit the activity of 5 alpha reductase. Azelaic acid was also shown to be a potent inhibitor of 5 alpha reductase. Inhibition was detectable at concentrations as low as 0.2mmol/l and was complete at 3mmol/l. When zinc, vitamin B6, and azelaic acid were added together at very low concentrations, which had been ineffective alone, 90% inhibition of 5 alpha reductase was achieved" (Source: *British Journal of Dermatology*, November 1988, pages 627–632). However, there is no other research showing azelaic acid to be useful for hair regrowth. Even the Web sites that claim there are numerous studies list no other sources.

Copper peptides are a group of ingredients that have caused excitement at several companies, who are now making noisy and serious claims about their hair-growth potential. According to a Reuters newswire story (April 4, 1999), the "ProCyte Corporation said that it obtained statistically significant results in an initial study of its hair growth compound, in a group of men, ranging in age from 18 to 40 years old, with male pattern hair loss. The early-stage Phase II clinical study of the company's investigational compound, trade-named Tricomin solution, enrolled 36 men with early to mid-stage androgenetic alopecia [male pattern balding]. Treatment with 2.5% PC1358 [alanine/histidine/lysine polypeptide copper hydrochloride] resulted in a statistically significant increase in the total hair count when compared to vehicle [placebo] treatment over the course of the study. Appreciable increases in total hair weight were not found over the treatment phase of the study." While this research is interesting, it has not convinced the FDA to approve copper peptides for hair regrowth, and no other research supports these results. In fact, neither ProCyte nor Skin Biology have additional research duplicating the same results. Of course, this hasn't stopped ProCyte and Skin Biology from selling several product lines that include forms of copper peptide. ProCyte owns Tricomin, and Skin Biology sells Folligen. These two companies are discussed further in Chapter Ten, "Product Reviews."

Tagamet (active ingredient cimetidine) is an oral medication commonly used for acid indigestion and to treat stomach ulcers and other digestive discomforts. However, Tagamet has been shown to have an anti-androgenic effect, meaning it blocks the binding of DHT, and that can in turn reduce hair loss (Source: *International Journal of Dermatology*, March 1987, pages 128–130). However, for women, there is research showing that cimetidine can also induce hair loss (Sources: *Therapie*, March-April 1995, pages 145–150; and *The Journal of Clinical Endocrinology & Metabolism*, January 2000, pages 89–94).

Ketoconazole is a topical and oral antifungal medication. It is used topically to reduce the presence of fungus that might be triggering dandruff, and orally to reduce systemic fungal infections. It has been observed that oral doses of ketoconazole can lower serum testosterone and thereby reduce the presence of DHT (Source: *Hormone and Metabolic Research*, August 1992, pages 367–370). However, there are serious side effects to taking ketoconazole orally, including dizziness, nausea, and headaches. Due to the associated problems with taking ketoconazole orally, there are those who think that applying it topically, in the form of the anti-dandruff shampoo Nizoral, can produce the same testosterone-lowering effect as the oral dosage. However, there is no research of any kind demonstrating this to be the case.

Hormone blockers (such as spironolactone, cyproterone acetate, and flutamide) are oral drugs that specifically reduce the production of testosterone by the adrenal glands and can thereby prevent DHT from having an effect on the hair follicle. But these are serious drugs and are not a consideration for men due to their feminizing effects (Source: *The Journal of Clinical Endocrinology & Metabolism*, January 2000, pages 89–94).

Birth control pills definitely affect hormones, and there are many conflicting opinions about their effect on hair loss or hair regrowth. Regrettably, there are few scientific studies on female pattern baldness, and even fewer when it comes to the effect of birth control pills on this condition. The small amount of research that does exist shows that some birth control pills have more testosterone-like activity, which can possibly promote hair loss by increasing the likelihood of testosterone being converted to DHT. That would cause a number of hair follicles to lapse into the telogen phase (shedding) and then not begin the anagen phase (growth) again. Further, the presence of testosterone can increase secondary male sex characteristics such as facial hair growth. It can also increase the likelihood of acne, because acne is frequently caused by androgen activity involving testosterone and DHT, the same hormones that trigger hair loss.

Many birth control pills also contain minimal amounts of testosterone, or have anti-androgenic properties (meaning they inhibit testosterone). These formulas can therefore reduce hair loss and may actually help hair growth on the head, while also reducing the risk of acne. When birth control pills contain estrogen, they can help reduce hair loss because estrogen makes hair stay on the head longer.

Because there are so many other complicated and significant health issues related to taking birth control pills, hair loss and hair growth should not be the primary reason for taking them. It is essential for you to discuss all the pros and cons of these drugs at length with your physician (Sources: *Obstetrics and Gynecology*, May 2003, pages 995–1007; *Drugs*, 2003, volume 63, issue 5, pages 463–492; and *American Journal of Clinical Dermatology*, 2002, volume 3, issue 8, pages 571–578).

Melatonin is an herbal supplement. One study, published in the *British Journal of Dermatology* (February 2004, pages 341–345), stated that because melatonin has been reported to have a beneficial effect on hair growth in animals, it was of interest to evaluate the effect of melatonin on hair growth in women with male pattern baldness. The double-blind, randomized, placebo-controlled study was conducted in 40 women suffering from diffuse alopecia or androgenetic alopecia. Either a 0.1% melatonin solution or a placebo was applied on the scalp once daily for six months. The results showed melatonin led to a significantly increased growth rate in comparison to the placebo group. However, this is the only study that indicates melatonin has this effect.

The FDA cited Texas hair-care marketer **Pride & Power** for anti-baldness claims made for their Don't-B-Bald Hair Care Treatment and Don't-B-Bald Scalp Stimulate. The claims made include lines such as "has many natural ingredients we believe help the process of keeping your hair healthy and aiding in growth" and "has been formulated to stimulate the scalp hair follicle, allowing blood cells to circulate." These statements classify Pride & Power hair products as unapproved new drugs. As such, the products are not recognized as safe and effective, and their continued sale is a violation of the Food, Drug, and Cosmetic Act. According to the FDA's Hair Grower and Hair Loss Prevention Products final monograph, over-the-counter products are prohibited from making any anti-baldness claim without prior FDA approval. A similar citation was issued to hair-care company Farouk, for their anti-baldness Power Plus products, and caused the manufacturer to change their hair-loss recovery claim to "hair thickening" (Source: *The Rose Sheet*, April 14, 2003, page 4).

HAIR TRANSPLANTS

Mention hair transplants to someone and it will immediately conjure up images of obvious, unsightly plugs of hair dotting someone's scalp like bad patches of grass on a lawn. Hair transplants from a decade ago did use grafts containing several hairs, and the results appeared like rows of planted hairs growing from a black plug on the scalp. Fortunately, those days are over, and new techniques in hair transplants create a completely natural look. Today's techniques implant only one to four hairs, with no detectable base in sight. This state-of-the-art procedure is called the follicular-unit grafting technique, a process that relies on microscopic dissection at the back of the head to produce the hair grafts. It is an expensive, complicated procedure, but the results are remarkable and the hair does grow with minimal to no risk of further hair loss or thinning (Sources: *Archives of Facial Plastic Surgery*, September–October 2003, pages 439–444; *Plastic and Recon-*

structive Surgery, January 2003, pages 414–424; *Dermatologic Surgery*, September 2002, pages 783–794; International Society of Hair Restoration Surgery, www.ishrs.org; and Hair Transplant Medical, www.hairtransplantmedical.com).

Before you decide to consult a physician for a hair transplant procedure of any kind, keep in mind that *any* licensed physician in the United States and Canada can perform hair surgery. That means a doctor who was previously a gynecologist, without taking one course, could hang out a shingle tomorrow declaring him- or herself a hair transplant specialist. It is that easy, and it happens all the time. This lack of licensing or coursework requirements means that it's easy for the consumer to end up with disappointing and inferior results, such as visible scarring, patching, fuzzy hair, or even more hair loss. Before you book an appointment, find out if the doctor you are considering is in good standing with the International Society for Hair Restoration Surgery (ISHRS); contact them through their Web site at www.ishrs.org, or contact the American Academy of Facial Plastic and Reconstructive Surgery at (800) 332-3223 or www.plasticsurgery.org.

HAIR GROWTH—SCAMS OR SOLUTIONS?

The number of hair-growth products on the market is literally hair-raising! Sadly, however, very few actually grow hair, though the companies that sell them are taking in a lot of your money. Several products and product lines make claims about hair growth, including Avacor, BioFolic, Fabao 101, Folliguard, Folligen, Hair Factor PX-2000, Hairgenesis, Hair Prime, Helsinki Formula, Nioxin, Nisim, Nutrifolica, Proxiphen, Pro-Genesis, Regenix, Revivogen, Shen Min, and I'm sure dozens—perhaps hundreds—more. I address some of these in Chapter Ten. But please, before you fall for the fraudulent or exaggerated selling tactics of any hair-growing product (even those products that *can* affect hair growth often exaggerate their claims), keep in mind the following information from www.keratin.com by Kevin McElwee:

"[First,] most alopecias are not a gradual progressive hair loss. Most, including androgenetic alopecia, develop in spurts and then stop. There may even be some improvement for a short time before the hair loss begins again. Someone using a hair growth product might falsely attribute this slowdown or temporary reversal to the use of the [product they purchased].

"Second, people who want to believe will believe. When real drug companies test products for hair regrowth they run at least two methods of analysis side by side. One method is entirely empirical evidence. They mark an area on the volunteer's head and count the hair density in the area before and after treatment to see if there is improvement. The other analysis method they run is more subjective. They give a questionnaire to the volunteer and ask how the volunteer tester perceives the drug is working. Most human trials of drugs for alopecia are classic double-blind studies involving a group that receives the drug and another control group that receives an innocuous placebo compound. No one knows whether they are using the drug or placebo. **Frequently what is found is that volunteers on the drug or placebo indicate they believe they have re-growth of hair, but when comparing their positive comments to the hair count/density data it is revealed there is no actual improvement and there may even be a deterioration.** Call it optimism or an overactive imagination, it is an important factor for professional scam artists [because they can tell you a product works when it only appears to work due to a placebo effect]." (Emphasis added.)

CHAPTER FOUR

Hair-Care Formulations

WHAT DO THEY MEAN WHEN THEY SAY...?

What startles me most in the world of hair care is how incredibly repetitive the formulations are. Despite the claims, the differences in formula composition between shampoos, conditioners, and styling products are minor. To compensate for the missing variety, an immense amount of marketing language is created to help support the illusion that there are amazing differences, when in fact there are little to be found.

So what *is* the difference between a product that builds body and one that builds volume? Are they one and the same or is there a difference? How *does* a product build volume or add body to the hair? Is a product designed for color-treated hair really very different from one designed for permed or damaged hair? What makes a product good for color-treated hair but not for dry hair, or vice versa? Can a hair-care product that claims to put curl back into the hair or to revitalize a perm really do that? Good questions!

One of the more confusing aspects of reviewing the hair-care industry is trying to keep the terminology and claims straight. Names for product types, descriptions of what they do, and the results they promise are not consistent from line to line or even within lines. As my reviews show, products claiming to clarify or deep-clean hair may contain ingredients that add more buildup, or be formulations that can't deep-clean. A shampoo claiming to be good for oily hair may contain conditioning agents that will only add up to a greasy feel. One line may have a host of products claiming they can add volume to the hair, but those products may have nothing in common with those from a different line that claim to do the same thing.

It is difficult to wade through this morass of contradictions and inconsistencies. The following general guidelines can help you get started.

Most products designated either separately or in combination for permed, color-treated, coarse, chemically processed, dry, damaged, porous, or sun-bleached hair tend to contain similar ingredients. These products all tend to be more emollient and conditioning than other product types, and generally there is little difference in how the products in this group are formulated. The reason these formulations can be the same and still function well is easy to understand. Although the cause of each of these hair problems is different, their effect on the hair shaft tends to be the same. Hair damaged by the sun, hair dyes, perms, or styling tools suffers the same injury regardless of the source.

Dry hair is a result of the hair losing its moisture content, often because damage has destroyed the hair's own ability to keep moisture in the hair. But it also can happen to healthy hair just because it's in a dry environment (in that case your hair could be dry without being damaged). Either way, the product you use to make your hair manageable, soft, and silky calls for the same formulation, even if the source of the problem is different (Sources: *Cosmetics & Toiletries*, May 2003, pages 28–32, and May 2004, pages 64–68).

Products that claim to add body, volume, or thickness to the hair almost always contain the same ingredients. A combination of lightweight water-binding agents such as glycerin, propylene glycol, amino acids, panthenols, and proteins, along with a small amount of styling agents (film formers and plasticizing agents) such as acrylates, PVP, and PVM/MA (polyvinyl methyl ether/maleic anhydride) are standard in products professing to make hair fuller and thicker. These styling agents are the same as those often found in hairsprays and especially in styling gels. The water-binding agents keep water in the hair to prevent dehydration and thus keep the hair swollen, helping to add a feeling of thickness. The styling agents cover the hair shaft with an almost imperceptible layer that adds to its thickness. None of these ingredients or products is in any way capable of changing the actual structure of hair; they merely add a coating that creates an illusion and feel of thickness.

Many products in many different forms claim to reduce frizzies. Anti-frizz products almost always contain some form of silicone, emollients, film formers, and detangling agents. These ingredients put an emollient layer over the hair, changing the way it feels to the touch by binding the cuticle down and slightly sticking the hairs together without making them feel as bonded as they do with hairspray, gel, or mousse.

What about products that say they can add shine to the hair? When the cuticle lies flat it has a smoother, more even surface that can reflect light. For example, think of a lake. When the surface is smooth, you can see your reflection shining back at you. When a breeze picks up, the surface becomes rough and uneven and its reflecting qualities are broken up. So how can you make the cuticle lie flat and appear smoother? There are three major ways— shampoo, conditioner, or styling product—all of which involve adding a low-pH product over the hair to make the microscopic layers of the cuticle close tight. As it turns out, most shampoos and conditioners these days have the right pH to create this effect.

But no matter what the pH of the product happens to be, if the hair is damaged it still won't look smooth and shiny, because the cuticle is so worn and chipped there is no even surface there to reflect the light. Adding ingredients to hair that fill in the chips and gaps is a wonderful way to give the image of shine and the feel of smoothness. Products that say they impart shine generally contain silicone, various oils, and conditioning agents, though silicone is by far the preferred ingredient for shine. Silicone is an outstanding hair-care ingredient and the unsung hero of the hair-care world. Not only does silicone add reflection and sheen, it also imparts an unbelievably sensual, silky feel. The only trick with these types of products is to not get carried away thinking more is better—too much can build up to a greasy mess that looks more wet and sticky than shiny.

Conditioners vary according to the amounts of emollients, water-binding agents (for moisturizing), detangling agents (for comb-ability), film formers (for volumizing), antistatic ingredients (for manageability), silicones (for shine, detangling, and a silky feel), and oils (for dryness) they contain. When a conditioner contains only small amounts of these, it is best for someone with normal, limp, fine, or oily hair. When a conditioner includes more of these, it is best for someone with any level of damaged or dry hair.

Styling products, with their film-forming ingredients and silicones, are the perfect adjuncts for imparting the most shine and silky feel to hair.

WHAT'S IN ALL THIS STUFF?

The average hair-care product is composed of 50% to 90% water. Thickeners, cleansing agents (detergents/surfactants), styling ingredients, and conditioning agents, which make the product look and perform the way we expect it to, comprise almost everything else. Less than 1% of the product contains the buzzword ingredients that we think we're buying, such as protein, panthenol, vitamins, and plant extracts. Some of these, such as proteins and panthenol, have merit for hair, but not when they are present in meager amounts. Regardless of the formulas and the marketing, there are no secrets when it comes to whether or not a product works for your hair. You can tell immediately if your hair feels clean, soft, is defrizzed, easy to style, and whether or not it stays put.

One way to demystify hair-care products is to learn what is in them, what those ingredients can and can't do for the hair, and how they can affect your hair despite the claims on the label. Cosmetics companies can say practically anything they want on their labels, brochures, advertisements, and in their sales presentations. They can tell you that their product restructures, builds body, reconstructs, mends, restores, rebuilds, nourishes, or revives the hair, and they don't have to prove or verify any of it because hair products are cosmetics, and cosmetics, according to the FDA, don't have to prove their claims. Even if a hair-care company can substantiate a claim, the results are often evident only with the aid of an electron microscope that blows up the image of a hair shaft to countless times its original size. That's great from a scientist's point of view, but it might not have anything to do with how a product or a specific ingredient will affect your hair.

The labels on hair-care products are almost absurd in their descriptions and explanations of what their products will do for your hair—except for the ingredient list. Legally, the ingredient list is the only part of a cosmetic's label that is strictly regulated. The more familiar you are with this part of the product, the less likely you are to be led astray by frivolous, flimsy, superficial information designed by marketing experts who want you to believe their products can do the impossible. The ingredient list is the best indicator of what you are buying. It is by far more accurate than anything else on the label. With that in mind, let's get a better sense of what we are putting on our heads.

Hair Note: The long list of plant extracts at the beginning of many hair-care ingredient labels may look appealing, but the notion that this "tea water" is providing some benefit for your hair is just not true. If plant extracts could take care of hair, couldn't you just make your own "plant tea" to create the same effect as the pricey stuff you're buying? Unfortunately, there isn't a plant or group of plants in the world that can clean hair, make it feel silky soft, or keep it in place after styling (Sources: *Cosmetics & Toiletries*, May 2003, page 130, and May 2004, pages 57–63; and *Cosmetic Dermatology*, February 2003, pages 71–76, and May 2003, pages 32–36).

SHAMPOO

First things first—and the first step is cleaning your hair. Get this step right and you are halfway home. You'll be relieved to learn that it is hard to get this step wrong. Most shampoos are kind to the scalp and do a good job removing oil, styling products, conditioning agents, mineral deposits, and dirt from the hair. For all their purported differences, all shampoos (especially the good ones) contain primarily water, detergent *surfactants* (**SURF**ace **ACT**ive Age**NTS**), lather builders, humectants (ingredients that attract water to the hair), thickeners (ingredients that give the shampoo a pleasing consistency), and preservatives, plus whatever fad "natural" ingredient or fragrance is added to make you think you're buying something special.

Shampoos (whether labeled as two-in-ones, moisturizing, volumizing, restructuring, and on and on) contain varying concentrations of conditioning agents, which range from quaternary ammonium compounds (antistatic and detangling agents) to panthenol, collagen, protein, elastin, silicones, amino acids (conditioning agents), and film-forming or holding ingredients (these are hairspray-type ingredients) to oils and other emollients. These conditioning ingredients are meant to stay on the hair even after it is rinsed clean. Using a shampoo that contains silicones, film formers, emollients, and detangling agents can have an impact on your hair, an impact that is both good and bad. **The good part is that they can help some hair types feel, look, and behave wonderfully; the bad part is that because they keep getting redeposited on hair and never really get washed out, they can build up, eventually making hair look flat and feel heavy.**

In general, if you are concerned with dry scalp or irritation, you may want to *avoid* shampoos that contain drying surfactants (cleansing agents) such as sodium lauryl sulfate, TEA-lauryl sulfate, sodium C14-16 olefin sulfonate, and alkyl sodium sulfate, especially if they are the second or third ingredient listed. (**Reminder:** Don't confuse sodium *lauryl* sulfate with sodium *laureth* sulfate. They are not the same thing. Sodium laureth sulfate is a mild surfactant. Just to be clear, although I discuss this in more detail in this section, ammonium lauryl sulfate and ammonium laureth sulfate are also standard surfactants used in shampoos and are considered gentle surfactants, though some would suggest ammonium lauryl sulfate is not all that gentle.)

As drying as some surfactants can be, there are lots of natural ingredients that are also drying and irritating to the scalp, such as lemon, grapefruit, orange, menthol, peppermint, lime, balm mint, oregano, essential oils (which are really just fragrance, a major source of skin sensitivity), avocado, horseradish, papaya, and a long list of other plant extracts.

You cannot tell the quality of a shampoo (or any hair product for that matter) by its color or fragrance. Those are all emotional qualities and not in any way relevant to the product's performance. As pleasant smelling as shampoos and other hair-care products can be, the fragrance serves no purpose. If anything, the fragrant ingredients in hair-care products—which often appear on ingredient lists as essential oils or plant extracts—can be skin irritants (Source: www.naturaldatabase.com).

Shampoos do vary according to the hair type listed on the label; however, market segmentation tends to create more categories than are really justified by the slight differences between products. For example, even though you will find many different shampoos that claim to be for different hair types—color-treated, permed, dry, dehydrated, brittle, damaged, sun-bleached, and straightened—they actually differ very little because all of these hair types need the same ingredients to look their best.

Hair Note: You will notice as you read this chapter that there is some overlap of ingredients between shampoos, conditioners, and styling products. That is because it's possible for all three product types to contain many of the same types of ingredients, and still do their respective jobs.

Surfactants/detergents and lather builders, in combination, are the essence of every shampoo you buy. The terms surfactant and detergent cleansing agent are often used interchangeably by chemists and researchers. I refer to these substances throughout this book as "detergent cleansing agents." And don't let the term detergent concern you, even though it may sound harsh. Most detergents are actually far gentler than soap. Soap solutions are alkaline, and that can damage the hair's cuticle and cortex, while detergents generally have a hair-friendly pH of 4.5 to 7. Aside from the damage soap can cause to hair, the ingredients that keep it in its bar form are difficult to rinse off and can leave a residue that makes hair hard to comb and difficult to manage. Detergents effectively degrease and emulsify oils and fats and suspend soil, allowing them to be washed away without leaving any residue—and, for the most part, they do this quite gently (Sources: Food and Drug Administration, *Office of Cosmetics and Colors Fact Sheet*, February 3, 1995, www.fda.gov; *Dermatology*, 1995, volume 191, number 4, pages 276–280; *Tenside, Surfactants, Detergents*, 1997, volume 34, number 3, pages 156–168; and http://surfactants.net.)

Interestingly enough, surfactants do not lather. They have no foaming ability. Lather builders, on the other hand, are what form suds into a bubbly mass over the hair. Yet all the lather in the world won't clean one hair on your head! It is strictly the surfactants that clean the hair and scalp. However, lather can indicate how well a hair-care product is working. When oil or styling agents build up on hair or are not removed, it will prevent lather agents from working. Therefore, seeing copious bubbles on the head is a good sign, indicating that your hair is clean or is getting clean.

The detergent cleansing agents used in almost every shampoo being sold are sodium laureth sulfate, ammonium lauryl sulfate, ammonium laureth sulfate, cocamidopropyl betaine, cocoamphodiacetate, sodium cocoglyceryl ether sulfonate, sodium lauryl sulfate, and sodium lauryl sarcosinate. There are many more, but these are the most common. The ingredients used to create lather are cocamide MEA, lauramide MEA, lauric DEA, lauramine oxide, cocamidopropyl hydroxysultaine, and polysorbate 20, among others.

The following detergent cleansing agents are also common and considered extremely gentle. However, they do not have good cleansing ability: cocamidopropyl betaine, cocamphocarboxyglycinate-propionate, sodium lauraminodipropionate, disodium monoleamide MEA sulfosuccinate, disodium monococamido sulfosuccinate, disodium cocamphodipropionate, disodium capryloamhodiacetate, cocoyl sarcosine, and sodium lauryl sarcosinate.

There is much discussion in the industry about which surfactants are the most gentle or the most problematic. On the problematic side, sodium lauryl sulfate, TEA-lauryl sulfate, sodium C14-16 olefin sulfonate, and TEA-dodecylbenzene tend to be far more drying and potentially irritating to the scalp than other cleansing agents.

Sodium lauryl sulfate (SLS) is a common cleansing ingredient in shampoos, and a large amount of misinformation about it is still being circulated on the Internet. SLS can be derived from coconut, and is used primarily as a detergent cleansing agent. Although it is a potent skin irritant, it is not toxic or dangerous for skin. However, in concentrations of 2% to 5%, SLS can cause allergic or sensitizing reactions in lots of people. It is so well-recognized for this that it's used as a standard in scientific studies that compare the irritancy or sensitizing properties of other ingredients (Sources: *European Journal of Dermatology*, September–October 2001, pages 416–419; *American Journal of Contact Dermatitis,* March 2001, pages 28–32; and *Skin Pharmacology and Applied Skin Physiology*, September–October 2000, pages 246–257).

Being a skin irritant, however, is not the same as saying that it may be linked to cancer, which is what erroneous warnings on the Internet are falsely claiming about this ingredient!

According to Health Canada, in a press release on February 12, 1999 (www.hc-sc.gc.ca), "A letter has been circulating the Internet which claims that there is a link between cancer and sodium laureth (or lauryl) sulfate (SLS), an ingredient used in [cosmetics]. Health Canada has looked into the matter and has found no scientific evidence to suggest that SLS causes cancer. It has a history of safe use in Canada. Upon further investigation, it was discovered that this e-mail warning is a hoax. The letter is signed by a person at the University of Pennsylvania Health System and includes a phone number. Health Canada contacted the University of Pennsylvania Health System and found that it is not the author of the sodium lauryl sulfate warning and does not endorse any link between SLS and cancer. Health Canada considers SLS safe for use in cosmetics. Therefore, you can continue to use cosmetics containing SLS without worry." Further, according to the American Cancer Society Web site (www.cancer.org), "Contrary to popular rumors on the Internet, Sodium Lauryl Sulfate (SLS) and Sodium Laureth Sulfate (SLES) do not cause cancer. E-mails have been flying through cyberspace claiming SLS [and SLES] causes cancer … and is proven to cause cancer…. [Yet] A search of recognized medical journals yielded no published articles relating this substance to cancer in humans."

Quaternary ammonium compounds are a wide range of ingredients, called "quats" for short, that share a unique molecular structure that makes them strongly attracted to hair. When one end of the quat grabs the hair, the other end sticks out, providing a handle for another quat molecule to grab onto. This linking creates a lineup on the hair that resembles a temporarily smooth surface, allowing combs and brushes to more easily glide through hair. Found primarily in shampoos, rinse-off and leave-in conditioners, and any product that claims to detangle the hair, these less-than-poetic-sounding ingredients are essential for having manageable hair. Typical quats on an ingredient list include guar hydroxypropyltrimonium chloride, dicetyldimonium chloride, dihydrogenated tallow benzylmonium chloride, behentrimonium chloride, behenalkonium betaine, benzalkonium chloride, quaternium 18, stearalkonium chloride, cetrimonium chloride, and many more.

Humectants/water-binding agents help keep water in the hair to prevent dehydration and thus keep the hair expanded to its natural shape, providing a feeling of thickness and softness. Glycerin, sorbitol, glycols, mucopolysaccharides, hyaluronic acid, sodium PCA, propylene glycol, and glycosphingolipids, among others, attract water from the air to the hair shaft and help keep it there, giving hair bounce and a feeling of fullness. Humectants work in conjunction with quats and conditioning agents to keep static cling at a minimum and give hair a softer, thicker feel. These also help keep the hair's natural water content intact, particularly in dry climates. Glycerin and propylene glycol, among other glycols, are inexpensive and effective protective agents for hair.

Conditioning agents such as collagen, protein, amino acids, silicone, panthenol, and triglycerides are often included in shampoos for the same reasons they are included in conditioners: They help make hair easier to comb, softer, shinier, and more silky feeling. The only problem with most conditioning agents, except for silicone, is that they can't stand up to water and tend to get washed or rinsed away. That's why conditioning shampoos rarely work well for damaged, dry, or coarse hair, because the shampooing process doesn't allow enough conditioning agent to be deposited to make that kind of hair manageable.

I wish there were more to tell you about protein and other conditioning agents, but there just isn't. Whether it comes in the form of wheat germ triglycerides, silk protein, or some other enticingly named ingredient, it brings no added benefit (such as strengthening) to the hair shaft. It simply provides a protective coating that is washed away the next time you wash your hair.

Whether conditioning agents can penetrate the hair shaft is open to much debate. What we do know, however, is that there are no unique ingredients with a special molecular structure that can do this. Even if conditioning agents could penetrate hair they would have a hard time staying there, because how would that happen and what would occur to cause the hair to hold onto the conditioning agents? It is important, however, not to shortchange what conditioners can accomplish: clinging and attaching to the layers of the cuticle. The cuticle is as important as the cortex, if not more so. What all conditioning agents can do, and do quite effectively, is *temporarily* protect and reinforce the hair's structure, mostly on the outside, and to some extent (how much and for how long is unknown) on the inside (Sources: *Journal of Cosmetic Science*, September–October 2001, pages 63–83 and January–February 2003, pages 265–280; *Cosmetics & Toiletries*, May 2004, page 130; and *Consumer Reports*, September 2000, pages 18–21.)

Plant extracts show up in hair-care products claiming to perform miracles for hair. The list of such ingredients is literally endless, and their individual merits and hypes are mostly way too complex to deal with in this book. I will do my best to explain briefly in Chapter Ten, "Product Reviews." Generally speaking, while some plant extracts do have antioxidant, anti-inflammatory, and antimicrobial properties for skin, when they are used in products such as shampoos and conditioners, the benefits are just rinsed off the scalp. Antioxidant benefits from plant extracts could help hair in terms of environmental protection, but again, these ingredients don't cling to hair very well and they don't remain stable when hair is being rinsed in the shower. For the most part, plant extracts have little benefit for hair. It is also important to remember that just because an ingredient comes from a plant doesn't automatically make it good for skin or for hair. There are plenty of natural ingredients that have the potential to irritate skin (Source: www.hairscientists.org/article7.htm; and www.naturaldatabase.com).

Volumizing ingredients. See the section *Volumizing Shampoos* below.

Thickeners are responsible for the texture, appearance, and movement of the final product you use. Literally hundreds of thickening ingredients are used in shampoos, conditioners, and styling products. Typical thickening agents you'll see on ingredient lists are cetyl alcohol, stearyl alcohol, hydrogenated lanolin, glycol stearate, palmitic acid, and so on. All of these, and many more, have soft, waxy textures and are responsible for the viscosity and weight of the final product. For styling products such as gels, the typical thickening agents used in almost every product are carbomer and/or guar. These gelatin-like substances create the appearance you associate with gels. The list of thickening agents is too long to include in a book of this kind, but the effects of these agents are the major reason you find a product desirable (Source: *Cosmetics & Toiletries*, October 2000, pages 67–73).

Vitamins are perhaps the most overhyped ingredients in hair care. When it comes to hair, even though it's dead, we still want to believe vitamins can somehow feed or nourish it. They can't. There is no research proving their effectiveness for hair. Panthenol and biotin are vitamin B derivatives that work topically on hair, but it's because of their consistency, not because of their nutritional value. There can be benefit in taking vitamins for hair growth, but the extremely complex internal digestive process just doesn't translate to topical application. Besides, even if vitamins could somehow affect the hair via the scalp—from the outside in—vitamins are present in hair-care products in such tiny amounts they couldn't cover even one hair shaft of your hair, much less your entire head.

Preservatives are an integral part of every hair-care formula because hair-care ingredients are combined together in a very liquid solution, and this wet environment is a perfect breeding ground for bacteria, fungi, and microbes. It is therefore of primary importance that we include preservatives in all formulations to prevent this normal, though potentially harmful, growth from taking place. To that end, antibacterial, antifungal, and antimicrobial agents are included to keep contamination to a minimum. The most popular preservatives used in hair-care products are methylparaben, propylparaben, phenoxyethanol, DMDM hydantoin, methylisothiazolinone, methylchloroisothiazolinone, and imidazolidinyl urea. For more specific information about these ingredients, please visit my Web site at www.cosmeticscop.com and refer to the Cosmetics Ingredients Dictionary.

WHAT ABOUT pH-BALANCED SHAMPOOS?

Cosmetics companies are notorious for bragging about the pH level of their products. A decade or so ago that would have been a good selling point, but today it's irrelevant. pH stands for "power [of] hydrogen," and indicates how acid or alkaline a formulation is. If a hair-care product is too alkaline (pH 8 and over) it can cause the hair shaft to swell and damage the cuticle and cortex. The consequences of high-pH ingredients on hair are seen most clearly in those who use hair dyes and perms. These products have a pH ranging from of 8 to 14, which can drastically and permanently alter the structure of hair. If a hair-care product is more acid (pH 3 to 5.5), it can tighten and flatten the cuticle, making the hair feel softer and look shinier. When the cuticle scales are lying flat and tight against each other, the hair reflects light better and the hair shaft is better protected from damage. What you should know is that for the past several years most hair-care companies have formulated their products with a pH of approximately 4.5 to 6.0 (keep in mind that water has a *neutral* pH of 7). That is considered standard in the industry and is very helpful for hair. If a shampoo has a low pH, lower than about 4, it won't lather well, and there are those who think the cleaning ability of the surfactant in it is also diminished. If you want to test the pH of your shampoos, you can purchase pH testing strips or litmus paper from a science supply store or on the Internet.

MOISTURIZING SHAMPOOS

If you have dry, damaged, or coarse hair, a moisturizing shampoo can be your best friend. In essence, moisturizing shampoos are similar to the two-in-ones discussed below. A well-formulated moisturizing shampoo should contain gentle detergent cleansing agents, conditioning agents, water-binding agents, and silicones. The good news is that's exactly what most of them do contain. For those with dry, damaged, or coarse hair it is still important that you follow up with a leave-in conditioner. Even for other hair types a leave-in conditioner is a great follow-up product.

VOLUMIZING SHAMPOOS

Most hairstyles require some fullness, as flat hair is rarely considered aesthetically desirable. If you happen to have fine, thin, limp, or fragile hair you have probably used or considered using shampoos labeled as volumizing to impart a feeling of thickness and fullness. Most volumizing shampoos contain a group of ingredients that are essentially just standard styling agents, such as acrylates, PVP, and PVM/MA. Styling agents, also referred to as film formers and plasticizing agents, are used in hairsprays, gels, and mousses to hold hair in place. When used in styling products, depending on the type and amount of film former or plasticizing agent, the hair can feel either rigid and impervious to movement or flexible and pliable with a slight amount of hold.

When film formers are used in small quantities in shampoos, these ingredients (which are resistant to shampoo and rinsing) remain on the hair shaft, covering it with an imperceptible layer that adds to its thickness. The amount of styling agent left behind on a single strand of hair doesn't amount to much, but multiply that microscopic layer by the 100,000 hairs on your head and it can give your hair a slight impression of feeling and looking thicker. It can also easily feel heavy—after all, an imperceptible layer is still a layer, and if this layer isn't shampooed off every time you wash your hair it can easily build up, resulting in hair feeling heavy and looking limp, not full. Because volumizing shampoos are designed to deposit film-forming ingredients on the hair and those ingredients don't wash out easily, it is essential to alternate your volumizing shampoo with a shampoo that doesn't contain any of those ingredients. Doing this at least every second or third shampoo will ensure that you remove all the buildup (Source: *Cosmetic and Toiletry Formulations*, second edition, volume 8, 2000, Ernest W. Flick, Noyes Publications).

TWO-IN-ONES

A shampoo and conditioner all in one was thought to be the ideal product for the new woman of the 1980s, who barely had time to cook dinner and feed her family, much less spend time grooming her hair with a battery of products. With this in mind, Procter & Gamble was in the right place at the right time with new research proving that you could wash your hair and condition it with the same product. Procter & Gamble's Pert (and later Pert Plus) two-in-one shampoo/conditioner was launched, and today Pert and its own spin-offs (ranging from Pantene to Vidal Sassoon, Physique, and Aussie among others) make up almost 20% of the shampoo market. Now nearly every line has a shampoo-and-conditioner-in-one to sell, though most of them are still based on Procter & Gamble's landmark research.

The conditioning agent in Procter & Gamble's two-in-one products is silicone (specifically, dimethicone). Silicone has an amazing attraction to the hair shaft and the spaces between the cuticle layers. Not only does silicone want to nestle in between damaged, lifted cuticles, but it is also relatively impervious to the force of rushing water trying to wash it down the drain. If anything, the water drives the silicone deeper into the cuticle while the shampoo is being rinsed away. From this perspective, two-in-ones work quite well, particularly for someone with normal to moderately dry or slightly damaged hair (Source:*Cosmetics & Toiletries*, November 2001, pages 55–64).

Two-in-ones come up short, however, for someone with seriously damaged or dry hair or someone who has an oily scalp but still needs conditioning on dry or chemically treated ends.

For someone with coarse, dry, or chemically treated hair, two-in-ones just don't have a wide enough variety of conditioning agents to deal with the amount of damage. While silicone does have a beautiful feel and texture, many other conditioning agents that don't hold up well in shampoo formulations can also help improve hair quality.

For someone with an oily scalp, two-in-ones pose a placement problem. Because of the way two-in-ones work, you can't control how much silicone conditioning agent gets deposited on the hair, or where it goes. Shampooing takes place all over the head, so that means the silicone is going to be left in places where you might not want it, for example, near the scalp, where more emollients (or a coating of any kind) are neither required nor wanted. Instead, you need a conditioner you can put on just the ends, where it is most likely to be needed.

Another problem with two-in-ones is buildup. The very action of two-in-ones means that the conditioning agent (silicone) is being deposited every time you wash your hair. Even though the surfactants can wash some of that away, it is impossible not to leave some of the old conditioner layer behind because it is made from ingredients that are designed to *hold up* under washing. It is unrealistic to expect two-in-ones not to build up. However, there are some hair types where buildup of silicone is not necessarily a bad thing. For example, two-in-ones work great for those with completely normal, healthy, straight to wavy hair, regardless of the length, if there is no great need for fullness. If anything, the continual deposition of silicone conditioning agent can help hair lay flatter against the head. For that very reason, two-in-ones also work well for short hair if it needs less fullness rather than more. (Interestingly, two-in-ones sell very well in Asian countries where the appearance of flat, smooth hair is preferred.)

CLARIFYING SHAMPOOS

A clarifying shampoo—or any shampoo claiming it can deep-clean hair—is simply a shampoo that does not contain any ingredients other than detergent cleansing agents and possibly a small amount of detangling agents (or at least that's all they should contain). By omitting the moisturizing, conditioning, and volumizing ingredients, clarifying shampoos leave no deposit on the hair, so there is no risk of buildup. If you are using a shampoo that does contain moisturizing, conditioning, and volumizing ingredients, these ingredients can build up because you are depositing and redepositing them every time you wash your hair, weighing it down. Using a clarifying shampoo every other time (or every two or three times) you wash your hair will eliminate the buildup from these other types of shampoos and help hair retain a feeling of fullness and softness.

BABY SHAMPOO

Baby shampoos are definitely gentler than most shampoos designed for adults, but as gentle as baby shampoo can be, there is truly no such thing as a "tearless" shampoo. Just a few drops of plain water in the eyes will cause enough irritation to produce discomfort and tearing. A product can be made friendlier to the eyes by using gentler surfactants, but it can still cause some irritation, and for some kids, that will cause tears.

When it comes to cleansing agents, the group of ingredients considered the most gentle are amphoteric surfactants. As stated in the *Hair and Hair Care, Cosmetic Science and Technology Series* (volume 17, 1997), amphoteric surfactants do not cleanse or foam as well as other surfactants, but their one unique property is their very low irritation potential. Amphoterics are so gentle that they can even reduce the irritation of other surfactants known for their sensitizing potential, such as sodium lauryl sulfate. It also stated that, "The skin irritancy of sodium lauryl sulfate in the presence of cocamidopropyl betaine [an amphoteric surfactant] is reduced substantially."

This explains why Johnson & Johnson's Baby Shampoo was such a phenomenal success when it launched in the 1960s. Johnson & Johnson's 1967 patent established the mild, nonirritating capacity for the amphoteric group of cleansing agents. As it turns out, the primary ingredient in Johnson & Johnson's baby shampoos is cocamidopropyl betaine. This also explains why, when you try to use baby shampoo on your own head, it doesn't work very well. The amphoteric surfactants just can't clean like other surfactants can, and given the styling products and conditioners most adults use it is essential to use a shampoo with good cleansing properties. Nowadays most baby shampoos contain a combination of cleansing agents to lower irritancy and improve cleansing, but they are still almost always more gentle than adult shampoos.

SHAMPOOS FOR SWIMMERS

Whether you swim in a swimming pool or in the ocean, or you happen to live in a home that uses well water, you're likely to have hair problems. Swimming pools can cause copper and chlorine buildup on the hair; salt water can cause dryness, breakage, and hard-to-remove tangles; and well water can deposit calcium, magnesium, and iron salts on the hair.

We tend to blame the chlorine in swimming pools for turning blonde hair green, but chlorine isn't the culprit in this case. Chlorine does dry out the hair by breaking through the cuticle, staying put, and tearing at the cuticle every time you brush. But the green discoloration comes from the copper leached from copper pipes into pool water (Source: *Cutis*, July 1995, pages 37–40).

Salt water, if left to dry on hair and combined with sun, wind, and sand, can leave the hair in a tangled, dried-out, frazzled state. These hazards are especially significant for someone whose hair is already damaged. Damaged hair is more porous and, therefore, more susceptible to the invasion of salt, chlorine, and copper.

To battle swimmer's hair in either situation (pool or ocean), and if a swimming cap isn't in your fashion forecast, you might want to consider loading your hair up with silicone serums **each time** before you go into the water. The silicone can cling to hair even in the presence of water and can act as a barrier to the copper in the pool and the salt in the ocean. When you're done playing in the water, if at all possible, be diligent about washing the hair (most of the silicone washes away with shampoo). It also helps to rinse the hair like crazy with fresh water **each time** you leave the pool or ocean, the sooner the better. Do not, and I repeat, *do not*, comb or brush through your hair until you've shampooed and applied conditioner. Wet hair is far more prone to damage, and hair that is wet and laden with salt or other minerals is that much more prone to injury.

When you wash your hair after being in the water, or if you live in a house that uses well water, be sure to use a shampoo that contains disodium or tetrasodium EDTA. These chelating agents help by attracting the minerals away from the hair shaft and making them easier to rinse away. Then apply a generous amount of conditioner to the ends. Never comb through your hair without the aid of a conditioner. Trying to smooth out tangles after a swim without conditioner is just asking for damage. The cuticle is already in a vulnerable position—wet and laden with minerals—which makes driving a brush or even a wide-toothed comb through it a highly risky procedure that can easily rip apart the hair shaft.

DANDRUFF SHAMPOO

See the section on dandruff in Chapter Five, "Hair Problems versus Scalp Problems."

CONDITIONERS

Conditioners and conditioning ingredients used in shampoos are nothing less than amazing. Made from fairly simple ingredients, conditioners can make hair feel and act like the hair you've always wanted, or at least a close facsimile. All conditioners, regardless of the price tag, deposit ingredients on the hair shaft and create an imperceptible, smooth layer over and between the cuticle layers. This invisible layer strengthens the cuticle, giving hair more flexibility, helping protect hair from the damage caused by styling tools, improving texture, making it easier to comb, and eliminating tangles. When hair is dry, conditioners help to seal moisture into your hair, keeping it from becoming dry and fragile, and also help reduce static electricity.

For all the claims about conditioners penetrating, restructuring, regenerating, and rebuilding hair, they have no ability to do any of that, at least not permanently. Conditioners can make hair *feel* repaired, restructured, and revitalized, but that benefit is gone once those ingredients are washed out of hair. Thankfully, the benefit returns every time you reapply the conditioner. Generally, conditioners temporarily modify the cuticle layer of hair. The scaled layers of cuticle covering the hair shaft need to be held down tightly to make the hair feel silky and soft. To that end, conditioners need to "glue" the cuticles down onto the hair shaft or fill in the damaged spaces, acting like a bandage over the tears and breaks in the cuticle that make hair feel rough and dry. This "bandaging" is done by ingredients that are attracted to the cuticle and have the ability to bond with it. Cuticles are like any dead, inanimate surface—not everything wants to stay put on them. Only certain substances have the physical properties to attach themselves and link to the unique physical features of the hair.

Can conditioning agents penetrate into the hair shaft? The answer is, "Possibly." There is some research showing that certain ingredients can be absorbed into the cortex of the hair shaft, but how much and to what benefit isn't clear. Once absorbed, conditioning agents do not necessarily remain in the cortex. They can get out as easily as they get in, and they end up not staying very long. But that isn't necessarily bad, because as I noted above, protecting the cuticle is of vital importance to the health of the hair. The whole purpose of the cuticle is to protect the cortex, and that means preventing things from getting inside. Think about it this way: Tiny molecules of hair-dye ingredients need a very elaborate, strong, chemical process to get the new hair color into the hair shaft and keep it there. It also takes a very elaborate, strong, chemical process to get your existing hair color stripped out of the hair's interior, which is what occurs when you dye your hair from brown to blonde. Hair likes to hold onto what it has, it doesn't want to let anything in and it doesn't want to let what is naturally inside out. The less permeable and more intact the cortex is, the better off it will be.

Conditioning agents stay mostly on the outside of the hair shaft, which is a good thing, because that's where you need them. Conditioning ingredients migrate and cling to the hair's cuticle layers, helping to shore up what's there and fill in (temporarily) what might be missing; that is, the gaps (damage) between the layers. To help facilitate this attachment, to get as much of the conditioning agents to migrate over, around, and under the cuticles, it is best to leave the conditioner on the hair for as long as possible so the conditioning ingredients have as much time as possible to get to where they need to be.

When you buy a conditioner, you will find one or more of the ingredients described in the paragraphs below on the ingredient list. They are found in different combinations in a long roll call of products whose names and descriptions defy the imagination: creme rinses, finishing rinses, deep conditioners, hair moisturizers, light conditioners, detangling conditioners, equalizing conditioners, reconstructors, and hair moisturizers. Regardless of the name, conditioners have far fewer differences than similarities, and none of them can repair, mend, reconstruct, or restructure hair.

Proteins are long-chain molecules that cannot be absorbed into the hair shaft. Proteins are often partially hydrolyzed to help them cling better to hair. Regardless, the best thing that proteins can do is coat the outside of the hair, filling in gaps between the cuticles, which can protect the hair and add a soft feeling. Proteins are ingredients that originate in and include plant and animal by-products. Even though proteins are an elemental building block of the hair, adding protein to hair-care products does not restructure or add to the hair's composition. To imply that any protein can somehow repair hair or permanently attach to hair is sheer alchemy and fantasy.

Many conditioners claim to contain protein derived from keratin, which they suggest will therefore bind and merge with the keratin in your hair (hair is mostly keratin) and restructure and restore your hair. There is no truth to this in the least. First, you can't get protein from hair keratin because it cannot be chemically broken down. Other forms of keratin that come from plants are just fine as conditioning agents, but that's it—they still can't repair hair. If anything, keratins and proteins are not the best conditioning ingredients. Chemically, keratins don't like to bind to surfaces, and the rinsing process wouldn't leave them much chance of attaching to the cuticle. Even leave-in conditioners do not significantly bind to the hair (Sources: *Hair and Hair Care*, Dale H. Johnson, 1998; *Conditioning Agents for Hair and Skin*, Marcel Dekker, 1999; and www.keratin.com).

Collagen and elastin are proteins that like to cling to hair. They serve several important roles in conditioning, and both nicely coat the outside layer of the hair, filling in the gaps of the damaged cuticle and adding a slight feel of thickness. Collagen and elastin also have water-binding properties, which are delivered mostly to the surface, and that is good for the hair.

Collagen and elastin can be broken down with water (hydrolyzed) to create a smaller molecular form that has a better chance of getting in and around the cuticle. (We're talking a microscopic level of penetration, so don't get excited or carried away thinking hydrolyzed collagen or elastin will repair your hair or somehow mend it. They won't.) Unfortunately, very little of the specially treated collagen or elastin can penetrate and be absorbed, because after they have been hydrolyzed—partially broken down with water—they are more prone to being washed away. Hydrolyzed collagen and elastin work best when given time to penetrate a dry or slightly damp hair shaft (Source: *Cosmetics & Toiletries*, November 1998, pages 69–73).

Silk protein is a popular ingredient that often shows up in conditioners. Perhaps it is the relation to silk that makes this protein sound like it is better for hair. It isn't (Source: www.hairscientists.org/article7.htm).

Amino acids are what make up proteins. There are 16 amino acids in hair—cysteine, serine, glutamic acid, threonine, glycine, leucine, valine, arginine, aspartic acid, alanine, proline, isoleucine, phenylalanine, histidine, tyrosine, and methionine—with the most prevalent being cysteine (Source: www.keratin.com). Proteins are assembled from amino acids, and in theory amino acids have a better affinity for hair because they are smaller and have a better chance of penetrating the cuticle layer and providing water-binding properties deeper inside the shaft. But that's only theory. Most cosmetics chemists believe that because amino acids are so small, they are also quite unstable and easy to rinse away and, therefore, they never get a chance to penetrate and do their thing.

Humectants and water-binding agents are included in conditioners for their thickening and slip properties. Slip properties are the properties of the polysaccharides in these agents that excel when it comes to grabbing onto hair, smoothing easily over the surface of the hair shaft, and staying put. They also have a side benefit of adding viscosity to a product. Several types of polysaccharides are used in hair-care products, including cellulose, glycosaminoglycans, hyaluronic acid, mucopolysaccharides, chitin, and chitosan PCA.

Glycerin, sorbitol, propylene glycol, and butylene glycol are all excellent water-binding agents, among many others. These ingredients help reduce the amount of damage done to hair by styling tools and brushing.

Fatty acids and fatty alcohols are lubricants and emollients that are often less oily or greasy than plant or mineral oils and, therefore, give the hair a soft, velvety feel without making it feel heavy or thick. Common members of this group include cetyl alcohol, stearyl alcohol, triglycerides, myristyl alcohol, caprylic acid, lauric acid, oleic acid, palmitic acid, and stearic acid.

Vegetable oils, lanolin, plant oils, castor oil, and mineral oil do for the hair pretty much what they do for the skin—leave a protective barrier that prevents dehydration. They are also extremely emollient and slippery, providing good moisture retention, but they also add oil to the hair, which can be problematic for hair that is normal to fine or thin, or for those with an oily scalp. Regardless of how exotic or earthy the oils may sound—such as jojoba, wheat germ, carrot, evening primrose, and babassu—they still function as oils, and they're no better for hair than any other less impressive sounding oils such as safflower or canola.

Though there are positive aspects of adding oils or lanolin to hair-care products, on balance there are more aesthetic negatives. The downside of all these ingredients is that they can leave a greasy, thick residue on the hair. This is particularly true for products designed for African-American hair, as these often contain large amounts of lanolin, petrolatum, and castor oil. All of these ingredients, by virtue of their sticky feel, also tend to attract dirt and increase the chance of styling products building up on the hair. The hair must be washed thoroughly, as these ingredients are hard to remove. **Products with oils and lanolin listed among the first ingredients are best used only occasionally, if at all, and then only in styling products that you use on the ends of hair to smooth over the most damaged areas, not all over.**

Vitamins can't feed hair because hair is dead. But can vitamins prevent free-radical damage to the hair or scalp the way they claim to work on the skin? Possibly. The problem is getting those ingredients to cling to the hair shaft or be absorbed into the scalp, and then getting them to stay there. When included in a rinse-off conditioner, the vitamins (or plant extracts) that have antioxidant properties are just rinsed down the drain. Included in a leave-in conditioner, they must be in direct contact with the scalp to be absorbed and impart their antioxidant benefits. That is an option, but it could make hair far too heavy and limp to be acceptable during styling. Most hairstyles do not benefit from applying conditioning ingredients (emollients or film formers) to the scalp because they can make hair heavy and limp. For the hair shaft, there is no research showing that vitamins can stick to the cuticle and afford the benefits they provide to skin.

Panthenol, biotin, and other derivatives of the B vitamin complex. Unlike other vitamins, the popular conditioning ingredient panthenol has an affinity for hair and is considered to have decent penetration into the hair shaft. Does that mean it can mend hair or perform any of a vast array of miracles, as claimed by hair-care companies? Can it really thicken hair up to 10%, stop hair loss, regrow hair, prevent damage caused by perms or dyes, or strengthen hair, as you've seen in brochures for hair-care products? All such claims are completely unsubstantiated. Panthenol does work as a conditioning agent, but no better or differently from lots of other great conditioning ingredients. What panthenol can do is give the hair a more substantial, smoother feel, keep moisture in the hair better if the hair is dry, improve movement if hair is stiff or brittle, and impart luster to the hair (Source: www.roche.com/vitamins/pdf/ethylpanth.pdf).

Biotin, as several chemists and dermatologists told me, is one of those hair-care ingredients that have little function, although women believe that it can help hair (and hair-care companies reinforce the notion). Biotin has minimal ability to hold up under water and it doesn't cling well to the cuticle. Companies make it sound as though it's strong, but it ends up being a small, weak molecule. Perhaps the confusion about biotin began because, when taken orally, biotin is a vitamin that directly impacts hair growth. Yet the way biotin works internally, in the complex chemical and biological system, to generate hair growth is impossible to duplicate topically (Sources: *Seminars in Dermatology*, March 1992, pages 88–97; *Journal of the American Academy of Dermatology*, July 1985, pages 97–102; and http://yalenewhavenhealth.org).

Quaternary ammonium compounds. See the description of these in the *Shampoo* section above.

Balsam is in limited use these days, so even mentioning it is almost unnecessary, but just in case there are those who remember it as a popular conditioning agent in the 1970s and 1980s, it's worth a quick comment. Balsam is a tree resin that has substantial ability to stick to the hair and coat it. Balsam also has a potent, but pleasant, herbal fragrance. Why then has balsam fallen out of the limelight? Despite balsam's positive attributes, it has overwhelming negative points—specifically, it makes hair feel sticky, and, because it builds up, can make hair brittle. It is best avoided in any hair-care formulation.

Thickeners and emulsifiers are the ingredients responsible for the consistency of all hair-care products. Thickeners also function as emollients in hair-care products, but primarily they help produce the feel and texture of the formulation. Emulsifiers help the ingredients (such as oil and water) stay mixed together. Without thickeners and emulsifiers, you would find most hair-care products would be watery mixtures that separate, similar to an oil and vinegar salad dressing.

Preservatives. Refer to the information on preservatives in the *Shampoo* section above.

Alpha hydroxy acids (AHAs) are very popular in skin-care products used to exfoliate skin. Recognizing their popularity, hair-care formulators tried to capitalize on the acceptance of AHAs by adding them to shampoos and conditioners. AHAs are effective in concentrations of 5% or greater at a pH of 4 or less. However, any hair-care product formulation that contains effective concentrations of AHAs at an effective low pH should never be used on the hair. (As it turns out, there are no hair-care products with effective AHA concentrations at effective pH levels.) This warning makes sense if you remember that hair is dead. If AHAs performed on the hair the same way they perform on the skin (as exfoliants removing dead skin cells) they would denature and destroy the hair shaft—since it's essentially dead skin (keratin).

Plant extracts and other natural ingredients such as honey, milk, various extracts, herbs, and essential oils may all have a healthy, vibrant sound and may even have some benefit for hair, but their value (if any) in shampoos and conditioners is lost, either in the rinse-out or the formulation. How can plant extracts and milk cling to hair under water pressure? They can't. Besides, the amount of these ingredients in a product is usually negligible to nonexistent. Just for the record, it is my opinion—and the opinion of countless cosmetics chemists I have interviewed—that these types of ingredients have limited to no benefit in hair-care products and are there mostly to entice the consumer (who almost always thinks natural ingredients are best).

Volumizing ingredients in conditioners are exactly the same as the volumizing ingredients in shampoos and styling products, all claim to add volume to hair. Covering the hair shaft with an extremely thin layer of film-forming ingredients, they can add an appearance of fullness and thickness. If you are using both a shampoo and conditioner that contain volumizing ingredients, that can definitely add too much weight to hair that is fine or thin, or even to normal hair. And because you are adding them to hair in two steps, not one, it is even more difficult to wash these ingredients out. To prevent this kind of buildup from making your hair heavy, limp, or stiff, it is essential that you use only one product that contains volumizing agents, either the shampoo or the conditioner. I vote for using a conditioner with volumizing ingredients rather than a shampoo because then the shampoo will wash the film-forming ingredients away each time, greatly reducing the chance of buildup (Source: *Cosmetic and Toiletry Formulations*, second edition, volume 8, 2000, Ernest W. Flick, Noyes Publications).

RINSE-OFF OR LEAVE-IN CONDITIONERS

Rinse-off conditioners are applied to the hair in the shower after shampooing and then rinsed off. Leave-in conditioners are applied after the hair is shampooed and towel dried, or added with a spray-on applicator that spreads a light mist over the hair shaft. On the surface, all conditioners leave the hair easier to comb, moisturized, somewhat protected from assault with blow dryers, and smoother to the touch, using practically the same ingredients. Leave-in and rinse-off conditioners perform these functions equally well because they often contain many of the same ingredients. Yet there are a few differences in consistency and in the amounts of emollients or film-forming ingredients that distinguish leave-in and rinse-off conditioners from one another.

Leave-in conditioners have a far thinner, less emollient texture than rinse-off conditioners. Leave-in conditioners also don't contain most of the emollient ingredients, such as the fatty acids, fatty alcohols, and thickening agents found in rinse-off conditioners. Because leave-in conditioners usually don't include heavy lubricating emollients or thickeners, they rarely weigh down hair and are, therefore, often recommended for women with thin, limp, or fine hair to add body and soft control. Leave-in conditioners often contain small amounts of styling ingredients such as PVP, PVP/VA, and acrylates/acrylamide copolymer to give the hair form and an impression of thickness by holding it slightly in place (as opposed to falling limp). These styling ingredients have different and distinct effects on hair, both positive and negative. These hairspray/styling-type ingredients place a light, slightly sticky substance on the hair that can build up, leaving the hair with a brittle, stiff feeling. Of course, most leave-in conditioners don't advertise this problem, and unless you know how to read an ingredient list you would never know what was making your hair feel unpleasant. Because of this problem, leave-in conditioners with film formers are best for someone who wants only minimal or extremely light, controlled styling and who washes her hair on a regular basis with a shampoo strong enough to remove the buildup. Leave-in conditioners that don't contain these styling ingredients vary for different hair types, and there are several excellent options chronicled in Chapter 10, "Product Reviews".

Rinse-off conditioners have many of the same properties as leave-in conditioners, but they differ in thickness. Because rinse-off conditioners are applied in the shower just after shampooing they need to contain ingredients that can remain in contact with hair despite the presence of so much moisture. They generally contain more thickening agents, emollients, and silicones to help maximize retention on the hair shaft. This is also what makes rinse-off conditioners far better for those with thicker, drier, or damaged hair. There are lightweight rinse-off conditioners that contain minimal amounts of emollients and easily rinsed-off thickening ingredients and that include more detangling agents than anything else. These formulations are excellent for thin, fine, and normal hair.

SILICONES

Silicones are barely a blip on most people's hair-care radar, but they are the primary ingredients in most conditioners and styling products—particularly those for dry, damaged, coarse, brittle, permed, or dyed hair—that make hair feel remarkable and behave beautifully. Even though silicones are merely conditioning ingredients, they have such amazing properties for hair that they deserve a section all to themselves.

Silicones are a vast range of ingredients typically listed on an ingredient list as dimethicone, phenyl trimethicone, or cyclomethicone, but there are many more. All of these are so vital to hair care and are used so widely in the hair- and skin-care industries that they deserve more praise than they receive. These unsung hair-care marvels have an incredible capacity to cling to and spread over, under, and around the cuticle. Silicone's unsurpassed ability to maneuver effortlessly over the hair shaft and hold up under water pressure or styling routines makes it superior for smoothing any rough edges on the cuticle. Even more astonishing is silicone's luxuriant, velvety texture. Silicone can impart the most wonderful, silky-smooth feel to the hair. It is impossible to comprehend how awesome silicone feels unless you buy one of the laminate or anti-frizz serums that have become so popular in styling products and feel it for yourself. Those types of styling products are usually pure silicone, which allows you to feel directly how sensational the texture is.

Silicone not only provides temporary renewed smoothness to the hair, but also is the subject of an enormous amount of research (that fills several folders in my office) demonstrating its extraordinary safety (I can't imagine who could be allergic to these benign substances). There almost isn't a downside, except that if you use too much of this stuff it can leave a greasy, rather than silky, feel on your hair. There is more to say about silicones and I discuss them more in Chapter Nine, "Styling Hair," but for now consider it your dry, coarse, frizzy, damaged, brittle, overstyled, wiry, rough, hard-to-comb hair's best friend (Sources: *Household & Personal Products Industry*, HAPPI, April, 2003; The First International Conference on Applied Hair Science, June 2004, Princeton, New Jersey; *Global Cosmetic Industry*, April–May, 1999, pages 44–55; *Soap, Cosmetics, and Chemical Specialties*, June 1998, pages 55–60; and *Cosmetics & Toiletries*, April 1996, pages 67–72).

Oils such as mineral oil, petrolatum, and plant oils perform in a manner similar to silicone, but they have a far more greasy or sticky feel, and they lack silicone's ability to spread evenly over the hair, to impart a glossy (rather than greasy) shine, and to provide a silky feel. Silicones have incredible movement, leaving a thin, even layer wherever you place them; oils don't have this ability.

MASKS, PACKS, AND SPECIALTY TREATMENTS

These supposedly intensive, specially formulated conditioning treatments are nothing more than standard, and sometimes relatively unimpressive, conditioners, just like the one you use every day in the shower. It takes only a quick look at the ingredient lists to notice how similar specialty treatments are to regular conditioners. The principal difference between regular conditioners and specialty hair treatments is that a container of the latter costs far more than daily conditioners, and there is far less product in the container. The other difference is that specialty hair treatments are intended to be left on longer, and they are more effective when you use them along with a hair dryer with only minimal heat (less than 100°F). Can you do the same thing with the conditioner you use every day and get the exact same results? Absolutely!

Every time I've gotten my hair dyed at a salon I've been told that I need to have a hair mask treatment or buy a hair mask to use at home to undo or prevent any damage from the chemical process. It simply isn't true. There are no ingredients in these treatment products that can perform any function over and above what is delivered by a traditional conditioner.

Perhaps most shocking are the hair masks that contain clay! What is clay doing in a hair-care product of any kind? Clay is a drying, absorbent substance with no other function. Plus, as the clay dries, it can actually chip away at the cuticle. What were they thinking?

You may have read that mayonnaise or vegetable oil, right out of your cupboard and heated up, is good for the hair. Almost without exception, hair-care products are infinitely superior to anything you can cook up in your kitchen because most hair-care products are designed and formulated to be water soluble. Mayonnaise and vegetable oils must be thoroughly washed out of the hair, and that isn't easy to do because they are so greasy (not to mention the smell). Using food-type oils means that you'd have to repeatedly lather up to be sure you got all the oil off your hair, and that excessive washing would damage your hair.

LAMINATES, SERUMS, HAIR POLISHERS, AND SPRAY-ON SHINE PRODUCTS

Laminates, hair serums, hair polishers, hair smoothers, defrizzers, and spray-on shine products are all designed to smooth away frizzies and add shine to the hair. They come in small bottles that hold from 1 to 4 ounces, and they look like a thick, viscous, clear oil (though the spray-on versions are far more watery in appearance). The major—if not the only—ingredients in all of these products are silicones, usually in the form of dimethicone, cyclomethicone, or phenyl trimethicone. As you become more familiar with ingredient lists, you will notice that these three ingredients show up in just about every hair-care product you use. Can silicones eliminate frizzies? To some extent they can, but definitely not even remotely as well as they appear to in the advertisements for these products, and absolutely not without the help of styling tools, particularly blow dryers, curling irons, or flat irons. What these laminates, serums, and polishers do superbly is add a gorgeous silky feel to the hair, along with a highly reflective shine.

Some of these products also contain plant oils, but you will notice that they are at the end of the ingredient list and that the silicones are almost always at the beginning. When it comes to imparting shine and incredible texture, there isn't a plant oil or emollient that can compete with the silicones. On occasion, these products also throw in a sunscreen just for good marketing measure, but it is only a gimmick; there is no SPF number and there is no way to know how much or how long your hair will be protected, if at all, from the sun.

The prices for these products are astounding, ranging from $6 for 4 ounces to $28 and above for 1 ounce. The high end of this wide price range is nothing more than marketing chicanery, because the ingredients and formulations are so standard and basic it is almost laughable.

POMADES AND STYLING WAX

These are the original frizz busters, the products that once were just a plain, sticky, wax that kept hair matted down and in place. As a result of innovative styling demands, many recent incarnations of pomades no longer resemble the earlier formulas. Far from being just sticky or waxy, pomades now have an elaborate range of forms, textures, and consistencies. Regardless of the packaging or the company's impressive name on the label, pomades can range from a greasy mixture of petrolatum, wax, and lanolin to a far less heavy mix of thickeners, silicone, plant oil, and film-forming agents. Why would you want any amount of this wax in your hair? Depending on the formula, pomades can fulfill a variety of styling needs. When accompanied by good styling techniques, pomades can help reduce flyaway ends, smooth down coarse hair, impart a lustrous shine with minimal sticky after-feel, and diminish frizz. And if you are interested in creating hairstyles that look chunky, textured, or matted, pomades are one of the only ways to achieve it.

Despite modern variations in formula and application, it's important to keep in mind that most pomades are still heavy and should be used sparingly. For the most part, pomades, waxes, and greases are best used on the ends of hair or over the surface, not all over as you would use a styling lotion or mousse. Women with limp or thin hair should proceed cautiously.

STYLING GELS, SPRAYS, AND MOUSSES

Here's where we start getting sticky (pun intended), but hopefully not too sticky. Gels, spray gels, mousses, volumizing sprays, curl revitalizers/boosters, and styling lotions are ingeniously formulated products designed both to help the hair and to make it stay put in ways it wouldn't otherwise.

Mousses, with their lighter-than-air texture, spread easily through the hair, melting into place and providing soft styling control and fullness. Styling gels are clear, viscous substances that move easily through the hair (but not as easily as mousses) and tend to offer more control and potential for fullness. For the most part, spray-on gels are diluted versions of the thicker gels, providing a softer degree of hold. Curl revitalizers/boosters and volumizing sprays are relatively light, almost like water, with small amounts of conditioner and styling ingredients. Sculpting and molding gels tend to be stiffer than mousses and styling gels, giving a range of control over where the hair finally ends up.

What these products all share is a tendency to dry slowly and allow the hair to move until the liquid dries, which allows you time to style your hair and control the end results. Regardless of the nuances (and there are an almost limitless number of names and formulas), what these products have in common, line to line, is pretty much the same array of ingredients. Often the only difference between products is the amount of film-forming agents they contain—or the price.

Regardless of the extraordinarily elaborate claims companies make about their styling products, there are only a limited number of ingredients that can mold and hold in this film-forming, plasticizing manner, and they are not unique or rare in the least. These standard film-forming/plasticizing ingredients, which show up in styling product after styling product, are called polymers. If you've skimmed almost any styling product ingredient list (other than pomade-type products and some softer-hold products), you've probably seen the ingredients PVP (short for polyvinylpyrrolidone), PVP/VA copolymer (VA is short for vinyl acrylate), acrylates/vinyl isodecanoate crosspolymer, acrylamide/ammonium acrylate copolymer, acrylic/acrylate copolymer, vinyl acetate, polyvinyl acetate, and styrene/acrylamide copolymer.

All of the above are varying forms of polymers. Polymers are long molecular chains of synthetic compounds, usually with high molecular weights (meaning they can't be absorbed into the hair or easily broken down) and with millions of repeating linked units. Yet despite the high molecular weight, each is a relatively light and simple molecule. It is the linking and lightweight nature of polymers that makes them so hair-friendly. Polymers can bind to the hair, creating a consistent film between and around two or more hair shafts with barely any detectable weight, and give the hair strength, resilience, and hold.

Alone or in combination, all of these styling ingredients provide a profusion of product choices. But again, as you get used to reading the ingredient list, you'll notice that beneath the surface of the marketing language lies a glaring similarity between styling products, regardless of price range or designer image.

Hair Note: Detangling agents (called quats for short) are sometimes included in styling products, but not often because they do the opposite of what you want the hair to do when you are trying to get it to stay in place. Detangling agents are meant to separate the hair, while styling products are meant to keep the hair together. Styling products also sometimes contain conditioning agents (most typically silicone) to provide protection from styling tools.

HAIRSPRAYS, SPRITZES, FREEZES, AND SCULPTING SPRAYS

The styling products described above are meant to be worked through an entire head of hair to give it form and shape while styling with blow dryers, curling irons, flat irons, or just your fingers. At the other end of the styling spectrum is the need for hairsprays and their counterparts that set and dry quickly, holding the hairstyle in place, preventing it from returning to its natural appearance, and, most important, helping as much as possible to limit the impact on hair of weather conditions such as wind and humidity. Hairsprays, no matter what they're called, work by building consistent, continuous bonds between hair fibers. Hairspray ingredients are identical to those in other styling products, only there is less (and sometimes zero) water and generally higher concentrations of film-forming/plasticizing agents such as acrylates, acrylamides, styrene, crotonic acid, and methylacrylate copolymer.

What about holding power? Generally, I find that hairspray and most styling product labels come relatively close to the truth about how well they hold the hair. If the label says "super hold" it means super hold; if it says "soft hold" it will do just that. There are exceptions, but I'll get to those in Chapter Ten, "Product Reviews."

Should you use aerosol hairsprays or nonaerosol hairsprays? That issue is primarily personal preference. The major difference between them is the way the spray is dispersed. Aerosols discharge a featherweight mist, while nonaerosols are apt to go on more heavily. It takes some skill to get nonaerosol sprays to go on lightly and sparsely.

The other aspect of using aerosol or nonaerosol is more an environmental concern than an aesthetic one. Aerosol hairsprays use volatile organic compounds (VOCs) to disperse the hairspray ingredients over the hair, and VOCs negatively impact the earth's atmosphere. "VOCs are released into the air from automobile exhaust and consumer products. While automobiles may seem to be a far greater source than a little can of hairspray, in California alone, the annual emissions of 176 million pounds of VOCs from 30 million Californians using consumer products are the same as if 20 million cars were added, each driving an additional 10,000 miles that year" (Source: Air Quality Resources, www.aqs.com/iaq/vol_org_compounds.asp).

Hairsprays containing ethyl alcohol (ethanol, listed as SD alcohol followed by a number), hydrocarbons, isobutane, and butane all release vapors into the air that generate ozone in the lower atmosphere. While other human-made pollutants deplete the ozone in the upper atmosphere, emitting VOCs into the lower atmosphere produces an additional ozone layer that traps heat and ultraviolet radiation nearer to the earth's surface, adding to the levels of smog in cities caused by automobiles and other industrial pollution. California and New York have been the leaders in setting environmental standards for VOCs, and since 1998, they have not allowed the sale of any hairspray containing more than 55% VOC. No other state since has established such strict regulations. In the meantime, if you've noticed changes in the hairsprays you're buying, they are changes for the better, at least for the environment.

Hair Note: Aside from environmental concerns, is alcohol a problem in hair-care products such as gels, mousses, and hairsprays? There are many types of alcohols, fatty alcohols, and emollient waxes in hair-care products and they're not a problem at all. It's true that SD-alcohol or grain alcohol is extremely drying and can be a problem for hair (which is why it is rarely, if ever, used in shampoos, conditioners, or specialty products). Otherwise, alcohol is a staple in most hairsprays. But there is no real need for concern because the amount of alcohol in hair-care products is likely not a problem for most hair types. In reality, alcohol in hairsprays evaporates too quickly to impact the moisture content of the hair. And water really can't substitute for alcohol because dispensing too much water onto hair will destroy a hairstyle (Sources: *Cosmetic and Toiletry Formulations*, volume 8, second edition, E. W. Flick, 2001, William Andrew Publishing/Noyes; Health Canada, www.ec.gc.ca/nopp/DOCS/consult/voc-cov/cons-2003/en/dp5.cfm; and *Drug & Cosmetic Industry*, April 1, 1997).

SUNSCREEN IN HAIR-CARE PRODUCTS

No question about it, hair needs to be protected from the sun! Sun damage destroys hair by breaking down the bonds that keep hair's structure intact. Where brushing and combing chip away at the outer cuticle, energy from the sun destroys the interior of hair, which explains why hair color fades with sun exposure. Yet despite this desperate need for protection, sunscreens in shampoos and conditioners are nothing less than a waste of time and money. Unfortunately, there is no way that these formulations can provide adequate sun protection for the hair because shampoos and conditioners are meant to be rinsed out, and consequently there is no way to know how much, if any, sunscreen remains on the hair. In fact, given the water-solubility of most sunscreens, they are probably rinsed away almost immediately. Creating water-resistant sunscreens is the logical solution, but to do so requires ingredients that are not substantive to hair, thus consumer acceptance of such products is bound to fail. After all, would you use a water-resistant sunscreen on your hair if you knew it would make it feel coated, look greasy, or cause your hairstyle to go flat?

Leave-in hair-care products that contain sunscreen are a better bet, but only slightly. Although the sunscreen's ability to stay on the hair shaft increases when it's included in a leave-in product, there is no way to know or measure whether any of the sunscreen remains on the hair after brushing or styling. What's foremost when considering this issue is that hair-care products are not allowed to have SPF numbers because the FDA does not consider hair-care products with sunscreen safe or reliable for sun protection. And without an SPF number (or even if there is an SPF number, which is illegal), there is no way to determine how long the hair shaft will be protected, or indeed if any sunscreen is left behind at all. If you don't know the SPF, you have no idea if the product is an SPF 2, SPF 8, or SPF 15. Moreover, with the skin we know that sunscreen must be reapplied after swimming or long exposure to the sun, but what about the hair? After two hours of bike riding, are you going to reapply your leave-in conditioner with sunscreen and get your hair gooped up all over again?

I'm not saying that sunscreen ingredients can't protect hair from sun damage, because they can. There are plenty of studies in which a swatch of hair is covered with sunscreen ingredients, then placed under UVA/UVB light, and after a period of time measured for deterioration. The sunscreen ingredients absolutely prevented damage. However, until there is a solution to the application and adherence issues, it is a huge mistake to rely on sunscreen in hair-care products. Until the FDA gives its SPF blessing to hair-care products, wear a hat when spending long periods of time in the sun. That's the only real way to prevent sun damage to your hair.

NATURALLY BAD

In the world of natural ingredients, some consider all things bright and beautiful. Many women believe that if they use a product labeled "natural," "pure," or "organic," their hair will be healthier than if they use products that contain synthetic ingredients. Nothing could be further from the truth: Natural doesn't ensure quality, or even safety. But that doesn't stop consumers or the cosmetics companies.

Many natural ingredients pose problems for the skin. While I can't stop the craze for natural ingredients, I can at least try to keep reality in the picture. I thought it would be a good idea to provide a list of the more popular, but possibly irritating or photosensitizing, natural ingredients found in cosmetics.

All of the following can cause skin irritation and/or sun sensitivity: almond extract, allspice, angelica, arnica, balm mint oil, balsam, basil, bergamot, chamomile, cinnamon, citrus, clove, clover blossom, coriander oil, fennel, fir needle, geranium oil, grapefruit, horsetail, juniper oil, lavender oil, lemon, lemongrass, lime, marjoram, melissa, oak bark, orange oil, papaya, peppermint, rose, sage, thyme, and wintergreen.

The label might say "pure and natural," but you could be buying a purely irritating product. It won't irritate the hair shaft, because the hair is dead, but if it rinses off onto your face or makes contact with your scalp, you could have problems. Even if natural ingredients were all beneficial to hair, they would work only if they were in leave-in products; in a shampoo, most of them would be rinsed down the drain.

You may have noticed lately that several cosmetics lines are using descriptive terms to identify either the source or the purpose of the ingredient. For example, Aveda lists polyquaternium-10 as "plant cellulose" and polyquaternium-16 as an "antistatic agent." Aveda and other companies that provide this more specific, apparently consumer-under-standable information are disclosing only what they want you to know about their ingredients. Polyquaternium-10 (and -16) are not plant cellulose, as the description implies; rather they are *derived* from plant cellulose. That is not just a technicality. How it is derived isn't quite as pure sounding as it reads. Very *un*natural ingredients are used to take the plant cellulose and turn it into polyquaternium-10. Does that change the acceptability or effectiveness of the polyquats as antistatic agents or surfactants (cleansers)? Not in the least. It is just another way the cosmetics companies help encourage the consumer to think more highly of natural ingredients than is necessary or warranted.

The pressure from consumers to have natural-sounding ingredients is so powerful that there is a new bit of deception taking place on ingredient lists. For example, rather than listing mineral oil or petrolatum in a product, some companies list the trade names instead, namely Protol and Protopet. Because many consumers erroneously believe mineral oil and petrolatum are bad for skin or hair, cosmetics companies use these other names to cloak the ingredients on the label.

One more point: The next time you hear a hair-care company proclaiming that their products are natural, give them a skeptical nod of your head and then read the ingredient list. You'll note that the amount of plants used in any hair-care product is negligible in comparison to the amount of chemical-sounding ingredients. Concentrating on natural is one way to get yourself duped.

ALLERGIC REACTIONS OR CLOGGED PORES

When it comes to hair products, as opposed to cosmetics, the chance of allergic reactions is greatly reduced, for the obvious reason that very little of the product actually stays on your skin for very long. Conditioners and shampoos have minimal contact with the scalp because there are copious amounts of water being used at the same time. Furthermore, because hair is dead as a doornail, you can put all kinds of irritating ingredients on it that would normally cause havoc on the skin and never be aware of the difference. The exceptions to this are AHAs and BHA (salicylic acid), which can, when used in an acidic base, denature the hair shaft. The problems start when the ingredients in hair-care products come in contact with the skin. Hair covered in conditioning or styling agents can come in contact with your hairline, face, neck, or shoulders, and that can cause irritation, allergic reactions, or breakouts.

Hair-care ingredients in most styling products, pomades, and conditioners (especially those designed for damaged, dry hair) can cause skin problems, including breakouts and allergic reactions (*all* styling products with film-forming agents can end up being fairly strong skin irritants). Although it is essential to experiment with products to find which ones won't be a problem for you, hair-care products are so similar that changing products may not be much help. The best option is to be careful about what gets on your skin.

When you apply hairspray, be sure you don't get any on your face. If you are using styling products and you often wear your hair brushed forward and you are breaking out in the areas where the hair touches the face, consider wearing your hair off the face for awhile or temporarily not using the styling products, and see what happens. The same is true for shampoos and conditioners. Conditioners don't often contain irritating ingredients (although there are several nowadays with some of the irritating ingredients I mentioned in the "Naturally Bad" section above that can cause allergic reactions), but they almost always contain emollients and conditioning agents that can clog pores. One way to avoid such problems is to be careful when rinsing off a conditioner; be sure to bend forward or backward to avoid getting it on your skin.

You can use the same trick for rinsing off shampoos to keep them away from the skin, but that won't help the scalp where the cleansing agents must do their job. There is a definite concern that some surfactants and other irritating ingredients can cause allergic or irritating skin reactions on the scalp. If your skin or scalp is particularly sensitive, or if you notice flaking or irritation, you may want to avoid shampoos that list sodium lauryl sulfate, TEA-lauryl sulfate, and alkyl sodium sulfate as the second or third ingredients, and avoid all of the irritating ingredients listed in the "Naturally Bad" section above.

YOU GOTTA HAVE A GIMMICK

You've probably noticed that many hair-care lines have divided their products into increasingly segmented groups, with each group further broken down into hair types, such as dry/delicate, normal/healthy, and fine/thin. Talk about getting specific! Every line has its own angle, with divisions formed according to the ingredients and how they are to be marketed. You'll see chamomile versus ginger, or proteins versus panthenol, or scalp type versus hair condition. Or conditioning goals such as more curl, less curl, enhanced smoothness, wave, and fullness, or whether or not you have long or short hair. Are these important differences? Regardless of what the products tell you, there is little basis for these divisions other than to create marketing niches. Dry, permed, color-treated, or damaged hair types need the same treatment. And whether hair is thin, limp, fine, fragile, or delicate, their treatment is similar, too. Sure enough, when you read the labels on products designed for dry, permed, color-treated, or damaged hair, they almost always have comparable ingredient lists. Product segmenting may seem helpful, but it ends up being more confusing than useful.

Similarly, specific ingredients alone do not guarantee the value of any given product. Panthenol may be a good conditioner, but, by itself and without the addition of quaternary ammonium compounds, emollients, and other conditioning agents, it won't perform the way you expect it to. Awapuhi and burdock root may sound healthy, but they (along with myriad other natural-sounding ingredients) won't produce healthy hair; they are nothing more than window dressing for the other, more chemical-sounding ingredients that make hair-care products effective. Proteins in conditioners may sound like they will help reinforce hair, but they actually do so poorly and unreliably. Focusing on one or two ingredients is a waste of time and energy when shopping for any hair-care product.

CHAPTER FIVE

Hair Problems versus Scalp Problems

NORMAL? OILY? DRY? DAMAGED?

We tend to treat the scalp and hair as if they were the same, or at least closely related, when that is not always (if ever) the case. Before you shampoo, condition, or style your hair it is necessary to differentiate between what the hair requires and what the scalp requires, and then make sure that each is getting what it needs. Your scalp type, the condition of your hair, and what you want the final results to look like determine what you should be using.

The four traditional categories of hair type—normal, oily, dry, and damaged (generally meaning chemically treated or overstyled hair)—are useful. However, they are too narrow and don't take into consideration many of the subtle distinctions and variations, and they don't explain how to actually use products. For example, your hair can be oily in places (mostly at the roots for curly hair, or all over for straight hair, or just on the scalp) and dry in places (the ends of longer hair, or all over for bleached blonde hair). The same is true for the scalp; it can be partly oily but still have dry flakes or be itchy and oily, or be just dry.

In addition, the hair and scalp are not static; seasonal changes can affect the hair, as can hormonal changes. Hair can be normal in the summer and dry in the winter, or it can be cooperative or uncooperative depending on the humidity. If you dye your hair you could have dry, damaged ends with frizzies, and an oily scalp with healthy hair near the base where new growth has been less processed than the rest of the strand. Moreover, hair care is greatly influenced by the movement of your hair. Straight hair has very different needs from wavy hair, curly hair, or kinky hair.

Often the hair and scalp types we think we have are really a result of the products or implements we use and not the true state of our hair. We might complain that our hair is flyaway and unmanageable or that our scalp is dry, and then go to the store wondering which products will correct the problem. What we don't realize is that the issue may not be about using different products, rather it may require a simple change in the way we take care of our hair. Flyaway hair can be caused by overbrushing, using a conditioner that isn't emollient enough to coat hair, overstyling, or using a rinse-out rather than a leave-in conditioner.

A dry scalp might not really be dry, but could be the result of overwashing the hair or not rinsing it well enough, using products that contain extremely drying cleansing agents, or using products that contain irritating plant extracts. An oily scalp might not be as oily as it appears, but rather the conditioner you're using may be making the scalp feel greasy or thick, or the root volumizing styling product you are applying may be adding a slick feel to the scalp. Before we can decide what our hair needs or doesn't need, we must first determine what kind of hair and scalp we really have and how what we are presently doing affects them.

Aside from the differences between hair and scalp, the quality of hair on any one head is not uniform. If your hair is long, the hair closest to the scalp is likely to be far healthier than the length of hair around your shoulders or beyond. The longer ends have been putting up with blow dryers, brushes, weather, swimming pools, styling products, and chemical treatments such as dyes or perms for a longer period of time. New hair does not need the same attention or product as the ends. Combination hair of this kind is even more typical than combination skin, yet the hair-care companies virtually ignore this condition.

Normal hair and normal scalp (usually straight or wavy). This is the dream head of hair. If your hair feels soft to the touch, has good body and manageability (and doesn't require a conditioner to feel that way), has not been color-treated or permed, and your scalp is neither dry nor oily, then you have "normal" hair and scalp. This hair type needs minimal attention. However, normal hair can quickly become damaged hair if you over-use styling implements or drastically change your hair color. Also, overwashing can dry out the scalp.

It is easy to get seduced by perms or extreme changes in hair color, especially when you have healthy, normal hair. You're told it will just bring a little more life to your hair—and no damage. I've seen it happen over and over. A woman with beautiful healthy hair is convinced that it could be *more* beautiful (we are so easily convinced we can be more beautiful with help from the cosmetics industry) with a few highlights or lightening the color a few shades. Now the normal hair is damaged and conditioner is mandatory, with no return to normal until the hair grows out—all for the sake of a "beautiful" change. Sometimes the best policy is to do as little as possible.

A shampoo for normal hair or a shampoo with a minimal amount of either rinse-off or leave-in conditioner does just fine for this hair type.

Oily hair and oily scalp (usually straight hair) or oily scalp and dry ends (usually curly or kinky hair that may or may not be color treated). Technically, hair itself is not oily; the scalp produces too much oil that makes its way along the hair shaft, causing the hair to become heavy and matted. This is especially a problem for those with straight hair and an oily scalp because the oil has a straight path down the hair shaft with no resistance. Curly hair, on the other hand, has more twists and turns, so even if the scalp is producing the same amount of oil as the scalp of someone with straight hair, the person with curly hair experiences it far differently.

The major questions most women have about their oily hair are how often you can wash it and how do you stop the oil? Essentially, you can wash your hair as often as you like. The only problem would be washing with shampoos that contain strong detergent cleansing agents, or that contain irritating ingredients. Both of these elements can dry out the scalp and hair. What you can't do is stop the oil from being produced. Shampooing or trying to dry up the oil won't stop or alter oil production in the least because you can't control or change oil production from the outside in. Oil production is controlled by hormonal activity, which cannot be influenced topically. So wash your hair as often as you like with shampoos that contain gentle cleansing agents (they will be enough to clean hair without causing dryness) (Sources: *Journal of the American Academy of Dermatology*, March 2004, pages 443–447; and *Seminars in Cutaneous Medical Surgery*, September 2001, pages 144–153).

For oily hair, it is essential to never use shampoos with conditioning agents (especially those designated as two-in-ones) because these deposit ingredients that add to the greasy feel of the hair, especially on the scalp. If the hair is hard to comb but not excessively dry, damaged, or coarse after washing, then use the lightest-weight conditioner possible and keep it away from the scalp. If the hair length is dry, damaged, or coarse, it needs a more emollient conditioner, but it should absolutely be a separate product from the shampoo and you should condition only the ends or dry sections of hair. As much as possible, never place conditioner on the scalp or anywhere near the root area close to the scalp.

Oily scalp and short hair. This scalp and hair combination can be a blessing because a simple shampoo with minimal to no conditioners, used as often as you want, is probably all you need. You probably produce enough natural oil to have enough of your own built-in conditioner. Since your hair is short, even if you color your hair it probably doesn't need a conditioner because you are constantly cutting or trimming away the damaged length. If you do need a conditioner, use the least amount possible and keep it away from the root area and off the scalp.

Very dry hair (regardless of the cause) and dry, itchy scalp (usually with straight, fine, or thin hair). Working with this type of hair is very tricky because if you apply an emollient conditioner all over, it can make your hair go limp, although it will help moisturize the dry scalp. But if you avoid an emollient conditioner or shampoo, your scalp can flake and your hair can be flyaway. And a two-in-one product won't provide enough conditioner to the dry hair. Another problem is the concern about overwashing. Someone with dry hair and dry scalp can go several days between shampoos, but that allows dead skin cells and old styling products to build up on the hair, making it look dull and lifeless.

The best thing to do is shampoo at least twice a week to prevent buildup and use an emollient conditioner that rinses easily off the scalp and hair. Avoid getting greasy conditioners and hair treatments near the scalp, even though they promise to take care of the dryness! If a product lists lanolin, vegetable or plant oils, cocoa butter, mineral oil, castor oil, or petrolatum among the first four to five ingredients on the ingredient list, it is considered fairly greasy. These ingredients are also difficult to wash out of the hair and tend to sit on the scalp, trapping dead skin cells. Shampoos and conditioners must be rinsed off well. Massage your scalp gently and thoroughly when shampooing and conditioning, but don't overmanipulate the hair.

Do not use leave-in conditioners; they are rarely emollient or moisturizing enough for this kind of dryness. Instead, apply a drop of silicone serum to the very dry ends of the hair before styling (see the *Laminates, Serums, Hair Polishers, and Spray-On Shine Products* section in Chapter Four, "Hair-Care Formulations"). This will make a big difference in the feel of your hair.

The best way to deal with a dry scalp is to treat it as you would dry skin anywhere else on your body. Consider using the lightweight moisturizer you are presently using for your face or body and apply it to your scalp at night, but only if you plan to shampoo the next morning. It may seem a little strange at first, but it can make a real difference in the condition of your scalp, particularly during the winter. When you shampoo in the morning, take extra care to massage and wash the scalp, rinsing generously.

If your scalp feels very itchy, a little over-the-counter cortisone cream massaged into the scalp the night before you wash your hair the next morning can easily take care of that problem.

Dry hair (regardless of cause) and dry, itchy scalp (usually with wavy, curly, coarse, or kinky hair). In many ways this hair type is easier to care for than the one above because wavy, curly, coarse, or kinky hair doesn't become as limp or heavy when you apply the emollient conditioners that these hair types really need. To this end, the main difference between this and the hair type above is that you can be more liberal with emollient products and less concerned about weighing hair down. You can also be more generous with the laminates, serums, or hair polishers. All of the other suggestions for the very dry hair type above still pertain.

Combination scalp and all hair types. If your scalp is both oily and flaky at the same time, but the flaking is not caused by dandruff or some other scalp condition (see the sections below on treating dandruff, seborrhea, and psoriasis), you've got a condition that's tricky to contend with. It might be caused by overwashing (causing dryness) or by not washing often enough (causing buildup of dead skin or styling products). The flaking can also be caused by irritation or an allergic reaction to the hair-care products you are using, or it can result from styling products that flake. As a general rule, it is best to use a shampoo that contains minimal to no conditioners and to be sure to gently massage your nails over your scalp to help exfoliation when shampooing. A lightweight conditioner that you use all over, but carefully rinse out, won't weigh the hair down and should help. If you have hair that's more coarse or dry, generously apply conditioner to those areas, avoiding the scalp.

If you suspect any of the flaking is a result of allergic reactions or irritation from the products you're using, simply change to another product and see if that eliminates the problem, although it may take some experimenting to find which solutions work for you. Massaging an over-the-counter cortisone cream into the scalp the night before you wash your hair can help reduce the itching.

Flaky dry scalp and all hair types. If the flaking is caused by dandruff or you suspect some other scalp dermatitis, see the sections below on dandruff, seborrhea, and psoriasis. If the flaking is not related to these disorders, there can be several causes and solutions. The flaking may not be related to a dry scalp, but could be a buildup of styling products coming off in sheets. Cutting back on the amount of styling products you use and keeping them away from the scalp will take care of the problem if it is related to buildup.

If your scalp is truly dry and it's not the result of irritating ingredients in your shampoo or conditioner, consider applying a moisturizer (the one you use daily for your face or body is great) to your scalp the night before you plan to wash your hair in the morning. Doing this on a regular basis can really make a difference in the condition of the scalp.

After shampooing and conditioning always rinse well; residue from shampoos can cause irritation and make matters worse. Two-in-one shampoos are a good option for this hair type because they avoid overconditioning normal hair but provide enough conditioner for the scalp.

Dry hair ends and oily scalp. If the entire hair shaft is dry and the scalp is oily, it is usually because the hair has been overprocessed or styled to death. In that case, you should first get a haircut to cut off the dry ends, which will improve the appearance of your hair almost immediately. Cut back on curling irons, blow dryers, and extreme changes in your natural hair color or you will only continue the cycle of dry ends. Use a shampoo designed for normal hair, one that contains no conditioning agents. Wash your hair as often as you like, but concentrate on your scalp and not on the length of hair. If you can, cut back on how often you wash your hair; that can be helpful because washing the hair too often also means more frequent use of blow dryers, curling irons, or flat irons, which further damage the hair. Select an emollient conditioner for dry, damaged hair and use it only on the ends, being sure to leave it on for as long as possible, then rinsing well. The longer you leave the conditioner on your hair, the more opportunity there is for the conditioning agents to be deposited on the hair shaft and/or absorbed around the cuticle. Applying a silicone serum to the ends can be incredibly helpful.

Fragile, dry hair and dry scalp. This combination is typical of African-American hair. For specific details and a thorough discussion of this unique hair type, please see Chapter Eight, "For Women of Color."

Fine, thin hair and normal scalp. Follow the basic guidelines for normal hair and normal scalp. It's best not to use overall conditioners or two-in-one shampoos for this hair type, as they can weigh down the hair. Lightweight, spray-on conditioners can be applied after washing to help with combing and to add a feeling of fullness, and with spray-ons it's easy to control where and how much you apply, keeping in mind that the less you use the better for thin hair, to avoid weighing it down. It is tempting to get caught up in using more and more products in the belief that the volume will just keep adding up, but thin hair can only take so much before it begins to fall. (Many products make claims about adding body, but you can't add body without risking adding weight to the hair.)

Chemical treatments such as perms or hair color (preferably not both; do one or the other because the combination can cause extreme damage) can add body and fullness because of the swelling effect these chemical processes have on the hair shaft. However, in time, with repeated coloring and perming, the fullness can change quickly to noticeable damage. What styling products you use always depends on the kind of look you want, but, as much as possible, you are better off with lightweight styling products to keep the hair from getting weighed down.

Fine, thin hair and dry scalp. Follow the basic guidelines for normal hair and dry scalp. Chemical treatments such as perms or hair color (not both; do one or the other) can add body and fullness as long as you don't make an extreme change, which will cause excessive damage. If you choose to perm, do not let your stylist use small rods. Large rods will add body and smoothness; small rods can make kinks and frizz.

Fine, thin hair and oily scalp. Follow the basic guidelines for normal hair and oily scalp. Chemical treatments such as perms or hair color (not both; do one or the other) can add body and fullness as long as you don't make an extreme change, which will cause excessive damage. If you choose to perm, do not let your stylist use small rods. Large rods will add body and smoothness; small rods can make kinks and frizz.

Coarse hair and dry scalp. Follow the basic guidelines for dry hair and dry, itchy scalp, usually with wavy, curly, coarse, or kinky hair. It is almost impossible to overcondition coarse hair, so don't be afraid to use emollient products generously; let them stay on as long as possible, and then rinse. Silicone serums are dream products for this kind of hair.

Avoid leave-in conditioners—they tend to make hair brittle because they usually contain styling agents such as acrylates, acrylamides, or PVP. Pomades are an option for this hair type, but be careful, as they can get greasy and tacky and leave a slick, messy finish when what you really want is a soft, smooth appearance. Use them sparingly and only in areas where they're needed, not all over. In general, avoid styling gels and hairsprays that leave a hard finish on the hair; they may hold better, but they can also make the hair feel more coarse.

Coarse hair and oily scalp. Use a "clarifying" shampoo that contains no conditioning agents or volumizing ingredients. Generously apply an emollient conditioner, but concentrate it on the length of hair, avoiding contact anywhere near the scalp. Silicone serums are wonderful to apply to the ends and dry areas of coarse hair. In general, avoid styling gels and hairsprays that leave a hard finish on the hair; they may hold better, but they can also make the hair feel coarser and rougher.

Chemically treated, damaged hair, regardless of scalp type. Essentially, it is best to use a shampoo for your scalp type and a separate conditioner for your hair, paying particular attention to the ends. Do not overwash or overmanipulate the hair. Be good about protecting your hair from exposure to the weather and sun by wearing a hat if you are going to be outside for long periods of time. As I explained earlier in this book, don't trust products that contain sunscreen to protect your hair from environmental damage.

Feel free to overuse conditioner and keep it on the hair (but away from the scalp) for as long as possible. Silicone serums work beautifully to make hair feel silky-soft. Pomades and styling waxes can help ends look smooth.

Sparse hair. Little can be done to handle sparse hair, at least when it comes to shampoos, conditioners, and styling products. If sparse hair is being caused by breakage from overperming, radical changes in hair color, or styling tools, you must address these issues. However, if sparse hair is a result of hair loss, refer to Chapter Three, "Hair Growth—Hair Loss."

FLAKY SCALP

When it comes to scalp problems, almost nothing is as annoying as dandruff or dandruff-like conditions. No matter how much you clean your hair, the flakes fall from your scalp in a virtual snow shower, leaving your shoulders messy and your scalp looking greasy and matted. What a pain! There is a difference, however, between dandruff and dandruff-like conditions. Dandruff-like conditions can happen for several reasons, such as when dead skin cells build up on the scalp and don't have the opportunity to slough off. This can be related to overuse of conditioners, infrequent hair washing, inadequate rinsing after shampooing (which can leave a flaky residue on the scalp), using a shampoo that contains cleansing agents that cause your scalp to flake, and/or a buildup of styling products on the hair shaft. Each of these things by itself, or several in combination, can cause the scalp to flake, and that can look a lot like dandruff. Another indication that you have dry scalp and not dandruff is that dandruff conditions often respond to dandruff treatments, but a flaky, dry scalp does not.

Dandruff-like conditions can be dealt with easily. Avoid heavy, concentrated conditioners and use them sparingly, if at all, near the scalp because these can build up on the scalp and hold down dead skin cells, causing excessive accumulation. After shampooing and conditioning, be sure to rinse well for at least a minute or more. Even if your hair and scalp are dry, don't go long periods of time between shampooing. If you have dry flakes, shampoo at least twice a week, concentrating your attention on the scalp. Give yourself a thorough scalp massage and gently use your nails to help exfoliation. Depending on your scalp's sensitivity, some surfactants (or several in combination) can cause flaking. In that case, all you need to do is change the shampoo you are using to stop the scalp from flaking. Also, avoid styling products that flake because they can resemble dandruff.

Dandruff-like conditions can also be seasonal. Dry heat and cold temperatures outdoors can leave the scalp hungry for moisture, yet you may not want to wash your hair too often for fear of drying out the scalp and hair even more. Shampooing infrequently is not the answer. You wash your face to keep the skin clean and remove dead skin cells, and you must do the same for your scalp; that is, treat a dry, flaky scalp the same as you would dry flaky skin on your face or body. Massage a moisturizer (the one you use on your face or body will work fine) on your scalp the night before you plan to wash your hair in the morning. Doing this on a regular basis can help get rid of dry scalp.

DANDRUFF, SEBORRHEIC DERMATITIS, AND SEBORRHEA

According to the American Academy of Dermatology patient information sheet on seborrhea (www.aad.org), there are distinct differences between dandruff, seborrheic dermatitis, and seborrhea. Dandruff appears as scaling on the scalp without redness or inflammation. Seborrheic dermatitis has the same flaking as dandruff, but with pronounced redness, inflammation, and itching. Seborrhea is similar to both dandruff and seborrheic dermatitis in regard to flaking, but there is no redness or inflammation. Instead, an extreme, thick oiliness is present that creates a matted, rough, crusty appearance where the lesions occur. A baby's cradle cap—called tinea capitis—is classic seborrheic dermatitis. The size of the eruption, the texture of the oil, and the tendency toward flaky skin are what differentiate seborrhea from plain, flaky dandruff.

Though subject to debate, most research indicates that dandruff and seborrheic dermatitis are both triggered by the presence of yeast organisms in the hair follicle, where there's sufficient oil production to promote growth. In fact, *Malassezia* fungi have been suspected as the cause of dandruff for more than a century. (Previously referred to as *Pityrosporum ovale* or *P. orbiculare*, these fungi are now believed to be a species of the genus *Malassezia*).

Other factors have also been suspected of causing dandruff or seborrheic dermatitis, but there is no research proving they are involved: too much oil production, abnormal skin cell growth inhibiting healthy cell turnover, poor diet, too much shampooing, too little shampooing, hair dye, cold weather, genetic disposition, and hormonal imbalances. However, if you have dandruff or seborrheic dermatitis there is a possibility some of these factors can make matters worse.

First and foremost, treating either dandruff or seborrheic dermatitis involves reducing the presence of the *Malassezia* fungi as well as creating a scalp condition that doesn't provide a favorable environment for their growth. For example, it's especially helpful to keep the scalp as free of oil as possible to reduce the environment the fungi prefer.

Unfortunately, while these scalp conditions tend to come and go, for the most part they are not really curable. However, they can be controlled, and some people do outgrow the condition (Sources: *Skin Pharmacology and Applied Skin Physiology*, November–December 2002, pages 434–441; *Skin Research and Technology*, August 2002, pages 187–193; *Journal of Clinical Microbiology*, September 2002, pages 3350–3357; www.emedicinecom, "Seborrheic Dermatitis," June 4, 2003; *Dermatology*, 2000, volume 201, issue 4, pages 332–336; and *Archives of Dermatological Research*, July 2002, pages 221–230).

TREATING DANDRUFF, SEBORRHEIC DERMATITIS, AND SEBORRHEA

Everyone knows dandruff when they see it. Small white flakes are dusted or clumped over and through the hair, congregating primarily on the scalp. Thankfully, dandruff is not contagious and the myth about dandruff causing hair loss is just that, a myth; there's no scientific basis or evidence for the notion.

As a first line of defense, dandruff shampoos are the best place to start. These shampoos generally contain one of the following ingredients to deal with the problem: **zinc pyrithione** (Head & Shoulders); **selenium sulfide** (Selsun Blue); or **ketoconazole** (Nizoral—available in both prescription strength and over the counter).

Zinc pyrithione, **selenium sulfide**, and **ketoconazole** each have a good deal of research showing they are effective in treating dandruff. They act as potent and proven antimicrobial agents, helping to decrease the amount of yeast present. These ingredients are an optimum way to control dandruff because they don't just tackle the symptom—they attack the organisms that are the underlying cause of the problem. A small amount of research indicates that ketoconazole is more effective than zinc pyrithione or selenium sulfide; nonetheless, it still requires experimentation to see which treatment works best for you (Sources: *Skin Pharmacology and Applied Skin Physiology*, November–December 2002, pages 434–441; *Journal of the American Academy of Dermatology*, December 2001, pages 897–903; *Dermatology*, 2001, volume 202, issue 2, pages 171–176; and *International Journal of Cosmetic Science*, 1997, volume 19, issue 3, pages 1467–2494).

Coal tar (Ionil-T, Pentrax, T-Gel, and Tegrin) slows the creation of skin cells and is an antimicrobial agent. It works by reducing the number of flakes present on the scalp and eliminating the yeast in the hair follicle that cause the condition. This is helpful for those with chronic or extremely stubborn dandruff or seborrhea that doesn't respond to other over-the-counter options. Regrettably, coal tar is a controversial ingredient for dandruff control because there is evidence that in large concentrations it can be a carcinogen, particularly for causing skin, lung, and scrotum cancer. However, there is no research showing that the use of coal tar in dandruff shampoos has this effect. The research showing coal tar to be a possible carcinogen was from studies carried out in industrial settings where workers were exposed to concentrated solutions over long periods of time (20 to 25 years) and from studies on animals. But the lack of research related to hair-care products doesn't mean there isn't an unknown risk factor to take into consideration, something even the FDA acknowledges.

Coal tar also produces photosensitivity, a skin reaction that occurs with exposure to sunlight. Residual amounts of coal tar may remain on the scalp, hair, or surrounding areas after use, which means that if you're going out in the sun after shampooing with these products, you need to take extra precautions. Due to the significant risks associated with coal tar, it should be considered a last-resort treatment after all other options have been exhausted (Sources: *Dermatology*, 2000, volume 200, issue 2, pages 181–184; www.mayoclinic.com; *Drug Safety*, December 1996, pages 374–377; www.fda.gov; and National Library of Medicine, Specialized Information Services, Coal-tars and Derived Products, www.toxnet.nlm.nih.gov/).

Piroctone olamine is a relatively new antifungal ingredient that is in the process of being approved by the FDA for use in dandruff shampoos. It has been available in Europe for such use and has been shown to be very effective (Sources: *International Journal of Cosmetic Science*, December 2003, page 1467; *Cutis*, January 1997, pages 21–24; *Fundamentals and Applied Toxicology*, January 1991, pages 31–40; and www.fda.gov).

Tea tree oil (also called melaleuca) is derived from a tree native to Australia. A study published in the *Journal of the American Academy of Dermatology* (December 2002, pages 852–855) found that "daily shampooing with 5% pure tea tree oil reduces the severity and extent of dandruff. Overall improvement is similar to topical treatment with ketoconazole [found in Nizoral].... Tea tree oil... has antifungal activity against *Pityrosporum ovale*, which is thought to be the causative agent of dandruff." Keep in mind that just because tea tree oil is a plant doesn't mean you can't have an allergic or sensitizing reaction to it (Source: *Medical Journal of Australia,* February 21, 1994, volume 160, page 236). As promising as this is, there are no hair-care products reviewed in this edition that have a 5% concentration of tea tree oil. Regrettably, every hair-care product claiming to contain tea tree oil has less than a 1% concentration. That may make the product smell nice, but it won't be helpful for the scalp. However, you can buy pure tea tree oil at health food stores and apply that to your scalp.

Salicylic acid (Ionil Plus, Salac, Sal-Clens) has keratolytic (skin exfoliating) and antimicrobial properties that help with skin-cell turnover. It can also reduce the presence of the fungi residing in the hair follicle that cause dandruff or seborrheic dermatitis. It is sometimes used in combination with **sulfur** (Sebulex), which can be effective for alleviating the symptoms of dandruff and seborrheic dermatitis. However, sulfur can damage the hair shaft and should be used only after other treatments have proven unsuccessful (Sources: *Journal of Dermatologic Treatment*, June 2002, pages 51–60; and Medline Plus, www.nlm.nih.gov/medlineplus/druginformation.html).

GETTING THE BEST RESULTS

As successful as dandruff and seborrheic dermatitis treatments can be, the problem with all the active ingredients is that they can have irritating, sensitizing, and drying side effects. Moreover, ingredients such as selenium sulfide and sulfur, in the amounts used in dandruff shampoos, tend to have a terrible smell and can damage hair.

What a dilemma! The very ingredients that can help dandruff can also cause scalp problems and make hair hard to manage! To reduce the drying effect of these products, it is often best to add a conditioner to the length of your hair or to alternate your dandruff shampoo with a regular shampoo. Fighting dandruff can take experimentation, so be patient. Also, don't think you are better off fighting the problem with salon products than with drugstore products. Most of the major dandruff research is being conducted by the pharmaceutical industry or the major hair-care companies, not by smaller contract manufacturers.

In general, the best option for those with true dandruff or other dermatitis-like scalp conditions is to start with products that contain zinc pyrithione. If zinc pyrithione isn't effective, the next step is to consider ketoconazole (Nizoral), which is available in drugstores or in prescription strength from your physician.

If you find Head & Shoulders and Nizoral aren't effective, the next step is a product that contains salicylic acid, followed by experimenting with sulfur, and finally coal tar.

Aside from experimenting with which product works for you, remember that how you use these products also affects the results you obtain. Research clearly shows that the longer you can keep the ingredients in contact with your scalp the more effective they will be in suppressing the growth of the fungi.

It is also important not to avoid washing your hair. A clean scalp has an easier time shedding unwanted skin cells and removing the oil that provides the perfect environment for the fungi. For many, it's not necessary to use a dandruff shampoo every time you wash your hair, rather you can alternate a dandruff shampoo with a regular shampoo, which may reduce some of the irritating side effects and aesthetic styling problems associated with these treatments. You can start by using the anti-dandruff product frequently, and then when the flaking is minimized or eliminated, you can alternate the dandruff shampoo with a shampoo for your scalp type, which can be anything from normal to dry. Don't avoid conditioner, but be careful to apply it only to the length of your hair and to keep it off your scalp because the emollients in a conditioner just add to the oil on the scalp, not a good idea since that just enhances the environment the fungi prefer.

Words of warning: If you color your hair, avoid dandruff products that contain sulfur or selenium sulfide because these ingredients can strip hair color. Many dandruff shampoos use irritating, drying ingredients such as menthol, sodium lauryl sulfate, and TEA-lauryl sulfate. These do not help deal with the cause of the dermatitis, but they can irritate and dry out the scalp.

Regardless of how you deal with dandruff, seborrheic dermatitis, or seborrhea, stay realistic about what works and be prepared to experiment to find what is best for your head. Nothing is guaranteed when it comes to dandruff, and as natural as tea tree oil sounds, it doesn't provide any more benefit than ingredients that sound more chemical. And if you've exhausted all the over-the-counter options, see your doctor about prescription options.

PSORIASIS

The most common type of psoriasis that occurs on the scalp is plaque psoriasis, a chronic, recurring disease of the skin, identified by the presence of thickened, rough skin covered by silvery white scaly areas with areas of pronounced redness. Often papules are present, small, solid, often inflamed bumps that, unlike pimples, do not contain pus or sebum. These bumps are usually slightly elevated above the normal skin surface, sharply distinguishable from normal skin, and red to reddish brown in color. The extent of the disease can vary from a few tiny lesions to generalized involvement over a good deal of the entire scalp. Counting all the various forms of psoriasis, it affects over 4 million people in the United States alone. For most people it tends to be mild and unsightly rather than a serious health concern.

It is now believed that psoriasis is an autoimmune disorder in which, to put it simply, the skin overproduces both normal and abnormal skin cells. A normal skin cell matures in 28 to 45 days, while a psoriatic skin cell matures in only 3 to 6 days.

Sadly, there is no cure for psoriasis, but there are many new treatments, both topical and systemic, that can clear it for periods of time. Experimenting with a variety of options is essential to find the treatment that works for you, but all require a doctor's attention.

Treating psoriasis can be similar to treating dandruff, seborrheic dermatitis, and seborrhea, and coal tar and salicylic acid can be helpful. Unique treatments for psoriasis include topical steroids and sun exposure, which are standard therapies that have been used in the past, as has **anthralin**, a form of coal tar and a dye. **Calcipotriene**, a synthetic vitamin D3 analog, has also been used to treat mild to moderate psoriasis. It is a prescription medication with few side effects. (This is not the same compound as the vitamin D in commercial vitamin supplements.) Calcipotriene is sold in the United States as a topical, odorless, nonstaining ointment and cream under the prescription brand name Dovonex. Other topical agents such as retinoids in the form of tazarotene (Tazorac) have also had success.

More serious systemic medications for severe psoriasis include **methotrexate**, which blocks a specific enzyme the cell needs to live. This drug can also interfere with the growth of cancer cells, which are eventually destroyed, but methotrexate may also affect the growth of normal body cells and cause additional side effects. **Oral retinoids** such as **Accutane** and **Soriatane** can have a considerable effect on psoriasis by reducing hyper, abnormal skin cell growth, along with producing normal growth and triggering anti-inflammatory activity in the skin.

Cyclosporin, **Pimecrolimus**, and **Tacrolimus** are medications, known as immunosuppressive agents, that slow the overproduction of psoriatic skin cells. There is a good deal of research showing them to be effective in the treatment of psoriasis (Sources: *International Journal of Clinical Practice*, May 2003, pages 319–327; *Journal of Allergy and Clinical Immunology*, May 2003, pages 1153–1168, and August 2002, pages 277–284; and *Journal of Investigative Dermatology*, October 2002, pages 876–887).

Photochemotherapy uses a combination of UVA light and a photosensitizing drug such as **methoxsalen**. This combination decreases skin-cell growth. Repeated treatments take place two to three times per week until lesions are cleared, with almost an 85% chance of remission. However, adverse effects of photochemotherapy include nausea, pruritus (itching), and burning. Long-term complications include increased risks of photodamage to the skin and skin cancer.

Discovering whether any of these treatments will work for you, alone or in combination, takes patience and a systematic, ongoing review and evaluation of how your skin is doing. As is true with all chronic skin disorders, success requires diligent adherence to the regimen and a realistic understanding of what you can and can't expect. It is also important to be aware of the consequences of the varying treatment levels. Each treatment has its pros and cons, and you must discuss these with your physician (Sources: www.emedicine.com, "Psoriasis, Plaque," May 20, 2004; *Dermatology*, 2004, volume 208, issue 4, pages 297–306; *Journal of Investigative Dermatology Symposium Proceedings*, March 2004, pages 131–135; *Skin Pharmacology and Physiology*, May–June 2004, pages 111–118; *Journal of European Academy of Dermatology and Venereology*, March 2004; pages 169–172; *Journal of Dermatologic Treatment*, January 2004, pages 8–13 and 14–22; *Journal of the American Academy of Dermatology*, February 2002, pages 228–241; and www.psoriasis.com).

CHAPTER SIX

Hair of a Different Color

REAL COLOR

Before you decide how you want to change your hair color, it's extremely helpful to understand the composition of the hair color you were born with. Everyone's hair follicles contain pigment producing cells that, depending on their genetic background, create two types of melanin (melanin is also the pigment found in skin cells), called eumelanin and pheomelanin. Eumelanin is a black-dark brown pigment, pheomelanin is a red pigment. Together, eumelanin and pheomelanin in varying combinations and concentrations create the endless variety and the shades of black, brown, red, blonde, and gray hair color.

Hair color is determined by the amount of each pigment in the hair follicle. As the amount of eumelanin decreases, the hair color turns from black to lighter shades of brown, and then to blonde. Almost every hair color contains some amount of reddish pigment. For darker shades of hair, the reddish pheomelanin is largely masked by the darker eumelanin pigment. Lighter shades of brown, however, are unable to cover the pheomelanin and thus reflect tones of warm gold or red (Source: www.keratin.com). This pheomelanin pigment explains why your hair often becomes some shade of red or copper when you try to lighten or dye it because lightening the darker hair color reveals the underlying red pigment in all hair color.

People with darker hair colors have more eumelanin, while those with light brown to blonde hair have less eumelanin. People with true red hair have far more pheomelanin pigment. Along with producing less of the dark eumelanin hair pigment, people with red hair have skin that also produces far less of the skin-related pigment of melanin, which is why true redheads are generally pale and especially prone to sunburn.

A study that analyzed the amount of eumelanin and pheomelanin in human hair suggested that "black hair contains approximately 99% eumelanin and 1% pheomelanin, brown and blonde hair contain 95% eumelanin and 5% pheomelanin; and red hair contains 67% eumelanin and 33% pheomelanin" (Source: *Analytical Biochemistry*, March 2001, pages 116–125).

The absence of pigment creates pure white hair and hair color usually changes with age. Most children who have whitish blonde hair end up with some shade of brown as adults, and as we age and lose pigment, hair becomes gray.

DOES SHE?

"Does she or doesn't she? Does she or doesn't she? Does she or doesn't she? Only her hairdresser knows for sure," echoes a deep male voice in the well-known 1956 Clairol television ad. What a powerful message that must have been back then! An attractive, elegantly dressed woman lights a candelabra, pausing long enough to admire her image in the mirror, then strokes her perfectly styled blonde tresses. Apart from the supercilious marketing, what women wanted almost 50 years ago for their hair is what they still want today, an easy-to-use, professional-quality, reliable product that can alter hair color yet still leave it looking natural and lustrous.

Before that ad appeared, only 7% of the adult female population in the United States dyed their hair. Today, depending on whose statistics you use, that number has increased to around 50%, and if you include the entire U.S. population, one out of every five people color their hair (Source: *Drugstore News*, March 26, 2001). The question now, as it was back then, still is: How do you get your hair to look like what all the ads have been promising? That's what you're about to find out.

Hair Note: Throughout this book, I use the words "color" and "dye" interchangeably to refer to a change of any kind from the natural color of the hair as the result of applying any salon or drugstore product. I've been told that "dyeing," like the word "beautician," is an old-fashioned term and that "coloring" and "tinting" are the more current terms. Well, they might be more current, but they also conveniently provide a way for companies and stylists to imply that the consumer won't be doing anything radical or damaging to her hair if she "colors" it rather than "dyes" it. There are indeed some hair-coloring processes that aren't at all damaging, such as the temporary or semi-permanent methods, but the demi, level 2, mid, intermediate, and permanent hair dyes, no matter how gentle they sound, do damage the hair. Furthermore, cosmetics chemists call those little molecules that affect hair color "dyes," and the dictionary makes the same connection, so I use the word "dye," too (Source: *Journal of Cosmetic Science*, July–August 2003, pages 379–394).

WHY COLOR?

Without question, there are unmistakably positive reasons for coloring hair. Hair dyes and color treatments can make the hair appear thicker, enliven otherwise drab hair, and create the perfect hair color. But by far the biggest reason most women (and men) dye their hair is because they don't want to show they are graying. In days gone by, the desire to be blonde drove the hair-color market; today, it is mostly the desire to be anything but gray.

When those gray strands start popping up, no matter how a woman feels about any other issue surrounding age, she is not happy about the prospect of losing her original hair color and becoming gray. Case in point: How many coloring products are on the market to change your hair *to* gray? None, although a small handful will brighten gray or reduce the yellow cast of the gray you already have—but those are few and far between. When it comes to changing hair to a precise or distinct shade of blonde, brown, black, or red, there are literally hundreds of options.

For those under the age of graying (assuming that you aren't graying prematurely) there is a huge incentive to change color just for the fun of it or for the sake of a new style or fashion statement. While most baby boomers want to cover gray without making any radical changes to their hair, women between the ages of 14 and 35 want to play with color the way they might try on a trendy, fun outfit. For those younger women, color is about making a statement, being glamorous, adding flash and excitement.

Regardless of the hair color you desire, hair-care companies would love for you to believe that changing the color of your hair won't cause damage, or at least not very much damage. But that isn't the truth. All the claims about moisturizing ingredients or gentle formulations can't alter the fact that dyes that change hair color must penetrate the cortex of the hair and stay there. That process is damaging, plain and simple. And it is especially damaging to make an extreme change from dark to light color, for example.

HAIR COLOR FOR WOMEN OF COLOR

A much smaller but growing portion of the hair-color market involves dyes for the ethnic market. Previously, women of color usually only accented their natural dark tresses with deeper or subtle tones of red, amber, or copper. Rarely did you see a woman of color with blonde or red hair. More recently, celebrities and models have started sporting golden and red locks. The problem is that celebrity hairdos often end up in the mainstream, and that translates into a lot of women dyeing their hair blonde or red. Regardless of race, anytime you make an extreme color change you run the risk of seriously damaging your hair, but this is of even more concern to African-American women because their hair is already fragile. When, as often happens, hair is chemically treated or harshly styled with blow dryers, curling irons, and hot combs, it adds up to extremely damaged hair. Adding color to fragile hair that is permed, as well as subjected to high-heat styling tools, almost guarantees compounding hair problems to the point of breakage.

The exception to this is for women of color with short, natural, nonstraightened hair. This virgin hair can handle the transition from dark to light far more easily. That doesn't mean with no damage, it just means less of it to get the color you want (see Chapter Eight, "For Women of Color," for more information).

DRUGSTORE VERSUS SALON HAIR COLOR

In 2003 the most popular brands of hair dye were L'Oreal Preference (15.7 million products sold); Clairol Nice 'n Easy (14.9 million); L'Oreal Excellence (13.2 million);

Revlon Colorsilk (12.3 million); Just For Men (10.3 million); Clairol Natural Instincts (9.6 million); L'Oreal Feria (9 million); Garnier Nutrisse (7.6 million); Clairol Hydrience (5.3 million); and L'Oreal Couleur Experte (2 million). Although there are no similar statistics for products used in hair salons, the vast majority of women, whether they are hiding gray, improving lackluster natural hair color, or simply treating hair to a fashion statement, are using products from the drugstore rather than paying to have it done at the hair salon.

Beyond the difficulty of some popular but technically demanding services (such as highlighting), turning dark hair blonde, or getting rid of unwanted color from a poor dye incident, there are good reasons to do the simpler processes at home yourself, the most compelling of which are saving time and money. If you get your hair dyed 6 to 12 times a year at a salon, you could save $400 to $2,000 or more by doing it at home. What you might not know is that the hair colors you buy at the drugstore are superbly formulated.

The ways hair dyes function and the ingredients that create the dyes do not differ between inexpensive products and those found in salon products. The major difference, and this is fairly major, is that a professional colorist can custom blend a specific color and control the amount of peroxide used.

If there are ingredient differences, no one in the industry, and none of the ingredient manufacturers or cosmetics chemists, seem to know about it. The myth that salon products are better than the ones at drugstores is asserted as a fact by every hairdresser I've ever interviewed, despite the lack of evidence or sources. The same ingredients that change hair color are used repeatedly throughout the industry. In fact, all makers of the major drugstore color lines also make the hair-coloring products widely used by salons.

There are also many reasons to get your hair colored at a hair salon, including the mess (it's theirs and not yours), the skill of the technician, and, perhaps most important of all, the benefit of your stylist's experience. It is great to just have the stylist make the decisions and do the work while you sit back and read a magazine. Professional hair-coloring products can be blended in myriad combinations and in multiple processes to create unique and attractive colors. Hairstylists can perform coloring techniques that would be impossible at home. For example, a talented technician can dye your hair a particular color and then put in a corresponding highlight with a foil. I would never in a million years suggest a woman try that at home herself.

Regardless of whether you dye your hair yourself or have it done at the salon, achieving exactly the color you want can be tricky, even with the most talented colorist. It is so easy to make a mistake. Even at the salon, all it takes is misjudging how porous or nonporous your hair is, underprocessing or overprocessing the hair, choosing the wrong color so your hair is too dark or not light enough, or adding the wrong tone so your hair is more orange than golden. And you can make all the same slip-ups as the salon experts.

You may be pleasantly surprised to learn that statistics indicate women who color their hair at home are as pleased (or displeased) with their results as women who have their hair dyed at a salon. A quick review of any chat room or Web site bulletin board about hair care will find lots of people sharing salon horror stories. I have a few of my own! That isn't surprising given how very tricky dyeing hair is.

To summarize, there are five major situations where a salon experience is preferred over dyeing hair yourself: (1) you want to lighten your hair more than three shades, (2) you have dark hair and want to dye your hair red, (3) you're a redhead or you have blonde hair and want to dye it red, (4) you're trying to fix a problem, and (5) you have light hair and want to make it darker.

You want to lighten your hair more than three shades. Regardless of how dark your hair is, if you want to have significantly lighter hair, think twice, and then think again before shopping at the drugstore for a dye product. Even if your hair doesn't appear to have any red or copper tones in it, don't be fooled: all dark hair contains at least some red pigment and it can become evident in the lightening process if you don't know how to correct for it. It is also difficult to lighten your hair in a one-step process. Making hair lighter requires a "double process," first removing the existing color from your hair and then toning, or adding the shade of color you want it to be. Those two distinct processes are difficult to get right and your odds are far better with an experienced hair colorist.

You have dark hair and want to dye your hair red. This is one you shouldn't do at the drugstore *or* salon, but at least someone at the salon will tell you not to do it and give you some better alternatives. There is no way around this one: It is impossible to make black or very dark brown hair red or even dark red without ending up with a very strange hair color, usually some shade of orange. It even says so on the side of the hair-dye boxes at the drugstore.

You're a natual redhead or you want to be a redhead. It doesn't matter what color you have or what color you want to be, it is hard to dye hair red. To figure out whether or not your hair can end up the shade you want or resemble some natural hair color, it is essential to discuss this with a professional colorist.

You're trying to fix a problem (whether you messed it up or your hairstylist made a mistake). You can always call the hair color consumer hot line at L'Oreal, Clairol, or Revlon, but you should also seriously consider getting help from a professional. The risk is that on your own you will only make matters worse. You can actually get to the point of no return, because the more chemicals you put on your hair the more damage occurs, and no matter the amount you can't fix overly damaged hair.

You have light hair and want to make it darker. In theory, this is not a difficult process to do yourself, as lighter hair will easily grab a darker shade. Rather, the difficulty is in trying to not end up with hair that looks like something from a Gothic novel or like Morticia Addams from *The Addams Family*.

WHICH TYPE OF HAIR DYE IS BEST?

There is a quagmire of confusing product choices, names, and misleading information out there that makes it almost impossible to discern the important differences between products. Conceivably the most confusing part of the entire hair-color business is that the names of the products are meaningless. Is L'Oreal's Excellence preferred over L'Oreal's Preference? Is Clairol's Hydrience better for hair than Clairol's Ultress, and does Clairol's Herbal Essences contain plant extracts that help hair, and if so, why aren't they in Clairol's other hair-dye products?

To make matters worse, and supposedly to help us understand what kind of hair dye we are purchasing and how long it will last, the companies have created phrases like "harmonizing color," "tone-on-tone," "oxidation" and "nonoxidation," "permanent" versus "intermediate" or "midcolor," or "level 2" and "demi color"—but what does any of that mean? (Thanks for the help, guys, but thanks for nothing.)

Even more confusing is that the terms for hair dyes in salons do not match the terms used for drugstore products. Salons have a language for hair color all their own. For example, drugstore products use the term "level" to identify three specific *categories* of hair dye: Level 1 for semi-permanent, Level 2 for demi or intermediate, and Level 3 for permanent. Salons use the term "level" to indicate the *depth* of your hair or the dye's color, ranging as follows: 1. Black; 2. Very Dark Brown; 3. Dark Brown; 4. Brown; 5. Medium Brown; 6. Light Brown; 7. Dark Blonde; 8. Light Blonde; 9. Very Light Blonde; and 10. Light Platinum Blonde.

This is not a user-friendly situation. If you are to go safely into the arena of hair color, you need to be armed with a cheat sheet and some straightforward facts so you can make informed decisions.

COLOR CATEGORIES AND TERMS

Essentially, there are five primary types of hair-coloring options available at the drugstore, and most of these—except for progressive dyes—are performed at salons as well. The five categories of hair color dyes are:

1. **Temporary**
2. **Semi-permanent** (also referred to as Level 1)
3. **Demi** (also called Level 2, Mid, Tone-on-Tone, Intermediate, Longer-Lasting Semi-Permanent or Shorter-Lasting Permanent, or In-Between color)
4. **Permanent** (also called Level 3, Bleaching, Blonding, Highlighting, Balliage)
5. **Gradual or progressive dyes** (also called metallic dyes; products called progressive dyes, marketed exclusively to men, can also be Demi, Level 2, Intermediate, and Permanent dyes, although these names are rarely used on the label)

Temporary hair colors coat the outside of the hair shaft with nonpenetrating dyes, so no physical change of any kind takes place within the hair. They are not alkaline and contain no peroxide, which is why these are also referred to as nonoxidizing hair color. Temporary hair colors are available in shampoos, conditioners, and mousses, and, generally, wash out after one or two shampoos.

Semi-Permanent or **Level 1** hair colors have the least amount of ingredients that can affect the internal composition of your hair color. They contain minimal dye content, have low alkaline levels, and contain no peroxide. Because they don't contain peroxide they are also referred to as nonoxidizing. They are not very stable and can often wash out after a few shampoos.

Demi, **Level 2**, **Mid**, and **Intermediate** hair colors are applied to either the entire head of hair or, when doing touch-ups, just the roots, and they come in gel, cream, or paste forms. Demi hair dyes contain ingredients identical to permanent hair color, only at much lower concentrations (particularly reducing the amount of peroxide and the degree of alkalinity) and are intended to make only subtle changes in your hair color and/or to cover some gray. You can't use this type of hair dye to go from brown to blonde or even from dark brown to light brown, and it is effective only if your hair is less than 40% gray (and for some resistant hair types, less than 30% gray). On the other hand, because you can't make a drastic change in your hair color there is little risk of getting terrible results, or suffering extremely noticeable grow-out. Despite the low concentration of peroxide, these are still referred to as oxidizing dyes because they can't work without that process.

Permanent, **Level 3**, **Bleaching**, **Blonding**, **Highlighting**, **Balliage** dyes are available in creams, lotions, and gels, and are shampooed into the hair, or applied just to the roots when doing touch-ups. They can make a considerable, permanent change in hair color, cover large amounts of gray, and will require touch-ups based on fading and grow-out. These dyes contain the highest concentrations of peroxide, have high degrees of alkalinity, and use penetrating dye molecules. There are single-process, double-process, and special-effects permanent dyes.

Progressive hair colors most frequently refer to products that contain lead acetate. Lead acetate gradually accumulates on the outside of the hair shaft or just under the cuticle, altering the hair shade with a blanket of color. For men this is an easy way to completely cover gray with a simple shampooing and without a radical overnight change. There's also no need to worry about grow-out because the color fades gradually when you stop using it. However, lead acetate can also give a strange greenish cast to the hair that is far from natural in appearance, and there are also health concerns.

Within this group of progressive colors are products marketed to men that can be demi or permanent hair colors. These are shampooed in for 5 minutes and then rinsed off. The repetitive, 5-minute applications are meant to gradually build up the color on the hair. Some amount of processing occurs with each successive shampoo. Unlike lead acetate-based progressive colors that cover the outside of the hair shaft, these are standard dye products. If you are wondering if men can use a dye product aimed at women, the answer is an indisputable yes! Why don't men use women's products? Because most men are unwilling to take the time to go through the 20- to 40-minute process, preferring the ease of getting rid of gray in the least amount of time possible. Can women use men's products? Again, the answer is yes, but with a caveat. These progressive permanent or intermediate dyes work only when the hair is short. If you constantly shampoo in color over longer hair, it will eventually saturate the length of hair with too much color and you will no longer get the color you want.

Two more terms will just about complete your hair-dye vocabulary: developer and developer volume.

Developer is another name for peroxide. Peroxide is the ingredient in semi-permanent and permanent hair dyes that removes some of your own color so the color pigment you are adding to your hair has room to get in.

Developer volume refers to the concentration of peroxide. The higher the volume, the more effect it has on your own hair color. Generally, 10- to 20-volume peroxide is used for semi-permanent dyes and 20- to 30-volume peroxide is used for permanent dyes (Sources: *Journal of the Society of Dyers and Colourists*, July–August 2000, pages 193–196; and *Cosmetic Dermatology*, December 2002, pages 47–48).

HOW DO DYES WORK?

Temporary and semi-permanent hair colors are strictly limited in what they can do, and they only coat the outside of the hair (the cuticle layers) with color. This color can be plant-based like henna or can be a synthetic coloring agent. They do not penetrate past the cuticle and do not change the structure of the hair shaft in any way.

In order for demi, level 2, mid, and intermediate or permanent/level 3 hair dyes to work, they require what is often referred to as a double process. They do this using the same basic ingredients, and cause the same remarkable chemical process to take place:

1. The first step involves using an alkaline base (almost always at a pH of 10 to 11) to swell the hair shaft, opening it up to make the cortex permeable so the precursor hair-dye molecules can penetrate and remain in the heart of the hair.

2. Hydrogen peroxide in some amount (the amount varies depending on how the product was formulated) lifts your existing color from the cortex.

3. Once the precursor dye molecules are in the cortex, they go through a chemical process that is turned on by the peroxide, and form large molecular chains of color that are now big enough to remain in the hair and are less likely to wash out. It is the action of the peroxide that gives these demi and permanent hair-coloring products the name oxidative hair dyes.

On a microscopic level, the dye molecules in permanent hair colors are capable of a limitless variety of tones, hues, tints, and intensities. Cosmetics chemists with computer simulation programs have concocted thousands upon thousands of potential color combinations for the hair. These dye molecules are a matter of pride for each of the companies that make hair-coloring products. Whether the product is a cream, lotion, gel, or foam, the product's pH level (it must be alkaline), the molecular structure of the dye, and the volume (concentration) of peroxide are what determine the outcome. Regardless of the claims, no matter how natural, organic, or moisturizing the product says it is, demi and permanent hair dyes are damaging to the hair. However, they can create magnificent color changes that are simply to dye for (Source: *Journal of Cosmetic Science*, July–August 2003, pages 395–409).

NON-AMMONIA HAIR COLOR

Some demi and permanent hair-coloring products claim to contain no ammonia. Although that may sound healthier for the hair, the claim is misleading. For a demi or permanent hair color to work, it must contain ingredients that can raise the pH of the product enough so that when it is applied to the hair it can swell the hair shaft so that the hair dyes can penetrate. If the pH is too low, say less than pH 9, you won't get acceptable penetration of color. Demi and permanent hair dyes need a pH of around 10 or 11 to work, and at least pH 10 if you want to make an extreme change in hair color. Ammonium hydroxide is one of the ingredients used to raise the pH of a product. The so-called non-ammonia-based permanent hair colors simply use a different alkaline ingredient, such as ethanolamine, to raise the pH of the product, and that can cause the same amount of damage to the hair shaft as ammonia. It is true that ammonium hydroxide or ammonia has a stronger odor than ethanolamine, but that doesn't translate into being better for the hair. A high pH is damaging to hair no matter what ingredient causes it.

It takes only about 1% of an alkaline ingredient to raise the pH of the dye to an acceptable level to allow the color to penetrate the hair shaft. The more the hair shaft swells, the better the penetration of the hair color. The more the hair shaft is expanded, the fuller it appears afterward. If your hair is already coarse and frizzy, a more swollen hair shaft can make that condition worse. But if your hair is thin, fine, or limp, that extra swelling can add welcome volume. Unfortunately, it can also add extra damage.

The only real benefit of non-ammonia-based hair colors is their more pleasant odor.

TEMPORARY HAIR COLOR

Temporary hair colors or color rinses are designed to be short-lived. The colors are deposited directly on the hair shaft and, because they don't penetrate the hair shaft, they are washed out the next time you shampoo your hair. Do not expect temporary hair colors to hide more than a few strands of gray, and even then they don't do it very well. They offer a sheer, translucent veil of color over the hair, but that's about it. The color of the dye you see in the container is the color your hair will be. These dyes are meant to be a fun, noncommittal way to improve hair tone or add subtle (and I mean really subtle) highlights, similar to trying on a see-through blouse (not exactly what you would call a full cover-up).

Temporary hair colors are a way to try exceedingly minor, almost inconsequential color variations in your hair without risk. They are also a good way to neutralize the yellow in white and gray hair or tone down the brassiness in certain shades of blonde and frosted hair for a day or two. They can also stretch the time between demi or permanent hair colorings by helping to disguise grow-out slightly. Some temporary hair colors are formulated with conditioners so they are less likely to cause frizzies or dryness. Despite this, the coating of dye over the hair shaft can be somewhat drying and can cause the hair to become flyaway.

All of these limitations explain why many temporary, color-enhancing shampoos, conditioners, and mousses have come and gone over the past few years. Major brands that remain are **Redken**, **ARTec**, **Aveda**, **Goldwell** (a leave-in mousse), **Graham Webb**, **Jason Natural**, **Nexxus**, **Bumble and bumble**, and **Paul Mitchell**.

Different hair types can have better or poorer results with these shampoos, but in general porous or lighter shades of hair, such as blonde or red, will show the most change and darker shades the least.

Even if you do not normally use a conditioner, it is best to do so when using color-enhancing shampoos because of the way the dye is deposited on the hair shaft. One of the drawbacks of color-enhancing shampoos, besides dryness and flyaway hair, is that the dyes do not stand up well to the entire shampooing process, so coverage can be uneven or disappointingly inadequate. A few companies have tried to correct this problem by creating conditioners with temporary colors. Conditioners are a better vehicle for wash-in, wash-out colors because they contain no detergent cleansers, and the conditioning agents, like the dyes, are meant to be left on the hair shaft. The only negative is that someone with an oily scalp or normal, thin hair will not be happy putting a conditioner all over the head or on the scalp. Conditioners with temporary coloring agents are best for someone with a normal to dry scalp and/or normal to coarse hair.

The best uses for temporary hair color are to blend away a very teeny amount of gray hair, deepen faded hair color in between using more permanent types of hair color, subtly brighten or highlight your own natural hair color, and reduce ash or red tones in the hair, both natural and those caused by demi or permanent hair dyes.

Hair Note: Lighter shades of hair will pick up temporary hair color more noticeably than darker shades, much the same way a white surface shows color more vividly than a black surface.

TEMPORARY PLANT-BASED HAIR COLOR

Plant-derived hair colors such as henna ebb and flow from the hair-market scene, but they never completely go away. They hold on because these colors come from natural sources, and the public believes natural must be better. Henna is by far the most popular temporary vegetable dye available; others are available, but their use is statistically insignificant and they offer minimal or even unpleasant color. By contrast, henna, produced from a shrub indigenous to North Africa and the Near East, has the requisite exotic background that is so intriguing to cosmetics consumers. On the hair, over several uses, henna deposits a stain, although it can create only a reddish orange shade (and not a very attractive shade, either).

Depending on your own hair color, henna can eventually turn more orange than red. Henna also has a few other problems. It tends to leave a sticky film over the hair that can dry out the hair shaft, making it a problem for most hair types. However, someone with fine, thin hair may want to try a product with colorless henna powder to add some thickness to the hair. Be careful, though, because henna buildup can make hair heavy and hard to manage. For the most part, henna should probably be avoided. (If you are using a henna product and it works for you, that's great. Just bear in mind that it might not contain much henna, or that your results come from using it once in a while instead of on a regular basis.)

Any henna product claiming it contains "black henna" or that it can impart darker shades of brown or black to the hair without synthetic ingredients is not telling the truth. Henna has either a reddish orange cast or no color at all. To achieve a darker color that adheres to hair it must also contain a synthetic ingredient.

Do not use henna products for at least a week or two before using a different hair-color product or perming the hair.

Hair Note: A clear, noncoloring form of henna is sometimes added to shampoos and conditioners in the name of improving the feel of the hair. It can add a certain amount of body or feeling of thickness to the hair, but when used repeatedly it can build up and become heavy and sticky. If you want to try a clear, noncoloring henna conditioner or shampoo, consider using it every other time you shampoo or only once a week to prevent hair problems.

SEMI-PERMANENT OR LEVEL 1 HAIR COLOR

Formulated to stay on the hair for 6 to 12 washings, semi-permanent, level 1 hair colors are more substantial than their temporary cousins. While temporary hair colors coat only the outside of the hair shaft, semi-permanent, level 1 hair colors have some ability to embed themselves into the top layers of the cuticle and diffuse into the cortex, although the primary effect is still more of a temporary hair stain than anything else. Over the past couple of years, fewer and fewer of these products have been available, either at the drugstore or at the salon. With consumers of all ages desiring dramatic changes in hair color (dark to light), vibrant hair-color improvement, and complete coverage of gray, there is little demand for semi-permanent, level 1 products.

The actual dyes used in semi-permanent, level 1 products are pre-formed, meaning they don't require peroxide or ammonia to be assembled, developed, or embedded into the cuticle. Despite the dye's limited capacity for making its way into the cuticle, temporary hair colors can make your hair only a little brighter or darker, adding subtle highlights of red, copper, or ash. Do not expect them to make the hair much more than a fractional amount lighter. Semi-permanent products can camouflage only up to 10% gray. That means if more than 10% of your hair is gray, semi-permanent colors won't hide it even a little. If you are graying in clumps, these products will also be ineffective. Semi-permanent hair colors are for blending or veiling minimal gray. When there is too much gray in one area, the veiling is less convincing. Much like temporary hair colors, which are gone after one shampooing, semi-permanent colors fade a bit with each washing, so there is no discernible grow-out. Instead, the color fades away until all that remains is your own color.

Semi-permanent hair colors do not contain any peroxide or ammonia, so they cause no damage to the hair shaft; however, the dyes can cause some detachment of the cuticle, resulting in minor damage and possibly dryness.

The best uses for semi-permanent hair color are to blend away a tiny percentage of gray hair, to test the effect of a new shade, or to make subtle (almost imperceptible for darker hair shades) changes in hair color before using a demi, level 2, mid, and intermediate or permanent hair dye. They also brighten or faintly highlight your natural hair color (to soften or intensify ash or red tones in your natural hair color), and can make your permanent or demi, level 2, mid, and intermediate hair color last longer between touch-ups.

Glazing or Glossing is a popular use of semi-permanent color. It involves applying the color on the hair for about 15 to 30 minutes to enhance the tone of hair, as opposed to affecting the depth or shade of the color.

Hair Note: Just as with temporary hair colors, lighter shades of hair will pick up semi-permanent hair color more noticeably than darker shades, much the same way a white surface shows color more vividly than a black surface.

SEMI-PERMANENT HAIR COLORS: Clairol Loving Care (34 shades); and L'Oreal Soft & Sheen Carson Dark & Lovely Reviving Colors (4 shades).

DEMI, LEVEL 2, MID, TONE-ON-TONE, OR INTERMEDIATE HAIR COLOR

Forgive this long section header, but these are the various names companies attach to their not-quite-but-almost-permanent hair dyes. It could have been even longer because this type of hair dye can also be called "longer-lasting semi-permanent," "shorter-lasting permanent," or "in-between colors." That is, while they do permanently change the color of hair, they also have lower concentrations of peroxide and dye molecules, and so they can only effect subtle changes in hair color. That means you are far less likely to make a mistake with these dyes because they aren't capable of radically changing hair color. They can alter the color only a shade or two and can cover gray, so it's almost impossible to end up with strangely colored hair. For the rest of this book I will refer to this type of dye as "demi."

Demi dyes last as long as permanent dyes (that is, until the hair grows out and the roots show up), but demi dyes cannot produce as great a change as permanent dyes. Demi colors contain a small amount of hydrogen peroxide, while permanent hair dyes contain twice as much. On the other hand, demi dyes have the same degree of alkalinity as permanent dyes, either from ammonia or ammonia-type (alkaline) ingredients.

Demi dyes can cover up to 30% gray. That means if more than 30% of the hair on your head is gray, demi dyes will be ineffective. If you are less than 30% gray but you are graying in clumps or in concentrated areas, demi color also won't work. In those cases, you need to consider the next step—permanent hair color.

Demi dyes *do* contain a small amount of peroxide and an alkaline base. Even when the label claims the product contains no ammonia, it just means they've included a different alkaline ingredient, such as ethanolamine, to raise the pH level of the product, and that can cause damage to the hair shaft.

Hair Note: All of the products in this group of hair colors claim boldly on the package that the color will last through at least 24 shampooings. That is incredibly misleading. These are not wash-out dyes; the color stays in the hair shaft *permanently*, period. You have to consider coloring your hair again after you see grow-out (meaning the gray roots are showing up). Grow-out happens after four to six weeks, which is what 24 shampoos add up to, because on average most women wash their hair four times a week. Demi dyes don't fade any more than permanent dyes, the difference is in the amount of color change you can obtain. Because demi dyes change the hair color only a shade or two, you won't notice different-colored roots as much, aside from the gray. That is a nice benefit of demi dyes, but it has nothing to do with the permanence of the color. Demi dyes are permanent, regardless of what the packages seem to assert.

DEMI, LEVEL 2, MID, TONE-ON-TONE, AND INTERMEDIATE HAIR COLORS: The choices in this group are Clairol Lasting Color (34 shades); Clairol Men's Choice (7 shades); Clairol Natural Instincts (31 shades); Clairol Natural Instincts for Men (7 shades); and L'Oreal ColorSpa Moisture Actif (18 shades).

PERMANENT OR LEVEL 3 HAIR COLOR

As the name implies, these traditional hair-coloring products permanently change your hair color to almost any color or shade you want. Black to blonde, red to brunette, and gray to brown are just a few of the awesome color change possibilities. And, most important, they can cover almost any amount of gray hair. Permanent hair colors (which involve the process of stripping hair color known as bleaching) are also known as oxidative colors, and contain about 20 to 40% (by volume) hydrogen peroxide in an alkaline base with a pH of about 10 to 11.

Permanent and bleaching hair-coloring products come in different forms, such as gels, foams, shampoos, and lotions. No one form has any particular advantage over another; it's a matter of personal preference. I find the gels easiest to work with, but I know other women who swear by the lotion formulas. Given that you will be dyeing your hair more than once, this is an area where you can experiment for yourself.

When trying to choose a product line, think about the color you want and ignore claims about the color being natural, gentle, or having a hair-strengthening formula. All of that marketing language is completely bogus. All hair-dye products in each category are shockingly similar and all have virtually identical instructions. Since they perform equally well, the major difference is the color choice. In the long run, color choice and experimentation should be your main considerations in making a final selection because all of the other stuff amounts to nothing more than gimmicks that try to get your attention, regardless of the facts.

Permanent hair-coloring products rely on three basic methods of application: shampoo-in, single-step process, and two-step process.

Shampoo-in permanent hair colors are the easiest and quickest, and can be used on dry, damp, or wet hair. With this type of product, the hair tends to fade slightly and you will see grow-out after four to six weeks. When you color your hair again, the dye is again shampooed in over the entire head all at once. Shampoo-in products are one of the standard methods used for men's coloring products. The most popular line is **Combe International Just for Men** (8 shades). Because most men keep their hair short and because these products are less potent than other permanent dyes, they can be reapplied in subsequent applications all over the head without the need to do roots first and then the length. Ease of application, quick processing time (most of these products require only 5 minutes on the hair), and the small range of color selections make it an uncomplicated purchase for men, whose comfort level with cosmetics is often somewhere between embarrassed and painful.

Single-step permanent hair colors (shampoo-in and root application) involve a first-time application for virgin hair with an overall shampooing-type application of the hair dye all over the head, which is left on for approximately 20 to 45 minutes. Subsequent colorings require sectioning the hair, applying the color only to the roots, and letting the roots process for the longest period of time (again, about 20 to 45 minutes). The dye can then be pulled through, via a shampooing motion, to the length of the hair, letting the color develop there for a shorter period of time, say 5 minutes or less, to refresh the previous color.

As the hair grows out, the gray or natural color of the roots becomes apparent if you have changed your hair color by more than two shades or if you were covering gray. That means the roots require the same amount of processing time the hair needed the first time you colored it, while the length needs less processing time because it has already been dyed and is at least close to the color you want.

Sectioning the hair and gauging the different processing times of the roots and the length of the hair makes this type of at-home coloring a bit tricky. Sectioning the back of the hair can be extremely tricky, and determining how long to leave the color on the length of the hair is a matter of judgment. Balancing the processing time of the roots and the ends is at first somewhat of a guessing game, but it does get easier with experience and a strand test. For some hair color, especially if you don't have a problem with fading, it isn't necessary to pull the color through to the ends each time—you can just color the roots and then shampoo it out when you're done.

Both shampoo-in and single-process hair-coloring products are the best choice when you are trying to cover more than 40% gray and/or you want to change your hair color by more than two shades.

Two-step permanent hair colors, **blonding**, and **bleaching and toning** are all variations on a theme, and essentially do the exact same thing. First, the natural or existing hair color is lifted out and removed from the hair with 20- to 40-volume peroxide. The next step is to add the color you want. The second step does not have to be performed; that is, you can strip (bleach) your hair and not add color, but that can leave the hair a straw-white color.

Two-step hair color is the process to choose when you want a radical change from any shade of brown or black to any shade of blonde (even someone with light brown hair must go through this routine to become blonde), or from red or blonde to black (though not very many people go that direction). Either way, this process requires bleaching (stripping) out your natural hair color (step one) so that when you apply the color you want (step two) it has a clear path ahead, with no dark or opposite colors to get in the way.

Two-step processing is very damaging, and there is no way around that. A dramatic change from dark to light may constitute a fashionable glamour statement or supposedly have more sex appeal, but up close, especially after a few applications, the hair looks and feels like straw instead of soft, healthy hair. If you also use blow dryers, curling irons, rollers, brushes, and/or styling products, you compound the damage even more. And then, if you run your hand through your tresses, you are likely to get stuck or break off brittle strands by the hundreds.

For that reason, I strongly suggest that radical color changes be handled at first by your hairdresser, or not done at all. There are just too many things that can go wrong along the way, such as the timing, the mess, judging the color saturation, applying the color evenly, and choosing the right color. But don't think that having your hair dyed blonde at the hair salon is any less damaging than doing it yourself at home, because it isn't. As I said before, changing the hair color radically, and doing it repeatedly, is damaging—period. What the stylist can provide is a better color tone, more accurate processing time, and more options for becoming blonder without dyeing the whole head of hair, such as frosting or foiling.

Highlighting is a process that requires selectively choosing which hairs will be altered. This can be a one- or two-step process. The one-step process first uses bleach to lift away the natural hair color, leaving varying degrees of lighter color depending on the processing time. That can be all you need to achieve the color you want. But highlighting can also be a two-step process in which the hair color is lifted (bleached) and stripped out completely, and then a second color (often called a tone) is applied to create a specific, more controlled color to the hair.

Low lights are similar to highlighting, except that the goal is to feather in a darker shade along with the lighter shade. This way you achieve a more natural look because it is never really one color, but rather variations on a theme.

The original method used in salons for highlighting was to place a plastic cap over the entire head through which strands of hair were pulled and then bleached. Pulling the hair through the cap was a fairly painful process, and the cap still prevented application of the dye close to the root area, making the highlights look like two months of grow-out as soon as you were done. Having the immediate appearance of grow-out and suffering the discomfort of yanking the hair were the primary reasons hair foiling became the preferred method for adding highlights in salons. Foiling is a process in which strands of hair are separated from larger sections, placed on precut sheets of tinfoil, painted with bleach or the color of hair you are trying to achieve, and then wrapped up in the little foil packet. Foiling is a more sophisticated way to place subtle-to-dramatic highlights throughout the hair, and closer to the root. Unfortunately, foiling can be accomplished only at the salon.

Balliage is a technique in which bleach is painted onto sections of hair to create noticeable layers and lines of lighter color. Generally, balliage is not applied to the roots, leaving obvious grow-out.

SHAMPOO-IN AND SINGLE-STEP PERMANENT HAIR COLOR: L'Oreal Feria (38 shades); L'Oreal Excellence (32 shades); L'Oreal Preference (45 shades); L'Oreal Soft Sheen Carson Dark & Lovely (16 shades); L'Oreal Garnier Nutrisse (30 Shades); L'Oreal Garnier Lumia (30 Shades); Clairol Hydrience (36 shades); Clairol Ultress (33 shades); Clairol Balsam Color (20 shades); Clairol Herbal Essences True Intense Color (32 shades); Revlon ColorSilk (40 shades); and Revlon High Dimension (29 shades).

BLONDING: Clairol Herbal Essences Intense Bleach Blonding; Clairol Maxi Blonde; Clairol Born Blonde Ultimate Lightening Kit; Clairol Born Blonde Natural Lightening Kit; Clairol Summer Blonde; Clairol Ultra Blue Hair Lightening Kit; Clairol Summer Blonde Shampoo-In Lightener; Revlon Frost and Glow Blonding Kits (2 shades); Revlon High Dimension Beach Blonde Lightening Kit.

HIGHLIGHTING: Clairol Nice 'n Easy with Built In Highlights (40 shades); Clairol A Touch of Sun (2 shades); Clairol Frost & Tip, Original, Permed, and Creme formulas; Clairol Nuances; Clairol Herbal Essences Highlights (3 shades); L'Oreal Feria Colour (8 shades); L'Oreal Feria Hi-Lifts Browns (3 shades); L'Oreal Couleur Experte (18 shades);

L'Oreal ColorSpa Moisture Actif Highlighting Kit; Revlon High Dimension Highlighting Kit (3 shades); Chattem Lab Solar Streaks; Chattem Labs Sun-In Spray-in (2 shades).

DO-IT-YOURSELF HIGHLIGHTING KITS

If the notion of spending anywhere from $75 to $200 getting your hair highlighted in a salon makes you dizzy, there are lots of new options available at the drugstore for doing this yourself at home. Clairol (now owned by Procter & Gamble), Revlon, and L'Oreal all offer a variety of products claiming to give you salon-like highlights.

Many highlighting products are a two-step process in which you apply your all-over color on the hair and then comb or brush in hair highlights. Spray-in products that distribute bleach randomly over the hair are very difficult to control, which is why there are so few available. Only one highlighting product stands out as having a one-step application: Clairol's Nice 'n Easy with Built-In Highlights. For some reason the color deposits lighter over some strands of hair and covers the rest of the hair with a different all-over color. Very unique and worth a try if that's the look you want.

To one degree or another, all of the highlighting kits claim they are easy to use, not messy, and deliver natural-looking, beautiful results. Spending $10 to $20 is a lot less painful than $200, but not if the savings means you end up with a hair disaster. You might not end up with a disaster, but none of these highlighting kits are a slam dunk. In fact, they can be anything but easy, especially if you don't follow the instructions exactly. And even then you can be easily confused by the color selection, how to place the color, or how long to process the hair. I strongly recommend considering the following *before* you decide to try this at home on your precious head of hair!

Highlighting can be done in one step by simply using a bleach that is artistically and randomly applied to your existing hair color, and letting it stay on until your hair is "lifted" to the color you want your highlights to be. If you want specific shades of highlights in your hair you may need to use a two-step process, which means bleaching the hair you want highlighted (removing hair color) and then applying the color you want over it. You need not worry about the deeper color of your hair being affected by the tone of blonde you apply all over because the lighter shade you are using can't impact your darker hair color, it can only affect the color of the highlights. You must also use a two-step process if you are more than 20% gray.

Practice before you begin. For the products that direct you to apply the highlights with a comb, brush, or applicator tips, trying the technique on a paper towel can help you figure out how to control the color. If you apply too much in one spot, you will get a swatch of color instead of the narrow strands of highlights you were hoping for.

Read the instructions carefully, and then read them again. Do not get started until you absolutely understand each step. Watching the videos or slides on the Web sites for L'Oreal, Clairol, and Revlon is even more helpful!

Have a plan. Before you apply anything to your hair, have a plan of action plotted out. What kind of highlights do you want? Sparse or dense streaks? Feathered-in color? More in the front, less in the back? With this in mind you will be better able to control the application.

Work section by section. Large hair clips are great for separating sections of hair so you can work in smaller areas rather than larger ones. Again, this offers better control over where the dye is placed.

Check your timing. To see if the product has been left on your hair long enough to lift or change your color, you need to wipe off a small section and see how it looks. Don't worry about affecting the color in that area—by the time you check, the dye molecules are already doing their thing inside the hair shaft, so wiping away a small section won't change the results in that area.

Don't do it alone. Getting the back of your head to look even is tricky unless you have a mirror setup that allows you to see what you are doing, and that means one that still allows you to work with both hands. A patient, somewhat artistic friend is even better to serve as eyes in the back of your head.

Don't do a dramatic change without calling. If you want to radically change your hair color, or your hair has been previously dyed or highlighted, call the company's hot line first. Do not make a dramatic change without getting some good advice about the specific products and color options available to help you obtain the results you want.

If you have shoulder-length hair or longer, buy two boxes. You don't want to get through the first package of dye and only then realize that it isn't enough for your application needs!

MEN'S HAIR COLOR AND PROGRESSIVE DYES

Simply put, men don't want anyone to know they are coloring their hair. **Grecian Formula** is probably the best-known men's hair-coloring product. It is a progressive hair-coloring product and because of its popularity the product line has been expanded to include **Grecian Cream** and **Grecian Plus** (a foam-in product). All Grecian Formula products contain lead acetate, a metallic dye. After several washings or applications, the lead acetate will accumulate on the outside of the hair shaft or just inside the cuticle, altering the hair shade with a blanket of color. For men this is an easy way to completely cover gray with a simple shampooing and without a radical overnight change. There's also no need to worry about grow-out because the color fades gradually when you stop using it.

While the change in color over time may be somewhat subtle (though a greenish cast to the hair is an inevitable, noticeably unattractive side effect), the change in hair quality is far from subtle. Metallic hair dyes can dry out the hair, leaving it brittle and stiff. But aside from the aesthetic problems, there are more serious questions with regard to these products.

First, there is controversy over the lead acetate in progressive dyes. After the first edition of this book was published, Combe Incorporated, the makers of Grecian Formula, a lead acetate-based progressive dye, provided me with extensive information demonstrating the safety of lead acetate, and the FDA concurs (Sources: U.S. Food and Drug Administration, Center for Food Safety and Applied Nutrition, *Office of Cosmetics and Colors Fact Sheet*, January 9, 2002, www.fda.gov; and *Food Chemistry and Toxicology*, July 1991, pages 485–507). There is limited research demonstrating that lead acetate can be absorbed into the bloodstream when applied to skin, but there are also sources that raise red flags. (Sources: *Science of the Total Environment*, May 1994, pages 55–70; *Environmental Health Perspectives*, "Lead Acetate and Lead Phosphate," http:// ehp.niehs.nih.gov/; Hazardous Substances Data Bank, National Library of Medicine, "Lead Acetate," June 12, 2000; and National Toxicology Program, "10th Report on Carcinogens, Reasonably Anticipated to be a Human Carcinogen," http://ntp-server.niehs.nih.gov/ NewHomeRoc/AboutRoC.html.)

Aside from the health issues, when it comes to creating a desirable hair color, far better options are available in traditional demi or permanent dye products than in shampoo-in type products aimed at men. When used in a shampoo-in-and-rinse-out-after-5-minutes kind of product, the color builds up gradually with each application and can cover a good amount of gray over time without radically changing natural hair color. The differences between men's products and those for women are in how they are applied and how long they are kept on. Men's products also have a limited color selection, offering less drastic changes. The application process for men is always done all over the head, with no sectioning or root application, as women often need to do for touch-ups. Men who keep their hair short (and this is true for women with short hair as well) don't have to worry about getting the ends too dark or too bleached if they are always cutting off the damaged length, which is why the repeated shampoo-in process can be successful for them.

Like all demi, level 2, mid, and intermediate and permanent, level 3 coloring products, shampoo-in colors do not wash out, and the roots grow out, showing the original hair color.

GETTING THE COLOR YOU WANT

For demi and permanent hair dyes, there is only one, ultimate, and definitive hair-coloring principle and five fundamental corollaries you must keep in mind if you want to dye your hair yourself. The definitive hair-coloring principle is:

Your hair color + **purchased hair color (dye) product**
= new hair color

Your own hair color (real or dyed) will directly affect the color you end up with. Do not rely on the model or celebrity on the cover of the dye box! She has nothing to do with the color you will end up seeing on your own head of hair. What the picture on the box depicts is only the color you will be putting on, and that will inevitably combine with your own hair color to create the final result. You must look at the chart on the side or back of the package to see how your natural hair color will mix with the shade in the box to determine approximately what color you will end up achieving.

Let's build on this principle of your hair color mixing with the hair dye you buy to create the color you get. It can be further understood and refined with a few corollaries.

Your hair color + what the color you purchased is
+ processing time
= new hair color

Your hair color + what the color you purchased is + processing time
+ how porous your hair is
= new hair color

Your hair color + what color you purchased is + processing time
+ how porous your hair is
+ the amount of gray you have
= new hair color

Your hair color + what the color you purchased is + processing time
+ how porous your hair is
+ the amount of gray you have
+ how different the color you purchased is from your own hair color
= new hair color

Your hair color + what the color you purchased is + processing time
+ how porous your hair is
+ the amount of gray you have
+ how different the color you purchased is from your own hair color
+ whether your roots or grow-out are a different color from the length
= new hair color

Processing time is how long you leave the dye on your hair, and it directly affects the end results. Instructions on dye packages call for ranges from 10 to 50 minutes (and no more than 1 hour) of processing time. You need to figure out what the right amount of processing time is to give the peroxide time to lift your hair color enough to make room for the dye molecules to penetrate into the cortex, so they can link together and produce a new stable hair color for you.

How porous your hair is affects how long you should leave the dye on your hair. If your hair is porous, then the peroxide and dye molecules will have an easier time getting in to change your hair color. The less porous your hair is, the longer it will take to get the same results. How can you tell if your hair is porous? It isn't easy, because hair can be deceiving. As a rule, the thicker, shinier, smoother, straighter, and healthier your hair is, the less porous it will be. The thinner, less reflective, coarser, curlier, and more damaged your hair is, the more porous it will be. Because it is so easy to misjudge how porous your hair is, it is best to check your hair along the way while the color product is on your hair. Wiping off a section to see at what color stage your hair is will give you the best information as to when it's time to rinse.

If you have long hair that has never been dyed, that can complicate matters because the length is often far more porous than the newer growth. That's because the length of the hair has been around much longer and has been subject to more damage from styling and repeated sun exposure. (If it has had numerous applications of dyes, the length will be even more porous.) The first time you dye your hair, you may apply the dye just to the root area, let it process for about 10 to 15 minutes, and then pull it through to the ends to finish the processing for another 15 minutes.

Gray hair adds another curve to your decision-making. How much gray hair you have determines the type of product you need. If your hair is about 10 to 20% gray, a demi hair color can work great. If your hair is about 30 to 40% gray you can try a demi hair color, but it may or may not cover all the gray. If your hair is more than 40% gray, only a permanent dye will guarantee complete coverage.

A **dramatic change** in hair color presents perhaps the most difficult aspect of hair dyeing. If you have dark hair and you want it to be lighter by five shades or more you should seriously consider getting it done at a salon. If you decide after all to do it at home, a single-step permanent hair color won't work. You will need to bleach the hair to the lightness you are looking for and then add the tone or shade you want that light color to be. Blonding kits were designed to create this kind of change.

If you are **touching up grow-out,** you must carefully apply the color to the root area only, and for a far longer amount of time than you apply it to the length. In fact, your length of hair might not need to have any dye placed on it at all. Once your roots are the right color (matching the rest of your hair length) you can either wash the dye out or decide that the length of hair needs a boost of color. Such a boost would require spreading the dye that is on the roots through the rest of the hair and letting it process for about 2 to 5 minutes.

GRAY CAMOUFLAGE

If you want to color your hair to cover gray, you should know how much gray you have before selecting a hair-coloring product because the percentage of gray affects the coverage of the different kinds of hair dye.

How do you know how gray you are? Single gray strands that pop up individually in no discernible concentration mean you are probably somewhere between 5 and 15% gray. Temporary and semi-permanent hair dyes are perfect for you, and can create an incredible highlight effect by turning the gray a lovely shade of copper or golden brown.

If you have a discernible amount of gray woven through your hair, but it still appears to be random and in no specific concentration, you are probably about 15 to 20% gray, and demi hair colors should cover the gray nicely, with minimal discernible grow-out.

If your gray hair has areas of concentrated gray where it is quite noticeable against your original hair color, you are about 30 to 40% gray. In this situation a demi hair dye may or may not work, but it is worth giving it a try to see how it works for you.

If you have clumps of gray hair, or you notice you have far more gray hair in some areas than your original hair color, then you are probably more than 50% gray. At this point only a permanent hair dye will be able to adequately cover the gray.

SPECIAL RULE FOR REDHEADS

For some unknown hair-chemistry reason, hair dyed any shade of red will fade faster than other colors—and getting the color right is just plain tricky. Keeping the hair from being too orange or copper, or too magenta or reddish brown isn't easy. If you want truly convincing red hair, do your hair a favor and have it done the first time at the salon before you try it yourself at home.

BASE COLOR AND TONE

Before you select a specific hair-coloring product, particularly one of the demi or permanent hair dyes, it is best to understand some of the common terms and concepts, which will help you determine what color to use on your hair. The first thing to ascertain is the hair color that you are starting with. Your own **base color** (ranging from blonde to black) is the basis for establishing how a particular dye color will affect your hair and no one else's (not Cindy Crawford's, Beyonce Knowles', Heather Locklear's, or any other celebrity gracing the ads for a hair product—just yours).

Your base color is determined by the **depth** and **tone** of your hair. The depth (also referred to as level) is the actual color of your undyed hair. The **depth** of your hair color is identified by whether it is light, medium, or dark. Once you have a sense of the depth of your natural hair color, such as dark brown, medium brown, or light brown, you need to determine the **tone** of your hair color. Tone refers to how warm or cool the color is. **Warm** is the amount of red, copper, auburn, or gold that appears in your hair. **Cool** is the amount of ash or the muted, more drab shade of your hair. (Cool is synonymous with drab in the world of hair color.)

Tones in all hair-coloring products affect the highlights that radiate from the hair along with the shade of brown, red, blonde, or black being used. Before you choose a hair color, you must determine not only what color you want your hair to be, but also what tone you want it to have. That can be relatively simple, but it does take forethought.

In terms of choosing which shade and tone would look best on you, the general rule is that warm shades are best for someone with warm (sallow) skin tones, and cool tones are best for someone with cool (blue) or fair skin tones, but this is only a general rule. You may have heard the recommendation that you choose the tone according to the color highlights in your eyes. I have no words to describe how limiting and silly that notion really is! If you have blue eyes, you are never going to have red highlights in them unless your eyes are bloodshot. Most brown or black eyes aren't going to have any highlights, and lots of eyes have multiple hues in them. What do you do then? Eye color has nothing to do with choosing hair color.

After you've done your best to choose a depth and tone of color that you think will be perfect, the tone may sometimes appear to be more red, yellow (brassy), or drab than you were hoping. Trying to achieve soft, warm (golden) highlights in your hair can pan out instead as red highlights. In trying to correct for this, you can compensate (but don't overcompensate) with an ash or cool color. The same thing can happen in the other direction; a fear of going too ash can leave you with highlights that look too red. How to compensate? It takes experimentation. Start with colors that have the least amount of red or ash tones (neutral) and see what happens. You're only committed to that color from application to application, so don't overreact if it isn't exactly right the first few times. Jumping in and re-dyeing your hair immediately will damage the hair more. Remember, the less often you process your hair, the healthier it will be.

Try some short-term steps and wait until the next time you color your hair. For example, if you use a permanent hair color and you feel the color looks too red, you can use a demi hair-coloring product to soften it. An ash or drab shade can reduce the red color. The same is true if you feel your hair appears too yellow or brassy. A demi color in a cool tone can reduce the yellow or brassy color (Source: *Haircoloring in Plain English, A Practical Guide for Professionals*, Roxy Warren, Milady/SalonOvations Publishing, 1998).

MIXING YOUR OWN CUSTOM COLOR

One of the more interesting and creative ways to get the color you want is to mix different containers of dye together. As long as you stay within the same brand (don't mix Clairol products with L'Oreal products) and the same product grouping (don't mix L'Oreal Feria with L'Oreal Excellence), you can control how dark, light, red, gold, ash, or dramatic the color is. If you are looking at the color shades on the front of the box and you don't see exactly the color you want, or the color you see is darker or lighter than what you were hoping for, you don't need to settle for one shade. You can select the next darker or lighter color and mix them together. This is also one way to improve your color results. If the shade you are currently using is a bit too light, for example, but the next shade is too dark, you can add some of the darker color to modify the original shade to your needs. It also works if you find the shade you are using is too dark; in which case, you'd mix in some of the next lighter shade.

Mixing colors is also a great method for modifying the color tone. If you want to add warm tones to your current dye color, mix in a hair-dye color with the word "reddish" or "golden" in its description. If you want to reduce the red or gold in your color, mix your current dye color with another similar color that has the word "ash" in its name (Source: www.clairol.com).

There are several ways to go about mixing colors. You can mix the two products together in equal amounts, using half of each one; or, for a subtle change, mix together one part of the adjusting hair dye to three parts of the primary hair dye you want to use. Always promptly dispose of any leftover hair dye that has been mixed. Keeping it around or storing it always ends up backfiring because the volatile mixed chemicals will eventually cause the container to burst.

STRAND TESTING

The choice between coloring hair yourself and having it done at a salon is a matter of preference, and is most assuredly open to debate. What is not debatable is the necessity of performing a strand test. Unless you want to play Russian roulette with your hair color, a strand test before you go about coloring your entire head of hair with either a demi or permanent dye is the only way to protect your hair's best interests.

Strand testing is recommended on every box of hair color I've ever seen, at the hair salon as well as at the drugstore, and yet it is probably the most overlooked step. I understand the reluctance to take the time for this tedious procedure. Not only do you have to go through an entire coloring process on a small section of hair, but also for demi and permanent products, it is recommended that you cut a tiny section of hair from your head to perform the test. What woman wants to do that? Yet there is absolutely no better way to avoid problems. Yes, a strand test is essential, but it isn't necessary to cut the hair from your head; there are two other viable options you should consider.

One way to perform a strand test is to create your own hair swatch by collecting hair from your brush or comb for several days. Bundle the hairs neatly with tape, and then use your "swatch" to check the color. You can also section off a tiny area of hair directly on your head and perform the strand test there. The most important thing is to keep track of the time, and to check for changes in the hair after 10 to 15 minutes.

CONSUMER HOT LINES

L'Oreal, Revlon, and Clairol all have consumer hot lines that field hundreds of thousands of calls a year. The overwhelming majority are from women who didn't get the color they were hoping for, but the customer service experts on the hotlines can also help you get started. With help from the consumer hot line (or a trip to the hair salon), you may be able to get close to the color you want without problems along the way.

Don't be alarmed to read that hundreds of thousands of women a year call consumer hot lines for help with drugstore hair-color products. When you consider that *millions* of women are coloring their hair at home every year, a few hundred thousand questions and complaints amount to only a fraction of the total picture.

L'Oreal (also owns Garnier products): (800) 631-7358

Clairol: (800) 252-4765

Revlon: (800) 473-8566

DEALING WITH GROW-OUT

As hair grows, the difference between your real hair color and the color of your dyed hair will show in contrast at the roots. It takes some skill when touching up your roots to get the color to go just where you want it—on the roots—not all over your hair. If you are using the same hair color as you used before, you will get the best results by sectioning the hair into small segments and spreading a thin strip of dye just on the area where the grow-out is, and avoiding the previously dyed area. If you get too much dye on the portion of your hair that was previously dyed, you can make it too dark.

Depending on how much fading has taken place, the color on the length of hair may also need refreshing. In that situation, dye the roots first and then 5 minutes before the color is ready to be washed off, spread the color all over the hair and let the processing go for another 2 to 5 minutes.

How often you touch up your roots depends on your tolerance for having a noticeable difference in color between the length of your hair and the roots. For some women the emergence of any gray or different color at the roots requires immediate attention, while others can wait for weeks. There are a few ways to prolong the time until you need to re-dye your hair. One is to use **hair mascara**. Hair mascaras are similar to regular eyelash mascara, except that the ones for your hair are lighter weight, less sticky, and do not change the length of the hair. Applying hair mascara at the hairline or along the area where you part your hair, using a color that matches the length of your hair, can put off the need to re-dye for at least a week. Wearing your hair with an uneven part can also help camouflage grow-out, and the fuller or curlier your hair is, the less obvious your grow-out will be.

How often can you dye your hair? Every two weeks if you like. There is no added risk to dyeing your hair more often because if you are doing it right, you are applying the dye only to new growth and not over previously dyed hair. So dye away. Just be sure you control the application of the color you're using.

CRITICAL RULES REMINDER

If your hair is damaged, naturally porous, or chemically treated, it will take **less time** for the hair to grab the color of the dye. The healthier or thicker the hair, the **more time** it will take to grab the color. Texture is one way to judge how porous your hair is. Curly, coarse, fine or fragile, and already processed or damaged hair tends to be more porous, while straight, thick, heavy hair tends to be less porous.

If you've been using henna or gradual dyes, **never** apply any color treatment until after several washings to be sure it is shampooed out of your hair.

Never add color to bleached hair without specific advice from a stylist or from the company whose product you decide to use.

Always do a strand test to be sure you will be getting the color you want. No matter how resistant you feel about this process, do it anyway; it will save you from struggling through several weeks or months of bad hair days.

Follow the directions of the product you are using *exactly,* or at least closely (I'll mention exceptions later). If you have any questions at all, are making a radical change in your hair color, are changing products, are coloring over a different type of product, or if you just want someone to talk to about the products you are using, thinking of using, or thinking of changing to, call the company's consumer hot line for help.

As I state several times throughout this book and will state several times more, **it is best not to both dye and perm the hair**, even if you wait between treatments. You can do one or the other, but doing both is risky and asking for trouble. (Exception: If you have extremely strong, resilient hair, you can consider doing both, but don't expect the texture of your hair to feel anything like normal, especially after additional perms and dyes.)

Demi and permanent red or light brown or blonde hair colors (especially red) **can fade,** regardless of what you do to prevent it from happening. Cosmetics chemists are not sure what makes these hair dyes less stable—it could be they are more affected by sunlight or shampooing—but regardless of the reason, fading is part of the struggle of hair coloring.

You can't make dark hair color more than four shades lighter without bleach. Whether it is your natural color or a dyed shade, if you want to lighten the color of your hair significantly you must strip (bleach) out the darker shade you are trying to change. You can't change a dark shade of hair color, natural or dyed, to a lighter shade without first performing this fundamental step.

Understanding tone variations is a significant part of getting the shade you want. Color theory is what hair color is all about, and those nuances establish whether the shade you get looks rich and vibrant or fake and contrived.

According to the FDA, "reactions to hair dyes can severely harm the eye and even cause blindness. Inadvertently spilling dye into the eye could also cause permanent damage. [The] FDA prohibits the use of hair dyes for eyelash and eyebrow tinting or dyeing even in beauty salons or other establishments." (Source: U. S. Food and Drug Administration, Office of Cosmetics and Colors Fact Sheet, August 1, 2001, www.cfsan.fda.gov/~dms/cos-821.html).

There is also a high incidence of **allergic reactions to hair-dye products.** Before getting started, it is essential to perform a patch test on your arm or behind your ear to be sure you don't have problems (Source: www.cfsan.fda.gov/~dms/qa-cos18.html).

KEEPING THE COLOR YOU WANT

Most hair-care companies want you to believe they have special shampoo and conditioner formulas that have the ability to keep your hair color around longer than if you were to use other products. "Color Hold," "Color Stay," "No Fade Shampoo and Conditioner," and "Protects Hair Color" are some of the more typical claims. But except for color-enhancing shampoos and conditioners, and other temporary or semi-permanent coloring products, there are no shampoos, conditioners, or styling products that can keep hair color in your hair. These so-called specially formulated shampoos and conditioners are anything but. They contain the exact same ingredients as regular shampoos and conditioners that don't profess to save your hair color.

Shampoos and conditioners that contain dye colors are a horse of a different color. These do add a topical layer of coloring agents to the outside of the hair shaft, giving the impression that there is a tad more color, but they cover poorly (to not at all) over roots or gray hair.

What makes hair color fade? In reality, the shampoo or conditioner you're using is the last thing to worry about because those that are well-formulated can't help *or* hurt hair color. However, exposure to the sun and air does play a big role in lifting color from your hair. Sun damage actually causes the structure of the hair to break down, and that allows the hair-dye molecules to break down and degrade. But despite the influence of sun and other factors that damage the hair, the truth is no one is exactly sure why some dyes fade faster than others or why some hair types lose color faster than others.

What can help is to protect your hair from the sun. That means wearing a hat because sunscreens in hair products cannot be relied on, but that still doesn't guarantee much. You could stay inside and not touch your hair until new growth required another dye job and it could still fade slightly, especially if you underwent a radical change in hair color or if you used any shade of red. In other words, fading is inevitable.

Some of the suggestions in the following sections can prevent poor product application (which can result in the color not grabbing well), but that is a technique problem, not an issue of fading.

GETTING RID OF THE COLOR YOU DON'T WANT

It is inevitable that at some point you will find the dyed hair color you have isn't the color you want. In this situation you really have only two options, or at least only two options that can possibly prevent more serious problems or mistakes. You can go to a salon and have a color technician rescue you, or you can call the company's consumer hot line and consult the customer service expert, who will understand the variables that affected your untoward outcome. Then you can receive very specific instructions based on your very specific circumstances.

DOING IT YOURSELF

Before you start applying dye to your hair at home, it is important to get an application system in place. Being well organized can make everything go more smoothly and reduce the likelihood of errors. The following is a great system for getting the best results:

- If you have **permed or extremely damaged hair, do not consider highlighting** or making an extreme hair color change. That is only asking for trouble.

- Don't proceed with an all-over hair color until you've done a **strand test and a patch test for allergic reaction.**

- **If you are highlighting, preselect the areas you want to color.** Having a game plan ahead of time can prevent mistakes and disappointments.

- **Assemble everything you need.** You can keep a carrying tray with all the things you need on it, including hair clips, extra plastic gloves, a comb with a pointed end (typically called a rat-tail comb), a small portable clock, hand mirror, comb, portable radio, scented candle, magazines, an extra package of dye in case you run out, and, depending on the product type, a small pair of scissors. A comfortable chair you don't mind getting stained will ensure that you have a place to sit other than the edge of the bathtub or the toilet seat. **Purchase a hose extension** for your sink or tub so you don't have to get in an awkward position to get your head under the faucet.

- Choose the bathroom with the **best light and largest mirror.** For demi and permanent hair dyes, use the bathroom with the best ventilation. Even non-ammonia products can have unpleasant fumes. Open the window or turn on the exhaust fan to keep the air moving.

- Set up a small **portable clock** on a shelf so that is clearly visible.

- Take four to six large towels that won't cause you stress if they get stained, and arrange them on the floor and over the countertop.

- Take a large portable mirror (an inexpensive lightweight one is best) and place it directly across from the mirror you will be facing, so that the hair on the back of your head is clearly visible with only minor head movements.

- **Be sure your hair is completely dry.** Dye is rarely applied to wet hair.

- Apply **Vaseline or thick cold cream** to your hairline; this prevents the dye from staining your skin or causing irritation on the face.

- Put on an **old lightweight outfit** that won't cause you stress if it gets stained.

- Use a pair of **good latex gloves** from the drugstore. The plastic gloves that come packaged with hair dyes tear easily.

- Before you get started, inform your family or roommates that you are not to be bothered for the next hour or so (unless they plan to help) and they had better use the bathroom now if they need to!

- Light the **scented candle** (this isn't for lighting purposes; the candle is to help mask the chemical scent and to set a pleasant mood), turn on your favorite radio station or pop in a favorite CD, set the chair in the most convenient position, and get ready to begin.

- If this is a touch-up application, **section the hair** with clips into five or six different areas to keep your product application organized. Release one area at a time and work only with that section, separating the hair into quarter-inch to half-inch parts. **Apply the color to the roots using a finger to spread the color on the gray areas.**

- If this is a first-time application, start with the same sectioning process, but work the color through to the ends.

- Be patient with the back area. That's what the mirror behind you is for. You should be able to apply the product and see what you are doing. It takes a while to get used to working with the mirrored image, but it is better than not seeing what you are doing at all. (Because the back area can be so tricky to do, consider having a friend help with this area.)

- Processing time varies, so **check the color at 15-minute intervals.** That means wiping the hair color off a strand of hair and checking to see if the color is what you want. For timing purposes, check the area of hair where the dye was first applied.

- When you are done, if this is a touch-up, you may need to **pull the color from the roots to the ends** and let it stay there for 2 to 5 minutes. Sometimes color on the length of your hair fades, and allowing it to process with the dye for a few minutes can help even out and refresh the color. Hair that is already dyed never requires as much processing time as the roots, which are virgin growth. For some hair types, pulling the color through to the ends can saturate that area with too much color. If you notice that the length of hair is darker than the root area after dyeing, do not pull the color through next time.

- When you are finally ready to rinse the color out of your hair, take your time and try not to splash. **Rinsing thoroughly is essential.** Keep a hand towel nearby to wipe away any drips that may get on your face or near your eyes.

- **Keep a chart** of everything you do to your hair and what the results were. Write down how long you kept the dye on the roots, how long you kept it on the ends, the name and color of the product, and how you felt about the results. That way you will have a clear record of what you need to change or what you want to keep the same next time.

CANCER AND HAIR DYES?

You have probably seen the news headlines echoing the question "Does dyeing your hair cause an increase in certain cancers?" This is a complicated question that has no easy answer, despite investigative work by the FDA, the National Cancer Institute (NCI), the National Institutes of Health (NIH), and several independent studies conducted by universities and laboratories around the world. Regrettably, there is no absolute consensus from any of these sources on whether or not a risk really exists. It turns out that the research is confusing and conflicting.

Some early epidemiological research in the 1990s showed a relation between hair dyes and bladder cancer, myeloma, and non-Hodgkin's lymphoma (Sources: *Journal of the National Cancer Institute*, 1994, volume 86, pages 941–943; and *Environmental Health Perspectives*, June–July 1994, pages 6–7).

Subsequent research noted problems with the results from those earlier findings (Sources: *European Journal of Cancer Prevention*, February 1995, pages 31–43). An article in *Cancer Investigation* (2000, volume 18, issue 4, pages 366–380) stated that "Although there are some reports of positive associations, overall the evidence linking personal use of hair dyes to various leukemia and MDS subgroups [myelodysplastic syndromes] is weak."

Recent research has thrown still another curve. A paper published in the *International Journal of Cancer* (April 2004, pages 581–586) stated that "studies have found an increased risk of bladder cancer among hairdressers and barbers who are occupationally exposed to hair dyes. However, the carcinogenic risk associated with personal use of hair dyes remains uncertain since several large case-control and cohort studies did not find an association between personal hair dye use and bladder cancer."

The *American Journal of Epidemiology* (January 2004, pages 148–154) found that "An increased risk of non-Hodgkin's lymphoma was observed among women who reported use of hair-coloring products before 1980…. On the other hand, the authors found no increased risk of non-Hodgkin's lymphoma … among women who started using hair-coloring products in 1980 or later. It is currently unknown why an increased risk of non-Hodgkin's lymphoma was found only among women who started using hair-coloring products before 1980."

Does that mean the hair-dye products developed after 1980 changed in some way that reduced the incidence of lymphoma, or did some other lifestyle change account for the difference? Or have women who started dyeing their hair after 1980 not been dyeing their hair long enough for it to result in problems? These questions have yet to be answered.

Further, a study in the *European Journal of Cancer* (August 2002, pages 1647–1652) "found no increased risk associated with the overall use of hair dye products or exclusive use of permanent or temporary types of hair dye products. There was also no increased risk of breast cancer associated with exclusive use of dark or light hair colouring products, or use of mixed types or colours of hair dye products. We also found no increased risk of breast cancer associated with hair dye use based on an individual's reason for using a hair colouring product, such as to cover grey or to change natural hair colour. These data suggest that the use of hair colouring products does not have a major impact on the risk of breast cancer."

Yet there are still more questions than answers. According to the FDA, "In 1978, FDA proposed to require a warning on the labels of hair dyes containing the compounds 4-methoxy-m-phenylenediamine (4MMPD) or 4-methoxy-m-phenylenediamine sulfate (4MMPD sulfate), two coal-tar ingredients. These followed findings by researchers at the National Cancer Institute in Bethesda, Maryland, that rodents fed either of the chemicals were more likely to develop cancer than animals not fed the substances .... Some researchers say that extrapolating results from ingested hair dye studies to absorbed hair dye use cannot accurately assess cancer risk because the compounds being tested are altered or are absorbed differently in the gut than they are when applied to the scalp" (Sources: www.fda.gov; and *FDA Consumer*, April 1993, Hair Dye Dilemmas).

In addition to 4-MMPD, other hair-dye ingredients are reported to be able to penetrate human and animal skin, and to cause cancer when fed to laboratory animals. These other ingredients include 4-chloro-m-phenylenediamine, 2,4-toluenediamine, 2-nitro-p-phenylenediamine, 4-amino-2-nitrophenol, paraphenylenediamine, p-phenylenediamine, 4-phenylenediamine, 1,4-phenylenediamine, 4-benzenediamine, 1,4-Benzenediamine, para-diaminobenzene, and para-aminoaniline.

What does all this mean for the consumer? In essence it means there is no definitive proof one way or the other. According to the FDA, "The findings so far are inconclusive. The studies raise some questions about the safety of hair dyes, but at this point there's no basis for us to say that hair dyes pose a definitive risk of cancer. In the final analysis, consumers will need to consider the lack of demonstrated safety when they choose to use hair dyes." (Source: www.fda.gov).

There is nothing definitive about any of this information and research. As a woman who does dye her hair, I am concerned. I wish there were something more conclusive to tell you but there isn't, and there are no alternatives I can offer other than to tell you not to dye your hair, but that is unrealistic. What is absolutely certain, however, is that "natural" hair dyes are not the answer. The products claiming to use natural dyes to permanently alter hair color and thereby eliminate any cancer risk are lying. They aren't "natural" because if they were, they couldn't affect hair color with anything more than a temporary coating.

HAIR-DYE PROBLEMS? HAIR-DYE SOLUTIONS!

Fundamental obstacles can get in the way of obtaining the color you want. If any of the following apply to you, be very careful about the next step you take when it comes to dyeing your hair.

Problem: The ends of your hair turned out darker than you expected.

Possible Reason: Hair that is damaged is more porous. When hair is porous, it can grab more of the dye color than virgin or undamaged hair. How can you tell if your hair is damaged? If you use heat-styling implements every day, have been dyeing your hair on a regular basis, spend a lot of time outdoors without covering your hair, have a lot of split ends, or your hair is shoulder length or longer, you can be reasonably certain the longer part of your hair is quite damaged and porous. Hair that has been around the longest is always more damaged than the newer hair near the roots.

Solution: Before coloring your hair, get a haircut that trims off the ends so the more damaged part of your hair doesn't grab more color. You can also try conditioning the ends that are damaged to coat the length of hair and prevent some absorption of the dye. Another option is to dye the root area first, let that process for about 10 to 15 minutes, and then apply the rest of the color to the length of your hair for the rest of the processing time.

Problem: The root area of your hair looks lighter than the rest of your hair.

Possible Reason: This generally happens only when you are dealing with grow-out and the hair is gray at the root, or a lighter color than the length. If you thought your hair was looking too dark you may have thought that if you applied a lighter color over the grow-out area and the length, that it would also lighten the length. That isn't possible.

You may also have processed the roots and then pulled the color through at the end of the processing time, and some hair doesn't require this pull-through technique.

If you didn't apply any color to the length, but applied it only to the root area, you may not have left the color on long enough.

Solution: If you want to lighten the length of your hair, applying a lighter one-step permanent dye won't do it. One-step dyes lift some of the color out of your hair but they can't lighten the length the same as the roots. The color of the hair reacts differently to one-step dyes. If you need to lighten your hair to bring it all up to the same color before you add the color you want, it requires two steps, and probably the help of a professional, or at the very least the consumer hot line of the company whose product you are using.

If you applied the color only to the root area (the same color as the length) and it turned out lighter, a longer processing time is probably needed.

Problem: The overall hair color turned out darker than you expected.

Possible Reason: Aside from the explanation above, if your hair isn't damaged, you may have chosen the wrong color. Lighting in drugstores isn't the best, and we are not always as familiar with our actual hair color as we like to think. This is one of the major shortcomings of shopping for a hair color at the drugstore. However, this can also be a problem at the hair salon, even with a very experienced hairstylist. Color swatches are only representations of hair-color potential. Your hair's condition could be another factor. As I've said before, more porous and damaged hair absorbs more color. Also, your natural color or previously dyed color affects the color you put on each time, making the correct processing time more difficult to determine.

Solution: If you can live with the color until the next time you color your hair, work with it, and then go a shade or two lighter later on, being sure to do a strand test. If you can't live with the color, consider seeing a hairstylist who can remove the offending hair color and hopefully add the right one. Stripping out the color is the last and least desirable move to make because it can be so damaging to the hair.

Problem: **The ends of your hair turned out lighter than you expected.**

Possible Reason: If your hair is seriously damaged, the color won't remain in the cortex of the strands. Serious damage can make your hair so porous that it prevents it from retaining any color. When hair is this damaged, it can't grab the color, which may explain why the ends remain lighter (or darker), depending on the original color of your hair and the color you were going after.

Solution: The only solution for this is to cut off the damaged ends or the entire damaged length or to wait patiently for the hair to grow out. All the conditioner in the world cannot rebuild (or even fake the appearance of rebuilding) a cuticle and cortex that is so damaged. If there is no place for dye to be deposited, it will just rinse right off your hair.

Problem: **The hair color you used went on unevenly.**

Possible Reason: This is primarily a problem with application technique.

Solution: Make sure you are sectioning your hair and applying the product in a continuous line along the part, spreading it with your fingers so it expands up evenly on the grow-out, and (if needed) the length of hair.

Problem: **The hair color you chose seems to have given you too many red highlights.**

Possible Reason: Most women, regardless of their hair color, have naturally red pigments in their hair that they weren't aware of. As a result, they may end up with reddish highlights they weren't counting on when they color their hair. This occurs most frequently with shampoo-in or single-step hair-coloring products. There just isn't enough peroxide in these products to lift the natural reddish color out of the hair. Also, you may have chosen a color that provides red highlights when you really didn't need any.

Solution: If you want to avoid red highlights, be very careful to choose hair colors described as ashy or golden. That should take care of the problem.

Problem: **The hair color you chose has too many ash or drab highlights.**

Possible Reason: Lead acetate progressive-dye products can leave a greenish cast on the hair. Alternatively, for other types of dye, you may have chosen a hair color that was too drab. This often happens when you overreact to the concern about making your hair too red, and then decide to use a color with a strong ash tone.

Solution: Avoid drab colors. In the meantime, use a semi-permanent or demi dye that has just a hint of red or a neutral tone. That can help improve the situation. The next time you dye your hair, think about using colors with a bit more red or copper color.

Problem: You followed the directions exactly, took time to match your natural hair color exactly, yet a good deal of the gray you were trying to cover was still there when you were done.

Possible Reason: You used the wrong type of hair-coloring product. Temporary hair colors barely cover any gray; semi-permanent hair colors realistically cover a little more, and demi hides 30% of the gray. The percentage of coverage also depends on the way you are graying. If you have concentrated patches or areas of gray, even if the ratio is less than 40% all over, the dyes mentioned here won't work over the area where you need color the most.

Solution: Rethink your product choice and consider a permanent hair color next time you color your hair. Permanent dye can cover 40% or more of gray. You may also not have left the color on long enough, as most product instructions recommend the shortest amount of time. Healthy hair may take longer to grab the color than the minimum time listed. Of course, you did remember to do a strand test, didn't you?

Problem: You finally gave in and used a permanent hair color to cover the gray, but it didn't work and the gray is still evident.

Possible Reason: Permanent hair color can be a big step for some women, and the fear of causing damage may have made you overly cautious so you didn't leave the color on long enough. Gray hair can be pretty resistant, so be patient.

Solution: Let the dye stay on for up to 45 minutes to cover the gray. What would work best is for you to leave it on for the same amount of time as the strand test took to develop the color you wanted.

Problem: The color you chose looked a shade or two lighter than your own hair color, but you ended up with a color much darker than you expected.

Possible Reason: If your hair is porous, damaged, previously color-treated, thin, fine, or permed, it can grab the color quickly, making it darker despite the lighter color on the box. You also likely did not do a strand test, which would have given you an indication of just how dark the particular dye you chose would go, and how long it would take for that to occur.

Solution: Certain hair types require shorter processing times than others. If you did a strand test and still didn't get the expected results, you may have tested an area of hair (usually from the nape of the neck) that was healthier than the rest of your hair, and it produced a different color. If your hair is naturally porous or damaged, has been repeatedly color-treated, or is thin, fine, or permed, you will want to reduce the amount of time the color stays on your hair. Keep in mind that different sections of hair can have different timing requirements.

Problem: Your hairline always ends up darker or too red after you dye your hair.

Possible Reason: The hair around your face may have a finer, thinner texture than the rest of the hair, making it more susceptible to grabbing the color.

Solution: If you don't want to change the color of the hair at the hairline (if there's no gray in this area), you can protect the hairs around your face with Vaseline. The goal is to cover the hair with something that will keep the dyes off that area. If the hairline has gray that you want to cover, apply the hair dye over this area 15 minutes after you apply it to the rest of your hair. The fine hair in this area probably needs less time to process.

Problem: The hair around your face shows gray roots sooner than the hair on the rest of your head.

Possible Reason: Gray hair appears for no rhyme or reason; it grows wherever it wants to. Some women gray at the crown first, some at the hairline, while others gray randomly in strands all over the head, though most typically women gray from the front of the hair nearest the face to the back. If you gray at the hairline, it will be more obvious as soon as you have any grow-out.

Solution: There is no reason not to dye just the hair around your hairline as soon as you see the gray, particularly if you are doing it at home yourself. That's true for any area that shows gray faster than elsewhere, such as a specific heavy patch of gray. Simply apply the hair color to the precise spots only and process as usual without pulling the color through to the ends. However, you can also use brow or hair mascaras over the hairline; this works wonderfully and takes only seconds to apply.

Problem: Your permanently dyed hair is fading, but you don't want to dye it again for another two weeks.

Possible Reason: The more porous, damaged, or gray the hair is, the more likely it is to fade. This is especially true in the summer or for outdoor enthusiasts, but it can happen any time of year if your hair is very gray. Gray hair and shades of red dye (and some shades of blonde) fade more quickly and may require a longer processing time than you have been using, or a stronger depth of color.

Solution: Color-enhancing shampoos, temporary colors, and semi-permanent colors are great ways to extend the time between re-coloring your hair, and they can conceal the fading. But be careful not to use these products in the last shampoo or two before you color your hair again because the dyes from these temporary coloring products lie on the hair shaft and can block the absorption of your normal hair-coloring product. Also, if your hair has become grayer over the years and you've noticed increased fading, you may want to do a strand test and see if your hair now requires a longer processing time.

Next time you dye your hair, instead of a soft strawberry blonde, go with a more vivid red shade. You may also be grayer than you think, and that may require you to use a longer processing time or a permanent dye instead of a demi dye.

Problem: **Your hair is extremely damaged from being dyed blonde and you don't want to damage it any more, but it is in desperate need of coloring.**

Possible Reason: Hair gets damaged mostly by brushing and by styling with blow dryers or curling irons, but absolutely the most harmful thing you can do to the hair is to repeatedly dye it with a bleaching color process. Turning darker hair blonde, particularly if you are keeping it long, destroys hair when the process is performed repeatedly to maintain the color.

Solution: There isn't an easy solution for this problem because there is no way to dye hair without causing further damage. You can try temporary or semi-permanent dyes that coat only the hair shaft until the damage grows out, but those products have extremely limited coverage. Growing out the damage and starting again is sometimes the only answer. Otherwise you will just be compounding the problem, never allowing the healthy roots to come out and shine. Your only option may be to cut off the damage and go short. Then when you dye your hair again, consider a less dramatic hair-color change.

Problem: **You hate the hair color you ended up with when you dyed your hair.**

Possible Reason: Either you went after too extreme a change, you misjudged your natural hair color, or the color of your dyed hair conflicts with the color of your roots. Often women think their hair is darker than it is, or they choose a darker color because they think it will look more dramatic or cover gray better. It's also possible you left the color on too long.

Solution: This is a difficult situation because you'll want to run out and try another color to get rid of the one you hate. But you can't just dye the hair a different color over a permanent hair color. First, the wrong hair color must be removed or lifted with bleach, and *then* a different color can be added. You need to either seek professional help from a trained hair colorist or call the consumer hot line of the company whose product you used.

While you are getting used to the process of dyeing your hair, it is best to start out with demi dyes to get a sense of how different colors look on your hair. These semi-noncommittal hair dyes wash out after a period of time, so the risk of making a glaring mistake is minimal. Once you find the color you are most comfortable with, you can start using permanent hair colors. You did remember to do a strand test, didn't you?

Problem: **You tried dyeing your hair red, but it just looks brown.**

Possible Reason: If your hair is damaged or porous, the hair might not have been able to hold onto the red dye. Dyeing hair red is difficult even for a professional.

Solution: Call the consumer hot line of the company whose product you used, or get this type of dye job done professionally at the salon.

Problem: You've been coloring your hair at the salon and you want to change to a drugstore product.

Possible Reason: It's getting too expensive or too difficult to schedule. You've also noticed that your friends who color their hair at home look pretty good, and you're tired of the expensive coloring mistakes that happen at the salon.

Solution: First, ask your stylist what coloring product and color he or she has been using on your hair. With that information in hand, you can call the consumer hot line of the drugstore product you are thinking of trying. This is the best way to avoid mistakes. Revlon, L'Oreal, and Clairol all have highly trained advisors who will direct you to the right product, color, and instructions for your specific situation.

Problem: Whenever you color your hair, you end up with dye under your fingernails or on your skin.

Possible Reason: Keeping those gloves on is difficult when you're trying to do two things at once. Also, the gloves often tear and you might not notice until you are almost done.

Solution: You can double up on the gloves, wearing two pairs instead of one or—even better—use plastic or latex gloves you buy at the drugstore instead of the gloves that come packaged in the hair-coloring kits. If you still have problems, there are products on the market designed to lift the color off the skin or from under the nails, such as Andre No Rub Hair Color Remover Wipes, Color Gone Hair Color Stain Remover, or Roux Clean Touch. All of these and other versions are available at most beauty supply stores.

Problem: You want to make your hair feel better after dyeing it. You've heard conditioners or botanicals in hair dyes will make hair feel better and reduce damage, but those products don't seem to make any difference.

Solution: Conditioners in hair dyes can make the hair feel better after being processed, but a product that contains conditioners isn't inherently better for the hair than one that doesn't contain conditioners. Botanicals don't improve a hair-coloring product in any way, and the little fragrance packets that are mixed in are useless and don't improve the end results. For a hair color to do what it has to do, the dye must get into the hair and stay there, and the ingredients making that happen can damage the hair. The only way to prevent the damage from the chemical assault on a hair shaft is to keep the chemicals off, and adding natural ingredients to the mixture can't change that fact.

Problem: How can you keep your hair color from looking fake?

Possible Reason: The most common cause of fake-looking hair color is choosing a dye that is too light or too dark, followed closely by choosing a shade that is too warm (golden/copper) or cool (ash) for your skin tone. Neglecting to perform a strand test or not checking the dye as it is processing can also lead to artificial-looking results.

Solution: Most pros suggest going one or two shades lighter instead of darker. Darker hair colors tend to look unnatural and fake. Also, the more dramatic the change, the less realistic the hair color will look. If it's too light or too dark, going too long between color treatments makes the roots stand out, which always makes any hair color look fake. In some circles, roots are considered a fashionable alternative to, and I quote, "looking like you're a slave to fashion." Now that's a creative rationale if I've ever heard one! I'm not in the circle that believes roots look natural. Even the *Sex & the City* women gave up that look early on in the series.

Problem: **How can you be blonder without using anything extreme on the hair?**

Solution: It depends on what is meant by extreme. If you just want your hair to be one shade lighter than it is, demi dye is the gentler way to achieve that result. If you want to become two or more shades lighter, permanent dyes are the only way to go. If you want to change your hair color by several shades in order to be blonde, there is no way to achieve that without using an extreme process, which is primarily bleaching the hair color and then adding the blonde shade you want.

Problem: **The light in drugstores is terrible; I feel like I'm poking around in the dark trying to match my hair color. Is there anything I can do to discern the color better?**

Solution: Great question, but I don't think the answer is that great. It is probably best to shop for a new hair color only during the daytime. Take a few color possibilities that you are interested in and ask the store clerk if you can take the boxes outside (or stand near the store entrance) and check them in the daylight. Other than that, there is no way to compensate for store light—or the light in the hair salon either. If your hairstylist is choosing a new color for you, check the hair samples in the daylight.

Problem: My eyebrows are a different color from my new hair color. Do I need to dye my eyebrows to match my hair?

Solution: Not all blondes have blonde eyebrows, so it's not necessarily more natural to have blonde eyebrows to accompany a head of artificially blonde hair. Another problem, particularly for women with dark brows who prefer low-maintenance beauty regimes, is that eyebrow grow-out can look strange. There are ways to cope when the brow does grow out and the roots become evident, such as brow powders, brow coloring gels, and mascara, but in general there is little reason to go through the hassle unless the difference in hair color is very light blonde with dark brown brows.

CAN LEMON JUICE LIGHTEN HAIR?

Over the years I've seen articles show up in fashion magazines describing the value of lemon juice for lightening hair. Don't believe it. Neither through a chemical reaction nor a physical process can lemon juice lighten or bleach hair. You can squeeze the stuff on your hair day and night for weeks and all you will end up with is dried-out, stiff, and eventually rather damaged hair.

Why does lemon juice have this reputation of being able to bleach hair? I suspect it's from the way women experience using the stuff, because it's certainly not about the lemon itself. Typically, women squeeze lemon juice on their hair during the summer months, soaking their strands and then sitting in the sun. Without question, unprotected sun exposure on the hair (meaning no hat or cover-up) definitely produces a loss of pigment by breaking down the hair's healthy protein bonds, leading to a loss of color. And lemon's acidity (pH of around 2) damages the hair's protective cuticle layer, making it more vulnerable to the sun's deleterious effect, resulting in color loss. When hair is damaged it becomes more porous and that degrades your natural or dyed color. You do end up with lighter hair after a great deal of effort (lots of lemon juice and lots of sun exposure), but it comes along with a good deal of damaged hair, including split ends and breakage.

Anything you do that encourages the breakdown and impairment of the hair shaft is not a good thing, at least not if you want healthy hair. One of the best things you can do for your hair (especially if it is dyed) is keep it out of direct sunlight. If you want to have highlighted, shinier, and healthier hair, there are plenty of more controlled and less time-consuming ways to do it.

CHAPTER SEVEN

Perms and Relaxers

WHAT'S NEW

The world of making hair straight changed a few years ago with the introduction of "thermal hair straightening." Thermal hair straightening is a highly specialized, lengthy, extremely expensive, technical process performed only at salons. I will discuss this new system and process after explaining how hair shape (curly or straight) works, and describing the typical perms and relaxers found at every drugstore and the types of services performed at most salons around the world.

THE SHAPE OF HAIR

Your hair's natural shape is the result of the arrangement of the hair's protein structure, in combination with an extensive, complex matrix of lipids, fatty acids, and other organic and inorganic matter. Under the microscope, you can see how protein is assembled like a twisting ladder throughout the hair shaft. Disulfide bonds are the strongest links in this protein ladder, and these are what hold the hair in its normal configuration. To change the shape of your hair, you must break these disulfide bonds, re-form them (either curly to straight or straight to curly), and then put them back together. Surprisingly, re-forming and putting the bonds back together isn't the difficult part of a perm; rather, what's most troublesome for the hair is the process that's used to break the disulfide bonds.

As mentioned above, disulfide bonds are incredibly strong and difficult to break, and it takes serious (meaning potent) chemicals to break them so you can modify their shape. However, after the disulfide bonds have been softened and split apart, they can be transformed into degrees of straight or curly hair. Restructuring hair in this manner requires specific substances to achieve the desired results. Permanents meant to curl hair or relaxers needed to straighten hair use formulas that are similar, if not identical. Only the choice of technique—either curling the hair with rods or combing the hair straight—differentiates these processes from one another.

SALON OR HOME PRODUCTS?

If you decide to try a permanent wave or relaxer, then my heartfelt suggestion is to get it done at the hair salon and not do it at home. It's not that permanent wave or hair relaxer products from a salon are any better than the ones you buy at the drugstore—these products are all the same whether they are purchased at a drugstore or performed at a hair salon. The issue is one of risk during the processing procedure, and how the hair is manipulated. If you wind the hair too tightly around the rod for the curly perms you can lose chunks of hair; if you comb hair in the wrong direction for a relaxer you can also destroy hair; or if you leave the chemicals on too long, you can end up with scalp burns and hair loss. Seeing an experienced professional reduces your risk immeasurably over doing this yourself.

I know many of you would like for me to recommend the perfect at-home permanent-wave or hair-relaxer kit or the exact method for getting foolproof results, but the truth is, there aren't any. Again, it's not that the product formulations are different, because they aren't. The basic principle is that permanent waving is simply hard on the hair, whether it's done at the salon or at home. Doing it yourself is riskier because so many details go into creating an attractive perm that it is hard for even the most experienced technician to get all the elements right.

For perms, the following factors must be considered carefully:

1. Protecting the skin (Vaseline is best)
2. Choosing the kind of permanent wave best for your particular hair type
3. Timing the processing exactly
4. Choosing the right rods
5. Winding the rods into the hair using the correct amount of tension
6. Handling the endpapers
7. Saturating the rods evenly
8. Rinsing the relaxer thoroughly
9. Neutralizing the hair thoroughly
10. Shampooing and conditioning hair

For relaxers, the following factors must be considered carefully:

1. Protecting the skin (Vaseline is best)
2. Choosing the kind of relaxer best for your hair type
3. Timing the processing exactly
4. Saturating the hair evenly with the relaxing ingredients
5. Combing through hair with equal, consistent tension
6. Keeping hair straight
7. Rinsing the relaxer thoroughly

8. Neutralizing the hair thoroughly
9. Shampooing and conditioning hair

SHOULD YOU PERM?

Before you make a final decision about perming or straightening your hair, the first questions to ask are whether or not you are truly a good candidate for a perm or relaxer, and whether you want to risk the outcome. If you have damaged hair, particularly if it has been dyed from black or brown to blonde, highlighted from sun exposure, or if your hair is extremely thin and fragile, you are not someone who should get a perm.

I cannot stress enough that perming and hair relaxing is ultimately damaging if you both color and perm your hair, even a few weeks apart from each other. All the permanent-wave kits on the market (and the ones at the salon) say you should **never** perm hair that has been double-processed, streaked, highlighted, colored with metallic dyes, or sun-damaged. I think they stop short of saying not to perm over permanent or demi-dyed hair because that would exclude millions of women who use these coloring products, leaving a very tiny group of women to buy perm and relaxer products. But the absolute truth is that perming or relaxing is hard on hair, and it is ruinous if you also color it. You may not want to hear this, but it will save you a lot of heartache if you know when not to perm.

After mulling this over, if you still think you have a knack with hair, can time all the chemical processes correctly, and can implement the combing or rolling portion properly, you may after all want to try it at home.

Are the risks less dire if you have healthy, non-color-treated hair that isn't porous, too curly, or too straight? Yes, the risks are greatly reduced (assuming, of course, the processing is done right). However, once you have your hair relaxed or curled, it is no longer healthy and you then run the same risks the next time around.

TYPES OF PERMS AND RELAXERS

No one will be shocked when I say that permanent waves (and hair relaxers, which are merely permanent waves with a different name and shaping technique) are not permanent, for the simple reason that they do not affect how hair grows. Ultimately, this impermanence is easily rectified because you can always apply another perm to take care of the grow-out. As easy as this sounds, in the long run it isn't easy to do, and it is assuredly not easy on the hair. Any chemical process that alters hair shape is going to be damaging.

There are three types of permanent waves—alkaline, acid, and neutral—each one using different reducing agents. Alkaline perms generally contain lye or sodium hydroxide, but there are "no-lye" versions that contain calcium hydroxide mixed with guanidine carbonate to form guanidine hydroxide. Acid perms contain forms of thioglycolic acid, and neutral perms contain sodium sulfite. All three types call for the same steps and basic formulation requirements, and they are all based on sulfur chemistry. The first step is to place the hair in the shape you want it to have. If you want the hair curly, rods are used to wrap the hair; if you want the hair straight, combing techniques or weights are used to hold the length of the hair elongated and vertical. The wave solution (reducing agent) is then applied to break the disulfide bonds. After a period of time, that solution is rinsed off to stop the action of the reducing agent. Finally, a neutralizing ingredient is applied (oxidizing agent) to relink the disulfide bonds and set the new hair shape.

As I go over the various formulations that go into the making of permanent waves and hair relaxers, the ingredients will sound a bit daunting. **But remember, the varying components are actually not as significant as the resulting pH of the product.**

Alkaline perms and relaxers contain various ingredients to create a product with a pH of 12 to 14. To achieve the desired pH requires an alkaline ingredient such as sodium hydroxide or guanidine hydroxide (formed by calcium hydroxide and guanidine carbonate). These ingredients are extremely caustic, but that's what it takes to curl or straighten some hair types. (For information about no-lye perms, see the "No-Lye is a Lie" section in Chapter Eight, "For Women of Color".

Acid perms and relaxers contain derivatives of thioglycolic acid, such as glyceryl monothioglycolate, sodium thioglycolate, or ammonium thioglycolate. Sodium thioglycolate is considered more damaging than the relatively gentler ammonium thioglycolate, while not enough is known about glyceryl monoythioglycolate to verify its gentleness compared to the other thioglycolates (Source: Hair and Hair Care, edited by Dale H. Johnson, 1997).

Although it's called an "acid" perm, it is still far more alkaline than it is acid, with a pH of 9 to 11, because the alkaline solutions are necessary to break the disulfide bonds that create hair shape so they can be re-formed. While the lower pH of the acid perm is indeed less damaging to the hair than the higher pH of the alkaline version (remember, alkaline perms and relaxers have a pH of 12 to 14), it also is limited in its effectiveness in straightening or curling hair.

Neutral or bisulfite perms or relaxers are even milder and less effective than acid perms, and have a pH of around 8 to 9. Bisulfite perms use sodium sulfite to break the disulfide bonds of hair. Bisulfite breaks the disulfide bonds using a lower pH than both the acid and alkaline perms, but the mildness of the neutral or bisulfite perms means they don't work very well, and they are inadequate when it comes to making much of a change in the shape of the hair.

There are hair relaxers that make claims of being effective at an extremely low pH (see Chapter 8, "For Women of Color"), but their low pH of 3 to 3.5 does not affect the shape of hair nearly as much as the higher-pH products do. Plus, the notion that a pH of 3 isn't at all damaging to hair is not substantiated (there is very little research on this issue). A pH of 3 is quite acid and can theoretically denature hair (Sources: Cosmetic Dermatology, March 2004, pages 303–306; and Cosmetics & Toiletries, February 2000, pages 47–52).

HOW TO CHOOSE

The more resilient the hair, the stronger the perm or relaxer must be, and the stronger versions are always more alkaline. However, a strong perm or relaxer that is not watched carefully or is used on damaged, porous, or color-treated hair can cause frizzy, broken-down, mushy hair. It can also cause severe irritation and inflammation of the scalp.

If you just want extra body, softer curls, or less-than-complete straightening, you can use a gentler product. All at-home perm kits are grouped by shape preference (soft curl, tight curl, or straightened) or hair type (thin, fragile, or color-treated; hard-to-curl; normal; and soft body wave are the most typical classifications). These hair-type categories are fairly accurate determinants of how your hair will react to a permanent-wave solution.

Alkaline perms or relaxers are the best choice for perm- and relaxer-resistant hair (such as stick-straight hair or thick, heavy hair), resistant gray hair, Asian hair, generally hard-to-perm or hard-to-relax fine hair, and normal, healthy hair, and these products are the ones you find most typically at the drugstore.

Acid perms and relaxers are not available at the drugstore. It isn't clear why, but perhaps it's due to their reduced performance. Acid waves are milder than alkaline perms. Because they work at a lower pH, they cause less swelling of the hair during the perm process, thus reducing the chance of damage to fragile or thinner hair types. Yet at the same time, they are limited in the amount of change they can produce.

Bisulfite perms are rarely used, and there are actually very few of these on the market. They don't take well and the result is minimal curl or hardly any straightening.

In summary, alkaline perms are by far more popular than acid perms, thanks to the quality of the results, which seem to be the results most women are seeking. Acid perms are far less effective, but if the consumer isn't looking for extremely straight or extremely curly hair, they are an option. Bisulfite perms are even less effective than acid perms and, therefore, far less useful for those looking to change the structure of their hair. For more specifics about hair relaxers, see Chapter Eight, "For Women of Color."

THE PERM/STRAIGHTENING PROCESS

Once a product type is chosen, on the basis of the desired results, the hair is either combed straight or curled around rods to fashion it into the intended shape. To say that the wrapping process for permanent waves or the combing method for hair relaxers is of vital importance is an absolute understatement! Keep in mind that it is critical to wrap the hair around the right-size rollers. Winding the rods and papers evenly and symmetrically—not too tight or too loose—all over your head, or alternating the various size rods to get the best look for your hair type and haircut, is a complicated, precise effort. For hair relaxers, the placement of the product at the root, and then a gentle combing procedure to cover the length of hair is crucial. Combing in the wrong direction can cause serious damage or less than desirable results.

For perms, once the rods are in place holding sections of hair, the reducing solution is poured over the hair and left there for a period of time, making the disulfide bonds malleable. Time is the key here. Some hair is stubborn and doesn't take to the solution very well, requiring more processing time, while other hair is more pliant and easier to reshape, requiring less processing time. For those with previous damage, the hair soaks up the alkaline solution like a sponge, causing it to practically dissolve. This is particularly true of African-American women who repeatedly perm their hair (and color it) and then use high-heat curling irons to create straight hairdos. This amount of damage is a disaster in the making.

When the processing time is up, a neutralizer is used (often hydrogen peroxide or potassium bromate formulated at a low pH) to stop the reducing solution from acting on the hair. Then the disulfide bonds realign, hopefully into the new style dictated by the size, placement, and number of rods used, or the combing method used for the now-straightened contour of the hair.

THE RODS

OK, you've decided you can handle all the steps I've listed and you still want to do your perm at home. You must now consider some other issues that I haven't yet discussed. There are different techniques for rolling the rods. For example, you can do a root perm if you want fullness at the roots only and not all over. In that case, only the root of the hair is rolled and the rest of the hair is covered in a thick cream or conditioner to prevent contact with the solution. You can create a spiral or ringlet effect if you place the rods at an angle to the head instead of parallel. The number of rods is also a factor in the perm you get. Too few rods and the hair will not take on an attractive shape or the perm will not hold well.

The various types of perms are:

- ✂ **Traditional perms** are rolled horizontally and evenly around the head, using the same size rod all over.

- ✂ **Body perms** create looser, softer curls by using large rods.

- ✂ **Root perms** add lift and volume to the root area only.

- ✂ **Spiral perms** involve rolling the hair around the rod vertically instead of horizontally to create corkscrew-type curls.

- ✂ **Spot perms** are those used only in areas where the hair needs more lift or shape.

How thickly you wrap each strand of hair around the rod determines how fast and how much of the perm solution is absorbed by the hair. If the wrapped hair has a thick structure (as opposed to thin or fragile) or if more hair is wrapped around each rod, more time is needed for processing. The less hair or the thinner the hair shaft is, the shorter the processing time. If the hair is also porous, the processing time must be reduced because porous hair absorbs the chemicals faster.

No matter how you look at it, perming is complicated, and I just don't have the heart to send you to the drugstore to risk your lovely tresses. It is enough of a risk at the hair salon.

CHECKING AND TIMING

Once you have chosen the right perm for your hair type to achieve the results you desire, rolled the right-size rods with neatly wrapped endpapers uniformly on your head, and applied the solution evenly and thoroughly, you must check the perm at 10-minute intervals to see how it is taking the curl or how the straightening process is being set in (this is true at home or at the salon). Undo a rod and test the curled hair for buoyancy, or manipulate straightened hair to see if it is retaining its straightness.

Some perm products are designed with their own internal "stopwatch." These products complete the processing of the chemical reactions within a set period of time. This minimizes the risk of overprocessing the hair, which could lead to disaster. However, the inherent problem with this kind of product is self-evident: How does the product know when your hair is done? If the product's preset processing time is 30 minutes, but your hair needs 20 minutes or 40 minutes, you're out of luck.

Many hair-care companies make a great to-do about how you can use products to prep the hair before or after you perm or relax. The truth is you can't prevent damage, although you can minimize it by using products judiciously and with skill. After you're done, you can absolutely reduce dryness by using emollient conditioners—although none of these will change or alter the damage one iota!

THERMAL HAIR STRAIGHTENING

Thermal hair straightening is more typically called Thermal Hair Reconditioning or Japanese Hair Reconditioning. The words "relaxing" and "straightening" sound far more intimidating than the term "reconditioning"; in fact, reconditioning not only sounds less damaging, but also actually makes it seem like you're doing something good for hair. Nevertheless, by any name, this process can result in smooth, silky-looking, absolutely straight hair. It is a relatively new technical service offered at hair salons around the country. With a large number of women envying the stick-straight coifs of celebrities and models, it isn't surprising that this new "relaxer system" would catch on. Thermal hair straightening definitely works, with impressive results that defy even the curliest of locks, and it lasts and lasts, at least until you cut it off or it grows out.

However, the procedure is neither easy nor cheap. Are you sitting down? It's a multi-step process that can take anywhere from four to six hours or longer, depending on the length and thickness of your hair, and the cost is between $500 and $1,000. That's enough to curl anyone's hair!

The process starts with a preconditioner that is meant to protect your hair from the damage caused by the heat and chemicals used during the treatment (the very process that the stylist will insist isn't damaging to your hair). Next, an ammonium thioglycolate-based relaxer with a pH of around 10 (traditional alkaline hair relaxers have a pH of 12 to 14) is meticulously applied to tiny sections of hair. After this has processed, the hair is dried to some extent and then flat-ironed. Depending on the appearance of your hair, the processing can be repeated and the hair dried and ironed once again. At this point, the hair is neutralized to lock in the shape. And voilà! You have unbelievably straight hair that requires little styling time to maintain the appearance.

As wonderful as the results sound (except for the time and cost), there are drawbacks. Despite the claim that this system doesn't damage hair (some go as far as to suggest that it essentially repairs hair), that simply is not the case. Anything that alters the structure of your hair (and this definitely does) is damaging and limits what else you can do to your hair. Flat irons can reach temperatures of 300°F to 400°F, and that isn't easy on hair. However, the smooth, straight appearance of the hair does look far healthier when compared to hair that is curly or frizzy (just as it does if you style your hair straight with styling tools and products). But *looking* healthier is not the same as *being* healthier.

As is true with any perm, you have to deal with grow-out. Depending on how fast your hair grows, the new growth that appears will need to be straightened as well, though this is generally less time-consuming and less expensive than the original treatment.

Most hair types will have success with the thermal hair straightening process, except for some hair of African descent, or hair that is highlighted. African hair is generally too fine and too fragile to handle the chemicals and heat, and excessive breakage and damage can result. For highlighted hair, the varying textures (healthy and dyed—the dyed parts being far less healthy) require different processing times, which cannot be accommodated using the thermal straightening system.

Perhaps the one negative result (or possibly the one positive, depending on your outlook) is that you must be prepared for your hair to be really, really straight! Be ready for your hair not to hold a curl. For some, perfectly straight hair can seem lifeless, and you may finally find out what your friends with straight hair have been complaining about every time you've coveted their smooth, orderly locks. Straight hair can be hard to get used to, but for those with arms tired from endlessly blow drying and round-brushing or using a flat iron, this may well be worth the trouble, risk, and expense.

If you are looking for a salon to perform thermal hair straightening for you, the most important thing to ask is how long have they been performing the procedure. All salons will claim that the products they use are the best, but that is irrelevant, because the formulations do not vary all that much, at least not in a way that your hair would notice. Experience is what counts in this case, and you don't want to be anyone's guinea pig.

For more information about thermal or Japanese hair straightening or reconditioning, visit http://thermalreconditioning.com or www.yukosystemorder.com.

CHAPTER EIGHT

For Women of Color

THE KITCHENS

For African-American women the term "kitchen(s)" is well known. If a black woman has long hair, more often than not, the hair at the nape of the neck tends to be a jangled, tangled group of knots that is almost impossible to comb through. This snarly area is referred to as the kitchens. How did it get this name? While many black women know the term, it took some time to find someone who knew the history behind it. According to several women I spoke to, the term kitchens seems to have originated from the way African-Americans used to style their hair before the advent of electricity. Hairstyling was done in the kitchen in order to be conveniently close to the stove, using it to heat up the curling irons, combs, and hot oil that were used to smooth through and straighten hair. The most difficult part was struggling with this area of hair at the nape of the neck. For young children, the notion of going to the kitchen and getting your hair done was a painful one, especially when you got to the back of the neck.

The kitchen was also associated with other disagreeable hair-styling techniques. In many ways, going to the kitchen for hair care could even be frightening. Using hot oil with a hot comb was a popular way of mechanically straightening black hair prior to the turn of the last century. The hotter the oil, the longer it would stay hot on the hair. Higher temperatures help make the hair as straight as possible when a hot comb is run through it. To say the least, this wasn't an easy process. Hot oil could easily drip onto the skin, causing serious burns. If it got on the scalp or forehead, a frequent occurrence, it would leave a scar that could prevent hair growth in that area. It was clearly a matter of history and slang that coupled the location of the kitchen as a hair salon with the most frustrating part of styling hair.

What makes this folklore significant is the notion that African-Americans have been grappling with their hair for quite some time. As writer Veronica Chambers explained in the June 1998 issue of *Vogue*, "Because I am a black woman, I have always had a very complicated relationship with my hair ... the politics of hair and beauty in the black community [is that] ... 'Good' hair is straight and, preferably, long ... 'Bad' hair is thick and coarse, a.k.a. 'nappy' and often short."

Following fashion trends and the pressure to have hair that is 180 degrees different from what is predetermined genetically is not easy. It is especially arduous and frustrating when obtaining the desired results causes damage and the upkeep generates a lot of trouble and inconvenience. As Chambers described it, "the sound of a hot comb crackling as it makes its way through a thick head of hair makes me feel at home; the smell of hair burning is the smell of black beauty emerging like a phoenix from metaphorical ashes."

Suffice it to say that the natural state of black hair is currently not an acceptable fashion statement for women of color. Even if it were, unless black hair is kept short, it isn't easy to work with. Meanwhile, the quest for smooth hair can be a never-ending problem, and "solving" it causes hair to become brittle, broken, and mushy, and scalps to be dry, flaky, and itchy. Over and above the issues of hair and scalp problems, there's the excessive amount of time, trouble, and expense it takes to deal with the styling. I doubt there is going to be a return to the short "Afro" anytime in the near future, but hopefully there are some beautiful alternatives to straight hair that just might be an option for women of color. These definitely can save hair, time, and money, while reducing the number of products required to take care of the destruction chemical processes leave in their wake.

The following information is not meant as a treatise on fashion or style. Every woman must decide for herself what she is comfortable with and how she wants to approach her beauty needs. Through a good deal of research I've uncovered some fascinating hair facts and I will try to present that information as concisely as I can. What you determine for yourself is certainly a personal decision, but hopefully that decision is based on reality and not the hype and hope concocted by a hair-care industry that, more often than not, avoids telling consumers the truth about its products.

STRUGGLING WITH NATURE

Most African hair is exceptionally fragile and delicate. Each bend, curve, and coil of African-American hair is a weak link that is likely to break even before it's been touched, let alone styled. Unlike any other hair type, it is prone to breakage and damage, whether or not braids are twisted into the tresses, hot irons are pressed through to flatten out the kinks, or straightening products are used to permanently generate smooth, shiny locks. Of course, any of those procedures make matters worse for fragile hair.

To facilitate and atone for the damage caused by the straightening process, the ethnic hair-care market is overflowing with product choices. The statistics are mind-boggling, and African-American spending power in the world of hair care is nothing less than extraordinary, representing more than 30% of the entire industry. Shampoo purchases by African-Americans totaled $8 million in 2003 and conditioners accounted for more than $20 million. Not surprisingly, 85% of African-American women have their hair chemically straightened and they do this at home themselves, with hair relaxer sales totaling $34 million (Source: *Household and Personal Products Industry*, www.happi.com, April 2004, pages 86–98).

With all that buying power and product selection, there should be a plethora of great options for creating attractive hairstyles for women of color. Yet nothing could be further from reality, at least in terms of healthy, state-of-the-art hair options.

Many of the products and hairstyles designed for African-American hair are unsuitable for that kind of hair. Even if the chemical processes used to straighten black hair weren't severely damaging, they would still be intolerable for African hair. African hair can barely survive simple brushing. Yet the ads in magazines aimed at black women suggest that all it takes is a change of shampoo, conditioner, perm, or relaxer for the hair to appear resilient and bouncy, without any negative side effects. That is absolutely not the case, and in fact, it is physiologically impossible. In truth, the options are limited; there are no perms or relaxers that can make fragile African hair smooth without causing damage (and there are assuredly no herbal or plant-based ones either). To top it all off, a great number of the products designed to correct or at least alleviate the damage caused by hair straightening, such as pomades, greases, and oils, can create even more problems.

Somewhere along the way, the cultural myth that greased-up, oiled, slicked-down hair was healthier hair became the norm for many black women. Too often, product after product for black hair is just another version of grease or oil. Yet all the grease, oil, and emollients in the world won't produce longer, thicker, or healthier hair. It simply is not possible. If anything, just the opposite is true. Grease and oil can clog hair follicles. What happens when follicles get blocked? The circulation is literally choked off and, as a result, the natural hair growth can become stunted. The products used most frequently by black women to handle the consequences of hair straightening or hot combing are the very products that can hamper hair growth, causing the hair to eventually become more fragile, weak, brittle, and damaged.

SHAMPOOING AND CONDITIONING

To complicate matters, many of the hair-care products used by African-Americans are extremely greasy or oily, and often sit on the scalp for long periods of time. The oil holds down the hair along with the skin cells that would normally be shed from the scalp, which, along with the grease, can cause a flaky, oily-looking scalp. The need to shed those skin cells is even greater when the hair has been chemically straightened. Any chemical process can temporarily dry out (actually burn) the scalp, resulting in more skin cells that need to come off. But what usually takes place after a chemical process is the application of hair treatments that grease up the dried-out scalp and fried hair. Just when the scalp needs to breathe and exfoliate, it gets suffocated with grease.

Ingredient lists on many hair-care products designed for African-American women are shockingly repetitive. Petrolatum, lanolin, waxes, oils, wax-like minerals, and emollients fill almost each and every one. While those can be good for the hair shaft (though there are lighter-weight ingredients such as silicones that can produce the same effect with far less stickiness or greasy feel), they are terrible for the scalp.

And then, despite the need to effectively remove these emollient conditioners from the scalp, the fact is that most shampoos designed for women of color are usually mild, so as not to further dry out the hair or scalp. That means the emollients in the hair-treatment products do not get washed off properly. Leaving any amount of grease on the scalp for long periods of time causes problems for hair growth.

Perhaps the most disastrous beauty advice directed at women of color is to wash their hair as infrequently as possible. If it weren't for this dilemma of emollients choking off the hair follicle, I would agree that less is better, because the more often you wash the hair, the more often you have to restyle it with curling irons, hot combs, and blow dryers. And the more you style and manipulate hair, especially African hair, the more you damage it—when avoiding damage was the very reason given for the reduced frequency of shampooing.

Unfortunately, that trade-off isn't a viable option. Taking more time between shampoos might leave a style in place longer, but if the hair-care products that are being used are loaded with grease, and many of them are, it renders the hair sticky and greasy, with split ends sticking out in a fuzzy mess. It can also make hair mat together in sections, and it creates a real potential for increased dandruff-like flakes.

Washing the hair at least once every four to five days is probably the best way to keep the scalp and hair healthy, along with choosing a hairstyle that requires the least amount of manipulation. Hair that is washed more frequently and styled carefully can have more movement, look less matted and greasy, and stay healthiest in the long run. Styling carefully is the crux of the matter, and that takes rethinking how the hair is handled.

HOW MUCH TO RELAX?

The first thing you need to know is that smoothing out tightly curled hair is relatively safe when the hair has some strength to it, though that isn't usually the case given the way most African-American women style their hair and the number of times they've had it straightened. Many hair relaxers for African-American women have extremely high pHs, somewhere between 12 and 14. If left on too long, this can burn the scalp and skin and fry the hair. Damage may not be evident the first time the hair is straightened, but any subsequent straightening after several weeks of grow-out will leave the hair begging for mercy. Add styling with overly hot hot-combs and curling irons to that and, in time, you won't have even a close facsimile of the soft, bouncy, smooth hair you were hoping for.

I know I'm not telling the African-American women reading this book anything they haven't heard before or don't know from experience. But, while the idea of using a chemical process that takes less time and preferably contains a lower pH (usually found in perms for Caucasian or Asian hair) instead of a highly alkaline perm is hardly new, it isn't mentioned or followed very often. And that is the only alternative to the same old merry-go-round of burnt, greased-up, stiff-looking hair.

This means that using a texturizing perm, as opposed to a hair-straightening perm, is the safest, healthiest, and easiest alternative for fragile African-American hair. Texturizing perms can create curls with fullness, length, softness, and bounce, and cause the least amount of damage. If you decide to go this route, remember to have a texturizing perm only once every three months; more often than that and you're back at the beginning with baked-to-a-crisp hair. I know this isn't an easy suggestion. To get to the point of doing a texturizing perm, you must grow out the damage you already have or cut it off and let it grow out. You can't do a texturizing perm over a straightening perm, as the hair will rebel and break off. Growing out damaged hair is a painful experience for any woman, but once you get through it, the hassle of struggling with your hair may be over forever.

To minimize the potential risks of perming, you should evaluate your hair for yourself. Before you choose a perm, pull out three strands of hair from the root from various areas of your head. Hold the hair tightly between two fingers and tug gently. If two of the three strands break, your hair is in no condition for any kind of perm. Another variation of this test that can help determine what kind of perm your hair can handle is to take strands of hair and run your nails over it in a pinching fashion, as if you were curling a ribbon. Again, if two of the three strands break, your hair is in no condition to be permed. If the hair curls easily in a wave or curls up tightly, you can handle a stronger, high-alkaline solution (but leave it on for no more than 20 minutes). If your hair doesn't curl up much or feels inelastic, you should use a gentler perm.

Judging the length of time of the application is perhaps the most critical part of any relaxing process. But where to place the solution, and being sure to wash it out of the hair when you're done, are also critical. To avoid damage or scalp irritation, regardless of the product, follow these guidelines:

- If you have fine or previously damaged hair, leave the solution on for no longer than 13 minutes.

- If you have medium-strength or slightly damaged hair, leave the solution on for no longer than 15 minutes.

- If you have coarse, resistant, and minimally damaged hair, leave the solution on for no longer than 15 minutes.

- If you are perming or relaxing over new growth, it is imperative to not get any of the solution on the previously permed or relaxed section of hair. This is tricky but it's essential to prevent serious damage.

- When you are finished with the main solution you must be certain all the chemicals are completely washed out of your hair. It is okay to shampoo and rinse the hair several times to be sure every last drop has been cleansed off the hair.

NO-LYE IS A LIE!

Well, at least it's a fib, depending on which products you're referring to, but even when it's true, it is meaningless when it comes to helping a consumer know if the product she's getting is going to be less damaging than another one might be.

Lots of perms and relaxers claiming to be lye-free and, therefore, more gentle for the hair are being promoted at salons and drugstores these days, with a large number aimed at African-American consumers looking for hair relaxers. There are two main issues here. First, is the product really "lye-free"? And second, is it better to use a lye-free product? Unfortunately, it turns out that the lye-free claim is more a matter of marketing language than it is of any benefit to a consumer.

Traditionally and technically, perms have used sodium hydroxide (lye) to raise the pH of the reducing solution, since a high pH is the best and most effective way to relax hair. However, there are lots of ways to significantly raise the pH of a product without sodium hydroxide. No-lye products often use calcium hydroxide mixed with guanidine carbonate to create guanidine hydroxide, which does the exact same thing as sodium hydroxide, and it can be just as irritating to the scalp and damaging to hair. I know lye-free products sound like they should make your hair happier, with less damage and dryness, but that is not automatically the case!

Think about it this way: The pH range is 1 to 14, with 1 the most acid (sulfuric acid has a pH of 1), 7 neutral (water has a pH of 7), and 14 the most alkaline (typically sodium hydroxide, meets this definition). But as you will see from the list below, many of the no-lye perms actually have a pH of 13 or 14, and that is just as damaging and irritating as a lye perm with the same pH. Regardless of the ingredient, a pH of 13 or 14 can burn your scalp and skin.

The history of using sodium hydroxide in perms and hair relaxers has not been a pleasant one, because these products almost guarantee damage and scalp irritation. What African-American woman wouldn't love to believe she could have straight hair without any negative side effects? So, because sodium hydroxide is (accurately) perceived by the consumer as being bad for hair, the hair-care industry created a bit of a ruse to make things appear nicer, even though the pH of the product still needed to be high to be effective. It turns out that lye-free relaxers have a pH that is almost as high as the pH of most sodium hydroxide relaxers!

Don't let the hair-care industry fool you with this one. There are no hair-restoring, more natural, or damage-free results with a no-lye perm if the pH is high! High-alkaline perms, even though they work better than lower-pH perms, still damage hair, and misrepresenting the ingredients doesn't change that. The following list of hair-straightening products and their pH might curl your hair, especially the product marketed toward children that has a pH of 14, and that is no lye!

- ✄ Africa's Best No-Lye Dual Conditioning Relaxer System Super ($5.99), pH 13

- ✄ African Pride Miracle Deep Conditioning No-Lye Relaxer System Regular, Super ($9.29), pH 13 (Regular), pH 14 (Super)

- ✄ At One with Nature Botanical Strongends Sensitive Scalp Relaxer No-Lye, Regular with Herbs and Moisturizers ($6.49), pH 14

- ✄ Dark & Lovely Beautiful Beginnings No-Mistake No-Lye Children's Relaxer System ($8.99), pH 13

- Dark & Lovely No-Lye Relaxer System, Regular ($6.39), pH 13

- Fabu-Laxer No-Lye Relaxer Kit Regular ($5.99), pH 13

- Gentle-Treatment No-Lye Conditioning Creme Relaxer, Regular for Fine or Normal Hair, Super ($5.49), both pH 13

- Isoplus No-Lye Conditioning Relaxer System Regular, Super ($6.39), pH 13

- Just for Me No-Lye Conditioning Creme Relaxer, Children's Regular Formula ($8.49), pH 14

- Lustrasilk Moisture Max Conditioning Relaxer Super Free from Lye ($5.98), pH 13

- Raveen No-Lye Conditioning Creme Relaxer with Multiple Conditioners ($4.99), pH 14

- Raveen Sensitive Scalp No-Lye ($6.99), pH 13

- Revlon Creme of Nature No Lye Relaxer System, Super ($8.99), pH 13

- Revlon Creme of Nature Creme Relaxer Sodium Hydroxide Formula, Super ($8.99), pH 12

- Revlon Realistic No-Lye Relaxer System, Regular, Super ($6.99), both pH 13

- Soft & Beautiful Botanicals Texturizer Coarse ($4.99), pH 12

- Soft & Beautiful Super No-Lye Conditioning Relaxer Regular, Coarse, and Super ($9.49), all pH 14

- SoftSheen Carson Optimum Care No-Lye Relaxer Regular, Super ($6.79), both pH 13

- TCB Naturals No-Lye Relaxer, Regular Extra Body ($6.29), pH 14

THE RIO HAIR DISASTER

A number of African-Americans are aware of the class action lawsuit against Rio Hair Naturalizer System. For those who aren't familiar with this saga, here's what happened. Going back two or three years, many women saw an infomercial for a do-it-yourself, at-home hair-relaxer called Rio Hair. The commercial claimed that, with supposedly no chemicals (it was "all natural") and no muss or fuss, Rio Hair could transform tightly curled African-American hair into silky Caucasian-like hair without any kinks, dryness, breakage, oil buildup, or any of the other hair problems that can plague black women.

For any woman of color who has coveted Oprah Winfrey's bouncy, smooth, flowing locks, Phyllicia Rashad's curl-free tresses, or Janet Jackson's sexy mane, this infomercial was mesmerizing. Even more difficult to ignore was the parade of apparently satisfied African-American women smiling as they shook their soft, pliable dos. How could this work, particularly sans chemicals? Is there actually a blend of plant extracts or vegetable oils that can "de-corkscrew" ultra-tight curls like no other products have before?

The answer was and still is an incontrovertible No, it isn't possible; there aren't any natural ingredients that can produce results like those shown on television. Not only did Rio products contain almost exclusively a concoction of very unnatural ingredients, the pH of the relaxer was between 1 and 2, acidic enough to eat through hair and scalp, which is exactly what it did (Source: *Archives of Dermatology*, September 2000, pages 1104–1108).

The following information is from the FDA: "Two types of hair relaxers, valued at almost $2 million, were destroyed last fall after thousands of consumers reported problems with them. It was the largest number of complaints [the] FDA had ever received about a cosmetic product" (Source: www.fda.gov).

The destruction was one of several measures the hair products' distributor, World Rio Corp. of Los Angeles, agreed to take in a consent decree entered in the U.S. District Court for the Central District of California on September 1, 1995.

In 1994 and early 1995, more than 3,000 people reported to the FDA that their scalp itched or burned and that their hair broke off or fell out—and, in some cases, turned green—after using the Rio Hair Naturalizer System and Rio Hair Naturalizer System with Color Enhancer.

Based on the complaints and an FDA investigation, the agency alleged that the hair products were being sold illegally in the United States because the adverse effects experienced by consumers were consistent with those seen with harmful substances. Their labeling was false. The products' labeling listed an acid pH level of 3.4, but FDA and California State analyses of the product found a pH range below 2. In addition, the FDA alleged the labeling falsely described the products as "chemical free," even though the ingredient labels listed substances commonly recognized as chemicals.

"On Jan. 23, 1995, at FDA's request, U.S. marshals seized the entire lot of products at Product Packaging West in California. On Jan. 24, an investigator with FDA's San Francisco district office went to Addressing and Mailing to inspect the firm and found more than 8,000 cases of the Rio hair relaxers, worth about $500,000 in retail value. FDA notified the State of Nevada Division of Health, which, in turn, embargoed the products, thus preventing their sale."

Relying on the hair-care industry to give you the whole story about any product is rarely wise. Rio Hair is perhaps the extreme, but it is not the only case involving blatant misinformation, lack of information, or misleading explanations about chemical content or product performance.

The reality is that there are always downsides to permanently altering the hair. The more gentle the product, the less effective it is. The more caustic, the more damage it causes; but the potential for straighter hair is better. Until that changes, and there is ongoing research into this issue, buying into exotic claims of all-natural ingredients giving you perfect hair is about the same as trying to buy the Brooklyn Bridge.

THEN THERE WAS COPA

Copa Natural Curl Release System ($19.95 for 1 application) followed Rio as the miracle hair-straightening product being sold to African-Americans, and when you hear the claims in the brochure, your hair will stand up and curl: "Copa Natural Curl Release System is not a straightener, but naturally releases tightly curled hair. Curl release is not instantaneous, but a natural process which requires some patience as the Copa system works naturally with your hair's chemistry and texture. Depending on the type of hair you have (and how permeable it is), it can take from one to five applications to achieve the level of curl control you desire. In our testing, the average number of applications required was three. With each successive application you will see a difference." Doesn't that sound a lot like Rio (who also said you could perm your hair several times, one after the other, to receive the desired results without causing damage)?

Copa is very aware of the similarity between its product claims and those of Rio's because they take some effort to pinpoint the major differences between the two companies: "Copa uses sodium thiosulfate and Rio used acid and cupric chloride; [Rio had a] different active pH (Copa at 3.5, and Rio as low as 2; and Copa and Rio have different reactions in the hair (Rio [affected] the disulfide bonds directly and Copa has salt bonds)."

First, Rio did not use "acid." Rio used ammonium chloride, cetrimonium bromide, and sodium thiosulfate, quite similar to Copa's ingredients. Rio did have a very low pH, but the hair doesn't have anything called "salt bonds"; the only molecular bonds that affect hair shape are disulfide bonds. If you don't break those and re-form them, you can't change the shape of hair, period. And there is nothing natural in the least about sodium thiosulfate. Rather, sodium thiosulfate is the salt form of thioglycolic acid, and is used in perms and straightening products—and in depilatories. So much for being special and different.

Copa's pH of 3.5 is indeed more gentle than Rio's, but it is still low and can denature hair. The real point is that you can't gently straighten your hair! As I explained above, the lower the pH, the less effective the hair-straightening product is. There is no way around this one.

In 2003, marketers of Copa Hair System agreed to settle a Federal Trade Commission (FTC) charge of unsubstantiated claims by paying $100,000 in civil penalties and $200,000 in consumer redress (Source: www.ftc.gov/opa/2003/08/goodtimes.htm).

"The FTC alleged that Copa was falsely marketed as having unique hair-strengthening properties. Its active ingredient, however, according to the FTC, may weaken hair while it straightens it. Further, through the use of before and after pictures, the defendants allegedly implied that consumers would experience hair straightening with just one use. The FTC charges that, instead, multiple applications may be necessary to achieve the depicted results." (Source: www.ftc.gov/opa/2003/08/goodtimes.htm).

For more information about Copa, visit //www.copahair.com/homepage.asp or call 1-800-516-7108.

WHATEVER HAPPENED TO CURLY PERMS?

There was a time during the 1980s when curly perms for African-Americans were all the rage. Curly perms used a process in which the hair was first straightened with an alkaline hair relaxer and then wrapped around rods to create soft, tendril-like curls rather than stick-straight hair. The concept was great because the curls required less aftercare than straightened hair. Straightened hair requires styling tools to create the desired look, while curly hair has minimal need for any further styling time. Using fewer styling tools also means there would be less additional damage to the hair. A curly perm was a truly carefree style, but unfortunately it had its problems, which caused the market to slowly decline to the point where this hairstyle is rarely seen. What went wrong?

Curly perms require a two-step process, and that means more damage. Each successive perm was like adding two treatments to the hair. That produced a lot of damage and dryness, despite the ease of styling. And in order to maintain the softness of the curls, a good deal of hair conditioning was required. These rich, emollient conditioning products easily built up on hair, producing a notoriously greasy, oily look that eventually became fodder for African-American comedians. A major problem for curly perms also happened at the salon level. According to *Hair and Hair Care*, "to offer economy to the hair stylists, manufacturers packaged the professional perm components in bulk sizes. The large, bulk-size cremes and lotions containing ammonium thioglycolate could not be packaged air-tight and they started to decrease in pH…. Therefore, at the salon level, permanent wave products were subject to inconsistent performance." (Source: *Hair and Hair Care*, Dale Johnson, 1997, Marcel Dekker). The demise of curly perms was also a result of a major fashion change for African-American women. Sleeker hairstyles became popular as more African-American models and actresses appeared in the media sporting smooth, flowing coifs.

BRAIDING, CORNROWING, AND WEAVING

Hair straightening isn't the only precarious hair fashion for women of color. Braiding (including extensions), cornrowing, and weaving designs into the hair may be alluring, but the expense, time, grow-out, maintenance, and potential harm to the hair make it almost a life-altering project. On the surface, braiding appears to be a pragmatic, utilitarian option because the braids can be washed and the hair requires no styling between weaves. As long as the braids aren't put in too tightly (which can cause pressure on the follicle that can make the hair fall out before its time and cause thinning or bald spots), the ease of maintenance is a benefit. However, all too often the weight of the braids and the tension on the connecting hair causes hair to fall out. Eventually, the effects can be seen in a continually receding hairline and bald spots. (Sources: *Dermatologic Therapy*, June 2004, page 164; *Dermatologic Clinics*, October 2003, pages 629–644; www.emedicine.com/derm/topic895.htm; and *Practitioner*, May 1986, pages 401–402.)

Over the past several years there has been a trend in black hair fashion for braiding extensions to become even thicker and longer—and, therefore, heavier. This extra weight only compounds the problem of hair loss.

Again, for women of color this is not new information—the results are blatantly obvious. Yet for some reason there is an overwhelming feeling that this is the price you must pay to be fashionable. I do not set trends, but I do frequently ask women to think more critically about how they allow themselves to become a slave to fashion styles that are either harmful or at the very least expensive and time-consuming. What are we willing to give up, and why are we willing to give up so much for a hairstyle? I can't answer that. This one is for the individual to think about and decide for herself what direction makes the most sense.

BACK TO BASICS

Regardless of the hairstyle you choose, all of the following suggestions can help prevent breakage and further damage:

- Do not run a brush through the entire length of your hair all at once.

- As much as is realistically possible, avoid brushing the length of your hair.

- When you do brush, use the softest-bristled brush you can find. If it tugs or tears at your hair the least little bit, it is not a good brush for your hair. Concentrate your brushing efforts on the scalp and minimally on the ends.

- Use your fingers to gently separate strands of hair and distribute the natural oil of the scalp through the hair with short, gentle, stroking motions.

- Massage your scalp twice a day. You can do this with your fingers or a very soft brush. Section the hair and gently stroke the scalp, then move on to the next section.

- The less pressure on the scalp, the better. Avoid tying your hair back in tight buns or ponytails. If you set your hair on rollers, don't wind them too tightly.

- Roller sets are safer for African-American hair than heat-producing tools. If you do use rollers, set them in hair that is just beyond damp but not yet dry. This will afford a shorter setting time. Avoid rolling hair up tightly.

- Consider sleeping on a satin pillowcase instead of a cotton one. The cotton fibers cause friction, grabbing the individual hairs and breaking them.

- When drying the hair, avoid using a terry-cloth towel. The hooked weave can catch on African-American hair and break it off. Try using a towel with a smooth, velvet-type surface.

- When you wash your hair, concentrate on the scalp and wash in one direction only. If you tousle your hair, it can easily become knotted, making styling more difficult and encouraging breakage.

✂ Rather than styling the hair perfectly straight, consider a looser natural curl as an option. It takes less effort and can save your hair.

✂ When using a blow dryer and a round brush, keep the heat moving over the hair; avoid concentrating the heat in one place for too long.

✂ Avoid thick, heavy styling products that contain petrolatum, lanolin, cocoa butter, or shea butter. If you do use pomades or rich cream treatments, use them sparingly, concentrating the application on the hair shaft, not the scalp.

What about the product choices for women of color? I think you would find it shocking how similar hair-care products are, regardless of who they are supposedly designed for. I'll get into that more in the product reviews, but in general, when there are differences in products, it is usually in favor of adding grease to damaged hair, but that isn't helpful. All the lubrication in the world can't repair hair or prevent damage. If you overlook the greasy pomades and hair treatments (as you definitely should), there is no discernible difference between hair-care products for women of color and those in other lines.

CHAPTER NINE

Styling Hair

IT ISN'T ALWAYS FAIR

A great haircut, the right styling products, and good styling tools are, without question, indispensable assets to creating a head of hair that looks and behaves the way you want it to. Well, almost indispensable. If your hair falls into place with just a shake of your head or a simple scrunching to arrange curls and then you're done, you probably need read no further. However, for most of us, it takes a lot more effort than that. Where most of us get snared is in the search for the right products. Yet all the best styling products in the world are worthless without the ability to proficiently handle styling implements. Knowing how to use a blow dryer, brushes, and a curling iron is integral to getting your head out of bad hair days, at least most of the time.

Aside from experimenting, finding a hairstylist who is willing to help teach you how to use styling tools is the wisest investment you could ever make. Learning the techniques, developing your own skill and talent, and then practicing until you get it right adds up to the totality of great looking hair.

Styling aptitude is of vital consequence for your hair, but your haircut is the structure and framework everything else is based on. Exactly how those locks of yours are trimmed, shaped, layered, or patterned is the basis for how your hair will look. Telling you exactly what haircut, style, silhouette, or hair color would look good on you is not within the scope of my work. But I can help point you in the right direction so you have an idea of how to get the look you want or need.

WHICH HAIRSTYLE TO CHOOSE?

Most women love looking at fashion magazines. The dazzling, alluring pictures are always exciting and fun to peruse. Admiring these photos is one thing, but basing a hairstyle choice on pictures of celebrities or models with great heads of hair more often than not has *nothing* to do with your lifestyle or what your hair can actually do. It rarely even has anything to do with the model or celebrity in their real life! Before their hair is meticulously styled, celebrities and models usually don't have perfect or even great-looking hair. Without the aid of an expert stylist, their hair is hardly worth looking at or emulating. What a picture represents is almost never reality. Model or celebrity pictures are just pretty pictures created by makeup artists, hairstylists, good lighting, and expert photography (plus some amount of digital retouching)—not what you would call low maintenance or easy to reproduce on your own. When it comes to finding a haircut appropriate to your needs, at least in terms of time and convenience, celebrity and model pictures are probably not very helpful.

So how do you get an idea of what hairstyles are workable for you? Look for someone you know who has a similar or identical hair type, face, and body shape, and who also has a haircut you admire. It would also be wise to select someone who is successful in the career or social track to which you aspire. Why is it better to emulate someone you know when it is so much more interesting to take the lead from someone famous or drop-dead gorgeous? You may think you want to look like a particular celebrity, but her style may be completely inappropriate for what you want to do in life. Also, assuming that the way a hairstyle or dress looks on your favorite star has nothing to do with how it would look on you (unless you look like that person), it requires a leap of faith that most of us would be foolish to make.

Bottom line: There isn't an easy answer to the right haircut or hairstyle, because there are so many options. There are, however, some basic rules you can follow:

- **Long faces** should consider wearing their hair cut above their shoulder in long layers with a side part; this keeps your hair from accentuating the length of your face and enhances your eyes and cheekbones instead. Avoid short haircuts.

- **Square faces** also benefit from a side part to take the emphasis away from the edges of the jaw, but the length of hair can depend on how wide the face is. If your face is wide rather than narrow, consider wearing your hair longer—just at the shoulder; if it is more narrow consider wearing it shorter, around the nape of the neck. Avoid bangs, which can add even more square dimensions to your face.

- **Oval faces** are considered classic and able to wear almost any style. It is best to avoid severe haircuts of any kind, so geometric patterns or asymmetrical cuts are not for you.

- **Round faces** can wear their hair in soft long layers, but do best without full bangs. Avoid styling hair so it is full at the sides of the face; rather, keep hair sleek and smooth over that area.

- **Heart-shaped faces** look best with hair that is just above shoulder length with long, full layers feathered through the length. Soft bangs can look quite nice, too.

One of my favorite Web sites for checking out styles is www.lhj.com (*Ladies Home Journal*). A section on their site allows you to upload your own picture and put different hairstyles and hair colors right on your own image.

HAIRSTYLE BASICS

Although I said I wasn't going to discuss hairstyles in depth, I want to go over a few of the basics to help you formulate some ideas when you start thinking about changing the way you wear your hair. There aren't many rules, but here are a few I encourage you to consider.

Bangs that are too long or too thick de-emphasize the eyes, accentuate the nose, and generally make your face look smaller. If you wear long, thick bangs that conceal your forehead and eyes, the next feature in line is your nose. Lighten up on the bangs and make sure they don't ride heavily below the eyebrows.

Parting your hair in the middle is another way to give the nose center stage (although it isn't as bad as dense bangs). A center part divides the face severely in half. This median line creates a linear movement down the face. The next feature that lines up with this central lineup is the nose. Center parts also tend to look childish or pubescent, instead of sophisticated and polished. Either no part or a side part will correct these problems.

Brushing hair away from the center of the face is, nine times out of ten, the best fashion advice. This is a hard one to convince women of because so many stylists love brushing hair into the face. Yet when fashion designers or advertisers showcase their latest looks or products, or when hair designers want to advertise their newest products, the models almost always have their hair blown away from the face. Let's say you don't want that flowing, wind-blown look. Even a short, styled hairdo can be brushed off the face or at least arranged in a way that doesn't hide the sides of the face. Hair that lies directly on the face cuts the cheekbone in half, making the face look rounder and fuller (so much for the hollowed-out cheekbone look), and if you wanted your eyes to look bigger, you've just cut off at least an inch of length. Style the hair away from the face, upward and out. Your hair will not only look fuller, but your facial features will look softer and yet more defined.

Extremely short hair looks best on thinner women with great bone structure. The same is true for extremely long hair. Layering is good for someone with hair that is neither too thin nor too thick. If the hair is too thin, layers hang obviously off the head in steps; if the hair is too thick, the layers can lift away from the head like a balloon. Full is good, but too full and you'll look like "Here comes the hair!"

Bilateral haircuts, where one section of hair is short and the other long, and etched haircuts, where one section of hair looks radically different from the other, are fashion statements you should avoid. They are trendy, hard to maintain, and make the hair look like it's been "cut." They are too severe and prevent a soft flowing look, making the head look like sculpted artwork.

Farrah Fawcett bangs from the '70s are out of style (and will remain so for eternity, I hope). Flipped-back bangs were fun once, but so were go-go boots and Nehru jackets; those days are long gone, too, and hopefully not coming back.

If you want your long hair to look fuller, cut it to just about the shoulders. The buoyancy created when hair resettles just above the shoulder will almost always make it appear fuller. Never allow your hair to get so long that it breaks at the shoulder, with some hair falling forward and some falling back.

TALKING TO YOUR STYLIST

Perhaps the most important tool for getting the look you want is recognizing how to make decisions about your hair and communicate them to your stylist. That isn't as easy as it sounds because your hairstylist may have a different agenda than you do. Some hairstylists are inspired by the latest trends being presented by their high-tech contemporaries who work for companies such as Sebastian and TIGI. One way that salon-only hair-care companies get the attention of hairstylists is by producing hair shows or semi-annual hair books that showcase the most outrageous or difficult-to-maintain styles. These also keep hairstylists interested in the latest styling products.

Sometimes hairdressers like to change your hair to satisfy their own artistic needs, rather than favoring *your* needs. While the latest hair trends may be right for you, I encourage you to consider whether or not that is really the direction you want to go. The design may be interesting for the hairstylist, but it may not be good for you. Think about whether or not getting a great cut is about convenience, your career, fashion, or fun. Choosing between these factors can help you communicate your needs to your stylist.

What makes a good hairstylist? Ah, now there's a loaded question! It depends on your tastes. Probably the best definition of a good stylist is one who has the training and experience to work with your head of hair. On your part, that means research and, for your budget, it is the one area where you should not cut corners. Talented hairstylists are worth the cost.

How do you find a trained and experienced stylist? Through referrals and by learning about the stylist's credentials, training, and amount of experience. Referrals are probably the most typical way we choose a stylist. A friend whose hair you admire goes to this wonderful stylist and the friend can't say enough about how much they love this person and how she wouldn't go to anyone else. Or you read a fashion magazine and discover an article that hails the talents of a local stylist. Those are probably the two most reliable ways to choose a hairstylist. Certainly they are more reliable than using a stylist because a hair salon ran a special for $25 off a perm and cut!

So why do referrals sometimes end up badly? You may have admired your friend's perfectly beautiful blunt cut, but you need a carefully blended layered cut, and the stylist may be a whiz at blunt cuts, but can't handle the difficulties of a long layered cut. To make personal referrals work well for you, look for someone whose hair is similar to yours. Similarly, the fashion magazine recommendation can also be a good referral option. Frequently, stylists do gain some recognition in your city (and that rarely happens accidentally); but, alas, what that stylist sees for you might not be what you want. Sometimes it's your lack of communication skills or unwillingness to be assertive about what you want, or maybe your inability to hear what the stylist is telling you—for example, about the limitations of taking naturally tight, curled hair and making it straight in a humid climate.

If referrals haven't panned out for you or you simply don't know anyone with hair like yours that's cut in a style you admire, then the only way to gauge a stylist's ability before you sit down in the chair is to check out his or her credentials and training. That means finding a stylist who has attended advanced hair schools or seminars—not just beauty school, but training above and beyond, as well as ongoing education. How do you find that out? You ask. "What training besides beauty school have you had?" is a more than valid question, and the answer you get is significant. A stylist whose only training is from beauty school has only rudimentary knowledge of what it takes to cut, style, color, or perm hair, or choose products for a client. It would be like going to a physician who just graduated from medical school; a doctor who hasn't done a residency has no experience. You want a stylist who has had at least some advanced training and does continuing education above and beyond the beauty school's state licensing qualifications.

Hair Note: Don't try to save money on a hairstylist. You can save *lots* of money on product choices and coloring your hair at home (if you aren't making a radical change) by following some of my advice, but don't scrimp on what you pay a hairstylist. That doesn't mean you have to spend a fortune, but it does raise your chances of finding the right stylist. (On the other hand, just because a stylist charges $50 and up for a cut doesn't guarantee he or she is automatically going to be proficient or best for you.) What it does mean is avoiding those places that advertise $10 or $20 haircuts. Some women have hair that can look great with a bargain haircut, but not many. Accomplished stylists charge more; it is an issue of skill having more value. For your head of hair, that is one area worth the expense.

WHY CAN'T YOU MAKE IT LOOK LIKE THE HAIRSTYLIST DOES? ... AND WHAT YOU CAN DO ABOUT IT

Why can't you get your hair to look like it does just after you leave the salon? You use the same styling products your hairdresser uses, the same blow dryer (the new one with the cool-air button), and soft brushes that can hold onto the hair. Yet, even so, it doesn't look the same. There are four basic reasons why the hairstylist is capable of doing what you aren't: **technique**, **tenacity**, **tools**, and **talent**.

Hairstylists are trained to make your hair look good. Cutting is one piece of their work, the other is the finishing work.

Technique refers to the fundamental skills hairstylists acquire to make hair look good. Which brush is best, how much tension to put on the hair, how to put lift on the root, how to control the direction of the hair, how much heat to use, and on and on, are all variables that a stylist is trained to understand for many different hair types. With practice you can acquire most of the skills you need to get salon results. It doesn't hurt to pay for a session with your stylist to have her show you how to work with your hair.

Tenacity is all about patience, taking the time to style each small section of hair until it performs just so. Stylists not only spend more time on your head than you do (which makes a vast difference both in the final appearance of your hair as well as in how long the style will stay in place), but also they are in a better position to get the right angle, pressure, and heat direction on your hair. Standing over your own head is something you simply can't do. That's why a salon style can have incredible movement and durability versus an at-home effort that falls out or is still fuzzy after you're done. Styling the back of your own hair will always be a challenge, but taking the time to make sure each section of hair is done to perfection (and is perfectly dry) will get you closer to the professional look you're trying to achieve.

Using the right **tools** is far more important for getting hair smooth and reducing frizz than almost any other aspect of styling hair. But not only do the right blow dryers, flat irons, curling irons, and diffusers make a huge difference in your final results, the right brushes are also needed to complete the picture. This means going shopping, and the simplest list of all is to buy the tools your designer uses. That takes the guesswork out of which brushes, blow dryer, or flat iron is best for your hair.

Bringing all these skills together is the embodiment of **talent**, an intangible dynamic, but it is the essence of what separates most of us from a capable and, ultimately, gifted stylist. You may never get to the point where you would consider yourself a "talented" stylist, but you can be talented with your hair by learning how to control it and finding the time to make it happen.

One thing to notice is what *doesn't* play a role in re-creating what your stylist does to your hair, and that's the choice of products. Many stylists have their favorites, but all the products in the world can't replace technique, tenacity, tools, and talent. Taking home salon products won't produce salon results, so don't buy into that myth.

Because of all those varying elements, there are some tricks of the trade that can get you closer to salon results. It just takes patience and experimentation to find out which techniques work best for you. The suggestions that follow will minimize damage but maximize style. And please notice that in most cases, as you might expect, less is more.

TRICKS OF THE TRADE

Never overuse a styling product. Too much or too many styling products that are too heavy or stiff (or even lightweight ones) can make the hair limp, heavy, stiff, greasy, and/or hard to manage. Almost without exception, the less you use the better. **Rule of palm:** Apply only enough gel, mousse, hair serum, or heat protection to *minimally* cover your palms and fingers in a thin layer. Then smooth this in an even layer through your hair, or just in the areas where your hair needs it. If you need more, add it only to the areas you know need more control.

What should you do with spray-on styling products? Be careful. Spray-on products are generally formulated to be lighter than those you apply to the hair with your hands, as a result, you aren't touching your hair as much, so it's harder to tell how much product you've applied, and whether or not you've applied it evenly. Spray-on gels don't guarantee thinner coverage. If you are trying to beat the frizzies, it is essential to cover every hair on your head, but if your hair is fine or limp, less coverage is better than more.

Use different products for different needs. One type of styling product is probably not enough, especially if your hair is thick, coarse, dry, or damaged. Your hair may need a silicone serum to make it smooth and silky, and a gel or styling lotion for hold, but you may also need a pomade or wax for the ends or the more damaged parts of your hair to lie smooth, and a hairspray to keep it all in place when you're done.

Hairstyling products often don't mean what they say, so don't take them seriously. Styling products with labels indicating they provide a "firm" or "medium" or "soft" hold aren't always accurate. Following my recommendations from Chapter Ten, "Product Reviews," always consider the lighter-weight styling products for all over the hair, and use firmer or heavier-hold products on stubborn areas only.

Gently move your wet hair into the shape you want it to be, with the least amount of brushing, combing, or manipulation. The less brushing, the less damage you will cause. A vent brush or a wide-toothed comb is best for arranging wet hair.

Do not begin styling your hair with a blow dryer and brush when it is sopping wet. Hair is at its most vulnerable and is most prone to damage when it is wet. Either let your hair air-dry for a period of time first or blow dry some of the moisture out using a diffuser or a medium heat and medium air setting before you begin to create a specific style. This is called rough-drying (even though you should never do it roughly). To rough-dry the hair, use either direct heat that you quickly move over the hair (including the root area) or a diffuser, always working the hair in the pattern or movement you want it to go. You can begin to use your fingers to scrunch your hair if you are going after a curly, natural look.

Use your fingers instead of a brush when you first begin to remove moisture from your hair. Never try to style dripping wet hair with a brush. Using your fingers instead of a brush can prevent a lot of damage to the hair's cuticle. It is very important to avoid dragging a brush through soaking wet hair. Wait until your hair is somewhere between not damp but not yet dry; that's the time to pick up the brush and start setting the style in place.

First style the roots by lifting and moving them against the direction you want them to go. After you've removed some of the excess moisture from your hair, concentrate on styling the root area before the length of your hair. For the most lift, direct the heat on the roots first, either with your fingers **lifting** the roots away from the scalp in a **forward angle** or **in the opposite direction** from where you ultimately want it to go. This will set in a good deal of fullness. You can also do the same thing by bending and turning your head upside down and blowing the hair dry from underneath first.

Treat the length of hair differently than you treat the roots. The roots get blown in an angle up and away from the head or slightly against the direction you want the hair to go. The length of hair is blown dry as much as possible in the direction of the cuticle, down along the hair shaft. Blowing across or against the downward-facing structure of the hair shaft can make the hair fuzzy or encourage frizzies by roughing up the cuticle.

Aim the heat on the length of the hair in the direction you want the hair to go, following the hair. As basic as that sounds, I've seen women at the gym just aim the heat on their hair without any rhyme or reason. Blowing high heat on the hair without controlling it with your fingers or a brush can cause damage (by roughing up the cuticle) and tangles. If you want the hair to curl under, move the heat along the top of the hair shaft in a downward motion, following the brush or your hand. To prevent damage, keep the heat moving and avoid holding it in one place for too long.

If your hair is coarse or frizzy, blow it dry on a hotter setting. It would be great if low heat could shape hair, but it can't. Altering the natural shape of your hair, particularly if you are going from curly to straight, requires a high-heat setting—the higher the better. Heat helps mold and re-form hair. If you want to blow dry away the frizzies or smooth coarse, kinky, or curly hair, higher heat is the only way to accomplish it. High heat is more drying and damaging to the hair, but there is no way around it if you are going after a specific style.

If your hair is thin, blow it dry on a lower setting. High heat can blow the life out of hair. To maintain some amount of thickness and fullness, and to prevent blowing out all the hair's natural movement, use lower heat.

After you're done rough-drying your hair, work systematically, blow drying each area of your hair. In essence, you are making sure you are not laying dried hair over wet hair, which can destroy the smooth or softly curled style you were trying to create. Wet hair can make a style go flat or frizzy. It may be helpful (though more time-consuming) to securely clip sections of hair so they don't get in the way of the hair you are working on. But always be sure your hair is thoroughly dry if you want a style to last the entire day.

The right brush can make a tremendous difference in the finished look of your hair. For styling purposes, a vent brush is best for creating the most fullness, but it isn't great at smoothing out frizzies when your hair is coarse. A round, circular-bristled brush is best for making hair smooth and even. A round brush with pliable wire bristles inserted into a metal base can grab hair better and is good if you aren't adept at getting a bristled brush through your hair. On the other hand, wire bristles aren't the best for smoothing coarse hair—for that, the best choices are boar-bristled brushes that are firm but not hard.

Use the brush and blow dryer together as a unit. Keep the brush moving through the hair in tandem with the blow dryer. Roll the hair up into the brush, hold the dryer in this position for a few seconds, take the blow dryer away from the hair and allow the hair to cool, and then pull the brush through the hair, following with the blow dryer along the length of the hair. Some blow dryers have a button that provides a shot of cool air on the hair for that purpose. Heat temporarily re-forms the molecular bonds that give the hair its shape, so you can mold it into the shape you want; cool air resets those bonds to keep the new shape in place. To get this technique down, have your hairdresser give you a lesson, even if you have to pay for the extra time, this is money well spent.

A good blow dryer is lightweight and produces a concentrated gust of high heat. In general, if a blow dryer doesn't yield high-enough heat, it won't be able to smooth or form thick, coarse, or curly hair. If a blow dryer is too heavy, you won't be able to hold it in position (usually up and over your head) as long as necessary to get the hair completely dry while styling. Too much power and it will be hard to control your hair. If your hair is thin, fine, or normal thickness and straight or slightly wavy, a 1600-watt blow dryer will work great, or an 1875-watt blow dryer used on a low-heat setting. For thick, coarse, curly, frizzy, or extremely wavy hair, an 1875-watt blow dryer on the high setting works best.

Heat is everything. I know I've already said this, but let me repeat: Hot, direct heat is the best way to reconfigure hair. Almost everything you've read about blow dryers says to hold them between six and nine inches away from the hair. Although that is a great way to reduce damage, it is unrealistic for styling hair. It takes high heat to change the shape of hair and smooth frizzies. It helps to keep the brush and blow dryer moving over the hair. **To minimize damage when working on your own, try to never hold the blow dryer in one spot for more than a few seconds.** Spray-on styling products or rich conditioners can reduce the damage from high heat, but all in all, this part of hairstyling has more cons than pros. The only advantage is that your hair will look the way you want it to.

If you're in a hurry, which most of us are, and you don't have the time to make sure your entire head of hair is dry before you leave the house, concentrate your blow drying efforts on the front of the hair. The back can fall or frizz a little bit without causing a serious bad hair day, but you cannot ignore the front.

Hair diffusers are good for setting in curls. You will still want to rough-dry the hair first, scrunching the curls as you go to save time. When the hair is no longer damp but not yet dry, start concentrating the diffused air equally on the roots and the length of your hair. Directing your attention on the length only can make the hairstyle go flat. Also, aim the diffuser equally on the top of the hair as well as underneath.

Use your fingers or a wide-tooth comb as much as possible to separate and move the hair. The less you use brushes, the less you damage the hair.

When using regular rollers, set the hair when it is nearly dry to prevent long dry-ing periods. Spray the hair with a mist of hairspray, spray gel, or volumizing spray (which is nothing more than a lightweight hairspray with more water), then roll it up, but not too tightly. You don't have to roll the whole head to get the benefits of curlers.

When you are using a flat iron or curling iron, your hair must be absolutely dry before you begin. You must remove every last drop of moisture from your hair before you touch a flat iron or curling iron to your hair. Any moisture that is left in your hair can literally explode when in direct contact with the heat from a flat iron or curling iron, and that can cause extreme damage.

Smaller-circumference curling irons and hot rollers are great for setting in soft curls. The trick is to use them as a finishing tool when the hair is completely dry. If you wish, use a light styling spray to get the style to last longer. Do not use firm-hold styling products with heat-producing implements, as they can make the hair sticky and brittle. Firm-hold styling products are best for natural air-drying, not heat styling.

Larger-circumference curling irons and flat irons are great for straightening hair. These tools are the absolute standard for making hair look stick-straight. Smooth these slowly over small sections of the hair, starting at the root area, using even pressure over the length of the hair. Never hold a curling iron or flat iron on any one section of the hair for more than a few seconds or you will fry your hair.

TOOLS OF THE TRADE

Great technique means little without the right tools. Poor tools will leave your hair open to more damage and make your style look second-rate. You will be relieved to know that there are more good styling tools than bad. If that's true, you may be wondering, why doesn't a specific brush or curling iron work for my hair? It might not have anything to do with the quality of the implement, and everything to do with the type of hair you have. A brush that is great for coarse, thick hair may be the worst for thin, straight hair, while a brush that can smooth away frizzies might make some hair types go limp. Even the size of the styling tool can make a huge difference. A small-circumference brush will make hair curlier, while a large-circumference brush will smooth out the curls. Purchasing the right styling tool means knowing your hair type and knowing which brush, curling iron, blow dryer, or hot rollers work best with that kind of hair.

Do you have to spend a lot of money on styling implements? Absolutely not. There are great options available at the drugstore. Unfortunately, at least when it comes to inexpensive brushes, you can't often touch or feel the bristles to help you make a decision about how the brush will work in your hair. I've made a few brush recommendations on the next page.

When it comes to blow dryers, flat irons, and curling irons, there are great ones available at the drugstore. The following sections will help you find the right tools for your hair type. But when in doubt, given that you should need to buy hair brushes only once in a great while, just get the ones your stylist uses on your hair. It might be more expensive, but wasting money on brushes that don't work will only add to your collection of brushes, and it won't help your hair.

BRUSHES

The number of brush styles that exist, and the wide array of types and sizes they come in, is nothing less than astonishing. But to begin, you should be familiar with a few basic types of brushes.

Half-round brushes are basic for styling and brushing through the hair. As the name implies, the bristles go only halfway around the brush. Generally, this all-purpose brush is difficult to get wrong, but there are brushes of this type that have very pointed, sharp, or stiff plastic bristles that can hurt the scalp and chip away at the cuticle. If the bristles are too soft they won't smooth through hair. Half-round brushes are best for rough-drying or brushing hair after it is styled. Traditional half-round brushes are the **Denman Classic Styling 7-Row Medium Size Hair Brush** ($7.59) and **Bozzi Styler Brush** ($6.39).

Vent brushes are recognizable by their wide bristle spacing, rubber-tipped ends, and, often large spaces in the base of the brush. Vent brushes and standard half-round brushes generally have rubber handles and bases with plastic bristles inserted in a plastic cushion. They are great for arranging wet hair or brushing through already styled hair to refresh it. They can also work well when the goal is to blow fullness into the hair, particularly thin, limp, or fine hair. Because the vents allow heat to blow through the brush (and then through the hair), instead of capturing the heat, which helps smooth hair, they are a poor choice for eliminating frizzies. When it comes to blowing hair dry, it is best to use vent brushes in conjunction with natural-bristle round brushes (see below). Use a vent brush during the rough-drying stage and a natural-bristle round brush for the smoothing stage of the drying process. Typical vent brushes are the **Denman Tunnel Vent Hair Brush** ($9), **Bozzi Style Vent Brush** ($5), **Spornette Vent Brush** ($3.99), or **Conair Velvet Touch for Blow-Dry Styling** ($4.77) (though I wouldn't recommend the Conair brush for its stated purpose).

Brush Note: It is best when the handle and base of half-round brushes are made out of rubber because this material reduces static. Regardless of the brush type, always avoid nylon-bristled brushes unless they have rubber tips. Nylon is just too scratchy and stiff to be good for the scalp or hair.

Round brushes are easily recognizable because the bristles go all the way around the brush. Round brushes come in varying widths to accommodate tighter or smoother curls, and offer different bristle density. Large, natural-bristled round brushes are great for smoothing out frizzies and adding fullness to the hair. The smaller the width of a round brush, the better it is for shorter hair or, if you use it on longer hair, the tighter the curl it produces. If you have fine, thin, or limp hair, the softer-bristled round brushes work best. If you have thick, coarse, or extremely frizzy hair, a firmer-bristled brush is best. Bristles that are too stiff can break or increase damage to the hair. Round brushes should have enough flexibility to move through the hair, but be stiff enough to grab the hair and hold it while you move a blow dryer over it.

Round brushes also come with wire bristles attached to a metal cylinder. These are slightly less effective at blowing out frizzies for coarse hair, but great for adding fullness to thinner hair. The metal part retains heat from the blow dryer, working somewhat like a curling iron. Some round brushes have rubber bristles with rubber tips, which can be good for someone with thin, fine, or limp hair as a way to add fullness and waves. Because this type of brush tends not to grab and hold the hair well, and the rubber doesn't retain heat, it also tends to blow in frizzies. Classic round brushes are the **Conair Professional Hairbrush with Aluminum Barrel Round** ($4.99) and **Phillips Round Brushes** ($4.99 to $19.99, depending on the size of the brush).

Flat or paddle brushes are another tool for straightening long wavy or curly hair. These generally come with wire or nylon bristles set into a rubber cushion (similar to a pin cushion) on a wide, flat, oval or square base. Paddle brushes grab hair well and are best for straightening out stubborn curls, rather than for smoothing out frizzies. To smooth out the hair and get rid of frizzies, use a paddle brush in conjunction with a round natural-bristled brush. Typical paddle brushes are the **Denman Paddle Brush** ($8.99) and **Spornette Paddle Brush** ($4.99).

BRISTLES

Hairstylists are fond of bragging about natural boar bristles being the best for use on any hair type. It takes only a quick peek in any stylist's utensil drawer, however, to reveal a selection of brushes ranging from boar bristles (natural bristles) to synthetic versions. Boar bristles are not necessarily any easier on hair than synthetic bristles. Natural bristles do not reduce friction or stress on the hair, and they do not distribute oil or styling products through the hair better than other bristles. And boar bristles can differ—they range from so hard they can hurt the hair and scalp to so soft that you can't get the brush through the hair.

Regardless of the material, a brush should never scratch or scrape at the scalp or tug and tangle the hair. A good brush should easily smooth through hair without pulling or tearing at the hair, and the bristles should be long enough to easily grab and hold the hair and still easily release as you pull it through to the ends.

Nylon or plastic quill brushes (typically found in vent, paddle, or half-round styles) are great for brushing dry hair or for rough-drying hair. Select the ones where the ends are soft or have rounded tips to prevent damaging the hair or hurting your scalp.

Boar bristles are best for round brushing as you style your hair with a blow dryer. Boar-bristled brushes should not be used for general everyday brushing, and they should never be used for brushing through wet hair.

Wire quills are often used on round brushes that have metal bases. The metal bases help deliver more intense heat to hair and can improve drying time and styling control. Wire-quill round brushes are another alternative to boar-bristled round brushes—there is no advantage in using one over the other, it is merely a matter of preference.

Boar-bristled and nylon or plastic quill brushes often have rubber pads, and these impart an anti-static property that can be helpful if you tend to have flyaway hair.

HOT ROLLERS

Over the past twenty years, hot rollers have taken a back seat to curling irons and blow dryers. Hot rollers are considered less convenient because they have to sit in the hair for awhile, while curling irons do their job immediately. There are few models available, but all in all, when you do have the time, hot rollers are a relatively quick, easy way to smooth out frizzies and put in soft or tight curls. To get the most mileage out of any hot roller, be sure you smoothly and evenly roll the rods into neatly parted hair sections. Too much hair, bunched-up hair, or loose ends will get you the worst results from any hot roller set.

Dry-heat rollers are more efficient and faster than steam-heat or damp-heat rollers. Steam-heat rollers are a viable option if you have more time, and you'll need it, since both the steam rollers and the hair must dry completely before you remove the rollers so you don't get frizzies. Because of the moisture they provide and the soft sponge part of the curlers, steam-heat rollers are considered less damaging than dry-heat rollers, and better for hair that isn't frizzy or coarse. Steam-heat rollers may also reduce static.

Dry-heat roller options include the **Helen of Troy HotSetter Ceramic 14-Piece Hairsetter** ($44.95); **Remington Tight Curls Hot Rollers** ($24.95); **Hot Spa Professional Fast Heat Hairsetter** ($43.99); and **Conair Instant Heat Hairsetter** ($37.95). Steam-heat roller option: **Caruso SalonPro 30 Molecular Steam Hairsetter** ($41).

Step-by-step hot roller use suggestions:

- Plug in the hot rollers.

- Blow dry your hair while the rollers are heating up. Use your fingers to get lift at the root, but smooth the length straight.

- Apply a styling spray lightly over hair. Do not make hair too wet.

- Separate the hair into sections with clips and work on only one section at a time.

- Be sure hair has no knots or tangles before you begin.

- Wrap a roller around a two- to three-inch section of hair and secure it with the correct pin.

- Roll the hair in the direction you want the curl. Rolling the hair over the top of the roller curls the hair up. Rolling the hair under the roller creates a pageboy style. If the hair is styled back, roll away from the face; if hair is styled forward, roll toward the face.

- For straight hair, spray the hair with a light-hold hairspray while the rollers are in place and still warm.

- Depending on how much curl you want, let the rollers remain between 10 and 30 minutes.

✁ After removing the rollers, style the hair as desired, but do not overbrush or you will lose the curl.

CURLING IRONS

A hairstyling staple for decades, curling irons are a fast, relatively easy way to style hair once it is has been completely and thoroughly dried. It takes practice to become adept with them, but there are some great curling irons on the market that make experimentation easy. Most of the better ones come with variable heat settings and tips that don't get hot, and it is best if they come with a spring-clamp closure on the barrel. Variable heat means you can learn how to use the iron on the lowest setting, which reduces the chances of burning yourself or destroying your hair. The cylinders also come in a range of sizes; the wider the cylinder, the smoother the curl and the easier it is to use. Begin after your hair is completely dried, in small sections at the base of the neck, and work toward the top of the hair. Clamp and roll sections of hair from the ends up, hold for no more than 5 seconds, and then release. Repeat if necessary.

Some suggestions for a great curling iron are the **Hot Tools 2 Inch Curling Iron** ($29.95); **BaByliss Professional Computerized Curling Iron** ($59.95); **Belson Gold'N Hot Curling Iron-Spring Grip** ($27.95); and **Conair Satin Finish Instant Heat Ceramic Curling Iron 1-Inch Barrel** ($14.99).

Hot-air styling brushes with curling irons are situated somewhere between curling irons and blow dryers. They look like curling irons, but the metal cylinder extension blows diffused, low-force hot air out of the center instead of just generating heat. The heat is practically instantaneous, unlike curling irons, although the metal cylinder cools off quickly once it is turned off. These tools are an option for smoothing out the hair. Unlike hot rollers and curling irons, which should not be used until the hair is completely dry, hot-air styling brushes and curling irons can be used when the hair is still slightly damp. The diffused air helps dry the hair, and the metal cylinder heats up enough to ease away the frizzies—just don't expect the same smoothness you can achieve with a regular curling iron.

Options for hot-air styling brushes are the **Helen of Troy Tangle-Free Thermal Hot Air Brush** ($24.99), and **Ceramic Tools 1¼" Hot Air Brush** ($34.99).

BLOW DRYERS

Blow dryers are the most fundamental of styling tools. A good blow dryer is the cornerstone for getting the style you want as well as drying your hair in an efficient manner. Despite the need for a superior blow dryer, the best blow dryers for in-home use are not the same as the professional ones your hairstylist uses. You and your hairstylist have different needs. Perhaps one of the most critical elements to take into consideration is weight. If a blow dryer feels heavy in the store, it will feel like a ton when you've been holding it over your head for 15 minutes or more. Hairstylists can use a more heavy-duty blow dryer because they stand over your head, keeping their elbows at their sides, which reduces stress on the arms—but they also build up strength in their arms from using heavy dryers so often.

Two more crucial components for a blow dryer are the heat settings and the wattage. Most blow dryers have between 1200 and 1875 watts of power, with the power affecting the air speed. Most stylists consider 1875 watts essential for concentrating enough air and enough heat to get the hair dried and styled. With less than 1875 watts, it is hard to get enough heat to control and shape hair, although if you have short or thin hair a 1600-watt blow dryer is fine.

Be sure to check the heat settings; if they are hard to figure out or difficult to manipulate, you won't use them, and they are essential for blowing your hair dry. Full air with medium or high heat is great for rough-drying, medium to full air with high heat is best for smoothing out frizzies, and low air with medium to high heat is great for setting in curls.

Many blow dryers have a cool-shot button in the handle that delivers a blast of cool air to the hair. If you have the time, this is a decent way to set in the style, because as long as hair stays hot it is vulnerable to changing shape.

Be sure the cord of the blow dryer is at least 6 to 9 feet long. Any shorter and you won't have the flexibility you need to reach your head from all angles after you've plugged the dryer into the wall socket. Some blow dryers are designed to stay on only if you depress a trigger on the handle. When you release the handle they turn off, preventing accidental immersion in water while on. Although this safety device makes sense, it can be extremely difficult on your hand and arm to keep the trigger depressed the entire time you're styling.

A straight-nozzle blow dryer is the only kind to consider. The long, vent-style blow dryers might be OK for men's hairstyles, but they won't give you the control and concentrated heat you need to smooth and shape hair with a brush. Some blow dryers come packaged with attachments such as diffusers, combs, and pick-like implements. For the most part, the only useful attachment is the diffuser, which is great for gentle drying or setting in natural curls. Combs and pick-like implements can't replace fingers or natural-bristled and vent brushes. As a rule, the best routine is to have the brush move through the hair as the heat moves down and over the brush. When the heat blows *through* the hair, you can get frizzies.

There are myriad great hair dryers to consider. A few reliable favorites include the **Vidal Sassoon Professional 1875 Watt Dryer with Metal Finish** ($19.95); **BaByliss Professional Hair Dryer 1875 Watt** ($49.95); and **ConairPro Plimatic Turbo Hair Dryer** ($24.95).

CERAMIC FLAT IRONS

When used correctly, a flat iron is the ideal tool for temporarily making your hair perfectly straight. Flat irons come with a variety of different coatings, depending on the plating—from chrome to gold (well, metal with a gold color) to ceramic. Originally, all hairstylists used gold-plated irons because it was believed they delivered concentrated heat to the hair evenly and smoothly. Over the past few years, gold-plated flat irons have been replaced in most professional hairstylists' tool drawers with ceramic-plated versions.

Despite the claims that ceramic flat irons can seal moisture in the hair or repair hair, neither is true in the least. What truly makes ceramic the preferred material is that the surface is incredibly smooth. There is no pulling or tugging at the hair, and that prevents breakage and greatly reduces damage. Ceramic flat irons also allow the surface area of the iron to get uniformly hot, and even, high heat makes it possible to make hair remarkably stick-straight.

Some flat irons have teeth as a way to help you remove knots or tangles as you smooth the flat iron over the hair. That is an option, but the trick is to be sure the teeth are aiming downward so they comb through the hair ahead of the ceramic-plate part of the flat iron.

Before you touch any flat iron to your hair, it is critical that your hair is completely dry. If hair is wet, the heat from the flat iron will literally steam the water inside the hair shaft, bringing it to a boil, and that can rupture the hair in those areas. It is also imperative to keep the iron moving over the hair at all times. Never allow the iron to rest on any one part or you will fry the area.

There are so many ceramic-plate flat irons to recommend that the list is almost endless. You can get great results from those in all price ranges. Some to consider are the **Hot Tools Ceramic Flat Iron** ($39); **Wigo Professional Ceramic Flat Iron** ($39); **BaByliss Pro Vented Ceramic Hair Straightening Iron** ($79); **Ceramic Tools Professional Flat Iron** ($35); and **Vidal Sassoon Ceramic Hair Straightener** ($23).

Crimping irons are similar to flat irons except that they have an undulating surface that creates tight horizontal waves throughout the hair. This is a difficult tool to use on hair because it can be so damaging. To obtain the best results you have to hold the crimping iron on the same section of hair for several seconds, and even longer if hair is thick or coarse, which is far longer than you would a flat iron, and that amount of time is plainly enough to cook the hair. For an occasional fun look it is an option, but it's best for your hair to use it as infrequently as possible.

Crimping iron options are the **Hot Tools Professional Hair Crimper** ($29) and **BaByliss Professional Texturizing Iron** ($79).

PROTECTING HAIR FROM HEAT

Lots and lots of products claim they can protect hair from the damaging heat generated by styling tools such as blow dryers, curling irons, and flat irons. To some extent, that is true. If the hair has a coating of conditioners, silicone serums, or styling lotions (when they contain silicones, glycerin, emollients, or water-binding agents), it can indeed reduce the damage caused by the heat from styling tools. But this protection is in no way absolute or complete, not by any stretch of the imagination. Blow dryers, curling irons, and flat irons can heat up to well past the boiling point. If those tools can burn skin (which they indeed can), they can damage hair. Styling products help protect the cuticle to some degree, but do not assume for one second that this buffering layer is a guarantee of no damage. As seductive as the claims of hair-protecting products sound, they cannot eliminate heat damage caused by styling tools. Nevertheless, they can reduce problems, and that can keep damage at bay for longer than if you had used nothing on your hair at all.

HAIR WANDS

There are several product catalogs and Web sites selling a device called the Ionic Hair Wand ($39), claiming that when this product is stroked through the hair, it "bathes each strand in ions, which adds body and volume; calms dry, brittle, or windblown hair; ... removes such odors as cigarette smoke; ... [and] reduces bacteria on the hair and scalp, while removing particles such as dandruff flakes; ... [and it] actually smoothes the hair by causing hair cuticle shafts to lie flat. It also unifies the charge, so hair strands no longer clump together."

If you've taken one or two chemistry courses you'll see enough scientific lingo here to sound almost convincing, but just almost, because you would also have enough information to know that other parts sound almost laughable. I guess you can put a price on anything, including static electricity, which is the issue at hand for the Ionic Hair Wand.

Ions are nothing more than groups of atoms that have a positive, negative, or neutral electric charge. They can't repair anything, despite the claims in the catalogs selling these implements. Hair itself has a negative electrical charge and is attracted to things with a positive charge. (Two positives repel each other and two negatives repel each other, but a positive and a negative attract.) Hair becomes flyaway when positive ions (static electricity) are conducted through the body (electricity can pass through people) and build up. The negatively charged hair responds to this positive charge moving up through the body and out the top of the head by standing on end. If you diminish or eliminate the static charge flowing up through the hair (that is, stop the flow of the positive ions), your hair will calm down. It's just that simple. Of course, if the air is cold, the second you shuffle over a carpet or some other fabric, static electricity will be generated again. And if the wand isn't nearby, your hair will take off again.

The information for this device also asserts that damaged or roughed-up scales on the hair shaft can be smoothed down by the wand's ion output. I assume that the same static charge that makes hair lift can get under the scales and make them lift and that negating that charge can reduce some frizziness. However, other things can also cause the hair to be frizzy, including humidity, curly hair's growth pattern, and the relative thickness of the hair, and none of these can be affected by ions.

The possibility that dandruff and bacteria will jump off the hair and scalp and grab the wand is much more suspect. If the electrical charge of the dandruff and bacteria is different from that of the wand, I suppose they would be attracted to the wand and cling to that instead of to the hair or scalp. However, you would never get all the bacteria and dandruff off the hair or scalp, nor would you be changing the environment under the skin of the scalp (where the wand's ions can't reach), which is causing the dandruff in the first place. In other words, don't rely on these hair wands as a dandruff remedy.

HAIR TIPS FROM TOP TO BOTTOM

This section just includes some reminders, a summary of the more salient points discussed throughout the entire book. They aren't the whole story, but they are standard operating procedures for getting your hair to behave and survive the latest hair fashion. If you want to convince your hair to do what it would rather not do, these concepts are basic.

- ✂ **When you wash your hair, take more time washing your scalp than the ends of your hair.** Hair ends don't get all that dirty (unless you've got large doses of styling products layered over them), but the scalp can get oily and can accumulate dead skin cells that need to come off. In addition, the scalp almost always can benefit from a massage, which will increase healthy circulation and help the hair that's developing in the follicles.

- ✂ **Conditioners that claim to deeply penetrate work only if there's enough time and heat for them to be absorbed into the hair shaft.** Most women who apply a conditioner in the shower never leave it on for longer than 1 or 2 minutes. That's fine, but don't expect the hair to soak it up. If you have damaged hair, it is very important to leave the conditioner on for as long as possible.

- ✂ **Too much conditioner or conditioner that isn't thoroughly rinsed out can make hair go limp.** Using a shampoo that contains conditioning agents plus a conditioner can result in buildup on the hair, making it heavy and lifeless. Generally, a shampoo with minimal or no conditioning agents at all is best, and then use your conditioner only where you need it, not necessarily all over or near the roots and scalp.

- ✂ **Be careful to thoroughly rinse shampoo out of your hair.** Leaving traces of detergent cleansing agents behind can make hair sticky and flat.

- ✂ **The longer you leave a dandruff shampoo on your hair, the more effective it will be.**

- ✂ **Apply shampoo and conditioner by first spreading it over your hands and then smoothing it over the hair.** Placing one big dollop in the middle and then working it through the hair wastes product and roughs up the hair more than necessary.

✄ **When in doubt, use products designed for your hair type.** Unless you have truly normal hair, undesignated products are not for everyone. There is no such thing as a one-size-fits-all hair-care product. Someone with coarse, dry hair has very different needs from someone with thin, healthy hair.

✄ **Every now and then, take your brush and comb into the shower with you and give them a good shampooing.** Styling products, conditioners, and your own oil can cling to brushes and combs, transferring some of the grime back to your clean hair. Remove the excess hair and go for it. For a more thorough cleansing, or if you have dandruff, soak them in a solution of diluted bleach; about three table spoons to a quart of water should be enough to kill whatever may be lurking around or between the bristles.

✄ **When using a blow dryer, hair is easier to style and control when it is damp but not wet.** When it comes to blow drying, hair can be fickle. It takes some experi- mentation to find out how damp your hair needs to be to get the best smooth ness. It is also less damaging to hair to blow it dry with a styling brush when it is slightly dry; wet hair is more vulnerable to damage than dry hair.

✄ **Always dry the root area first.** This will provide the most fullness and control the basic shape of the style you're trying to achieve.

✄ **Never use a curling iron on wet or damp hair.** The heat from a curling iron can easily exceed the boiling point of water. The water content inside the hair shaft can actually boil if you apply a hot curling iron to it, and cause serious breakage and damage in that spot.

✄ **When blowing your hair dry, go after the roots first.** Drying the roots up and away from the direction you want will achieve fullness and create the foundation for the rest of the hairstyle. Once the roots are done, you can smooth or curl the rest of the hair. If you leave the roots until last, they may already have dried in a direction you didn't want them to go, making them harder to shape. The length of the hair is easier to manipulate even if it is somewhat dry.

✄ **Wet or damp hair is more vulnerable to losing its shape.** It is best to blow your hair all the way dry and not leave any wetness, not even a little. Unless partial natural movement is what you are after, blow the entire head completely dry in order to keep the style in for as long as possible.

✄ **If you have the time, alternate using hot air and cool air while blow drying.** Heat forms the curl or smoothness, and the cool air helps keep it there.

✄ **To help prevent hairspray from flaking off in white specks, apply it at least six inches away from the hair.** A concentrated blast can make the polymers and resins go on too thickly, causing a stiff, matte bond that can lead to flaking.

✂ **Never backcomb or tease hair.** It is damaging, plain and simple, and there is no way around this one.

✂ **Do not use rubber bands.** Use only soft fabric tie-backs for your hair. Rubber bands or anything that pinches hair is chipping away at the cuticle, and when you remove a rubber band, it takes lots of hair with it.

GETTING IT STRAIGHT

For straightening hair, your best friends are either a blow dryer and a round brush, or a ceramic-plated flat iron. Both are great options, and deciding which to use is completely a matter of preference. However, a combination of both a blow dryer, round brush, and a flat iron can produce optimal results. Using a blow dryer and round brush first gives the hair lift and fullness. Then you can finish over the ends or areas that need smoothing with a flat iron, providing the best of both worlds.

✂ First you need to use a good emollient conditioner on the length of your hair. Depending on your hair type, both leave-in and rinse-out types are just fine. Leave-in is best if your hair is hard to control or very thick and frizzy.

✂ Towel-dry well by dabbing and blotting; avoid tousling or rubbing, which can damage the hair shaft.

✂ If you have dry, damaged, thick, or coarse hair, apply silicone serum to the length of hair, avoiding the root area (it can weigh hair down and make it look greasy). Adding silicone serum to the length adds a silky feel, helps start the smoothing process, and provides a small amount of heat protection.

✂ Then apply a hair-straightening gel or lotion, though almost any gel or mousse for your hair type will work.

✂ Next, use your blow dryer all over to remove excess moisture, lifting the hair at the root and smoothing the length of hair as you proceed from section to section. Be sure to get the underneath part of the hair, where water loves to hide and hold on.

✂ Use a ponytail holder or large clips to partition your hair. Start with the bottom layer near the neck and work your way up. If you have full hair, be sure to lift the roots up and concentrate the heat in that area, over every section. If you have flatter hair, pull the roots down and concentrate the heat there.

✂ The best tools are boar-bristled round brushes with wood handles, or metal-framed round brushes with plastic handles and synthetic quills. Vent or half-round brushes tend to make hair frizzy, so they work best on hair that tends to be naturally smoother. Both wood- and metal-framed round brushes work well, but, as a general rule, metal-framed brushes are better for slightly wavy hair that is fine or thin, and boar-bristled round brushes are better for coarse or thick curly hair. The larger the brush, the straighter your hair will be.

✂ You may have to round-brush several times over each section, following the blow dryer as you use the brush to smooth out the hair. Be sure to apply heat to the hair on top of the brush as well as the underside to get each small section entirely dry, and to distribute the heat evenly over the hair. You need to be patient on this step, because this is the only way to go about it.

✂ Be sure the hair is 100% dry. Any amount of dampness, no matter how slight, can change your hair from straight to frizzy or curly.

✂ After you are done blow drying and round-brushing your hair, go over the length of hair in small sections with a ceramic-plated flat iron for even smoother and straighter results.

✂ A small amount of pomade or styling wax can be used over the frizziest areas to get control and extra smoothness.

Tension and heat are the keys to getting hair straight. The tighter you pull your hair and the better able you are to get heat on it, the straighter it will be. The reason stylists can get your hair so straight is because they are in the perfect position to apply the necessary tension to make hair behave, and their styling tools generate intense heat. Another trick stylists use is to keep the blow dryer moving instead of leaving it in one spot. Aiming the heat at the roots and making sure the roots are going in the direction you want—up for more fullness, down for straightening—is the best way to get control of your locks. Another styling essential is to move the blow dryer down along the hair shaft instead of back and forth.

When Not to Straighten? Anytime humidity is in the air (which is not the same as a rainy day) it is best to let your curls or waves rule. It is impossible to keep humidity out of your hair, and once the moisture in your hair exceeds the normal amount that healthy hair contains, it will lose the shape you created and revert to its natural state, regardless of the products you use and the all-day, anti-humidity claims they advertise.

PRETTY CURLS

In some ways, curly hair is harder to control—but there is so much you can do with it! A tousled messy look, soft flowing curls, big looping tendrils, or twisted tresses are all options. Curling irons, hot rollers, and blow dryers with diffusers are all great ways to control curl. If you have straight hair and want to create curls, review the section above on hot rollers and curling irons. For those of you with natural curl, following are some suggestions to get everything moving in the right direction:

✂ Use an emollient conditioner on the length of hair, avoiding the roots, so you don't weight your hair down.

✂ Apply a silicone serum or spray over the dry areas of your hair, avoiding the scalp.

✂ Apply a light-hold mousse or styling gel over damp hair.

- ✂ Using a wide-tooth comb, separate the hair to eliminate tangles and knots.

- ✂ Then use your fingers to tousle the hair and bring out the curls you have.

- ✂ Using a blow dryer on medium heat and medium air speed with a diffuser, twist your hair into the shape of curl or tousled look you want to create, lifting at the root as you do.

- ✂ As the hair becomes dry, touch your hair as little as possible except for scrunching or lifting.

- ✂ When hair is completely dry, apply a lightweight, gel-style pomade with no holding agents to keep frizzies at a minimum without adding stiffness or stickiness to hair.

PRODUCT APPLICATION

You're looking at all the varied product options for styling hair—gels, laminates (silicone serums), pomades, styling sprays, and hairsprays—and wondering which to apply when. That's a good question. The only universally agreed upon order of things is that hairspray is applied last, after you are done styling. When to apply all other styling products depends on what hairstyle you are trying to create and your own personal preference. For example, if you have particularly coarse, curly hair and you are trying to get it to appear straighter and smoother, then it may be best to first apply a silicone serum all over the hair to get the silky-smooth feeling down first. Then you can apply a styling gel, styling spray, or mousse to begin the styling process of blowing the hair dry and/or using a curling iron. When you are done with that, you can apply a pomade or styling wax over stubborn ends to tame them. On the other hand, some hairstylists like to apply styling gels, sprays, or mousses first and then add silicone serum. It all depends on what works best for your hair.

For those with fine or thin hair, layering on styling products can be a problem. A leave-in conditioner with hairspray-type ingredients (film formers) may be enough and eliminate the need for any other styling product, although you can add a styling spray over stubborn areas. But be careful: Fine, thin hair gets weighed down easily by styling products.

FIGHTING HUMIDITY AND DESERT HEAT

Hair loses its shape at the extremes—when there is too much moisture in the air or when there's no moisture in the air. All the hair products and hair tips in the world can't convincingly counteract what I call Hawaii hair or Arizona hair.

Hawaii hair refers to what happens to hair when it is bombarded by high humidity. Some very stiff, firm-hold hairsprays can keep humidity off the hair, but then you sacrifice movement and your hair looks like a helmet, and even that isn't a guarantee.

Arizona hair occurs when extremely dry air sucks moisture from the hair shaft. You can load up the hair with conditioning agents, but then you end up with heavy, limp, or greasy hair, and even that can only do so much to keep some amount of moisture in your hair.

Myriad products try to combat all this, and their claims could fill a library, but the end results, as you will see from my reviews, are limited. You can fight physics, chemistry, and biology with hair-care products and styling tools only up to a point. After that, for the most part, genetics and the environment win.

If you still want to wage war against humidity (or lack of it), the following may give you a fighting chance:

- Shampoo and condition your hair as always.

- When the hair is wet, apply a lightweight silicone serum or silicone spray to the parts of your hair that tend to be frizziest or driest.

- Next apply a styling lotion or spray gel.

- Blow dry your hair smooth with a boar-bristle round brush. Be sure the hair is 100% dry, and then finish with a flat iron over the length of hair to seal in as much straightness as you can.

- Smooth pomade over the ends, flyaways, and the surface of the hair.

- Follow with a light application of medium-hold hairspray (regular or aerosol).

- Keep the pomade with you to smooth frizzies as they occur during the day.

STYLING PROBLEMS? STYLING SOLUTIONS!

Question: I have used lots of conditioners but they all seem to weigh my hair down. Is there a solution?

Answer: There are many reasons why conditioners are weighing your hair down. You may not be using the right conditioner for your hair type. If it's too rich and emollient it can be extremely heavy for fine, thin, or normal hair. You may be using the right conditioner but using too much of it, which can weigh hair down. You may also not need conditioner all over your hair, which is often the way it's applied, but rather only over the length of hair, far away from the root area. Applying too much conditioner at the root can make most hair types go limp. One other possibility is that you may not be rinsing your hair well enough; a thorough rinsing is essential to get the best results.

Question: Does diet affect my hair?

Answer: Popular theory has long suggested that vitamin A, vitamin B6, vitamin B12, folic acid, biotin, vitamin C, copper, iron, and zinc are hair-healthy vitamins and minerals, but there is little research showing that to be fact. One study (*Clinical Experimental Dermatology*, July 2002, pages 396–404) stated that "little is known about nutritional factors and hair loss. What we do know emanates from studies in protein-energy malnutrition, starvation, and eating disorders. There is no evidence to support the popular view that low serum zinc concentrations cause hair loss. Excessive intakes of nutritional supplements may actually cause hair loss and are not recommended in the absence of a proven deficiency." A healthy, balanced diet rich in antioxidants and a good multiple vitamin should cover all your bases and concerns.

Question: My hair is always frizzy. What should I do?

Answer. Many great silicone-based products are available that can help start the process of smoothing away your frizzies. Pomades and gel-style pomades are the next step to add a bit of weight and creaminess to ends and flyaways. The trick with both pomades and silicone serums (serums are best for coarse, thick hair) or sprays (sprays are better for fine, thin hair) is to use them sparingly. Applying too much can make hair look heavy and greasy.

Problem: What can I do about my dull hair?

Solution: First, make sure your hair is not a victim of product buildup from your shampoo. When a shampoo contains conditioning ingredients or volumizing ingredients, they are repeatedly deposited on the hair and are never really washed off. You can solve that problem by washing with a shampoo that contains none of these ingredients. Then follow up with a conditioner for your hair type, applied only where hair is dry. After that, the best way to add shine is, in one word, silicone, in the form of sprays or serums. Silicones offer almost foolproof results every time. If your hair's dullness stems from the color you dyed it, chances are you need to dye your hair again because the original color has faded, which greatly diminishes your hair's vibrancy.

Problem: What can I do about my dry hair?

Solution: Be sure you are using one of the gentle shampoos and conditioners for dry, damaged hair recommended in Chapter Ten, "Product Reviews." Also, be sure you are using styling lotions and gels that list silicone as one of the main ingredients. This will immediately add a silky, smooth feel to hair.

Problem: What can I do about my oily scalp?

Solution: There really isn't anything you can do for oily scalp, at least not in terms of controlling it. Oil production is controlled by your hormones and there isn't anything you can apply topically on the scalp (or anyplace on the skin) that can affect that. What you can do is wash your hair more frequently. Don't be afraid to clean your hair every day or every other day as long as you use a gentle shampoo. It doesn't take harsh or extra-strong shampoos to clean oil away; gentle shampoos are just as effective. Also, never use a two-in-one shampoo, because the conditioning agents in this type of shampoo will get deposited on the scalp *and* at the root, adding to your own oil. If you do use a conditioner, keep it far away from the scalp area. Take the same precautions with styling products, too, because many of these contain emollients or silicones that can make the scalp area or hair look oilier.

CHAPTER TEN

Product Reviews

THE PROCESS

You may well be wondering how I go about deciding what distinguishes a terrible product from an OK one, or a good product from a fantastic one. Above all, I want you to know that I do *not* base my decisions on my own personal experience and I do *not* let my personal feelings about a particular company blur my judgment. In other words, I know that just because I happen to like the way a shampoo or conditioner feels on my hair doesn't mean that someone else will feel the same way about their experience with that product. I base my decisions on the individual product's formulation, using published research about the ingredients and their possible resulting interactions with the hair and scalp. Further, every styling product reviewed in this book was tested for feel, texture, performance, weight, and intended function. Whether or not I think a company is absurdly overcharging for its products or is exceedingly dishonest in its claims and literature, and no matter how unethical I find it, that won't prevent me from saying a product is good for a particular hair type (though I do often say something like, "This is a good product but what a shame the price has to be so absurd and the claims so offensive and deceptive!").

I also asked the following questions to determine if a product could hold up to its claims, based on established research: (1) Given the ingredient list, could the product do what it promised? (2) How did the product differ from other products? (3) If a special ingredient or ingredients were showcased, how much of them were actually in the product, and was there independent, substantiated research verifying the claims for those ingredients? (4) Did the product contain problematic preservatives, fragrances, coloring agents, plants, or other questionable ingredients? (5) How farfetched were the product's claims? (6) If a product said it was good for sensitive skin or scalp, did it in fact actually contain irritants, skin sensitizers, or drying ingredients?

I wish I had the space to challenge and explain every single exaggerated claim and lofty explanation that accompanies the products reviewed in this chapter, but there is just not enough room (or time) to tackle that prodigious task. For this book, I wanted to include all the information I could to provide you with as much information as possible to help you understand the sales pitches so you can focus on a product's quality, realistic performance, and "feel," and not be taken in by deceptive marketing and advertising practices.

For those of you who are familiar with my reviews, you may notice that in this edition I am much more cautious about hair products that contain any amount of irritating ingredients, particularly those products containing lemon, grapefruit, mint, peppermint, menthol, camphor, eucalyptus, ivy, fragrant oils, overly drying detergent cleansing agents, or excessive amounts of useless plant extracts. These can all cause a flaky, itchy scalp—and some of them can dry out and damage hair.

My reviews of hair-care products, with a few exceptions, are organized in the following categories within each line: shampoos, conditioners, styling products, and specialty products such as hair masks or special conditioning treatments.

THE INGREDIENTS FOR HAIR CARE

Although I want to emphasize to what extent companies portray their hair-care products in misleading and disingenuous ways, I also want to underscore that great products *do* exist for all hair types. Yet, even when a product receives a good rating, that doesn't mean I agree with the claims or descriptions attributed to that product or with the hair type for which it is recommended. My positive recommendations are still often accompanied by comments about outrageous pricing, or the fact that the formula is best for oily hair and scalp even though it is labeled as being for dry or damaged hair. You will also find that I never go along when a product makes impossible claims. For example, I make it clear that it is a physiological impossibility for any hair-care product to repair or restructure hair.

Every hair-care product was first evaluated on the basis of what it contains (the ingredients) and then on how it performed. This was especially true for styling products; a real-life version of every styling product reviewed in this book was tested for whether it was greasy, sticky, stiff, or flaky. However, the ingredients and product application are always the basis for whether a claim can be verified. Remember that the relative amounts of the ingredients in a product always correspond to the order in which the ingredients appear on the ingredient list. Also, ingredients listed from about the midpoint to the end of the ingredient list are typically present in only trivial traces.

When reading ingredient lists, it is also important to note that the closer a specific ingredient's position on the list is to a preservative (such as methylparaben, propylparaben, ethylparaben, imidazolidinyl urea, or quaternium-15) or a fragrance (listed as fragrance or often as an individual essential oil like lavender or bergamot oil or as parfum) and the closer it is to the end of the ingredient list, the less likely that that ingredient is present in any significant amount.

Some ingredient groups, such as thickening agents, conditioning agents, and emollients, can overlap in function. All of these are technically interchangeable, but I refer to a specific type of ingredient according to its most typical function in a formulation. The same is true for detangling agents and film formers, whose functions can also overlap, though I describe them according to their predominant use in the product. This is also the case for some lather agents and detergent cleansing agents, which are often listed in conditioners and styling products, but the amounts used indicate they are meant to function as emulsifiers, ingredients that keep other ingredients mixed together. I did not indicate these occurrences in the product summaries.

When an ingredient is included in a product primarily for its cleansing ability I use the general term **detergent cleansing agent**. Ingredients in this category include sodium lauryl sulfate, sodium laureth sulfate, cocamidopropyl betaine, sodium cocoyl isethionate, sodium cocoamphoacetate, TEA-lauryl sulfate, cocamide DEA, ammonium laureth sulfate, and ammonium lauryl sulfate, to name a few (though these are the most common). Because sodium lauryl sulfate, TEA-lauryl sulfate, sodium C14-16 olefin sulfonate (and the lesser used sodium dodecyl sulfonate and alkyl benzene sulfonate) are very strong, drying, and irritating detergent cleansing agents, I warn against using a product that contains these ingredients when they are listed in the first part of the ingredient list. For those who dye their hair, using a product with sodium C14-16 olefin sulfonate, sodium dodecyl sulfonate, or alkyl benzene sulfonate can potentially strip hair color.

Lather agents are ingredients added to shampoos strictly to create a healthy dose of foaming suds on the hair. Most women don't feel that their hair is getting clean unless there is foam, yet the amount of foam is completely unrelated to the effectiveness of the detergent cleansing agents, and these agents are added strictly for aesthetics and consumer appeal.

Conditioning agents or **emollients** are designations I give to ingredients that are noted for their ability to coat hair and help improve its feel, perceived thickness, smoothness, and tensile strength. Some are better at this than others, but they are not the ones you immediately notice on an ingredient list. Proteins, amino acids, collagen, elastin, panthenol, and other hair healthy-sounding ingredients do an OK job, but they don't perform as well as you might expect given their names. However, the range of other conditioning and emollient ingredients, from silicones to quats (see detangling agents below), all do a very good job and help a conditioner provide the feel you want for your hair.

Silicone is an exceptionally hair-friendly ingredient that shows up repeatedly—it's in almost 80% of all hair-care products sold. This standard conditioning agent deserves special mention because it has unique properties and benefits for hair. Silicone's chemical components, technically speaking, are related to fluid technology, and they give an exquisite, silky, somewhat slippery feel to the hair. Its popularity in formulations reflects its versatility and the finish it gives. It is standard in all kinds of cosmetic products in all price ranges. In hair-care products, it is by far one of the fundamental conditioning agents, and is unequalled at producing shine, while also helping to protect hair during heat styling. It can cause buildup when overused, but just the tiniest amount can impart phenomenal smoothness, comb-ability, and luster to hair.

Castor oil and **mineral oil** are also typical conditioning ingredients that show up in many hair-care products. Castor oil's unique properties warrant an explanation about the way it affects a product's performance. Castor oil is a seed extract (there is actually a castor bean plant), an oil that, when dried, imparts a shiny look and smooth feel to hair; it can also be greasy and have a slightly sticky feel. The combination of shine and stickiness makes this an interesting, worthwhile styling agent for stubborn frizzies or curls. Mineral oil gets a bad rap in the cosmetics industry for being harsh or unnatural, when in fact it is neither. Mineral oil is one of the most benign of all cosmetic ingredients, rivaling even water in terms of lack of irritation potential. Regardless of the myths, for the hair it is a good conditioning agent, providing slip and conditioning effects on all degrees of dry hair.

When I use the term **thickener**, I'm referring to those ingredients that add texture, thickness, viscosity, spreadability, and stability to a product. Thickeners (when used as emulsifiers) are vital for their ability to help keep other ingredients mixed together. They also have a waxlike texture or a creamy, emollient feel, and can be great lubricants or conditioning agents. There are literally thousands of ingredients in this category, and they are the staples of every hair-care product out there.

A wide range of technical and chemical-sounding ingredients are used in shampoos and conditioners to make hair more comb-able, and I refer to these as **detangling agents**. This group of ingredients is known in the industry primarily by the abbreviated name "quats," derived from such common detangling agents as quaternium 18 or polyquaternium-11. Their unique molecular structure allows quats to cling to hair in a way that helps a brush or comb glide easily through the hair. Some detangling agents also function as film formers (see below).

Film formers are ingredients such as PVP, acrylates, acrylamides, styrene, crotonic acid, vinyl acetate/crotonates, vinyl neodecanoate copolymer, methacrylate copolymer, and polyglycerylacrylates, among many others that are the backbone of any styling product that pledges to provide some level of hold or control. This small but essential group of plastic resins holds hair in place, with relative comb-ability and firmness. These are also used in volumizing or thickening shampoos and conditioners to uniformly coat hair and add a feeling of thickness. What all film formers have in common is that they impart stiffness (of varying degrees) and leave a sticky feel on the hair. There is no way around this one because there are no film formers (and definitely not any one plant extract) that can hold hair in place without some firmness and a sticky feel. They also add weight to hair, which those with fine and thin hair may find heavy or flattening. What is most shocking about this group of ingredients is their redundancy; the same film-forming agents show up in product after product after product, and in all price ranges. Despite what you may emotionally think of less expensive products, the ingredients they contain to hold hair in place do not differ from those in the expensive ones.

Water can be given an elevated status by using an assortment of exclusive-sounding adjectives—deionized, purified, oxygenated, triple-purified, demineralized—to describe what is actually just plain water. These terms indicate that the water has gone through some kind of purification process, something that is quite standard for cosmetics and not the least bit special. You will also find phrases such as "infusions of" or "aqueous extracts of" followed by the name of one or a long list of plant extracts. I use the term **tea** when that type of concoction is listed; it merely means that you're getting nothing more than a tea concocted from a group of plants, or plant juice mixed with water. Is there any benefit to plant water? The hair-care industry would love you to believe there is—but water is water! The kind of water used does not affect the hair or the scalp, unless you happen to be allergic or sensitive to the myriad bouquets thrown into the product. As to the tea or plant water, even if the plant could be effective for hair care, after being combined with other ingredients, its original status is all but lost.

It is impossible to list all the individual **plant extracts** used in hair-care products. As far as the hair-care industry would have you believe, if it grows it can improve hair. Yet there is no consensus on which plant is the most amazing and there is no research demonstrating any hair-friendly properties for most plants. Of course, that's not what the hair-care companies want you to believe! As far as they are concerned plants from ginger to hemp, mango, pineapple, sambucus, horse chestnut, dandelion, oak bark, lemon, grapefruit, coffee, and on and on and on can all have the most astonishing merits. For hair, all of these are meaningless (Sources: *Encyclopedia of Shampoo Ingredients*, Anthony L. L. Hunting, 1998, Micelle Press, Port Washington, NY; and *Encyclopedia of Conditioning Rinse Ingredients*, Anthony L. L. Hunting, 1987, Micelle Press, Port Washington, NY). What is more significant for the scalp is that some of the plant extracts thrown into hair-care products to impress the consumer often are the actual cause of itching or irritation.

Plant oils (other than those called essential oils) are almost always beneficial as conditioning agents. The debate about whether or not sunflower, canola, olive, avocado, almond, or any of myriad other oils or blends of oils is superior is a marketing game to showcase a product; it has nothing to do with common sense about hair.

Some plant oils, often referred to as **essential oils**, are highly fragrant, volatile oils, and because these are usually irritants I indicate it when this is the case. However, I attribute no superiority to one over another, because none exists. Essential oils are nothing more than a way to get fragrance into a hair-care product. The hair-care industry knows that many women are aware that fragrance can be a strong source of skin irritation and sensitivities, so the companies use the term "essential oils" as a way to add fragrance to a product without saying "fragrance." Even though women know that fragrance ingredients are bad, they still want their products to smell nice. Caught between a rock and a hard place, the hair-care industry came up with essential oils as the way around the dilemma. But the notion that plants can save the hair is sheer fantasy and has no legitimate substantiation.

Vitamins in hair-care products are useless. Not only can they not feed dead hair, they also don't cling well to the hair shaft—so they aren't effective as conditioning agents either. Ingredients like panthenol and biotin do have vitamin origins, but their effectiveness for the hair has nothing to do with nutrients; they work because they cling to the hair shaft, improving feel and tensile strength just like any other conditioning agent.

For the scalp, vitamins would be rinsed off or brushed away before they had a chance to be effective. For skin care, most vitamins do perform well as **antioxidants**, but in hair-care products they just aren't around long enough to perform that function, especially under rinsing or the heat from styling tools. While there is impressive research pointing to the effectiveness of antioxidants for skin, there is no such research in regard to hair care.

Anti-irritants and **soothing agents** are ingredients known for their ability to reduce inflammation. A small group of ingredients, such as bisabolol, allantoin, burdock root, aloe, licorice root, and green tea, can perform this function. These ingredients work much better in skin-care products than in hair-care products because they need to be left on the skin (or scalp) to have an effect. In shampoos and conditioners, where they are typically found, such products are rinsed off before they ever have a chance to work.

Slip agents help other ingredients spread over or penetrate the hair's cuticle, and they have some moisturizing properties. Slip agents include propylene glycol, butylene glycol, polysorbates, and glycerin. They are as basic to the world of hair care as water.

Water-binding agents are known for their ability to help the hair retain water, but they have only minimal effectiveness because, with few exceptions, they are so easily rinsed or brushed away. These ingredients range from the mundane glycerin and propylene glycol to the more exotic hyaluronic acid, sodium hyaluronate, mucopolysaccharides, sodium PCA, collagen, elastin, proteins, amino acids (of which there are dozens), cholesterol, glucose, sucrose, fructose, glycogen, phospholipids, glycosphingolipids, and on and on. For the most part they all work equally well, and there is research indicating that the inexpensive standard ingredients such as glycerin and propylene glycol may be the most effective for clinging to hair and protecting from some heat damage. Despite this, looking for a specific ingredient is a waste of your time and energy. They are all what they are—good water-binding ingredients.

In the same way that the film formers mentioned above are fundamental to any hairstyling product, **propellants** are essential to aerosol-delivered hairstyling products, from mousses to hairsprays. Propellants such as butane and propane disperse a product over the hair in an aerated mist or a foaming lather. Whether you use an aerosol or a regular hairspray is personal preference. Some prefer the aerosol version because it sprays a fine, even mist, as compared to a regular hairspray that tends to concentrate the mist more and to cover less uniformly.

It is typical for aerosol and some nonaerosol hair sprays (as well as hairstyling gels) to contain **alcohol** as the main ingredient (I'm not referring to stearyl alcohol or cetyl alcohol, which are just benign thickening agents), usually listed as SD alcohol, isopropyl alcohol, or denatured alcohol. As drying as alcohol can be for the skin and hair, in hairsprays or styling products it evaporates before it has a chance to affect the hair negatively. In this regard, alcohol is a blessing for the hair, because liquid alternatives would quickly wreck a hairstyle! For gels and spray gels, the alcohol is slightly more problematic for hair, but not much. Its job is truly to evaporate before it has much of a chance to affect the hair, although it also helps the styling ingredients set faster on the hair without oversaturating it with more water.

Almost every single hair-care product in this book contains **fragrance**. Fragrances are used in cosmetics either to mask the smell of a product's ingredients or to add a specific fragrance. They have no other benefit. I clearly indicate the few instances when a product is truly fragrance free, and also indicate the many instances where the fragrance-free claim is in error.

The controversies surrounding the use of some **preservatives** in cosmetics, such as quaternium-15, 2-bromo-2-nitropane-1, 3-diol, dmdm hydantoin, methylparaben, and Kathon CG (methylisothiazolinone and methylchloroisothiazolinone) are explained at length on my Web site at www.cosmeticscop.com.

However, aside from specific issues for some specific preservatives, *all* preservatives can be a problem for many different types of skin, so, with the exception of Kathon CG (which should not be used in leave-in products but is fine in rinse-out products), it would be unfair and misleading to say that any one specific preservative is a problem. If you are concerned, you can avoid all of these ingredients. However, as several cosmetics chemists warned me, products with a reliable preservative system are better for the skin because without it microbial contamination could cause more problems for the eyes, lips, skin, and scalp than the risk of a reaction to a preservative.

Coloring agents are mentioned when pigments are added to a product to change the product's color. The term **dye agent** is used when hair colorants are added to change the actual color of the hair, however temporarily.

Antimicrobial agents are ingredients included to combat certain microbes that may cause dandruff or other scalp dermatitis. More often than not, I refer to these by their specific names. Most typically, they include zinc pyrithione, ketoconazole, coal tar, sulfur, and tea tree oil.

Chelating agents are ingredients added to shampoos to prevent minerals from binding together in the product and to prevent hardening or coupling of ingredients. When chelating agents appear high up on the ingredient list they are present in sufficient quantity to prevent most minerals in tap water, ocean water, or pool water from binding to the hair.

THE RATINGS

The following are the rating symbols for the products reviewed in this book. These simple, but succinct (albeit cute), symbols graphically depict my approval or disapproval of a specific product.

☺ This smiling face indicates a great product that I recommend highly and that is also low in price compared to its competition. It means the product is definitely worth checking into and potentially worth buying.

☺ $$$ This designates a great product that I would recommend without a doubt were it not so absurdly overpriced, either in comparison to similar products or in relation to what you are getting for the money. Still, if your hair-care budget is not restricted, they are worth checking out.

☺ This neutral face indicates an OK but unimpressive product or an OK product that can cause problems for certain hair or scalp types. I often use this symbol to portray a dated or old-fashioned product formulation. Depending on your personal preferences, products rated with this face may be worth checking out, but are nothing to get excited about.

☺ $$$ This symbol indicates an ordinary, boring product whose excessive price makes it ludicrous to consider. Why pay more for ordinary when you can pay less for extraordinary?

☹ This symbol indicates a product that is truly bad from almost every standpoint, including price, performance, application, texture, potential for irritation, scalp reactions, stiffness, or sticky feel.

Prices: Because the cost of drugstore and salon products fluctuates from store to store (and state to state), and because hair-care companies change prices frequently, the prices listed in this book may not be what you find at the store, on a company's Web site, home shopping channel, beauty supply store, drugstore, or salon where you shop. Use the prices in this book as a basis for comparison, but realize that they may not be precisely what you find when you go shopping.

Up-to-date information: My staff and I spend a vast amount of time and resources to make sure all the information we have is accurate and current. However, hair-care companies frequently and without notice change and reformulate their products, sometimes in a minor way and sometimes extensively. To help you keep abreast of these changes I report about the major revisions and new-product launches that occurred after this book went to press in my newsletter *Cosmetics Counter Update* and in my free online *Beauty Bulletin*.

No endorsements: Neither the information nor the evaluations included in any of my work are to be misconstrued as endorsements, nor do they represent a particular company's sponsorship. None of the companies listed paid me for my remarks or critiques. All the "Best Products" are nothing more than choices, with the final decision left to you.

Order of presentation: The lines are listed alphabetically by brand name, so the order in which they appear does not represent my preference. There is no implied winner among any of the hair-care companies included; no one line has all the answers or the majority of great products (even my own). Almost every line has its strong and weak points.

THE CRITERIA

Each product group has different elements that I consider essential for establishing a single product's desirability. These criteria are very specific and perhaps not something with which everyone would automatically agree, particularly the people who sell the products. But then again, I don't expect them to agree with me very often anyway. (Although they tend to strongly agree with me when I recommend one of their products, they vehemently disagree when I suggest that one of their products doesn't live up to its claims.)

I assigned each category of products specific standards and guidelines for evaluations.

- Shampoos for normal to oily hair and scalp needed to be practically free of emollients and oil, as well as lack irritating ingredients that could possibly cause a rebound effect.

- Conditioners for normal to oily hair had to have a minimal amount of conditioning agents and no heavy waxes or oils.

- Shampoos and conditioners designed for coarse hair needed to contain smoothing agents.

- Shampoos and conditioners claiming to be good for dry, damaged, chemically treated, or fragile hair needed to contain conditioning agents, emollients, detangling agents, silicone, and water-binding agents, and these ingredients had to be listed in the first part of the ingredient list, well before the preservatives or fragrance. (If they were listed after the preservative or fragrance, the amount would be negligible and have minimal effect on the hair.)

- If a company made claims about plants and their effectiveness on the hair, but did not supply substantiation, those assertions were considered invalid.

- Styling products needed to live up to their claims about hold, stickiness, and allowing the user to run a brush through his or her hair after using them.

- If a product claimed it was unique or superior and the ingredient list was the same as that of any other product in the same category, the claim of superiority was considered not substantiated.

- Shampoos, conditioners, and styling products were all rated as to how they were either similar or dissimilar to other products in their category.

Although shampoos and conditioners are usually labeled by companies to be used (and purchased) together, they do not have to be used that way. Sometimes, using shampoos and conditioners that are seemingly designed to work together can cause problems. Too much of one ingredient isn't always best for hair. For example, if a shampoo contains the same conditioning agents as its matching conditioner, and you use both, it can make hair heavy and limp. For this reason, I grouped the products in each line primarily by type; all the shampoos are listed together, then the conditioners, then the styling products, and then the specialty products.

I think you will be shocked when you notice how stunningly similar products are from line to line. The differences lie not in spectacular ingredient lists but rather in the amounts (how much protein or panthenol does a product really contain?) or in the specifics (is the detergent cleansing agent one that can strip color from the hair?).

Important cautions:

1. Any shampoo with conditioning agents, silicones, or film formers can cause buildup on the hair with repeated use. I tended to specifically point this out only if I thought the concentrations of these ingredients were high enough to make it a problem.

2. Any conditioner that contains emollients (conditioning agents) or film formers, as well as most styling products, can cause buildup. To eliminate this problem, it is essential to wash your hair with a shampoo that does *not* contain conditioning agents or film formers.

3. Shampoos and conditioners with film formers were almost always recommended only for those with normal to fine or thin hair. Film formers add a layer over the hair shaft that can add a feeling of thickness, which someone with coarse, thick hair normally would not want.

YOU DON'T HAVE TO AGREE

You're probably reading this section only after you've picked up this book and quickly looked up the products you are presently using, have used in the past, or are thinking of using in the future. You went to those sections first for a good reason—because my credibility often hinges on whether you agree with my assessments of the products you are using. However, be aware that you need not agree with all my reviews to obtain benefit from this book. As you read my comments, you may indeed find yourself disagreeing with me. That is perfectly understandable, as it should be, because the criteria you use to evaluate cosmetics may differ from mine. Or, for any one of a dozen reasons (personal preference, different expectations, actual usage—once a week versus twice a day, for example), a product I dislike may work well for you. Or just the opposite can be true: you may hate a product I love. What I cannot account for is how millions of different women will feel about a particular product or the nuances in usage or specific preferences.

What I present in the following pages are merely guidelines, based on my extensive research and experience about what works and what doesn't. If you decide to follow any of my suggestions, be aware that my recommendations are not a guarantee, but rather suggestions as to how to narrow down the endless options the hair-care industry sells and how to approach their relentless, deceptive marketing language more realistically. It is my earnest desire to help you choose from this very crowded field so you can make the best choices possible, but the final choice is yours.

Hair Note: For all the reviews that follow, it is assumed that chemically treated hair is not automatically a hair type. Most chemically treated hair, meaning dyed or permed, can be dry and damaged, but that is not always the case. How damaged your hair is has as much to do with the chemical process you used as well as with how you style your hair and how much sun exposure your hair gets. Further, how hair becomes dry or damaged is irrelevant and, as it turns out, shampoos and conditioners labeled for chemically treated hair contain ingredients that are identical to the ingredients for those labeled as being for dry or damaged hair. In more instances than you may think, shampoos for color-treated hair contain ingredients that can promote dry hair or potentially strip hair color. It is therefore unwise to purchase a shampoo simply because it is labeled as being for color-treated hair.

ABBA

Not to be confused with the 1970s singing group, ABBA is a line of salon hair-care products that has been around for quite some time, and has almost been relegated to the status of a second-class Aveda. There are many similarities between the two lines, primarily their emphasis on aromatherapy and on plant extracts being able to perform hair miracles they claim cannot be achieved by ordinary ingredients. For the most part, the flora and fauna ABBA uses, in reality, add only fragrance to their products, which, aromatherapeutic or not, is far better for your nose than for your scalp.

As far as the beneficial plant extracts—primarily soy and wheat proteins—they're certainly not unique to this line. ABBA claims to use "a unique tri-molecular weight protein system" comprising ultra-small molecules of hydrolyzed soy, wheat, and hair keratin proteins. According to ABBA, this protein system and the molecular delivery make it capable of penetrating each layer of the hair shaft to "completely condition and correct hair damage." None of that is possible—there is simply no way, short of magic and a good haircut, to repair hair damage. Proteins are good conditioning agents, but that's about it, and ingredients with a low molecular weight wouldn't hold up under washing, rinsing, or hair styling.

You don't have to use ABBA products to reap the benefits of protein because it's used in most hair-care lines, but ABBA still has enough worthwhile products to make taking a closer look a good idea. Unlike Aveda, few salons carry the entire ABBA line, so you may end up shopping Aveda for the sake of convenience. That's fine, because Aveda is not only comparable to ABBA, but also often offers more thoughtful formulations and similar pricing. For more information about ABBA, call (800) 848-4475.

What's Good About This Line: The styling gels and lotions offer various levels of hold with some beneficial conditioning agents.

What's Not So Good About It: Most of the products are highly scented and tend to be more perfume-like than aromatherapeutic.

☹ **AlphaWorks, Hair & Body Exfoliating Shampoo** *($12.25 for 12 ounces)* contains TEA-lauryl sulfate as its main detergent cleansing agent, and also contains peppermint oil, which make it too drying for the hair and irritating to the scalp. It also contains malic and glycolic acids, but while exfoliating the scalp may be helpful, exfoliating the hair shaft is a bad idea. Thankfully, the pH is too high for exfoliation to occur either on the hair or scalp.

☺ **Complete, Shampoo for All Hair Types** *($8.99 for 10 ounces)* is a very good shampoo for all hair types and poses no risk of buildup. The molecular weight of the proteins in this shampoo does not give them an edge, it just makes them good conditioning agents, similar to those in many other shampoos.

☺ **Creme-Moist Luxury Nourishing Shampoo** *($11.99 for 10 ounces)* is a good shampoo for hair that is normal to dry, coarse, or thick. It poses a slight risk of buildup and is best alternated with a shampoo that contains no conditioning agents.

☺ **Moisture Scentsation Shampoo for Moisture Starved Hair** *($11.99 for 10.1 ounces)* isn't all that moisturizing, especially if your hair is very dry, but it is a good shampoo for normal to dry hair of any thickness. It contains mostly plant tea, detergent cleansing agent, conditioning agents, film-forming agent, thickeners, fragrance, and preservatives.

☹ **Molasses Purifier** *($11.50 for 10 ounces)* is sold as a swimmer's shampoo, and it can indeed remove chlorine and mineral deposits from the hair, thanks to the chelating agents, not the molasses. Unfortunately, this shampoo contains a rather strong detergent cleansing agent, and also contains sodium bicarbonate (baking soda) and pentasodium pentetate, which are alkaline and can be drying to the hair and scalp. Still, for occasional use, this shampoo will definitely remove mineral buildup from the hair, be it from styling products or swimming.

☺ **Volumizing Shampoo, Botanical High** *($10 for 10 ounces)*. Botanical high? Is this supposed to be a selling point to compete with Clairol Herbal Essences? This conditioning shampoo is a good option for normal to dry hair of any thickness. It contains mostly plant tea, detergent cleansing agents, lather agents, thickener, several conditioning agents, preservatives, and fragrance.

☹ **Moisture Scentsation Conditioner Two-Minute Care for Moisture Starved Hair** *($13.99 for 10.1 ounces)* is a very good conditioner for normal to dry (but not moisture-starved) hair. Its main conditioning agents are silicones, accompanied by a standard detangling agent.

☺ **Nourishing Leave-On Moisturizer for Hair & Skin** *($11.99 for 10.1 ounces)*. While this is not nourishing in the least, nor a product I would recommend at all for skin care, it is a standard leave-in conditioner for normal to dry hair (though not for damaged or very dry hair) that can make hair soft and easy to comb through. It contains mostly plant tea, conditioning agents, detangling agent, plant extracts, preservatives, and fragrance.

☺ **Recoup, Intensive Reconstructor** *($15 for 10.1 ounces)* won't reconstruct anything, but can be an excellent conditioner for normal to very dry hair that is coarse or thick.

☺ **Thickening Conditioner, Volumetherapy for Fuller, Thicker, Shinier Hair** *($12 for 10.1 ounces)* works well for normal to dry hair that has a normal to fine texture. The film-forming agents can coat hair and lend a feeling of fullness, but they will build up with repeated use, so make sure you use this with a shampoo that does not contain conditioning agents.

☺ **TruMint Light Daily Conditioner** *($11.99 for 10.1 ounces)* is a very light conditioner whose primary benefit is as a detangler. The plant tea, while diluted, does contain balm mint, arnica, and peppermint, so keep this away from the scalp.

☺ **Botanical Finish, Maximum-Hold Finishing Hair Spray** *($11.50 for 10.1 ounces)* is a standard, alcohol-based nonaerosol hairspray that offers a strong hold that leaves hair stiff, though you can still brush through it thanks to the conditioning agents and silicone.

☺ **Botz** *($12.25 for 5.5 ounces)* contains mostly plant tea, film-forming agent, emollient, glycerin, conditioning agents, fixative, plant oils, antioxidant (which has no effect on hair), thickeners, preservatives, and fragrance. This semi-creamy styling gel offers a light hold that can be easily brushed through—a good combination of soft hold and conditioning agents for normal to dry hair with a normal to thick texture.

☺ **Exacting Medium-Hold Working Hair Spray** *($11.50 for 10.1 ounces)* is nearly identical to the Botanical Finish, Maximum-Hold Finishing Hair Spray above, but this one offers an even stronger hold. Otherwise, the same comments apply.

☹ **Forming Polish, Anti-Humectant** *($10.25 for 1.8 ounces)* is a sticky, goopy pomade that has a paste-like texture and stringy application. Doesn't sound too appealing, does it? It isn't, and although this helps mold hair into place, there are dozens of pomades whose textures are more user-friendly.

☺ **Gel-Lotion** *($13 for 10.1 ounces)* contains plant tea, film-forming agent, thickener, conditioning agents, preservatives, and fragrance. It offers a light hold with minimal stiffness that can be easily brushed through. It's a good option for all hair types.

☺ **Gelsential Maximum Support Styling Gel** *($11 for 10.1 ounces)* has a formulation similar to the Gel-Lotion above, but uses an acrylate-based holding agent, which provides a stronger hold and stickier feel, though it can still be brushed through. This is an option for all hair types if you prefer a strong-hold gel.

☺ **Instant Recall, Curl Activator & pH Balancer** *($12 for 10.1 ounces)* contains nothing that can activate curls, nor can it balance the hair's pH. It's just a standard styling spray that contains mostly plant tea, alcohol, film-forming agents, conditioning agents, preservatives, and fragrance. It offers a firm hold that's slightly sticky.

☺ **Molding Paste** *($10.25 for 1.8 ounces)* is aptly named because it does resemble paste. As such, it can be tricky to apply to the hair, but can keep ends in place and tame frizzies.

☺ **Pomade** *($12.75 for 2 ounces)* is a standard, water-soluble pomade. It can add texture and shine to the hair, but it can also look greasy if it's not used sparingly.

☺ **Sets Spray Gel** *($12.75 for 10.1 ounces)* is a standard, light-hold spray gel that is a good option for all hair types and can be easily brushed through.

☺ **Straightening Balm, Smooth & Control** *($12 for 5.5 ounces)* won't straighten hair without the help of a heat-styling implement and a good brush. Otherwise, it's a standard gel that has no holding agents, and the alcohol is not the best when using heat to style your hair. Still, with the right tools, this can produce decent results.

☺ Weightless Styling Gel, Volumetherapy for Fuller, Thicker, Shinier Hair *($13 for 10.1 ounces)* isn't weightless—it's actually a thicker-than-average gel that offers a strong, sticky hold that leaves hair feeling somewhat stiff. The Gel-Lotion reviewed above is the one to choose for a truly weightless gel. This option works best for hair that's difficult to manage.

☺ Zeroscent, Firm-Hold Fragrance-Free Hair Spray *($11.50 for 10.1 ounces)* contains alcohol, plant tea, thickener, silicones, and fragrance, so forget the "Fragrance-Free" claim in the name. The fragrance is cleverly disguised by the trade names of the scents used: lylial and lyral (Source: International Flavors and Fragrance, Inc., www.iff.com). As a hairspray, this lacks significant holding agents, and doesn't offer much benefit for the hair other than slight hold and some shine from the silicones.

☹ Mica, Hair Luminescent *($17 for 4.2 ounces)* is a standard silicone spray that contains the mineral mica for extra shine, but it also contains black pepper, juniper, rosemary, and peppermint oils, which can be very irritating to the scalp and skin. Even without the irritating fragrant plant oils, there is no reason to spend this much money when lines such as Citré Shine and John Frieda offer the same benefit for a lower price tag.

ADORN

For more information about Adorn, call (800) 575-7960.

What's Good About This Line: Workable aerosol hairsprays at an affordable price.

What's Not So Good About It: Inaccurate claims that Adorn hairsprays don't build up on hair.

☺ Hair Spray, Extra Hold *($3.99 for 7.5 ounces)* claims its special touch-top cap helps provide an even spray that won't feel stiff or sticky. However, as a standard, medium-hold aerosol hairspray, this is indeed sticky and can make hair feel stiff, though it can be brushed through. For a really strong hold, it is an option.

☺ Hair Spray, Frequent Use No Build Up *($3.99 for 7.5 ounces)* is nearly identical to the Hair Spray, Extra Hold above and the same comments apply. The film-forming agent in this hairspray can, without a doubt, build up on hair regardless of how frequently it's used.

☺ Hair Spray, Unscented Extra Hold *($3.99 for 7.5 ounces)* is nearly identical to both of the Adorn hairsprays above, and the same basic comments apply. This is unscented, but it's not fragrance-free. It contains a masking fragrance used to disguise the smell of the other ingredients.

AFRiCAN PRIDE

All AFRiCAN PRIDE products guarantee "miracle results" and make all sorts of claims that appeal to African-American consumers, whose natural hair texture tends to be coarse and dry. Yet nothing in any of the products reviewed below can repair split ends, prevent breakage, completely protect hair from heat, or rejuvenate hair that has been chemically processed. This line hasn't changed much since I last reviewed it, and remains a standard collection of overly emollient, dated products for dry to very dry hair. Although many of these products are recommended for treating dry scalp conditions, the heavy, greasy ingredients can create a waxy, oily layer capable of clogging the hair follicle and retarding hair growth. Moisturizing the scalp is one thing, but not while sacrificing the health of your hair.

The "African herbal complex" in these products is about as far removed from Africa as you can get. It is simply tea water made of hemp, nettle, rosemary, burdock, birch, rose hips, carrageenan, coltsfoot, wild cherry bark, dandelion, *Sambucus nigra* (black elder), horsetail, and coneflower. Even if these plants were harvested in Africa (which they are not) that wouldn't automatically make them better for tightly curled hair. My concern about a long list of plant extracts is the risk they pose of an allergic or sensitizing skin reaction. If you have problems with an itchy scalp, that may be the source of the itch.

AFRiCAN PRIDE is owned by the Colomer Group, the same company that owns the American Crew, mop (modern organic products), d:fi, and Revlon Realistic lines reviewed in this book. For more information about AFRiCAN PRIDE, call (800) 223-2339 or visit www.thecolomergroup.com.

What's Good About This Line: Gentle shampoos and many rich, emollient products for dry to very dry hair.

What's Not So Good About It: Rather dated formulations that leave hair and scalp too greasy.

☺ **Spray On Braid Shampoo** *($3.99 for 8 ounces)* is a very gentle shampoo that contains the same cleansing agent present in most baby shampoos. While that's great for babies, for adults who use hair-styling products and emollient conditioners it doesn't cleanse well enough. This is an OK spray-on shampoo (it still needs to be rinsed), but it simply is not up to the task of breaking down and washing away excess scalp oil or product buildup. However, if you have a dry scalp and don't use a lot of heavy hair-care products, this type of shampoo can be a good option, whether your hair is braided or not.

☺ **Shampoo & Conditioner 2-In-1 Formula** *($3.99 for 12 ounces)* is a good shampoo for normal to dry hair of any thickness, but those with dry hair will still need to use a separate conditioner.

☺ **Leave-In Conditioner** *($3.99 for 12 ounces)* is a very good, lightweight conditioner for normal to dry hair that is fine or thin, but use it sparingly until you can gauge how much is needed for your hair to feel soft and silky without looking greasy.

☺ **Wonder Weave Moisturizing Styling Gel** *($3.99 for 8.5 ounces)* is a good, lightly moisturizing gel with a soft hold. This gel works well to lightly condition while holding hair in place.

☺ **Braid Sheen Spray, Extra Shine** *($3.99 for 12 ounces)* won't add as much sheen to braids as a silicone serum or spray-on product would, but it does add a soft luster that is not sticky and leaves hair conditioned. It can work well to keep braids, twists, and weaves looking smooth and well-groomed. This product claims to reduce scalp itching, but if anything, the plant and herbal extracts in this product's tea water *can cause* the scalp to itch. Finally, nothing about this product can make braids tighter—that is strictly dependent on how the braids were done originally. If your braids have come loose or are unraveling, this product won't do a thing to stop it.

☺ **Braid Sheen Spray, Regular** *($3.99 for 12 ounces)* is nearly identical to the Braid Sheen Spray, Extra Shine above, except this product contains a bit more silicone, and as such is really the one to choose for extra shine. Otherwise, the same comments apply.

☹ **Braid Sheen Spray, with Tea Tree and Peppermint Oil** *($3.99 for 12 ounces)* is similar to both Braid Sheen Sprays above, but adds peppermint oil to the mix, which makes this too irritating for the scalp. Women with braids tend to shampoo their hair infrequently, which means the peppermint oil stays on the scalp for longer than it should, thus compounding the irritation and possibly causing itchiness.

☺ **Castor & Mink Oil with African Shea Butter** *($3.99 for 5.3 ounces)* is an exceptionally greasy concoction of Vaseline, mineral oil, plant oils, thickener, lanolin, plant extracts, fragrance, and preservatives. It can make hair feel heavy, though it can certainly condition all manner of dry hair. Using this on the scalp can lead to clogged hair follicles, which can stunt the growth of healthy hair. Contrary to claim, this product cannot repair split ends or stop breakage; also, despite the product's name, it doesn't contain any mink oil.

☺ **Easy Out Spray Braid & Weave** *($3.99 for 8 ounces)* is a good, basic, leave-in conditioner, but it lacks the detangling agents necessary to facilitate braid and weave removal. It can work to some extent, but there are better options available, including Johnson's No More Tangles Spray-On Detangler ($3.39 for 10 ounces).

☺ **Grooming Tools for Men Oil Moisturizing Spray** *($3.29 for 8 ounces)* is similar to the Braid Sheen Spray, Extra Shine above, and the same basic comments apply. This product does have a strong scent that can easily become overpowering if used in excess.

☺ **Grooming Tools for Men Oil Sheen Finishing Spray** *($3.49 for 13 ounces)* is a lightweight spray that can condition hair, but not without creating a waxy buildup. This also isn't much for shine; it produces a smooth matte finish on the hair that is far removed from the type of high-gloss shine you can get from an oil or silicone spray.

☺ **Hair & Scalp Spray** *($3.99 for 8 ounces)* has a formula that's nearly identical to the Braid Sheen Spray, Extra Shine above, and the same basic comments apply. Supposedly, this is an "ancient African recipe," but hundreds of years ago, silicone technology did not exist, nor were other helpful options like propylene glycol, acetamidopropyl trimonium chloride, or biotin around! Nothing about this product will guarantee a "problem-free scalp." Chances are much greater that the plant extracts it contains will cause scalp dryness and itching.

☺ **Hair, Scalp & Skin Oil** *($3.99 for 8 ounces)* consists of a blend of seven oils (mineral and plant), plant tea water, emollient, fragrance, and preservatives. It does a very good job of moisturizing the hair, scalp, and skin, but it can be quite greasy and is best used on very dry areas only. To avoid potential irritation from the plant tea or fragrance, your skin and scalp would be better off if you used plain olive, safflower, almond, or sesame oil from your kitchen cupboard.

☺ **Heat Protector Spray** *($2.99 for 7.5 ounces)* works well as a non-sticky, light-hold, watery styling spray, but cannot come close to providing "maximum protection against curling iron and blow dryer damage." Even low heat would cause this product to lay down its meager defenses and surrender!

☺ **Instant Oil Moisturizing Hair Lotion** *($3.99 for 12 ounces)* is a good water- and mineral oil-based conditioner for dry hair, but can be slightly greasy. It contains mostly plant tea water, mineral oil, thickeners, film-forming agent, fragrance, preservatives, and coloring agent. But this is definitely a less greasy option than any of the Magical Gro products below.

☹ **Magical Gro, Maximum Herbal Strength** *($4.99 for 5.3 ounces)* is an incredibly greasy concoction of Vaseline, mineral oil, plant oils, plant extracts, shea butter, lanolin, castor oil, fragrance, and preservatives. Nothing in this product can prompt hair to grow, nor can these ingredients rejuvenate chemically treated hair. This can moisturize dry, very dry, and damaged hair, but it is difficult to rinse or shampoo out, and using this on the scalp can clog the hair follicle, impairing healthy hair growth. This is best used sparingly to smooth the ends of dry hair.

☹ **Magical Gro, Rejuvenating Herbal Formula** *($4.99 for 5.3 ounces)* is nearly identical to the Magical Gro, Maximum Herbal Strength product above, minus the extra castor seed oil, and the same comments apply. If this is an "ancient African recipe," then where did they find the Vaseline and mineral oil, the backbone of this formulation?

☹ **Magical Gro, Rejuvenating Oil Formula** *($4.99 for 5.3 ounces)* is nearly identical to the Magical Gro products above, and the same comments apply.

☺ **Miracle Magical Gro, Regular** *($4.99 for 5.3 ounces)* contains mostly mineral oil, plant oils, plant extracts, lanolin, emollients, fragrance, and preservative. It is similar to, but less greasy than, the Magical Gro, Maximum Herbal Strength above, and the same basic comments apply.

☺ **Miracle Cream, Creme Hair Dressing** *($4.99 for 5.3 ounces)* shares a formula similar to the Magical Gro products above, but has a less greasy, creamier texture. Although this is a lighter option for dry, very dry, and damaged hair, it can still be greasy and difficult to rinse, and is best used only for dry ends. It's interesting to note that the herbs and plant extracts are described as "newly discovered," yet they're the same ones that show up in all of the AFRiCAN PRIDE products, where they are referred to as "ancient." Ah, the caprices of marketing!

AFRICAN ROYALE

Designed for African-American hair, AFRICAN ROYALE products contain the same mix of ingredients seen in the majority of other ethnic hair-care lines being sold at drugstores. That means you'll find gentle shampoos that aren't all that adept at removing the greasy, oily residue the heavy styling and conditioning products leave behind. AFRICAN ROYALE's products don't break any new ground, though they do offer a couple of silicone-based products that are a nice change of pace from the heavier Vaseline-laden offerings. AFRICAN ROYALE is nearly identical to AFRiCAN PRIDE, especially when it comes to claims for repairing or healing damaged hair. Both use combinations of plant extracts in their products that serve no purpose for the hair or scalp but, at least on the label, help reinforce each company's "ingredients from nature" marketing angle.

AFRICAN ROYALE mentions that its G.R.O. formulas contain the same "herbal secrets" known to attendants who served the kings and queens of Egypt, but that's sheer fantasy created solely to appeal to consumers' sense of ancestry and history. None of the Egyptian kings or queens were using products like these, primarily because ingredients such as Vaseline, mineral oil, and silicones were not available. The source of the Vaseline (petroleum) was present in the earth, but the technology to develop it was millennia away from being invented. So much for finding common ground with royalty! For more information about AFRICAN ROYALE, call (800) 241-6151 or visit www.bronnerbros.com.

What's Good About This Line: Gentle shampoos and many rich, emollient products for dry to very dry hair.

What's Not So Good About It: Rather dated formulations that leave hair and scalp too greasy.

☺ **BRX Braid & Extensions Spray On Shampoo** *($3.99 for 12 ounces)* contains mostly water, detergent cleansing agent, lather agents, thickeners, preservatives, film-forming agent, plant oil, plant extracts, and fragrance. This is a good, gentle shampoo for all hair types that poses minimal to no risk of buildup. Nothing about this shampoo makes it particularly useful for braids or extensions, save for the convenience of its spray-on application.

☺ **Soft As Me Herbal Shampoo** *($3.55 for 8 ounces)* is a standard shampoo that is a good option for normal to dry hair of any thickness, and poses minimal risk of buildup. The plant extracts have no effect on the scalp or hair.

☹ **Castor G.R.O.** *($4.59 for 6 ounces)*. The G.R.O. part stands for gelatin-rich oils, but none of the oils in this product contain gelatin, though it is one of the ingredients. Gelatin is used in hair-care products as a thickener and film-forming agent because it can help ingredients like proteins cling to the hair better. This greasy mix of Vaseline, plant oils, gelatin, vitamins (which have no effect on hair), silicone, and plant extracts works on very dry hair, but the walnut shell pieces (and they're quite large) can flake off and resemble dandruff on the scalp. What was AFRICAN ROYALE thinking?

☺ **Daily Doctor Maximum Strength Leave-In Conditioner** *($4.49 for 12 ounces)* has a great name and can be a good spray-on, leave-in conditioner for normal to dry hair that is fine or thin.

☺ **Extra Light Creme of Ginseng** *($3.99 for 6 ounces)* isn't "extra light" in the least. It's a fairly greasy conditioner that contains mostly water, mineral oil, film-forming agent, castor oil, thickeners, aloe, slip agent, silicone, plant extracts (including ginseng, which has no proven benefit for hair), preservative, and fragrance. This is a decent option for dry, coarse hair, but should be used sparingly and kept away from the scalp.

☺ **Extra Light Super G.R.O.** *($4.69 for 6 ounces)* is horribly misnamed. There is nothing "extra light" about this product. It contains mostly Vaseline, plant oils, gelatin (which serves only as a thickener), vitamins, silicone, plant extracts, and fragrance. It can leave hair feeling heavy and greasy, and can impede healthy hair growth when applied daily to the scalp. This is best for use on the ends of very dry hair, and for this use only is worthy of a happy face rating.

☺ **Maximum Strength Super G.R.O.** *($4.59 for 6 ounces)* is nearly identical to the Extra Lite Super G.R.O. above, but contains more Vaseline and less oil, so it has a thicker, more emollient texture. Regardless of thickness, the same comments apply.

☺ **M.O.M. Miracle Oil Moisturizer** *($4.49 for 12 ounces)* beckons you to "put a miracle in your hair," but aside from moisturizing dry to very dry or damaged hair, there are no miracles to be found here. It is much lighter than the Super G.R.O. products above, but can still make hair feel greasy if it is not used sparingly.

☺ **Super G.R.O.** *($4.59 for 6 ounces)* is nearly identical to the Maximum Strength Super G.R.O. above and the same comments apply. For some reason, this G.R.O. product contains coloring agents while the others don't.

☹ **Mink Oil Gel for Hair and Scalp** *($3.99 for 6 ounces)* is less a gel and more a thick, greasy emulsion that contains walnut shell pieces that can flake off and make your scalp look as though it has brown dandruff.

☺ **Royale Mist Natural Fro Spray for Hair & Scalp** *($3.99 for 12 ounces)* is a very lightweight spray-on, leave-in conditioner that is a good option for normal to slightly dry hair. It can also aid with detangling.

☺ **BRX Braid & Extensions Sheen Spray** *($3.99 for 12 ounces)* is supposed to reduce itching, but there are no ingredients in this product that can do that. Other than that, it's a good lightweight spray to add a little bit of shine that won't appear greasy.

☺ **Diamond Drops** *($4.99 for 2 ounces)* is a standard silicone serum that also contains plant oil, plant extracts, and fragrance. This can smooth frizzies and leave hair with a dazzling shine, but it should be used sparingly to avoid a greasy, limp appearance. This is a far more elegant way to condition and add shine to the hair than any of the G.R.O. products above.

☺ **Hot Six Oil** *($4.79 for 8 ounces)* can be a good conditioning oil treatment for dry to very dry hair, but if you intend to leave this in the hair it should be applied sparingly.

It contains mostly plant oils, vitamins, silicone, plant extracts, and fragrance. Given the amount of oils this waterless product contains, it is quite a bargain!

☹ **Hot Six Oil, Hair & Body Mist** *($4.79 for 8 ounces)* is a spray-on, lighter-weight version of the Hot Six Oil above. It loses points and a happy face rating by omitting most of the excellent plant oils used in that product and instead adding irritating eucalyptus, rosemary, and geranium oils.

ALBERTO VO5

Illinois-based Alberto-Culver has been a mainstay in the hair-care aisles of drug and mass-market stores for decades. They offer some wonderful products whose prices are almost a steal for what you get, but this line also suffers from a disproportionate amount of poor formulations (especially their shampoos) and a preponderance of repetitive products whose only major difference is a change in fragrance. I could more easily justify the need for a hair-care line to offer more than 20 shampoos if each one was a thoughtful, purpose-driven formulation specific to the needs of a wide variety of hair types and conditions. But Alberto simply rehashed the same basic formula almost two dozen times, and follows the same routine for its conditioners and most of its hairsprays. Besides crowding the shelves, all this really does is create consumer confusion. How many women have tried to shop Alberto but have been overwhelmed by the sheer volume of choices for something as straightforward as shampoo? Believe me, I get frustrated, too. The good news is that after you read the reviews below you will be able to walk away from the line with some outstanding products whose prices fit almost any consumer's budget, with money to spare! For more information about Alberto VO5, call (708) 450-3163 or visit www.alberto.com.

What's Good About This Line: Great prices and effective formulations for conditioners and basic styling products.

What's Not So Good About It: Every one of Alberto's shampoos contains sodium lauryl sulfate as its main detergent cleansing agent. The plant extracts and vitamins are merely window dressing and add no benefit for the hair or scalp.

☹ **Balsam & Protein Shampoo** *($1.29 for 15 ounces)* contains sodium lauryl sulfate as its detergent cleansing agent, which makes this shampoo (which, despite the name, contains no balsam) too drying for all hair and scalp types.

☹ **Blueberries & Cream Replenishing Shampoo** *($1.29 for 15 ounces)* is similar to the Balsam & Protein Shampoo above, and the same comments apply. Blueberries are nutritional powerhouses when eaten, but have no effect on the hair or scalp.

☹ **Blushin' Apple Shampoo** *($1.29 for 15 ounces)* also contains sodium lauryl sulfate and is nearly identical to the Blueberries & Cream Replenishing Shampoo above, save for the use of apples rather than blueberries. Otherwise, the same comments apply.

☹ **Creamy Citrus Healthy Shine Shampoo** *($1.29 for 15 ounces)* is, save for the use of orange peel instead of apples, identical to the Blushin' Apple Shampoo above, and the same comments apply.

☹ **Creamy Fresh Peaches Revitalizing Shampoo** *($1.29 for 15 ounces)* is, save for the use of peaches instead of apples, identical to the Blushin' Apple Shampoo above, and the same comments apply.

☹ **Cucumber Melon Crush Shampoo** *($1.29 for 15 ounces)* is, save for the use of melons instead of apple, identical to the Blushin' Apple Shampoo above, and the same comments apply.

☹ **Deep Cleansing Shampoo** *($1.29 for 15 ounces)* contains sodium lauryl sulfate as its main detergent cleansing agent, and that makes this standard shampoo too drying for the hair and irritating to the scalp.

☹ **Extra Body Shampoo** *($1.29 for 15 ounces)* is similar to the Deep Cleansing Shampoo above, and the same comments apply.

☹ **Free Me Freesia Moisturizing Herbal Shampoo, for Normal Hair** *($1.29 for 15 ounces)* is yet another standard shampoo that contains sodium lauryl sulfate as its main detergent cleansing agent. This shampoo can be drying to the hair and irritating to the scalp, and is not recommended.

☹ **Fresh Vanilla Bean Nourishing Shampoo** *($1.29 for 15 ounces)* is nearly identical to the Free Me Freesia Moisturizing Herbal Shampoo above, and the same comments apply.

☹ **Fruitsation Shampoo, for All Hair Types** *($1.29 for 15 ounces)* is nearly identical to the Free Me Freesia Moisturizing Herbal Shampoo above, and the same comments apply.

☹ **Jasmine Tease Volumizing Herbal Shampoo** *($1.29 for 15 ounces)* is nearly identical to the Free Me Freesia Moisturizing Herbal Shampoo above, and the same comments apply.

☹ **Kiwi and Lime Squeeze Herbal Shampoo** *($1.29 for 15 ounces)* is nearly identical to the Free Me Freesia Moisturizing Herbal Shampoo above, and the same comments apply.

☹ **Luv Me Lavender Herbal Shampoo, for Normal Hair** *($1.29 for 15 ounces)* is nearly identical to the Free Me Freesia Moisturizing Herbal Shampoo above, and the same comments apply.

☹ **Pear Mango Passion Herbal Shampoo, for Color Treated Hair** *($1.29 for 15 ounces)* is nearly identical to the Free Me Freesia Moisturizing Herbal Shampoo above, and the same comments apply.

☹ **Pina Colada Moisturizing Shampoo** *($1.29 for 15 ounces)* is nearly identical to the Free Me Freesia Moisturizing Herbal Shampoo above, and the same comments apply.

☹ **Punchy Pomegranate Herbal Shampoo, Volume Boost** *($1.29 for 15 ounces)* is nearly identical to the Free Me Freesia Moisturizing Herbal Shampoo above, and the same comments apply.

☹ **Shampoo for Normal Hair** *($1.29 for 15 ounces)* is nearly identical to the Free Me Freesia Moisturizing Herbal Shampoo above, and the same comments apply.

☹ **Strawberries and Cream Smoothing Shampoo** *($1.29 for 15 ounces)* is nearly identical to the Free Me Freesia Moisturizing Herbal Shampoo above, and the same comments apply.

☺ **Sun Kissed Raspberry Herbal Shampoo, for Normal Hair** *($1.29 for 15 ounces)* is nearly identical to the Free Me Freesia Moisturizing Herbal Shampoo above, and the same comments apply.

☹ **Tangerine Tickle Herbal Shampoo** *($1.29 for 15 ounces)* is nearly identical to the Free Me Freesia Moisturizing Herbal Shampoo above, and the same comments apply.

☹ **Volumizing Shampoo** *($1.29 for 15 ounces)* is nearly identical to the Free Me Freesia Moisturizing Herbal Shampoo above, and the same comments apply.

☺ **Balsam & Protein Conditioner** *($1.29 for 15 ounces)* doesn't contain any balsam, but that's a good thing because it can quickly build up on the hair making it feel stiff and sticky. This is a very standard conditioner that contains mostly water, thickeners, detangling agent, conditioning agents, a teeny amount of vitamins (which have no effect on hair), panthenol, fragrance, more thickeners, preservatives, and coloring agents. It works well for normal to dry hair that has a normal, fine, or thin texture.

☺ **Blueberries & Cream Replenishing Conditioner** *($1.29 for 15 ounces)* is nearly identical to the Balsam & Protein Conditioner above, but has fewer conditioning agents; otherwise, the same basic comments apply.

☺ **Blushin' Apple Conditioner** *($1.29 for 15 ounces)* is nearly identical to the Balsam & Protein Conditioner above, but has fewer conditioning agents; otherwise, the same basic comments apply.

☺ **Creamy Citrus Healthy Shine Conditioner** *($1.29 for 15 ounces)* is nearly identical to the Balsam & Protein Conditioner above, but has fewer conditioning agents; otherwise the same basic comments apply.

☺ **Creamy Fresh Peaches Revitalizing Conditioner** *($1.29 for 15 ounces)* is nearly identical to the Balsam & Protein Conditioner above, but has fewer conditioning agents; otherwise the same basic comments apply.

☺ **Cucumber Melon Crush Conditioner** *($1.29 for 15 ounces)* is nearly identical to the Balsam & Protein Conditioner above, but has fewer conditioning agents; otherwise the same basic comments apply.

☺ **Detangle & Shine Lightweight Leave-In Conditioner All Hair Types** *($3.99 for 10 ounces)* is indeed very lightweight and is appropriate only for normal to fine hair that needs minimum conditioning and a little bit of help for comb-ability.

☺ **Dry Ends, Daily Rinse-Out Conditioner** *($5.99 for 7.5 ounces)* is similar to the Balsam & Protein Conditioner above, but this one contains a larger amount of detangling agents, which makes it somewhat more appropriate for longer hair. Otherwise, the same comments apply and the price discrepancy is unwarranted.

☺ **Extra Body Conditioner** *($1.29 for 15 ounces)* is identical in every respect to the Balsam & Protein Conditioner above, and the same comments apply.

☺ **Free Me Freesia Moisturizing Herbal Conditioner, for Normal Hair** *($1.29 for 15 ounces)* is nearly identical to the Balsam & Protein Conditioner above, but with slightly fewer conditioning agents listed, which makes it better for normal hair with minimal conditioning needs.

☺ **Fresh Vanilla Bean Nourishing Conditioner** *($1.29 for 15 ounces)* is nearly identical to the Balsam & Protein Conditioner above, but with slightly fewer conditioning agents listed, which makes it better for normal hair with minimal conditioning needs.

☺ **Fruitsation Conditioner, for All Hair Types** *($1.29 for 15 ounces)* is similar to all of the Alberto conditioners above, but contains an appreciable amount of plant oil, which makes this one preferred for dry hair of any thickness.

☺ **Jasmine Tease Herbal Volumizing Conditioner** *($1.29 for 15 ounces)* is nearly identical to the Balsam & Protein Conditioner above, but with slightly fewer conditioning agents listed, which makes it better for normal hair with minimal conditioning needs. There isn't much in the way of volumizing help in here, so think of this as an extremely lightweight conditioner.

☺ **Kiwi & Lime Squeeze Herbal Conditioner** *($1.29 for 15 ounces)* is nearly identical to the Balsam & Protein Conditioner above, but with slightly fewer conditioning agents listed, which makes it better for normal hair with minimal conditioning needs.

☺ **Luv Me Lavender Herbal Conditioner, for Normal Hair** *($1.29 for 15 ounces)* is nearly identical to the Balsam & Protein Conditioner above, but with slightly fewer conditioning agents listed, which makes it better for normal hair with minimal conditioning needs.

☺ **Mend & Defend Conditioner, for All Hair Types** *($4.36 for 6 ounces)* is similar to the Dry Ends, Daily Rinse-Out Conditioner above, and that makes it particularly helpful for dry ends.

☺ **Pear Mango Passion Herbal Conditioner, for Color Treated Hair** *($1.29 for 15 ounces)* is nearly identical to the Balsam & Protein Conditioner above, but with slightly fewer conditioning agents listed, which makes it better for normal hair with minimal conditioning needs. There is nothing in this product that makes it helpful for someone with color-treated hair.

☺ **Pina Colada Conditioner** *($1.29 for 15 ounces)* is nearly identical to the Balsam & Protein Conditioner above, but with slightly fewer conditioning agents listed, which makes it better for normal hair with minimal conditioning needs.

☺ **Punchy Pomegranate Herbal Conditioner** *($1.29 for 15 ounces)* is nearly identical to the Balsam & Protein Conditioner above, but with slightly fewer conditioning agents listed, which makes it appropriate for normal hair with minimal conditioning needs.

☺ **Strawberries and Cream Smoothing Conditioner** *($1.29 for 15 ounces)* is nearly identical to the Balsam & Protein Conditioner above, but with slightly fewer conditioning agents listed, which makes it better for normal hair with minimal conditioning needs.

☺ **Sun Kissed Raspberry Herbal Conditioner, for Normal Hair** *($1.29 for 15 ounces)* is nearly identical to the Balsam & Protein Conditioner above, but with slightly fewer conditioning agents listed, which makes it better for normal hair with minimal conditioning needs.

☺ **Tangerine Tickle Herbal Conditioner** (*$1.29 for 15 ounces*) is nearly identical to the Balsam & Protein Conditioner above, but with slightly fewer conditioning agents listed, which makes it better for normal hair with minimal conditioning needs.

☺ **Conditioning Hairdressing, Extra Body for Fine Hair** (*$3.79 for 1.5 ounces*) is basically a standard, old-fashioned pomade in a squeeze tube. It contains mostly mineral oil, water, Vaseline, thickeners, lanolin, waxes, fragrance, surfactant, preservatives, and coloring agents. This greasy product is inappropriate for fine hair, but can smooth frizzies and tame flyaway ends of dry to very dry hair that is coarse or thick.

☺ **Conditioning Hairdressing, for Gray, White & Silver Blonde Hair** (*$3.79 for 1.5 ounces*) contains mostly mineral oil, Vaseline, lanolin, thickener, wax, fragrance, preservatives, and coloring agents. It is a heavier, greasier pomade than the Conditioning Hairdressing, Extra Body for Fine Hair above, and is best used sparingly to smooth the ends of dry, damaged hair. The coloring agents in this pomade can help (to a minor extent) reduce the sometimes brassy tones of silver or white hair.

☺ **Conditioning Hairdressing, for Normal/Dry Hair** (*$3.79 for 1.5 ounces*) is nearly identical to the Conditioning Hairdressing for Gray, White & Silver Blonde Hair above, only this does not contain any coloring agents. Otherwise, the same basic comments apply.

☺ **Conditioning Hairdressing, Unscented** (*$3.79 for 1.5 ounces*) is identical to the Conditioning Hairdressing, for Normal/Dry Hair above, and the same comments apply. This product does contain fragrance, though it is less pervasive than the fragrance in the other Conditioning Hairdressing products.

☺ **Crystal Clear 14 Hour Hold Hair Spray, Unscented Hard to Hold** (*$2.99 for 10 ounces*) is a standard nonaerosol hairspray with a firm hold that remains sticky, making it tricky to brush through. Save it for times when you need a firm-hold hairspray and have no intention of brushing through your hair later.

☺ **Crystal Clear 14 Hour Hold Hair Spray, Hard to Hold** (*$2.99 for 8.5 ounces*) is a standard, nonaerosol, alcohol-based hairspray that provides a light hold that can feel stiff, but that can easily be brushed through.

☺ **Crystal Clear 14 Hour Hold Hair Spray, Extra Body Hard to Hold** (*$2.99 for 8.5 ounces*) is identical to the Crystal Clear 14 Hour Hold Hair Spray, Hard to Hold above, and the same comments apply. The minute amount of collagen added to this formula does not make it conditioning for hair, nor does it provide extra body.

☺ **Brush Out Hair Spray, Extra Hold** (*$2.99 for 8.5 ounces*) is similar to both Crystal Clear Hair Sprays above, but includes enough conditioning agents to leave hair less stiff and very easy to brush through. The drawback is that it has a weaker hold, but this is a good hairspray for keeping hair softly in place.

☺ **Crystal Clear 14 Hour Hold Hair Spray, Silver Hard to Hold** (*$2.99 for 8.5 ounces*) is identical to all of the Crystal Clear Hair Sprays above, except this adds a violet dye to help counteract brassy tones in silver hair. The effect is too subtle to notice, and this remains a standard, aerosol hairspray with a light, brushable hold.

☺ **Crystal Clear 14 Hour Hold Hair Spray, Super Hard to Hold** *($2.99 for 8.5 ounces)* is a standard, alcohol-based aerosol hairspray similar to all of the Crystal Clear versions above, except this one provides a stronger hold, which is better for hard-to-manage hair.

☺ **Crystal Clear 14 Hour Hold Hair Spray, Unscented Hard to Hold** *($2.99 for 8.5 ounces)* does contain fragrance—clearly indicated on the label. It has as much scent as the Crystal Clear Hair Sprays above, as well as an almost identical formula, and provides a light hold that can be easily brushed through.

☺ **Free Me Freesia Non-Aerosol Hair Spray, Extra Hold** *($2.99 for 8.75 ounces)* is a nonaerosol hairspray that goes on somewhat wet, which can be a problem for those fighting frizzies, though it does have a medium hold with no flaking and can be easily brushed through. The fragrance is rather intense, so be sure you like it before purchasing.

☺ **Hairdressing Gel for Men** *($3.79 for 4.5 ounces)* contains nothing that makes it special for a man's hair, other than a masculine, soapy fragrance. It is a standard, light-hold styling gel.

☹ **Multi-Vitamin Non-Aerosol Hair Spray, Extra Hold** *($2.99 for 8.75 ounces)* is similar to, but less fragrant than, the Free Me Freesia Non-Aerosol Hair Spray above, and the same basic comments apply, except for one important issue: this one flakes. The formulas are similar, but several A/B tests found that this version consistently flaked while the Free Me Freesia did not.

☺ **Sheer Hairdressing, Lightweight Leave-In Anti-Frizz & Shine Creme** *($5.99 for 4 ounces)* is a remarkable styling cream that makes hair feel incredibly silky while imparting shine. It is excellent when used with heat and a round brush to straighten the hair, and the silicones can provide some protection from heat damage. Use sparingly for best results; those with fine or thin hair will want to apply this product only on the ends of hair.

☺ **Straight Hair, Straightens, Smoothes and Shines** *($5.99 for 4 ounces)* is a clear, slightly thick gel that can work with heat and the proper styling tools to straighten curly or wavy hair. It does not contain film-forming agents, so it won't add any hold or stiffness to the hair. This is a good product to mix with the Sheer Hairdressing above to straighten hair and help a little to protect hair from heat damage.

☺ **Sun Kissed Raspberry Non-Aerosol Hair Spray, Maximum Hold** *($2.99 for 12 ounces)* is identical to the Free Me Freesia Non-Aerosol Hair Spray, Extra Hold above, and the same comments apply. This is not a maximum-hold hairspray.

☺ **Sun Kissed Raspberry Styling Gel, Mega Hold for Shaping** *($2.99 for 12 ounces)* is a very standard but good styling gel that offers strong hold with a sticky feel that can be easily brushed through.

☺ **Hot Oil Hair Treatment, Color Keeper** *($3.99 for two 0.50-ounce tubes)* contains mostly water, detangling agents, thickeners, plant extracts, conditioning agents, slip agents, preservatives, and fragrance. There is no oil in this liquidy product, and the overall ingredient roster isn't impressive enough to make this worth using as a special treatment.

There is nothing in this product that can prolong the life of color-treated hair or protect it from fading. At best, this is a lightweight detangling conditioner that can work well for normal to slightly dry hair that is normal to fine or thin.

☺ **Hot Oil Hair Treatment, Moisturizing** *($3.99 for two 0.50-ounce tubes)* is nearly identical to the Hot Oil Treatment, Color Keeper above, and the same basic comments apply. This product is minimally moisturizing or conditioning.

☺ **Hot Oil Hair Treatment, Smoothing** *($3.49 for two 0.50-ounce tubes)* is nearly identical to the Hot Oil Treatment, Color Keeper above, and the same basic comments apply. Nothing about this product gives it an edge for creating smoother hair.

☺ **Hot Oil Hair Treatment, Strengthening** *($3.99 for two 0.50-ounce tubes)* is nearly identical to the Hot Oil Treatment, Color Keeper above, and the same basic comments apply.

☺ **Hot Oil Shower Works Hair Treatment, for Color Treated Hair** *($5.99 for 2 ounces)* is nearly identical to the Hot Oil Treatment, Color Keeper above, and the same basic comments apply. This does contain less detangling agent and more panthenol than those reviewed above, but that does not make it preferred for color-treated hair.

☺ **Hot Oil Shower Works Hair Treatment, Moisturizing** *($5.99 for 2 ounces)* is nearly identical to the Hot Oil Treatment, Color Keeper above, and the same basic comments apply.

☺ **Total Hair Recovery** *($6.49 for 1 ounce)* is an extremely standard conditioner that is a good option for normal to dry hair of any thickness. Do I have to mention that nothing in this product can help damaged hair make a total recovery? The only way to correct damaged hair is to cut it off and then be as gentle as possible to your hair.

ALTERNA

I don't quite know where to begin describing this overly expensive and overly extensive salon/spa hair-care line, other than to wonder why they needed 67 hair-care products, many of which contain the same standard assortment of cleansing, conditioning, and styling ingredients merely packaged in different containers. From a marketing standpoint, such an enormous assortment of products means that Alterna appears to have at least one item to meet just about any hair-care need you can imagine, though many of their claims are anchored in fantasy rather than reality.

Alterna (short for "alternative") was launched in 1997. According to their Web site, the company's goal is "to continually push the envelope by revealing the latest in hair-care ingredients and technologies in order to shape the future of professional hair care." I must admit, as far as ingredients go, Alterna does use a dizzying and dazzling array of "goodies"—from amino acids and antioxidants to minerals, polypeptides, and on and on to exotic plant oils. To its credit, Alterna has included enough uncommon, novel, and fairly expensive ingredients to justify its prices, especially for consumers who are intent on believing that vitamins and other nutrients can fortify their hair.

Alterna's major philosophy, which is unique and of course is used heavily in their marketing and the claims for all of their products, is their belief in enzyme therapy for the hair follicle. Alterna believes that adding enzymes (as well as other ingredients) to hair-care products allows the nutrients in the products to absorb better into the hair follicle (where hair growth takes place) and into the hair shaft. Once in (and on) the hair, these enzymes supposedly serve as the catalyst that allows hair to use ingredients such as fatty acids, vitamins, and minerals in a completely new way. The company's enthusiastic belief is that enzymes applied topically can quite literally change your hair for the better. It's an interesting theory, but allow me to get scientific for a moment. Enzymes are protein molecules that cells use to dissolve nutrients and to create molecules that the cell subsequently uses to survive and reproduce. Enzymes also enhance or create chemical reactions between cells. Each enzyme has a unique shape that determines its function; that is, one enzyme works only on one related material. For example, the enzyme amylase acts on starches in the foods we eat, turning it into glucose, which is used for energy. Actually, food itself is essentially just a mixture of chemicals that are broken down by enzymes. Vitamins and nutrients cannot work in the body by themselves; they require myriad enzymes to transport them throughout the body to serve their unique purposes. Enzymes unlock the benefits of vitamins, minerals, proteins, and hormones so these compounds can do their work in our bodies.

With this basic understanding of enzymes, Alterna claims that their "advanced liposomal delivery system allows bio-active enzymes to stimulate the breakdown of essential hair-care building blocks at the matrix (life source) of the hair. If the matrix is supplied with both the fundamental building blocks of keratin and the specific enzymes required to break them down, there is an increased opportunity for stronger, healthier keratin formation." This statement definitely has some basis in science, but it takes a leap of faith in terms of what can actually occur in the hair follicle. Hair growth is an extremely complicated process that is pre-set by genetics and depends on an intricate mix of chemical interactions. Hair grows in cyclical phases, affected primarily by hormones. Hair keratinization alone—the conversion of amino acids and other substances into hair protein—is exceedingly complex (Source: *Journal of Investigative Dermatology*, volume 110, February 1998, pages 158–164). And if that isn't complicated enough, consider that a type of hair keratin has been identified that is created by 450 amino acids (Source: *Journal of Investigative Dermatology*, volume 116, January 2001, pages 157–166). This is far beyond anything Alterna or any hair-care product is capable of delivering to the hair shaft. There is also no proof that adding enzymes to hair-care products can have an impact on the hair's rate of growth, tensile strength, or outward appearance. (The only evidence that does exist comes from a small number of experiments on mice, but these experiments did not use hair-care products.) The claims do sound appealing, but adding enzymes to hair-care products, regardless of the delivery system, is unlikely to change how your hair grows, and it definitely cannot change damaged hair in any way. That means the fancy ingredients are useless in styling products. One more point: Even if enzymes did have merit for hair, we don't know how much of any particular enzyme is needed to produce results, or what combination works best.

Most of the products also contain a few state-of-the-art antioxidants, though most often just trace amounts. While we have a good understanding of the benefit antioxidants have on skin in regard to sun damage, reducing inflammation, and improving cell production, there is little to no information about how they help hair. What's certain is that antioxidants cannot hold up under normal styling conditions of high heat and repetitive brushing, nor can they protect hair from ultraviolet light or preserve hair color.

Alterna deserves credit for creating a hair-care line that, for the most part, performs well and offers consumers many (actually, too many) options, especially for styling products. Few hair-care lines have such an abundance of pomades, waxes, putties, and texturizers. The line has four subcategories and I describe their unique properties in the respective reviews below. As you may have guessed already, what makes these subcategories special are only minor differences. Either they include ingredients that have no proven benefit for hair, or they feature costly ingredients that, functionally, can easily be replaced by less expensive options without hair being deprived of something claimed to be amazing. The majority of Alterna's products will be helpful for hair, producing results that should not disappoint if your expectations are within reason. What's important to keep in mind is that it is the classic, tried-and-true hair-care ingredients that are responsible for the results you get, not the newfangled and "age-old" ingredients boasted about on every Alterna product. For more information about Alterna, call (888) 4-ALTERNA or visit www.4alterna.com.

What's Good About This Line: The styling products are a diverse collection capable of helping you create any hairstyle imaginable; Alterna's formulations tend to use state-of-the-art ingredients, though many of these have questionable benefits for hair.

What's Not So Good About It: The prices are steep; many products contain wasabi (Japanese horseradish) extract, which can cause acute scalp irritation. The hair-care industry is full of overblown claims, and Alterna's Caviar line is a prime example; a few of the products contain ingredients whose effect is undocumented and may even be dangerous.

☹ **Clarifying Shampoo** *($18 for 16.9 ounces)* contains sodium lauryl sulfate (SLS) as its main detergent cleansing agent, which makes this shampoo too drying for all hair and scalp types. Without the SLS, this would have been a fine shampoo for all hair types, one that poses minimal to no risk of buildup. Alterna's claim that Clarifying Shampoo will not strip hair color is completely untrue because SLS is a strong cleansing agent that can cause the hair shaft to swell, which increases the likelihood of pigment being released from color-treated hair.

☺ **$$$ Nutritive Leave-In Conditioner** *($15.60 for 10.1 ounces)* is a very lightweight, standard, leave-in conditioner that contains mostly water, conditioning agent, silicones, film-forming agent, wax, plant extracts, vitamins, amino acids, thickeners, preservatives, and fragrance. It can make hair easy to detangle and provide some protection from heat-styling implements, but it cannot completely prevent heat damage, as Alterna claims.

☺ $$$ **Volumizing Spray Leave-In Conditioner** *($16.50 for 8.5 ounces)* is a good, very light leave-in conditioner that contains mostly silicone and no film-forming agents, at least compared with the Nutritive Leave-In Conditioner above. This spray is a fine post-shampoo option for normal to fine hair, and will help to detangle and add some softness and smoothness.

☺ $$$ **Hard Hold Styling Gel** *($15.30 for 8.5 ounces)* is as standard as it gets for styling gels. In the backbone of this firm-hold gel are the same ingredients you'll see in countless other (often less expensive) styling gels, namely water, PVP/VA copolymer (film former), alcohol, PVP (film former), and carbomer. Alterna wants to sell you on its belief in enzyme therapy as hair's saving grace, but enzymes are of little use to hair because hair is not living protein. Therefore, enzymes in hair-care products do not serve as an "activated" ingredient to enhance the penetration of nutrients and conditioning agents into the hair. It's an enticing hook, but nothing to take seriously when comparison-shopping between hair-care lines. Hard Hold Styling Gel has a sticky after-feel, but the hair can still be brushed through. This gel works best for creating lift and strong hold on short, textured, or spiked hairstyles.

☺ **Maximum Hold Finishing Protectant** *($13.80 for 8.5 ounces)* is a strong-hold, nonaerosol hairspray that contains polyurethane as its holding agent, which can indeed provide hold, though not without making your hair feel stiff and coated. As a finishing product, this spray has a rather heavy feel, and it takes longer to dry than most hairsprays. It does contain plant oil and silicone for conditioning, and these make it possible to brush through the hair without causing breakage while using this product.

☺ $$$ **Styling & Nutritive Creme Gel** *($15.30 for 8.5 ounces)* works well as a medium- to firm-hold styling gel, and has a formula that is akin to combining a standard, water-based styling gel formula with a lightweight silicone serum. The result when styling is that hair maintains the desired style while staying smooth and relatively frizz-free. This is a good styling gel for medium to thick hair, but can be a bit too heavy for normal to fine hair.

ALTERNA CAVIAR

The first thing you may notice about Alterna's Caviar products is that they cost considerably more than the other Alterna products. With the Caviar name, did you expect anything else? This line of products is targeted to the baby-boomer generation and beyond, using the notion that, as we age, hair loses the ability to hold onto nutrients, thus becoming dry and brittle. Following this reasoning, Alterna developed the Caviar line to supply aging hair with what it is missing, which (according to Alterna) is omega-3 fatty acids. Omega-3 fatty acids have been in the medical and health news quite a bit lately, and for good reason. Research has shown these polyunsaturated fatty acids have an important effect on our overall health and well-being, particularly in regard to reducing cellular inflammation within the body, a condition that can lead to serious problems commonly associated with aging (Source: www.drweil.com/app/cda/drw_cda.html). Alterna's marketing conceit comes into question, however, when you consider the fact that there is zero substantiated evidence that topically applied omega-3 fatty acids can have an antiaging effect on the skin—much less on hair. Besides, despite Alterna's claims, caviar extract is not "the richest provider of omega-3," that distinction belongs to flaxseed oil (Source: www.drweil.com). And there is nothing about omega-3 fatty acids, or any other ingredient, that can prevent hair from turning gray, which is the most significant aspect of aging hair. I guess the elite *Caviar* name was likely too good to pass up, especially given caviar's association with the finer things in life. If the caviar Alterna uses is from salmon, that would bode well for its omega-3 content, but the source of the caviar is not revealed, and there's still the fact that applying omega-3 oil to the hair won't rejuvenate it (though any oil can condition the hair). All told, these are relatively standard hair-care products whose claims are not based in reality, but rather are used to justify the higher prices. None of the Caviar products can make your hair young again, but they all serve their purpose in terms of cleaning, conditioning, and styling the hair.

☺ **$$$ Caviar Shampoo with Age-Control Complex** *($19 for 12 ounces)* is a standard shampoo that contains mostly water, detergent cleansing agents, conditioning agents, film-forming agent, caviar extract, plant extracts, vitamins, preservatives, and fragrance. This is a good shampoo for all hair types, though there is a chance of buildup if it is used exclusively. Nothing in this product will help control the aging of hair.

☺ **$$$ Caviar Conditioner with Age-Control Complex** *($19 for 12 ounces)* claims to "rebalance moisture levels in the hair" while protecting it from aging, yet nothing in this product can stop hair from aging (no hair-care product can), and any good conditioner can change the moisture level of your hair for the better. As for the caviar, it and a lengthy list of other intriguing ingredients are listed after the mineral pigments mica and titanium dioxide, which add shimmer and opacity to this conditioner, but won't help make hair smoother or softer. At best, this is a decent, though overpriced, conditioner for normal to dry hair with a normal to thin texture.

☺ **$$$ Caviar Treatment Conditioner with Age-Control Complex** *($24 for 8.5 ounces)* is nearly identical to the Caviar Conditioner with Age-Control Complex above, but this product gives you greater amounts of caviar extract, plant oil, various plant extracts, and vitamins. Although the plant extracts and vitamins have negligible benefit for the hair, at least you're getting them in amounts that help to justify this conditioner's overinflated price tag. This is a good conditioner for normal to dry hair that has a normal to thin texture.

☺ **$$$ Caviar Age-Free Protectant Defining Lotion** *($15.30 for 3 ounces)* is a lightweight conditioning styling lotion that contains a small amount of film-forming agent for a soft, flexible hold that isn't stiff or sticky. Alterna took an "everything-but-the-kitchen-sink" approach to this formula, tossing in all manner of plant extracts, vitamins, amino acids, enzymes, plant oil, even melanin (which has no effect on hair color when used in hair-care products). They don't add anything significant to the formula, but at least you're not paying a double-digit price for a bare-bones basic product. Alterna claims the neroli and hazelnut oils can protect hair from free-radical damage and preserve hair color—feats these two ingredients simply cannot do. In fact, most of the fancy ingredients in this product can't hold up under the use of heat in styling or brushing. This styling lotion provides minimal hold and is an option for all hair types.

☺ $$$ **Caviar Age-Free Protectant Smoothing Creme** *($18.90 for 8.5 ounces)* is a very good finishing cream for normal to very dry hair that is also coarse or thick. This creamy lotion contains rather commonplace conditioning agents, but they do the job to smooth hair and minimize frizzies without making hair feel heavy or greasy.

☹ **Caviar Age-Free Protectant Styling Tonic** *($20.10 for 8.5 ounces)* is a water-based styling product that ups the ante in terms of how much caviar extract is included. Although it can be a good conditioning agent for hair when used in this amount, it won't reverse what happens to your hair as it ages, though it can make it temporarily look and feel better. What's problematic about this spray-on styler is the inclusion of wasabi extract. A form of horseradish, this ingredient can be a potent scalp irritant, and in a spray-on product like this, it's nearly impossible to keep the product off of your scalp. As such, this is not recommended.

☺ $$$ **Caviar Mousse with Age-Control Complex** *($19 for 14.1 ounces)* is a standard, propellant-based, alcohol-free styling mousse that contains the same film-forming and holding agents found in countless other mousses. This product does contain a nice blend of conditioning agents, including panthenol and silicone, along with a long list of antioxidants. Regrettably, the antioxidants don't have the same benefit for hair that they do for skin or in the diet, though some antioxidants do have mild conditioning properties. It provides a light hold that is slightly sticky but can be brushed through, and is a good option for normal to fine hair.

☹ $$$ **Caviar Styling Lotion with Age-Control Complex** *($18.50 for 3 ounces)* contains a holding agent that provides a stronger hold than you might expect from a styling lotion, but it can also feel a bit sticky. The long list of vitamins, minerals, and amino acids present in the other Caviar products is here, too, but, at best this ingredient cocktail has minor conditioning and water-binding benefits for the hair. Caviar Styling Lotion does contain the problematic wasabi extract, in a lesser amount than the Caviar Age-Free Protectant Styling Tonic above, which is why this product earns a neutral rating rather than a sad face.

☹ **Caviar Styling Spray with Age-Control Complex** *($24 for 8.5 ounces)* is more a spray-on, weightless, leave-in conditioner than a styling spray. It provides no hold whatsoever, but does contain a high amount of wasabi extract, which spells trouble (in the form of irritation) for your scalp. It is not recommended.

☺ **\$\$\$ Caviar Working Hairspray with Age-Control Complex** *(\$24 for 15.5 ounces)* is a very good, though fairly standard, aerosol hairspray. It provides medium hold and contains enough silicone to leave hair shiny without weighing it down. Hair is held in place but remains brushable should you wish to restyle. The only drawback is the potent fragrance.

☺ **\$\$\$ Caviar Rapid Repair Spray with Age-Control Complex** *(\$28 for 4 ounces)* does not repair the hair in the least, and the notion that these Caviar products can somehow control the hair's aging is silly, especially since this product is nothing more than an aerosol silicone spray that contains more alcohol than it does of the extolled caviar. Like all silicone sprays, this one will give your hair a dazzling shine on application, but there is no need to spend almost thirty dollars when you can get the same (and I do mean *same*) effect from much less expensive silicone sprays available at the drugstore from lines such as Citré Shine, Pantene, and Jheri Redding.

ALTERNA HEMP SEED

All of the products below contain varying degrees of hemp seed oil or a hemp seed derivative. Because both hemp and marijuana are from the same genus (*Cannabis*) they are often thought (incorrectly) to have the same properties. However, hemp does not contain any THC (delta-9-tetrahydrocannabinol), the active ingredient in marijuana, and is not considered a drug. That means as an ingredient it has no drug-like effects. In the hair-care products below, hemp is used as a conditioning agent, and it can indeed moisturize dry, damaged hair thanks to its makeup of multiple fatty acids. Hemp is not exclusive to Alterna, nor is it a must-have ingredient, but, like all nonvolatile plant oils, it can have a positive effect on the hair.

☺ **Hemp Seed Anti-Dandruff Shampoo** *(\$16.50 for 10.1 ounces)* contains 1% salicylic acid as its active ingredient, which can help exfoliate the scalp and eliminate flakes, provided the pH is low (acidic) enough. That's not the case with this product, however, so this is merely a standard but good shampoo that contains gentle detergent cleansing agents and minimal conditioning agents, which means the risk of buildup is low. This shampoo does contain a long list of irritating fragrant plant extracts, though the amounts are likely too small to be a problem for the scalp.

☹ **Hemp Seed Hydrating Shampoo, for Dry/Damaged Hair** *(\$19.25 for 16.9 ounces)* is a standard shampoo that contains gentle detergent cleansing and lather agents, along with a few problematic plant and food extracts (such as ivy and wasabi extracts) in amounts great enough to cause scalp irritation.

☹ **Hemp Seed Scalp Therapy Shampoo** *(\$16.50 for 10.1 ounces)* is supposedly therapeutic for the scalp because it contains peppermint and menthol. But, as I have mentioned countless times before, these two ingredients can do nothing but cause irritation while imparting no special benefit for the scalp. This shampoo is not recommended for any hair or scalp type.

☹ **Hemp Seed Shampoo, for Chemically Treated Hair** *($19.25 for 16.9 ounces)* is nearly identical to the Hemp Seed Hydrating Shampoo, for Dry/Damaged Hair above, and the same comments apply. The amount of hemp seed oil in this shampoo is minuscule, so if you were hoping for some special benefit from hemp, you won't get it from this product.

☹ **Hemp Seed Shampoo, for Normal to Dry Hair** *($19.25 for 16.9 ounces)* is nearly identical to the Hemp Seed Shampoo, for Chemically Treated Hair above, and the same comments apply. Contrary to claim, this shampoo cannot balance the hair or scalp.

☺ **Hemp Seed Shine Shampoo** *($18 for 16.9 ounces)* is one of the few Alterna Hemp shampoos that leaves out the irritating wasabi extract. This is a standard conditioning shampoo that contains gentle detergent cleansing agents and a mix of irritating and non-irritating plant extracts, all in amounts too small to be of much benefit or detriment, though they do contribute to the shampoo's fragrance. This is a good shampoo for normal to dry hair (the shine comes from silicone), but it should be alternated with another shampoo to prevent buildup.

☹ **Hemp Seed Anti-Dandruff Conditioner** *($18.50 for 10.1 ounces)* contains willow bark extract as its anti-dandruff agent, presumably because of its relation to salicylic acid, a proven anti-dandruff ingredient. Although willow bark is a plant extract and, therefore, more appealing to many consumers than salicylic acid, it is simply not an effective anti-dandruff agent. But where this conditioner really goes astray is with the inclusion of sulfur, a strong antimicrobial agent that is also a potent irritant and damaging to hair. Adding more irritation are several volatile plant extracts, none of which are helpful for the scalp. There is no reason to consider using this product when lines like Head & Shoulders sell less expensive options with effective active ingredients and without such an array of unnecessary irritants.

☺ **$$$ Hemp Seed Deep Conditioner** *($23.75 for 8.3 ounces)* costs a pretty penny, but at least you do get an above-average conditioner that contains a dry-hair-helping blend of silicone, emollients, plant oil, detangling agents, protein, panthenol, and water-binding agents. The wasabi extract makes a return appearance here, but in an amount that's too small to cause irritation. Hemp Seed Deep Conditioner is recommended for normal to very dry hair of any thickness.

☺ **$$$ Hemp Seed Chemically Treated Hair Restorative Conditioner** *($19.25 for 10.1 ounces)* isn't quite as elegant as the Hemp Seed Deep Conditioner above, and includes wasabi extract in a greater amount, which increases the risk of causing scalp irritation. This is an OK conditioner for normal to slightly dry hair, but doesn't distinguish itself from dozens of less expensive conditioners at the drugstore, from Clairol to Pantene.

☺ **$$$ Hemp Seed Normal to Dry Hair Restorative Conditioner** *($19.25 for 10.1 ounces)* is a redundant formula that is nearly identical to the Hemp Seed Chemically Treated Hair Restorative Conditioner above, except that this product leaves out the castor oil, which makes it less emollient. Otherwise, the same comments apply.

☺ $$$ **Hemp Seed Shine Conditioner** *($19.25 for 10.1 ounces)* actually contains an appreciable amount of hemp seed oil compared to the other Alterna Hemp conditioners, though the result is still an ordinary formula that contains the same conditioning agents used by countless other lines. This is a good, emollient option for normal to dry hair that is thick or coarse.

☺ $$$ **Hemp Seed Hair Concrete** *($18 for 2 ounces)* is one of a new and increasingly common type of pomade, those that use standard waxes and oils along with clay for a textured look with a matte finish. In contrast to similar products from Matrix and KMS, this product still leaves hair with a slight sheen. The thick, putty-like formula takes some getting used to (and should be used sparingly), but is excellent for use on dry hair when you want to create a chunky or piece-y look that lasts through the day.

☺ $$$ **Hemp Seed Modeling Clay** *($17.70 for 2 ounces)* is a water-based pomade with a low wax content and that uses avocado oil in place of more common ingredients such as mineral or castor oil. The second ingredient is a holding agent that is typically used in hairsprays, and that gives this a sticky feel that is slightly offset by the avocado oil. This is an OK product for short hairstyles when you want the molding capabilities of a pomade combined with the strong hold of a hairspray. Do keep in mind that although your hair will remain pliable, the sticky feeling does not dissipate.

☺ **Hemp Seed Polishing Gloss** *($14.10 for 2.5 ounces)* is a standard, but very good, silicone gel that contains some SD-alcohol, but not enough to cause irritation. This waterless gel should be used sparingly, and works on wet or dry hair to add a glossy shine and tame frizzies or flyaways. It works best on normal to dry hair that is not too thin or fine.

☺ $$$ **Hemp Seed Sculpting Putty** *($17.70 for 2 ounces)* is a water-based pomade-gel hybrid that has a thick, semi-solid texture and is slightly stringy, which can make initial application unexpectedly messy. It works well as a smoothing pomade that adds medium hold and soft shine to hair. For best results, use it sparingly on the ends of dry hair.

☺ $$$ **Hemp Seed Sheer Pomade** *($16.76 for 3 ounces)* is a water-based, water-soluble pomade that is also wax-free. This does contain plant oils, so it should still be used sparingly. It is a good option for normal to dry hair with a normal to fine texture. This adds shine and control without the tackiness of products like Alterna's Hemp Seed Modeling Clay above, and rinses out with one shampoo.

☺ **Hemp Seed Shine & Texturizing Catalyst** *($10.75 for 3.4 ounces)* is a thinner version of the Hemp Seed Polishing Gloss above, and would be a better option as a silicone finishing product for normal to fine-textured hair. This product contains a tiny amount of hemp seed oil, and relies instead on coconut oil for increased shine and emollience. The small amount of alcohol is unlikely to be a problem for the scalp, especially because products like this are best used on the ends of hair for smoothing.

☺ $$$ **Hemp Seed Spray Wax** *($23.70 for 4.7 ounces)* is an aerosol spray-on pomade that is thin-textured, almost liquidy, but also quite greasy. It goes on wet and takes several moments to dry, leaving a thin layer of wax and oil on the hair. Hemp Seed Spray

Wax contains no holding agents, but can provide weight to the hair so it lies in place smoothly and stays groomed. This product is best for normal to dry hair that is also coarse to thick.

☺ $$$ **Hemp Seed Straightening Balm** *($15.30 for 8.3 ounces)* is a lightweight styling lotion with a soft, non-sticky hold and enough hemp seed oil to moisturize dry or damaged hair. It works well to straighten wavy or curly hair when used with a heat-styling device. As with any straightening product, using it alone (without heat and tension) will not make curly hair straight.

☹ $$$ **Hemp Seed Straightening Starch** *($20 for 8 ounces)* is essentially an aerosol hairspray with a blend of silicones to make hair smooth and shiny. This product is meant to be used with a blow dryer to make hair "stick straight." It dries quickly, and the type of tacky hold it provides is not conducive to getting a brush through wavy or curly hair to straighten it with heat. It can be done, but not without some snags along the way, and that can cause cuticle damage that is only compounded when you add the high heat needed to make hair straight.

☺ $$$ **Hemp Seed Styling Mud** *($19.80 for 4 ounces)* is a thick styling compound that behaves like a pomade, offering light to medium hold depending on how much you use. It can easily make hair feel heavy and look greasy if not used sparingly, but can smooth the hair and tame frizzies. This product is too heavy for thin or fine-textured hair.

☺ $$$ **Hemp Seed Styling Souffle, Medium Hold** *($18 for 2 ounces)* looks creamy in the container but emulsifies into a clear liquid that works very much like a standard styling gel, though this is slightly thicker than most. As its name implies, it provides a medium hold, but it can also make hair feel slightly stiff and sticky. The formula includes plant oils and silicone for conditioning, and these also allow hair to be easily brushed through. This is a good styling product for medium to thick or coarse-textured hair.

☹ **Hemp Seed Texturizing Glaze** *($18.90 for 8.3 ounces)* performs well on curly or wavy hair if you are looking for a conditioning styling product with a soft, light hold. The problem is that the formula tends to ball up and flake off the hair, especially if you use more product than your hair can handle. I suspect this may happen because of an incompatibility between the holding agent (polyquaternium-46) and the beeswax, but the bottom line is that the flaking is a disappointment and deterrent.

☺ $$$ **Hemp Seed Thickening Compound** *($18.60 for 5.1 ounces)* won't thicken even one strand of hair, at least not any more than similar water- and silicone-based gels can. This lightweight styling gel contains more silicones than holding agent, so you get a smooth, groomed look without any stickiness, ideal for all casual styles on all but fine hair. This would also work brilliantly, with heat and the proper styling tools, to straighten curly or wavy hair. Contrary to claim, the fennel extract in this product cannot prevent hair color from fading. Trust me, if it could do that, every hair-care company would be using copious amounts of fennel in their styling products and I would be eating the stuff daily!

☺ **$$$ Hemp Seed Ultra Hard Hold Jelly for Max Hold** *($15.30 for 4 ounces)* has a texture akin to Jell-O mixed with rubber cement, and requires you to "dig" the product out of its jar container. Emulsifying this gel takes some time. Rather than smoothing easily between your palms, it tends to ball up and break apart before finally (with concerted effort) breaking down into a clear film, ready to apply to your hair. If you're willing to put up with this gel's quirks, you'll be rewarded with a rock-hard, immovable hold, perfect if your hairstyle is extreme or your hair is stubborn about holding a style. The holding agents in this gel are normally seen in hairsprays and hair freezes, and they definitely make the hair feel stiff.

☺ **$$$ Hemp Seed Maximum Hold Volume Lock** *($21.60 for 14.1 ounces)* really does provide maximum hold, and this aerosol hairspray does so with the accompaniment of silicones and plant oils for added conditioning and noticeable shine. The light mist is ideal as a finishing spray for all hair types desiring a strong hold that can still be brushed through. Yes, there are less expensive hairsprays that provide the same effect as this, but if you prefer to purchase salon products, and want gravity-defying hold, you won't be disappointed with this one.

☺ **$$$ Hemp Seed Damage Control** *($15 for 3 ounces)* uses silicones to smooth and fill in chips on the cuticle of the hair shaft, which can temporarily allow it to behave as if it were not damaged. This product provides no hold, but can make hair feel silky and look sleek. Due to the inclusion of wasabi extract near the top of the ingredient list, this product should be kept away from the scalp. For the money, any of the silicone products from Citré Shine or John Frieda would have the same effect on the hair as this product, and without concern for irritation from the wasabi.

☹ **Hemp Seed Oil Hair Therapy** *($17.70 for 5.1 ounces)* would have been an excellent spray-on conditioning oil for dry, damaged, or chemically treated hair, but Alterna opted to include irritating spearmint oil. Probably they chose to so that consumers would feel the tingle (which is irritation) and think this specialty product was "working." What a shame, because this product has an otherwise intelligent blend of plant oils, silicone, panthenol, and proteins that are all helpful for abused or weather-beaten hair.

☻ **$$$ Hemp Seed Split Ends Repair** *($12.69 for 2.5 ounces)* cannot repair split ends—no product can; the only way to remedy split ends is to cut them off. This water-based product contains an acrylic film-forming agent along with wax, silicone, and protein to form a protective bandage around the hair shaft. To some extent, this can improve the appearance of split ends because they are coated and easier to smooth out. However, this is a temporary fix that in no way can take a split end and restore it to healthy hair, though the claims surrounding this and similar products are certainly tempting! Ignoring the split ends claims, this product isn't as well-formulated as the Hemp Seed silicone products above, such as the Shine & Texturizing Catalyst.

☺ **$$$ Hemp Seed Spray Shine** *($18.60 for 4 ounces)* is a standard and effective silicone spray that, like others of its ilk, can impart a halo of shine to the hair. The alcohol in this formula prevents the silicone from going on too heavily, which means this product can be an option for those with fine or thin hair. One caution: Hemp Seed Spray Shine has an intense orange/citrus fragrance that you should be sure you like before purchasing the product.

ALTERNA LIFE PRODUCTS

Alterna's Life products are positioned as their "total well-being" hair-care line. Yet how can products you apply to your hair significantly affect the rest of your being, unless your hair is the sole champion of your spirit? In short, they can't. The Life products are subdivided according to formulas, some meant to volumize hair, others to address the needs of thinning hair, and yet others to nourish chemically straightened hair, all through a combination of "Western technology with age-old Eastern wisdom." The Western technology comprises standard hair-care ingredients found in all of the other Alterna products and in every hair-care line in existence, while the Eastern wisdom comes from a plethora of exotic plant extracts whose benefits are based in folklore. (Eastern wisdom was not interested in making hair look thicker or in the problems associated with styling curly hair straight.) There are lots of buzz-worthy ingredients in these products, but what is really making a difference for your hair and scalp are the tried-and-true detergent cleansing agents, conditioning agents, and modern synthetic ingredients such as silicones and polymers.

☺ $$$ **Life Curls Shampoo** *($20 for 12 ounces)* contains mostly water, detergent cleansing agents, lather agents, fragrant plant extracts, vitamins, amino acids, conditioners, thickeners, and preservatives. Not one ingredient makes this product specific for curly hair. Several of the plant extracts can cause scalp irritation, but they will be rinsed away before they can cause problems; just be sure to rinse thoroughly. This shampoo is an option for all hair types, although someone with a sensitive scalp would fare better using one without all the plant extracts.

☹ **Life Restore Shampoo for Thinning Hair** *($26 for 12 ounces)* is a basic shampoo that contains a fairly high amount of acrylate copolymer, an extremely standard film-forming agent that is deposited on the hair shaft and can add a feeling of fullness. Since it can also build up with repeated use and leave fine, thin hair feeling dry and brittle, it is best to alternate this product with a shampoo that does not contain film-forming agents. Alterna claims that the azelaic acid in this shampoo can stop DHT (dihydroxytestosterone, the hormone responsible for male pattern baldness) activity by "acting on receptor sites" and blocking the enzyme (5-alpha reductase) that converts testosterone to its more potent form, DHT. Research shows that azelaic acid does indeed have this blocking effect, but so far this has been shown to be true only in a petri dish, not on real hair (Source: *British Journal of Dermatology*, November 1998, pages 627–632). What Alterna doesn't discuss is how long the azelaic acid (along with zinc) needs to be left on the scalp to inhibit 5-alpha reductase enzyme. Putting azelaic acid in a shampoo would not be the preferred way to reap its potential benefit because the shampoo is rinsed away before it can have an effect.

What is of concern with this product is Alterna's inclusion of the ingredient Calphostin-C. While there is a small amount of research showing this ingredient can increase the growth phase of the hair follicle (Source: *Skin Pharmacology and Applied Skin Physiology*, May–August 2000, pages 133–142), it is considered toxic to healthy cells (Source: www.kamiyabiomedical.com/04LifeScienceResearchProducts/PackageInserts/2/AP-0004%20Calphostin%20C%20082703%20.pdf).

☺ **$$$ Life Straight Shampoo** *($20 for 12 ounces)* has no special benefit for chemically straightened hair, beyond being a fairly gentle shampoo that will not cause buildup with repeated use.

☺ **$$$ Life Volumizing Shampoo** *($17 for 12 ounces)* does not cause buildup, nor is it effective for creating volume. This standard, but good, formula produces a rich lather that rinses easily, while the detergent cleansing agents leave hair free from styling product residue and excess oil.

☺ **$$$ Life Curls Conditioner** *($22 for 12 ounces)* is a lightweight conditioner that contains plenty of silicone, which makes it a good choice for dry, damaged, thick hair, whether straight or curly. Silicone is relatively impervious to water, so it is a good ingredient for smoothing the hair shaft and minimizing frizziness, two common issues associated with naturally curly or wavy hair. This conditioner contains enough plant oil to make it a consideration only for medium- to thick-textured hair; those with normal to fine hair will likely find this product makes hair (straight or curly) seem flat and limp, especially after repeated use.

☹ **Life Restore Conditioner for Thinning Hair** *($29.70 for 12 ounces)* contains Calphostin-C, which can be toxic to healthy cells. It is not recommended for any hair or scalp type due to the unknown risks of using this ingredient topically, especially with its limited ability to have any effect on hair growth.

☺ **$$$ Life Straight Conditioner** *($22 for 12 ounces)* is nearly identical to the Life Curls Conditioner above, except this product contains grape seed oil rather than palm oil and uses fewer detangling agents, which makes it somewhat lighter but still capable of leaving hair soft, hydrated, and manageable. Nothing about this conditioner makes it especially responsive to the needs of chemically straightened hair.

☺ **$$$ Life Volumizing Conditioner** *($18 for 12 ounces)* is a very light conditioner that is an excellent choice for normal hair that is fine or thin. The hydrolyzed pearl, flower, and herbal extracts are plentiful enough to open an exotic apothecary, but your hair won't be transformed (or volumized) by these ingredients at all.

☺ **$$$ Life Volumizing Leave-In Conditioner** *($16.50 for 8.5 ounces)* has a good formula, a reasonable price (at least compared to many Alterna products), and will do its job by making hair soft and easy to detangle while improving manageability. This does contain some film-forming and anti-static agents that can build up on hair over time, but this is a non-issue if you are using a shampoo that can effectively remove product buildup. Life Volumizing Leave-In Conditioner is recommended for all hair types.

☺ **$$$ Life Curls Detangler, for Naturally Curly Hair** *($18 for 8.5 ounces)* contains little to condition the hair other than amodimethicone (a form of silicone) and a tiny amount of panthenol. That is helpful for normal to dry hair, but it isn't special for keeping hair curly, though it can smooth frizzies.

☺ **$$$ Life Curls Shape Activator, for Naturally Curly Hair** *($20 for 5.1 ounces)* is a lightweight styling spray for all hair types that goes on wet and can add soft hold and body to the hair without feeling sticky.

☺ **Life Pliable Molding Paste** *($14.10 for 3 ounces)* is a creamy, water- and wax-based pomade whose formula is cut with a small amount of SD-alcohol to offset the heaviness of the waxes. As an alternative to traditional pomades, this product adds soft shine and texture to hair without weighing it down, though it should still be used sparingly. Hair is left feeling slightly bulked up and coated, but this shampoos out easily and is worth trying if you have normal to fine hair and want the texture, control, and separation without the heaviness of typical pomades and styling waxes.

☺ **$$$ Life Straight Radiant Finishing Lotion** *($26 for 2.6 ounces)* is a standard water- and silicone-based styling lotion that must be used sparingly to avoid a slick, greasy look. Alterna's Hemp Seed Thickening Compound, reviewed above, costs less for twice as much product, has a similar formula that is less greasy, and is easier to work with. This product should be used only by those with normal to dry hair that is thick or coarse.

☺ **$$$ Life Volumizing Flex-Hold Hair Spray** *($19.50 for 8.5 ounces)* is a very standard, nonaerosol hairspray that provides a medium hold that can be easily brushed through.

☹ **$$$ Life Volumizing Spray Gel** *($16.50 for 8.5 ounces)* is a fairly thin, alcohol-free spray gel that provides a firm hold with a sticky feel that can be difficult to brush through. There isn't much else to say about this overpriced product.

☹ **$$$ Life Volumizing Spray Mousse, for Fine and Thin Hair (Aerosol)** *($19 for 10.5 ounces)* is dispensed like an aerosol hairspray, which can make for messy application. The product mists out forcefully and then foams, but the foam can quickly clog the nozzle, which causes the product to "spray" onto countertops or your mirror as well as the palm of your hand. This mousse has a medium hold that isn't too stiff or sticky.

☹ **Life Restore Scalp and Follicle Extra Strength Serum for Thinning Hair** *($27.75 for 4.4 ounces)*. Alterna does not explicitly claim this product stops hair loss or cures baldness, but instead uses the word "combats," which only means "fights"—it doesn't mean this product will *win* the fight against hair loss. However, most consumers will interpret Alterna's claim to mean that this product can stop hair loss, and it cannot. This is primarily water and alcohol mixed with Calphostin-C (for information about this ingredient read the comments for Life Restore Shampoo for Thinning Hair above).

☹ **Life Restore Scalp and Follicle Stimulating Treatment, for Thinning Hair** *($33 for 4.4 ounces)* is mostly water and mild detergents mixed with lather agents and amino acids. This product also contains Calphostin-C (for information about this ingredient read the comments for Life Restore Shampoo for Thinning Hair above).

ALTERNA LUXURY

☺ $$$ **White Truffle Luxury Shampoo, Private Reserve** *($72 for 10.1 ounces)* is, first and foremost, not worth even a fraction of its ludicrous price tag. This shampoo contains a standard detergent cleansing agent coupled with a lather-enhancing ingredient and several conditioning agents, so it works well on normal to very dry hair, but not any better than lots of shampoos that cost a whole lot less. The big deal ingredient in this product is white truffle, although it has no distinctive benefit for hair, and its inclusion doesn't make this a shampoo to consider over others, luxury or not. White truffles are a gourmet indulgence, and are indeed expensive (0.9 ounce of whole white truffles sells for $163.95 online). However, this indulgence is one that does not translate to healthier, stronger, or shinier hair. Alterna claims white truffles are "the planet's richest source of B vitamins," yet even if white truffle were the top source of B vitamins, they would be useless to the hair because hair is dead and cannot absorb vitamins from foods (not to mention that the truffles would be rinsed down the drain. What a waste!).

Aside from the tiny amount of truffles in this product it also contains a cocktail of plant-based anti-inflammatories (such as nettle and cassia), although their positive effect is canceled by the inclusion of irritants like arnica and olibanum (frankincense). To Alterna's credit, they did create a premium-positioned shampoo that does contain a long list of rather expensive ingredients—it's just that there's no research showing these ingredients have benefit for hair, and even if they did there aren't enough of them to have any positive effect on the hair or scalp. In addition, few of them can cling to hair, so the ingredients you're paying for are rinsed away with the suds.

☺ $$$ **White Truffle Luxury Conditioner, Private Reserve** *($102 for 10.1 ounces)* contains the same main ingredients found in dozens of conditioners that cost 90% less than this overpriced concoction. This conditioner does contain several plant oils, and the high wax content makes it a suitable choice for those with normal to dry hair that is thick or coarse. The same pro and con plant ingredients present in the White Truffle Luxury Shampoo above appear here, too, but are of little benefit, and the truffles needlessly add to the cost of what is, at its core, a standard conditioner.

AMERICAN CREW

American Crew is one of the few comprehensive hair-care lines marketed exclusively to men, and its presence in salons sends a strong message that it's OK for men to shop for hair-care products. You can't help but notice this line's masculine, no-frills packaging, straightforward product names, and potent aromas favoring the outdoors that range from mint to citrus or forest-like scents. Yet for a company that "strives to build the best men's grooming products available" American Crew has made many wrong moves, though most men aren't likely to notice. Be forewarned that many of the American Crew products contain menthol, peppermint, spearmint, or eucalyptus, all ingredients that can be irritating to the scalp for both men and women. Ingredients that tingle are used in products to give the impression the product is "working," when in reality they offer no benefit for the scalp or hair. If these mint oils and derivatives were nixed, this line would be much easier to recommend to men. For now, there are some great products to be found here, but you'll need to shop with caution. For more information about American Crew, call (800) 598-CREW or visit www.americancrew.com.

What's Good About This Line: A plentiful selection of mid-priced styling products with scents, packaging, and a marketing angle that should be appealing to the average guy.

What's No So Good About It: Shampoos and conditioners contain too many needlessly irritating ingredients, primarily peppermint oil and menthol.

☹ **Anti-Dandruff Shampoo** *($10.99 for 6.76 ounces)* is a standard dandruff shampoo that contains zinc pyrithione as the active ingredient, the same one you'll find in several Head & Shoulders shampoos, all of which cost proportionately less than this option. American Crew unwisely added menthol and spearmint oil to the mix, which can cause irritation and increase itching, an even more convincing reason to consider Head & Shoulders if dandruff is a concern.

☺ **Daily Moisturizing Shampoo** *($9.49 for 8.45 ounces)* is a standard but good shampoo that contains only a tiny amount of conditioning agents, which helps prevent buildup, and it works well on short hair. This product also contains small amounts of irritating plant extracts, but likely not enough to actually cause irritation. This shampoo works well for normal to dry hair that is not fine or thin.

☺ **Daily Shampoo** *($8.49 for 8.45 ounces)* is a fine shampoo for normal to dry hair of any thickness, and is similar to the Daily Moisturizing Shampoo above.

☺ **Sport Tea Tree Shampoo** *($9.49 for 6.76 ounces)* doesn't contain anything that makes it particularly suited to men who play sports. It's just a standard shampoo that contains enough film-forming agents to cause buildup with repeated use, though that's not a problem for those with short hair. The tea tree oil present could have been an option for treating dandruff, but not when present in this low amount. The small amount of peppermint oil can cause irritation, so rinse well.

☹ **Daily Conditioner** *($13.49 for 8.45 ounces)* contains menthol and peppermint oil, two ingredients that have no business being in any hair-care products, let alone those marketed for daily use.

☹ **Leave-In Conditioner** *($8.49 for 8.45 ounces)* contains a flurry of ingredients that will serve only to make your scalp dry and itchy. Thyme, rosemary, peppermint, eucalyptus, and clove may impart a fresh, invigorating fragrance to this conditioner, but they are all scalp irritants. However, you don't purchase a conditioner to smell it, you purchase it for how well it will work on your hair or scalp.

☺ **Classic Wax, Pliable Styling Wax** *($14.95 for 3.53 ounces)* is less waxy than most pomades and is actually a workable, slightly water-soluble pomade that can impart a smooth, groomed look to hair. It definitely has a greasy texture and should be used sparingly to avoid weighing the hair down. Perhaps what's most impressive is that American Crew finally opted to leave out the peppermint and menthol present in most of their shampoos and conditioners!

☺ **$$$ Fiber** *($16.99 for 3.53 ounces)* is as thick as butter but has a harder texture that must be softened in your hands before you apply it to the hair. This water- and lanolin wax-based pomade offers substantial moisture and a low-gloss finish that works well to create a natural, groomed look on hair that is coarse or thick. Although American Crew recommends using this on towel-dried hair, it works best when used sparingly on dry hair.

☺ **Forming Cream, High Hold** *($14.99 for 3.53 ounces)* is a creamy water- and Vaseline-based pomade with a texture akin to cake frosting. This is heavy-duty stuff that contains spiderweb-like fibers that become stringy in the hair if manipulated too much. Therefore, if you opt to use this, make sure it's for a structured style you don't intend to touch. The reward will be a style that lasts all day long with high shine (though not with the matte finish the product claims to provide).

☺ **Grooming Cream** *($12.49 for 3.53 ounces)* is a lighter pomade than the Classic Wax, Fiber, and Forming Cream above. This one is a fairly straightforward pomade that can smooth frizzies and add texture to hair when used sparingly. The lanolin definitely makes it greasy, but it is an excellent ingredient for dry, coarse hair.

☺ **Grooming Spray** *($9.75 for 8.45 ounces)* works well as a light-hold hairspray that is minimally sticky and that can easily be brushed through hair. There is more alcohol than water in this product, but in a hairspray it evaporates before it has a chance to cause dryness, and it helps keep your hairstyle from falling apart.

☺ **$$$ Pomade** *($15.99 for 3.53 ounces)* is more of a thick gel than a true pomade, and works well for softly groomed hairstyles where a smooth appearance with some shine is more important than a strong hold. Compared to American Crew's other pomade-style options, this product is the most water-soluble, which means it shampoos out easily.

☺ **Spray Gel, Medium Hold** *($11.49 for 8.45 ounces)* is a basic spray-on styling gel that contains mostly water, holding agents, slip agent, silicone, and small amounts of protein and plant extracts, along with fragrance and preservatives. The absence of alcohol means that this goes on wet and takes some time to dry. It provides a medium hold that is slightly sticky but can be brushed through.

☺ **Styling Gel, Light Hold** *($11.49 for 8.45 ounces)* is a very basic, but good, styling gel that has a thinner texture than the Styling Gel, Medium Hold above but still provides medium hold with just a slight stickiness.

☺ **$$$ Styling Gel, Firm Hold** *($18.99 for 15.2 ounces)* is similar to the Styling Gel, Light Hold above, and the same comments apply.

☺ **$$$ Texture Creme** *($18.99 for 8.45 ounces)* combines a light-hold gel with conditioning agents for a smooth, non-sticky finish. This is a great finishing cream for all but fine hair types, particularly slightly dry or coarse hair.

☺ **Shine Tonic** *($11.99 for 1.7 ounces)* is a very good, though standard, silicone serum for hair. This product contains additional conditioning agents, which makes it preferred for normal to dry hair that is thick or coarse. As with all silicone serums, this should be used sparingly to avoid a greasy appearance.

AMERICAN CREW CITRUS MINT

☹ **Citrus Mint Active Shampoo** *($10.49 for 8.45 ounces)* lists orange, lime, peppermint, and spearmint oils rather high up on the ingredient list. The only "active" thing about this shampoo is the scalp irritation these unfriendly ingredients can cause.

☹ **Citrus Mint Cooling Conditioner** *($10.49 for 8.45 ounces)*. For the most part, when you see the word "cooling" used to describe a product, you can count on it containing irritating ingredients that are there to create the cooling effect. This standard conditioner is no exception. With a medley of citrus and mint oils, it is bound to be problematic for your scalp, and is not recommended.

AMERICAN CREW CLASSIC GRAY

☺ **Classic Gray Shampoo** *($9.99 for 8.45 ounces)* claims to contain "balancing properties which help remove brassy, yellow tones from gray and graying hair," and it does, in the form of synthetic coloring agents. These can tone down undesirable tones in gray or silver hair, but in a shampoo the dye agents don't cling to the hair that well, so their effect is minimal. This is otherwise a standard, gentle shampoo that contains a small amount of film-forming agents that can cause buildup with repeated use.

☺ **Classic Gray Conditioner** *($9.99 for 8.45 ounces)* contains mostly water, emollient, thickeners, conditioning agents, plant and food extracts, plant oil, dye agents, and preservatives. Because the ingredients in conditioners are better able to cling to the hair than the ingredients in shampoos, the coloring agents can help (to a minimal extent) to counter gold or brassy tones in gray or silver hair. This is a good, basic conditioner for normal hair of any thickness.

☺ **Classic Gray Styling Conditioner** *($9.99 for 8.45 ounces)* is a lightweight styling cream that does not contain the coloring agents found in the Classic Gray Shampoo and Conditioner above, so it can't impart any color-enhancing effect. This product offers a soft, flexible hold and works well for all but fine hair types. The played-up ginseng and sage extracts in this product have no effect on hair, and even if they did, they're present in an amount that's too minuscule to matter.

AMERICAN CREW LIQUID LINE

☺ **Liquid Line Groom, Pliable Styling Lotion** *($12.99 for 6.76 ounces)* is a conditioning styling lotion whose holding agent leaves hair feeling unexpectedly stiff and sticky, though it can be easily brushed through for a softer look and feel. This is a good, versatile, medium-hold styling lotion for all hair types.

☺ **Liquid Line Structure, Firm Hold Styling Lotion** *($12.99 for 6.76 ounces)* is nearly identical to the Liquid Line Groom, Pliable Styling Lotion above, except it contains lanolin wax instead of silicone, which lends a thicker texture that is preferred for dry hair that is coarse or thick. Otherwise, the same comments apply.

☺ **Liquid Line Texture, Thickening Texture Spray** *($10.99 for 6.76 ounces)* contains mostly water, magnesium sulfate (that's Epsom salt), surfactant, sea salt, plant oil, plant extracts, and preservative. This can create texture on fine or thin hair, but that's only because the salt roughs up the cuticle layer. You will have fuller hair, but with long-term use it will also be damaged and dry, so don't make it part of your daily routine.

AMERICAN CREW REVITALIZE
REVITALIZING HAIR SYSTEM FOR THINNING HAIR

☺ **Revitalize Revitalizing Daily Moisture Shampoo, for Normal to Dry Hair** *($12.99 for 12 ounces)* claims it is "formulated to maximize the life cycle of each hair strand and infuse each follicle with our patented Nutri-Rich Copper Complex." Applying copper to the scalp has limited, if any, effect on the life cycle of hair, especially not the tiny amount in this product, not to mention that in a shampoo it would just be rinsed down the drain anyway. Copper peptides may have potential for stimulating hair growth, but the research has either been done on animals (Source: *Journal of Investigative Dermatology*, July 1993, pages 143S–147S) or was conducted and paid for by companies that sell the ingredient or the products that contain it. Even taking that into consideration, the positive results were noted for copper concentrations above 2.5%—much more than the concentration in this standard shampoo. This product not only won't stimulate hair growth, but also contains a small amount of menthol, which can be stimulating, but also irritating.

☺ **Revitalize Revitalizing Daily Shampoo, for Normal to Oily Hair** *($12.99 for 12 ounces)* is similar to the Revitalizing Daily Moisture Shampoo above, but this product does not contain menthol, and that makes it a fine, though standard, option for all hair types. The comments about copper made above apply here, too.

☺ **Revitalize Revitalizing Daily Conditioner, for All Hair Types** *($16.99 for 12 ounces)* contains mostly water, thickeners, plant extracts, panthenol, slip agent, fragrance, and preservatives. The small amount of copper peptide will have no effect on hair, for better or worse. This is merely a basic conditioner for normal hair of any thickness. It contains several plant extracts that should be kept away from the scalp to avoid irritation.

☹ **Revitalize Serum** *($17.75 for 1 ounce)* lists alcohol as the second ingredient, plus a potent dose of peppermint oil. It will make the scalp tingle but that's it. This absurdly expensive waste of money is a watery serum that won't revitalize anything, though it will cause scalp itching and irritation.

☺ **$$$ Revitalize Revitalizing Spray Solution** *($31.99 for 6 ounces)* is a lightweight, spray-on conditioner for hair that contains mostly water, alcohol, copper peptides, detangling agents, conditioning agents, fragrance, and preservatives. Although the amount of copper peptide is not disclosed (it's just described as being "highly concentrated"), there is still no proof that copper peptides can stimulate hair growth or stop hair loss. It sounds promising, but is still just theory. For the money, there is good research to show that Minoxidil (either generic or Rogaine) has a vastly better chance of growing hair. As it is, this is a decent though minimally moisturizing, leave-on conditioner for normal to fine hair.

AMERICAN CREW THICKENING

☹ **Thickening Shampoo** (*$7.49 for 8.45 ounces*) contains a high amount of menthol, which may make you feel like something is happening, except that the real effect is one of irritation and dryness. This shampoo is not recommended, and contains nothing that can thicken even one strand of hair.

☹ **Thickening Conditioner** (*$8.99 for 8.45 ounces*) is a very standard conditioner that lists menthol rather high up on the ingredient list, and that means it can be a problem for causing scalp itching and irritation.

☺ **Thickening Lotion** (*$10.49 for 4.2 ounces*) promises to make hair look its thickest while providing excellent hold, but it cannot thicken hair any better than most other leave-in conditioners or lightweight, low-wax pomades. The film-forming agent provides a strong hold that's slightly sticky, but the conditioning agents allow hair to remain relatively soft and brushable. This does contain a small amount of eucalyptus, so try not to get it on the scalp.

ANTHONY LOGISTICS

Anthony Logistics is primarily a skin-care line whose packaging and presentation are designed to appeal to men. The majority of this line's skin-care products are either ordinary formulations carrying extraordinary prices or they contain at least one potent irritant. Neither option is helpful for a man's skin, especially when the irritation occurs after shaving. Unfortunately, Anthony Logisitcs' small collection of hair-care products follows suit. There are no breakthrough or unique products to be found, but plenty of irritation from the shampoos. The styling products are OK, but quite ordinary for the money. Other than the fragrance, there is nothing about this line that makes it preferred for men. For more information about Anthony Logistics, call 866-Anthony or visit www.anthony.com.

What's Good About This Line: Standard styling products that perform as promised.

What's Not So Good About It: Shampoos and conditioners that contain peppermint oil and/or camphor, which only serve to cause scalp itching and irritation.

☹ **Everyday Shampoo, for Normal to Dry Hair** (*$16 for 8 ounces*) contains peppermint oil, which makes it too irritating to the scalp. With the wealth of gentle shampoos from readily available hair-care lines, men are often better off avoiding lines whose marketing caters to them because the formulations are usually as problematic as this one.

☹ **Everyday Shampoo, for Normal to Oily Hair** (*$16 for 8 ounces*) is nearly identical to the Everyday Shampoo above, and the same comments apply. This one contains peppermint oil and camphor, which only increase scalp irritation while offering no benefit for oily hair.

☹ **Everyday Conditioner, for All Hair Types** *($18 for 6 ounces)* is a very basic detangling conditioner that is made problematic by the inclusion of peppermint oil. Any conditioner from L'Oreal or Pantene costs much less and offers an improved formulation without irritants.

☺ **$$$ Stronger Than Usual Conditioner, for Normal to Dry Hair** *($18 for 6 ounces)* doesn't contain peppermint oil, but does have more fragrance than anything uniquely beneficial for the hair. This is as basic as conditioners get, and contains mostly water, thickeners, detangling agent, fragrance, emollients, plant extracts, preservatives, and plant oils. It's an OK option for normal to slightly dry hair.

☺ **$$$ Hair Cream, for All Hair Types** *($18 for 4 ounces)* is mostly water, thickeners, squalene (an emollient), detangling agent, honey (which has water-binding properties for hair), preservatives, slip agent, conditioning agents, plant oils, and panthenol. The intriguing ingredients are listed after the preservative, but this can still be an OK, leave-in conditioner for normal to slightly dry hair of any thickness.

☺ **$$$ Hair Gel, for All Hair Types** *($15 for 4 ounces)* is an extremely standard gel that offers a smooth, light hold that is minimally sticky and can be easily brushed through. Still, for the money, almost any styling gel at the drugstore will perform similarly without this one's high price tag.

AQUA NET

Aqua Net has been around for decades, and I dare say many baby-boomer women had their inaugural hairspray experience with one of Aqua Net's products. Though the formulas have changed over the years, what remains the same is that Aqua Net delivers on its promise of all-day hold that does not flake. Don't discount this line just because it has been around forever, or because the same holding ingredients show up in all hair sprays—the prices are bona fide bargains and the hairsprays themselves perform admirably. For more information about Aqua Net, call (800) 626-7283.

What's Good About This Line: Workable aerosol hairsprays at an affordable price.

What's Not So Good About It: These formulas dry so fast there is little to no time to play with your style after you apply them, so these are strictly style-holding sprays, not styling sprays.

☺ **2 Super Hold All Day All Over Hold, Fresh Fragrance** *($2.59 for 14 ounces)* is a standard aerosol hairspray that contains mostly water, propellant, alcohol, film-forming/holding agents, preservative, silicones, and fragrance. It offers a strong hold that remains slightly sticky, making hair a bit difficult to brush through. Yet if you don't plan to brush through your hair, this hairspray works well to maintain your hairstyle, be it simple or complex.

☺ **2 Super Hold All Day All Over Hold, Unscented** *($2.59 for 14 ounces)* contains a masking fragrance that does impart scent, so this is not a fragrance-free hairspray. It is otherwise identical in every respect to the 2 Super Hold All Day All Over Hold hairspray above, and the same comments apply.

☺ **3 Extra Super Hold All Day All Over Hold, Fresh Fragrance** *($2.59 for 14 ounces)* is nearly identical to the 2 Super Hold All Day All Over Hold, Fresh Fragrance hairspray above, but with a slightly stronger hold that is, surprisingly, less sticky. This can be difficult to brush through with ease, but it's great for locking your style in place or controlling flyaway strands.

☺ **3 Extra Super Hold All Day All Over Hold, Unscented** *($2.59 for 14 ounces)* is identical to the 3 Extra Super Hold All Day All Over Hold hairspray above, except that it contains a much softer fragrance, and the same basic comments apply. Unscented, however, does not mean fragrance-free; it has a scent to mask the smell of the alcohol.

ARTEC

ARTec was one of the first and is still one of the best lines to offer temporary color-enhancing shampoos and conditioners. Since the last edition of this book, they have nicely organized their selection of 12 options into simple categories of blonde, brunette, and red hair. Of course, they still want you to believe it is their "pure and natural" ingredients that are responsible for the color-enhancing effect. But just a cursory look at the ingredient list reveals that what's doing the work are the same basic, synthetic dyes you'll find in all shampoos and conditioners claiming to affect the color of hair. Regardless, these products are still worthy options to subtly (and I mean very subtly) brighten or enhance the color of your hair.

ARTec has expanded considerably over the last few years. I wish I could say that the latest additions are all wonderful, refreshing options, but in the world of hair-care formulations, there is rarely anything new under the sun—though the marketing language always paints a novel picture. For the most part, ARTec's expansion has only increased the number of potentially irritating products. These tend to cloud the fact that, beneath all the hype and potent fragrances, there are some outstanding ARTec products, at prices that are a step above what you'll pay at the drugstore but less than what many salon lines (particularly those from designer hairstylists) are charging. For more information about ARTec, call (800) 443-7763 or visit www.artecworldwide.com.

What's Good About This Line: A very good selection of color-enhancing shampoos and conditioners (with the conditioners being the preferred product to deposit color on the hair) and a wide selection of styling products for just about any hairstyle you care to create.

What's Not So Good About It: The entire Pure Hair line is rife with problematic essential oils (though some products do fare better than others); the claims for the Kiwi Coloreflector line being able to seal and prolong hair color are without proof.

ARTEC BLONDES

☺ **Blondes Color Depositing Shampoo** *($11.80 for 8 ounces)* is a fairly standard, gentle shampoo, available in four different formulas that differ only in the dye ingredients each contains. All of them would be great options for blonde hair of any thickness, be it natural or color-treated. The plant extracts have no effect on hair color. Rather, the unnatural coloring agents in each natural-named formula are responsible for depositing color on the hair. Keep in mind, though, that in a shampoo these dyes do not cling too well, so the effect tends to be barely discernible. *Note: This shampoo and the corresponding conditioner below come in Ginger Root, Lemon Flower, Sunflower, and White Violet.*

☺ **Blondes Color Depositing Moisturizer** *($11.80 for 8 ounces)* is a better option for depositing color on the hair than the shampoo above because you leave the conditioner on the hair longer and the conditioning agents allow the dyes to cling better to the hair shaft. This conditioner is available in four different shades for blonde hair and is good for normal to dry hair of any thickness.

ARTEC BRUNETTES

☺ **Brunettes Color Depositing Shampoo** *($11.80 for 8 ounces)* is similar to the Blondes Color Depositing Shampoo above, except that the dye agents are meant to enhance all shades of brown hair. Again, four shades are available; which one to choose depends on the depth and tone of your brown hair, though the effect of the dye agents in this shampoo is minimal. *Note: this shampoo and the corresponding conditioner below come in Blue Orchid, Coco Bean, Mahogany, and Walnut.*

☺ **Brunettes Color Depositing Moisturizer** *($11.80 for 8 ounces)* is available in four shades for enhancing various tones of brown hair. With the exception of the dye agents used, the formula is nearly identical to the Blondes Color Depositing Moisturizer above, and the same comments apply. The coffee extract in these conditioners can help enhance the effect of the synthetic dyes.

ARTEC REDS

☺ **Reds Color Depositing Shampoo** *($11.80 for 8 ounces)* also comes in four shades for enhancing red to auburn hair, and has a formula that, save for the dye agents and a couple of plant extracts (which have no effect on hair color), is identical to the Blondes Color Depositing Shampoo above, and the same basic comments apply. *Note: This shampoo and the corresponding conditioner below come in Cherry Bark, Orange Marigold, Red Clover, and Strawberry.*

☺ **Reds Color Depositing Moisturizer** *($11.80 for 8 ounces)* is available in four shades for enhancing red or auburn tones in hair, and, aside from the dye agents and plant extracts, is nearly identical to the Blondes Color Depositing Moisturizer above, and the same basic comments apply.

ARTEC KIWI COLOREFLECTOR

The Kiwi Coloreflector line is positioned as being able to seal in hair color, yet it contains the same standard hair-care ingredients as the rest of ARTec's products (and the entire hair-care industry, for that matter). The styling products cannot protect color from fading. A few of the products do contain sun-protecting ingredients, but it's impossible to gauge how much protection they provide because there are no official standards of measurement. Plus, sunscreen ingredients do not hold up under rinsing, blow dryers, or flat irons. What's most troubling about this subcategory is the use of drying detergent cleansing agents and a film-forming ingredient that can strip hair color. Proceed with caution.

☹ **Kiwi Coloreflector Shampoo** *($8 for 8 ounces)* contains sodium C14-16 olefin sulfonate as its main cleansing agent, which can be too drying for all hair and scalp types. There are some plant oils that can have a conditioning effect on the hair, but that is compromised by the drying detergent cleansing agent. Nothing about this shampoo makes it a good option for color-treated hair.

☺ **Kiwi Coloreflector Conditioner** *($10 for 8 ounces)* is a very standard conditioner that works well for normal to slightly dry hair. It has no special benefit for color-treated hair. If anything, those with color-treated hair will find this not moisturizing or smoothing enough.

☺ **Kiwi Coloreflector Hydrating Treatment** *($9.60 for 8 ounces)* is a good, slightly emollient conditioner for normal to dry hair that is not fine or thin. Calling it a treatment is a misnomer because nothing in this product is radically different from what's found in most standard conditioners.

☺ **Kiwi Coloreflector Blaster Spray, Fast Drying Super Hold Hairspray** *($12 for 10 ounces)* is a standard aerosol hairspray with medium hold that is slightly sticky, but it can be easily brushed through.

☹ **Kiwi Coloreflector Blow Up Volume, Adds Density and Volume** *($11.55 for 8 ounces)* is meant to be used with a blow dryer for adding volume to hair, but the small amount of conditioning agents it contains makes it a poor choice for offering hair some protection from heat. As if that weren't enough, this gel contains sodium polystyrene sulfonate as the main film-forming agent, an ingredient that can strip hair color with repeated use. What's that doing in a product meant to help *preserve* hair color?

☺ **Kiwi Coloreflector Blow Serum, Smoothes and Repairs Stressed Hair** *($10.60 for 8.5 ounces)* is a lightweight, almost no-hold styling liquid that can make hair easy to brush through while styling, though it offers minimal protection from heat. That means it's best used with a silicone gel or serum. This absolutely does not repair hair, no matter how stressed it is.

☺ **Kiwi Coloreflector Detailer Spray, Fast Drying Power Hold Hairspray** *($11.50 for 10 ounces)* is nearly identical to the Kiwi Coloreflector Blaster Spray above, and the same comments apply. This does provide a bit more hold than the Blaster Spray, but not enough to make one or the other a better choice.

☺ **Kiwi Coloreflector Manipulating Wax** *($12.50 for 3 ounces)* is one of the newer breed of aerosol pomades, or "wax in a can." It allows you to add texture and definition to hair without much weight, and provides a natural, non-sticky finish with minimal shine.

☺ **Kiwi Coloreflector Piecing Paste, Power Hold to Piece and Shape** *($13.80 for 4 ounces)* is a conditioning gel-pomade that offers a thick texture capable of a firm, non-stiff hold, but not without a lot of stickiness. This is a good option for those who wish to exaggerate or add strong texture to short, spiky hairstyles.

☺ **Kiwi Coloreflector Rock-It Spray, Rock-Hard Hold** *($10 for 8 ounces)* is a standard nonaerosol hairspray that offers a strong, stiff, slightly sticky hold that can be brushed through, though it is best reserved for creating gravity-defying hairstyles you don't intend to touch once they're in place.

☺ **Kiwi Coloreflector Root Elevator, Power Hold Foam Gel Root Lifter and Detailer** *($12.75 for 9.5 ounces)* is akin to a pressurized styling mousse, but has a special applicator nozzle that allows you to spray this lightly foaming product directly onto the roots of your hair. It tends to go on quite wet, and will be too runny if you spray too much (which is easy to do), but it does provide a medium hold that will indeed give lift and support to roots when used with heat-styling tools. This does have a tacky after-feel, but it can be easily brushed through.

☺ **Kiwi Coloreflector Shaping Foam, Shapes and Conditions Hair** *($8.50 for 7 ounces)* is a standard styling mousse that offers a good medium hold that is stickier than most, but can still be brushed through (which will help to lessen the stickiness).

☺ **Kiwi Coloreflector Shine Wax** *($12 for 2 ounces)* is traditional pomade that is primarily water, castor oil, and wax. The small amount of film-forming agent provides a hint of hold, but hair still remains soft and pliable. This should be used sparingly and works best on thick, coarse hair to smooth the ends or calm frizzies.

☺ **Kiwi Coloreflector Blow Silk, Silk Shine for Dry and Wet Styling** *($11 for 2 ounces)* is a runny silicone serum that contains some alcohol, which helps to thin the silicone and distribute the fluid evenly over the hair. This can make hair feel silky-smooth, but should be used sparingly and on dry, thicker hair for best results.

☺ **Kiwi Coloreflector Kiwi Detangler, Leave-In Styling Conditioner** *($10.60 for 8.4 ounces)* contains mostly water and detangling agent. The rest of the formula is plant extracts (which have no conditioning effect on hair) and tiny amounts of panthenol, soy protein, and plant oil. This can indeed detangle the hair but offers no hold, so it's best used for natural hairstyles you allow to air dry.

ARTec Pure Hair

The Pure Hair line is clearly ARTec's attempt to compete with (and some might say copy) Aveda. Right on the bottles, ARTec proudly states these products use "Pure organic plant and flower aromatherapy" and that they contain 100% pure essential oils—no artificial fragrance or color. Of course, the essential oils are nothing more than a fancy, roundabout way to include fragrance, so why advertise that these products contain no artificial scents or coloring agents when the rest of the ARTec line does? Should you avoid buying their other products because they lack this feature? It turns out the Pure Hair products have more problems than benefits for hair because several of the essential oils are potent scalp irritants.

☹ **Pure Hair Mandarin Bodifying Shampoo** *($10.65 for 9 ounces)* is a standard conditioning shampoo that would have been a fairly gentle option if it didn't feature rosemary, lemon, and mandarin orange oils high up on the ingredient list. These may make this shampoo smell divine, but will only cause scalp itching and irritation.

☹ **Pure Hair Patchouli Balancing Pure Shampoo** *($10.65 for 9 ounces)* contains a startlingly high amount of potent scalp irritants, including clove, cardamom, lavandin, orange, rosemary, and geranium oils. This shampoo is not recommended for any hair or scalp type.

☹ **Pure Hair Rosemary Purifying Shampoo** *($10.65 for 9 ounces)* contains eucalyptus and rosemary oils, and both can cause scalp irritation. This shampoo is not recommended, and won't purify anything (though it can clear your sinuses if you smell it!).

☹ **Pure Hair Sweet Fennel Hydrating Shampoo** *($10.65 for 9 ounces)* contains several plant oils that are irritating to the scalp, including geranium, silver fir, lavender, and patchouli. This shampoo also contains balsam oil, which can quickly build up on the hair and make it feel dry and brittle.

☹ **Pure Hair Basil Mint Detangling Elixir** *($10.65 for 9 ounces)* is a basic conditioner that is not recommended due to the inclusion of wild mint, rosemary, and peppermint oils, along with menthol. My scalp is hurting just thinking about it!

☹ **Pure Hair Chamomile Aloe Moisturizing Balm** *($14.85 for 9 ounces)* is a standard detangling conditioner that is a poor option for your scalp thanks to the inclusion of clove, cardamom, lavandin, and a slew of other fragrant oils rather high up on the ingredient list.

☹ **Pure Hair Geranium Replenishing Tonic** *($12.75 for 9 ounces)* lists geranium oil as the second ingredient, followed by balsam, which can irritate the scalp and dry out the hair. This is about as replenishing for hair as drinking Tabasco sauce is for a sore throat.

☺ **Pure Hair Borage Supporting Liquidgel** *($14.30 for 9 ounces)* is a spray gel with a medium hold that is slightly sticky but can be easily brushed through. It works well to style normal to fine hair.

☺ **Pure Hair Cornflower Working Spray** *($12.75 for 12 ounces)* is an alcohol- and water-based nonaerosol hairspray that stays wet longer than most hairsprays, so you have extra time to manipulate your hairstyle. It offers a light, flexible hold that can be easily brushed through.

☺ **Pure Hair Grapeseed Finishing Pureshine** *($14.85 for 2 ounces)* is a standard pomade that can easily make hair feel heavy and look greasy if you use too much. Used sparingly it does smooth ends and add shine.

☺ $$$ **Pure Hair Jasmine Volumizing Fixative** *($15.95 for 9 ounces)* is a good, though extremely ordinary, medium-hold styling spray that is overpriced unless jasmine is a fragrance you must have on your hair.

☺ **Pure Hair Meadowfoam Seed Styling Mousse** *($13.80 for 7 ounces)* is similar to Aveda's Phomollient ($12 for 6.7 ounces), but Aveda does not include the irritating essential oils ARTec chose for this liquid styling foam. Geranium, patchouli, silver fir, and balsam are just a few of the potent offenders in this product, which makes Aveda's option, along with those from other lines, all that much better. The neutral face rating assumes you will not use this product near the scalp, because the essential oils in it will cause problems.

☺ **Pure Hair Sandalwood Finishing Spray** *($10 for 12 ounces)* is a nonaerosol, alcohol-based, firm-hold hairspray that can be easily brushed through.

☺ **Pure Hair Soybean Bodifying Puregel** *($12.75 for 8 ounces)* is a standard styling gel with a thin texture and a slightly sticky medium hold that can make hair feel stiff but is easily brushed through.

☺ **Pure Hair Watercress Finishing Purehold** *($14.85 for 2 ounces)* is similar to, but less waxy than, the Pure Hair Grapeseed Finishing Pureshine above. This is a good pomade for all but fine hair types, and works best when used sparingly on dry hair.

☺ **Pure Hair Neroli Reflecting Sprayshine** *($12.99 for 4 ounces)* is an alcohol-based, waterless silicone spray that is light enough to be used as a finishing touch by those with fine hair. The small amount of holding agent this contains does not make the hair feel sticky or stiff.

ARTEC TEXTURELINE

Textureline comprises the bulk of ARTec's vast product selection, and has been around the longest. Out of all the ARTec subcategories, this one offers the most options with the fewest causes for concern. Gone are almost all of the scalp-irritating essential oils that are a concern for many of the Pure Hair products, and the Textureline products do not contain the drying detergent cleansing agents found in the Kiwi Coloreflector line. The Textureline subcategory is not without problems, but for the most part these are the ARTec products that deserve the most consideration.

☺ **Textureline Smoothing Shampoo** *($10.10 for 12 ounces)* is a standard conditioning shampoo that is good for normal to dry or chemically treated hair, although it can cause buildup with repeated use.

☺ **Textureline Volume Shampoo** *($10.10 for 12 ounces)* is nearly identical to the Textureline Smoothing Shampoo above, only this one contains less conditioning and film-forming agent, and is recommended for all hair types. This will not cause buildup, so it is an option to alternate with the Smoothing Shampoo above.

☺ **Textureline Smoothing Conditioner** *($9.99 for 8 ounces)* is a very good moisturizing conditioner for dry to very dry hair of any texture except fine or thin.

☺ **Textureline Volume Conditioner** *($9.50 for 8 ounces)* is a good lightweight conditioner for normal to slightly dry hair that is fine or thin.

☺ **$$$ Textureline Adhesive, Radical Hair Glue** *($15.95 for 5.75 ounces)* comes in a bottle reminiscent of Elmer's Glue, an apt feature for this clear styling gel that offers an incredibly strong hold that remains sticky and can make hair difficult to brush through. This gel is best for hair that resists staying in place when using conventional styling products, and it also works well on short, textured hair when a high degree of hold is required.

☺ **Textureline Aeromousse, Spray-On Mousse Gel (Aerosol)** *($10.60 for 10 ounces)* is an aerosol, spray-on mousse whose application method holds no advantage over a traditional mousse. It is a lightweight product that contains cornstarch as the main holding agent, an OK option for a light, non-sticky hold that can be combed through. This offers no significant protection from heat, so it's best paired with a silicone product if you intend to use a blow dryer or flat iron.

☺ **Textureline Control Gel, Exceptionally Strong All Day Hold for Curly and Wavy Hair** *($10 for 8 ounces)* is a standard, firm-hold styling gel that can make hair feel slightly stiff and sticky, though it can be brushed through. It works well for all hair types, though someone with curly hair may not appreciate this gel's stiffness.

☹ **Textureline Magnifier, Adds Substance and Hold for Blow Drying** *($11.95 for 8 ounces)* contains sodium polystyrene sulfonate as the main film-forming agent, and that can be drying to hair and strip hair color, too. This product offers no protection from heat-styling implements.

☺ **Textureline Material, Pliable Material for Matte Finishes on Dry or Wet Hair** *($11.75 for 2 ounces)* is a heavy-duty pomade that contains mostly water, lanolin wax, mineral oil, thickener, alcohol, film-forming agents, beeswax, preservatives, and fragrance. It can smooth the hair and add texture with a low-gloss shine, and is best for thick or coarse hair that is dry to very dry. This does leave hair in a pliable state, so it can be manipulated as often as needed.

☺ **Textureline Smoothing Serum, Exceptional for Blow Drying Smooth and Straight Styles** *($12.75 for 8 ounces)* is a lightweight, minimally sticky styling lotion that functions primarily as a leave-in conditioner. The amount of plant oils it contains means that it can provide some protection from heat styling. This product is best for normal to dry hair that has a normal to coarse or thick texture.

☺ **Textureline Straight Spray, for Straight Styles and Flat Iron** *($9.95 for 5.3 ounces)* is an alcohol-based aerosol hairspray that offers a firm, stiff hold that can be brushed through. This is not the best product to use with flat irons, or blow dryers, for that matter, and is not preferred to a product like the Textureline Smoothing Serum above, which conditions hair and offers some protection from heat. It works best after heat styling as a finishing spray.

☺ **$$$ Textureline Texture Creme, Weightless Volume for Moisture Deprived Hair** *($15.70 for 8.4 ounces)* is basically a styling cream with holding agents, similar to what you'd get if you mixed a leave-in conditioner with a standard styling gel. It offers a medium hold that is slightly sticky, but the hair stays relatively soft and can be easily brushed through. This works well for normal to dry hair that has a normal to thick or coarse texture.

☺ **Textureline Texture Freeze, Super Fast Drying Hair Spray with Shine (Non-Aerosol)** *($8.20 for 8 ounces)* does not dry "super fast," but actually takes longer to set than most hairsprays. It works well as a standard, light-hold hairspray that is minimally sticky. The alcohol- and water-based formula contains enough silicone to add shine, while the plant and vegetable oils help make hair easier to brush through.

☺ **Textureline Texture Gel, Weightless Finishing Gel** *($9.95 for 8 ounces)* is a very standard styling gel. Although lightweight, it can leave hair feeling stiff and sticky. It offers a medium hold that is somewhat difficult to brush through.

☹ **Textureline Texture Mousse, Non-Aerosol Liquid to Mousse Technology** *($12 for 8.5 ounces)* contains sodium polystyrene sulfonate as the main film-forming agent. It can be drying to hair and strip hair color, and this is not recommended.

☺ **Textureline Texture Paste, Shaping, Piecing, Defining** *($14.95 for 4 ounces)* isn't really a paste, it's more of a conditioner with film-forming/holding agents for extra control. This is a good styling cream for normal to dry hair that is thick or coarse. The product remains moist, though the holding agents do add a slightly stiff, sticky feel.

☺ **Textureline Texture Shine** *($12.75 for 2.64 ounces)* is a very good, though slightly heavy, water-soluble pomade. It contains mostly water, thickeners, plant oil, lanolin, glycerin, more thickeners, fragrant plant extract, film-forming agent, slip agent, preservatives, mica, and fragrance. The mica adds shiny particles to this pomade that can add extra shine to the hair, and these do not flake off. This is best used sparingly on dry hair, and is not recommended for those with fine or thin hair.

☺ **Textureline Texture Shine Spray, for Weightless Finishing and Blow Drying (Non-Aerosol)** *($12.75 for 4 ounces)* is a lightweight silicone spray whose main ingredient is alcohol. This allows the silicone to go on lighter, while still imparting shine. It works well as a finishing touch for all hair types, though it should be used sparingly by those with fine hair.

☺ **Textureline Texture Spray, Fast Drying Spray for Weightless Hold (Aerosol)** *($11.75 for 10 ounces)* is a standard aerosol hairspray that dries quickly after application and still goes on very light, providing shine and a medium hold that can be brushed through.

☺ **Textureline Texture Spray Firm, Fast Drying Hairspray for Firm Hold (Aerosol)** *($11.75 for 10 ounces)* is nearly identical to the Textureline Texture Spray above, though this option is slightly less sticky. Otherwise, the same comments apply.

☺ **Textureline Volume Gel, Weightless Gel for Blow Drying** *($9.95 for 8 ounces)* doesn't contain anything that makes it preferred for blow drying, and it lacks ingredients that can provide even limited protection from heat. It is just a standard lightweight styling gel with a good medium hold that is slightly sticky, though hair can still be brushed through.

☺ **Textureline Inner Structure Treatment, Restructurizing Leave-In Treatment** *($10.95 for 12 ounces)* takes the prize for the ARTec product that makes the most unrealistic claims. This spray-on detangler is supposed to help repair the cuticle while equalizing and adjusting its porosity so your hair will be healthier from the inside out. Considering this product is primarily water, silicone polymer, detangling agents, and water-binding agents, the best it can do is make hair easier to comb through while providing light conditioning and making hair feel a bit softer. None of these ingredients can repair the cuticle or affect the porosity of the hair. This product works well for all hair types, provided you keep your expectations based in reality.

☺ **Textureline Shine & Frizz Repair, Weightless Shine Drops** *($12 for 2 ounces)* is a standard silicone serum that works as well as any to make hair look sleek and smooth while providing a high-gloss shine.

AUBREY ORGANICS

The Aubrey Organics hair-care line has been preaching pure and natural ingredients for over 30 years. Aubrey Hampton literally wrote the book on natural ingredients. His publications, which include *What's in Your Cosmetics?* and *Natural Organic Hair and Skin Care*, are proof he takes the study of natural ingredients and their applications in personal care products seriously. Foremost is his company's philosophy "All Aubrey Organics® products are completely natural, made with herbals, essential oils and natural vitamins. No synthetic chemicals of any kind are ever found in any of our formulas. We use liquid coconut oil in our soaps and shampoos and coconut fatty acids and essential fatty acids in our creams and lotions, and a natural preservative of citrus seed and vitamins A, C and E." What's not explained, however, is the very synthetic process that these ingredients undergo to make them work in cleansers and shampoos or the fact that vitamins are not the best preservatives, largely due to their inherent instability over the long term. Because Hampton doesn't reveal the specific forms of the vitamins he uses (even though he is required to by the FDA), we can't be sure just how stable his preservative system is. In fact, Hampton's ingredient lists don't comply in the least with FDA standards, so trusting them at all is a leap of faith.

The company is also keen on promoting the use of organic ingredients, but this, while helpful for the environment, has no effect on the final product's performance. Also, keep in mind that although an Aubrey product (and products in other lines as well) may start out organic, by the time it's in a product formulated to clean, condition, or style hair, it isn't organic anymore. After all, when was the last time you saw a shampoo or hairspray growing from the ground?

The ingredient lists and the company's noncompliance with regulations regarding claims made for over-the-counter products (including those for hair care) have led the FDA to issue warnings to Aubrey Hamilton (Source: www.fda.gov/foi/warning_letters/m2393n.pdf). Clearly, Hampton did little to heed the warnings, particularly in regard to full disclosure of product ingredients. For example, his Jojoba & Aloe Hair Rejuvenator & Conditioner lists its ingredients as organic jojoba oil, organic aloe vera, and "a natural coconut fatty acid base." Not only is the last part of the ingredient statement noncompliant with the FDA and Cosmetics, Toiletries, & Fragrance Association (CTFA) labeling regulations, but this product also has a potent floral-musky fragrance that does not match how any of these ingredients should smell. In other words, something's missing here, and for all Hampton's "natural = safe" for consumers posturing, this is an inexcusable omission that keeps consumers in the dark about what is really in these products. The icing on the dishonest cake is reading on Hampton's Web site that the company prides itself (and has for years) on "Full Label Disclosure."

Another point to ponder is that, according to the Web site, his products are sold worldwide in over 4,500 stores. Yet despite this massive distribution, all of his 140+ products are supposedly handcrafted in small batches. Having toured many facilities that handle raw ingredients and manufacture skin- and hair-care products, I can tell you that this claim is completely implausible. Does Hampton want consumers to believe that his recipes are cooked up in kitchens, using fresh herbs from an adjacent garden? That can work in small batches, but when was the last time you tried to make enough cakes (for example) to send to 4,500 locations? And that's assuming each locale wants only one cake, not dozens. The freshness and tender loving care aspect is nice imagery, but in reality, if these products are to be sold worldwide, they are being manufactured in the same manner as all cosmetic products, meaning in enormous batches with automated machinery.

The hair-care products reviewed below have changed little since I last reviewed this line. Although most lines have their share of good and bad products, Hampton's line has a disproportionate amount of hair-care products to avoid, due either to poorly chosen cleansing agents or to problematic plant oils, such as balsam and lavender. The good products are nothing exceptional, but can work well enough to appease consumers intent on believing in Hampton's all-natural hype. For more information about Aubrey Organics, call (800) 282-7394 or visit www.aubrey-organics.com.

What's Good About This Line: For fans of natural products, the prices for most of the items are more than reasonable.

What's Not So Good About It: Every shampoo contains a drying soap cleansing base, the fragrance is knock-your-socks-off potent, and the too-natural-to-be-true ingredient lists for many products are highly suspect.

☹ **Aloe Essence Clarifying Shampoo for Oily Hair** *($8.95 for 11 ounces),* **Aloe Essence Everyday Shampoo for Normal Hair** *($8.95 for 11 ounces),* **Aloe Essence Moisturizing Shampoo for Dry Hair** *($8.95 for 11 ounces)* **Aloe Essence Revitalizing Shampoo for Damaged/Treated Hair** *($8.95 for 11 ounces),* **Blue Camomile Shampoo** *($8.95 for 8 ounces),* **Blue Green Algae Hair Rescue Vegetal Protein Shampoo** *($10 for 8 ounces),* **Calaguala Fern & Cade Tar Scalp Treatment Shampoo** *($10 for 8 ounces),* **Camomile Luxurious Herbal Shampoo** *($7.50 for 8 ounces),* **Green Tea Hair Treatment Shampoo** *($9.50 for 8 ounces),* **Honeysuckle Rose Conditioning Shampoo** *($7.75 for 8 ounces),* **Island Naturals**

Island Butter Shampoo *($8 for 8 ounces)*, J.A.Y. (Jojoba/Aloe/Yucca) Desert Herb Shampoo *($10.50 for 8 ounces)*, Mandarin Magic Ginkgo Leaf & Earth Smoke Shampoo *($7.75 for 8 ounces)*, Polynatural 60/80 Shampoo *($9.25 for 8 ounces)*, Rosa Mosqueta Rose Hip Herbal Shampoo *($8.75 for 8 ounces)*, Sea Buckthorn Egg Conditioning Shampoo *($8.90 for 8 ounces)*, Selenium Natural Blue Shampoo *($8.75 for 8 ounces)*, and White Camellia & Jasmine Conditioning Shampoo *($8.50 for 8 ounces)* all have a coconut-oil soap base, which can be extremely drying to the hair and irritating for the scalp. Almost all of these shampoos also contain fragrant oils that can cause scalp irritation, and despite the inclusion of protein and randomly dispersed conditioning ingredients, they cannot overcome the dryness caused by this soap base. None of these are recommended.

☹ Egyptian Henna Shampoo *($8 for 8 ounces)* doesn't list coconut oil soap, but rather lists coconut oil, which you have to assume is the saponified soap form because coconut oil by itself cannot clean hair, would not rinse easily out of hair, and would make it impossible to obtain any lather. Once again, Aubrey Hampton's ingredient lists are not as structured or as accurate as they should be. This shampoo can be even more drying than the ones above because it also contains henna, which can build up on the hair with repeated use and make it feel brittle.

☹ Natural Baby and Kids Shampoo *($7.95 for 8 ounces)* is similar to all of the shampoos above that use drying coconut oil *soap* as their base, though it is incorrectly labeled as just coconut oil. This shampoo's inclusion of balm mint and mistletoe makes it completely inappropriate for use on kids and babies. Adults would also do well so stay away from this shampoo!

☹ Primrose & Lavender Herbal Shampoo *($7.25 for 8 ounces)* contains a coconut-oil soap base, incorrectly listed as just coconut oil. This product also contains grain alcohol, balm mint, lavender oil, and balsam oil, which can cause considerable scalp irritation and contribute to the drying effect that coconut soap has on all hair types.

☹ QBHL Quillaya Bark Hair Lather *($7.50 for 8 ounces)* uses less coconut oil-based soap than the other shampoos in this line because the cleansing effect is supposed to come from the quillaya bark, which is a source of saponins, ingredients that have a mild cleansing effect, among other traits. This is still too drying for all hair and scalp types, and the balsam in it only makes that worse.

☹ Saponin A. A. C. Herbal Root Shampoo *($9.95 for 8 ounces)* contains both coconut-oil soap as well as castile soap, which uses olive oil instead of animal fat. This is just another problematic soap-based shampoo that contains minimal conditioning agents. It's nice that the balsam and irritating essential oils are not present in this product, but the soap base still spells trouble if your goal is healthy, smooth, manageable hair.

☹ Swimmers Shampoo *($7.25 for 8 ounces)* contains soy soap as its main cleansing agent, which has no special benefit for swimmers, so this shampoo's name is a bit perplexing. The dryness the soap base can cause makes it a problem for all hair types, just like all of the shampoos above.

☺ **Blue Green Algae Hair Rescue Vegetal Protein Cream Rinse** (*$12.25 for 8 ounces*) contains mostly fatty acid emollients, water, aloe, plant extracts, lavender oil, fragrant water, and preservatives. This is a good, though exceedingly basic, conditioner for coarse, dry hair, but, for the money, it offers nothing special other than the lure of natural ingredients.

☹ **Calaguala Fern & Cade Tar Hair Thickener and Conditioner** (*$10.25 for 8 ounces*) is an unusual conditioner because it uses plant gums and a plant resin to coat the hair. The tiny amounts of plant extracts and other conditioning agents have no effect on the hair, which means you're counting on the gums and resin to keep your hair smooth and combable. That may work initially, but with repeated use these natural ingredients will build up on the hair and make it feel stiff and dry.

☹ **Egyptian Henna Hair Rinse** (*$8.25 for 8 ounces*) contains henna (who knows if it's from Egypt or not, but the country of origin doesn't matter to your hair), which can eventually build up on the hair, making it feel brittle. With witch hazel, alcohol, and peppermint oil along for the ride, there is no logical reason to consider this liquidy, drying conditioner. If you're keen on using henna, you would be better off purchasing it in powder form and using it (occasionally, not daily) to enhance your hair color.

☺ **GPB (Glycogen Protein Balancer) Hair Conditioner and Nutrient** (*$9 for 8 ounces*) contains mostly water, emollient, alcohol, conditioning agent, plant oil, plant extracts (including balsam oil, which can make hair feel sticky and brittle), more plant oils, and small amounts of the irritants rosemary oil and sage oil. This ends up being a basic conditioner with more problematic ingredients than you should have to accept for smoother, softer hair. It's an option for normal to dry hair of any thickness, but not a great one.

☺ **Green Tea Herbal Cream Rinse** (*$10 for 8 ounces*), according to the label, contains mostly fatty acids. That's not an FDA-accepted ingredient disclosure because there is no way to know which one of the many fatty acids is being used, and they each have varying benefits for hair. It also contains aloe, plant powder, and plant oil. Almost all of the plant extracts can be problematic for the scalp, but this rinse can make dry hair of any texture feel smooth and soft, though not to the same extent that a conditioner with silicones can.

☺ **Honeysuckle Rose Hair & Scalp Conditioner** (*$9 for 4 ounces*) contains mostly fatty acid emollient, flowers, plant oils, plant extracts (including sage and rosemary oil, so keep this off of the scalp), and preservative. It's a good, though basic, conditioner that works well for normal to slightly dry hair that has a normal to thick texture.

☺ **Island Naturals Island Spice Cream Rinse** (*$8 for 8 ounces*) can be a rich conditioner for dry to very dry hair. This is a good option to condition the ends of curly or wavy hair.

☺ **Jojoba & Aloe Hair Rejuvenator & Conditioner** (*$13.50 for 4 ounces*) is a basic conditioner of plant oil, emollient, and aloe—though I suspect there is more to this formulation than what is revealed on the ingredient list. For one thing, this conditioner is similar to many of the options above, but lists no preservatives (the others do). This is still a good option for dry to very dry hair that is normal to coarse or thick.

☺ **Polynatural 60/80 Conditioner** *($10.75 for 4 ounces)* contains mostly emollients, aloe, plant extracts (most of which are scalp irritants), plant oil, and preservatives. It is similar to the Jojoba & Aloe Hair Rejuvenator & Conditioner above, and the same comments apply.

☺ **Rosemary & Sage Hair & Scalp Rinse** *($7.75 for 8 ounces)* doesn't offer much to condition the hair. It's a very lightweight liquid conditioner that contains mostly water, witch hazel, plant extracts, amino acids (water-binding agents), and preservative. At best, this is a mediocre detangler for hair.

☹ **Rose Mosqueta Rose Hips Conditioning Hair Cream** *($18.25 for 8 ounces)* contains a high amount of coltsfoot extract, an irritant and potential carcinogen (Sources: http://www.naturaldatabase.com; and *American Journal of Health-System Pharmacy*, January 1999, pages 125–138) that should not come in contact with the skin or scalp.

☺ **Sea Buckthorn Egg Cream Rinse** *($9.60 for 8 ounces)* contains mostly water, emollient, alcohol, conditioning agents, plant extracts (including balm mint, so keep this off the scalp), essential oils of rosemary and sage (both are scalp irritants), water-binding agents, vitamins, and nonvolatile plant oils. The alcohol cuts this conditioner's moisturizing ability, and makes it best for normal to dry hair that has a normal to thin texture.

☺ **Swimmers Conditioner** *($8.50 for 8 ounces)* contains nothing that makes it preferred for swimmers. It is similar to the Green Tea Herbal Creme Rinse above, and the same comments apply.

☺ **B-5 Design Gel** *($10.75 for 8 ounces)* is a silky, minimally sticky gel that provides a soft, light hold that can be brushed through with ease. Balsam oil can build up on hair with repeated use, but so little of it is present in this product that buildup would not be a problem for quite a while.

☺ **Mandarin Magic Ginkgo Leaf & Ginseng Root Hair Moisturizing Jelly** *($10.75 for 8 ounces)* is essentially an alcohol-free version of the B-5 Design Gel above, and the same basic comments apply. This gel does not contain any balsam oil, and the other plant extracts used have no effect on hair.

☺ **Natural Body Highliter Mousse, Chestnut Brown** *($8 for 8 ounces)* isn't a mousse because it doesn't foam and it's not dispersed by propellants (or air, as is the case with many mousses today). Rather, this is a styling gel that provides a light hold that's slightly sticky but can be brushed through. It contains caramel coloring to minimally enhance brunette shades of hair.

☺ **Natural Body Highliter Mousse, Golden Camomile** *($8 for 8 ounces)* is similar to the Natural Body Highliter Mousse, Chestnut Brown above, except this contains turmeric for color instead of caramel.

☺ **Natural Body Highliter Mousse, Soft Black** *($8 for 8 ounces)* is similar to the Natural Body Highliter Mousse, Chestnut Brown above, only this contains an indigo dye to minimally enhance black hair.

☺ **Natural Missst Herbal Hairspray, Regular Hold** *($9.95 for 8 ounces)* provides a very light, natural hold that doesn't make hair stiff and can be easily brushed through. The balsam oil may build up on hair after repeated use, which can cause it to feel dry and brittle.

☺ **Natural Missst Herbal Hairspray, Super Hold** *($9.95 for 8 ounces)* has a formula that's nearly identical to the Natural Missst Herbal Hairspray above, only this contains more gum arabic for a stronger hold. Unfortunately, this also makes the hair feel sticky and the stickiness does not dissipate, which can make hair difficult to brush through. For a firm-hold, nonaerosol hairspray, it works OK, as long as you're not planning to brush very often.

☺ **Primrose Tangle-Go Hair Conditioner, Lusterizer and Styling Spray** *($7.25 for 4 ounces)* can be a good, very basic detangling spray, but it does not contain ingredients that can protect hair from heat, nor does it add much shine to the hair.

☺ **Sea Buckthorn Leave-In Conditioner & Curl Activator** *($9.15 for 4 ounces)* is a lightweight, spray-on conditioner that contains a nice array of conditioning agents and, surprisingly, no irritating plant oils or extracts. This works well on normal to fine hair to make it easier to comb and to provide a small amount of protection from heat.

☺ **White Camellia and Jasmine Shine Conditioner Spray** *($7.25 for 4 ounces)* is a less elegant option than the Sea Buckthorn Leave-In Conditioner & Curl Activator above. It can still work as an extra-light, alcohol-free spray-on detangler for normal to fine hair. The small amount of film-forming agents can make hair feel slightly sticky.

☺ **Blue Green Algae Hair Rescue Conditioning Mask** *($13.75 for 4 ounces)* is a basic, emollient conditioner that contains shea butter, so this is best for dry to very dry hair that is normal to thick or coarse-textured. The plant extracts are decent for the scalp, but in a rinse-out conditioner they are rinsed away before they can have an impact.

☹ **Ginseng Shampoo, Men's Stock** *($9 for 8 ounces)* is similar to almost all of the Aubrey Organics shampoos above in that it contains coconut-oil soap as its main cleansing agent. The cleansing agent is drying enough, but it also contains pine extract, which has the potential to cause scalp irritation.

☺ **$$$ Biotin Hair Repair, Men's Stock** *($14.80 for 4 ounces)* is a standard emollient conditioner that does contain biotin (and some other conditioning agents), but none of them are capable of repairing the hair, nor are they specific to a man's hair-care needs. This isn't much different from most of the conditioners in this line, and is an OK option for normal to dry hair of any thickness.

☺ **Ginseng Hair Control, Men's Stock** *($7.25 for 4 ounces)* is similar to the Natural Missst Herbal Hairspray Super Hold above, only this has a "masculine" fragrance and is slightly (just slightly) less sticky. Otherwise, the same comments apply.

AUSSIE

This Australian-themed line debuted in 1979, and although the products are made in the United States by Procter & Gamble, the line was originally inspired by the flora and fauna of southwest Australia. Does an infusion of kangaroo paw flower or wild cherry bark make a noticeable difference in your hair? Not in the least. These plant, flower, and food extracts are strictly window dressing to gussy up the standard hair-care ingredients that comprise every single product below (and hair-care products industry-wide, for that matter). Almost all the Aussie products reviewed below have strong fragrances that are floral-sweet, so, if possible, be sure you can live with the scent before purchasing. For the most part, Aussie has some wonderful products, especially in the category of hairsprays. The shampoo and conditioner selection has dwindled, but that's not such a bad thing when you realize that what was offered was never more than ordinary in the first place. For more information about Aussie, call (800) 947-2656 or visit www.aussie.com.

What's Good About This Line: Generous sizes and great prices; excellent styling products, especially if you are a fan of aerosol and/or nonaerosol hairsprays.

What's Not So Good About It: All of the shampoos contain sodium lauryl sulfate; the fragrant plant and flower extracts can be a problem for those with sensitive scalps.

☹ **Color Mate Shampoo** *($3.99 for 16 ounces)* contains sodium lauryl sulfate as one of its main detergent cleansing agents, and that makes this shampoo inappropriate for all hair types, but especially for color-treated hair. The eucalyptus oil in this shampoo is also a problem for the scalp.

☹ **Mega Shampoo, Everyday Cleansing for Normal Hair** *($3.99 for 16 ounces)* is similar to the Color Mate Shampoo above, minus the eucalyptus oil, and the same basic comments apply.

☹ **Moist Shampoo for Dry/Damaged Hair** *($3.99 for 16 ounces)* is sold as a "moisture-infusing formula for thirsty hair"—but with sodium lauryl sulfate as one of the main detergent cleansing agents, this won't moisturize hair in the least. The Australian plant extracts add exotic appeal (and aroma), but this shampoo is a bad choice for dry or damaged hair.

☹ **Real Volume Shampoo for Fine, Limp Hair** *($3.99 for 16 ounces)* is similar to the Color Mate Shampoo above, minus the eucalyptus oil, and the same basic comments apply.

☺ **3 Minute Miracle Reconstructor Deep Conditioning for Damaged Hair** *($4.49 for 8 ounces)* has been in the Aussie line for years, and remains a basic, but good, conditioner for normal to dry hair that is thick or coarse. Regardless of how long you leave this on the hair, it is neither a miracle nor a "deep" conditioner.

☺ **Color Mate Conditioner for Colored or Permed Hair** *($3.99 for 16 ounces)* is a basic, but good, conditioner for normal to dry hair of any thickness.

☺ **Hair Insurance Leave-In Conditioner for Weak, Distressed Hair** *($3.99 for 8 ounces)* works well if you're looking for a good, lightweight detangler with minimal conditioning properties. The who's who list of vitamins cannot fortify weak, distressed hair (the minimal amounts present can have no effect on hair at all). This works best on normal to fine-textured hair that needs light conditioning without weight.

☺ **Mega Conditioner, for Everyday Conditioning for Normal Hair** *($3.99 for 16 ounces).* There is nothing "mega" about this product, though the rest of the name fits nicely. This is an exceptionally basic conditioner that contains mostly water, thickeners, detangling agent, Australia-oriented plant extracts, more detangling agents, slip agent, fragrance, preservatives, and coloring agents. It works well as a daily conditioner for all hair types that are normal to slightly dry.

☺ **Moist Conditioner for Thirsty/Distressed Hair** *($3.99 for 16 ounces)* is almost identical to the Mega Conditioner for Normal Hair above, and the same basic comments apply. The plant and flower extracts have no effect on the hair, though they do add fragrance.

☺ **Real Volume Conditioner for Fine, Limp Hair** *($3.99 for 16 ounces)* is nearly identical to the Mega Conditioner for Normal Hair above, but it has a much shorter list of plant and flower extracts so it is somewhat preferred if you have a sensitive scalp or plant allergies. Otherwise, the same basic comments apply. This is an OK option for fine or limp hair, but many with this hair type will find it too heavy.

☺ **Slip Detangler for Tangly Hair** *($3.99 for 12 ounces)* contains far fewer plant extracts than all of the Aussie conditioners above, which is good news for your scalp. This is a great lightweight conditioner for normal to slightly dry hair that is normal to fine or thin.

☺ **12-Hour Hair Spray** *($3.99 for 12 ounces)* is a standard nonaerosol hairspray that promises and delivers a firm hold, though not without noticeable stiffness and stickiness. The film-forming agent does a good job of keeping hair from falling prey to humidity, but remember that no matter how strong the hairspray, at the end of the day humidity always wins.

☺ **AirDo Flexible Hold Styling Mist, Aerosol** *($3.99 for 7 ounces)* is an aerosol hairspray with an unusually light, flexible hold. What a great find for those seeking a weightless finishing product to add an extra touch of styling support. Those with fine or thin hair whose styles don't demand a firm hold should definitely try it.

☺ **Instant Freeze Super-Hold Hairspray, Aerosol** *($3.99 for 7 ounces)* is a standard aerosol hairspray that offers a strong hold with a minimally sticky feel that can be brushed through. This non-flaking formula is best used on dry hair.

☺ **Instant Freeze Super-Hold Hairspray, Non-Aerosol** *($3.99 for 8 ounces)* is the nonaerosol version of the Instant Freeze Super-Hold Hairspray, Aerosol above, and aside from a heavier application (which is characteristic of nonaerosol hairspray), this offers the same amount of hold and works well as a finishing spray for structured hairstyles.

☺ **Mega Hold Mousse, Extra Hold & Control** *($3.99 for 6 ounces)* is not mega hold in the least. This is a fairly standard, propellant-based mousse that provides a soft, brushable hold without stiffness or stickiness. This is a very good option for normal to fine hair that needs body and fullness.

☺ **Mega Spray Gel for Sculpting & Shaping, Firm Hold** *($3.99 for 12 ounces)* is a standard spray gel with enough food extracts to make a tasty salad, though ingredients like tomato, pineapple, and garlic have no effect on the hair. Over time, however, they can cause scalp itching and irritation. Still, they are present in meager amounts, and this remains a good, light-hold product that is non-sticky and can be easily brushed through.

☺ **Mega Styling Gel for Design & Hold** *($3.99 for 8 ounces)* is a very standard, but good, styling gel that provides medium hold with a slightly sticky after-feel. It works well for all hair types.

☺ **Mega Styling Spray, Aerosol** *($3.99 for 14 ounces)* is a standard aerosol hairspray that provides a light, touchable hold that can be easily brushed through. The plant extracts have no effect on hair, and the conditioning agents are present in such tiny amounts that your hair won't show a difference.

☺ **Mega Styling Spray, Non-Aerosol** *($3.99 for 12 ounces)* is a standard, firm-hold hairspray that can be easily brushed through. It has a stickier feel than the other Aussie hairsprays (both aerosol and nonaerosol), but can keep unruly hair in place, and it doesn't flake.

☺ **Natural Gel** *($3.99 for 7 ounces)* contains few natural ingredients, so don't be misled by the name. This standard conditioning gel offers a smooth, light hold that is minimally sticky and can be easily brushed through. This is a great gel to emphasize the texture of curly or wavy hair of any thickness.

☺ **Real Volume Body Lock Volumizing Hairspray, Aerosol** *($4.29 for 6 ounces)* is an excellent ultra-light hairspray that applies with a fine mist that won't weigh hair down or make it feel stiff. It provides a light hold that can be brushed through with ease, and does a good job adding body and fullness to hair.

☺ **Real Volume Root Lifter, Root Volumizing Styler** *($4.29 for 6 ounces)* is similar to the Mega Spray Gel for Sculpting & Shaping, Firm Hold above, only the applicator for this spray-on product helps to concentrate the product at the roots of hair. When applied in this manner and used with heat, this can indeed create extra body and volume, but that trait is not exclusive to this product. Otherwise, the same comments made for the Spray Gel above apply here, too.

☺ **Real Volume Styling Whip for Body and Control** *($4.29 for 6 ounces)* is nearly identical to the Mega Hold Mousse above, and the same comments apply. This does contain more conditioning ingredients, which can make it a slightly better choice for dry hair that is fine or thin.

☺ **Smoothy Gel, Medium Hold** *($3.99 for 8 ounces)* is a standard, alcohol-free styling gel that offers a strong (not medium) hold with a slightly sticky feel that can be easily brushed through. This is a great option for all hair types—just keep in mind that the plant and food extracts have no effect on hair.

☺ **Sprunch Spray, Aerosol** *($3.99 for 14 ounces)* is an aerosol hairspray that provides a firm hold that can leave hair feeling stiff and sticky. This is not the best to brush through, but when you need hold and want time to play with your style before your hairspray dries, this is a good option.

☺ **Sprunch Spray, Non-Aerosol** *($3.99 for 16 ounces)* is similar to the Sprunch Spray, Aerosol above, but offers slightly less hold (and also less stiffness and stickiness). This is a good working hairspray that allows you to arrange your hair into place rather than drying immediately. This also contains small amounts of conditioning agents, which add some shine and allow hair to be brushed through.

☺ **Sprunch Spray, Non-Aerosol, Unscented** *($3.99 for 12 ounces)* is identical to the Sprunch Spray above, only this has a less intense fragrance. It is not unscented, however; fragrance is clearly listed on the label, and this also contains fragrant plant extracts.

AVACOR

For more information about Avacor (distributed by GlobalVision, Inc.) call (877) 805-9743 or visit www.avacorusa.com. My strong recommendation, though, is to lose their number. For objective and well-documented research about hair loss, please visit www.keratin.com.

What's Good About This Line: If you're looking for a product with minoxidil (the active ingredient in Rogaine), you'll find an option here, as well as an herbal supplement containing saw palmetto.

What's Not So Good About It: See below for the full story of Avacor's claims and blatant misinformation.

Whether it's BioFolic, Fabao 101, Folliguard, Folligen, Hair Factor PX-2000, Hair Prime, Helsinki Formula, Nioxin, Nisim, Nutrifolica, Pro-Genesis, Regenix, Revivogen, or Shen Min, to name just a few of the product lines making claims about miraculous hair regrowth, their claims sound just like Avacor's. You'd think that with the abundance of such products it would be shocking to find anyone still experiencing hair loss. But clearly, that is not the case.

Avacor's claims are best described as questionable science. The study they showcase on their Web site was not performed double-blind, it was not peer reviewed, it was never published, and, not surprisingly, the only study that exists is their own. The claim on their Web site states, "the ingredients in Avacor hair re-growing formula have been extensively tested by medical doctors at the Hair & Skin Treatment Center and New York Hair Laboratories in New York City. Other studies have been performed at leading universities and clinics in both the USA and Europe, on the active ingredients in Avacor." That is true, but that's only because the ingredients in Avacor are found in lots of products being sold for hair regrowth that cost far less and don't make exaggerated, absurd claims and promises.

What is perhaps most disturbing is that Avacor does not disclose that one of their products contains minoxidil, the same ingredient present in hair regrowth products (most notably Rogaine) available at the drugstore for a fraction of the cost. Avacor lists minoxidil on their label as 2,4-diamino-6-piperidino-pyrimidine-3-oxide. That is not only misleading, but also blatantly deceptive (not to mention completely "unnatural" despite their "all natural" claim). To make matters worse, Avacor answers the question about whether or not their product is like Rogaine by stating on their Web site "No. Our system contains three parts…." Yes, there are three separate products, but one of those three parts is just like Rogaine.

Even more suspect is the question-and-answer page on the Web site, which states, "There are no known side effects with the use of Avacor." However, on their guarantee page they post the warning that you should stop using the products if you develop "Chest pain, rapid heartbeat, faintness, dizziness, suddenly unexplained weight gain, water retention, redness, or irritation." Obviously, they know that there are side effects, and these are the exact same warnings that accompany Rogaine and other products containing the drug minoxidil. Even the FDA sent Avacor a "Warning Letter" on April 3, 2003, stating that their products were in violation of unproven drug claims (Source: www.fda.gov/foi/warning_letters/g3938d.htm). For the price, you'd be better off buying generic 2% minoxidil at Costco or other wholesale outlets (Sources: UC Berkeley Wellness Letter, www.berkeleywellness.com/html/ds/dsAvacor.php and www.askdocweb.com/avacor.html).

Avacor's herbal supplement includes saw palmetto, an ingredient that is readily available at health food and larger grocery stores. Saw palmetto is known to be effective in inhibiting the action of 5-alpha reductase, which is the enzyme believed to be responsible for male pattern balding (Source: *Cosmetic Dermatology*, October 2000, pages 78–80). Whether saw palmetto is helpful for women is not known, but it is thought to be safe for women to take.

AVEDA

Aveda has been on the hair-care scene since 1978, and has always promoted its use of pure flower and plant essences. Of course, these plants and flowers (whether they are organically sourced or harvested by an indigenous tribe in the Brazilian rainforest) merely serve as the marketing lure for consumers hungry for anything natural, regardless of whether or not is it helpful for their skin and hair. Despite the claims, the truth is that there are no plant extracts, teas, or aromatic essences in nature that can even remotely take the place of standard, downright boring, but essential hair-care ingredients—the same ones used industry-wide in all manner of products. Aloe, lavender, and galbanum sound pure and exotic, but won't do a thing to keep hair in place, clean hair, remove product buildup, or help your hair feel smooth and silky after you wash it. Aveda tries to skirt this issue by claiming (often right on the product labels) that ingredients such as PPG-5-Ceteth-10 Phosphate and Polyquaternium-10 are actually just coconut and cellulose, but that kind of wishful thinking is akin to taking a piece of tree bark, calling it paper, and trying to write on it. In short, just because an ingredient may have a natural source does not mean that in its final state in a cosmetic it resembles anything remotely natural.

Aveda is owned by Estee Lauder, an alliance that has enabled them to launch dozens of new products since the last edition of this book. They remain a reliable hair-care line to shop; most of their greatly expanded product selection does an admirable job of cleansing, conditioning, and styling the hair, and for the most part, Aveda avoids the formulary repetition rampant in most large hair-care lines. Just keep in mind that it's not the fragrant plant extracts that make these products perform as they do; rather, just like other product lines, to extol the benefits of silicones and PVP (acrylate styling agents) just isn't as interesting to cosmetics companies or unsuspecting consumers. For more information about Aveda, call (866) 823-1425 or visit www.aveda.com.

What's Good About This Line: Excellent conditioners and styling products for just about every imaginable hair-care need; Aveda is an admirable company when it comes to environmental consciousness and using sustainable resources.

What's Not So Good About It: A garden full of problematic fragrant plant extracts that can cause dry, itchy scalp, although most of them are used as a plant tea, which means their irritant potency is significantly diluted. Aveda suffers from too many choices in each category, creating consumer confusion.

☺ **Black Malva Shampoo** *($8 for 8.5 ounces)* contains mostly plant tea, detergent cleansing agent, water-binding agents, silicone, fragrance, preservatives, and coloring agents. Aveda maintains that black malva enriches darker tones of hair and eliminates red tones, but what they don't mention are the number of artificial colorants in the product that actually do enrich the dark tones and eliminate the red tones. As a shampoo, this mostly unnatural formula (and that's not a bad thing) is a good option for all hair types, and the silicone poses little to no risk of buildup. The minute amount of lactic acid present does not exfoliate the scalp or, thankfully, the hair shaft.

☺ **Blue Malva Shampoo** *($8 for 8.5 ounces)* is identical to the Black Malva Shampoo above, save for a different plant tea concoction and violet coloring agent. Otherwise, the same comments apply.

☺ **Camomile Shampoo** *($8 for 8.5 ounces)* is identical to the Black Malva Shampoo above, save for a different plant tea blend and the absence of synthetic coloring agents. Pure chamomile can have a mild highlighting effect on blonde hair, but the tiny amount of it in this product will not affect blonde hair in the least. This is still a fine shampoo for all hair types.

☺ **Clove Shampoo** *($8 for 8.5 ounces)* is almost identical to the Black Malva Shampoo above, though this shampoo does not contain synthetic coloring agents. Clove and coffee have minimal to no effect on brunette hair colors, especially when used in the form of a plant tea, where the color-imparting extract is diluted.

☺ **Madder Root Shampoo** *($8 for 8.5 ounces)* is identical to the Black Malva Shampoo above, save for a different plant tea and no synthetic coloring agents. Otherwise, the same comments apply.

☺ **Color Conserve Shampoo** *($12 for 8.5 ounces)* claims that it can "extend the vibrance of color-treated hair—as only nature can. Our gentle plant-infused shampoo, with 100% organic aroma, helps do what harsher cleansers can't—resist fading. Keeps hair color vibrant longer. Protects color-treated hair from damaging effects of sun, water, and environmental stresses." It seems rather ironic to claim that nature can be a benefit for color-treated hair when it is nature, via the sun, that causes most of the fading in the first place. This rather standard, detergent-based shampoo is filled with a cornucopia of plant extracts that have no ability to help retain color in your hair. The cleansing agents in this product aren't any gentler than or different from what you will find in lots of good shampoos, from L'Oreal to TRESemme.

☺ **Hair Detoxifier** *($9 for 8.5 ounces)* cannot detoxify hair or scalp because the hair and scalp don't harbor toxins. It is still an excellent shampoo that will not cause buildup and can be used by all hair types. It contains mostly plant tea, detergent cleansing agent, lather agent, water-binding agents, vitamin E, and fragrance. One claim for Hair Detoxifier is that it can remove chlorine and other mineral deposits from hair, but without chelating agents (such as tetrasodium EDTA) it won't be very effective for this purpose.

☺ **Personal Blends Shampoo Formula** *($10.50 for 7 ounces)* is unscented, which makes it an excellent option for those with sensitive scalps. It contains mostly plant tea, detergent cleansing agents, water-binding agents, plant oil, soy protein, film-forming agent, and preservatives. Aveda's Personal Blends concept allows you to choose the scent for this product from several premixed options. That's fine if you want to add perfume to your shampoo, but given the lack of fragrance-free shampoos, this is quite a find. It is a great shampoo for all hair types, though the plant oil and film-forming agent can cause slight buildup.

☹ **Rosemary Mint Shampoo** *($8.50 for 8.5 ounces)* contains many ingredients that make it a wonderful shampoo that won't cause buildup, but there are too many irritants included, such as large amounts of rosemary, peppermint, camphor, and menthol. All of these mints and their derivatives create the "energizing" sensation (which is nothing more than irritation) used to market this shampoo, but they also mean that using it will, in the long run, be a mistake for your scalp.

☺ **Scalp Benefits Balancing Shampoo** *($12 for 8.5 ounces)* is a fairly gentle shampoo that is a good option for those with normal to dry hair of any texture. This does contain some silicones that can build up with repeated use, but the amounts used are small enough so that it would take quite some time for this to occur.

☺ **Shampure Shampoo** *($9 for 8.5 ounces)* is a relatively gentle conditioning shampoo that can be an option for all hair types except fine or thin. The small amount of plant oils should not be a problem for causing buildup, and the antioxidants, while great for skin, have no effect on the hair, and would be rinsed down the drain anyway.

☺ **$$$ Annatto Color Conditioner** *($16 for 8.5 ounces)* is a great way to boost fading auburn color between salon appointments, but the boost is courtesy of basic synthetic dyes, not from the played-up plant extracts. It also contains some henna, which can affect hair color, although repeated use of henna can cause buildup, creating dry, difficult-to-manage hair. This is otherwise a lightweight conditioner that contains some silicone and plant oil for moisture and smoothness. It is a good option for all but very dry or damaged hair.

☺ $$$ **Bixa Color Conditioner** (*$16 for 8.5 ounces*) is nearly identical to the Annatto Color Conditioner above except that this one does not contain henna, which makes it a safer bet for regular use on all but very dry or damaged hair. The colorants are best for auburn and orange-red hair shades.

☺ $$$ **Black Malva Color Conditioner** (*$16 for 8.5 ounces*) is, save for the coloring agents that make this product preferred for enhancing darker hair tones, identical to the Bixa Color Conditioner above, and the same comments apply.

☺ $$$ **Blue Malva Color Conditioner** (*$16 for 8.5 ounces*) is, save for the coloring agents that make this conditioner preferred for those with platinum blonde, silver, or gray hair, identical to the Bixa Color Conditioner above, and the same comments apply.

☺ $$$ **Camomile Color Conditioner** (*$16 for 8.5 ounces*) is, save for the coloring agents that make this conditioner preferred for those with golden blonde hair, identical to the Bixa Color Conditioner above, and the same comments apply.

☺ $$$ **Clove Color Conditioner** (*$16 for 8.5 ounces*) is, save for the coloring agents that make this conditioner preferred for those with all shades of brown hair, identical to the Bixa Color Conditioner above, and the same comments apply.

☺ $$$ **Madder Root Color Conditioner** (*$16 for 8.5 ounces*) is identical to the Annatto Color Conditioner above, and the same comments apply. The synthetic coloring agents in this conditioner make it preferred for red to strawberry blonde hair colors.

☺ $$$ **Cherry/Almond Bark Reconstructive Hair Conditioner** (*$18 for 8.5 ounces*) claims to prevent damage caused by styling, but it is incapable of protecting hair from heat damage, and how many of us style our hair without some type of heat source? Aveda also claims the plant extracts (mostly plant tea) "provide excellent detangling," but I challenge anyone to try and run a comb through their hair after applying aloe, wild cherry bark, marshmallow, or echinacea extracts to it! This is merely a good, though standard, conditioner that isn't very exciting once you realize the plants don't do anything for hair other than add fragrance. It is nevertheless a good option for normal to dry hair that is normal, fine, or thin.

☺ **Color Conserve Conditioner** (*$12 for 6.7 ounces*). Much like the Color Conserve Shampoo above, this product includes plant extracts that have no ability to prevent hair from losing color. However, this is a good, lightweight conditioner for someone with normal to dry hair.

☺ **Color Conserve Foaming Leave-In Conditioner** (*$12 for 6.7 ounces*) claims to protect hair from fading by preserving color with emollients and naturally derived sun filters. This liquid-to-foam product does contain several plant extracts, some of which have antioxidant benefits, but antioxidants can't hold up under the heat of styling tools, so they have no real function on hair. Doubtless, the claims about the product will arouse curiosity in women who routinely dye their hair. This ultralight, leave-in conditioner contains mostly plant tea, slip agents, antistatic agents, antioxidants, conditioning agents, fragrance, plant oils, more fragrance, holding agent, and preservatives. It is a good option for normal hair that is also fine or thin.

☺ **$$$ Deep Penetrating Hair Revitalizer** *($21 for 8.5 ounces)* doesn't penetrate hair any better than most other conditioners, but is nevertheless a fairly emollient, creamy conditioner for dry to very dry hair of any thickness. (Those with fine hair should use this sparingly and only on the ends of hair.) It contains mostly plant tea, emollients, thickeners, silicone, water-binding agent, fragrance, conditioning agents, and preservatives.

☺ **Elixir Daily Leave-On Hair Conditioner** *($9 for 8.5 ounces)* works beautifully as a leave-on conditioner for most hair types, but not very damaged or thick, coarse hair. Aveda avoided using heavy, drying, or film-forming ingredients so the hair is left soft, weightless, and easy to detangle. This liquidy formula contains mostly plant tea, conditioning agent, silicone, thickeners, wheat protein, panthenol, fragrance, and preservatives.

☺ **$$$ Personal Blends Conditioning Formula** *($19 for 7 ounces)* is an excellent emollient conditioner for normal to very dry hair, though unlike the Personal Blends Shampoo above, it is not fragrance-free.

☹ **Rosemary Mint Conditioner** *($8.50 for 8.5 ounces)* is a very light detangling conditioner that contains rosemary and peppermint as part of the plant tea, plus a small amount of peppermint oil. This can be a potentially irritating conditioner if it comes into contact with the scalp. Used with caution, it is a good option for normal to fine or thin hair—just don't count on the rosemary mint combination revitalizing your scalp.

☺ **Scalp Benefits Balancing Conditioner** *($12 for 6.7 ounces)* contains the same beneficial and potentially problematic plant extracts as the Scalp Benefits Balancing Shampoo above. It also contains several plant oils and silicone, which makes it a good conditioner for someone with normal to dry hair that is coarse or thick. This conditioner will make hair soft, smooth, and easy to detangle, but keep it off the scalp to avoid irritating it.

☺ **Shampure Conditioner** *($9 for 8.5 ounces)* contains mostly plant tea, conditioning agents, wheat and nut proteins, film-forming agents, panthenol, fragrance, and preservatives. This works well as a conditioner for normal to dry hair of any thickness. The ingredient list makes it look as though the cetyl alcohol, glyceryl stearate, and other commonly used ingredients are from coconut. However, despite their natural origin, the process used to create the actual ingredients from coconut is decidedly unnatural, and the result does not resemble anything akin to a coconut when mixed into a product.

☺ **$$$ Air Control Hair Spray** *($23 for 9.1 ounces)* is a standard, highly fragranced aerosol hairspray that provides medium hold with a slight amount of residual stiffness and stickiness. The propellant produces a forceful burst of hairspray—more of the hairspray goes into the air than onto your hair—so this can be more difficult to control than similar options. The film-forming agent is said by Aveda to come from pine, which may make you think this hairspray is a more natural, safer choice than competing products. Pine may have been used at some point as the ingredient to hold hair, but its final form, as VA/butyl maleate/isobornyl acrylate copolymer, is nothing you would ever see sprouting from the ground. Beyond this, the only disappointing aspect of this hairspray is its near-outrageous price.

☺ **$$$ Be Curly** *($16 for 6.7 ounces)* is a lightweight, silicone-based lotion with a small amount of film former that offers minimal hold but leaves a soft feeling on your hair. This pricey product offers no advantage over L'Oreal's Studio Line Lasting Curls, which also helps hair softly hold its shape.

☺ **$$$ Confixor Conditioning Fixative** *($15 for 8.5 ounces)* is a soft-hold styling liquid that contains enough conditioning agents to make hair feel smooth and be easy to brush through. Confixor is a good styling aid for hair that's normal to fine or thin, including curly hair. A portion of the plant tea is lavender, white oak, rosemary, and peppermint, so be careful not to get it on the scalp. This product does have a potent fragrance, more so than many other Aveda styling products.

☹ **$$$ Control Granules Hair Texturizer** *($29 for 0.35 ounce)* is a white, powdery substance that is one of the most expensive styling products being sold (note that you get less than half an ounce of product). You dispense the powder onto your hands or hair and, once rubbed in, it liquefies and functions as a texture and volume enhancer. It's an interesting concept (and it does work), but it can leave hair feeling very dry and somewhat coated. Hair is also difficult to comb through without snags or snarls. This product is best used on dry (not damp) hair to add a messy "bed head" texture. There are other products for much less money that can achieve the exact same look without any concerns. But if you are someone who likes a novel approach to hair styling, this one will fill that need.

☺ **$$$ Control Paste** *($21 for 1.7 ounces)*. As the name implies, this fragrant, pomade-style buttery wax lives up to its claims of leaving hair pliable with a small amount of hold and a slight greasy after-feel. However, the price is unrealistic for what ends up being just a creamy, slightly heavy pomade.

☺ **$$$ Custom Control Styling/Finishing Emulsion** *($16.50 for 2.6 ounces)* is just a standard silicone gel with film-forming agents that leave the hair shiny and with a slightly stiff, sticky feel that helps keep hair in place with a light to medium hold. The deodorant-style wind-up dispenser is interesting, but not an improvement over a standard tube container. If anything, this type of packaging makes it very easy to "dial up" more product than you intend (or need) and there is no way to get it back in the container once dispensed. A little of this goes a long way!

☺ **Firmata Hair Spray** *($11 for 8.5 ounces)* doesn't have the same rigid, cement-like hold it used to, but is still a force to be reckoned with when it comes to firm-hold hairsprays. This contains mostly alcohol, plant tea, holding agent, conditioning agents, fragrance, and antistatic agent. Firmata works best when used as a finishing spray on dry hair.

☺ **Flax Seed/Aloe Strong Hold Sculpturing Gel** *($11 for 8.5 ounces)* is now an alcohol-free gel that contains the same film-forming and holding agents seen in hundreds of other styling gels. The only difference is the window dressing of plant extracts and Aveda's fragrance. This gel provides a medium hold that is barely sticky and allows hair to be easily brushed through.

☺ **Flax Seed/Aloe Strong Hold Spray-On Styling Gel** *($11 for 8.5 ounces)* is an excellent alcohol-based spray gel that provides a firm hold and a smooth, shiny finish. It can be easily brushed through, and this product works equally well on wet or dry hair. Fortunately, the alcohol will evaporate before it has a chance to affect the hair negatively. This does provide a slightly stronger hold than the Flax Seed/Aloe Strong Hold Sculpturing Gel above.

☺ **$$$ Hang Straight** *($16 for 6.7 ounces)*. This product won't help your hair be straight without the help of a blow dryer, round brush, or flat iron. However, it is a good silicone-based lotion with a good amount of film former to help keep unruly hair in place. It has a light to medium hold that can easily be brushed through.

☺ **Phomollient Styling Foam** *($12 for 6.7 ounces)* performs well as a light-hold, nonpropellant-based styling mousse, leaving hair soft and non-sticky. Phomollient contains mostly plant tea, thickeners, film formers, fragrance, water-binding agents, and preservatives. It is an option for all hair types, but especially those with fine or thin hair.

☺ **$$$ Self Control Hair Styling Stick** *($15.50 for 2.5 ounces)* is a stick pomade that includes the standard assortment of emollient and wax-like ingredients to smooth frizzies and add texture. But it also includes a film-forming agent for a firm hold that can make it difficult to brush through. This is best used sparingly to tame unruly sections of hair rather than all over.

☺ **Volumizing Tonic** *($12 for 3.4 ounces)* is a plant water-and alcohol-based styling spray that provides a soft, flexible hold that can be easily brushed through. As for the volumizing part, that has to come from skillful use of a blow dryer and brush—this product doesn't create volume on its own!

☺ **Witch Hazel Hair Spray** *($10 for 8.5 ounces)* is a very standard, alcohol-based hairspray that goes on light and provides medium hold with a slightly stiff feel. The tiny amount of plant oil present can add a touch of shine to hair.

☺ **Scalp Remedy Anti-Dandruff Styling Tonic** *($11 for 3.7 ounces)* contains 0.02% zinc pyrithione, which is the same active ingredient used to fight dandruff in Head & Shoulders products, although H&S uses at least a 1% concentration. Despite the higher price for this product, the benefit of being able to apply the active ingredient in lotion form that can remain on the scalp overnight is helpful when compared with a shampoo, in which case the ingredient is rinsed out (which explains why the Aveda product can contain a lower concentration of the active ingredient and still be effective—the concentration is less, but the duration the active ingredient is in contact with your scalp makes the difference). The minimal amount of film-forming agent in this product provides almost no hold, though the conditioning agents can lightly moisturize hair.

AVEDA ALL-SENSITIVE

☺ **$$$ All-Sensitive Shampoo** *($16 for 6.7 ounces)* is a very good conditioning shampoo for normal to very dry hair that is coarse or thick, but the fragrant plant tea this contains is not suitable for someone with a sensitive scalp. If the goal was to create a line of products ideal for sensitive scalps, it would have been better to avoid even small, diluted amounts of plant extracts. This shampoo also contains geranium oil, another problematic ingredient if the goal is to reduce sensitivity and soothe the scalp. Those without sensitivities should do well with this product, but it is best alternated with another shampoo to avoid buildup.

☺ **All-Sensitive Conditioner** *($10 for 6.7 ounces)* contains mostly plant tea, conditioning agent, detangling agent, water-binding agents, plant oil, thickeners, fragrant plant oil, and preservatives. This is a great conditioner for those with normal to dry hair of any texture except fine or thin. The plant tea and geranium oil are not appropriate for those with sensitive scalps.

☺ $$$ **All-Sensitive Styling Gel** *($16 for 6.7 ounces)* is a fluid, light-hold conditioning styling gel that features a plant tea similar to that in the All-Sensitive Shampoo and Conditioner above, only this one has more anti-irritant plant extracts. That can be beneficial in a styling gel, because it's meant to be left on the hair. The geranium oil is still present, though the amount is likely too small to be a problem for all but the most sensitive scalps. The gel can be easily brushed through and does not leave hair feeling sticky or stiff.

AVEDA BRILLIANT

☺ **Brilliant Shampoo** *($11 for 8.5 ounces)* is a textbook example of a basic shampoo, but that does not mean it isn't effective. Quite the contrary, the minimal amount of conditioning agents means this will not build up on the hair. It contains mostly plant tea, detergent cleansing agent, lather agents, fragrance, and preservatives, and is an option for all hair types.

☺ $$$ **Brilliant Conditioner** *($18 for 7.9 ounces)* contains mostly plant tea, water-binding agent, conditioning and detangling agents, plant oils, silicone, thickener, fragrance, plant extracts, and preservative. This is a great moisturizing conditioner for dry to very dry hair of any texture, but especially coarse, curly, or thick.

☺ $$$ **Brilliant Anti-Humectant Pomade** *($18 for 2.6 ounces)* is an emollient, wax-free pomade that can be quite slick and greasy, though it works well to smooth frizzies and create a sleek finish on straight hairstyles when used sparingly. The plant oils and silicones make this best for dry to very dry hair that is coarse or thick.

☺ **Brilliant Damage Control** *($14 for 8.5 ounces)* is a lightweight, water-based, spray-on conditioner that is a good conditioning/styling product that provides a light hold for all hair types—but nothing in this product can keep hair from being damaged by styling tools or sun exposure.

☺ $$$ **Brilliant Forming Gel** *($15 for 5 ounces)* is a thick, mildly conditioning styling gel that provides light to medium hold without being stiff or too sticky. This gel contains particles of mica, which do add shine—but they can also flake off throughout the day.

☺ **Brilliant Hair Spray** *($13 for 8 ounces)* is a great working hairspray that gives you time to play with and rearrange your hairstyle rather than instantly freezing it in place. It offers a light, natural hold that is very easy to brush through. While this is a good hairspray, it is not for someone looking for strong hold or all-day style support. It contains mostly alcohol, plant tea, film-forming agent, antistatic agent, silicone, and fragrance.

☺ $$$ **Brilliant Humectant Pomade** *($18 for 2.6 ounces)* is a versatile, water-based pomade that needs to be used sparingly to avoid a greasy look, and is an option for all hair types seeking a sleek, frizz-free style.

☺ **Brilliant Retexturing Gel** *($14 for 5 ounces)* is similar to the Brilliant Forming Gel above, offering a just slightly stronger hold and featuring greater amounts of plant oil and conditioning agents. This is a great alcohol-free gel for all hair types.

☺ $$$ **Brilliant Universal Styling Creme** *($15 for 5 ounces)* is a thick, slightly greasy styling cream that is best for dry to very dry, coarse, or thick hair. It must be used sparingly to avoid a weighed-down, greasy look, and it works best on dry hair because it doesn't emulsify well in wet hair.

☺ $$$ **Brilliant Emollient Finishing Gloss** *($23 for 2.5 ounces)* is a very standard silicone serum that works well to smooth and add high shine to dry, coarse, or thick hair. But unless you have an allegiance to Aveda, there is no reason to consider this silicone serum over the far less expensive options at the drugstore.

☺ $$$ **Brilliant Spray-On Shine** *($18 for 3.4 ounces)* is an alcohol-based silicone spray, and the alcohol means this goes on much lighter than the Brilliant Emollient Finishing Gloss above. It is a good option for adding shine to any hair type, including fine or thin, but use it sparingly.

AVEDA CURESSENCE

☹ $$$ **Curessence Damage Relief Shampoo** *($17 for 6.7 ounces)* lists peppermint leaf, rosemary leaf, and lavender high on the ingredient list, and these are all ingredients that can be scalp irritants. That's a shame, because this would otherwise be a very gentle shampoo. It poses minimal risk of buildup, but absolutely cannot prevent damage or repair damaged hair. At best, expect your hair to be clean, soft, and easy to detangle if you pair this with any good conditioner.

☺ $$$ **Curessence Damage Relief Conditioner** *($17 for 6.7 ounces)* is a repackaged, renamed, and slightly reformulated version of Aveda's former Curessence Intensive Repair Treatment. This version places greater emphasis on silicone (great for dry hair, though decidedly not natural) and replaces the formerly hyped human-hair keratin protein with Brazil nut and wheat protein, though your hair won't notice the difference. Curessence Damage Relief can't repair hair, but it is a good conditioner for dry to extremely dry and also coarse or thick hair.

☺ **Styling Curessence Hair Rejuvenator and Detangler** *($13 for 8.5 ounces)* is a good, spray-on conditioner with minimal hold. It works well as a curl enhancer or to provide some protection from heat-styling implements. It does not leave hair feeling stiff or sticky, but the conditioning agents can build up with repeated use.

AVEDA LIGHT ELEMENTS

☺ $$$ **Light Elements Finishing Solution** *($20 for 6.7 ounces)* contains certified organic lavender water, which sounds intriguing but won't do a thing for hair other than make it wet (it is water, after all) and add fragrance—and most of the ingredients are anything but natural. This Finishing Solution is essentially a lightweight styling lotion with a lavender fragrance. It contains a tiny amount of holding agent, and has a good mix of silicone, glycerin, and plant oils for shine and emolliency (glycerin is a great conditioner, too). In the end, this is an ordinary, but good, non-sticky styling lotion for all but very fine hair.

☺ $$$ **Light Elements Defining Whip** *($20 for 4.1 ounces)* is a styling cream whose texture is reminiscent of Cool Whip Dessert Topping. It offers a smooth finish with a light hold and is best for dry, very dry, coarse, thick, or damaged hair. The claim that this product is weightless isn't accurate—someone with fine or thin hair will quickly see their style fall flat using this type of conditioning styling product.

☺ $$$ **Light Elements Detailing Mist-Wax** *($21 for 6.7 ounces)* is a styling spray that promises "weightless detail with a natural finish," but the ingredients in here can definitely add weight to the hair, especially if it is fine or thin. Compared to a standard, wax-based pomade, this product is much lighter, and can work well to add texture, separation, and soft, non-sticky hold to most hair types.

☺ $$$ **Light Elements Reviving Mist** *($21 for 8.5 ounces)* is not positioned as a styling product but is instead supposed to be used between shampoos to refresh your scalp and revive your hairstyle. There are several plant extracts present that should not be sprayed directly on the scalp, and you can refresh your hairstyle by using plain water or a bit of diluted styling gel (but only if your hair isn't curly or frizzy). For a hefty price, you're getting primarily plant tea, alcohol, lavender water, silicone, and a small amount of conditioning agents. This unnecessary product is really meant for hair-care consumers with money to burn, or those who want to add plant perfume to their hair-care regimen.

☺ $$$ **Light Elements Smoothing Fluid** *($23 for 3.4 ounces)* is a standard, but very good, silicone serum that has a lighter feel and a more liquid texture than others in its class—though there are many similar products that are available for a quarter of this price at the drugstore. Rather than relying on one form of silicone, Light Elements Smoothing Fluid achieves a balance of shine without heaviness or a greasy appearance (when applied sparingly) by combining five forms of silicone with several lighter plant oils. This silicone serum is an option for all hair types.

AVEDA SAP MOSS

☺ **Sap Moss Shampoo** *($11 for 4.2 ounces)*. According to Aveda, "This concentrated shampoo is ideal for dry hair conditions, as well as color-treated hair. [It] … provides gentle cleansing through saponins including yucca, soapwort and quillaja. Use daily or as a weekly supplement—the longer the shampoo is left on the hair, the greater the conditioning effects." First, the amount of yucca and soapwort in this product is minuscule compared with the amount of the standard detergent cleansing agents—sodium cocoyl isethionate, sodium coco-sulfate, sodium methyl cocoyl taurate, and cocamidopropyl betaine. Synthetic ingredients come through again! However, do not leave detergent cleansing agents like these on your hair for any longer than it takes to clean it, and then rinse the shampoo away immediately. Aveda's advice is completely off-base, because even gentle cleansing agents (natural or otherwise) can quickly dry out the hair or irritate the scalp. And moss of any kind has no moisturizing impact on hair in any way, shape, or form.

☺ **Sap Moss Conditioning Detangler** *($11 for 6.7 ounces).* The amount of sap moss in this product is almost imperceptible in relation to the amounts of dipalmitoyl hydroxyethylmonium methosulfate, dimethicone (silicone), and behentrimoium methosulfate (along with lesser amounts of dicetyl dimonium chloride and centrimoium chloride), and that means it has an insignificant impact on conditioning the hair. This is still a good conditioner for normal to dry hair, but it is not unique, and the showcased natural ingredients are more hype than help.

☹ **Sap Moss Nourishing Concentrate** *($18 for 4.2 ounces)* is sold as a pre-shampoo "healing treatment" for dry hair, but it is just washed away once you shampoo your hair. Even more disappointing, it contains too few emollients and too many irritating plant oils to be of much help for dry hair. Finally, the lemon peel oil and peppermint oil can be irritating to the scalp, especially when left on for long periods.

☺ **Sap Moss Styling Spray** *($16.50 for 8.5 ounces)* does contain a small amount of moss extract, along with some sap and an Aveda-approved list of plant extracts. If you look past the plants, you will find the same synthetic hair-styling agents present in all hair-styling products, which make this an effective hairspray. It is a good choice for an alcohol-free spray gel for all but very fine hair, providing firm but surprisingly flexible hold, and it has only a slight stickiness. In addition, this can be easily brushed through and adds a nice shine without looking or feeling greasy.

AVON

With the August 2003 debut of their Advanced Techniques products, Avon revamped a large part of its hair-care line. This new collection comes with all sorts of enticing claims, from protecting and sealing hair color to using marine extracts to strengthen hair at the root and creatine to nourish hair on the inside. As usual, the claims make for interesting reading, but there is little to no substantiated science behind them. What you're left with is a group of incredibly standard (but mostly inexpensive) products that take good care of your hair. For more information about Avon, call (800) 367-AVON or visit www.avon.com.

What's Good About This Line: Basic but functional hair-care products, most of which are inexpensive and can be purchased in generous sizes.

What's Not So Good About It: Some shampoos include sodium lauryl sulfate; the Advanced Techniques line is not advanced at all, nor is it unique.

☺ **Echinacea Relief Shampoo** *($16 for 16.7 ounces)* is a very standard shampoo that is slightly marred by the inclusion of sodium lauryl sulfate. Although SLS is not the main cleansing agent, its presence can make this otherwise fine shampoo too drying and irritating for the scalp.

☺ **Lemon Lite Shampoo, for Normal to Oily Hair** *($16 for 16.7 ounces)* is nearly identical to the Echinacea Relief Shampoo above, and the same comments apply. The inclusion of balm mint extract does not make this any gentler for the scalp.

☺ **Lil' Hugs Gentle Body Wash & Shampoo** *($6 for 8 ounces)* is a very gentle shampoo that contains mild detergent cleansing agents, which are preferred for the hair and scalps of babies. It would have been better if Avon had left out the fragrance, except that for many mothers therein lies the whole appeal of baby shampoo. This would not be a good option for adults because it's too mild and would not be able to break down and wash away conditioner and styling product residue.

☺ **Rich Mango Moisturizing Shampoo** *($16 for 16.7 ounces)* is nearly identical to the Echinacea Relief Shampoo above, and the same comments apply. This shampoo is not rich in the least.

☺ **Soothing Seagrass Conditioner** *($16 for 16.7 ounces)* contains mostly water, thickeners, detangling agent, plant-oil fragrance, plant extracts (including eucalyptus, which can be problematic for the scalp), and preservative. It is an OK, though unexciting, option for normal to slightly dry hair that is normal to slightly thick.

☺ **Planet Spa Mediterranean Olive Oil Conditioning Hair Mask** *($6.50 for 5.9 ounces)* is a very good emollient conditioner for dry to very dry hair that is normal to thick or coarse. If that describes your hair type, this product would have the most benefit as a daily conditioner rather than as a hair mask you use once per week or less. The glycolic acid in this conditioner does not exfoliate the scalp, or, thankfully, the hair shaft.

AVON ADVANCE TECHNIQUES

All of the Advance Techniques products below contain creatine, which Avon claims strengthens the hair shaft from the inside. Creatine is a compound found naturally in our muscles, and the body uses it to form the adenosine triphosphate (ATP) molecule. ATP serves as a burst of fuel for our muscles when they are subjected to intense or strenuous use. In essence, creatine stimulates production of a molecule that makes our muscles perform more efficiently under stress. How this ever got parlayed to hair-care is anyone's guess, but with all the fad ingredients on the market today, I suppose Avon just wanted to put a new spin on things. The bottom line is that creatine does not strengthen hair at all, and at best serves as a water-binding agent. There is no substantiated research pertaining to creatine's benefits for hair, though there is anecdotal information that creatine supplements (meaning their consumption in the diet) causes hair loss!

☺ **Advance Techniques Color-Protection Shampoo** *($3.49 for 11 ounces)* is a standard, but good, shampoo for all hair types that poses minimal risk of buildup. Avon claims this shampoo protects hair color and keeps it vibrant twice as long as regular shampoos—but this product is just regular, ordinary shampoo! It contains the same basic ingredients as thousands of other shampoos, namely water, detergent cleansing agents, lather agent, water-binding agents, film-forming agent, silicones, fragrance, preservatives, and plant oil. None of these ingredients preserve color any better in this shampoo than they do in countless other shampoos.

☹ **Advance Techniques Curly & Chic Shampoo** *($3.49 for 11 ounces)* contains sodium lauryl sulfate as one of the main detergent cleansing agents, and can be too drying for all hair and scalp types.

☹ **Advance Techniques Daily Results Shampoo** *($3.49 for 11 ounces)* is nearly identical to the Advance Techniques Curly & Chic Shampoo above, and the same comments apply.

☹ **Advance Techniques Straight & Sleek Shampoo** *($3.49 for 11 ounces)* is nearly identical to the Advance Techniques Curly & Chic Shampoo above, and the same comments apply.

☹ **Advance Techniques Tress Therapy Shampoo, for Dry or Damaged Hair** *($3.49 for 11 ounces)* is nearly identical to the Advance Techniques Curly & Chic Shampoo above, and the same comments apply. This is a poor choice if your hair is dry or damaged, and given the blatant similarities between most of the Advance Techniques shampoos, the various hair types designated in the names have nothing to do with the formula and everything to do with marketing and selling more bottles of shampoo.

☹ **Advance Techniques Volumizing Shampoo** *($3.49 for 11 ounces)* is nearly identical to the Advance Techniques Curly & Chic Shampoo above, and the same comments apply. This also contains sodium polystyrene sulfonate, another drying ingredient that can potentially strip hair color with repeated use.

☹ **Advance Techniques Keep Clear Pyrithione Zinc Anti-Dandruff 2-in-1** *($3.49 for 11 ounces)* would have been a fine option for an anti-dandruff shampoo that lists 1% zinc pyrithione as its active ingredient. However, it contains sodium lauryl sulfate as one of the main detergent cleansing agents, and that makes it too drying to the hair and too irritating to the scalp.

☺ **Advance Techniques Color-Protection Conditioner** *($3.49 for 11 ounces)* works well to moisturize normal to dry hair of any thickness, and can make hair easier to comb. Those with coarse or damaged hair may not find this emollient enough.

☺ **Advance Techniques Curly & Chic Conditioner** *($3.49 for 11 ounces)* is a lightweight conditioner that contains mostly water, thickener, silicone, glycerin, water-binding agents, detangling agents, fragrance, and preservatives. It is a very good option for normal to fine hair that is normal to dry, but it has no particular advantage for curly hair.

☺ **Advance Techniques Daily Results Conditioner** *($3.49 for 11 ounces)* is similar to the Advance Techniques Curly & Chic Conditioner above, only without the same amount of silicone and minus the glycerin. That makes it an even lighter option that can hydrate and detangle normal to slightly dry hair that is normal to fine or thin.

☺ **Advance Techniques Straight & Sleek Conditioner** *($3.49 for 11 ounces)* is nearly identical to the Advance Techniques Curly & Chic Conditioner above, only with less glycerin. Otherwise, the same basic comments apply.

☺ **Advance Techniques Tress Therapy Conditioner, for Dry or Damaged Hair** *($3.49 for 11 ounces)* is similar to all of the Advance Techniques conditioners above, only this option contains more detangling agents. That can be beneficial for dry, damaged hair, because when the cuticle layer of hair is damaged it becomes very difficult to comb without the aid of a conditioner like this. This is a great option for normal to dry hair that is normal to thick.

☺ **Advance Techniques Volumizing Conditioner** *($3.49 for 11 ounces)* is the most basic and ordinary of all the Avon Advance Techniques conditioners. It is still a decent conditioner for normal to slightly dry hair that is normal to fine or thin.

☺ **Advance Techniques Curly & Chic Styling Gel** *($3.99 for 5 ounces)* is a standard styling gel that lacks moisturizing or conditioning agents that can help curly hair look its best. This water-based, alcohol-free gel can provide a firm hold that can feel somewhat sticky, though hair can still be brushed through.

☺ **Advance Techniques Daily Results Flexible Hold Finishing Spray** *($3.99 for 6.7 ounces)* is a standard, but good, nonaerosol hairspray that offers a light hold that doesn't make hair stiff but can leave it slightly sticky.

☺ **Advance Techniques Daily Results Flexible Hold Gel** *($3.99 for 5 ounces)* is a basic, but good, gel that provides medium hold that is minimally sticky and can be brushed through. It is not conditioning enough to use alone when styling hair with heat.

☺ **Advance Techniques Daily Results Flexible Hold Hair Spray** *($3.99 for 6.7 ounces)* is a nonaerosol alcohol-based hairspray, and it really does offer a flexible hold that is best described as light and barely sticky. If you need significant style support, this is not the hairspray for you, but this works well for a natural, touchable finish.

☺ **Advance Techniques Straight & Sleek Smoothing Balm** *($3.99 for 5.1 ounces)* is a conditioning, lightweight styling gel that provides a light, minimally sticky hold that can work well to smooth and straighten hair when used with heat and a round brush. For better protection from heat, pair this with a styling cream or silicone serum.

☺ **Advance Techniques Volumizing Volume Body-Building Mousse** *($3.99 for 6.7 ounces)* is a feather-light mousse that contains cornstarch as its main holding agent, and it does an OK job of providing soft, natural style support without being sticky or making hair feel stiff. There isn't much else to this mousse other than preservatives and fragrance. The silicones and conditioning agents are present in such small amounts they have little to no impact on hair and do not provide a suitable amount of heat protection. This is a decent option for normal to fine or thin hair.

☺ **Advance Techniques Volumizing Volume Root-Lifting Texturizer** *($3.99 for 6 ounces)* is an incredibly standard styling spray that offers medium hold. It can leave hair feeling sticky but it can still be brushed through. The conditioning agents are present in amounts too small to matter for hair.

☺ **$$$ Advance Techniques Curly & Chic Anti-Frizz Capsules** *($4.99 for 18 capsules for a total of 0.58 ounce)* ends up being a costly way to use what amounts to silicone serum packaged unnecessarily in capsule form. This is an inconvenient way to apply silicone serum because you may not need to use as much serum as each capsule provides, and what's left must be discarded unless you want to risk the mess when the remaining contents ooze out. As a silicone serum to smooth hair, add shine, and calm frizzies this works splendidly, but there are equally impressive options that cost the same but offer two to eight times as much product.

☺ **Advance Techniques Straight & Sleek Dry Ends Serum** *($3.49 for 1 ounce)* is a standard, but effective, silicone serum that contains a small amount of alcohol, which aids with the evaporation of the silicones and can keep this serum from being too heavy (though it should still be used sparingly). This is an inexpensive way to smooth frizzies and add shine to finished hairstyles.

☺ **Advance Techniques Straight & Sleek Shine Spray** *($4.99 for 3.4 ounces)* is an alcohol-based silicone shine spray that works beautifully to add smoothness and gloss on normal to fine hair. This mists on lightly and doesn't feel greasy, but use it sparingly until you learn how much product you need to achieve the results you want without making hair look slick or greasy.

☺ **Advance Techniques Tress Therapy Active Replenishing Mask, for All Hair Types** *($4.99 for 5 ounces)* is nothing more than a creamy, thick conditioner that is very good for normal to very dry hair that is normal to coarse or thick. It can (and should be) used daily, rather than as a special weekly treat for hair.

☺ **Advance Techniques Tress Therapy Hot Oil Treatment, for Dry or Damaged Hair** *($4.99 for 1 ounce)* contains no oil at all. It's just a fluid, water-based solution with silicone, creatine (which has no substantiated effect on hair), thickener, film-forming agent, water-binding agent, fragrance, and preservatives. It works well for light conditioning or to make normal to fine hair easier to comb through, but despite the name, it won't do much to impress those with dry, damaged hair.

☺ **Advance Techniques Tress Therapy Hydrating Spray Lotion, for Dry Hair** *($4.99 for 5 ounces)* is a spray-on, leave-in conditioner that has a silkening effect on hair and can aid in detangling, especially if hair is fine or thin.

BACK TO BASICS

Back to BASICS is a large hair-care line sold primarily in salons. Their tagline is "natural prescriptions for beautiful hair," but aside from token amounts of (mostly fragrant) plant extracts, nothing about these products is remotely natural. Throughout this extensive, often repetitive, hair-care collection, you will find products that contain the same basic ingredients used throughout the hair-care industry. Several items are bare-bones basic formulations that work well but simply don't have enough of the touted ingredients or conditioning agents to be of much help to your hair, at least beyond the duties of cleansing and making hair easier to comb through. That doesn't mean these products should be overlooked, just that their showcased special ingredients don't contribute much, if anything, to the products' performance. Although the majority of the products don't go above and beyond the norm, they shouldn't disappoint either, unless you're put off by potent fragrances. Graham Webb International owns Back to BASICS (for more information about Graham Webb and his far more expensive salon line of hair-care products, see the review for Graham Webb). For more information, call (800) 456-9322 or visit www.backtobasics.com.

What's Good About This Line: The prices are great and there is a nice variety of conditioners for various hair types.

What's Not So Good About It: Too many shampoos whose only major difference is a change of fragrance or fragrant plant extracts. Some of the hairsprays go on heavier and are stickier than the norm.

BACK TO BASICS AUTHENTIC MEN'S GROOMING COLLECTION

☺ **Daily Shampoo, for Men** *($5.95 for 8.5 ounces)* is an exceptionally standard shampoo that is good for all hair types. The small amount of film-forming agent poses minimal risk of buildup.

☹ **Volumizing Shampoo, for Men** *($5.95 for 8.5 ounces)* is similar to the Daily Shampoo, for Men above, but contains a small amount of eucalyptus, and that can be a problem for the scalp. This is not preferred to the shampoo above.

☺ **Daily Conditioner, for Men** *($6.95 for 8.5 ounces)* is a good, basic conditioner for normal to slightly dry hair of any thickness.

☺ **Finishing Spray, for Men** *($9.95 for 8.5 ounces)* is a standard, but good, aerosol hairspray that offers a medium hold with a minimally sticky finish that can be easily brushed through. The vitamins in this product have no effect on the hair, and the only thing that makes this specific for men is the fragrance.

☺ **Holding Paste, for Men** *($12.95 for 4 ounces)* is a thick styling cream that can easily feel heavy or look greasy unless used sparingly. It's a good smoothing and finishing product for those with thick, textured hair, and allows for flexible styling with a moist, slightly sticky feel.

☺ **Liquid Styling Gel, for Men** *($9.95 for 8.5 ounces)* is a very standard styling gel that offers a firm hold and can make hair feel stiff and sticky, but it can be brushed through.

☺ **Pomade, for Men** *($9.95 for 4 ounces)* is a water- and castor oil-based pomade that also lists lanolin as one of the main ingredients, which makes this best for dry to very dry hair that is thick or coarse. It works well to smooth dry ends and tame flyaway strands, while adding texture and shine when used sparingly.

☺ **Styling Fiber, for Men** *($9.95 for 4 ounces)* is a very heavy pomade that contains mostly water, lanolin wax, alcohol, and film-forming agent. It is difficult to shampoo out, but can be an OK option to smooth the ends of dry, textured hair while adding a low-gloss shine. The directions indicate that this is to be applied to towel-dried hair, but ignore that because this does not distribute well through damp hair and can easily clump.

☺ **Super Hold Gel, for Men** *($8.95 for 8.5 ounces)* is a standard, alcohol-free styling gel that offers a strong hold that feels sticky but can be brushed through without flaking. The conditioning agents can help make hair softer and provide a small amount of protection from heat.

BACK TO BASICS BASIC STYLE

☺ **Basic Style Curl Catalyst, Curl Activating Gel** *($9.95 for 6 ounces)* is a good, soft-hold styling gel that is minimally sticky and offers some conditioning benefits for hair. It won't activate curls where none exist, but can enhance the texture and shape of permed or naturally curly/wavy hair without making it feel stiff or brittle.

☺ **Basic Style Final Fix, Firm Hold Hair Spray** *($10.95 for 10 ounces)* is a standard, but good, aerosol hairspray that goes on heavier than most but provides a light hold that can be easily brushed through. The tiny amount of fruit oil can add shine.

☺ **Basic Style Liquid Lift, Root Amplifying Spray** *($9.95 for 8.5 ounces)* is a light-weight, non-sticky water- and alcohol-based spray gel that features a special nozzle so you can easily spray this on the roots.

☺ **Basic Style Sleek Creme, Anti-Frizz Straightening Balm** *($9.95 for 5.5 ounces)* can indeed make hair sleek, and works well (when used with heat and the proper brush) to straighten hair and add shine. This water- and silicone-based formula feels creamy and contains a low amount of film-forming agents, so it offers control without stiffness, though it can feel slightly sticky.

☺ **Basic Style Up Hold, Extra-Strength Styling Gel** *($9.95 for 7.5 ounces)* is an exceptionally basic styling gel that also has tiny mica particles that add shine with minimal flaking. This firm-hold gel offers a lightweight but sticky finish that can be somewhat difficult to brush through. It's best for slicked-back wet looks or for defining curls on hair that is not overly dry or damaged.

BACK TO BASICS GINGER COLLECTION

☺ **Ginger Therapy Shampoo** *($8.95 for 12 ounces)* does contain some ginger extract, but it mostly adds fragrance and has no effect on hair (though it can be a scalp irritant). Otherwise, this standard shampoo contains gentle detergent cleansing agents and enough film-former to cause buildup with repeated use. It is a good option for normal to dry hair that is normal to thin.

☺ **Ginger Scalp Therapy Shampoo** *($9.95 for 6 ounces)* is a vegetable oil-based shampoo that doesn't contain any water, so this is a very rich shampoo for dry to very dry hair that is coarse or thick. There isn't much to this beyond the oil and detergent cleansing agents. The small amount of alcohol won't be drying to the hair, and the salicylic acid has no effect on the hair (which is a good thing) because the pH of this shampoo is too high for it to exfoliate the scalp.

☺ **Ginger Therapy Conditioner** (*$8.95 for 12 ounces*) is a standard detangling conditioner for normal to dry hair that is normal to thin.

☹ **Ginger Therapy Masque** (*$10.95 for 4 ounces*) is a thick conditioner that lists clay as the third ingredient. Not only is clay unable to moisturize the hair, it can also chip away at the cuticle and make hair drier.

BACK TO BASICS GREEN TEA COLLECTION

☺ **Green Tea Daily Moisturizing Shampoo** (*$7.95 for 12 ounces*) can be a good shampoo for dry hair that is not fine or thin, but the film-forming agent will cause buildup, so alternate this with a shampoo that does not have that effect.

☺ **Green Tea Ultra Hydrating Shampoo** (*$9.95 for 12 ounces*) is indeed hydrating, and is an excellent shampoo for those with dry to very dry hair that is normal to thick. The film-forming agent it contains poses minimal risk of buildup.

☺ **Green Tea Daily Moisturizing Conditioner** (*$8.95 for 12 ounces*) is similar to the Ginger Therapy Conditioner above, and the same comments apply.

☺ **Green Tea Firm Hold Gel** (*$8.95 for 8 ounces*) is a standard, lightly fragranced styling gel that provides a medium to firm hold with a stiff, sticky feel. Hair can be brushed through, but this gel works best for wet looks or on short, closely cropped hair.

☺ **Green Tea Smoothing Elixir, Anti-Frizz Straightening Gel** (*$9.95 for 8.5 ounces*) is a styling and smoothing gel without hold, which means it does not make hair feel stiff or sticky. It works well to straighten hair when used with heat, but is best paired with a silicone serum for added heat protection.

☺ **Green Tea Spray Finish Firm Hold Hair Spray** (*$9.95 for 10 ounces*) is an effective aerosol hairspray that provides a firm hold and contains a small amount of conditioning agents, so hair doesn't get too stiff and remains easy to brush through. My only complaint is that the orifice in the container's nozzle tends to dispense too much hairspray at once, which can result in uneven or too heavy application.

☺ **Green Tea Texturizing Lotion** (*$8.95 for 6.8 ounces*) is a lightweight styling balm that contains softer-hold film-forming agents that can be easily brushed through (the addition of moisturizing agents helps, too). This slightly sticky balm works well for those with normal to dry hair that is not fine or thin.

☺ **Green Tea Thickening Serum** (*$8.95 for 8.5 ounces*) doesn't contain anything that can make hair thicker, and it's not a serum. Rather, this is a standard fragranced styling gel that has medium hold and leaves hair feeling sticky, so it's not the best if you want to brush through your hair.

☺ **Green Tea Volume Infusing Spray Foam** (*$10.95 for 9 ounces*) is a spray-on aerosol styling mousse that should still be sprayed into your palm rather than applied directly to the hair. It provides a firm, sticky hold that can be somewhat difficult to brush through. It's an option for all hair types, but the light foam texture works best on normal to fine hair.

☺ **Green Tea Reparative Conditioning Balm** *($10.95 for 6.8 ounces)* cannot repair hair. It's just a good emollient conditioner for dry to very dry hair that can make hair softer, smoother, and easier to comb.

BACK TO BASICS KIWI MELON COLLECTION

☺ **Kiwi Melon Body Boosting Shampoo** *($8.95 for 12 ounces)* is a very good shampoo for all hair types. The tiny amount of film-forming agent poses little to no risk of buildup.

☺ **Kiwi Melon Body Boosting Conditioner** *($9.95 for 12 ounces)* is nearly identical to the Ginger Therapy Conditioner above, only this omits the plant oil, so it's preferred for normal to slightly dry hair that is normal to fine or thin.

BACK TO BASICS MARINE COLLECTION

☺ **Marine Color Protection Shampoo** *($8.95 for 12 ounces)* claims to seal and protect hair color, but contains nothing that can do that (actually, it's not possible to seal color to prevent fading). It's just a standard, but good, shampoo that is a good option for normal to dry hair of any texture and that poses minimal risk of buildup.

☺ **Marine Color Protection Conditioner** *($9.95 for 12 ounces)* is a lightweight conditioner that is a great alternative to regular conditioner for someone with normal to slightly dry hair that is fine or thin. Nothing in this product will help color last longer or prevent the inevitable fading.

☺ **Marine Color Sealant** *($9.95 for 12 ounces)* is a standard, spray-on detangling conditioner. The "nutrient-rich Marine Complex" harvested "from the depths of the ocean" is supposedly what's responsible for protecting hair color, but seaweed and sea grass extracts absolutely cannot keep hair color from fading. This is a good, very lightweight conditioner that can make normal to fine hair easier to comb through, but that's it.

BACK TO BASICS POMEGRANATE PEACH COLLECTION

☺ **Pomegranate Peach Replenishing Shampoo** *($8.95 for 12 ounces)* is a very good conditioning shampoo for normal to dry hair of any thickness.

☺ **Pomegranate Peach Replenishing Conditioner** *($9.95 for 12 ounces)* works well as a lightweight conditioner for normal to slightly dry hair that is fine or thin, but don't count on substantial moisture replenishment.

BACK TO BASICS RASPBERRY ALMOND COLLECTION

☺ **Raspberry Almond Intensive Shampoo** *($8.95 for 12 ounces)* is similar to the Green Tea Daily Moisturizing Shampoo above, and the same basic comments apply.

☺ **Raspberry Almond Strengthening Shampoo** *($9.95 for 12 ounces)* is nearly identical to the Raspberry Almond Intensive Shampoo above, and the same comments apply. The fruit and plant extracts it contains cannot make hair stronger.

☺ **Raspberry Almond Strengthening Conditioner** *($9.95 for 12 ounces)* contains nothing that can strengthen hair. What makes this claim particularly absurd is that this product contains the same ingredients found in every other Back to BASICS conditioner! This is a good option for normal to slightly dry hair that is normal to fine.

BACK TO BASICS SUNFLOWER COLLECTION

☺ **Sunflower Moisture Infusing Shampoo** *($8.95 for 12 ounces)* is nearly identical to the Green Tea Daily Moisturizing Shampoo above, and the same comments apply.

☺ **Sunflower Leave-In Detangling & Conditioning Spray** *($8.95 for 8.5 ounces)* works as a detangling spray for all hair types. This is so watery and light that the conditioning benefits are minimal.

☺ **Sunflower Moisture Infusing Conditioner** *($9.95 for 12 ounces)* is similar to the Marine Color Protection Conditioner above, and the same comments apply.

☺ **Sunflower Creme Mousse** *($7.99 for 8.5 ounces)* is a standard, propellant-based mousse that provides a light-to-medium, slightly sticky hold that can be easily brushed through. The formula includes a good amount of plant oil, making it preferred for normal to very dry hair that is not fine or thin.

☺ **Sunflower Firm Hold Hair Spray** *($7.99 for 10 ounces)* is similar to the Green Tea Spray Finish Firm Hold Hair Spray above, and the same basic comments apply. This hairspray offers a bit more silicone and adds a small amount of plant oil, which makes it slightly better for drier hair and for heightened shine.

☺ **Sunflower Firm Hold Spritz** *($9.95 for 8.5 ounces)* is a nonaerosol hairspray that applies heavier than most thanks to its pump mechanism. It provides a strong, slightly stiff hold that can be brushed through, but not without some snags along the way. This is best used to set styles you don't intend to retouch later, and the holding power is such that you likely won't have to do that anyway!

☺ **Sunflower Spray Gel** *($9.95 for 8.5 ounces)* is a lightweight, alcohol-based spray gel that applies and holds more like a traditional hairspray. The film-forming/holding agent offers long-lasting style support but not without feeling somewhat stiff and sticky. This works well as a finishing spray on all hair types.

☺ **Sunflower Styling Gel** *($9.95 for 8.5 ounces)* is similar to the Green Tea Firm Hold Gel above, and the same comments apply.

BACK TO BASICS TANGERINE COLLECTION

☺ **Tangerine Grapefruit Clarifying Shampoo** *($8.95 for 12 ounces)* is a very standard shampoo that is an option for all hair types, and has no risk of buildup. Tangerine and grapefruit are not helpful for scalp or hair.

☺ **Tangerine Twist Daily Radiance Shampoo** *($8.95 for 12 ounces)* is similar to the Tangerine Grapefruit Clarifying Shampoo above, only with fewer potentially problematic citrus extracts. Otherwise, the same comments apply.

☺ **Tangerine Twist Daily Radiance Conditioner** *($9.95 for 12 ounces)* is similar to most of the Back to BASICS conditioners above, making it a basic, but effective, moisturizing conditioner for normal to dry hair of any thickness.

BACK TO BASICS VANILLA PLUM COLLECTION

☺ **Vanilla Plum Fortifying Shampoo** *($8.95 for 12 ounces)* is nearly identical to the Tangerine Twist Daily Radiance Shampoo above, only this shampoo does not contain citrus extract and instead uses vanilla and plum (which have no effect on the hair, but do add fragrance). It also offers slightly more conditioning effect from the proteins it contains, but it's doubtful your hair will notice.

☺ **Vanilla Plum Fortifying Conditioner** *($8.95 for 12 ounces)* is a lightweight, but hydrating and detangling, conditioner that contains enough silicone to make hair smooth and very silky. This is a very good option for normal to dry hair that is normal to thick or coarse.

BACK TO BASICS WHITE GRAPEFRUIT

☹ **White Grapefruit Clarifying Shampoo** *($10.99 for 12 ounces)* contains the drying detergent cleansing agent TEA-dodecylbenzenesulfonate as one of its main ingredients, and is not recommended for any hair type.

BACK TO BASICS WILD BERRY COLLECTION

☺ **Wild Berry Volumizing Shampoo** *($8.95 for 12 ounces)* is another standard, but worthwhile, shampoo that poses no risk of buildup and is a good option for all hair types.

☺ **Wild Berry Volumizing Conditioner** *($8.95 for 12 ounces)* works well as a lightweight option for normal to fine or thin hair and functions best to detangle and add some softness.

BAIN DE TERRE

The bain de terre line has made some changes since the last edition of this book, mostly in regard to the fragrance in the products, which has taken on an intensity that might just knock your socks off. Their marketing angle is similar to those of Aveda, Origins, and other so-called natural-ingredient hair-care lines. There are no plants in these products that are significantly helpful for hair—but that didn't stop bain de terre from capitalizing on the consumer's desire for anything natural sounding.

All bain de terre products contain what the company refers to as their "bio-renew complex." Although the ingredients in this complex are not clearly indicated, I suspect the name refers to the botanical, herbal, and spice extracts present throughout the line. Can any of these naturally derived ingredients "replenish, revitalize, and renew the hair"? Nope. Not a single one, though they all contribute to the product's fragrance, and a few of them can be good conditioning agents. For more information about bain de terre, owned by Zotos International, call (800) 242-WAVE or visit www.zotos.com.

What's Good About This Line: A few of the shampoos and conditioners are great options for those with dry to very dry hair.

What's Not So Good About It: Some drying shampoos, a peppermint oil-based "treatment" product, and the majority of the styling products have incredibly strong fragrances.

☹ **Green Meadow Daily Shampoo** *($10.49 for 13.5 ounces)* is a standard shampoo that contains both sodium C14-16 olefin sulfonate and sodium lauryl sulfate as the main detergent cleansing agents. That means this can be unduly irritating to the scalp and drying for hair, especially if used every day, and as such this shampoo is not recommended.

☺ **Jasmine Moisturizing Shampoo** *($10.49 for 13.5 ounces)* is a standard, but very good, shampoo that works well for normal to very dry hair that is coarse or thick. This poses a slight risk of buildup.

☺ **Kiwi Color Protecting Shampoo** *($9 for 13.5 ounces)* is a great shampoo for all hair types, particularly normal to fine or thin, and poses minimal to no risk of buildup. The tiny amount of wasabi extract (Japanese horseradish) is unlikely to be a problem for the scalp. Although this shampoo will not strip hair color, nothing in it is capable of protecting it either.

☹ **Lemongrass Volumizing Shampoo** *($10.49 for 13.5 ounces)* contains TEA-lauryl sulfate as its detergent cleansing agent, which makes it too drying for the hair and irritating to the scalp.

☺ **Cucumber Moisturizing Conditioner** *($11.89 for 13.5 ounces)* really does smell like cucumber, so if that appeals to you and your hair is normal to slightly dry, give this conditioner a try. This is a great option for thicker, drier hair textures.

☺ **Herbal Sea Mist Leave-In Detangler** *($9.19 for 6.7 ounces)* is a very lightweight detangler that contains mostly water, silicone, and plant extracts (which have no effect on hair's comb-ability). This is a good option for normal hair that is normal to fine or thin, and it affords some protection from heat styling.

☺ **Lavender Color Protecting Conditioner** *($10 for 13.5 ounces)* cannot protect color, at least no more than any other standard conditioner. This is a good option for normal to very dry hair that is normal to coarse or thick.

☺ **Watercress Volumizing Conditioner** *($11.89 for 13.5 ounces)* is simply a conditioner that works well for normal to slightly dry hair that is normal to fine or thin.

☺ **White Clover Daily Detangling Conditioner** *($11.89 for 13.5 ounces)* is similar to the Watercress Volumizing Conditioner above, except this has a larger amount of silicone, which makes it better for smoothing and detangling the hair. Otherwise, the same basic comments apply.

☺ **All Day Straight Safflower Smoothing Gel** *($8.99 for 6.7 ounces)* is more a leave-in conditioner than a styling product. All Day Straight contains no film-forming/holding agent, and can help make hair straight only when used with heat and the appropriate brush or flat iron.

☺ **Final Touches Goldenseal Dual-Purpose Styler** *($10.49 for 6.7 ounces)* is an alcohol- and water-based styling spray that provides medium hold when used on wet or dry hair, and either application method leaves hair slightly stiff and sticky. The small amount of silicone and conditioning agents help make brushing through the hair easier.

☺ **Firm Action Flax Seed Styling Gel** *($10.49 for 5.1 ounces)* is a standard, firm-hold styling gel that feels lighter on the hair than you might expect based on the relatively thick texture of the product. This non-flaking formula leaves hair a bit stiff and sticky, but can be easily brushed through. One caution: The henna extract has the potential to make hair feel drier with repeated use.

☺ **Infinite Hold Flax Seed Finishing Spray** *($13.19 for 10.2 ounces)* is a standard, but workable, aerosol hairspray that, despite being described as "unscented," contains fragrance. It provides a light hold that is minimally stiff and sticky, so hair is easily brushed through. Note: This product is available in two formulas, an 80% VOC formula not for sale in California, and a 55% VOC formula that is for sale in California.

☺ **Rise 'n Shine White Willow Volumizing Mousse** *($13.19 for 8.5 ounces)* is a liquid-to-foam styling mousse that features an alcohol-free formula with medium hold. It can leave hair feeling slightly sticky, but is easily brushed through. This is a good option for normal to fine or thin hair, but the fragrance is intense.

☺ **Spring Back Lemon Balm Texture Reviver** *($11.89 for 5.1 ounces)* is said to rejuvenate wavy, curly, or textured hair, but it doesn't contain anything to make these hair types do an about-face. It's merely a standard styling cream that offers light, conditioned hold that stays moist but can also make hair feel slightly sticky. The lack of silicones of any kind makes it hard to recommend because most of the competing products in this category contain silicone for its wonderful smoothing abilities.

☺ **Stay 'n Shape Lemongrass Shaping Spray** *($11.89 for 10.2 ounces)* is almost identical to the Infinite Hold Flax Seed Finishing Spray above, except this provides a slightly softer hold. Otherwise, the same comments apply.

☹ **Take Shape Mint Balm Spray Gel, Medium Hold** *($10.49 for 5.1 ounces)* works well as a light-hold spray gel with conditioning agents, but the amount of balm-mint leaf extract is great enough to cause scalp irritation (you'll feel a tingle as soon as this hits the scalp), so it is not recommended.

☹ **Whip Into Shape, Chamomile Cream Pomade** *($10.99 for 3.4 ounces)* contains sodium polystyrene sulfonate, a film-forming agent that can strip hair color and cause dryness. This is also a fairly sticky styling cream that just isn't easy to work with, at least in comparison to similar products.

☹ **Peppermint Patty Invigorating Scalp Treatment** *($13.19 for 4.2 ounces)* is in-vigorating, but in this case that also means irritating. With peppermint oil and menthol, too, this witch hazel- and water-based gel offers significantly more problems than benefits for your scalp. If the name appeals to you, try the York Peppermint Patty mints instead!

☺ $$$ **Recovery Complex Anti-Frizz Shine Serum** *($19.80 for 1.7 ounces)* is a standard silicone serum that works well to smooth frizzies and add shine, but there is no reason to spend this much when companies like Avon and Citré Shine offer nearly identical products for under $7.

☺ **Mega Masque White Ginger Hair Repair** *($13.19 for 5.1 ounces)* is nothing more than a conditioner parading as a special treatment for hair. While it can't repair even one strand of hair, it is still a very good, creamy conditioner for normal to very dry hair of any thickness except fine or thin. If your hair is dry to very dry, you'll get better results from daily rather than weekly use of this product.

BATH & BODY WORKS

Bath & Body Works offers an enormous assortment of products, ranging from skincare and makeup to body-care and home fragrance items. Their hair-care collection has been revamped and tweaked more times than I care to count, and the products below represent their latest efforts, which are mostly unoriginal creations inspired by other successful hair-care lines, particularly Aveda. Basically, the theme of aromatherapy and plant essences permeates each product, and the aromas of most of them could permeate your deepest sinuses! This is not to imply that Bath & Body Works hair-care products are bad, because there are many worthwhile products to consider; it's just that there are definitely some you'd be better off avoiding. Their products are not necessarily original, but isn't imitation the sincerest form of flattery? For more information about Bath & Body Works, call (800) 395-1001 or visit www.bathandbodyworks.com.

What's Good About This Line: On the best products, the prices are more than reasonable.

What's Not So Good About It: Many problematic shampoos that contain sodium lauryl sulfate and ammonium xylenesulfonate; some of the styling products contain the preservatives methylchloroisothiazolinone and methylisothiazolinone (Kathon CG), which are sensitizing and contraindicated for use in leave-on products. Most products are intensely fragranced, which may not be to everyone's liking.

BATH & BODY WORKS AROMATHERAPY

☹ **Aromatherapy Sensuality Hydrating Shampoo** *($9 for 10 ounces)* is a standard group of shampoos available in several different versions, each using an essential oil blend that not only adds fragrance but also can cause scalp itching and irritation. Even if the essential oils were completely benign ingredients, each of the Aromatherapy shampoos contains sodium lauryl sulfate as one of the main detergent cleansing agents. But wait—there's more: Each of these shampoos also contains ammonium xylenesulfonate, an ingredient that can cause further hair dryness and scalp irritation. If your goal is to avoid problematic shampoos, these should be near the top of your "ignore" list.

☹ **Aromatherapy Sensuality Volumizing Shampoo** *($9 for 10 ounces)* is also available in several versions, each containing a different essential oil blend for fragrance (and offering the unpleasant side effect of scalp irritation). The base formula is nearly identical to the Aromatherapy Sensuality Hydrating Shampoo above, and the same comments apply.

☹ **Aromatherapy Sensuality Hydrating Conditioner** *($9 for 10 ounces)* shares the same concept as the two Aromatherapy shampoos above, meaning one basic formula is available with several different essential oil blends for fragrance. This is an exceptionally standard conditioner for normal to slightly dry hair that is normal to fine or thin, but the amount of fragrance and added essential oils can conspire to cause potent irritation to the scalp, and these are not recommended.

☹ **Aromatherapy Sensuality Volumizing Conditioner** *($9 for 10 ounces)* shares the same essential oil concept as the Aromatherapy conditioner above, except the base formula is slightly lighter in texture. Otherwise, the comments made above apply here, too.

BATH & BODY WORKS BIO

The "Bio" in this Bath & Body Works hair-care subcategory stands for "beauty individualized organics." The name is meant to invoke a feeling that these products are personalized hair prescriptions filled with farm-fresh organic ingredients. Organic is a big buzzword that has permeated the cosmetics industry, even though there aren't any regulated standards regarding the use of organic ingredients in hair-care products. Until standards are set, there is no advantage to choosing hair-care products made with tiny amounts of organic ingredients. Moreover, the ingredient lists for the Bio products do not indicate the plant and fruit extracts are organic, nor is there any third-party certification on the product labels (which is the standard established for foods that are labeled organic). That means the natural ingredients may or may not be organic. In fact, the only thing you can count on with the Bio products is that they contain more synthetic fragrance than anything natural, and they use the same standard hair-care ingredients found industry-wide.

☹ **Bio Clarifying Shampoo, with Peppermint and Lemongrass** *($7.50 for 12 ounces)* contains sodium lauryl sulfate as one of its main detergent cleansing agent, which makes it too drying for the hair and irritating to the scalp. It also contains a hefty amount of peppermint, which increases the irritation factor.

☹ **Bio Color Protect Shampoo, Helps Protect Color and Revitalizes Its Shine** *($7.50 for 12 ounces)* contains sodium lauryl sulfate and ammonium xylenesulfonate—two very drying and irritating ingredients that won't do a thing to protect even one molecule of color.

☺ **Bio Curl on Cue Shampoo, Strengthens, Defines and Tames Curls** *($7.50 for 12 ounces)* has an enticing name (what was the runner-up, "Poof! Your Hair is Curly"?) and is a much gentler shampoo than all of the preceding options. Unfortunately, the inclusion of ammonium xylenesulfontate means this doesn't quite cross the finish line to earn a smiling face rating. The neutral face rating is for the mostly innocuous formula and the presence of the ammonium xylenesulfonate, even in a very small amount. By the way, nothing about this shampoo can strengthen, define, or tame curls, though the silicone can help them look somewhat smoother.

☹ **Bio Hydrating Shampoo, Helps Replenish Essential Moisture to Strengthen Dry Hair** *($7.50 for 12 ounces)* is similar to the Bio Color Protect Shampoo above, and the same comments apply. This shampoo is about as moisturizing as sand.

☹ **Bio Max Volume Shampoo, for Fine, Thin Hair** *($7.50 for 12 ounces)* is similar to the Bio Color Protect Shampoo above, and the same comments apply.

☺ **Bio Restorative Shampoo, Strengthens Damaged, Overstressed Hair** *($7.50 for 12 ounces)*. Finally, a Bath & Body Works shampoo to extol! This is a standard, but very good, shampoo that is excellent for all hair types. It poses no risk of buildup. After all of the disappointing options above, this is a breath of fresh air!

☹ **Bio Straight & Sleek Shampoo, Relaxes Curls and Fights Frizz for a Smooth, Shiny Finish** *($7.50 for 12 ounces)* contains ammonium xylenesulfonate, and in an amount that can be too drying for the hair and scalp. This shampoo is not recommended, and won't help frizzy hair.

☺ **Bio Color Protect Conditioner, Helps Protect Color and Revitalizes Its Shine** *($7.50 for 12 ounces)* is a good, though basic, conditioner for normal to dry hair that is normal to slightly thick.

☺ **Bio Curl on Cue Conditioner, Strengthens, Defines and Tames Curls** *($7.50 for 12 ounces)* is a good, though rather boring, conditioner for normal to dry hair of any thickness. The silicone helps make curly hair look smoother, but won't make it any stronger.

☺ **Bio Hydrating Conditioner, Helps Replenish Essential Moisture to Strengthen Dry Hair** *($7.50 for 12 ounces)* is nearly identical to the Bio Color Protect Conditioner above, and the same comments apply.

☺ **Bio Max Volume Conditioner, for Fine, Thin Hair** *($7.50 for 12 ounces)* is a very good, though standard, conditioner for normal to fine or thin hair that can make it softer and easier to comb through.

☺ **Bio Restorative Conditioner, Strengthens Damaged, Overstressed Hair** *($7.50 for 12 ounces)* is similar to the Bio Max Volume Conditioner above, except this option contains more detangling agent and includes silicones, which makes it preferred for normal to slightly dry hair that is normal to slightly thick but not coarse.

☺ **Bio Restorative Leave-In Conditioner, Strengthens Damaged, Overstressed Hair** *($7.50 for 12 ounces)* can't strengthen hair in the least, but it can be a good lightweight detangler for normal to fine hair. The film-forming agent can leave hair feeling slightly sticky and coated, so this may also be the only styling product you need.

☺ **Bio Straight & Sleek Conditioner, Relaxes Curls and Fights Frizz for a Smooth, Shiny Finish** *($7.50 for 12 ounces)* won't relax curls one bit, but it is a good conditioner for normal to dry hair that is normal to thick or coarse.

☺ **Bio Curl on Cue Defining Gel** *($8 for 7 ounces)* is a standard styling gel that holds no advantage for curly hair. It does have a rather masculine fragrance that will enter a room before you do, and it provides a medium to firm hold that stays sticky and is somewhat difficult to brush through.

The Reviews B

☺ **Bio Max Volume Finishing Spray** *($9 for 8 ounces)* is a standard aerosol hairspray that provides a light hold that is slightly sticky but can be easily brushed through. Compared to the Bio Curl On Cue Defining Gel above, the fragrance in this product is (thankfully) much softer.

☺ **Bio Max Volume Root Lifter** *($9 for 8 ounces)* contains more fragrance than film-forming agent, which gives this liquid styling product a very light hold that is barely sticky. This doesn't offer much style support, especially if your hair tends to fall flat too soon, but it can be a good all-over styling product for a natural look with minimum hold.

☹ **Bio Max Volume Volumizing Gelee** *($9 for 8 ounces)* is a below-average styling gel that, while being non-sticky and providing light hold, flakes terribly, even before it dries.

☺ **Bio Straight & Sleek Extreme Smoothing Creme** *($9 for 3.4 ounces)* contains the essential ingredients to help make curly or wavy hair straight and sleek! Of course, the product alone won't create this oft-coveted look. You still need to use this with heat and the appropriate brush. This water- and silicone-based cream is wonderfully creamy and can make hair feel very silky and look shiny. The film-forming/holding agent helps during styling and does not make hair feel sticky.

☺ **Bio Straight & Sleek Light Smoothing Lotion** *($9 for 5.5 ounces)* is similar to the Bio Straight & Sleek Extreme Smoothing Creme above, except this has a thinner texture and uses lighter silicones. It works well to create smooth, sleek styles when used with heat and the proper styling tools. Relative to the Smoothing Creme above, this works better on normal to fine hair.

☺ **Bio Curl on Cue Rejuvenating Mist** *($8 for 8 ounces)* is a very basic spray-on styling liquid that contains mostly water, film-forming/holding agent, fragrance, conditioning agents, thickener, slip agent, and preservatives. This won't rejuvenate hair, but it will provide a light hold with a slightly sticky finish that can be easily brushed through.

☺ **Bio Curl on Cue Shine Serum** *($10 for 3.4 ounces)* is a standard, but very good, silicone serum that contains alcohol to dilute the silicone's potency. This tactic can work to create a silicone serum that works for all hair types, but it can still look slick and greasy if not applied sparingly, a critical tip if your hair is fine or thin.

☺ **Bio High Shine Gloss** *($12 for 2 ounces)* is similar to the Bio Curl On Cue Shine Serum above, except this does not contain alcohol and as such is a richer silicone serum that's best for normal to very dry hair that is coarse or thick.

☺ **Bio Restorative 3-Minute Treatment Cream** *($8 for 5 ounces)* is so similar to all of the Bio conditioners above that calling it a "treatment" is almost funny. This is a good, though standard, conditioner that works well for normal to dry hair of any thickness. As with any conditioner, the longer you leave it on the hair, the better.

☺ **Bio Restorative Hair Treatment Capsules** *($10 for 12 capsules)* are just tiny capsules filled with silicones, slip agent, panthenol, vitamin E, plant oil, and plant extracts. These work well to smooth the hair, create shine, and eliminate frizzies but for the money, any of the other Bath & Body Works Bio silicone serums are preferred, are easier to use, and have the exact same effect on hair.

☺ **Bio Straight & Sleek Healthy Shine Serum** *($12 for 2 ounces)* is similar to the Bio High Shine Gloss above, but is not quite as good. However, it can still make hair look smooth, feel silky, and exhibit shine.

BATH & BODY WORKS BOTANICAL NUTRIENTS

The Botanical Nutrients collection uses the same hook (and often the same plant ingredients) as Aveda. Specifically, all of the unnatural-sounding ingredients are listed in parentheses as having a coconut oil source. Many of these ingredients really do come from coconut oil, but what it takes to convert coconut oil into decyl glucoside and cocamide MEA is not natural in the least, and the result is an ingredient that bears no resemblance to its original, natural source. That isn't a bad thing, but to position synthetic (and commonly used) hair-care ingredients as being natural is disingenuous, and that's not helpful for consumers. All told, the Botanical Nutrients line, which proudly touts "the pure power of plants," relies on the same standard ingredients everyone else does to create hair-care products that clean, condition, and style the hair.

☺ **Botanical Nutrients Rose Hips & Aloe Shampoo, for Color-Treated Hair** *($7.50 for 8 ounces)* is a standard shampoo that is a good shampoo for all hair types and poses no risk of buildup.

☹ **Botanical Nutrients Rosemary Mint Shampoo, for Fine/Normal Hair** *($7.50 for 8 ounces)* contains a plant tea of rosemary, peppermint, and eucalyptus, which, though not as potent as the oil form of these ingredients, can still cause scalp irritation and that makes this shampoo tough to recommend.

☺ **Botanical Nutrients Soyflower Shampoo, for Daily Use By All Hair Types** *($7.50 for 8 ounces)* is similar to the Botanical Nutrients Rose Hips & Aloe Shampoo above, and the same comments apply.

☺ **Botanical Nutrients Wheat Bran Patchouli Shampoo, for Dry Hair** *($9 for 5 ounces)* contains a plant tea of potentially problematic ingredients, even though they would be rinsed down the drain in short order. It's still a good shampoo for normal to dry hair types, although it can build up with repeated use. It contains mostly plant tea, detergent cleansing agents, lather agents, film-forming agent, glycerin, silicone, conditioning agents, thickener, fragrance, more conditioning agents, plant oil, chelating agent, and preservatives.

☹ **Botanical Nutrients Yucca Aloe Purifying Shampoo, for All Hair Types** *($10 for 8 ounces)* is similar to the Botanical Nutrients Rosemary Mint Shampoo above, and the same comments apply.

☺ **Botanical Nutrients Leave-In Creme Conditioner, for Damaged or Color-Treated Hair** *($7.50 for 6 ounces)* works to detangle and soften the hair, and is best for normal to slightly dry hair that is normal to thick.

☺ **Botanical Nutrients Rose Hips & Aloe Conditioner, for Color-Treated Hair** *($7.50 for 8 ounces)* is a very good conditioner for normal to dry hair that is normal to coarse or thick.

☺ **Botanical Nutrients Rosemary Green Tea Leave-In Conditioning Mist, for Fine/ Normal Hair** *($11.50 for 7.5 ounces)* is primarily plant tea, film-forming agents, and fragrance. It is a good, though basic, detangler that has little conditioning ability.

☹ **Botanical Nutrients Rosemary Mint Conditioner, for Fine/Normal Hair** *($7.50 for 8 ounces)* contains a plant tea of rosemary, peppermint, and eucalyptus, and that can be too drying and irritating for the scalp.

☺ **Botanical Nutrients Soyflower Conditioner, for Daily Use By All Hair Types** *($7.50 for 8 ounces)* is a standard conditioner that is good for softening normal to dry hair and making it easier to comb.

☺ **Botanical Nutrients Wheat Bran Patchouli Conditioner, for Dry Hair** *($9 for 5 ounces)* is similar to the Botanical Nutrients Rose Hips & Aloe Conditioner above, and the same comments apply.

☺ **Botanical Nutrients Wheat Germ Almond Hair Reconstructor, for All Hair Types** *($10 for 5 ounces)* is a great conditioner for normal to dry hair of any thickness, but it cannot reconstruct anything.

☹ **Botanical Nutrients Green Tea Conditioning Fixative** *($11.50 for 8 ounces)* is a standard styling lotion that provides a light hold, but it contains the skin-sensitizing preservative Kathon CG which is not recommended for use in leave-in products.

☺ **Botanical Nutrients Meadowsweet Flexible Hold Hair Spray** *($10.50 for 7.5 ounces)* is a standard nonaerosol hairspray that provides a light, brushable hold that does not get stiff or sticky. This does contain rather strong fragrance.

☺ **Botanical Nutrients Neroli Flaxseed Styling Foam** *($9.50 for 6.7 ounces)* is a lightweight, liquid-to-foam styling mousse that provides a soft hold with a lingering hint of stickiness. This is a good styling product for normal to fine or thin hair.

☺ **Botanical Nutrients Nettle Elderflower Sculpting Gel** *($10 for 6 ounces)* is a standard styling gel that provides a firm hold that can remain slightly sticky. When used on wet hair, it can make it stiff, but it's easily brushed through. The conditioning agents don't amount to much for helping the hair feel softer.

☹ **Botanical Nutrients Olive Sandalwood Styling Pomade** *($13.50 for 2 ounces)* contains the skin-sensitizing preservative Kathon CG and is not recommended.

☺ **Botanical Nutrients Watercress Hair Volumizer** *($12 for 3.4 ounces)* is similar to a hairspray and contains mostly alcohol, plant tea, film-forming/holding agent, water-binding agents, more film-forming agent, fragrance, silicone, and sunscreen (though sunscreen cannot protect the hair from sun damage). It provides a firm hold that is slightly sticky, but when brushed through leaves hair feeling silky.

☺ **Botanical Nutrients Willow Bark Firm Hold Hair Spray** *($10.50 for 7.5 ounces)* is nearly identical to the Botanical Nutrients Watercress Hair Volumizer above, except that this product offers a slightly stronger hold, but not enough to make a noticeable difference. Ounce for ounce, this product is a better value than the Volumizer.

☺ **Botanical Nutrients Thyme & Wheat Protein Intensive Hair Repair, for Damaged or Color-Treated Hair** *($10 for 5 ounces)* isn't intense at all; rather, it is just a thin-textured, basic conditioner for normal to dry hair that is fine or thin. Damaged hair deserves a richer conditioner than this.

BEAUTY WITHOUT CRUELTY (BWC)

Aside from some very good products, the best reason to shop the BWC hair-care line is their passion for completely avoiding ingredients that have been tested on animals. Beauty Without Cruelty is one of the few companies that has a strict, rigorously defined position concerning animal testing. Its products are not tested on animals and none of them contain animal by-products. However, the company's claim that none of the ingredients it uses has been tested on animals since the 1960s is disingenuous. Several of their skin-care products contain ingredients that have been shown to be effective through animal testing done in the 1990s, including sunscreen, vitamin C, and alpha hydroxy acids. For more information about Beauty Without Cruelty, call (800) 227-5120 or visit www.beautywithoutcruelty.com.

What's Good About This Line: Generous-sized products at prices that are more than reasonable; styling products with very light, nonintrusive fragrance.

What's Not So Good About It: The essential oils in a few of the products can be a source of scalp irritation and itching.

☺ **Daily Benefits Shampoo, Benefits All Hair Types** *($6.95 for 16 ounces)* is a standard shampoo that contains plant tea, detergent cleansing agent, lather agent, vitamins, water-binding agent, essential oils (fragrance), aloe, and preservatives. This is a good shampoo for all hair types, and it does not cause buildup. The essential oils pose a slight risk of scalp irritation.

☺ **Moisture Plus Shampoo, Benefits Dry/Treated Hair** *($6.95 for 16 ounces)* is aptly named, and works beautifully for dry to very dry hair that is coarse or thick.

☺ **Daily Benefits Conditioner, Benefits All Hair Types** *($6.95 for 16 ounces)* is a very basic conditioner that works well to smooth and detangle normal to slightly dry hair that is normal to fine or thin. The essential oils do pose a slight risk of scalp irritation, so focus application of this conditioner on the hair, not the scalp.

☺ **Moisture Plus Conditioner, Benefits Dry/Treated Hair** *($6.95 for 16 ounces)* is nearly identical to the Daily Benefits Conditioner above, except that this product contains fewer thickeners and different essential oils for fragrance. Otherwise, the same basic comments apply.

☺ **Revitalize Leave-In Conditioner, Benefits Dry/Treated Hair** *($6.95 for 8.5 ounces)* is a great leave-in conditioner for normal to dry hair that is normal to thick. Because this product is meant to be left on the hair, the essential oils pose a greater risk of irritation, so avoid the scalp area as much as possible.

☺ **Natural Hold Hair Spray** (*$6.95 for 8.5 ounces*) is a very good, light-to-medium-hold nonaerosol hairspray. It leaves hair with little to no stiff feel, though some stickiness is apparent. It can be brushed through, but works best to simply hold hair in place and tame flyaways. This also has a barely discernible fragrance—a nice change of pace considering the glut of highly perfumed hairsprays on the market.

☺ **Volume Plus Spray Gel** (*$6.95 for 8.5 ounces*) is an alcohol-free, light-hold spray gel that is great for creating natural hairstyles with flexibility and movement. This has no stiff feel and is minimally sticky, allowing hair to be easily brushed through. Like the Natural Hold Hair Spray above, this has a barely discernible fragrance.

BINGE

This small hair-care line was owned by pH-beauty, and is now owned by Freeman. According to the information on binge's Web site, "Binge's top-notch formulas give you exactly what you crave—salon quality performance and indulgence—at a price you can afford." I agree that these products are affordable, but nothing about binge is all that indulgent or salon-quality, primarily because the whole "salon-quality" term is just a marketing angle to try to convince consumers that these types of products have a distinctive edge. As it turns out, binge offers poorly formulated products in comparison to both salon lines and drugstore lines. Last, although it's alluring to think that "trend-setting hairstylists" created these products, they didn't. They may have had input while testing the various formulations, but it takes a skilled, talented cosmetics chemist to create the state-of-the-art products binge strives for. And I would be leery of hairstylists who approved hairsprays and straightening balms that flake like binge's do. For more information about binge, visit www.bingehair.com.

What's Good About This Line: Conditioners that address the needs of different hair types, and some very good, versatile styling products.

What's Not So Good About It: Shampoo that contains sodium lauryl sulfate; a couple of the styling products flake; use of the preservatives methylchloroisothiazolinone and methylisothiazolinone (Kathon CG) in a leave-on product.

☹ **Wet Your Appetite Nourishing Shampoo** (*$5.99 for 13.5 ounces*) contains sodium lauryl sulfate as one of its main detergent cleansing agents, which means this isn't nourishing in the least and can lead to hair and scalp dryness.

☺ **Comfort Food Nourishing Conditioner** (*$5.99 for 13.5 ounces*) is a standard, relatively lightweight conditioner that can make normal to fine or thin hair softer and more manageable.

☺ **2,500 Calorie Intensive Conditioner** (*$5.99 for 8.5 ounces*) is a standard conditioner that is very good for smoothing dry to very dry hair that is normal to thick or coarse. Binge claims this conditioner is "lavish with rich fats and proteins," but it does not contain protein of any kind, and although it does contain a fatty alcohol (almost all conditioners do), the silicones are the unsung heroes here.

☹ **Finish it off Extreme Hold Hairspray** *($5.99 for 6.8 ounces)* is terribly misnamed and is actually a poor product! This aerosol hairspray provides only a hint of hold, takes longer than usual to dry, and flakes easily. It is not recommended.

☺ **Give It a Swirl Curl Enhancer** *($5.99 for 8.5 ounces)* is a very good conditioning spray gel for normal to very dry hair that is normal to coarse or thick, including curly or wavy hair. It has an impressive blend of silicones and lightweight conditioners and provides a light, non-sticky hold that can be easily brushed through. This enhances curls beautifully and also provides some protection during heat styling.

☹ **Hair Jam Freezing-Hold Gel** *($5.99 for 8.5 ounces)* is a very standard gel that contains the sensitizing preservative Kathon CG. Because it can lead to scalp problems, this preservative system is not recommended for use in leave-on products.

☺ **Hair Pudding Texturizing Cream** *($5.99 for 5.1 ounces)* is a very good, slightly heavy, light-hold styling cream that works well to smooth the hair, tame frizzies, and add shine. Although Vaseline is the second ingredient, this product won't make hair look greasy if it is applied sparingly. It is best for normal to very dry hair that is not fine or thin. This can be a great alternative to a standard Vaseline- and wax-based pomade.

☺ **Ultimate Smoothie Straightening Balm** *($5.99 for 5.1 ounces)* is a fairly standard styling balm that can make hair straight when used with heat and the appropriate brush. It is a smooth, minimally sticky formula, but the film-forming agent has a slight tendency to flake, which makes this less impressive.

☺ **Whipped Cream Root Boost Mousse** *($5.99 for 6.8 ounces)* is a standard, propellant-based styling mousse that has slightly creamy foam and offers a firm, sticky hold that can still be easy to brush through. This works well for styling stubborn hair that is normal to thin or fine.

BioSilk

Not surprisingly, BioSilk is all about the supposedly miraculous properties of silk on hair. Their brochure extols its many benefits, which they say includes the ability to penetrate hair and permanently reconstruct it (not true in the least). In addition, they boast about the special botanicals and vitamins BioSilk has selected and that are also supposed to have the ability to renew hair from the inside out. Their logic hinges on the fact that silk is one of the strongest of natural fibers, and that it surely must convey that same attribute to human hair; so let's go with that and add some statements about silk being around for thousands of years (to establish, however fictional, an historic track record) so consumers will embrace silk as the be-all and end-all solution for their every hair-care woe. What a classic example of how hair-care companies (like many skin-care companies) focus on one ingredient as The Best for whatever the consumer's needs may be! Silk protein, which isn't the same thing as the silk fabric you wear, can be a good conditioning agent, but it is no better than others in this category that range from wheat and soy protein to panthenol. There is no substantiated information anywhere pertaining to the ability of silk (or silk amino acids or protein) to reconstruct hair, and there's nothing about it that can cause a permanent change in the hair shaft. BioSilk offers some wonderful products (along with more than their fair share of poor options), but if you were hoping this line has all the answers for your hair, you are bound to be disappointed. BioSilk is owned by Houston, Texas-based Farouk International. For more information about BioSilk, call (800) 237-9175 or visit www.farouk.com.

What's Good About This Line: Some wonderful silicone-based conditioners and styling products for straightening the hair, and a good selection of color-enhancing conditioners that rivals those of its competitor ARTec.

What's Not So Good About It: Several of the shampoos use drying/harsh detergent cleansing agents; many styling products contain the sensitizing preservatives methylchloroisothiazolinone and methylisothiazolinone (Kathon CG), and/or the drying film-forming agent sodium polystyrene sulfonate.

☹ **Dandruff Control Shampoo** *($10 for 11.6 ounces)* contains 1% zinc pyrithione, an over-the-counter drug that can have a positive effect on dandruff, but this standard shampoo also contains peppermint oil, which can cause further problems for the scalp. Put that together with the price of this product and there is no reason to consider it over the superior options from Head & Shoulders and Neutrogena.

☹ **Equinox Shampoo** *($9 for 11.6 ounces)* contains TEA-lauryl sulfate as its main detergent cleansing agent, and is not recommended for any hair type. This also contains lemon juice, which can be highly irritating to the scalp.

☹ **Hydrating Shampoo** *($10 for 11.6 ounces)* contains TEA-lauryl sulfate as its main detergent cleansing agent, and is not recommended for any hair or scalp type. The balm mint it contains is also a problem.

☹ **Shampoo Out** *($9 for 11.6 ounces)* can be too drying for all hair and scalp types. With sodium C14-16 olefin sulfonate as its sole detergent cleansing agent, this shampoo's mantra could be "shampoo out, dryness in."

☺ **Silk Therapy Shampoo** *($10 for 11.6 ounces)* is an excellent shampoo for normal to dry hair that is normal to slightly thick. It can build up with repeated use.

☺ **Silk Therapy Smoothing Shampoo** *($8.95 for 11.6 ounces)* is nearly identical to the Silk Therapy Shampoo above, except this has a thicker texture and contains some plant extracts that can be problematic for the scalp, although the amounts used are likely too small to cause trouble. Otherwise, the same basic comments apply.

☺ **Silk Therapy Thickening Shampoo** *($8.95 for 11.6 ounces)* is nearly identical to the Silk Therapy Shampoo above, except the increased amount of conditioning agents makes this one preferred for dry to very dry hair. Otherwise, the same basic comments apply.

☺ **Silver Lights Conditioning Shampoo** *($9 for 11.6 ounces)* contains a small amount of violet dye, which can minimally reduce yellow or brassy tones in silver, white, or gray hair. It is otherwise nearly identical to the Silk Therapy Hydrating Shampoo above, and the same comments apply. This is not nearly as conditioning as BioSilk's Silk Therapy Thickening Shampoo.

☹ **Volumizing Shampoo** *($9 for 11.6 ounces)* contains TEA-lauryl sulfate as its main detergent cleansing agent, and is not recommended for any hair or scalp type.

☺ **Conditioner-Moisturizer** *($9 for 11.6 ounces)* is a very standard conditioner that is a good option for normal to slightly dry hair that is normal to fine or thin.

☹ **Dandruff Control Conditioner** *($12 for 11.6 ounces)* contains menthol and peppermint, which can be irritating to the scalp and have no positive effect on controlling dandruff. The small amount of salicylic acid can't exfoliate the scalp or hair shaft because the pH of this shampoo is too high for exfoliation to occur.

☺ **Fruit Cocktail** *($12 for 11.6 ounces)* is an outstanding conditioner for dry to very dry hair that is coarse, textured, or thick. The fruit in this product has no effect on the hair, but at least it's used in amounts too small to irritate the scalp.

☹ **Hydrating Conditioner** *($11 for 11.6 ounces)* is a standard conditioner that is not recommended due to the senseless inclusion of menthol, peppermint, and balm mint. This triple threat of irritants can cause scalp itching and dryness, and they are present in amounts greater than the interesting, beneficial ingredients for hydrating the hair.

☺ **Pre Plus Detangler** *($10 for 11.6 ounces)* can detangle hair and make it easier to comb through, but avoid getting it on the scalp because this it contains several potentially irritating plant extracts, including balm mint and lavender.

☺ **Sealer Plus** *($10 for 11.6 ounces)* is sold as a specialty conditioner to be used after any chemical service, such as perms or coloring. However, there is nothing in this formula that can seal color or curls; it is just a standard, but good, lightweight conditioner. BioSilk's Fruit Cocktail conditioner above is significantly more helpful to use post-perm or color, when hair is often at its driest and could use more substantial ingredients to smooth roughed-up cuticles. Sealer Plus is best as a detangling conditioner for normal to slightly dry hair that is normal to fine or thin.

☺ **Silk Filler** *($12 for 11.6 ounces)* is a good conditioner for fine or thin hair because it detangles and adds softness without weight.

☺ **Silk Therapy Conditioner** *($12 for 11.6 ounces)* is an excellent emollient conditioner for dry to very dry hair that is normal to coarse or thick.

☺ **Silk Therapy Smoothing Conditioner** *($9.95 for 11.6 ounces)* is a good option for normal to dry hair of any thickness.

☺ **Silk Therapy Thickening Conditioner** *($9.95 for 11.6 ounces)* is similar to the Silk Therapy Smoothing Conditioner above, and the same basic comments apply. This product contains more silicone, which makes it preferred for normal to dry hair that is coarse or thick, but it can still work for normal to dry hair of any thickness.

☺ **Tone & Shine, Color Enhancing Conditioner** *($11 for 10 ounces)* is a standard conditioner available in nine colors and one Clear Shine (colorless) formula. All of the conditioners with color (basic dye ingredients) can add a slight hint of color to the hair, or, in the case of Silver Minx, minimize brassy tones. The base formula for each is a great conditioner for normal to dry hair that is normal to thick or coarse.

☺ **Finishing Spray Firm Hold (Aerosol)** *($10.50 for 10 ounces)* is a standard hairspray that does provide a firm hold that remains relatively stiff, though it can be brushed through with some effort. It is best used as a finishing spray on hard-to-hold sections of hair.

☺ **Finishing Spray Natural Hold (Aerosol)** *($10.50 for 10 ounces)* is similar to the Finishing Spray Firm Hold above, but provides a softer, more flexible, less sticky hold that can be easily brushed through. Both of these hairsprays contain a meager amount of silk.

☹ **Glazing Gel** *($9 for 11.6 ounces)* is an alcohol-free styling gel that is below standard because it flakes so easily.

☺ **Molding Silk Designing Paste** *($12.50 for 4 ounces)* is a heavy, thick styling paste that can be difficult to work with because the fibers in the product make it stringy. It can smooth and add textured hold to the hair, and it shampoos out well, but use it sparingly. This product is nearly identical to, but less expensive than, Sebastian's Molding Mud.

☺ **Rock Hard Gelee Hard Hold Gel** *($11 for 6 ounces)* is a standard styling gel whose name is to be taken seriously. This offers a very strong hold with a sticky after-feel, and is best for detailed or slicked-back styles when you want to sport a sleek, wet look.

☺ **Silk Mousse Medium Hold** *($10.50 for 10 ounces)* is a standard, propellant-based mousse that, true to its name, provides medium hold. This can be brushed through and is slightly sticky, but works well as a conditioning mousse for normal to fine-textured hair.

☺ **Silk Pomade Designing Finish** *($11 for 4 ounces)* is a water-soluble, gel-type pomade that can still be heavy, so use it sparingly. This product is best for smoothing the ends of dry hair, taming frizzies, and softly defining curls for those with coarse-textured hair. The holding agent provides style support without being sticky or stiff.

☺ **Silk Polish** *($11 for 4 ounces)* is a traditional Vaseline- and mineral oil-based pomade that can be quite greasy, though it works well to smooth the ends of dry hair or add a polished shine to very dry hair that is coarse or thick. This does not contain holding agents.

☺ **Silk Therapy** *($12 for 2.26 ounces)* is a standard, but very good, silicone serum that, like all silicone serums, can make hair feel incredibly silky and add amazing shine. This should be used sparingly, and is a bit too greasy for those with fine or thin hair.

☺ **Silk Therapy Hairspray** *($10 for 11.6 ounces)* is a standard, nonaerosol hairspray that provides a light hold that can be easily brushed through with only a slight feeling of stiffness and stickiness. The tiny amount of silicone can add a hint of shine.

☺ **Silk Therapy Gel** *($11 for 6 ounces)* is a standard styling gel that offers a medium hold that is slightly sticky but can be brushed through. The conditioning agents can make hair look smoother and feel soft.

☺ **Silk Therapy Smoothing Balm** *($8.95 for 6 ounces)* is a lightweight, soft-hold styling balm that works well to make hair look smooth and sleek.

☹ **Silk Therapy Smoothing Solution** *($14.95 for 8.5 ounces)* contains sodium polystyrene sulfonate, a film-forming agent that can be drying and possibly strip hair color with repeated use. This product is not recommended.

☹ **Silk Therapy Thickening Builder** *($9.95 for 11.6 ounces)* is a standard spray gel that provides a firm hold that remains unpleasantly sticky, and it contains the preservative Kathon CG, which can be highly sensitizing to the scalp. This product is not recommended.

☹ **Silk Therapy Thickening Creme** *($8.95 for 6 ounces)* contains the preservative Kathon CG, and is not recommended.

☹ **Silk Therapy Volumizing Foam** *($9.95 for 8.5 ounces)* contains sodium polystyrene sulfonate as its main film-forming agent, which can cause unnecessary hair and scalp dryness while potentially stripping hair color.

☹ **Spray Gel** *($11 for 11.6 ounces)* contains the preservative Kathon CG, and is not recommended.

☺ **Spray Spritz Firm Hold Styling Spray (Non-Aerosol)** *($10 for 11.6 ounces)* is a very good, light-hold hairspray that can keep hair supported without making it feel stiff or sticky. The small amounts of silicone and conditioning agents allow the hair to be brushed through while adding a touch of shine.

☺ **Fortifying Leave-In Treatment** *($12.95 for 8 ounces)* is a standard, but good, detangling conditioner for normal to slightly dry hair that is normal to fine or thin.

☺ **Recovery Treatment** *($12 for 6 ounces)* is the most basic, downright boring conditioner in the entire BioSilk line. This is sold as "an intense, deep penetrating reconstructor," but it doesn't even contain the silk amino acids that BioSilk maintains are the key hair-reviving ingredient in most of their product lineup. It isn't intense in the least, but it is an OK conditioner for normal to dry hair of any thickness.

☺ **Silk Strate** *($11 for 11.6 ounces)* is a styling balm meant to be used prior to straightening hair with heat. BioSilk recommends combining this with their other products, and if you interpret that to mean a silicone serum, that is a great option. This non-sticky, semi-fluid balm can make hair smoother and stay straight (with heat, of course).

☺ **Silk Therapy Shine On** *($12.50 for 5.3 ounces)* is a silicone spray in aerosol form. As such, it can dispense a very light mist of product, ideal for adding a glossy finish to fine or thin hair. Those with thicker hair can apply it more generously as a finishing touch for extra-shiny tresses.

☺ **Ultra-Hydrating Balm** *($14.95 for 8.5 ounces)* is a good, slightly emollient conditioner for normal to dry hair that is normal to thick. I wouldn't consider this ultra-hydrating, though; for that, BioSilk's Fruit Cocktail or Silk Therapy Conditioner are much better options.

BioSilk Kids BubbleGum Bubbles

☺ **BioSilk Kids BubbleGum Bubbles Fun Body Foam, BubbleBerry Blue** *($9 for 8 ounces)* is a liquid-to-foam shampoo whose packaging and candy-sweet fragrance are meant to appeal to kids. This is an gentle formula overall, but the fragrance is more than a child's skin should attempt to handle. I wouldn't consider this over Johnson & Johnson's Baby Shampoo, but it is an OK option.

☺ **BioSilk Kids BubbleGum Bubbles Fun Body Foam, BubbleGum Pink** *($9 for 8.5 ounces)* is identical to the Kids BubbleGum Bubbles Fun Body Foam, BubbleBerry Blue above, and the same comments apply.

☺ **BioSilk Kids BubbleGum Bubbles No Kink Conditioner** *($9 for 10 ounces)* is a very good conditioner that can easily detangle the hair while adding softness and moisture. It can be a bit heavy for fine hair.

☹ **BioSilk Kids BubbleGum Bubbles No Tangles Tangle Buster** *($9 for 8 ounces)* contains the preservative Kathon CG, which is not recommended for use in leave-on products, and is particularly not recommended for children.

☺ **BioSilk Kids BubbleGum Bubbles No Tears Shampoo** *($7.10 for 10 ounces)*. Despite the name, this shampoo does contain cleansing agents that can sting if they accidentally get into the eye. It's a shampoo that is better for adults, and it won't cause buildup, but you have to be willing to tolerate the bubblegum scent.

THE BODY SHOP

Many of The Body Shop's hair-care products have been around for years, and though they are decent, the formulations are often boring and mundane. As one of the first companies to espouse the wonders of natural ingredients (particularly plants and food), The Body Shop still uses only token amounts of those ingredients in their products. It would be nice if seaweed and peony really could make hair stronger, or if bananas had what it takes to make dry, damaged hair feel like silk, but these ingredients have little if anything to do with how your hair will feel and behave after using the product. For the most part, The Body Shop's natural ingredients are merely window dressing to make standard hair-care products seem more exotic than they are. They're on par with the company's marketing and image, but your hair won't notice the difference, and that's what counts most. For more information about The Body Shop, call (800) BodyShop or visit www.thebodyshop.com.

What's Good About This Line: Standard formulations that perform reliably, including some very good options in every category for dry to very dry hair.

What's Not So Good About It: Though not an expensive hair-care line, many of the formulations are exceptionally basic for the money; the Ice Blue products are problematic for the scalp.

☺ **Banana Nourishing Shampoo, for Normal to Dry Hair** *($8 for 8.4 ounces)* contains a good amount of banana pulp, which can slightly moisturize hair but can also make it feel slightly sticky, especially since it is used with a film-forming agent that can cause buildup with repeated use. This is still a good, gentle shampoo for normal to dry hair that is normal to thick or coarse.

☺ **Brazil Nut Damage Care Shampoo, for Dry, Damaged & Chemically Treated Hair** *($8 for 8.4 ounces)* is a standard conditioning shampoo that can be an option for normal to dry hair that is thick or coarse. But since the silicone and film-forming agents can build up on the hair, this is best alternated with another shampoo that won't cause buildup.

☺ **Chamomile Shampoo, for Dry or Blonde Hair** *($8 for 8.4 ounces)* is a very standard shampoo that is a good option for all hair types, and it poses no risk of buildup. The small amount of yellow coloring agent has no effect on blonde hair, nor is this shampoo preferred for dry hair (the Brazil Nut Damage Care Shampoo above would be much better).

☺ **Ginger Shampoo, Anti-Dandruff** *($8 for 8.4 ounces)* contains the anti-dandruff ingredient piroctone olamine. As this book goes to print, the FDA is still evaluating that ingredient for its effectiveness against dandruff. In other words, piroctone olamine is not part of the FDA's over-the-counter monograph for dandruff products (Source: www.fda.gov). However, there is research showing that piroctone olamine is an effective ingredient in controlling dandruff, though it's no more effective than zinc pyrithione (found in Head & Shoulders) or ketoconazole (found in Nizoral A-D) (Source: *International Journal of Cosmetic Science*, October 2002, page 249).

☺ **Hemp Daily Shampoo, for Normal to Dry Hair** *($12 for 8 ounces)* contains only the tiniest amount of hemp seed oil, so don't count on this to nourish dry hair. It is a very standard shampoo that is a good option for all hair types, and it does not cause buildup.

☺ **Honey Moisturizing Shampoo** *($8.50 for 8 ounces)* is a creamy, conditioning shampoo that contains gentle detergent cleansing agents. It is an excellent choice for those with dry hair that is normal to thick. It does contain an appreciable amount of honey, but other than being a water-binding agent, honey has no special properties that make it a must for dry hair. This can build up with repeated use.

☹ **Ice Blue Shampoo, for Oily Hair** *($8 for 8.4 ounces)* contains menthol and peppermint oil, which can be very irritating and drying to the scalp. Further, these ingredients have no effect on oily hair or scalp, so why bother using them at all?

☺ **Nettle Oil Balance Shampoo** *($8.50 for 8 ounces)* is a very standard, but good, shampoo that is an option for all hair types. It poses minimal risk of buildup, and contains far more fragrance than nettle, which is hardly a loss for your hair. This shampoo cannot balance an oily scalp, but it can nicely remove excess oil from the scalp and hair, same as many other shampoos.

☺ **Olive Glossing Shampoo** *($8.50 for 8 ounces)* is similar to the Nettle Oil Balance Shampoo above, except this adds glycerin and plant oil to the mix, which makes it preferred for slightly dry hair of any thickness. The conditioning agents can build up with repeated use, but it would take quite awhile for this to occur.

☺ **Seaweed & Peony Strengthening Shampoo, for Normal Hair** *($8 for 8.4 ounces)* is an incredibly standard shampoo that has no ability to make hair stronger (a feat attributed to the peony extract, which is used in the smallest amount imaginable in this shampoo). It is one more gentle but effective option for all hair types, and poses no risk of buildup.

☺ **Tea Tree Oil Shampoo Treatment** *($8 for 8.4 ounces)*. In one study, a 5% concentration of tea tree oil was shown to be effective in the treatment of dandruff (Source: *Journal of the American Academy of Dermatology,* December 2002, pages 852–855). However, this shampoo contains nowhere near that amount, which makes it more window dressing than a treatment for the scalp or hair.

☺ **Amlika Leave-In Conditioner, for All Hair Types** *($6 for 3.4 ounces)* works well as a lightweight, leave-in conditioner for all hair types, particularly normal to fine or thin hair.

☺ **Banana Nourishing Conditioner, for Normal to Dry Hair** *($8 for 8.4 ounces)* doesn't contain much in the way of conditioning agents, and isn't the best choice for treating dry hair. This is a good detangling conditioner for normal to slightly dry hair that is normal to fine or thin.

☺ **Brazil Nut Damage Care Conditioner, for Dry, Damaged & Chemically Treated Hair** *($8 for 8.4 ounces)* is a good, though basic, conditioner for normal to dry hair of any thickness.

☺ **Brazil Nut Deep Conditioning Hair Treatment for, Dry, Damaged & Chemically Treated Hair** *($8 for 8.4 ounces)* is a very good conditioner for normal to very dry hair that is normal to thick or coarse, and is indeed a good choice for chemically treated hair.

☺ **Chamomile Conditioner, for Dry or Blonde Hair** *($8 for 8.4 ounces)* is a good conditioner for normal to slightly dry hair of any thickness. There is nothing in this product that makes it preferred for blonde hair or very dry hair.

☺ **Hemp Daily Conditioner, for Normal to Dry Hair** *($12 for 8 ounces)* is a lightweight conditioner that works well for normal to slightly dry hair that is normal to fine or thin.

☺ **Honey Moisturizing Conditioner** ($8.50 for 8 ounces) combines the best qualities of the Banana Nourishing Conditioner and Brazil Nut Damage Care Conditioner above into one conditioner. As such, it is the preferred option if you have dry hair that is normal to thick or coarse and are considering purchasing a conditioner from The Body Shop. This does contain a fair amount of honey, but all it does is serve as water-binding agent and add a slightly sweet fragrance.

☹ **Ice Blue Revitalizing Conditioner, for Oily Hair** *($8 for 8.4 ounces)* is an exceedingly standard conditioner that is not recommended because it contains peppermint oil and menthol, which can cause serious scalp irritation.

☺ **Nettle Oil Balance Conditioner** *($8.50 for 8 ounces)* is a standard, lightweight conditioner suitable for someone with normal to slightly dry hair that is normal to fine or thin. It absolutely cannot balance an oily scalp, nor are the conditioning ingredients in here appropriate for use on oily hair.

☺ **Olive Glossing Conditioner** ($8.50 for 8 ounces) is similar to, but slightly heavier (more emollient) than the Honey Moisturizing Conditioner above, and the same review applies.

☺ **Seaweed & Peony Strengthening Conditioner, for Normal Hair** *($8 for 8.4 ounces)* is as basic as a conditioner gets, and contains mostly water, thickener, detangling agent, preservative, silicone, fragrance, panthenol, and plant extracts. This conditioner is incapable of making hair stronger, but it can make normal to fine or thin hair easier to comb through.

☺ **Beeswax Texturizing Wax** *($8 for 1.7 ounces)* is a thick pomade that contains enough plant oil to be considerably more greasy than waxy. It isn't a great option for adding texture and definition to hair, but it works beautifully to smooth dry ends and frizzies while imparting glossy shine. It is recommended for those with thick, coarse hair that is dry to very dry.

☺ **Define & No Frizz Styling Cream** *($10 for 3.4 ounces)* is a thin-textured, silky styling cream whose silicone and glycerin base can make hair look shiny and feel smooth. This works well for all hair types to smooth frizzies and flyaway hair, while adding soft, natural control. Those with fine or thin hair should use this sparingly, while someone with thick or coarse hair can be more liberal in their application.

☺ **for Men, Hair Slick** *($8 for 3.38 ounces)* contains mostly water, plant oils, film-forming/holding agent, preservative, fragrance, more film-forming agent, and vitamin A. It works well as a slightly greasy styling cream for styles that need conditioning with a flexible hold. The fragrance is potent.

☺ **Gloss Over Glossing Wax** *($8 for 1.7 ounces)* is a water-soluble pomade that maintains a thick, greasy feel that means this will work best for normal to very dry hair that is thick, curly, or coarse. It does not contain holding agents. This is best for smoothing the ends of hair or defining curls, but should be used sparingly.

☺ **Green Tea Fixing Gel** *($8 for 3.38 ounces)* is an exceptionally standard styling gel that provides medium to firm hold and a stiff, slightly sticky finish. It can still be brushed through, but is best for slicked back wet looks. The amount of green tea is too small to even mention, and of no benefit for hair or scalp.

☺ **Hold Still Styling Gel** *($8 for 3.4 ounces)* is an excellent light-hold styling gel that contains some conditioning agents for softness and is a cinch to brush through. This non-flaking, alcohol-free formula is a great option for all hair types, and is just barely sticky.

☺ **Wheat Protein Volumizing Mousse** *($10 for 6.75 ounces)* is a standard, liquid-to-foam mousse that offers medium hold and a flexible, yet sticky, finish that can still be brushed through. It does contain enough conditioning agents to help smooth and lightly moisturize hair.

BRECK

Breck is back. Why it came back is a mystery, though, because there are plenty of shampoos that could (and did) take its place. Yet for those old enough to revisit this line with a strong sense of nostalgia, these basic shampoos do work well to cleanse the hair without drying it. For more information about Dial-owned Breck, call (866) BreckShampoo.

What's Good About This Line: Simply formulated shampoos that do their job well.

What's Not So Good About It: Nothing, unless you were hoping for unique shampoos.

☺ **Beautiful Hair BRECK Shampoo for Normal Hair** *($3.39 for 12 ounces)* is a very standard shampoo that contains mostly water, detergent cleansing agents, lather agents, preservatives, fragrance, thickener, and coloring agents. This works well for all hair types and will not cause buildup.

☺ **Beautiful Hair BRECK Shampoo for Dry Hair** *($3.39 for 12 ounces)* is identical to the shampoo above, and does not distinguish itself, as its name implies, for dry hair. It certainly won't moisturize hair, but it cleanses gently and won't make hair drier, which makes this worth considering. Former Breck girls Kim Basinger, Brooke Shields, and 1980s supermodel Christie Brinkley would be proud.

BUMBLE AND BUMBLE

Estee Lauder–owned Bumble and bumble has grown quite a bit since the last edition of this book, which isn't too surprising given the infusion of capital that comes from being owned by one of the largest cosmetics conglomerates in the world. Bumble and bumble was founded in 1979 by hair designer Michael Gordon, and his New York City salon still stands today as a mecca for the urban fashion and social elite. The ever-expanding B&b product line is said to be the brainchild of brilliant hairdressers and session stylists, many of whom have worked on photo shoots for high-profile magazines such as *Vogue*. This line's pedigree is impressive, but do keep in mind that hairstylists, even brilliant ones, are not skilled in the art of hair-care formulations. It takes much more than good products to create the often fantasy-driven images you see in these magazines, and when the cameras are clicking you can be sure there is always a team of talented people on hand to make sure every last well-lit hair on the model's perfectly tilted head is as perfect as can be. A truly talented hairstylist can create awe-inspiring hairstyles using almost any products coupled with the right heat-styling implements and brushes. And Bumble and bumble is not the only hair-care line to show up at fashion shoots.

None of this is meant to imply that Bumble and bumble products aren't up to the task of helping you take better care of and easily style your hair. Quite the contrary: Almost all of the products reviewed below can do just that, though the prices are often out of line for what you get.

Looking through Bumble and bumble's marketing materials, it's clear that they are holding fast to the fact that celebrities and models use their products. Product descriptions mention which shampoo Natalie Portman is fond of, which products clutter the bathrooms of the actresses on *Sex & the City*, which conditioner Donatella Versace buys in bulk, and which product all of the latest supermodels have been converted to thanks to one of B&b's stylists. This information doesn't tell you anything about whether or not a particular Bumble and bumble product is right for you, but it does attract attention. Consumers are almost always interested in what their favorite celebrity is using, ostensibly because they are in a position to demand (and would deign to use) only the best. It's not true. Celebrities and supermodels can be just as fickle as the rest of us, often professing to love a new product whenever they're profiled in a fashion magazine, or just happen to be working with a new stylist or makeup artist. These tidbits of information are fun to read, but they shouldn't help you decide which products are best for your needs. Once you read my reviews below, you will have a much better understanding of what the Bumble and bumble products can and cannot do, and that's knowledge you can bank on! For more information about Bumble and bumble, call (800) 7-BUMBLE or visit www.Bumbleandbumble.com.

What's Good About This Line: A great selection of styling products, including several pomades and some hairsprays with unique qualities. Almost all of the shampoos and conditioners offer gentle, effective formulations, a few with enough bells and whistles to help justify the higher price points.

What's Not So Good About It: Some of the items have senseless price tags given their basic formulations; the Tonic products are a misstep that should be ignored; their Gentle Shampoo is anything but.

☺ $$$ **Alojoba Shampoo** *($17 for 8 ounces)* is a standard shampoo that is a great option for normal to very dry hair of any thickness. The conditioning agents pose minimal risk of buildup.

☹ **Gentle Shampoo** *($16 for 8 ounces)* contains sodium C14-16 olefin sulfonate as one of its main detergent cleansing agents, which makes it quite drying for all hair and scalp types. The addition of plant oil helps offset the drying effect to some extent, but why bother to use such a drying ingredient at all? This also contains film-forming agents that will build up with repeated use, and one of them (styrene/PVP copolymer) can make hair feel stiff.

☺ $$$ **Seaweed Shampoo** *($12 for 8 ounces)* is a standard shampoo that does not contain ingredients that cause buildup, so it is a good option for all hair types. Contrary to Bumble and bumble's claims, the algae, spirulina, and kelp in this product do not add elasticity, luster, or strength to the hair. They are good water-binding agents, but because they do not cling well to the hair they have little effect.

☺ $$$ **Sunday Shampoo** *($13 for 8 ounces)* is a great shampoo for all hair types, and it does not cause buildup. The name comes from the idea that at least one day per week you should use a shampoo that does not contain conditioning agents in an effort to help remove the buildup from hair-care products, a point with which I concur. This shampoo also contains a chelating agent, so it also removes minerals and chlorine from the hair.

☺ $$$ **Thickening Shampoo** *($16 for 8 ounces)* is a standard shampoo that contains gentle detergent cleansing agents and several film-forming/conditioning agents that can attach to the hair shaft and make hair feel slightly thicker. With repeated use, these helpful ingredients can build up on the hair, which means those with fine or thin hair will find their hair feeling heavy and looking limp. This effect can be mitigated by alternating this shampoo with a shampoo that does not contain conditioning agents.

☹ **Tonic Shampoo** *($16 for 8 ounces)* is positioned as a "love it or hate it" product, and although I don't hate it, I certainly don't recommend it. This shampoo contains menthol, peppermint oil, and peppermint extract, which can cause hair dryness and scalp irritation.

☺ **$$$ Alojoba Conditioner** *($18 for 8 ounces)* is a standard, but very good (and very overpriced), conditioner for normal to dry hair of any thickness.

☺ **$$$ Leave In (Rinse Out) Conditioner** *($16 for 8 ounces)* isn't a very exciting formula, but it serves its purpose as a leave-in conditioner by making hair softer, easier to detangle, and smooth without feeling heavy. This is a good option for all hair types, and can be mixed with styling products to give them a softer hold.

☺ **$$$ Seaweed Conditioner** *($12 for 8 ounces)* is a very standard conditioner that works well for normal to slightly dry hair that is normal to fine or thin, but its a basic formula that doesn't justify the price.

☺ **$$$ Super Rich Conditioner** *($17 for 8 ounces)* isn't that rich, though it is thicker than the Bumble and bumble conditioners above. It is a good option for normal to dry hair of any thickness.

☺ **$$$ Thickening Conditioner** *($17 for 8 ounces)* supposedly makes hair thicker because it contains silk powder. Although it's nice to think silk is capable of this, silk as a cosmetic ingredient simply does not cling well to the hair, at least not like the less enticing (from a marketing standpoint) ingredient polyquaternium-11 does. And that's what makes the hair feel thicker, though it can also build up with repeated use. This is a good conditioner for normal to dry hair that is normal to thick or coarse. The sunscreen ingredients in this product cannot protect hair from UV damage.

☺ **$$$ Brilliantine** *($15 for 2 ounces)* is a lightweight, slick styling cream that beautifully smoothes the hair and adds shine without looking greasy. It should be used sparingly, but it can be used by all hair types and is much lighter (and more water-soluble) than traditional pomades. Brilliantine does not contain holding or film-forming agents.

☺ **$$$ Classic Hairspray** *($15 for 10 ounces)* is a firm-hold aerosol hairspray that is slightly sticky, but the conditioning agents and silicone allow hair to be easily brushed through.

☺ **$$$ Does It All Styling Spray** *($19 for 10 ounces)* is a uniquely versatile aerosol hairspray that offers a light, flexible hold with barely a hint of stickiness or stiffness. Hair can be easily brushed through, re-sprayed, and restyled without feeling clumped or product-laden. This is an ideal product for hairspray-haters because it features most of the good qualities and has none of the bad (unpleasant) side effects of a traditional hairspray. It's nice to know that Nicole Kidman and Julia Roberts use this product to straighten their curly hair, but guess what? Next month, they'll be using (or said to be using) something else.

☺ $$$ **Extra Strength Holding Spray** *($15 for 8 ounces)* is a standard nonaerosol hairspray that provides a medium-to-firm hold with a hint of stickiness. This can be easily brushed through, but works best as a final styling step to help wayward strands stay put.

☺ $$$ **Grooming Creme** *($20 for 5 ounces)* works well to smooth the hair and create a polished finish, but should be used sparingly to avoid a heavy look and feel. This is much easier to shampoo out of the hair than a standard pomade.

☺ **Holding Spray** *($13 for 8 ounces)* is similar to the Does It All Styling Spray above, except this is a nonaerosol product and has a bit of stickiness. Otherwise, the same basic comments apply—this is a great hairspray for those who typically shun such products, but whose hair could use the extra help they provide!

☺ $$$ **Straight** *($20 for 5 ounces)* contains mostly slip agent/solvent, silicone, water, more silicones, wax, film-forming agent, conditioning agent, and preservative. This thick, silky gel works marvelously with heat and the proper styling tools to make hair smooth and straight with lots of shine. It's pricey for the amount of product, but it doesn't disappoint and is fragrance-free! What a find for those with allergies or a sensitive scalp!

☺ $$$ **Styling Creme** *($18 for 5 ounces)* is a styling cream with enough holding/film-forming agents to make hair feel somewhat stiff and sticky. This provides a medium hold that can be brushed through, but is best for use on thick, coarse, or highly textured hair that needs conditioned control without much movement.

☺ $$$ **Styling Lotion** *($18 for 8 ounces)* isn't a lotion, it's a standard water- and alcohol-based liquid styling spray that provides a light, flexible hold with minimal stickiness. The conditioning agents are a dusting at best.

☺ $$$ **Styling Wax** *($15 for 1.5 ounces)* promises "hold, separation, and texture that rinses right out," and, for the most part, this product delivers. This reasonably water-soluble pomade has a thick but easy-to-spread texture that can smooth the hair, add shine, and tame frizzies, but use it sparingly to avoid a greasy appearance. This works well to define short, close-cropped styles or to add definition to thick, curly/wavy hair.

☺ $$$ **Sumotech** *($19 for 1.5 ounces)* is an unbelievably thick paste/pomade hybrid that offers hold and texture with a low-gloss finish. This should be used sparingly and only on the ends of hair because it can easily build up and make hair feel gummy and sticky. It is ideal for someone with thick, coarse hair that has a mind of its own and needs a substantial product to keep it in place.

☺ $$$ **Sumowax** *($19 for 1.5 ounces)* is a fairly standard castor oil- and lanolin-based styling wax that is very good for adding texture without, surprisingly enough, a lot of weight or greasiness. As with all waxes, this should be used sparingly. Sumowax can be difficult to shampoo out, but its combination of plant oils, emollients, and waxes provide all-day smoothing with a natural shine.

☺ $$$ **Surf Spray** *($16 for 4 ounces)* is meant to add the sort of fullness you see in hair after a day of swimming in the ocean and frolicking on the beach. Ocean water is salt water, and salt is included in this product to rough up the cuticle. This can make hair feel and appear fuller, but in the long run continually spraying salt on the hair will cause it to become dried out and brittle. A product like this is an OK option for occasional, but not daily, use.

☺ **$$$ Thickening Spray** *($19 for 8 ounces)* is a standard styling spray that contains film-forming agents that can make hair feel thicker, though they can also build up with repeated use. This product provides a light, slightly sticky hold but doesn't distinguish itself from less expensive, similarly formulated options from the L'Oreal Studio Line.

☺ **$$$ Deeep Treatment** *($20 for 5 ounces)* could have contained several ingredients that would have justified the name, but instead it remains another standard conditioner that is a good option for normal to dry hair of any thickness.

☺ **$$$ Defrizz** *($18 for 4 ounces)* is a standard silicone serum that contains two forms of silicone—and nothing else. It doesn't get more basic than this, but it can work wonders to make hair feel silky and be amazingly shiny.

☺ **Gloss** *($13 for 4 ounces)* is an alcohol-based finishing spray that contains emollients and silicone to add a veil of shine to the hair. This works as well as most silicone sprays, but has the added benefit of conditioning agents beyond silicone, so it is a helpful product for dry to very dry hair of any texture, although someone with fine or thin hair should use as little as possible to avoid a greasy look.

☹ **$$$ Hair Powder** *($27 for 2 ounces)* is nothing more than a blend of cornstarch, clay, tapioca and oat starches, oat flour, silica, fragrance, and pigments. The idea behind this was to offer a way for jet-setting fashionistas to touch up their hair, absorb excess oil, and create full hair styles on the go, but the execution is messy and definitely not conducive to traveling or styling with convenience. The cornstarch base can absorb excess oil from the hair, but the directions say you should apply Bumble and bumble's Sumowax first, so the powder has something to adhere to. Since that only puts more oils on the hair, what you end up with basically turns your pomade into a thick, absorbent, matte-finish paste that can make hair look clumped and unkempt. If you're curious to try this effect at home, you can net the same results (minus the color, which can flake off onto clothing and get on your hands) by applying plain cornstarch mixed with flour to your hair. It costs pennies and will end up looking as bad as if you had overspent on this product.

☺ **Prep** *($13 for 8 ounces)* is a very lightweight, spray-on, leave-on conditioner that contains mostly water, plant extracts (water-binding agents), vitamins, conditioning agents, silicone, detangling agents, slip agent, preservatives, and fragrance. This is a decent detangler, but provides little style help to live up to Bumble and bumble's claim that it provides "the ultimate blow dry." Prep is an option for fine or thin hair.

☹ **Tonic** *($14 for 8 ounces)* should have been named "irritation," because that's what your scalp can expect. The instructions explain that you will "feel a tingle," but that sensation is the skin's response to irritation, and that's not a good thing. What a shame, because the amount of tea tree oil in the product gave it the potential to be effective as an alternative treatment for dandruff.

BUMBLE AND BUMBLE COLOR SUPPORT

☺ $$$ **Color Support Extra Mild Shampoo** *($18 for 8 ounces)* is a standard, color-enhancing shampoo that isn't capable of supporting color (as in preventing color loss or fading) anymore than any other color-enhancing shampoo, and the dye agents do not cling well enough to the hair shaft to have much impact. As a shampoo, each of the five shades is a good option for normal to dry hair, and pose minimal risk of buildup.

☺ $$$ **Color Support Extra Mild Conditioner** *($18 for 8 ounces)* is a stripped-down, basic conditioner whose primary benefit is detangling. It is a great option for normal to fine or thin hair, and the coloring agents impart a hint of color, nothing more. Five shades are available, each with the same base formula containing mostly water, detangling agents, thickener, glycerin, silicone, preservatives, and fragrance.

BUMBLE AND BUMBLE CURL CONSCIOUS

Curl Conscious debuted in late 2003 as Bumble and bumble's first group of products tailored to surprise those with curly hair. Supposedly, these products contain special in-gredients to "loosen and define curls at every step," a strange comment because the looser a curl becomes the less defined it is! Regardless, ingredient lists for the Curl Conscious products are not unique to Bumble and bumble (nor to the needs of curly hair), although each of the products contains the ingredient transglutimase, which the company refers to as""curl-building" and able to form "bonds to create humidity-resistant curls with defini-tion and hold." Transglutimase appears to be a natural component of human and plant tissues, but it has no special affinity for hair, curly or otherwise. As it turns out, Curl Conscious is a versatile line that can be considered by persons with any hair type.

☺ $$$ **Curl Conscious Shampoo, for Fine to Medium Hair** *($18 for 8 ounces)* is a very good shampoo for all hair types. The film-forming agents pose minimal risk of buildup.

☺ $$$ **Curl Conscious Shampoo, for Medium to Thick Hair** *($18 for 8 ounces)* is nearly identical to the Curl Conscious Shampoo above, except this adds squalane, which makes it a more emollient option for normal to very dry hair. Otherwise, the same basic comments apply.

☺ $$$ **Curl Conscious Conditioner, for Fine to Medium Hair** *($20 for 8 ounces)* is a very good conditioner for normal to dry hair of any thickness, and the silicone can make curly hair look smoother (though this ingredient is not unique to these products).

☺ $$$ **Curl Conscious Conditioner, for Medium to Thick Hair** *($20 for 8 ounces)* is nearly identical to the Curl Conscious Conditioner above, except this contains a greater amount of wheat proteins and starch, but these ingredients don't make this conditioner automatically better for medium to thick hair. Otherwise, the same basic comments apply.

☺ $$$ **Curl Conscious Curl Creme, for Fine to Medium Hair** *($25 for 8 ounces)* is a lightweight styling cream that contains some excellent conditioning ingredients, but nothing that justifies its high price. This can make curly hair (or any textured hair) look smooth, feel moist, and become manageable, and it provides a subtle hold that does not make hair feel stiff or sticky. However, its main ingredients are found in dozens of products that cost less. Curl Conscious Curl Creme is too heavy for very fine or thin hair, even if used sparingly.

☺ $$$ **Curl Conscious Curl Creme, for Medium to Thick Hair** *($25 for 8 ounces)* is similar to the Curl Conscious Creme above except that this option is actually better for normal to fine hair because it substitutes a lightweight silicone for the Vaseline and it contains fewer thickeners. This has the same traits and benefits as described above, but can be used (sparingly) by those with fine or thin hair who needs a good leave-in conditioner.

BURT'S BEES

Since Burt's Bees has gained in popularity, Burt's weathered face has taken a back seat to the more traditional and typical faces that grace other cosmetics lines. With all due respect to Burt, that's probably good news if selling hair-care products is the goal; the appearance of Burt's hair is not something most female (or male) consumers would want for their own hair! For more information about Burt's Bees, call (800) 849-7112 or visit www.burtsbees.com.

What's Good About This Line: The conditioner has merit, especially for fans of natural products.

What's Not So Good About It: Everything else!

☹ **Herbal Treatment Shampoo with Cedar Leaf & Juniper Oil** *($10 for 7.5 ounces)* contains several ingredients that can be a problem for the hair and scalp, including lemon water, peppermint leaf, cedar, lemon, rosemary, juniper, and peppermint oils. This is not recommended for any hair or scalp type.

☹ **Rosemary Mint Shampoo Bar with Oat Protein and Pro Vitamin B5** *($6 for 3.5 ounces)* is bar soap positioned as shampoo, and it is more difficult to work with than traditional liquid shampoos. This product contains rosemary and peppermint oils, which only make a poor product worse.

☺ **Avocado Butter Hair Treatment with Nettles and Rosemary** *($9 for 4 ounces)* is a rich conditioner that is a very good option for dry to very dry hair that is coarse, thick, or damaged. The orange oil can be a problem for scalp irritation (don't use this immediately after coloring or perming your hair), but if you focus it on the hair rather than the scalp, you can avoid problems.

CHARLES WORTHINGTON

Charles Worthington's first hair-care line, called Results, was originally sold at Bloomingdale's but was pulled and replaced with his upscale Dream Hair line (Source: *The Rose Sheet*, May 21, 2001). Results is now found at Target and Walgreens stores, where it was joined several months later by Worthington's Big Hair collection. Most consumers won't notice the change because die-hard Bloomies customers aren't about to shop for their hair-care or skin-care needs at a drugstore. They will most likely continue to assume that any product sold at an upscale store is better than one sold at a drugstore, even if that product is now selling at a drugstore! Other than the shopping experience and location, there is nothing about the Dream Hair line that is superior to the Results or Big Hair lines. Variations between them involve nuances amounting to less than 1% of most of these products' ingredients. The differences might make for good advertising copy that contrasts amino acids with keratin, but your hair won't notice or feel the difference.

This marketing accomplishment has been spun by United Kingdom-based hairstylist Charles Worthington. Worthington has an impressive celebrity clientele and owns five salons in London. His recognition as a hairdresser is well deserved, but whether or not hair-cutting and hairstyling skills equal hair-care formulation expertise is another kettle of fish altogether. For more information on Dream Hair and Results, call (800) 519-8121 or visit www.cwlondon.com.

What's Good About This Line: Excellent styling products, including two silicone serums whose prices are amazing; the Results and Big Hair lines are actually better than the more expensive Dream Hair, which contains so much fragrance it's akin to dousing hair with perfume, though Dream Hair's packaging is decidedly upscale.

What's Not So Good About It: The buzz-worthy ingredients in almost every product reviewed below show up on the ingredient list after the fragrance (which is quite potent, especially in the Dream Hair line) and/or preservatives; the claims for most of the products don't match what the actual formula is capable of doing.

CHARLES WORTHINGTON DREAM HAIR

☺ $$$ **Bright Future Shampoo, for Color-Treated and Dehydrated Hair** *($14 for 8.75 ounces)* is a standard, gentle conditioning shampoo that contains mostly water, detergent cleansing agents, lather agents, thickeners, film-forming agent, conditioning agents, fragrance, silicone, water-binding agents, and preservatives. This works well for color-treated hair of any thickness, although the film-forming agents can cause buildup.

☺ $$$ **Sensational Shampoo Oily/Combination Hair** *($14 for 8.75 ounces)* is as standard a detergent-based shampoo as it gets. It contains minimal conditioning agents so it won't cause buildup, and that's great for all hair types. The claims that it fortifies hair and reduces oxidation harm by 24% are completely without validity, as there are not enough antioxidants in this product to do that and even if there were, they would just be washed down the drain when you rinsed your hair. The teeny amount of amino acid in this product is not enough to have any real benefit for hair.

☺ $$$ **Heavenly Hair Wash Normal to Dry Hair** *($14 for 8.75 ounces)* is almost identical to the Sensational Shampoo Oily/Combination above, and the same comments apply.

☺ $$$ **Unbelievably Clean All Hair Types** *($14 for 8.75 ounces)* is almost identical to the Sensational Shampoo Oily/Combination above, and the same comments apply.

☺ $$$ **Seeing is Believing Outrageously Rich Conditioner** *($14 for 8.75 ounces)* is an extremely standard conditioner that works well for normal to dry hair of any thickness except fine or thin. This is also supposed to reduce oxidation harm by 21%. However, the ingredients have minimal antioxidant properties, they couldn't hold up after the conditioner is rinsed, and any traces that did remain couldn't hold up to styling. The claim sounds good but it won't hold up (literally) under water.

☺ $$$ **Out of This World Conditioner Oil-Free Conditioner, Oily/Combination Hair** *($14 for 8.75 ounces)* is similar to the Seeing is Believing conditioner above, only without the silicone, which makes it a good option for someone with normal to dry hair that is fine or thin.

☺ $$$ **Definite Difference Instant Repair Treatment All Hair Types** *($30 for 6.12 ounces)* is almost identical to the Seeing is Believing conditioner above, and the same basic comments apply. The silicone in it makes it appropriate for all hair types except fine or thin, though these hair types can use conditioners with silicone occasionally.

☺ $$$ **Stay True Moisture Surge Conditioner, for Color-Treated and Dehydrated Hair** *($14 for 8.7 ounces)* is very similar to the Dream Hair conditioners above, only this contains more silicone and has a thicker, slicker texture. It works best for normal to dry hair that is normal to coarse or thick.

☺ $$$ **Scalp Energizer All Hair Types** *($7 for 1.05 ounces)* is very similar to all of the Dream Hair conditioners above, and is not energizing for the scalp at all, so the tiny quantity you get for this price is bizarre, especially when compared to the products above. This does contain piroctone olamine, which is used in some hair-care products as an antimicrobial to combat dandruff. As this book goes to print, the FDA is still evaluating that ingredient's efficacy for dealing with dandruff. In other words, piroctone olamine is not part of the FDA's over-the-counter monograph for dandruff products (Source: www.fda.gov). However, there is research showing that piroctone olamine is an effective ingredient in controlling dandruff, though it's no more effective than zinc pyrithione (found in Head & Shoulders) or ketoconazole (found in Nizoral) (Source: *International Journal of Cosmetic Science*, October 2002, page 249), and those products cost far less than this one.

☺ **Feels Fabulous Supercontrol Mousse, Firm Hold for All Hair Types** *($10 for 5.25 ounces)* doesn't feel any more fabulous than most styling mousses, but it works well as a medium-hold mousse that is barely sticky and allows hair to be easily brushed through. This is a great option for all hair types.

☺ **Feels Fabulous Supercontrol Mousse, Light for All Hair Types** *($10 for 5.25 ounces)* has a formula similar to the Feels Fabulous mousse above, except it contains less film-forming/holding agent, so you get less hold and less stickiness. This works great for normal to fine or thin hair that needs little help with manageability but could use extra body.

☺ $$$ **Looks Amazing Invisible Control Blow-Dry Spray, Medium Hold for All Hair Types** *($15 for 5.1 ounces)* is an alcohol-based styling spray that does provide a medium hold. It can feel slightly thick and sticky in the hair, so use sparingly if your hair is fine or thin.

☺ **Perfect Reflection Wax, for Dark Hair Shades** and **Perfect Reflection Wax, for Blonde Hair Shades** *(both $12 for 1.7 ounces)* are standard, water-soluble pomades whose only difference is in the amount of mineral pigments used to impart shimmer and subtle color to hair. These have a thick, gooey texture that can feel greasy, so use them sparingly. They both work well to smooth and add shine (including shimmer) to the hair, and because the shimmer particles are in a moist base (that stays moist) they do tend to stay put.

☺ **$$$ Shining Star Spectacular Glossing Spray, for All Hair Types** *($15 for 1.75 ounces)* is a standard, alcohol-based silicone spray. It definitely adds shine to hair and works as well as any at the drugstore that cost far less.

CHARLES WORTHINGTON RESULTS

☺ **Moisture Seal Glossing Shampoo** *($5.99 for 10.9 ounces)* is a standard, detergent-based shampoo with conditioning and detangling agents, so it can cause buildup. It works well for someone with normal to dry hair of any thickness. To prevent buildup, it's best to alternate this shampoo with one that doesn't contain conditioning or detangling agents.

☺ **Everyday Shine Shampoo, for Dull Lifeless Hair** *($5.99 for 10.9 ounces)* is almost identical to the Moisture Seal Glossing Shampoo above, except this contains far less film-forming agent, which reduces the chance of buildup. Otherwise, the same comments apply.

☺ **Balancing Act Oil-Regulating Shampoo** *($5.99 for 10.9 ounces)* is almost identical to the Moisture Seal Glossing Shampoo above, except this contains less film-forming agent, which reduces the chance of buildup. Otherwise, the same comments apply.

☹ **No Flake Shampoo** *($5.99 for 10.9 ounces)* is a standard, detergent-based shampoo that contains the antimicrobial ingredient piroctone olamine. As this book goes to print, the FDA is still evaluating that ingredient's effectiveness against dandruff. In other words, piroctone olamine is not part of the FDA's over-the-counter monograph for dandruff products (Source: www.fda.gov). However, there is research showing that piroctone olamine is an effective ingredient in controlling dandruff, though it's no more effective than zinc pyrithione (found in Head & Shoulders) or ketoconazole (found in Nizoral) (Source: *International Journal of Cosmetic Science*, October 2002, page 249). This also contains tea tree oil, which can have some positive benefit for those with dandruff, but the amount present in this product is too small to have any effect on that scalp condition.

☺ **Gentle All in One Cleanse and Nourish, for All Hair Types** *($5.99 for 10.9 ounces)* is a standard shampoo that poses minimal risk of buildup and is appropriate for all hair types.

☺ **Superconditioner** *($5.99 for 10.9 ounces)* is a very standard, rather lightweight conditioner that is best for someone with normal to slightly dry hair that is fine or thin.

☺ **Daily Treat Conditioner, Normal Hair** *($5.99 for 10.9 ounces)* is similar to the Superconditioner above, only this one contains plant oil, which actually makes it slightly better for somewhat dry, not normal, hair.

☺ **Nourish as Needed Rebalancing Conditioner, Combination Hair with Oily Roots, Dry Ends** *($5.99 for 10.9 ounces)* is almost identical to the Daily Treat Conditioner above, except there is more fragrance than plant oil. Otherwise, the same comments apply.

☺ **Everyday Shine Conditioner for Dull, Lifeless Hair** *($5.99 for 10.9 ounces)* is nearly identical to the Nourish as Needed Rebalancing Conditioner above, and the same comments apply. Why this is marketed as "everyday" and the other "as needed" has everything to do with marketing and nothing to do with the formulation.

☺ **Hair Healer Intensive Leave-In Conditioner, for All Hair Types** *($1.99 for 1.7 ounces)*. Nothing in this product can "heal" hair. This is a very boring, leave-in conditioner that offers minimal moisture, although it can make almost-manageable hair easier to comb through. It does contain sunscreen, but because hair-care products are not allowed (by the FDA) to have an SPF rating, there is no way to know how much protection you are getting, or whether or not those ingredients are still present after you've finished styling your hair.

☺ **Extra Texture Hold and Shape Gel, Medium Hold All Hair Types** *($5.99 for 9.3 ounces)* is a standard gel with a medium hold that has a slight sticky feel, but it lets you easily brush through hair.

☺ **Body-Booster Silkening Mousse, Firm Hold All Hair Types** *($5.99 for 8.5 ounces)* is a standard mousse with a light-to-medium hold that has a minimal stiff or sticky feel, and it can easily be brushed through.

☺ **Invisible Hold Thickening Hairspray, Extra Hold, for All Hair Types** *($5.99 for 9 ounces)* is a standard hairspray that goes on a bit wetter than most, but offers a strong hold once it dries. Hair can be brushed through, but this works best as a finishing-touch setting spray.

☺ **Relax and Unwind Blow-Dry Straightening Balm for Curly, Frizzy, and Unruly Hair** *($5.99 for 9 ounces)* is a silicone-based balm that has a slight Vaseline-like feel but smoothes to a sheen over the hair and provides a light hold with minimal to no stiff or sticky feel. This provides some heat protection when straightening the hair.

☺ **Hair Makeover Blow-Drying Spray, Medium Hold for All Hair Types** *($5.99 for 9 ounces)* is a very light-hold styling spray (not medium in the least) that has minimal to no stiff or sticky feel. The silicone makes it better for someone with hair that's normal to dry but not fine or thin.

☺ **Lasting Impression Defining Wax** *($5.99 for 1.7 ounces)* is a traditional Vaseline- and mineral oil-based pomade that works great to smooth frizzies and adds shine to thick, coarse, or highly textured hair. Don't let the lighter texture of this fool you—it can still be greasy, so use sparingly.

The Reviews C

☺ **Stay in Shape Hair Superspray, Firm Hold All Hair Types** *($5.99 for 8.5 ounces)* is a standard aerosol hairspray that provides a light (not firm) hold with minimal to no stiff or sticky feel.

☺ **Shine, Shine, Shine Gloss and Refresh Spray, All Hair Types** *($5.99 for 5.9 ounces)* is a basic silicone spray that makes hair feel silky soft and adds shine. A silicone spray works best for normal to slightly dry hair that is normal to fine or thin.

☺ **Shine Silkening Serum** *($5.99 for 1.7 ounces)* is a very good silicone serum that can leave hair feeling silky soft and shiny. This contains a blend of silicones, which makes it a bit more versatile than most other silicone serums that use just one or two silicone ingredients.

☺ **Frizz Taming Serum** *($5.99 for 1.7 ounces)* is nearly identical to the Shine Silkening Serum above, and the same comments apply.

CHARLES WORTHINGTON BIG HAIR

☺ **Body Beautiful Shampoo for Fine, Limp, and Flyaway Hair** *($5.99 for 8.5 ounces)* contains no volumizing agents of any kind, so there is nothing about this formula that makes it better for creating big hair. This is merely a standard shampoo that won't build up on hair. The entire premise of Worthington's Big Hair line appears to be marketing more than anything else.

☺ **Full Volume Conditioner** *($5.99 for 8.5 ounces)* is a lightweight conditioner with some film-forming agents that can lend added volume to fine or thin hair, but can also build up with repeated use.

☺ **Great Body! Styling Spray** *($5.99 for 6.7 ounces)* is a standard styling spray that stays wet longer than most traditional hairsprays, which can negatively affect hair that is vulnerable to even the slightest presence of moisture. This provides light to medium flexible hold and is minimally sticky.

☺ **Lift-Off Ultra Fine Hair Spray** *($5.99 for 6.75 ounces)* is a standard aerosol hairspray that, despite the name, does not have an ultra-fine application. This applies rather heavily and creates a firm, fast-drying hold. It is an OK option for use as a finishing spray on dry hair.

☹ **Putty in Your Hands Push Into Shape Texturizer** *($5.99 for 2.5 ounces)* is a thick, Vaseline-based pomade that also contains clay to enhance hair texture and leaves a natural matte rather than a greasy-looking finish. This is heavy-duty stuff, and does not shampoo out easily. It works best to exaggerate short or spiked hairstyles. Those with longer hair should use it sparingly, if at all, as it is difficult to work through the hair evenly.

☹ **So Uplifting! Volumizing Mousse** *($5.99 for 6.75 ounces)* is an exceptionally standard, alcohol-based styling mousse. It's an OK option for medium hold, but its lack of conditioning agents leaves hair stiff and somewhat sticky. The price is attractive, but Pantene, TRESemme, and Vidal Sassoon offer better options for styling mousse.

CITRÉ SHINE

The tagline for Citré Shine is "nature's prescription for shine." Although their products all contain a medley of citrus extracts, these are not the ingredients responsible for giving your hair a brilliant shine. Rather, it is the assuredly *un*natural silicones found in most of these products that produce such favorable results. Actually, the citrus extracts are the only major drawback of this otherwise stellar hair-care line. Thankfully, they are present in such small amounts that they pose little problem for the scalp.

Since the last edition of this book, almost all of Citré Shine's poorly formulated shampoos and conditioners have been discontinued, and it is apparent Citré Shine's owner, Advanced Research Laboratories, decided to focus on creating styling products, which are (and always have been) the highlight of this hair-care collection. For more information about Citré Shine, call (800) 966-6960 or visit www.citreshine.com.

What's Good About This Line: A well-rounded selection of styling products, most of which offer exemplary performance at attractive prices; the Smooth Out Shampoos and Conditioners work well for textured hair.

What's Not So Good About It: One of the hairsprays contains acetone; the citrus extracts used throughout the line may cause scalp irritation.

☺ **Color Brilliance Shampoo** *($3.99 for 16 ounces)* is a standard shampoo that is an option for all hair types and poses minimal risk of buildup. Other than by having a gentle formula, this cannot preserve hair color better than similar shampoos, primarily because no shampoo can preserve hair color.

☹ **Daily Revitalizing Shampoo** *($3.99 for 16 ounces)* contains sodium C12-15 alkyl sulfate as its main detergent cleansing agent. Owing to this ingredient's similarity to sodium lauryl sulfate, it can have the same drying effect on the hair and scalp, and this product is not recommended.

☺ **Moisture Burst Shampoo** *($3.99 for 16 ounces)* is nearly identical to the Color Brilliance Shampoo above, and the same comments apply. This shampoo cannot moisturize the hair, but it won't cause dryness either, which is great.

☺ **Smooth Out Shampoo** *($3.99 for 16 ounces)* is a very good shampoo for normal to dry hair that is normal to coarse or thick. The silicone and film-forming agent can build up with repeated use.

☺ **Color Brilliance Conditioner** *($3.99 for 16 ounces)* claims to prolong the vibrancy of color-treated hair, but any good conditioner (which this is) can do that, provided you keep your hair away from water and sunlight, which isn't too likely! It works well for normal to dry hair of any thickness.

☺ **Daily Revitalizing Conditioner** *($3.99 for 16 ounces)* is a very good, though standard, conditioner that works well for normal to fine or thin hair if your scalp can take the fragrant citrus extracts.

☺ **Moisture Burst Conditioner** *($3.99 for 16 ounces)* is similar to the Color Brilliance Conditioner above, except this replaces the silicone with a detangling agent, and that makes it a slightly better option for normal to slightly dry hair that is fine or thin.

☺ **Smooth Out Conditioner** *($3.99 for 16 ounces)* is similar to the Daily Revitalizing Conditioner above, and the same comments apply.

☺ **Big Volume Styling Foam** *($4.99 for 8.5 ounces)* is a standard, propellant-based styling mousse that has a creamy texture and offers medium hold that is slightly sticky.

☺ **Clear Shine Style & Shine Gel** *($2.49 for 16 ounces)* is a very standard alcohol-free styling gel that offers a light hold that is slightly sticky but can be easily brushed through.

☺ **Curl Crunch Curling Creme** *($3.49 for 6 ounces)* is a creamy styling gel that contains enough silicone to help smooth hair, add shine, and provide some protection from heat-styling tools. This provides a medium hold that can be sticky, but it's easily brushed through. And it can indeed make it easier to define curls when hair is wet or dry.

☺ **Curl Define Style & Shape Gel** *($3.89 for 16 ounces)* is almost identical to the Clear Shine Style & Shine Gel above, and the same comments apply. Both of these gels can help define curls when used with a diffuser dryer set on low to medium heat.

☺ **Get Smooth Straightening Balm** *($4.99 for 3.3 ounces)* works beautifully to help straighten and smooth the hair with heat and the appropriate styling tools, and the price makes this almost a steal! This product is comparable to Bumble and bumble's Straight ($20 for 5 ounces) with the price being the only real difference.

☺ **Highly Polished Glossing Pomade** *($4.99 for 2 ounces)* is a water-soluble pomade that has a soft texture, though it can be quite greasy. It works well to smooth thick, coarse, or highly textured hair, and certainly adds a glossy shine, but use it sparingly for best results.

☺ **Making Waves Curl Booster** *($4.99 for 12 ounces)* is a standard styling gel that provides a light hold that is minimally sticky, so hair can easily be brushed through. Nothing about this product makes it preferred for those with curly hair—it works well for all hair types.

☺ **Mega Hold Style & Control Gel** *($2.49 for 16 ounces)* is a standard styling gel, similar to Citré Shine's Clear Shine Style & Shine Gel and Curl Define Style & Shape Gel above, but provides slightly more hold. The product advertises ultimate control and ultra-hard hold, but doesn't even come close to achieving that. Instead, this is a good light-hold gel for all hair types.

☺ **Taking Hold Styling Glue** *($4.99 for 6 ounces)* is packaged like Elmer's Glue, and provides a very strong hold that leaves hair feeling sticky and slightly moist. Several film-forming/holding agents are joined by Vaseline and standard thickeners to create a styling product that is best for thick or coarse hair that needs a high degree of control. This also works well for adding exaggerated texture and definition to short, spiky hairstyles.

☺ **Texture Play Chunking Creme** *($4.99 for 2 ounces)* is a surprisingly lightweight pomade that has a whipped texture and creamy application. This provides minimal hold but works well to create a smooth appearance on unruly ends with a natural, non-greasy shine. It does not work well to create a chunky, textured look. For that, turn to the Take Hold Styling Glue above. This product can be used sparingly on fine or thin hair, and more liberally on hair that's normal to thick or coarse.

☹ **Under Control Shaping Spray** *($4.99 for 8 ounces)* contains acetone, which can be very irritating to the scalp and damaging to the hair shaft. With so many other worthwhile aerosol hairsprays available (in all price ranges), why consider this problematic option?

☺ **Wound Up Curling Mousse** *($4.99 for 8.5 ounces)* is similar to the Big Volume Styling Foam above, except this has slightly more hold and contains plant oil for extra conditioning. Otherwise, the same basic comments apply.

☺ **Color Miracle Color Protecting Polishing Serum** *($6.99 for 4 ounces)* is a standard silicone serum and is also one of the more affordable silicone serums available. It is every bit as effective as pricier options from salon and designer lines. As is true for all silicone serums, this needs to be used sparingly to avoid a slick, greasy appearance and it cannot protect hair color. What it can do is smooth the hair's cuticle so it reflects light evenly, which will show off the nuances and vibrancy of color-treated hair.

☺ **Shine Miracle Anti-Frizz Polishing Serum** *($6.99 for 4 ounces)* is nearly identical to the Color Miracle Color Protecting Polishing Serum above, and the same basic comments apply.

☺ **Shine Mist Anti-Frizz Spray Laminator** *($4.99 for 3 ounces)* is a silicone spray that does not contain any water or alcohol to dilute the effect of the silicone. That means that even though it's a spray, it can go on heavier than you want, which can make hair look greasy. This is best for normal to very dry hair that is normal to thick or coarse, and should be sprayed on sparingly until you've gauged how much silicone your hair can handle.

CLAIROL

Clairol is one of the largest hair-care companies in the world. They are owned by personal- and home-care corporate giant Procter & Gamble, the same company that also owns globally distributed hair-care lines Pantene, physique, Head & Shoulders, Infusium 23, Pert Plus, and Vidal Sassoon. Where Clairol really excels is with their at-home permanent and semi-permanent color products. Brands include Ultress, Nice 'N Easy and Natural Instincts, and the technology that goes into creating these dyes is impressive. Sadly, the same cannot be said for their hair-care products, which now include two main lines—Daily Renewal 5x and Herbal Essences—and the dwindling Daily Defense line.

Daily Renewal and Herbal Essences offer an enormous assortment of products, but the redundancy between them is staggering, as you will see from the reviews below. A major problem is that the Herbal Essences shampoos were the top-selling shampoos of

2003, despite the fact that every one of them contains the drying detergent cleansing agent sodium lauryl sulfate. That is not good news, and it means that millions of consumers are causing their hair and scalp to be needlessly dry by turning to these heavily advertised shampoos. Presumably, many of you like the smell of the Herbal Essences products, and this is an area where we'll have to agree to disagree, because the entire Herbal Essences line is one of the most perfumed hair-care collections around. The olfactory experience may please you, but you're not doing your scalp any favors by cleansing, conditioning, and styling with such strongly scented products. OK, I'll stop harping about fragrance and simply let the reviews speak for themselves. For more information about Clairol, call (800) 223-5800 or visit www.clairol.com.

What's Good About This Line: The conditioners, though astoundingly repetitive, have merit for normal to dry hair of any thickness; most of the styling products perform well, though few offer the degree of hold advertised.

What's Not So Good About It: The strong sense of redundancy across product lines and types; almost all of the shampoos contain sodium lauryl sulfate as one of the main detergent cleansing agents; the Herbal Essences line has an overwhelming fragrance; several of the Herbal Essences styling products flake.

CLAIROL DAILY DEFENSE

☹ **Light Bloom Shampoo, for Fine/Oily Hair** *($1.19 for 13.5 ounces)* contains the strong solvent ammonium xylenesulfonate as one of its main ingredients, which means this shampoo can cause hair and scalp dryness.

☹ **Tender Apple Shampoo, for Dry/Damaged/Color-Treated Hair** *($1.19 for 13.5 ounces)* is similar to the Light Bloom Shampoo above. Although this contains less ammonium xylenesulfonate, it's still problematic for long-term use on hair.

☹ **Water Lily Shampoo, for Normal Hair** *($1.19 for 13.5 ounces)* is nearly identical to the Tender Apple Shampoo above, and the same comments apply.

☺ **Light Bloom Conditioner, for Fine/Oily Hair** *($1.19 for 13.5 ounces)* is a standard, lightweight conditioner that would indeed work well for fine hair, but it is not the best for oily hair, which traditionally doesn't need any conditioner.

☺ **Tender Apple Conditioner, for Dry/Damaged/Color-Treated Hair** *($1.19 for 13.5 ounces)* is identical to the Light Bloom Conditioner above, and the same comments apply. This would not be an ideal conditioner for dry hair, especially if it is coarse or thick.

☺ **Water Lily Conditioner, for Normal Hair** *($1.19 for 13.5 ounces)* is identical to the Light Bloom Conditioner above, and the same comments apply.

CLAIROL DAILY RENEWAL 5X

The claim that these products can make hair five times stronger is based on a test of the tensile strength of hair when the Daily Renewal products were used on hair versus leaving hair untreated with nothing on it at all. Clairol's research didn't compare their products to anyone else's. Truth be told, all hair is stronger when it is conditioned than when it is dry. Therefore, the claim makes for good copy but doesn't prove anything about the value of these products in comparison to other formulations.

☹ **Daily Renewal 5x Refresh Shampoo, for All Hair Types** *($2.99 for 13.5 ounces)* contains ammonium xylenesulfonate, which can be drying to the hair and irritate the scalp. Adding to this risk, your scalp will likely react to the orange and lemon oils used as fragrance, not to mention that the smell is reminiscent of furniture polish!

☹ **Daily Renewal 5x Replenishing Shampoo, for Dry/Damaged Hair** *($3.99 for 13.5 ounces)*, **Daily Renewal 5x Revitalizing Shampoo, for Color/Permed Hair** *($3.99 for 13.5 ounces)*, and **Daily Renewal 5x Volumizing Shampoo, for Fine Hair** *($3.99 for 13.5 ounces)* all contain sodium lauryl sulfate as one of the main detergent cleansing agents, and that makes these shampoos too drying and irritating for all hair and scalp types. They will not replenish, renew, or revitalize the hair, though words like that are sure to grab the attention of many unsuspecting consumers.

☺ **Daily Renewal 5x Daily Nourishment Creme, Leave-In** *($4.99 for 4.2 ounces)* is a standard, but good, leave-in conditioner that works well on normal to fine hair that is normal to slightly dry, although the film-forming agent can build up with repeated use.

☺ **Daily Renewal 5x Refresh Conditioner, for All Hair Types** *($2.99 for 13.5 ounces)* is a good conditioner for normal to dry hair of any thickness except fine or thin.

☺ **Daily Renewal 5x Replenishing Conditioner, for Dry/Damaged Hair** *($4.99 for 13.5 ounces)* is a basic, but good, conditioner that is a good option for normal to dry hair of any thickness.

☺ **Daily Renewal 5x Revitalizing Conditioner, for Color/Permed Hair** *($3.99 for 13.5 ounces)* is nearly identical to the Daily Renewal 5x Replenishing Conditioner for Dry/Damaged Hair above, and the same comments apply.

☺ **Daily Renewal 5x Volumizing Conditioner, for Fine Hair** *($4.99 for 13.5 ounces)* is nearly identical to the Daily Renewal 5x Replenishing Conditioner, for Dry/Damaged Hair above, and the same comments apply.

☺ **Daily Renewal 5x Hydration Therapy, Intensive Treatment** *($4.99 for 5.9 ounces)* is nearly identical to the Daily Renewal 5x Replenishing Conditioner, for Dry/Damaged Hair above, and the same comments apply. There is nothing intense about this product—it's just a name change to differentiate it from what it really is—a standard conditioner.

☺ **Daily Renewal 5x Restyle Extra Hold Extra Control Hairspray, 7** *($2.99 for 9 ounces)* is a standard, nonaerosol hairspray that provides a very soft, non-sticky hold. It is not a contender for "extra control," but is great for putting a finishing touch on hairstyles. This product's ultra-light finish is ideal for very fine or thin hair.

☺ **Daily Renewal 5x Restyle Extra Hold Extra Control Mousse, 7** *($2.99 for 9 ounces)* doesn't win points for originality, but few hair-care products do. This is just a standard, but good, propellant-based mousse with minimal to no hold and a smooth, non-sticky finish that can be brushed through easily.

☺ **Daily Renewal 5x Restyle Ultimate Hold Super Control Gel, 10** *($2.99 for 9 ounces)* is a watery, alcohol-free gel whose "ultimate hold" claim stops short at medium hold. This gel leaves hair slightly stiff and sticky, but it can be brushed through easily.

CLAIROL HERBAL ESSENCES

☺ **Herbal Essences Anti-Dandruff Shampoo, for All Hair Types** *($3.99 for 12 ounces)* contains salicylic acid, which can exfoliate the scalp, but the pH of this shampoo is too high for that to occur, and the amount of salicylic acid is not revealed. As a shampoo, this is a basic formula that is primarily water, detergent cleansing agent, lather agent, and fragrance, and it's unlikely to be of much help for those struggling with dandruff flakes.

☹ **Herbal Essences Clarifying/Residue Removal Shampoo, for Normal to Oily Hair** *($3.99 for 12 ounces)*, **Herbal Essences Extra Body Shampoo, for Fine, Limp Hair** *($3.99 for 12 ounces)*, **Herbal Essences Fruit Fusions Hydrating Shampoo, for Dry/Damaged Hair** *($3.99 for 12 ounces)*, **Herbal Essences Fruit Fusions Protecting Shampoo, for Colored/Permed Hair** *($3.99 for 12 ounces)*, **Herbal Essences Fruit Fusions Purifying Shampoo, for Normal to Oily Hair** *($3.99 for 12 ounces)*, **Herbal Essences Fruit Fusions Revitalizing Shampoo, for Normal Hair** *($3.99 for 12 ounces)*, **Herbal Essences Intensive Blends Moisturizing Shampoo, for Normal Hair** *($3.49 for 12 ounces)*, **Herbal Essences Intensive Blends Protecting Shampoo, for Colored/Permed Hair** *($3.99 for 12 ounces)*, **Herbal Essences Intensive Blends Replenishing Shampoo, for Dry/Damaged Hair** *($3.99 for 12 ounces)*, **Herbal Essences Moisture-Balancing Shampoo, for Normal Hair** *($3.99 for 12 ounces)*, **Herbal Essences Natural Volume Texturizing Shampoo** *($3.99 for 12 ounces)*, **Herbal Essences Rainforest Flowers Refreshing Shampoo for Normal Hair** *($4.29 for 12 ounces)*, **Herbal Essences Rainforest Flowers Replenishing Shampoo, for Colored/Permed/Dry/Damaged Hair** *($4.29 for 12 ounces)*, **Herbal Essences Rainforest Flowers Uplifting Shampoo, for Fine/Limp Hair** *($4.29 for 12 ounces)*, and **Herbal Essences Replenisher Shampoo, for Colored/Permed/Dry/Damaged Hair** *($3.49 for 12 ounces)* all have, save for a change in fragrance and fragrant plant extracts, nearly identical formulations. Each of these shampoos contains sodium lauryl sulfate as one of the main detergent cleansing agents, and that means all of them can be drying to the hair and irritating to the scalp. The various plant extracts chosen, organic or not, have no effect on the hair, but can contribute to scalp irritation.

☺ **Herbal Essences Clean-Rinsing Conditioner, for Normal to Oily Hair** *($3.99 for 12 ounces)* is a basic conditioner that works for normal to dry hair of any thickness.

☺ **Herbal Essences Dry Scalp Conditioner** *($2.99 for 12 ounces)* isn't all that beneficial for dry scalp (plain moisturizer, or even olive oil from your kitchen, massaged into the scalp the night before you wash your hair in the morning would be a far better choice). Still, this is a good, lightweight conditioner for normal to slightly dry hair that is normal to fine or thin.

☺ **Herbal Essences Fruit Fusions Hydrating Conditioner, for Dry/Damaged Hair** *($3.99 for 12 ounces)* is nearly identical to the Herbal Essences Clean-Rinsing Conditioner, for Normal to Oily Hair above, and the same comments apply. This is not emollient enough to use it for dry or damaged hair.

☺ **Herbal Essences Fruit Fusions Protecting Conditioner, for Color-Treated Hair** *($3.99 for 12 ounces)* is nearly identical to the Herbal Essences Clean-Rinsing Conditioner, for Normal to Oily Hair above, and the same comments apply. Nothing about this formula makes it the preferred choice for color-treated hair—that's just marketing language.

☺ **Herbal Essences Fruit Fusions Purifying Conditioner, for Normal to Oily Hair** *($3.99 for 12 ounces)* is nearly identical to the Herbal Essences Clean-Rinsing Conditioner, for Normal to Oily Hair above, and the same comments apply.

☺ **Herbal Essences Fruit Fusions Revitalizing Conditioner, for Normal Hair** *($3.99 for 12 ounces)* is nearly identical to the Herbal Essences Dry Scalp Conditioner above, and the same comments apply.

☺ **Herbal Essences Intensive Blends Restoring Conditioning Balm** *($3.99 for 12 ounces)* is a very good, though standard, conditioner for normal to dry hair that is normal to thick or coarse.

☺ **Herbal Essences Intensive Blends Creme Leave-In** *($3.99 for 12 ounces)* is, with the exception of the fragrant plant and flower extracts and the addition of panthenol, nearly identical to the Daily Renewal 5x Daily Nourishment Creme Leave-In above, and the same comments apply.

☺ **Herbal Essences Intensive Blends Moisturizing Conditioner, for Normal Hair** *($3.49 for 12 ounces)* is nearly identical to the Herbal Essences Clean-Rinsing Conditioner above, except this contains a longer list of conditioning agents. The amounts are too small for your hair to notice a significant difference between products, though, so the same comments apply.

☺ **Herbal Essences Intensive Blends Protecting Conditioner, for Colored/Permed Hair** *($3.99 for 12 ounces)* is a good, though basic, conditioner for normal to dry hair of any thickness.

☺ **Herbal Essences Intensive Blends Replenishing Conditioner, for Dry/Damaged Hair** *($3.99 for 12 ounces)* is nearly identical to the Herbal Essences Intensive Blends Moisturizing Conditioner, for Normal Hair above, and the same comments apply.

☹ **Herbal Essences Leave-In Conditioner, Lightweight Formula for All Hair Types** *($4.39 for 10 ounces)* contains the preservatives methylchloroisothiazolinone and methylisothiazolinone (Kathon CG), which are not recommended for use in leave-on products due to the risk of causing a sensitizing reaction. What a shame, because this is otherwise a well-formulated conditioner, and one of the more original options in the Clairol line.

☺ **Herbal Essences Light Conditioning, for Fine/Limp Hair** *($3.99 for 12 ounces)* is nearly identical to the Herbal Essences Clean-Rinsing Conditioner above, and the same basic comments apply.

☺ **Herbal Essences Moisturizing Conditioner, for Normal Hair** *($3.99 for 12 ounces)* is nearly identical to the Herbal Essences Clean-Rinsing Conditioner above, and the same basic comments apply.

☺ **Herbal Essences Natural Volume Weightless Conditioner** *($3.99 for 12 ounces)* is nearly identical to the Herbal Essences Clean-Rinsing Conditioner above, and the same basic comments apply.

☺ **Herbal Essences Protecting Conditioner, for Colored/Permed/Dry/Damaged Hair** *($3.99 for 12 ounces)* is as basic a conditioner as the rest of the repetitive Herbal Essences lineup, and although it can be good for normal to dry hair of any thickness, it has no special benefit for color-treated or damaged hair.

☺ **Rainforest Flowers Refreshing Conditioner, for Normal Hair** *($4.29 for 12 ounces)* is nearly identical to the Herbal Essences Intensive Blends Restoring Conditioning Balm above, and the same comments apply.

☺ **Rainforest Flowers Replenishing Conditioner, for Colored/Permed/Dry/Damaged Hair** *($4.29 for 12 ounces)* is nearly identical to the Herbal Essences Intensive Blends Restoring Conditioning Balm above, and the same comments apply.

☺ **Rainforest Flowers Uplifting Conditioner, for Fine/Limp Hair** *($4.29 for 12 ounces)* is nearly identical to the Herbal Essences Intensive Blends Restoring Conditioning Balm above, and the same comments apply. This conditioner is too heavy for fine or limp hair.

☹ **Herbal Essences Hairspray, Extra Hold (Aerosol)** *($3.99 for 8 ounces)* isn't extra-hold in the least. It's actually a light-hold hairspray that disappoints not because the hold is less than the name advertises, but because this product flakes.

☹ **Herbal Essences Hairspray, Flexible Hold (Aerosol)** *($3.79 for 8 ounces)* is nearly identical to the Herbal Essences Hairspray, Extra Hold above, and has the same flaking problem.

☹ **Herbal Essences Hairspray, Maximum Hold (Aerosol)** *($3.79 for 8 ounces)* is nearly identical to both of the Herbal Essences products above, except it does have a stronger hold, but it still flakes.

☺ **Herbal Essences Natural Volume Bodifying Foam** *($3.79 for 7 ounces)* is a standard, propellant-based mousse with a creamy-foam texture that provides a light, touchable hold that can be easily brushed through. The fragrance can be overpowering, but this is still a good styling mousse.

☹ **Herbal Essences Natural Volume Body Boosting Gel** *($3.79 for 7 ounces)* has a rather unusual formula, and by that I mean the ingredient list doesn't read like those of almost all of the other styling gels available. Perhaps this was an attempt to come up with a new gel formulation, but it wasn't a good one. This viscous gel can flake, especially when hair is brushed through, and it is not recommended.

☺ **Herbal Essences Natural Volume Root Volumizer** *($3.49 for 6 ounces)* is a standard styling spray with a special nozzle that allows you to focus application at the roots. It provides a very light, non-sticky hold that can work (with heat) to build body and volume into fine or thin hair. Unlike many of the Herbal Essences styling products above, this one does not flake.

☺ **Herbal Essences Natural Volume Weightless Hairspray** *($3.79 for 7 ounces)* is a standard aerosol hairspray that offers a light hold that can be easily brushed through. This fragrant hairspray works well for all hair types that need just a touch of hold without stiffness or stickiness.

☺ **Herbal Essences Non-Aerosol Hairspray, Extra Hold** *($3.49 for 8.5 ounces)* works well as a medium-hold hairspray for all hair types. It leaves hair slightly sticky, but the stiffness can be easily brushed through.

☺ **Herbal Essences Non-Aerosol Hairspray, Flexible Hold** *($3.79 for 8 ounces)* doesn't offer a flexible hold, it offers a strong hold that can leave hair feeling slightly stiff and sticky. This isn't as easy to brush through as the Herbal Essences Non-Aerosol Hairspray, Extra Hold above, and is best when you want to freeze your style in place and leave it alone.

☺ **Herbal Essences Non-Aerosol Hairspray, Maximum Hold** *($3.79 for 8.5 ounces)* offers a strong hold that leaves hair feeling slightly stiff and sticky, but it's easier to brush through than the Herbal Essences Non-Aerosol Hairspray, Flexible Hold above. That gives it more versatility for those who use hairspray for control, but who also want to brush through and redo their hair later.

☺ **Herbal Essences Spray Gel, Extra Hold** *($3.79 for 8.5 ounces)* is a standard spray gel that provides light (not extra) hold and leaves hair feeling moist and slightly sticky. The conditioning agent in this product can provide some protection from heat styling.

☺ **Herbal Essences Styling Gel, Extra Hold** *($3.49 for 8.5 ounces)* is an exceptionally standard styling gel that provides a light to medium hold that leaves hair feeling sticky. This can be brushed through, but the fragrance is so intense you may think you're applying perfume, rather than styling gel, to your hair.

☺ **Herbal Essences Styling Mousse, Extra Hold** *($3.79 for 8 ounces)* is a standard, propellant-based styling mousse with a thin texture that provides an incredibly soft hold. Hair is easily brushed through, and this simple formulation is a great option for fine or thin hair.

☺ **Herbal Essences Styling Mousse, Maximum Hold** *($3.99 for 8 ounces)* is nearly identical to the Herbal Essences Styling Mousse, Extra Hold above, and the same comments apply.

☺ **Herbal Essence Styling Spritz, Maximum Hold** *($3.99 for 8.5 ounces)* is a standard hairspray that is similar to most of the Herbal Essences Non-Aerosol options above, and it provides a light hold that is slightly sticky but not stiff, so hair is easily brushed through. This alcohol-in-water formulation does take longer to dry, which gives you more time to style your hair before it sets.

CLAIROL PROFESSIONAL SHIMMER LIGHTS

☹ **Shimmer Lights Shampoo** (*$9.95 for 16 ounces*) contains sodium lauryl sulfate as its sole detergent cleansing agent, and is not recommended. This is actually a very dated formula that offers more problems than benefits for those with silver, gray, white, or blonde hair.

☺ **Shimmer Lights Conditioner** (*$9.95 for 16 ounces*) contains mostly water, thickener, detangling agents, water-binding agent, fragrance, more thickener, preservatives, and coloring agents. The tiny amount of violet dye does little to counteract brassy or yellow tones. This is a very basic conditioner that is an OK option for normal to slightly dry hair that needs help with combing, but little else.

CLAIROL METALEX

☺ **Metalex Hair Conditioner 511** (*$12.99 for 4 ounces*) doesn't condition hair at all. Rather, this hard-to-find product contains a high amount of sulfated oil, which strips hair color. Metalex is a specialty product designed to remove hair color, such as from a dye job gone awry, either at home or in the salon. It does indeed remove hair color, allowing you to dye the hair again, but it also causes further hair damage. Nevertheless, the tradeoff—removing unwanted color or an undesired tone—can make it worthwhile. The happy face rating is because this unique product has the ability to successfully remove unwanted hair color, not because it does so in a gentle or harmless manner.

CLINIQUE

Talk about reinventing the wheel! These hair-care products from Clinique arrived with much fanfare but they are merely standard fare, and don't set a new standard or create a special benefit for hair of any type. The shampoos are pretty much just shampoo, the conditioners just conditioners, and the styling products just styling products. These products are easily replaced with products costing half as much. For more information about Clinique, call (212) 572-3800 or visit www.clinique.com.

What's Good About This Line: Gentle shampoos and basic, though effective conditioners, including a great option for very dry hair.

What's Not So Good About It: Despite the 100% fragrance-free claim, all but one of Clinique's hair-care products have fragrant plant extracts which definitely add a scent.

☺ **Daily Shampoo Everyday Cleansing** (*$11 for 6.7 ounces*) is a fairly standard, detergent-based shampoo that would work well for most hair types. It does contain some conditioning and detangling agents, which means it could cause buildup with repeated use and would need to be alternated with a shampoo without conditioning agents. It is interesting to note that the cleansing agents are fairly gentle, making this a good option for those with a sensitive scalp. The teeny amount of spearmint in here probably won't cause irritation.

☺ **Exceptionally Clean Clarifying Shampoo** *($11 for 6.7 ounces)* is almost identical to the Daily Shampoo Everyday Cleansing above only with stronger detergent cleansing agents, which makes it somewhat better for those who have an oily scalp. However, the conditioning agents in here can still cause buildup with repeated use.

☺ **Gentle Wash Moisturizing Shampoo** *($11 for 6.7 ounces)* is a standard shampoo that would indeed be a gentle shampoo, but the methyldihydrojasmonate is a fragrant additive which serves no other purpose for the hair or scalp.

☹ **$$$ Quick Detangle Light Conditioner** *($11 for 6.7 ounces)* is, just as the name implies, a detangler; this one uses behentrimonium chloride, a standard detangling agent, though if you have a sensitive scalp, the balm mint, cinnamon, and coriander in here can cause irritation. Other than that, this contains only a tiny amount of conditioning agents, which means it is best for someone with normal to slightly dry hair that is fine or thin.

☺ **Super Condition Restoring Conditioner** *($11 for 6.7 ounces)* is much like hundreds of other conditioners; the effective ingredients are silicone and detangling agents. Also in here, in far tinier amounts are some emollients, but the main ingredients are the workhorses, and they do a good job for someone with normal to dry hair of any thickness. This does contain fragrant plant extracts.

☺ **Dramatic Moisture Intensive Conditioner** *($11 for 6.7 ounces)* is almost identical to the Super Condition Restoring Conditioner above, except this has slightly more plant oil and less detangling agent. This one would work well for someone with normal to thick or coarse hair that is dry to very dry, as the name implies.

☺ **$$$ Defined Curls** *($14.50 for 5 ounces)* is a good lightweight styling gel with minimal to no sticky feel that has a very soft hold, so if you have stubborn or hard-to-hold hair this isn't the product to consider. It works best as a leave-in conditioner for normal to dry hair that is normal to slightly thick.

☺ **$$$ Extra Body** *($14.50 for 4.2 ounces)* is a basic, water- and alcohol-based styling spray that uses a standard film-forming agent to provide light to medium hold. That can make the hair feel fuller but it can also feel slightly sticky, though it can be brushed through.

☺ **$$$ Light Control Gel** *($14.50 for 5 ounces)* is a smooth, alcohol-free gel that feels weightless in the hair and provides light, brushable hold that is slightly sticky but not stiff.

☺ **$$$ Natural Hold** *($14.50 for 6.7 ounces)* is a standard aerosol hairspray that gives light to medium hold and minimal sticky feel. The silicone in here adds a touch of shine to the hair.

☺ **Non-Aerosol Hair Spray** *($11.00 for 8 ounces)* is similar to the Natural Hold, only with slightly more hold, and, as the name says, it's non-aerosol. This is completely fragrance-free.

☺ **$$$ Perfectly Straight for Fine or Medium Hair** *($14.50 for 5 ounces)* and **Perfectly Straight for Medium or Thick Hair** *($14.50 for 5 ounces)*. I don't have to tell those of you with curly or frizzy hair that there are no products that will make your hair perfectly straight without a great deal of work with a blow dryer and round brush, curling iron, or hair iron, and these very standard styling balms are no exception to that. The silicones and film former in here can help control hair but if you use too much, they can also make hair feel greasy and heavy. Less is best, but both of these are options for a good styling balm if you know how to use the tools to make hair behave. Perfectly Straight for Medium or Thick Hair has a much greater amount of silicones and few film-forming agents, while the Fine or Medium Hair option contains more film-forming agents, glycerin, and plant oils than silicones.

☺ $$$ **Strong Control Gel** *($14.50 for 5 ounces)* is an exceptionally standard gel with medium hold and minimal to no stiff or sticky feel. That's great but there's nothing here that's unique. This does contain fragrant plant extracts.

☺ $$$ **Shaping Wax** *($14.50 for 1.7 ounces)* is a very lightweight, gel-type pomade that isn't waxy in the least. Rather, it is extremely water-soluble and not at all heavy on the hair. This is more of a very thick traditional hair gel that has minimal hold and no stiff or sticky feeling.

☺ $$$ **Healthy Shine Serum** *($14.50 for 1.7 ounces)* is a standard silicone serum that includes cinnamon and coriander as the fragrance. The price isn't bad, but there are identical silicone serums at the drugstore for a quarter of the price (check out Citré Shine and Charles Worthington Results come to mind).

CONAIR

Conair hair-care products tend to come and go every year or two. When they do appear on the scene, the products typically impress, particularly when you consider the formulas and the low price tags. Their latest collection is Headcase, and it is a kicky, slightly irreverent line of styling products aimed at preteens and teens. However, adults looking for remarkable products would be remiss to let this inexpensive line sit on the shelves. Most of the products perform admirably, and the formulations contain ingredients touted by many expensive lines that use them in much smaller amounts than Conair. If you can get past the edgy names, you'll find some of the best all-around styling products that are available at the drugstore. The line is not without shortcomings, but for the most part shopping it will be time (and money) well spent! For more information about Conair, call (800) 326-6247 or visit www.conairhaircare.com.

What's Good About This Line: Most of the styling products contain an impressive blend of conditioning agents, and the variety (rather than repetition) is refreshing.

What's Not So Good About It: A few of the styling products contain the preservatives methylchloroisothiazolinone and methylisothiazolinone (Kathon CG), which are contraindicated for use in leave-on products due to a high likelihood of a sensitizing reaction.

☺ **Headcase Act Up, Gravity-Defying Spiking Glue** *($3.99 for 4 ounces)* is a thick, pasty styling gel that takes its name seriously—this will provide hold that makes hair stand on end and stay that way! It is tricky to work with, but for those who want to exaggerate and define short, spiky hairstyles, take note—this product delivers and is easy to shampoo out.

☺ **Headcase Bee Good, Shape & Define Spray Wax** *($3.99 for 4.5 ounces)* is an aerosol styling aid that contains more silicone than wax, so it works best to add shine (not texture) to the hair. This sprays on forcefully and heavily, which makes it best for those with hair that is normal to thick or coarse. Its primary benefits are adding shine and making hair look smoother.

☺ **Headcase Dense, Hair-Raising Root Lifter** *($3.99 for 6 ounces)* is a standard styling mousse whose packaging resembles an aerosol hairspray, but with a directional nozzle that allows you to reach the roots of your hair. This dispenses forcefully, so applying it directly to the hair can be messy. It works well as a light-hold, lightly conditioning styling mousse for normal to fine or thin hair. The formula is neither too stiff nor too sticky.

☹ **Headcase Dominate, Volume-Building Foaming Mousse** *($3.99 for 7 ounces)* is a liquid-to-foam styling mousse that has a lot going for it, except that it contains the preservative Kathon CG, which is not recommended for use in leave-on products.

☺ **Headcase Fixated, Relentless Hold Hair Spray** *($3.99 for 8 ounces)* is a standard aerosol hairspray. Despite the name, it offers a light, flexible hold that can be easily brushed through without leaving hair sticky.

☹ **Headcase Hodgepodge, Tousling Texturizer** *($3.99 for 4.5 ounces)* contains the preservative Kathon CG, and is not recommended for any hair or scalp type.

☺ **Headcase Mind Bender, Ruthless Hold Gel** *($3.99 for 5 ounces)* is a firm-hold styling gel that contains a hair-friendly array of plant oils and silicone conditioning agents. This is ideal for taming unruly hair that is coarse, curly, or thick; it's a bit too heavy for fine or thin hair. It can be brushed through easily, and works well on dry hair for extra hold and definition.

☺ **Headcase Motivator, Style Defining Pomade** *($3.99 for 2 ounces)* is a very water-soluble, gel-type pomade that contains a film-forming/holding agent. This is a good option for all hair types looking to smooth unruly ends, tame frizzies, or add a touch of control with shine. It is minimally greasy and distributes evenly through the hair, but use it sparingly until you know how your hair responds to it.

☺ **Headcase Out There, Beads-of-Shine Defining Gel** *($3.99 for 8 ounces)* contains tiny colored beads that break open when you massage this gel in your hands. Supposedly, the beads contain shine-enhancing ingredients. This standard, but very good, medium-hold gel contains plant oil, mineral oil, and silicone for shine, but that is hardly a unique combination. The beads end up being more of a clever visual lure than anything else. This liquidy gel is a wonderful option for all hair types. It's slightly sticky but can be easily brushed through, and also provides some protection during heat styling.

☹ **Headcase Quirky, Bodybuilding Curl Booster** *($3.99 for 8 ounces)* contains the preservative Kathon CG, which can be very sensitizing when used in leave-on products. Therefore, this otherwise fine styling product is not recommended.

☺ **Headcase Be Bright Frizz Serum Lusterizer** *($3.99 for 1.9 ounces)* is a spray-on glossing product that contains a mixture of emollients, slip agents, and silicones. It works well to add shine but the application is quite heavy, depositing a concentrated blast of liquid instead of a fine mist. That can be tricky to deal with, and this is recommended only for those with thick, coarse hair that is curly or wavy. You may want to try spraying this on your hand, then applying it to the hair where needed.

CURL FRIENDS

This small, niche hair-care line has big plans to be for curly hair what Head & Shoulders is for those with dandruff. At least, that's the forecast since Curl Friends was purchased by investment firm CP Baker & Company in 2003 (Source: *The Rose Sheet*, November 10, 2003). Sold primarily in salons and retail stores such as BeautyFirst, Curl Friends has some very good products, but they're no more special for curly hair than those from countless other lines, and the prices are absurd for such standard formulations. Curly hair needs products that keep curls smooth, moisturized, and easy to detangle. Yet because curly hair can be any thickness (from ultra-fine and stringy to a thick mass of tangled spirals or tight corkscrews), products marketed to curly hair should be able to meet the differing needs of this entire range of textures. That is not the case here. If anything, most Curl Friends products are middle-of-the-road options that work primarily for normal hair that isn't too thick, too dry, too thin, or too limp. For more information about Curl Friends, call (800) 621-CURL or visit www.curlfriends.com.

What's Good About This Line: Gentle shampoos and effective conditioners, though they're not intrinsically better for curly hair.

What's Not So Good About It: Needlessly pricey; two of the styling products contain the preservatives methylchloroisothiazolinone and methylisothiazolinone (Kathon CG), which are not recommended for use in leave-on products.

☺ **$$$ Clarifying Shampoo** *($18 for 8 ounces)* is an exceptionally gentle shampoo that is similar to most "tear-free" baby shampoos. This contains a tiny amount of chelating agent, though probably not enough to remove mineral buildup, but it will certainly cleanse the hair without drying or causing conditioner buildup. This is recommended for all hair and scalp types except oily, but it isn't the best if you use a lot of styling products.

☺ **$$$ Purify Shampoo** *($18 for 5.5 ounces)* is identical to the Clarifying Shampoo above, and the exact same comments apply. Why this shampoo provides less product for the same amount of money is a question worth asking, but don't expect a straight (pun intended) answer.

☺ **$$$ Shampoo** *($19 for 8 ounces)* is a standard, gentle shampoo that works well for normal to dry hair of any thickness (curly or not). The film-forming agent poses a slight risk of buildup.

☺ **$$$ Humidity Blocker Leave-In Conditioner** *($20 for 2 ounces)* contains the same assortment of thickeners and conditioning agents found in hundreds of other conditioners, but the others are usually the rinse-out variety. This is rather heavy for a leave-in product that isn't emollient enough for thick or coarse hair and is *too* heavy for fine or thin hair.

☺ **$$$ SOS Sea Essentials Conditioner** *($20 for 7 ounces)* is an OK conditioner for normal to slightly dry hair that is normal to slightly thick. The silt (sea mud) limits the moisturizing properties of this product.

☺ **$$$ Anti-Frenzy Smootherator** *($21 for 2 ounces)* has a strange name but ends up being a very good silicone serum for all hair types, thanks in part to its glycol- and water-based formula, which gives it a thinner texture that is less greasy and slick-feeling than many silicone products.

☹ **Curl Power Texturizing Mist** *($16.50 for 8 ounces)* contains the preservative Kathon CG, which is not recommended for use in leave-on products due to its high risk of causing a sensitizing reaction to the scalp.

☺ **$$$ Gooey-Goo Wonder Wax** *($18 for 2 ounces)* is a unique product that is a styling gel/pomade hybrid. It's unique because it has a gooey, icing-like texture, and it may take some experimenting before you know just how much to use for the best results. This ends up being a versatile product for all hair types except fine or thin. It provides smooth control with soft, flexible hold, and manages this without feeling too greasy or sticky.

☹ **High Humidity Gel** *($22 for 8 ounces)* is a standard styling gel that contains the preservative Kathon CG, and is not recommended.

☺ **$$$ All Weather Shine** *($24 for 2 ounces)* is a standard silicone serum that contains three types of silicone. It works as well as any, but for the money there is no reason to consider this over options from Citré Shine, Charles Worthington Results, or many, many others available at the drugstore.

☺ **$$$ Heat Beater Thermal Protectant** *($20 for 8 ounces)* is a light- to medium-hold styling spray that contains conditioning agents. The name implies this product can win the war against heat damage for your hair, but that is absolutely not the case. No product can prevent the heat from flat irons or blow dryers from damaging hair.

DARPHIN

Darphin is similar to Clarins and Decleor, two high-end cosmetics lines whose raison d'être is plants and essential oils, and the (allegedly) remarkable effects they have on your skin (including the scalp). The first thing I noticed about Darphin (whose small hair-care line is significantly better than its skin-care and makeup lines) was the preponderance of standard, synthetic ingredients. However, that's a good thing, because the exotic plant extracts and fragrant oils Darphin boasts about have little, if any, positive effect on your hair and scalp. Extolling the benefits of impossible-to-pronounce plants and flowers is alluring, but behind the scenes the same detergent cleansing, detangling, and condition-

The Reviews D

ing agents the rest of the hair-care industry uses are busy making hair look and feel amazing. They're the reason you should consider this line. Just be aware that the exorbitant prices are not bringing you benefits any more special than what you get from products you can find elsewhere for far less money. For more information about Darphin (owned by Estee Lauder), call (888) 611-3003.

What's Good About This Line: The shampoos and conditioners, though pricey, are (with minor exceptions) all excellent.

What's Not So Good About It: Many of the products contain lemon peel oil, which can be a scalp irritant; the treatment products for exfoliating the scalp and helping thin hair or an oily scalp are worthless and/or irritating.

☺ $$$ **Anti-Dandruff Shampoo with Sage, for All Hair Types** *($22 for 6.7 ounces)* is a standard, detergent-based shampoo that contains the antimicrobial ingredient piroctone olamine. As this book goes to print, the FDA is still evaluating the effectiveness of that ingredient against dandruff. In other words, piroctone olamine is not part of the FDA's over-the-counter monograph for dandruff products (Source: www.fda.gov). However, there is research that shows piroctone olamine is an effective ingredient in controlling dandruff, though it's no more effective than zinc pyrithione (found in Head & Shoulders) or ketoconazole (found in Nizoral) (Source: *International Journal of Cosmetic Science*, October 2002, page 249). For the money, I would consider the anti-dandruff shampoos at the drugstore before this option. By the way, sage has no effect on dandruff, though it can be a scalp irritant.

☺ $$$ **Cream Shampoo with Olive, for Dry, Damaged Hair** *($22 for 6.7 ounces)* is a rich, conditioning shampoo that works well for normal to very dry hair that is normal to thick or coarse. The detangling/conditioning agents can build up over time, so alternate this with a shampoo that does not contain conditioning agents.

☺ $$$ **Gentle Shampoo with Calendula, for All Hair Types** *($22 for 6.7 ounces)* is a standard, detergent-based shampoo that is similar to the Cream Shampoo with Olive above, except this contains fewer conditioning agents and omits the lemon peel oil, which does indeed make it a gentler option for normal to dry hair that is normal to thick or coarse.

☺ $$$ **Regulating Shampoo with Badian, for Oily and Combination Hair** *($22 for 6.7 ounces)* is nearly identical to the Gentle Shampoo with Calendula above, only this one contains Badian (or anise). Otherwise, the same basic comments apply. The only thing this shampoo can "regulate" is how clean your hair and scalp will be after using it, just like every shampoo.

☺ $$$ **Volume Shampoo with Gleditschia, for Thin and Dull Hair** *($22 for 6.7 ounces)* is similar to the Cream Shampoo with Olive above, except this adds silicone to the mix, and that makes it an excellent smoothing, detangling shampoo for longer hair that is normal to dry and coarse or thick. The silicone can build up with repeated use, and makes this shampoo a poor option if you have fine or thin hair and want to add volume. While gleditschia may have some anti-inflammatory and anti-allergenic properties (when given to mice) (Source: *Biological and Pharmaceutical Bulletin*, September 2002, pages 1179–1182), it has no known benefit for hair, and any possible benefit for the scalp would be rinsed down the drain.

☺ **$$$ Conditioning Care with Jojoba, for All Hair Types** *($22 for 4.4 ounces)* is a standard, but very good (albeit overpriced), conditioner for someone with dry to very dry hair that is normal to thick or coarse. This is too emollient for fine or thin hair types.

☺ **$$$ Cream Mask with Shea Butter, for Dry and Damaged Hair** *($45 for 7 ounces)* has an overall formulation that isn't all that different from the Conditioning Care with Jojoba above, although the higher amount of plant oil in this one and the addition of shea butter make it better for very dry or damaged hair.

☹ **$$$ Exfoliating Complex, for All Scalps** *($45 for ten 0.33-ounce doses)* is a waste of time and money. These "treatment" vials contain nothing that can exfoliate the scalp. What a "Why bother?" product!

☺ **$$$ Protective Shining Oil, for All Hair Types** *($25 for 1.6 ounces)* contains an intelligent blend of conditioning emollients, along with plant and nut oils. This will nicely take care of dry to very dry hair, particularly if it's coarse, curly, or thick. The price for this spray-on product is steep, but if you're inclined to overspend on hair-care, at least this won't be a misstep.

☹ **Regulating Complex, for Oily Scalp** *($45 for ten 0.33-ounce doses)* contains alcohol, which won't help an oily scalp, along with thyme and lavender oils, menthol, and thymol, all irritants. This pointless product is a scalp irritation problem waiting to happen, and the price is ludicrous.

☹ **Revitalizing Complex, for Thinning Hair** *($60 for ten 0.33-ounce doses)* contains nothing that can benefit thinning hair, but it does contain the irritating oils of lavender, rosemary, and cedarwood. This useless concoction is not recommended.

DENOREX

Talk about a problem line! Denorex has been on store shelves for decades, and has changed little since the last edition of this book. It has expanded slightly, but the new products contain the same problematic ingredients found in the original products, and it all adds up to making this line impossible to recommend to someone fighting dandruff. For more information on Denorex, call (800) 443-4908 or visit www.denorex.com.

What's Good About This Line: The active ingredients can help combat dandruff and control flaking.

What's Not So Good About It: All of the products contain either drying detergent cleansing agents, menthol, or both.

☹ **Advanced Formula Dandruff Shampoo, Daily Use** *($8.99 for 8 ounces)* would have been an excellent anti-dandruff shampoo, complete with 2% zinc pyrithione as its active ingredient. Unfortunately, it also contains menthol, which can cause unnecessary scalp irritation—not what someone trying to fight dandruff needs.

☹ **Extra Strength Medicated Shampoo** *($8.99 for 8 ounces)* offers a 3% salicylic acid formula to help loosen and remove dandruff flakes, but the shampoo base contains sodium C14-16 olefin sulfonate and menthol, which can be doubly drying and irritating to the scalp and won't help fight dandruff.

☹ **Extra Strength Medicated Shampoo and Conditioner** *($8.99 for 8 ounces)* is similar to the Extra Strength Medicated Shampoo above, except this adds silicone conditioning agents. However, these agents do not offset the dryness and irritation from the sodium C14-16 olefin sulfonate or menthol.

☹ **Medicated Shampoo, Dandruff Fighting** *($9.49 for 8 ounces)* is similar to the Extra Strength Shampoo above, except this contains 1.8% salicylic acid. Otherwise, the same comments apply.

☹ **Medicated Shampoo and Conditioner, Dandruff Fighting** *($9.49 for 8 ounces)* is similar to the Extra Strength Medicated Shampoo and Conditioner above, except this contains less salicylic acid. Otherwise, the same problems abound, and this is not recommended.

DEP

For more information about Dep, call (800) 326-2855 or visit www.dep.com.

What's Good About This Line: The styling products, though repetitive, perform well.

What's Not So Good About It: Every single Dep product contains the preservatives methylchloroisothiazolinone and methylisothiazolinone (Kathon CG), which are not recommended for use in leave-on products.

☹ **Botanicals Moisturizing Gel, Extra Super Hold Level 8** *($2.99 for 12 ounces)*, **Curl Defining Gel, Extra Super Hold Level 8** *($2.99 for 12 ounces)*, **Moisturizing Gel, Super Hold Level 6** *($2.99 for 12 ounces)*, **Shaping Gel, Extra Hold Level 7** *($2.99 for 12 ounces)*, **Sport Endurance Gel, Ultimate Xtreme Hold Level 10** *($2.99 for 12 ounces)*, **Sport Endurance Pomade, Non-Stop Hold Level 12** *($2.99 for 2.6 ounces)*, **Sport Styling Glue, Non-Stop Hold Level 12** *($2.99 for 6.4 ounces)*, **Sport Thickening Gel, Ultimate Xtreme Hold Level 10** *($2.99 for 8 ounces)*, **Texturing Gel, Ultimate Hold Level 8** *($2.99 for 12 ounces)*, and **Anti-Frizz Gel Serum with Shine Complex** *($2.86 for 4.8 ounces)* all contain the preservative Kathon CG, which has a high risk of causing a sensitizing reaction on the scalp, and is contraindicated for use in leave-on products (Sources: *Contact Dermatitis*, November 2001, pages 257–264, and *European Journal of Dermatology*, March 1999, pages 144–160).

D:FI

This Generation-Y positioned hair-care line doesn't offer anything unique or exciting other than its marketing angle, which encourages teens and early twenty-somethings to express themselves creatively through their hairstyles. Brochures for d:fi (which was derived from the word "modify") talk about changing one's attitude, environment, and fashion statement simply by reaching for a different styling wax or gel. They mention that today's teens must have "image consciousness born out of intelligence" if they are to set themselves apart—but choosing to do that with hair-care products is superficial at best, especially when this generation has so much more to offer than well-coiffed hair. Owned and distributed by American Crew, it's no surprise that the d:fi and American Crew styling products are remarkably similar, save for their fragrances. For more information about d:fi, call (800) 598-CREW or visit www.dfihair.com.

What's Good About This Line: The styling products, though not as edgy as their names, perform as stated, with most of the pomades being best for those with thick, coarse hair that is dry to very dry.

What's Not So Good About It: The shampoos contain drying detergent cleansing agents.

☹ d:tox Extreme Cleansing Shampoo *($6.95 for 12 ounces)* does provide extreme cleansing—too extreme, thanks to the drying detergent cleansing agents sodium C14-16 olefin sulfonate and TEA-dodecylbenzenesulfonate. This shampoo is not recommended for any hair or scalp type.

☹ Hydrate:d Shampoo *($6.95 for 12 ounces)* contains sodium C14-16 olefin sulfonate as one of its main detergent cleansing agents, and that makes this shampoo too drying for the hair and scalp. The cactus extract has no effect on hair's hydration level. Just because a cactus can hold onto water doesn't mean that it can transfer that benefit (unique to this plant when it is in soil, not when it's in a hair-care product) to hair.

☺ d:stroyed Daily Conditioner *($6.95 for 12 ounces)* is a very standard, rather boring, conditioner. It works well for normal to slightly dry hair that is normal to fine or thin. This has no special benefit for damaged hair—if anything, damaged hair needs more than this basic conditioner can provide.

☺ Beach Bum Texturizing Spray *($9.95 for 4.2 ounces)* is a lightweight, no-hold styling spray that contains an alkaline ingredient (magnesium sulfate) and sea salt to rough up the hair's cuticle layer. That can add texture but it is also damaging when done repeatedly. The coconut oil helps add shine and keep hair soft, but it's not enough to offset the damage that can occur with routine use of this type of product. For occasional use, this is an OK option for all hair types.

☺ d:struct Pliable Molding Creme *($9.95 for 2.6 ounces)* is a thick, creamy pomade with a slightly stringy texture, but it can smooth coarse, thick hair and help control frizzies. This is thick stuff, and capable of grooming hair while providing light hold that doesn't get stiff, but it can feel tacky if not used sparingly.

☺ d:tails Pomade for Hold and Shine *($9.95 for 2.6 ounces)* is a water-soluble, gel-type pomade that works well for all hair types except fine or thin. It provides moisture to hair and is excellent for molding and defining curls and waves without stiffness. Used sparingly, this calms frizzies and smoothes hair ends while adding a high-gloss shine.

☺ **Heavy Wax Firm Hold Hair Wax** *($9.95 for 2.3 ounces)* is a thick, pasty pomade that is only for those who have thick or coarse hair that is unruly and needs a heavy product to shape and define it. This can feel slightly sticky, even though it does not contain any holding agents. It works best on dry hair.

☺ **Hi:fi Firm Hold Gel** *($7.95 for 8.45 ounces)* is a very standard styling gel that, true to its name, provides a firm hold. This is a great option for all hair types, and although it remains sticky, hair can be brushed through.

☺ **Light Wax Medium Hold Hair Wax** *($9.95 for 2.3 ounces)* is another fairly heavy pomade that is a bit more greasy than the Heavy Wax Firm Hold Hair Wax above. This works great to tame frizzies and smooth hair that is thick, coarse, or highly textured. It is not recommended for those with normal to fine or thin hair.

☺ **Lo:fi Medium Hold Gel** *($6.95 for 8.45 ounces)* is nearly identical to the Hi:fi Firm Hold Gel above, except this offers slightly less hold and is less sticky.

☺ **Straighten Smoothing Serum** *($8.95 for 8.4 ounces)* is a lightweight styling cream with a soft hold. It can smooth and straighten hair, but doesn't contain enough silicone to protect hair from heat, so this is best paired with a separate silicone serum if you intend to heat-style your hair.

☺ **$$$ Thick Stick Thickening Lotion** *($14.95 for 1.5 ounces)* is a creamy styling gel that provides a medium hold plus conditioning agents that can keep hair from getting stiff and allow it to be easily brushed through. This works well to provide some protection during heat-styling, but the small amount of product you get for the price is a bit of a burn. If you have thick or coarse hair, this will be gone in a month!

☺ **Up Firm Hold Hairspray** *($8.95 for 8.4 ounces)* is a nonaerosol hairspray that provides a medium, flexible hold that lets hair be brushed through. There isn't anything exceptional about this product, but it works to keep hair in place without making it feel too stiff or sticky.

DHC

Aside from locations in a few California shopping malls, this Japanese cosmetics line is primarily mail order. They offer a huge assortment of products, the bulk of which fall into the skin-care category. The hair-care products are noteworthy because none of them contain coloring agents and two of them are completely fragrance-free, which is quite a rarity and definitely gives this line credibility. I wish the entire line was fragrance-free, but something is better than nothing. Actually, the rest of DHC's hair-care line isn't anything to get excited about, especially when you consider the higher-than-average prices. For more information about DHC, call (800) DHC-CARE or visit www.dhccare.com.

What's Good About This Line: One of only a handful of hair-care lines to offer a truly fragrance-free shampoo and conditioner.

What's Not So Good About It: A few of the products contain irritating essential oils, while the specialty products are fraught with irritants; given the basic formulations, the line is more expensive than it needs to be.

☺ $$$ **Baby Hair Shampoo** *($6 for 3.3 ounces)* is an exceptionally mild, fragrance-free shampoo that is an excellent option for babies and adults, though the detergent cleansing agents are not strong enough to cut through styling products, nor are they effective for those with an oily scalp. If you have a sensitive, itchy scalp, this shampoo is a marvelous option. It will not cause buildup, and, overall, the price is somewhat reasonable (at least in comparison to the other hair products in this line).

☹ **Head Shampoo** *($17.50 for 10.1 ounces)* contains sodium lauryl sulfate as one of its main detergent cleansing agents, and that makes this strangely named shampoo too drying for all hair and scalp types. The rosemary leaf oil can cause further scalp irritation.

☺ $$$ **Mild Shampoo** *($17.50 for 10.8 ounces)* isn't as mild as the Baby Hair Shampoo above, but is a good, basic shampoo for all hair types that will not cause buildup.

☺ $$$ **Hair Treatment** *($19.50 for 7 ounces)* is a good, though exceptionally standard, conditioner for normal to dry hair of any thickness. Calling this a treatment product is a gross exaggeration, though I suppose they needed to justify the steep price for what is essentially a basic hair conditioner.

☺ $$$ **Head Conditioner** *($16 for 6.7 ounces)* is fragrance-free and is a good conditioner for normal to slightly dry hair that is normal to fine or thin. It is a great option for someone with a sensitive, itchy scalp.

☹ **Hair Tonic** *($36 for 6 ounces)* is sold as an aid to free the scalp of impurities and fortify the cuticle with B vitamins, but this liquid is problematic on numerous counts, since it includes potent scalp irritants such as capsicum, menthol, and resorcinol, and fragrant plant extracts known for their potential as an irritant, not a benefit, for the skin (scalp).

☹ **Head Oil** *($17.50 for 1 ounce)* is primarily olive oil, which you probably already have in your kitchen cupboard. This product also contains vitamin E and plant extracts, but these won't help nourish the hair or scalp when applied topically. The inclusion of arnica and rosemary oil is a problem, and makes it even easier to recommend skipping this product in favor of plain olive oil. Your scalp and pocketbook will both be better off.

DOVE

Every time a hair-care line launches—especially from a known cosmetics line—I still have some hope that their formulations will truly be different from what's already crowding the shelves. After all, with so much competition, a hair-care line that can deliver on its promises or offer something no other line does has a good chance of winning consumer loyalty and may enjoy some longevity before it's superceded by the next impossible-to-resist hair-care claim. According to Joanne Crudele, senior development manager for Dove Hair Care, "The new line of Dove Hair Care products was formulated in response to the needs of women who have been looking for shampoos and conditioners that can deliver both moisture and body simultaneously…. Other products on the market today primarily focus on delivering one benefit, with all other benefits being secondary" (Source:

PRNewswire, Press Release, Dove Hair Care, January 28, 2003). Doesn't that sound like Dove Hair Care is the only line that goes beyond what other hair-care products provide *and* gives women precisely what they want? Nothing can be further from the truth. Dove's shampoos do contain a fair amount of glycerin, which can cling to the hair shaft and prevent moisture loss. However, every Dove shampoo also contains a small amount of ammonium xylenesulfonate, a detergent cleansing agent and solvent that can cause scalp irritation and dryness, and several products contain TEA-dodecylbenzenesulfonate, a drying detergent cleansing agent. The silk-derived amino acids, which look impressive on the label, are present in such small quantities that your hair won't even notice them, and the same comments apply to the fatty acids from the barely present borage extract.

Dove is owned by Unilever, one of the largest consumer product companies in the world. Unilever also owns the Finesse, Suave, Salon Selectives, and Thermasilk hair-care lines, which the Dove addition closely resembles. If anything, the Dove Hair Care line is simply capitalizing on a familiar, secure brand name and does little to diversify or improve your choice of hair-care products. For more information about Dove, call (800) 598-5005 or visit www.dove.com.

What's Good About This Line: The conditioners will detangle and make hair feel smooth and soft; the line is affordable for most consumers.

What's Not So Good About It: No great shampoo options, because all of them contain ammonium xylenesulfonate.

☹ **Shampoo, Beautifully Clean** *($4.29 for 12 ounces)* is a standard shampoo that also contains ammonium xylenesulfonate, which can cause unnecessary scalp dryness and irritation.

☹ **Shampoo, Extra Volume** *($4.29 for 12 ounces)* is nearly identical to the Shampoo, Beautifully Clean above, and the same basic comments apply.

☹ **Shampoo, Intense Moisture** *($4.29 for 12 ounces)* doesn't contain anything that makes it more intense than many other conditioning shampoos, including those from TRESemme, Thermasilk, and L'Oreal. The difference is that this formula contains ammonium xylenesulfonate, which is a shame, because this would otherwise be a very good conditioning shampoo for normal to dry hair.

☹ **Shampoo, Moisture Rich Color** *($4.29 for 12 ounces)* is virtually identical to the Shampoo, Intense Moisture above, and the same basic comments apply. With the exception of the ammonium xylenesulfonate, this is a gentle shampoo, but it's not in any way distinctive for color-treated hair.

☹ **Shampoo, Volumizing Color** *($4.29 for 12 ounces)* is virtually identical to the Shampoo, Moisture Rich Color above, and the same basic comments apply. There is too much silicone in this shampoo to create volume, especially for someone with fine or thin hair.

☹ **2 in 1 Shampoo and Conditioner, Beautifully Clean** *($4.29 for 12 ounces)* is nearly identical to the Shampoo, Volumizing Color above, and the same basic comments apply. If this is being sold as a two-in-one option, then several of Dove's other shampoos also fit this description. However, in addition to the ammonium xylenesulfonate, this particular shampoo also contains TEA-dodecylbenzenesulfonate, which can be doubly drying to hair and scalp.

☻ **2 in 1 Shampoo and Conditioner, Extra Volume** *($4.29 for 12 ounces)* is identical to the 2 in 1 Shampoo and Conditioner, Beautifully Clean above, and the same comments apply.

☻ **2 in 1 Shampoo and Conditioner, Intense Moisture** *($4.29 for 12 ounces)* is identical to the 2 in 1 Shampoo and Conditioner, Extra Volume above, and the same comments apply. The repetitiveness among these formulas is ridiculous! Why not just sell one formula that supplies moisture, volume, *and* clean hair?

☺ **Conditioner, Extra Volume** *($4.29 for 12 ounces)* is a very basic conditioner with a lightweight formula helpful for someone with normal to fine or thin hair.

☺ **Conditioner, Intense Daily Conditioning Treatment** *($4.29 for 12 ounces)* is a more elegant conditioner than the Conditioner, Extra Volume above, and better for normal to dry hair because it contains silicones. Still, this is a no-frills product and can't compete with similar conditioners from Pantene that include silicones with panthenol, an excellent hair-conditioning agent.

☺ **Conditioner, Intense Moisture** *($4.29 for 12 ounces)* is nearly identical to the Conditioner, Extra Volume above, and the same basic comments apply. Someone with dry, thick, damaged, or coarse hair will not find this conditioner intensely moisturizing in the least.

☺ **Conditioner, Moisture Rich Color** *($4.29 for 12 ounces)* is nearly identical to the Conditioner, Extra Volume above, and the same basic comments apply. There is nothing about this conditioner that makes it preferred for keeping color-treated hair moist.

☺ **Conditioner, Volumizing Color** *($4.29 for 12 ounces)* is nearly identical to the Conditioner, Extra Volume above, and the same basic comments apply. Again, there was no need for Dove to launch so many conditioners if they were going to rely on the same basic formulation for them all.

☺ **Foam Conditioner, Extra Volume** *($3.99 for 9 ounces)* is a very light conditioner dispensed by propellants as foam. It is a top choice for fine or thin hair that is dry. Note that this is a rinse-out rather than a leave-in conditioner.

☺ **Foam Conditioner, Volumizing Color** *($3.99 for 9 ounces)* is identical to the Foam Conditioner, Extra Volume above, and the same review applies. Nothing in this conditioner can protect color-treated hair from fading.

FINESSE

For more information about finesse, call (800) 621-2013 or visit www.finesse haircare.com.

What's Good About This Line: Affordable, well-formulated shampoos and basic, but effective, conditioners; overall excellent hairsprays for flexible, soft hold.

The Reviews F

What's Not So Good About It: The shampoos and conditioners are remarkably similar, despite the different hair types they're marketed toward; no conditioners for those with dry to very dry hair that is normal to coarse or thick.

☺ **Color Care Shampoo** *($3.79 for 15 ounces)* is a standard shampoo that is good for all hair types except fine or thin hair. The silicone in this shampoo makes it great for dry or damaged hair, but it can cause buildup with repeated use. Nothing about this shampoo makes it particularly special for color-treated hair.

☺ **Curl Hydrating Shampoo** *($3.69 for 15 ounces)* is almost identical to the Color Care Shampoo above, and the same basic comments apply.

☺ **Enhancing Shampoo** *($3.79 for 15 ounces)* is similar to the Color Care Shampoo above, except it contains much less silicone, so the risk of buildup is minimal. This is a great shampoo for all hair types.

☺ **Moisturizing Shampoo** *($3.79 for 15 ounces)* is nearly identical to the Color Care Shampoo above, and the same basic comments apply.

☺ **Volumizing Shampoo** *($3.79 for 15 ounces)* is nearly identical to the Enhancing Shampoo above, and the same comments apply.

☺ **Enhancing Shampoo Plus Conditioner** *($3.79 for 15 ounces)* is nearly identical to the Color Care Shampoo above, and the same basic comments apply. If finesse is serious about this shampoo being a "two-in-one" option, then so are most of the other shampoos in their line that contain this much silicone.

☺ **Moisturizing Shampoo Plus Conditioner** *($3.79 for 15 ounces)* is nearly identical to the Color Care Shampoo above, and the same comments apply.

☺ **Color Care Conditioner** *($3.79 for 15 ounces)* is a standard, but good, conditioner that contains mostly water, thickener, water-binding agents, detangling agent, silicone, sunscreen (which does not protect hair from UV damage because it is rinsed away), fragrance, anti-static agent, preservatives, and vitamins. This would work well for normal to slightly dry hair that is normal to fine or thin.

☺ **Curl Hydrating Conditioner** *($3.79 for 15 ounces)* is nearly identical to the Color Care Conditioner above, and the same basic comments apply.

☺ **Enhancing Conditioner** *($3.79 for 15 ounces)* is nearly identical to the Color Care Conditioner above, and the same basic comments apply.

☺ **Moisturizing Conditioner** *($3.79 for 15 ounces)* is nearly identical to the Color Care Conditioner above, and the same basic comments apply.

☺ **Volumizing Conditioner** *($3.79 for 15 ounces)* is nearly identical to the Color Care Conditioner above, and the same basic comments apply.

☺ **Touchables Hair Spray, Extra Hold, Scented (Aerosol)** *($3.89 for 7 ounces)* is a light-hold hairspray that is not stiff or sticky and is easily brushed through. The silicones add a touch of shine to the hair and aid with combing.

☺ **Touchables Hair Spray, Extra Hold, Scented (Non-Aerosol)** *($3.89 for 8.5 ounces)* is a great choice for a truly soft, brushable hold that does not make hair feel stiff and is barely sticky. This is another good option for those who hate standard "helmet head" hairsprays!

☺ **Touchables Hair Spray, Extra Hold, Unscented (Aerosol)** *($3.89 for 7 ounces)* is identical to the Touchables Hair Spray, Extra Hold, Scented (Aerosol) above, except this has a much lighter scent (which means it is not really fragrance-free). Otherwise, the same comments apply.

☺ **Touchables Hair Spray, Extra Hold, Unscented (Non-Aerosol)** *($3.89 for 7 ounces)* is identical to the Touchables Hair Spray, Extra Hold, Scented (Non-Aerosol) above, except this has a much lighter scent.

☺ **Touchables Hair Spray, Maximum Hold (Aerosol)** *($3.89 for 7 ounces)* doesn't offer maximum hold, but does offer more hold than the Touchables aerosol hairsprays above. This medium-hold option leaves hair feeling slightly stiff and sticky, but hair remains surprisingly easy to brush through and holds its shape well.

☺ **Touchables Hair Spray, Maximum Hold (Non-Aerosol)** *($3.89 for 8.5 ounces)* offers slightly more hold than the Touchables Hair Spray, Extra Hold (Non-Aerosol) options above, but not enough to make choosing this one imperative.

☺ **Touchables Mousse, Curl Defining** *($3.79 for 7 ounces)* is an extra-light-textured mousse with a light, conditioned hold that is not stiff or sticky. This is an excellent mousse for fine or thin hair, be it curly or straight.

☺ **Touchables Mousse, Extra Control** *($3.79 for 7 ounces)* is nearly identical to the Touchables Mousse, Curl Defining above, except this offers slightly more hold, which is enough to make a difference if your hair needs that bit of extra help to hold its style.

☺ **Touchables Mousse, Moisturizing** *($3.79 for 7 ounces)* is identical to the Touchables Mousse, Curl Defining above, and the same comments apply. All of the Touchables mousses can moisturize, just not very substantially.

FOLLIGEN

Folligen hopes to be the one and only company those who are suffering from hair loss and baldness will turn to for a solution. The company's claims revolve around the use of copper peptides to stimulate dormant hair follicles to become active again (thus regrowing lost hair), while also creating a healthier scalp so that new and existing hair has a more robust hair shaft, resulting in stronger individual hairs.

The line was started by Dr. Loren Pickart, who has been studying copper peptides since the early 1970s and founded ProCyte in 1985. While at ProCyte, Pickart parlayed his copper peptide technology into the Tricomin line of products, which are still sold today. Pickart left ProCyte after his original copper tripeptide complex failed FDA clinical trials for wound healing, and in 1994 began another company, Skin Biology, which markets the Folligen line. I assume some bad blood developed between Pickart and his colleagues at ProCyte because Skin Biology's Web site makes frequent reference to the inferior copper peptide products from ProCyte, noting Folligen's superior level of breakdown-resistant copper peptides, the absence of blue dyes (signifying that using a dye might make it appear that there is more copper in the formula than there actually is), and lower cost per ounce. Clearly, Pickart believes his latest copper peptide formulations are the best, never mind that they paid a lab to substantiate these claims and that there's little corroborating evidence from anyone other than those involved in selling products containing copper.

But for the whole picture, it is important to understand a little background about hair loss. It is estimated that about 95% of all cases of hair loss, even for women, are the result of male-pattern baldness, technically referred to as androgenetic alopecia. "Androgenetic" refers to male hormones such as testosterone and dihydrotestosterone, and "alopecia" is the medical term for hair loss. Many different types of hormones affect hair growth, but the hormones with the largest impact are the androgens, which are responsible for increasing the size of hair follicles early in life, and, ironically, for decreasing and shrinking the hair follicles later in life. Certain male hormones cause the growth cycle of hair to slow (decreasing the growth phase and lengthening the resting phase) and eventually stop altogether.

Technically, what is in part believed to be taking place in the hair follicle is that testosterone is being changed to dihydrotestosterone (DHT) by the enzyme 5-alpha reductase (5AR). DHT slows and ultimately stops hair growth. It is also believed that the effect of DHT is compounded or enhanced by an individual's genetic hair-follicle traits (Sources: www.emedicine.com; *Journal of Alternative and Complementary Medicine*, April 2002, pages 143–152; *British Journal of Dermatology*, April 2004, pages 750–752; *Journal of the American Academy of Dermatology*, May 2004, pages 777–779; and *Journal of Investigative Dermatology*, December 2003, pages 1561–1564).

Is there good science behind using copper peptides to combat hair loss? The theory is that copper peptides stimulate the growth of the blood supply, which reinvigorates the hair follicle. The "reawakened" follicle then ignores any alternative messages from the androgens and instead thrives again. Just how the blood supply stops the effect of androgens on the growth cycle of hair is the puzzle, because the blood supply is not the cause of hair loss in the first place. If it were, then baldness would be a diffuse, generalized problem, instead of occurring as a specific pattern on the head. Why does the blood-supply problem occur only at the front or center of the scalp and not at the back? Further, successful research on improving hair growth for male-pattern baldness over the past decade has involved blocking 5AR from creating DHT.

It is also important to realize that despite years of Pickart's professing that copper peptides can restore hair growth, not a single substantiated study on humans exists to support his claims. His product information still refers to studies performed in the early 1990s that examined the effect of copper peptide on hair growth on the backs of mice. These results, though initially promising, were never proven true for humans. Even the links on Pickart's own Web site to clinical and safety studies are not for his products. Rather, all of the studies he lists pertain to using copper in skin-care products and mention nothing about stimulating dormant hair follicles or promoting hair growth. For more information about Folligen, call (800) 405-1912 or visit www.folligen.com. Note: Folligen also sells their version of Rogaine, offering ☺ $$$ **2% Minoxidil for Women** (*$17.95 for 2 ounces*) and ☺ $$$ **5% Minoxidil for Men** (*$18.95 for 2 ounces*). These over-the-counter drugs contain the same active ingredient used in Rogaine, and there's every reason to expect they would work just as well.

What's Good About This Line: Achieving hair growth results from these products is sketchy at best, but a few can function as good leave-in conditioners.

What's Not So Good About It: Copper peptides are overhyped and unproven for stimulating hair growth and/or preventing hair loss.

☹ **Therapy Shampoo** (*$19.95 for 8 ounces*) contains sodium C14-16 olefin sulfonate as its main detergent cleansing agent, which can be drying for both scalp and hair.

☺ $$$ **Therapy Conditioner** (*$19.95 for 8 ounces*) contains mostly aloe, detangling agent, thickener, panthenol, copper peptides, conditioning agents, plant extracts, fragrance, slip agent, and preservatives. This can work as a detangling conditioner for normal to slightly dry hair that is normal to fine or thin. There is no solid evidence that copper peptides will help restore hair growth or prevent hair loss, and once rinsed away they don't have much chance to affect the blood supply in the hair follicle.

☺ $$$ **Cream** (*$21.95 for 2 ounces*) is recommended by Folligen as scalp cream to be used along the hairline to improve hair follicle health and scalp vitality. This is an emollient conditioner that can soften and smooth the hair, but, as stated above, there is no solid evidence that the copper peptides or the saw palmetto oil can slow hair loss or improve healthy hair growth. At best, this is a very expensive (but good) leave-in conditioner for normal to very dry hair that is normal to coarse or thick.

☺ $$$ **Emu Oil S Lipid Replenisher for Hair** (*$29.95 for 2 ounces*) is just emu oil with saw palmetto and vitamin E. Like all oils, it can moisturize dry, damaged hair, but emu oil isn't any better for replenishing lipids than most other oils, including jojoba, olive, and safflower. According to Folligen's web site, a Boston University study found that emu oil activated 80% of dormant hair follicles, causing them to revert to the growing stage again. However, this study was neither published nor substantiated; the only references to it appear on Web sites selling hair-growth products that contain emu oil. If emu oil could awaken dormant hair follicles, we would see very few people with receding hairlines and baldness! The smiling face rating is strictly for this product's ability to moisturize, not regrow, hair.

Saw palmetto has far more interesting properties relating to hair growth. There is research showing it can inhibit 5AR (the enzyme that converts testosterone to the hair-stopping DHT) when taken orally. However, no research has been done with saw palmetto in relation to hair growth. The studies that do exist have been concerned with use of saw palmetto in the treatment of benign prostatic hyperplasia (BPH). Both BPH and male-pattern baldness are affected by the production of DHT. This research has shown that saw palmetto can block the production of DHT by inhibiting 5AR, so it isn't a stretch to assume that saw palmetto may therefore be effective in the treatment of male-pattern baldness (Sources: www.naturaldatabase.com; *Journal of the American Medical Association*, November 1998, pages 1604–1609; *American Family Physician*, March 2003, pages 1281–1283; and *Urological Research*, June 2000, pages 201–209). But you don't need this product to gain benefit from saw palmetto. Saw palmetto supplements are available for far less money at health food and most major grocery stores.

☺ **$$$ Lotion** *($21.95 for 2 ounces)* is a lightweight version of the Cream above, and the same comments apply.

☺ **$$$ Solution Therapy Spray** *($36.95 for 8 ounces)* contains the same copper peptide complex as the Cream and Lotion above, but omits the saw palmetto oil. Because this product has minimal conditioning properties (it isn't even a good detangler), it is not rated as well as the Cream and Lotion products.

FRAMESI

Framesi prides itself on being a superior hair-care line for color-treated hair. Their main group of products is the Biogenol Color Care collection, and each features Framesi's Phycocorail Color Shield Protective Ingredient System. Phycocorail is not a registered ingredient with the Cosmetic, Toiletry, and Fragrance Association (CTFA) and appears to be a made-up name representing a blend of algae and coral extracts that appear in some of Framesi's products. Aside from the romanticized story of marine algae harvested from the sea, can this ingredient really keep hair color from fading? Absolutely not. At best, it can serve as a water-binding agent for hair, but any antioxidant benefits would be either rinsed down the drain or destroyed by blow dryers, curling irons, flat irons, or even brushing.

The Biogenol products also contain protein-bonded superoxide dismutase, an antioxidant that has no protective benefit for the hair, though it can be a good moisturizing ingredient for the scalp. In short, if you routinely color-treat your hair (and the majority of women do), Framesi is not the fail-safe solution you may be seeking. For more information about Framesi, call (800) 321-9648 or visit www.framesi.it.

What's Good About This Line: The Framesi Shine In line offers a fragrance-free shampoo and conditioner; for a salon line, prices are reasonable; some good conditioners and a few excellent styling products.

What's Not So Good About It: A few of the shampoos contain drying detergent cleansing agents; several styling products contain the sensitizing preservatives methylchloroisothiazolinone and methylisothiazolinone (Kathon CG).

FRAMESI BIOGENOL COLOR CARE SYSTEM

☺ **Biogenol Color Care System Bathe Moisturizing Shampoo** *($11 for 16 ounces)* is a very standard, but good, shampoo for all hair types. It poses a slight risk of buildup and holds no special benefit for color-treated hair—but it is by no means problematic for those who dye their hair, either.

☺ **Biogenol Color Care System Clarifying Shampoo** *($11 for 16 ounces)* is a good, basic shampoo that is an excellent choice for all hair types, and it does not cause buildup.

☹ **Biogenol Color Care System Nourishing Shampoo** *($11 for 16 ounces)* contains TEA-lauryl sulfate as its main detergent cleansing agent, which is hardly nourishing. This shampoo can be too drying for all hair and scalp types and is not recommended.

☹ **Biogenol Color Care System Replenishing Shampoo** *($11.50 for 16 ounces)* is nearly identical to the Biogenol Color Care System Nourishing Shampoo above, and the same comments apply.

☺ **Biogenol Color Care System Ultra Body Shampoo** *($11 for 16 ounces)* is a standard, but good, shampoo for fine or thin hair. The film-forming agent can attach itself to the hair shaft and create fuller, thicker-feeling hair, but it can build up with repeated use, making normal to fine or thin hair flat and limp. To avoid this, alternate with a shampoo that does not build up.

☺ **Biogenol Color Care System Violights Shampoo** *($11 for 10.1 ounces)* is the gentlest Framesi shampoo, and is an outstanding option for all but oily hair types. It poses a slight risk of buildup. The "Violights" in the name refers to the violet dye in this shampoo, which has minimal impact on highlighting silver/gray hair or softening brassy tones.

☺ **Biogenol Color Care System Leave-In Conditioner** *($10 for 10.1 ounces)* is a very good, leave-in, detangling conditioner for normal to slightly dry hair that is normal to fine or thin.

☺ **Biogenol Color Care System Moisture-Rinse** *($10 for 10.1 ounces)* is a standard conditioner that can work for normal to dry hair of any thickness.

☺ **Biogenol Color Care System Reconditioner for Dry, Damaged Hair** *($11 for 10.1 ounces)* is nearly identical to the Biogenol Color Care System Moisture-Rinse above, and the same comments apply. This is not an optimum choice for dry, damaged hair.

☺ **$$$ Biogenol Color Care System Anti-Frizz/Smoothing Cream** *($10 for 4.23 ounces)* is similar to a leave-in conditioner, but with a light hold that leaves hair smooth, soft, and minimally sticky. The tiny amount of superoxide dismutase in this product cannot prevent hair color from fading, but overall this is a good styling cream for normal to dry hair that is normal to coarse or thick.

☹ **Biogenol Color Care System Bodifying Foam, Strong Hold** *($12 for 9 ounces)* is a standard, propellant-based styling mousse that dries quickly and offers a medium hold with a slightly sticky finish that can be brushed through. However, it contains the preservative Kathon CG, which is too sensitizing for use in leave-on products if it gets on the skin.

☹ **Biogenol Color Care System Bodifying Spray, for Fine Hair** *($10 for 10.1 ounces)* contains sodium polystyrene sulfonate as one of its main film-forming agents, an ingredient that can dry the hair and scalp and potentially fade hair color.

☹ **Biogenol Color Care System Brash, Hard Gel** *($7 for 4.23 ounces)* contains the preservative Kathon CG, which is contraindicated for use in leave-on products due to the high probability of causing a sensitizing reaction on the scalp.

The Reviews F

☹ **Biogenol Color Care System Definition, Conditioning Creme Gel** *($15 for 8.5 ounces)* contains the preservative Kathon CG, which is contraindicated for use in leave-in products due to the high probability of causing a sensitizing reaction on the scalp.

☺ **$$$ Biogenol Color Care System Design Spray (Aerosol)** *($12 for 10 ounces)* is a standard hairspray that provides a light, flexible hold and gives enough play time so you can continue to style (and restyle) your hair as you use it. The minor amount of conditioning agents can help with comb-through, but it provides no protective benefit for color-treated hair.

☹ **Biogenol Color Care System Dew** *($12.50 for 2 ounces)* is water-soluble pomade that contains the preservative Kathon CG, which is a sensitizer if it gets on the skin. This product is not recommended.

☺ **Biogenol Color Care System Forming Glaze, Strong Hold** *($9 for 10.1 ounces)* contains mostly water, film-forming/holding agents, water-binding agents, conditioning agents, slip agent, fragrance, and preservatives. It's a typical, but workable, styling gel that offers a light (not strong) hold that leaves hair soft and smooth. This would work well for all hair types.

☺ **Biogenol Color Care System Snapp, Curl Rejuvenator** *($10 for 10.1 ounces)* is an exceptional styling spray that contains several very good water-binding and conditioning agents, along with a lightweight film-forming agent for a soft, non-sticky hold. This would be ideal for curly or textured hair to create natural definition while drying hair with a diffuser.

☺ **Biogenol Color Care System Spray Gel, Firm Hold** *($10 for 10.1 ounces)* is a standard, but very good, spray gel that provides medium hold that can feel slightly sticky, yet allows the hair to be easily brushed through. This contains an excellent blend of conditioning agents as well.

☺ **Biogenol Color Care System Stop-Frizz, Anti-Humectant** *($12.50 for 2 ounces)* is a thick styling cream that at first seems like it will feel heavier than it really does. Once applied to the hair, this becomes a lightweight balm that provides mild smoothing and shine-enhancing benefits without a trace of hold. It can work well for normal to dry hair that is normal to fine, and works equally well on wet or dry hair. Keeping moisture out of the hair shaft on a humid day is next to impossible, though most styling products that provide hold or coat the hair can help a little.

☺ **Biogenol Color Care System Thick & Body, Styling Gel** *($9 for 4.23 ounces)* is a standard styling gel with medium hold that tends to stay slightly sticky, though it can be brushed through. The conditioning agents can provide some heat protection, and the mica adds additional shine, though the shiny particles have a slight tendency to flake when you brush through your hair.

☺ **$$$ Biogenol Color Care System Ultra-Deep Masque** *($13 for 4 ounces)* isn't that deep at all. This is a standard conditioner that is similar to, but thicker than, the Biogenol Color Care System Moisture-Rinse above, and the same basic comments apply.

FRAMESI SHINE IN

☺ **Shine In Shampoo** *($11 for 10 ounces)* doesn't add more shine to the hair than any other standard shampoo with silicone. The best reason to consider this shampoo is that it is completely fragrance-free and would work well for all hair types. It poses a slight risk of buildup with repeated use.

☺ **Shine In Conditioner** *($10 for 10 ounces)* is a fragrance-free conditioner that is a good, basic option for normal to dry hair of any thickness.

☺ **Shine In Frizz Away, Frizz Eliminator and Straightener** *($10 for 2 ounces)* is nearly identical to the Biogenol Color Care System Anti-Frizz/Smoothing Cream above, except this one contains no film-forming/holding agent. Otherwise, the same comments apply.

☺ **Shine In Gelly, for All Hair Types** *($10 for 5 ounces)* is a very standard, firm-hold styling gel that has a liquidy texture and can leave hair feeling stiff and sticky.

☺ **Shine In Mousse, for All Hair Types** *($10 for 9 ounces)* is a propellant-based styling mousse with medium hold that can feel slightly sticky, though it can easily be brushed through. It would work for normal to fine hair that needs sufficient styling control.

☺ **$$$ Shine In Polishing Cream** *($16 for 5 ounces)* is a light-textured styling cream that can leave hair looking slick and slightly greasy. It's best for normal to very dry hair that needs light smoothing or help taming frizzies. Use it sparingly for best results.

☺ **Shine In Polishing Spray** *($17 for 8 ounces)* is an alcohol-based, no-hold shine spray that contains a blend of emollients, silicone, and plant oil. This works well as a glossing spray on dry to very dry hair that is normal to coarse, curly, or thick.

☺ **Shine In Take Hold (Aerosol)** *($10 for 10 ounces)* is a standard, light-hold hairspray that keeps hair soft and flexible, so you can easily brush through or restyle your hair. It leaves a minimally sticky finish with barely any stiffness.

FRÉDÉRIC FEKKAI HAIR CARE

Frédéric Fekkai is yet another hairstylist to the rich and famous who has created his own line of products. And, like hairdressers Vidal Sassoon and Jose Eber years before him and (more recently) Charles Worthington, Fekkai has written a book on the subject of hair care (along with other elements of style, from makeup to nail polish to luxurious living). His salon/spas are in some of the most chic locations, one presiding above a Chanel boutique in New York City and another filling a penthouse on Beverly Hills' fabled Rodeo Drive. Fekkai's talents are up to the status of his desirable locations, but how do his products measure up? Well, without the benefit of Fekkai's personal hands-on touch, it takes nothing more than a cursory look at his products' formulas to see that his shampoos, conditioners, and styling products are not at all unique, but are actually rather standard, ordinary formulations. The smattering of plant extracts and vitamins thrown in (carrot extract, vitamin A) are for the sake of making an impression on consumers and have no benefit for hair. Fekkai's claims about using naturally derived cleansing ingredients can be made for all cleansing agents in shampoos because they are all derived primarily from coconut. But they are far removed from the natural state—you wouldn't want to use them in your pina colada!

Choosing most of these pricey formulas over less expensive options is a bit like requesting chocolate decadence and receiving just plain old Duncan Heinz chocolate cake (which is great if you knew that's what you were really paying for). For more information on Frédéric Fekkai, call (212) 583-3359 or visit www.fredericfekkai.com.

What's Good About This Line: The line presents a wide variety of conditioners and styling products to meet the needs of every hair type and style; a few styling products go beyond standard to outstanding performance.

What's Not So Good About It: Many of these shampoos contain drying detergent cleansing agents; one of the styling products contains the problematic sodium polystyrene sulfonate; and the prices are high.

☹ **Apple Cider Clarifying Shampoo** *($18.50 for 8 ounces)* contains TEA-lauryl sulfate as its main detergent cleansing agent, and that makes this ordinary shampoo too drying and irritating to the scalp.

☺ $$$ **Baby Blonde Color Enhancing Shampoo with Chamomile** *($18.50 for 8 ounces)* contains a minuscule amount of chamomile, but it's the synthetic coloring agents that have the (minimal) enhancing effect on blonde hair. This is just a standard, but good, shampoo for all hair types that poses minimal to no risk of buildup.

☹ **Full Volume Shampoo** *($18.50 for 8 ounces)* is nearly identical to the Apple Cider Clarifying Shampoo above, and the same comments apply.

☹ **Brilliant Brown Color Enhancing Shampoo with Coffee** *($20 for 8 ounces)* contains TEA-lauryl sulfate as one of its main detergent cleansing agents, which makes it too drying for all hair and scalp types. What a shame, because otherwise this would be a great color-enhancing shampoo for brunettes.

☹ **Rio Red Color Enhancing Shampoo** *($20 for 8 ounces)* is, save for a change in dye agents, identical to the Brilliant Brown Color Enhancing Shampoo above, and the same unfortunate comments apply.

☺ $$$ **Gently Clean Extra Gentle Shampoo** *($18.50 for 8 ounces)* is indeed extra gentle, and is an excellent shampoo for babies and children, though it would be even better without the fragrance. The gentle detergent cleansing agents are from a group of ingredients known as amphoteric surfactants, and the trade-off for their mildness is that they aren't the best for washing away styling products.

☺ $$$ **Glossing Shampoo** *($20 for 8 ounces)* is a very good conditioning shampoo for dry hair that is normal to thick or coarse. This product has a softer scent than most other Fekkai shampoos.

☺ $$$ **Moisturizing Shampoo with Shea Butter** *($22.50 for 6 ounces)* is a standard, detergent-based shampoo that contains a minuscule amount of shea butter—and that's not enough to be much of a moisturizer for hair. It is a gentle shampoo that would work well for most hair types, but not so well for those who use heavy styling products. This does contain TEA-lauryl sulfate, but the amount used is likely too small to cause scalp and hair dryness.

☹ **Polished Platinum Brightening Shampoo** *($20 for 8 ounces)* contains TEA-lauryl sulfate as its main detergent cleansing agent, and, despite the moisturizing agents it also contains, it can still be too drying and irritating to the scalp.

☹ **Protein Rx Reparative Shampoo** *($20 for 8 ounces)* contains nothing that can repair the hair, because hair cannot be repaired—once it is broken (damaged), it can't be fixed, and especially not by a shampoo whose main detergent cleansing agent is the drying TEA-lauryl sulfate.

☹ **Technician Shampoo for Dry, Damaged, Color-Treated Hair** *($18.50 for 8 ounces)* contains sodium C14-16 olefin sulfonate as one of its main detergent cleansing agents, and that makes this shampoo a problem for all hair and scalp types. Those with color-treated hair, steer clear of this one!

☺ **$$$ Technician Shampoo for Normal Hair** *($18.50 for 8 ounces)* is an excellent shampoo that would work well for all hair types and will not cause buildup.

☺ **$$$ Apple Cider Clean Conditioner** *($18.50 for 8 ounces)* is a very lightweight conditioner that would work well for normal to slightly dry hair that is fine or thin. All of the showcased ingredients are listed well after the fragrance, however, which makes them nothing more than the merest window dressings. Its pH is 5, which means that the vinegar is not in the best acidic base to help the cuticle lay flat and reflect light.

☺ **$$$ Apple Cider Clearing Rinse** *($16.50 for 8 ounces)* is almost identical to the Apple Cider Clean Conditioner above, although the film-forming agent in this one can build up on the hair with repeated use—it won't remove "environmental and product residue" from the hair, as claimed.

☺ **$$$ Baby Blonde Conditioner** *($18.50 for 8 ounces)* is a fairly heavy conditioner that is an option for those with normal to very dry hair that is thick or coarse. Other than the coloring agents that give the product a blonde shade, there is nothing in this to make it preferred for blonde hair (and it's definitely not superior to John Frieda's Sheer Blonde products, which are half the price).

☺ **$$$ Full Volume Conditioner, Body Building Conditioner for Fine or Thin Hair** *($20 for 8 ounces)* is a good detangling conditioner for hair that is normal to fine or thin, but the film-forming agents can cause buildup.

☺ **$$$ Glossing Conditioner** *($20 for 8 ounces)* is a great conditioner for normal to dry hair of any thickness, though the film-forming agents may be too much for those with thick hair, and they will build up with repeated use.

☺ **$$$ Instant Detangler** *($18.50 for 8 ounces)* is an exceptionally lightweight conditioner/detangler that would work well for normal hair. There's not much to this, as all the interesting ingredients are listed well after the fragrance, but for a basic detangler, it will work as well as any.

☺ $$$ **Moisturizing Conditioner with Shea Butter** (*$22.50 for 6 ounces*) is a very good, emollient conditioner (the second listed ingredient is shea butter) for very dry hair. Other than that, it contains all the typical detangling and conditioning agents and would work well.

☺ $$$ **Protein Rx Reparative Conditioner** (*$20 for 8 ounces*) cannot repair anything. It is just a very standard, but good, conditioner that would work well for normal to dry hair of any thickness.

☺ $$$ **Technician Conditioner for Dry, Damaged, Color-Treated Hair** (*$18.50 for 8 ounces*) is a very good, very basic conditioner for normal to slightly dry hair of any thickness. The plant extracts don't amount to anything, but the tried-and-true conditioning agents are really doing all the work anyway. For dry or damaged hair, this doesn't hold a candle to Pantene conditioners!

☺ $$$ **Technician Conditioner for Normal Hair** (*$18.50 for 8 ounces*) is almost identical to the Technician Conditioner for Dry, Damaged Color-Treated Hair above, and the same comments apply.

☺ $$$ **Baby Blonde Hair Treatment** (*$22.50 for 5 ounces*) is a standard conditioner that features matricaria (chamomile) extract as one of the main ingredients. This is supposed to brighten color-treated blonde hair, but if it worked there would be no need for the standard synthetic coloring agents also present in this formula. This is a decent conditioner for normal to dry hair that is normal to fine or thin.

☺ $$$ **Hair Mask with Shea Butter** (*$22.50 for 5 ounces*) is a mixture of standard conditioning agents, plant oils, thickeners, and nut oils. It would work great for dry to very dry hair that is normal to coarse or thick, but it is still just a conditioner.

☺ $$$ **Finishing Polish** (*$20 for 1.7 ounces*) is a standard silicone serum that has a thick texture, which makes it preferred for those with coarse or thick hair. The addition of several plant oils sets this apart from many similar products, but doesn't justify the higher-than-average price.

☺ $$$ **Glossing Cream** (*$18.50 for 4 ounces*) is a water- and silicone-based styling cream that does not contain any holding agents, so it is best for smoothing dry hair, calming frizzies, and adding a lustrous shine. This can easily become too heavy and slick for those with fine or thin hair.

☺ $$$ **Full Volume Mousse** (*$18.50 for 5 ounces*) is a medium-hold, liquid-to-foam mousse that provides smooth, flexible control that is slightly sticky, but can be easily brushed through. It's a great (albeit expensive) option for fine or thin hair that is hard to hold.

☺ $$$ **Instant Volume Root Lifting Spray** (*$17.50 for 8 ounces*) is an alcohol-based styling spray that would work well on most hair types and has a minimally sticky feel and light hold.

☺ $$$ **Luscious Curls** (*$18.50 for 4 ounces*) has a texture similar to most standard conditioners, but it lists a film-forming/holding agent as the second ingredient, so it works more like a leave-in conditioner/styling product. It provides a light, moist hold that makes it easy to control and condition curly or wavy hair without feeling stiff, sticky, or flaking.

☺ $$$ **Pomade Cristal** *($18.50 for 2.6 ounces)* is a water-based, water-soluble pomade that is minimally greasy but can still smooth the hair (especially flyaways) and add shine. This contains tiny particles of mica for a crystalline shine that can look wet if this is overused, so be judicious with your application.

☺ $$$ **Sheer Hold Hairspray** *($22.50 for 5.8 ounces)* is a standard aerosol hairspray with a light application and a medium hold that still lets hair be brushed through with minimal stickiness. There is no reason to choose this over aerosol options at the drugstore, but you won't be disappointed if you decide to overspend on this product.

☺ $$$ **Smooth Hair** *($16.50 for 4 ounces)* is a lightweight styling cream with no stiff or sticky feel. It will help smooth the hair and cut down on frizzies, but use it sparingly, as too much can make the hair look and feel heavy.

☺ $$$ **Styling Gel** *($16.50 for 4 ounces)* is an exceptionally standard styling gel that provides a medium hold and a slightly sticky, stiff feel. Most of the conditioning agents are listed after the fragrance, so their presence is inconsequential for hair.

☺ $$$ **Straight Away Straightening Balm** *($16.50 for 4 ounces)* is a good, lightweight styling gel that has no stiff or sticky feel, but it only works when used with a blow dryer and the proper styling techniques that can help straighten and smooth hair.

☺ $$$ **Stylist Spray** *($17.50 for 8 ounces)* is almost identical to the Instant Volume Root Lifting Spray above, and the same comments apply.

☺ $$$ **Texturizing Balm** *($16.50 for 4 ounces)* is a standard styling gel that offers a light, flexible hold with minimal to no stiff or sticky feel. In fact, this makes hair feel quite soft. It would work well on all hair types and is a great alternative for consumers who typically shy away from gels.

☹ **Wave Spray** *($18.50 for 8 ounces)* contains sodium polystyrene sulfonate as its main film-forming/holding agent, which can dry the hair and potentially strip hair color. This product is not recommended.

☺ $$$ **Protein Rx Reparative Spray** *($18.50 for 4 ounces)* contains so little protein the name is almost a joke. What isn't so funny is that protein is not the prescription for repairing hair—actually, nothing can repair hair once it is damaged. This is a standard silicone spray that can add shine and help make hair a cinch to comb through, but that's about it. Avoid this product if you have fine or thin hair, because even a sheer application can be too greasy.

☺ $$$ **Protein Rx Reparative Treatment Mask** *($28.50 for 5.5 ounces)* is nearly identical to the Protein Rx Reparative Conditioner above, and the same comments apply. The addition of macadamia nut oil doesn't turn this conditioner into a special treatment for the hair.

☺ $$$ **Sun Protectant Spray** *($22.50 for 6 ounces)* contains nothing that can protect the hair from the sun, though it is a very good spray-on conditioner for all hair types. It does not contain film-forming agents, so stickiness should not be a problem, but the conditioning agents can build up with repeated use.

FEKKAI FOR MEN

☹ **Fekkai for Men Everyday Shampoo** *($20 for 7 ounces)* contains drying TEA-lauryl sulfate as one of its main detergent cleansing agents, and is not recommended.

☺ **$$$ Fekkai for Men Light Conditioner** *($20 for 7 ounces)* is nearly identical to the Protein Rx Reparative Conditioner above, and the same comments apply. Notice that the two products are the same price, but for some reason this one provides one ounce less product than the one above.

☺ **$$$ Fekkai for Men Grooming Clay** *($18.50 for 1.5 ounces)* is a traditional pomade packaged in a shoe polish tin–style container. This does contain clay, but it is used primarily as a thickener, and its drying effect is offset by the greater amount of Vaseline and beeswax in this product. Grooming Clay is best for dry to very dry hair that is coarse, curly, or thick. It can easily make hair look and feel greasy if not used sparingly.

☺ **$$$ Fekkai for Men Hair Gel** *($18.50 for 4 ounces)* is nearly identical to the Styling Gel above, except that this offers a bit more hold. Otherwise, the same comments apply. Why this formula costs two dollars more than the other is a mystery.

FREE & CLEAR

Minimalism can be a good thing, as is evidenced here by this small, but impressive, collection of products, each completely fragrance- and colorant-free and without a single unnecessarily irritating ingredient. Free & Clear, owned by Rochester, Minnesota–based Pharmaceutical Specialties, is sold in most major drugstores (ask your pharmacist). It is definitely worth seeking out if you have a sensitive scalp, itchiness, allergies, or have problems with commonly used preservatives, such as the parabens or phenoxyethanol. There are no frills or fancy ingredients in this line, but in a sea of hair-care products that take an everything-but-the-kitchen-sink approach to product formulation, this unique line is a wonderful change of pace! For more information about Free & Clear, call (800) 325-8232 or visit www.psico.com. **Note:** In Canada, the Free & Clear line is labeled Clinaderm, and their Web site is www.canderm.com.

What's Good About This Line: Every product is completely fragrance-free and formulated with gentle but effective ingredients.

What's Not So Good About It: Limited options for styling products; lack of conditioner options for those with dry to very dry or damaged hair.

☺ **Shampoo, for Sensitive Skin & Scalp** *($7.80 for 8 ounces)* is a standard, very basic shampoo that does not contain conditioning agents, so there is no chance of buildup. This works beautifully for all hair types (including color-treated), although someone with very oily hair or scalp may find they really do need to lather, rinse, and repeat.

☺ **Hair Conditioner, for Normal & Sensitive Skin** *($7.80 for 8 ounces)* is a no-frills, but effective, conditioner that is a good detangling conditioner for normal to slightly dry hair that is normal to fine or thin. Someone with thick, coarse, or damaged hair will need something more emollient.

☺ **Hair Spray for Sensitive Skin, Soft Hold** *($10.95 for 8 ounces)* is a standard, nonaerosol hairspray that offers a very light, touchable hold with no stiffness or stickiness. For natural, unstructured hairstyles, this is a great styling product.

☺ **Hair Spray for Sensitive Skin, Firm Hold** *($10.95 for 8 ounces)* is nearly identical to the Hair Spray for Sensitive Skin, Soft Hold above, except this offers slightly more hold. Otherwise, the same comments apply.

FRESH

The story of how Boston-bred "fresh" came to exist is full of compelling adjectives and phrases like "dynamic," "passions," "inspiration," and "destined to create." It seems that two happy newlyweds, both with artistic backgrounds, felt there was a void in the world of luxury bath soaps. They searched far and wide, but could not find a soap that met their criteria (it isn't exactly clear why they were searching for such a product). They began experimenting with their own formulas, gained local notice with what they developed, and yet another clone of The Body Shop was born. Of course, fresh didn't stop at soaps. They also sell "groundbreaking" products that capitalize on such innocuous-sounding, good-for-you ingredients as milk, rice, and soy, and fresh claims to "deliver these ingredients in abundance." fresh may want to double-check their ingredient lists (as you certainly should), since more often than not these "meaningful" ingredients are barely present, as is the case with most of their hair-care products.

Founders Lev Glazman and Alina Roytberg's success has led them from a single boutique in Boston to a series of shops in New York City, additional shops in Los Angeles, Chicago, and Paris, plus a presence in upscale department stores such as Bergdorf Goodman and Neiman Marcus. In 2000, fresh was purchased by luxury goods purveyor (and owner of Sephora) LVMH, a not-too-surprising alliance given fresh's price point and positioning.

The major issue I have with all of the fresh hair-care products is the potent scent wafting from each one. Fresh describes the fragrance in their products as "bright, beguiling" and as having the ability to "subtly remind you of its presence every now and then, like someone blowing gently in your ear." That romantic comparison would make sense if the fragrance were subtle, but all of the products are so fragranced you won't think someone has blown in your ear, you'll think they sounded an air horn right next to it! The scents may draw you in to visit fresh, but your scalp may not like it if you choose to stay. For more information on fresh, call (800) FRESH-20 or visit www.fresh.com.

What's Good About This Line: Despite the fragrance and fragrant plant extracts, many fresh hair-care products work well for their intended hair type, particularly the conditioners.

What's Not So Good About It: The potent fragrance, often present in amounts greater than the played-up plant extracts and oils; a mixed bag of effective and poor shampoos; entire line is overpriced given the container sizes and the overwhelmingly basic formulations.

☺ $$$ **Milk & Rose Shampoo** *($24 for 10 ounces)* is just shampoo, dressed up to appear more natural and pure by including rose-flower water and a tiny amount of milk protein, among other barely present plant extracts. This would work well for all hair types and does not cause buildup, but don't expect it to rejuvenate your hair as fresh says it will.

☺ $$$ **Rice Shampoo** *($24 for 10 ounces)* lists the film-forming acrylates/copolymers as the second ingredient, and that can quickly build up on the hair. Those with chemically treated hair may find that this shampoo makes their hair feel drier and brittle. This can be a good volumizing shampoo for fine or thin hair.

☹ **Soda Shampoo** *($22 for 10 ounces)* contains peppermint extract and lavender water as the main ingredients, and these are too irritating for the scalp. This also contains a large amount of fragrance. In fact, the fragrance is listed well before any of the back-to-nature ingredients fresh likes to include and boast about.

☺ $$$ **Soy Shampoo** *($22 for 10 ounces)* is just a standard shampoo for all hair types that has a lot more fragrance than soy, and a meager amount of ginseng root, which fresh incorrectly maintains can strengthen hair. There are also some conditioning ingredients, but the amounts are too small for them to have a noticeable effect on the hair.

☹ **Umbrian Clay Shampoo** *($24 for 5 ounces)* is based on fuller's earth (clay), which is drying for hair, so using it serves no purpose. This product also contains eucalyptus oil, which can be a scalp irritant, along with balm mint oil and enough potassium hydroxide to cause even more dryness. The clay-as-a-natural-remedy angle is enticing, but doesn't hold up in the real world.

☺ $$$ **Illipe Butter Conditioner** *($24 for 5 ounces)*. If your scalp can get past the lavender and bitter orange flower water, you will find this is a thick, creamy conditioner suitable for normal to very dry hair that is also coarse or thick. This very emollient conditioner works well for smoothing and detangling, but be sure you like the fragrance, because it can be overpowering.

☺ $$$ **Meadowfoam Cream Treatment Conditioner** *($32 for 5.1 ounces)* is recommended by fresh for extra dry, overprocessed, or disobedient thick hair, but it comes up a bit short for these hair types, which tend to do best with an emollient conditioner, which this conditioner is not. This could still work well for normal to dry hair that is normal to fine or slightly thick.

☺ $$$ **Pomegranate Conditioning Hair Rinse** *($22 for 8.8 ounces)* is a very basic conditioner for dry hair of any thickness. Pomegranate is considered effective as an anticarcinogen and antioxidant when taken orally, but there is no research showing what effect, if any, this extract has on skin or hair, especially when it is rinsed down the drain

(Sources: *Journal of Agricultural Food Chemistry*, January 2002, pages 81–86 and 166–171; and *International Journal of Oncology*, May 2002, pages 983–986).

☺ **$$$ Hair Cream, Extra Definition (All Hair Types)** *($20 for 3.5 ounces)* is more of a leave-in conditioner than a styling cream, as it does not contain any holding agents. It is appropriate for those with normal to dry hair that is not too fine or thin.

☺ **$$$ Hair Shine, Extra Polish (for Dull Hair)** *($24 for 1.8 ounces)* is one of the most expensive standard silicone serums around, but it does do the job of smoothing hair, adding a glasslike shine, and taming frizzies. Would I trade my Pantene or Citré Shine silicone serums for this? No, but for those who love to splurge on hair care this is a worthwhile product, and the fragrance isn't as penetrating as it is in the rest of fresh's hair-care products.

☹ **$$$ Hair Volumizing Tonic** *($22 for 5 ounces)* is almost identical to the Shaping Foam below, except this one sprays on instead of dispensing as a foam. It's just as highly fragranced, only this adds irritants like sage leaf and peppermint leaf, which have no purpose for hair or scalp and instead can cause irritation or a sensitizing reaction.

☹ **$$$ Shaping Foam** *($20 for 5 ounces)* is a liquid styling product dispensed as a foam, though no aerosols are used. The dispensing method is far more intriguing than what's inside, which is essentially eau de cologne with a firm-hold, slightly sticky film-forming agent. It's an option for all hair types, but not preferred to products like Aveda's Phomollient ($12 for 7 ounces) or TRESemme's Hydrology Moisture Mousse, Extra Hold ($3.99 for 8 ounces).

☺ **$$$ Styling Gel, Extra Control** *($20 for 3.5 ounces)* bestows hair-saving qualities on almost all of the plant- and food-based ingredients it contains, but cucumber can't restore hair and soy protein doesn't protect hair from the environment. Those make for good ad copy, but the heart of this product is a very standard, medium-hold styling gel that is a bit sticky, yet still allows you to brush through the hair.

☺ **$$$ Sugar Shea Butter** *($38 for 3.5 ounces)* is nothing more than fragranced shea butter, which can be a good emollient ingredient for dry scalp and hair, though it is not easy to rinse out when used in this amount. This expensive treatment can work well, but use it as an overnight treatment with the intent of shampooing it out the next morning, or as a 30-minute conditioner you apply before shampooing. For the record, Jason Natural Cosmetics also has a 100% pure Shea Nut Butter at $4.99 for 1.7 ounces that provides identical benefits and is fragrance-free.

FUDGE

For more information about Fudge, visit www.fudge.com.

What's Good About This Line: Fudge's prices and performance are often ahead of the curve; every category has praiseworthy products for almost all hair types.

What's Not So Good About It: There are no viable conditioner options for those with fine/thin or very dry hair; their Beach Bum Blonding products are a bust.

The Reviews F

☹ **Beach Bum Blonding Shampoo** *($12.96 for 10.1 ounces)* starts out as a standard, innocuous shampoo, but takes a turn for the worse by including a fairly high amount of lemon, grapefruit, and pineapple juices. All of these can be drying for hair while also irritating the scalp, not to mention the sting if this shampoo accidentally gets in your eyes. What's more, none of these juices can have a blonding effect on hair when they are going to be rinsed out. Bottom line: don't bother!

☺ **Oomf Shampoo, the Power Kick for Fine Limp Hair** *($10.20 for 10.1 ounces)* is a very good conditioning shampoo for normal to dry hair of any thickness. The conditioning agents can build up with repeated use, most noticeably on hair that is already fine or limp.

☺ **The Shampoo, Shampoo for Normal to Dry Hair** *($10.20 for 10.1 ounces)* is a great shampoo for all hair types except fine or thin. The conditioning agents and silicone are excellent for dry hair, but can build up with repeated use.

☹ **Beach Bum Blonding Conditioner** *($12.96 for 10.1 ounces)* is a below-standard conditioner that contains mostly lemon juice and a small amount of pineapple and grapefruit juices, all of which are very drying to hair and irritating to the scalp, not to mention they won't make hair blonde (or even enhance hair that's already blonde). There is nothing in lemon juice that facilitates lightening hair in the sun, and leaving hair exposed to sunlight is extremely damaging and unhealthy for hair, scalp, and skin.

☹ **Beach Bum Blonding Cream** *($12.96 for 4.2 ounces)* lists lemon juice as the second ingredient, along with lesser (but still problematic) amounts of grapefruit and pineapple juices. This also contains diluted hydrogen peroxide, which definitely can lighten hair, although the amount used is not enough to have a significant blonding effect unless your hair is already blonde or you use it day after day. It's far easier and cheaper to just buy an 89-cent bottle of hydrogen peroxide. As is, those with light to medium brown hair will end up with a copper to bronze or orange-y color because the peroxide isn't strong enough to lift their natural color to blonde. Add the lemon juice (as well as lemon peel oil) and it all makes this too drying to consider.

☺ **Oomf Conditioner, Extra Gutz for Fine Limp Hair** *($10.20 for 10.1 ounces)* contains too much silicone to make it appropriate for fine hair, but it can be an outstanding conditioner for normal to very dry hair that is normal to coarse or thick.

☺ **The Conditioner, Conditioner for Normal to Dry Hair** *($10.20 for 10.1 ounces)* is similar to the Oomf Conditioner above, except this contains fewer silicones and more detangling agents. This is a very good conditioner for normal to dry hair of any thickness, though someone with fine hair should alternate this with a lighter conditioner unless their hair is dry to very dry.

☺ **Creative Hair Cement, Very Strong Styling Mist** *($10.25 for 10.1 ounces)* is a standard, fast-drying nonaerosol hairspray that offers a very strong hold that leaves hair stiff and slightly sticky. This is not very easy to brush through, so it's best for freezing styles in place or adding lasting lift to specific areas.

☹ **Creative Hair Gum, Extra Strong Gel** *($10.20 for 4.2 ounces)* contains the preservative Kathon CG, which is contraindicated for use in leave-on products due to a high risk of sensitizing reactions to the skin (scalp).

☺ **$$$ De Frizz Polish and Control for All Types of Hair** *($16.96 for 1.69 ounces)* is a very standard silicone serum. It would work as well as any to smooth hair, add a glossy shine, and keep frizzies in check, but you may first want to check out the less expensive and similar (or identical) serums available at the drugstore.

☺ **$$$ De Frizz Polish and Control for Blond Hair** *($16.96 for 1.69 ounces)* is identical to the De Frizz Polish and Control for All Types of Hair above, except this contains dye agents to minimize brassy tones in blonde hair, even if their effect in this regard is, at best, minimal. Still, if that's a concern, this would be the preferred choice in the Fudge line.

☺ **$$$ Erekt, Non Chemical Hair Straightener Heat Sensitive** *($13.05 for 4.2 ounces)* is a water-based styling gel that contains enough silicone to allow you to smooth and straighten your hair—with heat and the proper styling tool. This does not offer any hold, so stickiness is not a concern, and it is light enough to use on all hair types except fine or thin.

☺ **Hair Licorice, Light Hold Factor 5** *($11.75 for 3.5 ounces)* is a creamy, soft-textured pomade that seems lighter than it is. This can work well to smooth dry ends and tame frizzies, but not without some greasiness that can make normal to fine or thin hair feel heavy and coated. It's best for dry to very dry hair that is coarse or thick.

☺ **Hair Putty, Medium Hold Factor 3** *($11.75 for 3.5 ounces)* isn't a putty—it's not nearly as thick as the name implies. Rather, this is a styling cream with holding agents, wax, and silicones. It provides a light to medium hold that remains slightly moist but is also a bit sticky. It's best for creating texture and hold on short hairstyles. This does an OK job at smoothing frizzies.

☺ **Hair Shaper, Firm Hold Factor 2** *($11.75 for 3.5 ounces)* is a thick, gummy pomade that is surprisingly easy to apply evenly through the hair and will add strong texture and definition with minimal hold. This would work well for normal to very dry hair that is coarse, curly, or thick.

☺ **Hair Varnish, Medium/Light Hold Factor 4** *($11.75 for 3.2 ounces)* is Fudge's thickest, greasiest balm, and most closely resembles a traditional Vaseline-based pomade. This is heavy-duty stuff and is best used sparingly on the ends of dry to very dry hair. It provides a very glossy finish.

☺ **Oomf Booster, Styling Muscle for Fine Limp Hair** *($10.20 for 10.1 ounces)* is a light-hold styling gel with enough silicone and conditioning agents to make it somewhat heavy for fine or limp hair. This is an excellent, minimally sticky smoothing gel for normal to dry hair that's normal to thick or coarse.

☺ **$$$ Pump Up, Alcohol Free Foaming Gel** *($20.25 for 7 ounces)* is a standard, propellant-based styling mousse that provides a medium hold that is slightly sticky but still allows hair to be brushed through.

☺ $$$ Skrewd, Enhances Curl and Eliminates Frizz Heat Responsive *($10.90 for 4.2 ounces)* is a standard, medium- to firm-hold styling gel that has no special benefit for curly hair.

☺ Skyscraper, Firm Hold Hairspray *($14.95 for 21.5 ounces)* is a light-hold aerosol hairspray that leaves hair soft and flexible. This is an ideal working spray during styling because hair remains pliable while staying in place. This is not a great option for gravity-defying styles. The silicones add a touch of shine and aid with combing.

☺ $$$ 1 Shot Hair Reconstructing Clinic in a Bottle *($12.35 for 4.2 ounces)* has an attention-grabbing name—this sounds like instant hair-repair in a bottle. One shot and your hair is cured of all its woes! The formula contains mostly water, silicone, detangling agents, thickener, water-binding/film-forming agent, slip agents, alcohol, preservatives, and fragrance. It won't reconstruct a single hair, but it will aid with combing, add soft-ness, and create shine. This is light enough to use on fine or thin hair, and provides a decent amount of heat protection when combined with styling products.

☺ $$$ Dynamite Deep Penetrating Hair Treatment *($10.35 for 4.2 ounces)* is a standard conditioner. It's labeled as a special hair treatment—and isn't—but it can be an emollient conditioner for normal to dry hair that is normal to thick.

☺ Head Polish Hair Shiner *($9.25 for 1.6 ounces)* is a water-based silicone serum that contains a tiny amount of film-forming/holding agent. This is a good silicone serum for all hair types, and the light texture makes it easier to use on fine or thin hair. Just use it sparingly for best results.

FUDGE UNLEADED

☺ Unleaded Shampoo 1, Mild Cleansing Shampoo for Everyday Use of Normal to Dry Hair *($13.55 for 16.8 ounces)* is nearly identical to The Shampoo, Shampoo for Normal to Dry Hair above, and the same comments apply. Ounce for ounce, this prod-uct works out to be a better bargain and is just as effective.

☺ Unleaded Shampoo 2, Everyday Shampoo for Tortured and Chemically Treated Hair *($13.55 for 16.8 ounces)* contains nothing that makes it a must-have for tortured or chemically treated hair. It's just a standard, but good, shampoo that is very similar to the Oomf Shampoo, the Power Kick for Fine Limp Hair above.

☺ Unleaded Conditioner 1, Everyday Conditioner for Normal to Dry Hair *($13.55 for 16.8 ounces)* is nearly identical to The Conditioner, Conditioner for Normal to Dry Hair above, and the same comments apply. Ounce for ounce, this product works out to be a better bargain.

☺ Unleaded Conditioner 2 *($13.55 for 16.8 ounces)* is a very good conditioner for normal to dry hair that is normal to coarse or thick.

☺ Unleaded Detangler, Leave-In Conditioner *($13.55 for 10.1 ounces)* is a water-light conditioner that can be moderately helpful for detangling the hair. This is really too watery to be of much use to most hair types, but it is OK for very fine hair, although the TEA-dodecylbenzenesulfonate can potentially cause scalp and hair dryness.

☺ **Unleaded Fat Hed** *($11.80 for 3.5 ounces)* is a thick, slightly gooey pomade. This heavy-duty, moderately greasy product is best for hard-to-manage hair that is thick, coarse, or curly. It provides a good degree of control while smoothing hair and adding shine, but use it sparingly or your hair will quickly feel overloaded with product.

GARNIER FRUCTIS

L'Oreal-owned Garnier has made a name for itself in the United States with its permanent hair color lines, Nutrisse and Lumia. In Europe, where Garnier generates three-quarters of its sales, the Fructis hair-care line has been available for some time. L'Oreal has begun a blitz of the U.S. market with ads for Garnier, with the goal of making it as much a household name as L'Oreal, Maybelline, and Lancome.

Fructis claims to make hair five times stronger and five times smoother with its combination of fruit acids, vitamins, and sugar derivatives. Of course, the test results to prove these claims are not available to the public, so we're left to believe Garnier's statements hold true to what they discovered in side-by-side brushing/combing tests with another (unnamed) shampoo and conditioner duo. The reality is that a dusting of vitamins and fruit extracts (which really just add fragrance) cannot make the hair stronger. Hair can be "fortified" with conditioners to make it less susceptible to breakage and the rigors of heat-styling damage, but it won't be any stronger than with any other conditioner. For more information about Garnier, call (800) 4-Garnier or visit www.garnierfructis.com.

What's Good About This Line: Mostly excellent, though standard, shampoos and conditioners; workable styling products that feature enough choices to create almost any hairstyle.

What's Not So Good About It: The shampoo and conditioner formulas are repetitive, with little to no difference between them, even though they're sold as being designed for different hair types.

☺ **Fortifying Anti-Dandruff Shampoo** *($3.99 for 13 ounces)* is a standard, but good, dandruff shampoo that contains 1% zinc pyrithione as the active ingredient. It's considered an effective over-the-counter remedy for some types of dandruff and is standard in most Head & Shoulders brand shampoo products. The shampoo is a gentle formula that contains some silicone, so it can build up with repeated use. The touted vitamins and sugar derivatives are listed after the fragrance, which gives you some idea of how important Garnier really thinks they are.

☺ **Fortifying Shampoo + Conditioner, for Normal Hair** *($3.99 for 13 ounces)* is a very standard "two in one" shampoo that uses mild detergent cleansing agents and a large amount of silicone to meet the needs of those who want the convenience of using only one product for their hair. Although this is an option, the silicone will build up on hair with repeated use, so this should be alternated with another shampoo that does not contain conditioning agents.

The Reviews G

☺ **Fortifying Shampoo, for Color Treated or Permed Hair** *($3.99 for 13 ounces)* is almost identical to the Fortifying Shampoo + Conditioner above, except this contains one less conditioning agent. Otherwise, the same basic comments apply. The vitamins and sugar extracts are listed after the fragrance.

☺ **Fortifying Shampoo, for Dry or Damaged Hair** *($3.99 for 13 ounces)* is nearly identical to the Fortifying Shampoo for Color-Treated or Permed Hair above, and the same comments apply. One of the reasons hair becomes dry is from chemical treatments, and either of these Fructis shampoos is a safe choice for color-treated hair.

☺ **Fortifying Shampoo, for Fine Hair** *($3.99 for 13 ounces)* contains mostly water, detergent cleansing agent, lather agents, silicone, thickener, pH-adjuster, fruit extract, fragrance, film-forming agent, and preservatives. This is a standard, but good, shampoo for all hair types, though the silicone can build up with repeated use.

☺ **Fortifying Shampoo, for Normal Hair** *($3.99 for 13 ounces)* is nearly identical to the Fortifying Shampoo for Color-Treated or Permed Hair above, and the same comments apply. Normal hair (meaning hair that has not been chemically treated and is not too coarse or too thin) does not need a primary-use shampoo with this much silicone. A conditioning shampoo like this is best alternated with a shampoo that won't cause buildup.

☺ **Fortifying Cream Conditioner, for Dry or Damaged Hair** *($3.99 for 13 ounces)* is a good, though completely standard, conditioner for normal to fine hair. It is similar to many of the other conditioners sold in L'Oreal's main line of Vive products. There is more fragrance in this product than there is of the supposedly hair-strengthening fruit acids and sugars.

☺ **Fortifying Cream Conditioner, for Color-Treated or Permed Hair** *($3.99 for 13 ounces)* is nearly identical to the Fortifying Cream Conditioner, for Dry or Damaged Hair above, and the same comments apply. There really was no need to add this product to compete with the dry/damaged version, since all color-treated and permed hair is already damaged and very likely dry, too.

☺ **Fortifying Cream Conditioner, for Normal Hair** *($3.99 for 13 ounces)* is nearly identical to the Fortifying Cream Conditioner, for Dry or Damaged Hair above, save for a few very minor ingredient changes. The same basic comments apply.

☺ **Fortifying Cream Conditioner, for Fine Hair** *($3.99 for 13 ounces)* is lighter than the three Fortifying Cream Conditioners above, and is appropriate for someone with fine hair. This conditioner is best for detangling, not moisturizing, and the only caution is that the film-forming agents can build up on fine hair, making it flat and limp.

☺ **Fortifying Deep Conditioner 3 Minute Masque** *($3.99 for 5 ounces)* may sound like a rich treatment product for hair, but it has essentially the same conditioner formula as the ones above, with additional amounts of thickener to give the product a creamier consistency. It isn't a bad choice if you have normal to fine hair, but those with dry, thick, or coarse hair will find this is not emollient enough to manage their hair.

☺ **Curl Construct Mousse Weightless Curls & Hold, Extra Strong** *($2.64 for 6.8 ounces)* is a very standard styling mousse that liquefies nicely and spreads evenly through the hair, although the holding agent (acrylate copolymer) can leave hair feeling somewhat stiff and sticky. I wouldn't consider this extra-strong hold—at best it provides a medium to firm hold.

☺ **Curl Shaping Spray Gel Curl Defining, Strong** *($2.64 for 8.5 ounces)* offers a soft, flexible hold that can nicely define curls and waves. What it lacks are any significant shine or anti-frizz ingredients, so if frizzies and a smooth feel are an issue, you'll want to pair this with a silicone spray or serum.

☺ **Fiber Gum Putty Pliable Molding, Extra Strong** *($2.64 for 5 ounces)* isn't a putty in the true sense of the word, but it is a gummy, slightly stringy styling gel that provides a fairly strong hold that can be easily brushed through. The formula is standard fare and, unlike true styling putty (which is similar to a pomade or wax), this product does not stay pliable. Rather, once it dries, it behaves like most styling gels. That means that if you want pliability with this product, you either need to re-wet your hair and restyle, or add more product.

☺ **Full Control Aerosol Hairspray All Day Firm Hold, Ultra Strong** *($2.64 for 8.25 ounces)* does not provide ultra-strong hold in the least and is therefore not a consideration if you want a firm, gravity-defying hold. If you want a light-hold aerosol hairspray that can be easily brushed through and is minimally sticky, this is a great product—just ignore the name, because nothing about this hairspray makes it firm or ultra-strong.

☺ **Full Control Aerosol Hairspray All Day Flexible Hold, Strong** *($2.64 for 8.25 ounces)* is nearly identical to the All Day Firm Hold, Ultra Strong above, only this product offers an even softer hold for when you need just a hint of control but still want your hair to have movement.

☺ **Full Control Non-Aerosol Hairspray All Day Flexible Hold, Strong** *($2.64 for 8.5 ounces)* continues the "holding pattern" of the two Fructis aerosol hairsprays above, only the Non-Aerosols apply a bit heavier because they're not aerosols. This provides a natural, flexible hold that's quite different from most hairsprays, especially if you're trying to avoid making your hair too stiff.

☺ **Full Control Non-Aerosol Hairspray All Day Hard Hold, Ultra Strong** *($2.64 for 8.5 ounces)* is nearly identical to the Full Control Non-Aerosol Hairspray All Day Flexible Hold, Strong above, except that this product has a stronger (but still flexible) hold. Otherwise, the same comments apply.

☺ **Shake Effect Liqui-Gel Intense Texture, Extra Strong** *($2.64 for 5.1 ounces)* is a thin liquid gel that comes in a spray bottle. The formula consists mainly of water, film former, and preservatives. It provides a strong, slightly sticky hold and works well on wet or dry hair. This mists on, so it lets you touch up or add texture to dry hair without making it look too wet.

☺ **Shake Effect Liqui-Gel Intense Volume, Strong** *($2.64 for 5.1 ounces)* is nearly identical to the Shake Effect Liqui-Gel Intense Texture, Extra Strong above, except this formula provides slightly less hold, which also means it's a bit less sticky. Otherwise, the same comments apply.

The Reviews G

☺ **Smoothing Milk Instant Smoothing & Frizz Control, Strong** *($2.64 for 5.1 ounces)* shouldn't be described as "strong" because this contains only a minimal amount of holding agents, meaning that hair is left with no stiffness or stickiness. This can work beautifully as a finishing cream to smooth and add shine to dry hair, or mix it with a gel (for hold) prior to heat styling. It would work well for all but fine or thin hair types. This contains enough silicone to warrant a "use sparingly" caution.

☺ **Super Stiff Gel Intense Structure & Hold, Ultra Strong** *($2.64 for 6.8 ounces)* must be mixed together in your hands to activate the fibers (which are part of the main holding agent) before use. This is one of the few Fructis styling products whose name accurately describes the type of hold the product provides. It would work well for extreme hairstyles or on stubborn hair, but as you might guess, it can be difficult to brush through without some snags along the way.

☺ **Volume Inject Mousse Weightless Body & Hold, Ultra Strong** *($2.64 for 6.8 ounces)* is a very light-textured, standard styling mousse that provides a soft, non-sticky hold that can be easily brushed through. Nothing about this product's hold is "ultra strong." If anything, this is an ideal mousse to emphasize curls or enhance waves without making hair feel the least bit heavy or coated.

☺ **Wet Shine Gel All Day Wet Look & Hold, Strong** *($2.64 for 6.8 ounces)* gets its wet-look features from the glycerin in the formula. Of course, that also means this gel dries more slowly than you might expect, but the payoff is smoother, hydrated hair (assuming you do not live in a low-humidity climate, in which case glycerin's hydrating abilities are compromised). This gel offers a light hold that can feel sticky if you overuse it. It's a fine choice for slicked-back wet looks, or for heat-styling your hair while it's still damp.

GARREN NEW YORK

Garren reigns as one of New York City's premier hairstylists. His reputation is about as close to perfect as you can get in the ultra-highbrow world of Manhattan's fashion and beauty scene elite. In addition to tending to the tresses of such luminaries as Cindy Crawford, Madonna, and supermodel Gisele Bündchen, Garren has a monthly advice column in *Allure* magazine.

How do Garren's years of haircutting experience and his celebrity client list translate to hair-care products? From a formulary standpoint, most of the products are very good, although they don't hold a single advantage over countless other, far less expensive lines. The Upper East Side mentality comes into play with Garren New York's prices, which are more on the outlandish side of the economic scale. No doubt most celebrities and supermodels wouldn't have an issue with paying almost $50 for a shampoo and conditioner, but they might if they knew that, beyond the gleaming gold Garren-approved initial on the minimalist bottles and tubes, there is nothing about these products that warrants even a fraction of the steep prices. As is most often the case, that does not mean these are not worthwhile products—almost all of them will do an excellent job of keeping hair feeling and (with the right styling techniques) looking good. Of course, so will many other hair-care products in every price range, which is why the decision on how much to spend to manage your hair is up to you; your hair won't even notice. The beauty- and fashion-conscious may flock to this product line, but Garren himself performs the real magic. Any talented hairstylist can use styling products of any price and, with the proper technique and tools, style hair magnificently. For more information about Garren New York, call (877) 441-9255 or visit www.garrennewyork.com. **Note:** All Garren New York hair-care products contain fragrant plant extracts.

What's Good About This Line: Almost every product has merit for hair and will perform as indicated, minus the occasional overblown claim.

What's Not So Good About It: High prices, especially given the smaller-than-average quantity held by each product container.

☺ **$$$ Anyday Shampoo** *($25 for 8 ounces)* is a very good, but very standard, shampoo that contains gentle detergent cleansing agents and a touch of silicone for a mild conditioning/detangling effect. This is a fine option for all hair types, including chemically treated hair. Just know that the price has nothing to do with this having a superior formula; it has to do only with Garren's New York fashion scene image.

☺ **$$$ Color Stabilizing Shampoo** *($30 for 8 ounces)* is meant to preserve and protect hair color, but nothing in the formulation can do that. If it could, then Garren would have to concede that hundreds of similarly formulated, much less expensive shampoos can also preserve hair color. This is a very good shampoo for all hair types that will certainly not make color-treated hair feel or look drier than it may already be, but it cannot make hair color last longer, not even one shampoo longer. The antioxidants in this formula are a nice touch, but, performance-wise, they are rinsed away or blown dry away before they can have an effect on hair.

☺ **$$$ Nourishing Creme Shampoo** *($32 for 7 ounces)* is an exceptionally gentle shampoo that does contain several conditioning agents, and that makes it appropriate for dry, coarse, or damaged hair. With repeated use, these conditioning agents can build up on the hair, so alternate it with a basic, no-frills shampoo to keep hair looking healthy and vibrant.

☹ **Volumizing Shampoo** *($23 for 8 ounces)* is Garren's least impressive shampoo, primarily because it is the only one that contains TEA-lauryl sulfate and sodium C14-olefin sulfonate, both drying detergent cleansing agents that can cause scalp irritation and strip hair color.

☺ **$$$ Light Volumizing Conditioner** *($22 for 6 ounces)* is recommended for daily use, and that would be appropriate if your hair is normal to fine or thin. This is a standard, but effective, conditioner that won't mend split ends (at least not in the curative sense), but it will make hair easy to comb through and leave it feeling soft. It's up to you to decide whether you want to spend $22 for the Garren name or get the same effect with a $3.99 bottle of conditioner from Pantene.

☺ **$$$ Nourishing Creme Conditioner** *($35 for 7 ounces)* lists drying isopropyl alcohol as the third ingredient, so any nourishing by this conditioner will be short-lived. Aside from the fragrant plant extracts and vitamins (which have no benefit for hair), this is one of the most overpriced, ordinary conditioners you're likely to find. There really is nothing to say about this product other than "Why bother?"

☺ **$$$ Designing Spray Tonic** *($26 for 6 ounces)* somewhat justifies its price by being an above-average styling spray. This alcohol-free formula goes on light and provides a natural hold that remains flexible rather than stiff or too sticky. Due to the absence of alcohol, this does air-dry slowly, but that won't be a problem if you are using it with a heat-styling implement.

☺ **$$$ Holding & Molding Gel** *($20 for 4 ounces)* is a slippery, thin-consistency styling gel that contains standard acrylate film-forming agents along with antioxidants and lightweight conditioners. It offers a light, flexible hold that lets hair be easily brushed through, and it's minimally sticky.

☺ **$$$ Straightening & Styling Gel** *($19 for 4 ounces)* has a slightly thicker consistency than the Holding & Molding Gel above and is also somewhat stickier. It doesn't break any new ground when it comes to styling gels, but it's still an effective option for a light hold and a sleek finish. This does contain some very good conditioning agents, but none of them are present in amounts sufficient to have a noticeable impact on the hair. Witch hazel extract is the second listed ingredient, and it can cause irritation, so be cautious of getting too much of this product directly on the scalp.

☺ **$$$ Styling Creme** *($25 for 4 ounces)* is sold with the claim of being an "ultra-conditioning formula"; however, the first several ingredients listed are not what any cosmetics chemist would call substantial conditioning agents. This is actually a lightweight product that dissipates quickly and leaves a slightly silky, barely moist finish. It is a good finishing product for normal to fine hair, be it straight or curly. Those with thick or coarse hair will likely prefer a styling cream (or pomade) that offers more weight and allows for more definition.

☺ **$$$ Hair Fragrance** *($35 for 0.04 ounce)* is nothing more than alcohol-based perfume for hair. Perhaps Garren thought his styling products were not fragrant enough (and compared to many others, his are indeed softly scented) and wanted to give his clients the option of adding a noticeable aroma to their coiffures. In any case, this is an indulgence for the hair. It will have no bearing on its style, but should help minimize unpleasant odors that can be absorbed by the hair, such as those from pungent foods or cigarette smoke.

GIGA.HOLD BY SALON GRAFIX

Giga.Hold is a line of styling products designed for young urbanites trying to create "styles that defy gravity." The line is owned by Michigan-based Salon Grafix, reviewed elsewhere in this book. For more information about Giga.Hold, call (248) 642-3041 or visit www.gigahold.com.

What's Good About This Line: Every product makes good on its claim of providing extreme hold. They're serious when they say "products for an impenetrable style"!

What's Not So Good About It: The high levels of film-forming/holding agents and acrylates are not easy to shampoo out, often requiring you to lather, rinse, and, yes, repeat.

☺ **Freeze Hair Putty** *($5.99 for 2 ounces)* is a water-based, gelatinous paste that provides a very strong hold and leaves hair feeling slightly stiff and very sticky. This works brilliantly to spike hair or exaggerate texture, but you already know that you won't be able to brush through your hair!

☺ **Freeze Hair Spray Ultra Intense, Aerosol** *($5.99 for 10 ounces)* is a standard aerosol hairspray that provides a very strong hold and leaves hair feeling stiff and slightly sticky. This is wind tunnel–surviving hold, and ideal for anyone who needs their finished style to last (and not move) all day.

☺ **Freeze Hair Spray Non-Aerosol Styling Mist** *($5.99 for 8 ounces)* is a great hairspray that goes on a bit heavier than most, but works well to freeze styles in place. Once dry, hair will feel slightly stiff, but this is less sticky than the Freeze Hair Spray Ultra Intense, Aerosol above.

☺ **Freeze Hair Spray Ultra Intense, Unscented** *($5.99 for 10 ounces)* is identical to the Freeze Hair Spray Ultra Intense, Aerosol above, and the same comments apply. Despite being labeled "unscented," this does contain fragrance, though the scent is subtle.

☺ **Spike & Freeze Gel** *($5.99 for 8 ounces)* is the styling gel to choose if every other gel you've tried has not been strong enough to manage your hair or create the style you want. This alcohol-free gel provides an incredibly strong hold that leaves hair feeling sticky, but delivers on its promise of "the most intense hold on the market." Beware, this gel is not for beginners!

GOLDWELL

Goldwell has been on the hair-care scene since 1948, when it launched in Germany with one product (a setting lotion). It has always been a line designed for and sold to salon professionals through a network of worldwide distributors, and the company remains well known in the salon industry for their educational leadership. Goldwell was purchased by Japan-based Kao Corporation in 1989. Although many of the products work quite well, this line, for all its history and education-oriented approach and the products' technically impressive names, is not all that innovative. And remember, just because a company is known for their education does not mean they're teaching hairstylists anything about how hair-care products are formulated or how the ingredients in the products function (beyond the hype and marketing language). Learning how to cut, color, perm, and style hair is vastly different from understanding what it takes to create excellent hair-care products and how various disparate ingredients work together to produce results that please consumers. For more information about Goldwell, call (800) 333-2442 or visit www.goldwellusa.com.

What's Good About This Line: The color-enhancing mousses are unique; most of the shampoos and conditioners are respectable formulas; styling products offer some fun (and effective) alternatives to traditional products.

What's Not So Good About It: A few of the shampoos and conditioners contain lime oil; a few styling products have issues with flaking or are simply too ordinary for the money; a lack of substantially emollient conditioners for dry to very dry hair.

GOLDWELL COLORANCE

☺ $$$ **Colorance Soft Color Foam Colorant** *($11.12 for 4.2 ounces)* is a color-enhancing, propellant-based mousse available in 21 shades, from ash blonde to copper red and violet. This very light mousse contains no holding agents, but does include conditioning agents to keep hair soft and smooth. The color-enhancing effect is achieved from basic dyes, which can do a decent job of adding color to the hair, but they will not provide noticeable gray coverage. These products are a convenient way to refresh or intensify your color between salon visits, and the dye agents shampoo out easily.

☺ **Colorance Color Styling Mousse** *($7.97 for 2.4 ounces)* is similar to the Colorance Soft Color Foam Colorant above, only this adds film-forming/holding agents so it behaves like a traditional light-hold, non-sticky styling mousse. Each of the 19 shades uses the same basic dyes as the Foam Colorant above, but in this product the colors are slightly softer. There is also a Refresher shade, which is a pale violet color meant for highlighted hair. This can, to a minimal extent, tone down yellow, golden, or brassy tones (which occur as highlights oxidize and fade. Its formula is slightly different from the Colorance Color Styling Mousse, yet its holding and non-sticky properties remain the same.

GOLDWELL DEFINITION

☺ **Definition Color & Highlights Shampoo** *($8 for 8.4 ounces)* is a very standard, but good, shampoo that has a small amount of film-forming agent. There's not enough of it to be concerned about buildup, so that makes this an option for all hair types.

☺ **Definition Dry & Porous Shampoo** *($8 for 8.4 ounces)* is nearly identical to the Color & Highlights Shampoo above, except this has a greater amount of plant oil, which makes it preferred for normal to dry hair that is normal to slightly thick.

☺ **Definition Kids Hair & Body Shampoo** *($10 for 8.4 ounces)* is fairly similar to the Color & Highlights Shampoo above, and it's not necessarily better for kids (the detergent cleansing agent can sting if it gets into the eyes). This is still a gentle shampoo, just not as mild as a product like Johnson & Johnson's Baby Shampoo. For adults of all hair types, this is a very good option and poses no risk of buildup.

☺ **Definition Permed & Curly Curl Care Shampoo** *($8 for 8.4 ounces)* is nearly identical to the Dry & Porous Shampoo above, except this one contains almond oil instead of avocado oil. Otherwise, the same basic comments apply.

☹ **Definition Shine & Vitality Shampoo, for Normal Hair** *($8 for 8.4 ounces)* is nearly identical to the Dry & Porous Shampoo above, but the formula takes a wrong turn and causes unnecessary scalp irritation by including an appreciable amount of lime oil.

☹ **Definition Shine & Vitality Intensive Shampoo** *($8 for 8.4 ounces)* is nearly identical to the Shine & Vitality Shampoo, for Normal Hair above, and the same comments apply.

☺ **Definition Color & Highlights Color Conditioning Foam, Leave-In** *($14 for 6.7 ounces)* is a standard, propellant-based styling mousse that offers almost no hold but does provide a conditioning, detangling benefit to hair. The lactic acid in this product cannot exfoliate the hair or scalp, which is a good thing, especially if your goal is to preserve hair color! If the AHA could exfoliate, it would denature the cuticle and cause your color to fade much sooner than it normally would.

☹ **Definition Shine & Vitality Conditioning Balm** *($12 for 8.4 ounces)* contains a large amount of lime oil, which can cause scalp irritation and itching, particularly if hair or scalp is exposed to sunlight. This product is not recommended.

☺ **Definition Color & Highlights Color Conditioning Intensive Treatment** *($8 for 5 ounces)* is a very standard conditioner that is not intense in the least. As it is, this is an OK conditioner for normal to slightly dry hair that is normal to fine or thin.

☺ **Definition Color & Highlights Color Stabilizer, Leave-In** *($5 for 0.6 ounce)* is a straightforward, basic, leave-in conditioner that works best as a lightweight detangler for normal hair. The AHAs in it will not exfoliate the hair or scalp, which is to your benefit.

☺ **Definition Dry & Porous Intensive Treatment, for Dry/Coarse Hair** *($8 for 5 ounces)* is a good, basic conditioner for normal to dry hair that is normal to slightly thick. I wouldn't consider this intense, especially if your hair is dry.

☺ **Definition Dry & Porous Repair Serum** *($5 for 0.6 ounce)* is a standard silicone serum that is actually not as nice as many other options, and the single-application packaging makes this more expensive than the silicone serum options from Citré Shine, Ion, göt2b, or Charles Worthington. And, of course, this product absolutely cannot repair hair.

☺ **Definition Dry & Porous Strengthening Treatment, for Fine & Stressed Hair** *($8 for 5 ounces)* is a very good, emollient conditioner that is inappropriate for fine hair. The combination of thickeners, mineral oil, plant oil, and water-binding agents is best for dry to very dry hair that is normal to coarse or thick.

☺ **Definition Permed & Curly Curl Care Foam, Leave-In** *($14 for 6.7 ounces)* is a propellant-based, light-hold styling mousse that works very well as a leave-in conditioner, though it contains nothing that makes it preferred for someone with curly hair. This can indeed moisturize and help softly define curls and waves, but it works well for those with any hair type looking for a non-sticky styling mousse.

☺ **Definition Permed & Curly Curl Care Intensive Care Treatment** *($8 for 5 ounces)* can be a great conditioner for normal to dry hair of any thickness, though it's not all that intense.

☺ **Definition Permed & Curly Curl Stabilizer, Leave-In** *($5 for 0.6 ounce)* is similar to the Definition Color & Highlights Color Stabilizer, Leave-In above, and the same basic comments apply.

☺ **Definition Shine & Vitality Volume Spray, Leave-In** *($8 for 5 ounces)* is a standard water- and alcohol-based styling spray that provides light to medium hold with minimal to no sticky feel.

GOLDWELL ELUMEN

☺ **$$$ Elumen Wash** *($12 for 8.4 ounces)* is a standard shampoo that can work well for all hair types; it poses no risk of buildup.

☹ **Elumen Care** *($12 for 5 ounces)* is supposed to be a leave-in conditioning spray, but it contains mostly water and alcohol, so don't count on much benefit from this overpriced, poorly formulated product. The minimal amount of conditioning and detangling agents means hard-to-comb hair will remain so.

☺ **$$$ Elumen Treat** *($12 for 4.2 ounces)* is a standard, almost boring conditioner that is an OK option for detangling normal to slightly dry hair that is fine or thin.

GOLDWELL FOR MEN

☹ **for Men Refreshing Gel Shampoo** *($11 for 8.4 ounces)* contains menthol and peppermint, which makes it too irritating for the scalp. Men's products do not need to tingle to fool guys into thinking they're doing something special on the scalp.

☺ **$$$ for Men Freestyler, Unlimited Effects** *($12 for 1.6 ounces)* is a very standard styling wax, packaged in a deodorant-style container. This has a hard texture and provides a natural, low-gloss finish. It can work well to smooth the ends of hair or add subtle texture to short or close-cropped styles.

☺ **$$$ for Men Power Gel, Extreme Wet Look** *($12 for 5 ounces)* is a great, relatively standard styling gel for naturally groomed or slicked-back hairstyles. The formula provides a light hold that is minimally sticky and can be easily brushed through. It contains some good conditioning agents to help keep hair smooth and soft.

GOLDWELL KERASILK

☺ **Kerasilk Rich Care Shampoo** *($8 for 8.4 ounces)* is a standard shampoo that is a good option for all hair types. The film-forming agent is present in such a small amount that there is no risk of buildup.

☺ **Kerasilk Ultra Rich Care Shampoo** *($9 for 8.4 ounces)* is nearly identical to the Kerasilk Rich Care Shampoo above, and the same comments apply. Neither of these shampoos is very rich, so don't count on them to moisturize dry to very dry or damaged hair.

☹ **Kerasilk Rich Care Conditioner** *($10 for 5 ounces)* is primarily a detangling product, and with alcohol as its second ingredient, is not "rich care" in the least. There is little else to say about this conditioner except that better options abound.

☺ **Kerasilk Ultra Rich Care Conditioner** *($11 for 5 ounces)* is similar to the Definition Dry & Porous Strengthening Treatment, for Fine & Stressed Hair above, and the same comments apply.

☺ **Kerasilk Ultra Rich Treatment** *($11 for 5 ounces)* is nearly identical to the Definition Dry & Porous Strengthening Treatment, for Fine & Stressed Hair above, and the same basic comments apply. The plant oils are present in somewhat higher amounts, so it is slightly better for very dry hair.

☺ **$$$ Kerasilk Rich Care Leave-In Silk Fluid** *($16 for 4.2 ounces)* is close to a standard silicone serum, and is an outstanding product to smooth the hair, improve its feel, and add tremendous shine. Use it sparingly, especially if your hair is fine or thin.

GOLDWELL TRENDLINE

☺ **Trendline Finish Spray, Extreme (Aerosol)** *($14.50 for 8.6 ounces)* is a firm-hold hairspray that goes on light and dries almost immediately. The silicone adds shine and allows hair to be brushed through with minimal snags.

☺ **Trendline Finish Spray, Strong (Aerosol)** *($14.50 for 9.2 ounces)* is identical to the Trendline Finish Spray, Extreme (Aerosol) above, and the same comments apply. This one gives you more product for the same amount of money.

☺ **Trendline Finish Spray, Strong (Non-Aerosol)** *($12.50 for 6.7 ounces)* is a very good, medium-hold hairspray that adds shine and allows hair to be brushed through.

☺ **Trendline Freeze Pudding, Extreme Hair Styling** *($14.50 for 4.2 ounces)* does have a pudding-like texture (and a pistachio green color) that can be tricky to work with at first, but may be worth it if you're looking for a gel-cream product that provides a very strong hold for complex styles. This does leave hair stiff and sticky, but it can be brushed through.

☺ **Trendline Gel Wax, Normal** *($14.50 for 3.3 ounces)* is a standard, water-soluble pomade that comes packaged in a bottle with a pump applicator, making it much neater than using your fingers to scoop out product. This is lightweight and works well to smooth the hair and add shine, but the mineral oil can make hair look greasy unless this is used sparingly.

☺ **$$$ Trendline Jelly Mousse, Extreme Experience** *($16.50 for 3.5 ounces)* is a mica-infused styling gel that dispenses as a foam, which is the only thing remotely "extreme" about this product. It offers more conditioning than hold, and is a good option for natural hairstyles of all hair types. It is non-sticky and does not flake.

☺ **Trendline Lagoom, Strong** *($12.50 for 5.7 ounces)* is a jellylike styling gel that dries quickly and provides a firm hold that remains stiff and sticky. It is worth considering for creating more complex styles, including root lifts or spiked dos. It is surprisingly easy to brush through and is light enough to work for all hair types. I have no idea what "lagoom" means, but I know it's doesn't have anything to do with an island in the South Pacific.

☺ **Trendline Liquid Gel, Strong** *($12.50 for 8.4 ounces)* is a fast-drying, light- to medium-hold styling gel that leaves hair slightly stiff and sticky, but it can be brushed through. The conditioning agents provide some protection during heat styling.

☺ **Trendline Matt Wax, Extreme** *($14.50 for 3.6 ounces)* is a very thick, difficult-to-use styling wax that leaves a matte finish on the hair. Used sparingly, this can work well to smooth the ends of hair or shape thick curls and waves while taming frizzies. This is way too heavy for anyone with normal to fine or thin hair.

☺ **Trendline Mello Goo, Extreme** *($14.50 for 4.4 ounces)* is similar to the Trendline Matt Wax above, except this has a creamier texture and replaces the lanolin and candelilla waxes with mineral oil, which provides shine but also feels greasier. The same how-to-use comments about the Matt Wax above apply here, too.

☺ **$$$ Trendline Shine Wax, Extreme Shine** *($16.50 for 3.1 ounces)* is a standard mineral oil- and wax-based pomade that adds shine while working to smooth frizzies and control flyaway strands. This dense-textured product is best for hair that is normal to thick or coarse, and should be used sparingly.

☹ **Trendline Straightener, Extreme** *($16.50 for 8.4 ounces)* is not as impressive as other straightening products, which typically contain more silicones and smoothing agents than this one. A major problem with this product is that it can chunk up on the hair, but it also flakes when dry, so this is one to ignore in the extreme.

☺ **Trendline Styling Gel, Strong** *($12.50 for 6.5 ounces)* is a standard styling gel that does indeed provide a strong hold, so it works well for hard-to-manage hair, although you do have to put up with a sticky, stiff finish that is somewhat difficult to brush through. For wet looks that you don't intend to brush through, this is a great option.

☺ **Trendline Volume Mousse, Extreme** *($14.50 for 10.2 ounces)* is an excellent, medium- to firm-hold, propellant-based styling mousse that contains an impressive blend of silicones, plant oil, and conditioning agents. This creamy foam leaves hair minimally stiff and sticky, allowing it to be easily brushed through.

☺ **Trendline Volume Mousse, Normal** *($14.50 for 10.2 ounces)* is similar to, but less impressive than, the Trendline Volume Mousse, Extreme above. This provides a light hold that is minimally sticky. For the money, though, it holds no advantage over styling mousses from L'Oreal or Aussie.

☺ **Trendline Shine Spray** *($12.50 for 3.7 ounces)* is an aerosol silicone spray that puts out a fine mist to add a finishing touch of shine to hair. This versatile product goes on light enough that it can be used without worry by all hair types.

GÖT2B

Drugstore line göt2b is owned by Advanced Research Laboratories, the same company that owns the Citré Shine, Thicker Fuller Hair, and Zero Frizz lines reviewed elsewhere in this book. Göt2b offers playful, kicky product names and colorful packaging to attract a younger, perhaps more experimental audience, but even adults whose hairstyles are more conservative should not let the many wonderful, reasonably priced options this line offers pass them by. For more information about göt2b, call (800) 966-6960.

What's Good About This Line: An array of styling products that can provide every level of hold and control imaginable, all at affordable prices; conditioners are mostly standard fare but there are still effective options.

What's Not So Good About It: All but one of the shampoos contain problematic ingredients; "emergency repair" and treatment products have better names than formulas.

☹ **Moisture Freak Smoothing Shampoo** *($5.99 for 12 ounces)* contains the drying detergent cleansing agent sodium C12-15 alkyl sulfate. This ingredient is similar to sodium lauryl sulfate, but has the ability to strip hair color, be it natural or dyed. This shampoo is not recommended.

☹ **Squeaky Clean Daily Cleanse Shampoo** *($5.99 for 12 ounces)* is nearly identical to the Moisture Freak Smoothing Shampoo above, and the same comments apply.

☺ **Instantly Gratified Instant Conditioner** *($5.99 for 8.5 ounces)* is a very standard, but good, conditioner that would work well for normal to dry hair of any thickness.

☺ **In Therapy Reconstructing Conditioner** *($5.99 for 8.5 ounces)* is nearly identical to the Instantly Gratified Instant Conditioner above, and the same basic comments apply. Neither of these conditioners can repair or rebuild the hair.

☺ **Curled-Up Curling Spray** *($5.99 for 6 ounces)* is a basic styling spray that provides a medium, slightly sticky hold and light conditioning. This can be used by all hair types—it offers no special advantage for someone with curly hair. If anything, those with curly hair may prefer a product that leaves their curls softer rather than rigid.

☺ **Defiant Define & Shine Pomade** *($5.99 for 2 ounces)* is a standard, water-soluble pomade with a thick, gel-like texture that belies how light this can feel on the hair, especially when used sparingly. The mica particles add shine and tend not to flake. This is a very good smoothing pomade for all hair types except thin.

☺ **Full of Yourself Volumizing Gel 2 Mousse** *($5.99 for 7 ounces)* is a propellant-based mousse that dispenses thicker than most, but not as thick as a standard styling gel. It provides a medium hold that remains slightly sticky, although it can be great for tousled or slicked-back wet looks that you allow to dry naturally.

☺ **Glued Spiking Freeze Spray** *($5.99 for 12 ounces)* is an aerosol hairspray that provides a firm hold and a stiff, sticky finish. It's not quite glue, but it does dry quickly and can support more outrageous hairstyles for those hoping to be noticed for their gravity-defying locks.

☺ **Glued Styling Spiking Glue** *($5.99 for 6 ounces)* has a name that deserves to be taken seriously—this is strong stuff! It's a thick, paste-like styling cream that is meant to be used on highly exaggerated or spiked hairstyles for all-day hold and lift. It fulfills this duty beautifully, though it can be difficult to shampoo out. The trade-off for this much hold is a slightly stiff and very sticky feel that does not dissipate.

☺ **In Control Hard-Hold Hairspray** *($5.99 for 9 ounces)* is an aerosol hairspray with a no-frills formula that provides a light to medium hold while keeping hair pliable. If you're looking for something to freeze hair in place, keep looking.

☺ **Kinky Curl Defining Curling Mousse** *($5.99 for 8 ounces)* has no special benefit for styling curly hair. It can define curls, but so can countless other propellant-based styling mousses, which is exactly what this product is. It provides a medium, slightly sticky hold, and the plant oil can provide some protection during heat styling.

☺ **Playful Weightless Creme Pomade** *($5.99 for 2 ounces)* isn't weightless, but this creamy pomade is much lighter than most water-soluble pomades. It is a great option for smoothing or adding soft texture to normal to fine hair. This provides a modestly shiny finish and, once dry, has just a hint of greasiness.

☺ **Roughed Up Spray Wax Pomade** *($5.99 for 3.3 ounces)* is an aerosol silicone spray that contains a small amount of wax for additional texture. This can go on heavy and quickly make hair look greasy, so use it sparingly. It's best as a glossing spray on normal to dry hair that is thick or coarse.

☺ **Shocking Firm-Hold Sculpting Gel** *($5.99 for 8.5 ounces)* is a standard, alcohol-free styling gel that provides a firm hold that leaves hair feeling slightly stiff and sticky, though it can be brushed through.

☺ **Smoothed Over Straightening Balm** *($5.99 for 4.2 ounces)* is a very well-formulated straightening balm that contains a nice balance of silicones, wax, and film-forming agent to allow you to expertly create smooth, sleek, straight hair with the aid of a blow dryer and round styling brush. This also works well when used in small amounts (after heat styling) to add extra shine to the hair.

☺ **Spiked-Up Max Control Styling Gel** *($5.99 for 8.5 ounces)* is similar to the Shocking Firm-Hold Sculpting Gel above, except this one offers a stronger hold.

☺ **Dazzling Shine Spray** *($5.99 for 6 ounces)* is a very good, lightweight silicone spray that contains some alcohol to cut the potentially greasy side effect of silicones.

☺ **Glossy Anti-Frizz Shine Serum** *($5.99 for 4 ounces)* is a simple, but excellent, silicone serum that would work beautifully to smooth frizzies, add a silky feel, and create incredible shine on the hair. A little of this goes a long way, and the price makes this a hair-care bargain!

GÖT2B SO BLONDE

☹ **So Blonde Highlight Enhancing Shampoo, Honey 2 Dark Blonde** *($5.99 for 10 ounces)* contains sodium polystyrene sulfonate, which can be drying and can potentially strip dyed hair color with repeated use. There isn't a great deal of it in this otherwise standard shampoo, but its inclusion in a color-enhancing shampoo is senseless.

☹ **So Blonde Highlight Enhancing Shampoo, Platinum 2 Ash Blonde** *($5.99 for 10 ounces)* is nearly identical to the So Blonde Highlight Enhancing Shampoo, Honey 2 Dark Blonde above, and the same comments apply.

☺ **So Blonde Highlight Revealing Conditioner, Honey 2 Dark Blonde** *($5.99 for 10 ounces)* is a good conditioner for normal to dry hair that is normal to coarse or thick, but the coloring agents have no effect on accentuating highlights.

☺ **So Blonde Blonde Aid Intensive Hair Repair** *($5.99 for 6 ounces)* is an excellent emollient conditioner for dry to very dry hair of any thickness except fine or thin. This won't repair the hair, but it can temporarily make hair feel silky-soft and look smoother.

☺ **So Blonde Highlight Revealing Conditioner, Platinum 2 Ash Blonde** *($5.99 for 10 ounces)* is identical to the So Blonde Highlight Revealing Conditioner, Honey 2 Dark Blonde above, except this contains fewer coloring agents (which have no effect on your highlights anyway). Otherwise, the same comments apply.

☺ **So Blonde Glamour Mist Shine Spray** *($5.99 for 4 ounces)* is a very good silicone spray for dry hair of any thickness, though someone with fine or thin hair should used this sparingly.

☺ **So Blonde Wanna Be Blonde Highlighting Gel** *($5.99 for 6 ounces)* is a water-based gel that contains enough hydrogen peroxide to lighten blonde to medium brown hair if used often enough, though it's not strong enough to produce more than a yellow/gold to golden bronze blonde tone on any hair type. It can be used in the sun or with heat to lighten hair, but is hardly different from buying an 89-cent bottle of 3% hydrogen peroxide and applying that daily to your hair.

☺ **So Blonde Wanna Be Blonde Highlighting Spray** *($5.99 for 6 ounces)* is similar to the So Blonde Wanna Be Blonde Highlighting Gel above, except this is a spray-on, water-based liquid. Otherwise, the same comments apply.

GÖT2B SO SMOOTH

☺ **So Smooth Creme Shampoo** *($5.99 for 8.5 ounces)* is a standard, detergent-based shampoo that is a great option for all hair types. This contains nothing to make hair any smoother than almost every other standard shampoo can. It contains a minimal amount of conditioning agents and so poses little to no risk of buildup.

☺ **So Smooth One Minute Emergency Repair Cream** *($5.99 for 16 ounces)* has an enticing name that is intended to set it apart from the other göt2b conditioners. A closer look at the formula, however, reveals that it is just another standard conditioner that can be a good choice for normal to dry hair of any thickness. Leaving this on for one minute, one hour, one day, or even one week will not repair hair in any way, shape, or form.

☺ **So Smooth Moisturizing Conditioner** *($5.99 for 10 ounces)* is nearly identical to the So Blonde Blonde Aid Intensive Hair Repair above, and the same comments apply. Notice that this conditioner provides four more ounces for the same amount of money compared to the So Blonde product.

☺ **So Smooth Creme Straightener** *($5.99 for 6 ounces)* is a very good straightening balm with a soft, touchable hold that helps keep hair smooth and prevents frizzies.

☺ **So Smooth Style It Smooth Shine Pomade** *($5.99 for 2 ounces)* is nearly identical to the Defiant Define & Shine Pomade above, except this contains more conditioning agents, which makes it preferred for drier hair. Otherwise, the same comments apply.

☺ **So Smooth Liquid Fixx Miracle Repair Treatment** *($7.99 for 4 ounces)* isn't a miracle, but it is a very good spray-on, leave-in conditioner for all hair types. It can be paired with other styling products without impeding their performance.

☺ **So Smooth Liquid Shine** *($5.99 for 4 ounces)* is similar to the Glossy Anti-Frizz Shine Serum above, only this one has more conditioning agents, which makes it a better choice for dry to very dry or damaged hair.

☺ **So Smooth Smoothing Serum Anti-Frizz Treatment** *($7.99 for 2 ounces)* is similar to the Glossy Anti-Frizz Shine Serum and So Smooth Liquid Shine products above, except this has a slightly more elegant formula that favors increased amounts of conditioning agents, including panthenol. Otherwise, the same basic comments apply.

GRAHAM WEBB

An ingredient referred to as Thermacore Complex is present in almost all of the Graham Webb line products. It sounds very scientific, but it is nothing more than a blend of panthenol, allantoin, and an ingredient to keep the two mixed together. The allantoin is a skin-soothing agent, but one that is rinsed away in a shampoo and that has little benefit for the scalp in styling products. Overall, this complex functions primarily as a standard conditioning agent, no better or worse than those found in hundreds and hundreds of products, although Webb has come up with an impressive name. And while it cannot protect the hair from the rigors of heat styling, many of the products below contain silicones and proteins (the same as most hair-care products) that can do a good job of protecting hair from heat. Just remember that no product can provide significant protection from heat damage. The best you can do is to choose products that minimize damage while helping you create and maintain your hairstyle. For more information about Graham Webb, now owned by Procter & Gamble, call (800) 470-9909 or visit www.grahamwebb.com.

What's Good About This Line: Overall excellent shampoos and conditioners; enough styling products to satisfy anyone's needs, from natural to extreme, including some unique options.

What's Not So Good About It: The Ice Cap product line is nothing more than a showcase for menthol; a few of the conditioners contain a high amount of clay, which is nothing but drying for hair; too many repetitive products—this line should be streamlined.

☺ $$$ **Classic Indulgence Pearl Enhanced Shampoo** *($13.90 for 8.5 ounces)* is a standard, creamy shampoo that would work well for normal to dry hair of any thickness. It poses little to no risk of buildup, and the pearl powder it contains is more frivolous than indulgent.

☺ **$$$ Cleanse Sheer, Shampoo for Normal Hair** *($13 for 16.9 ounces)* is a standard, but good, shampoo for normal to dry hair of any thickness.

☺ **Visibility Clarifying Shampoo** *($9.25 for 11 ounces)* contains salicylic acid, but the pH of this shampoo is too high for it to be useful as an exfoliant (and that's a good thing for your hair). This is otherwise a very standard shampoo that contains enough plant oil to make buildup an eventual problem. Still, this is a good option for normal to dry hair that is normal to coarse or thick.

☹ **Classic Indulgence Pearl Enhanced Conditioner** *($13.90 for 8.5 ounces)* lists clay as the third ingredient, and that can make it far too drying for the hair. This conditioner is not an indulgence, it's a problem.

☺ **Condition 30 Second Sheer Conditioner** *($11.11 for 11 ounces)* is a simple, lightweight conditioner that would work well to moisturize and help detangle normal to slightly dry hair that is normal to fine or thin.

☺ **Condition The Untangler Light Detangling and Conditioning Spray** *($11 for 8.5 ounces)* is a basic detangling spray that contains more plant extracts than beneficial conditioning agents. Still, it is an OK option for fine or thin hair. This does not contain film-forming agents, so there is no chance of buildup.

GRAHAM WEBB BRIT STYLE

☺ **Brit Style Energy Lock Hair Spray** *($10.18 for 10 ounces)* is a standard aerosol hairspray that provides a medium hold with a minimally sticky, stiff feel. Hair is easily brushed through, and the silicones add a touch of shine to your finished style.

☺ **Brit Style Exothermic Styling Gel** *($10.18 for 8.5 ounces)* is a very good light- to medium-hold styling gel that contains plant oil to provide some protection during heat styling. This gel does not leave hair feeling stiff, and it is minimally sticky.

☺ **Brit Style Finishing Spray** *($10.18 for 8.5 ounces)* is a good, firm-hold nonaerosol hairspray that pretty much freezes hair in place and makes it difficult to brush through. It is best reserved for times when you need long-lasting hold or support and do not intend to restyle your hair before your next shampoo.

☺ **Brit Style Flexible Hold Hair Spray** *($9.25 for 6.5 ounces)* is a standard aerosol hairspray that applies as a very fine mist, which allows it to provide light hold that leaves hair minimally stiff and keeps it easy to brush through.

☺ **Brit Style Hair Wax** *($9.25 for 2 ounces)* is a thick, greasy pomade that is not as modern-feeling as many others. This can certainly add shine and smoothness to the hair, but the greasiness makes it best for those with dry to very dry hair that is coarse, curly, or thick.

☺ **Brit Style High-Gloss Spray Gel** *($10.18 for 8.5 ounces)* isn't high-gloss at all. This is a standard water- and alcohol-based spray gel that provides a firm, sticky hold that can still be brushed through. For the money, this isn't much different from what you'd find in L'Oreal's Studio or Garnier Fructis lines.

The Reviews G

☺ **Brit Style Liquid Hold** *($12.97 for 4 ounces)* is positioned as being liquid hairspray that you apply with your fingers instead of the conventional spray-on method. It's essentially a watery styling gel that provides a firm, moderately sticky hold and is best used to control stubborn strands or for areas where you want or need exaggerated hold or lift.

☹ **Brit Style Liquid Pomade** *($9.25 for 2 ounces)* is less of a pomade and more of a styling gel that smoothes and adds shine to hair without being too heavy or greasy. Unfortunately, this contains sodium polystyrene sulfonate, which can cause unnecessary dryness and potentially can strip dyed hair color with repeated use.

☺ **Brit Style Magnitude Mousse** *($10.18 for 8.5 ounces)* is a standard, no-frills aerosol mousse capable of light hold that's not sticky, nor does it make hair feel stiff. It is a good choice for normal to fine or thin hair, but provides little in the way of heat protection.

☺ **Brit Style Moussing Wax** *($11.11 for 6 ounces)* contains the preservatives methylchloroisothiazolinone and methylisothiazolinone (also known as Kathon CG), which are contraindicated for use in leave-on products due to the risk of a sensitizing reaction, so keep this away from skin. Other than that, this is a thick mousse with a medium hold that can feel slightly sticky, although it can be brushed through.

☺ **Brit Style Sculptor** *($14.83 for 3.4 ounces)* is a very thick styling cream that contains a mixture of ingredients more typically seen in pomades, gels, hairsprays, and styling lotions. This isn't a confused product, it's actually quite versatile. It can provide texture and definition with a light to medium hold while adding a slightly greasy shine, it can tame frizzies or smooth flyaway hair, or it can be used with heat to create soft curls and waves. It can be too heavy for fine or thin hair, but every other hair type should experiment with a product like this, especially if you're tired of having to mix standard styling products to get the look you're after.

☺ **Brit Style Styling Paste** *($12.97 for 3 ounces)* is a thick, slightly creamy styling paste that is for use only on dry hair (it does not emulsify or distribute well through wet hair), and only then if the hair needs some heavy-duty smoothing or hold with stickiness. This is not as elegant as the Brit Style Sculptor above, but is an OK option for creating enhanced texture with hold for short, choppy hairstyles.

☺ **$$$ Brit Style Styling Putty** *($15.76 for 3.5 ounces)* is an incredibly thick pomade that is primarily water, lanolin wax, and thickeners. The lanolin wax is tricky to spread and lends a slightly sticky, coated feel to the hair along with a low-gloss shine. This type of product is best reserved for those with dry to very dry hair that is very thick or coarse as well as stubborn.

☺ **Brit Style Volumizing & Thickening Spray** *($10.18 for 8.5 ounces)* is a very good, alcohol-based styling spray that provides a light hold that leaves hair minimally stiff or sticky. The plant extracts have no effect on hair, but the added conditioning agents can provide a small amount of heat protection.

☺ **$$$ Brit Style Wax Pomade** *($17 for 1.7 ounces)* contains no wax at all, so the name is misleading. This is a standard, water-soluble pomade that adds a great deal of shine to the hair courtesy of plant oil and mica particles. It is a great smoothing product for all hair types except fine or thin, though someone with fine hair could get away with using a tiny dab of this on the ends of the hair.

☺ $$$ **Brit Style Shine Serum** *($15.76 for 2 ounces)* is a standard silicone serum that can add shine and make hair feel silky smooth, but there is no reason to spend this much when similar products are available at the drugstore for less than six dollars.

☺ **Brit Style Shine Spray** *($12.04 for 4 ounces)* breaks tradition by not including any silicones, instead relying on mineral oil and myristyl alcohol for shine. This can be a good glossing spray for those with dry to very dry hair that is normal to thick or coarse, but mineral oil and wax don't leave the same silky feel as silicone does.

GRAHAM WEBB COLOR CARE

☺ **Color Care Shampoo** *($13.25 for 8.5 ounces)* is a standard shampoo available in several shades that claims to enhance hair color. However, because the coloring agents in this product have minimal ability to cling to the hair shaft, the effect (if you notice one at all) is incredibly subtle. As a shampoo, this is a very good, detergent-based option for normal to dry hair of any thickness except fine or thin. The conditioning agents can build up with repeated use.

☺ $$$ **Color Care Conditioner** *($17.75 for 8.5 ounces)* is a better option than the Color Care Shampoo above for adding a subtle hint of color to the hair: the dye agents are better able to cling to the hair because of the conditioning agents found in this product. As a conditioner, this is a good option for normal to slightly dry hair of any thickness. Several shades are available to add a touch of temporary color.

☺ **Color Care Blonde Shimmer Cream** *($12.95 for 1.7 ounces)* is a thick finishing product that is essentially a way to add shimmer and smoothness to hair while adding a bit of texture. Any hair color can use this to add shimmer, but a product like this is best reserved for evenings or special occasions.

☺ **Color Care Mousse** *($11 for 8.5 ounces)* is a very standard, propellant-based mousse that offers a light to medium hold and allows hair to be easily brushed through. The conditioning agents provide a small amount of protection during heat styling.

GRAHAM WEBB ICE CAP

☹ **Ice Cap Revitalizing Shampoo** *($7.95 for 11 ounces)* is a standard shampoo that contains menthol, which is needlessly drying and irritating for the scalp.

☹ **Ice Cap Hypothermic Bonding Conditioner** *($12.95 for 11 ounces)* also contains menthol, and is not recommended.

☹ **Ice Cap Revitalizing Conditioner** *($9.95 for 11 ounces)* contains menthol, and is not recommended.

GRAHAM WEBB MAKING WAVES

☺ **Making Waves Curl Defining Shampoo** *($10.18 for 11 ounces)* is a very good shampoo for normal to dry hair of any thickness, and poses only a slight risk of buildup.

☺ **Making Waves Curl Defining Conditioner** *($11.11 for 11 ounces)* is a great option for normal to dry hair that is normal to thick or coarse. This provides no special benefit for curly hair.

☺ $$$ **Making Waves Curl Defining Gel** *($15.60 for 8.5 ounces)* is a moisturizing styling gel that provides medium hold, and it can work well to define and shape curls or waves without stiffness but with moderate stickiness.

GRAHAM WEBB SILK REPAIR

☺ **Silk Repair Super Silk Shampoo** *($10.95 for 11 ounces)* is similar to the Visibility Clarifying Shampoo above, except this contains token amounts of plant oil and thickeners. Otherwise, the same basic comments apply.

☺ **Silk Repair Pure Gold Conditioner** *($12.95 for 11 ounces)* is an emollient conditioner that is a great option for dry to very dry hair that is normal to coarse or thick.

☹ $$$ **Silk Repair Silk Protein Leave-In Conditioner** *($12.95 for 8.5 ounces)* is a below-average, do-nothing leave-in conditioner that contains mostly water, standard thickener, and preservative. All of the interesting ingredients are present in amounts too small to have an effect on hair, but this can be OK for normal hair that needs some moisture.

☹ **Silk Repair ThermaClay Hair Maximizing Conditioner** *($12.95 for 6 ounces)* lists clay as the second ingredient, which serves no purpose for hair other than to dry it out. Nothing about this product will maximize your hair, unless you're looking to make it as dry as possible.

☹ **Silk Repair ThermaCore Therapy Advanced Recovery Treatment** *($3.95 for 1 ounce)* is a two-part conditioning treatment said to have the ability to "instinctively detect and treat hair's most damaged areas, providing unsurpassed strength, body, and shine." The dual-sided packet features a standard conditioner on both sides. One side is acidic, the other alkaline. You're supposed to mix the two parts together, transforming this into an "active" product, before applying it to the hair. The only activity that occurs on mixing is the foaming action from combining an acid and a base. None of this has anything to do with advanced recovery for hair; it's just basic science hocus-pocus so you think you're using something special. At best, this is a basic detangling conditioner that is an OK option for normal to slightly dry hair of any thickness.

☺ **Silk Repair Thermal Care, Shampoo for Dry, Damaged Hair** *($10.95 for 11 ounces)* is a very good shampoo for all hair types, and poses minimal to no risk of buildup.

GRAHAM WEBB STICK STRAIGHT

☺ **Stick Straight Smoothing Shampoo** *($10.18 for 11 ounces)* is a very standard, detergent-based shampoo that is an option for all hair types, posing minimal to no risk of buildup. This shampoo offers no special advantage for those with straight hair (or those who wish their hair was straight).

☺ **Stick Straight Smoothing Conditioner** *($11.11 for 11 ounces)* is a standard conditioner for normal to slightly dry hair that is normal to slightly thick or coarse.

☺ **Stick Straight Smoothing Gel** *($12.04 for 6 ounces)* is a substandard straightening gel that lacks silicone or conditioning agents to adequately protect hair during heat styling. It contains no holding agents, but can make hair feel slightly smoother and add a bit of fullness.

☺ $$$ **Stick Straight Super Strength Smoothing Gel** *($16.69 for 6 ounces)* has what the Stick Straight Smoothing Gel above is missing, and is a superb option for use when straightening hair with heat. The multiple silicones help make hair smooth and shiny.

GRAHAM WEBB THICK INFUSION

☺ **Thick Infusion Thickening Shampoo** *($9.95 for 11 ounces)* is similar to the Making Waves Curl Defining Shampoo above, and the same basic comments apply.

☺ **Thick Infusion Thickening Conditioner** *($11.11 for 11 ounces)* contains mostly water, slip agent, thickener, silicones, detangling agent, film-forming agents, fragrance, panthenol, and preservatives. It's a good conditioner for normal to slightly dry hair that is normal to fine or thin. The film-forming agent can create a feeling of thickness, but builds up over time, and that can make fine or thin hair feel heavy.

☹ $$$ **Thick Infusion Root Volumizing Spray** *($15.76 for 8.5 ounces)* is a standard hairspray that comes in a container with a special nozzle that allows you to direct a concentrated blast of this product toward the roots of your hair. Unless you have a keen understanding of how to style your hair, this product's application can be a problem, if for no other reason than it provides a firm hold and sticky finish that isn't best to apply so close to the scalp.

GRAHAM WEBB VIVID COLOR

☺ **Vivid Color Color Locking Shampoo** *($10.18 for 11 ounces)* is similar to the Cleanse Sheer, Shampoo for Normal Hair above, and the same comments apply. This shampoo cannot lock in color, though the name certainly makes it tempting to believe.

☺ $$$ **Vivid Color Color Locking Conditioner** *($13.90 for 6.7 ounces)* is similar to the Making Waves Curl Defining Conditioner above, and the same basic comments apply.

☹ $$$ **Vivid Color Color Locking Leave-In Conditioner** *($13.90 for 6.7 ounces)* is similar to the Silk Repair Silk Protein Leave-In Conditioner above, except this formula is a bit more helpful for detangling hair. Otherwise, the same basic comments apply.

☺ **Vivid Color Color Locking Hair Spray** *($11.16 for 10 ounces)* is a standard aerosol hairspray that dries quickly and provides a light hold that is non-sticky and can be easily brushed through. This is a great working hairspray, but won't do a thing to protect or prolong color.

☺ **Vivid Color Color Locking Foaming Gel** *($10.18 for 6 ounces)* is a standard, propellant-based styling mousse whose texture is slightly thicker than most. This provides a firm, stiff hold that can be brushed through, but not easily. It remains sticky and is best for wet looks or mixing with a silicone serum before you heat-style your hair.

☺ **Vivid Color Color Locking Maximum Hold Gel** *($12.04 for 8.5 ounces)* provides a medium hold that has a slightly sticky, moist finish that lets hair be easily brushed through. This is a good styling gel for normal to thick or coarse hair, but contains nothing that can protect your hair color.

☺ **$$$ Vivid Color Reparative Shine** *($18.55 for 1.7 ounces)* is a standard, but very good, silicone serum that can work as well as any to smooth hair and add a dazzling shine. Still, you don't need to spend more than six dollars on a silicone serum from the drugstore to achieve the exact same effect you get from this product.

H$_2$O+

There isn't much to say about this hair-care line, other than H2O+ shines more with their skin-care products! The products reviewed below are mostly worthwhile, but the standard formulations and tiny amounts of exotic ingredients don't justify the salon-caliber prices. For more information about H2O+, call (800) 242-2284 or visit www.H2Oplus.com.

What's Good About This Line: The conditioners are all efficacious.

What's Not So Good About It: The shampoos are problematic, including either drying detergent cleansing agents or a plethora of menthol and mint extracts.

H$_2$O+ MILK

☹ **$$$ Milk Shampoo** *($15 for 12 ounces)* is a standard, detergent-based shampoo that contains sodium lauryl sulfate, though in an amount small enough that it may not be a problem for the scalp or hair, so this can still be an option for those with normal to oily hair that is fine or thin. Because this contains an acrylate-based film-forming agent, it should be alternated with a shampoo that does not cause buildup. The milk protein functions as a conditioning agent, although it's no different from countless other conditioning agents; milk just sounds more natural and healthier for hair, even though it isn't.

☺ **$$$ Milk Conditioner** *($16 for 12 ounces)* is a very good, though pricey, conditioner for normal to dry hair that is normal to coarse or thick.

☺ **$$$ Milk Silkening Hair Mask** *($17.50 for 6 ounces)*. If you were thinking this hair mask would be a rich, emollient treat for overstressed tresses, you would be wrong. At best, this is a good detangling conditioner for normal to dry hair that is fine or thin. There are too few emollient ingredients to make this worthy of being a conditioning treat for hair, especially not very dry or thick hair.

H$_2$O+ SPA

☹ **Spa Mint Ice Shampoo** *($15 for 11.5 ounces)* contains several irritating plant extracts, including peppermint, spearmint, and pennyroyal, plus a menthol kick for additional irritation. This shampoo may feel invigorating on the scalp, but that's just irritation occurring, and the long-term results are a problem for your scalp.

☹ **Spa Sea Marine Revitalizing Shampoo** (*$13 for 8 ounces*) contains sodium lauryl sulfate as one of its main detergent cleansing agents, and as such this shampoo is too drying for all hair and scalp types.

☹ **Spa Sea Plankton Restructuring Shampoo** (*$14 for 8 ounces*) is similar to the Spa Sea Marine Revitalizing Shampoo above, and the same comments apply.

☺ **$$$ Spa Hair Repair Seaweed Masque** (*$17.50 for 6 ounces*) is a very standard conditioner that would take good care of normal to dry hair of any thickness, but doesn't deserve the status of a specialty product with such an absurd price tag.

☺ **$$$ Spa Sea Marine Collagen Conditioner** (*$15 for 8 ounces*) is nearly identical to the Milk Conditioner above, and the same basic comments apply. The sea extracts serve as water-binding agents only, and have little impact on your hair's volume or manageability.

☹ **Spa Mint Ice Conditioner** (*$16 for 11.5 ounces*) contains peppermint oil along with several irritating mint extracts and, to top it all off, menthol. This conditioner is seriously irritating to the scalp, and is not recommended.

☺ **$$$ Spa Sea Plankton Restructuring Conditioner** (*$16 for 8 ounces*) is similar to the Spa Hair Repair Seaweed Masque above, only this contains some silicone, which makes it preferred for drier hair. Of course, this can neither restructure the hair nor rebuild the hair shaft, as H$_2$O+ claims.

HAYASHI

For more information about Hayashi, call (800) 448-9500.

What's Good About This Line: Almost all the shampoos and conditioners have merit for all hair types; styling products perform well, though a few contain scalp irritants.

What's Not So Good About It: Hayashi's overall philosophy that their products must be used together is faulty because their products contain the same fundamental ingredients used throughout the hair-care industry; Plus Hair and Scalp Revitalizer is nothing but a problem for the scalp.

HAYASHI SYSTEM 911

☺ **$$$ Shampoo Emergency Repair for Dry Damaged Hair** (*$13 for 10.6 ounces*) is a very good shampoo for normal to dry hair of any thickness, though the conditioning agents can build up with repeated use. This absolutely cannot repair damaged hair.

☺ **$$$ Daily Remedy Conditioner for Damaged Hair** (*$13 for 10.6 ounces*) is a standard, fairly lightweight conditioner that would work well for normal to slightly dry hair that is normal to fine or thin. The film-forming agents pose a slight risk of buildup with repeated use.

☺ **$$$ Emergency Pak Reconstructor for Damaged Hair** (*$17 for 6 ounces*) is a basic, but good, conditioner for normal to slightly dry hair that is normal to fine or thin. It won't reconstruct hair, and it's not a very good choice for damaged hair, so ignore the product's claims.

☺ **Protein Mist Leave-In Conditioner Detangler Body Builder** *($11 for 8.4 ounces)* is an excellent leave-in conditioner that can soften and detangle all hair types except coarse or very thick hair.

HAYASHI SYSTEM COLOR

☹ **Protecting Shampoo, for Color Treated Hair** *($9 for 8.4 ounces)* contains sodium C14-16 olefin sulfonate as its main detergent cleansing agent, which makes this shampoo too drying for all hair and scalp types. That cleansing agent also does not belong in a product designed for color-treated hair.

☺ **Protecting Conditioner, for Color Treated Hair** *($10 for 8.4 ounces)* is a good option for normal to slightly dry hair that is normal to fine or thin.

HAYASHI SYSTEM DESIGN

☺ **Freeze-It, Working Spray Fast Dry Strong Hold** *($11 for 8.4 ounces)* is a standard hairspray that provides light, flexible hold that is minimally stiff or sticky. The conditioning agents help hair stay soft and remain easy to brush through with no flaking.

☺ **Instant Replay, Shaping Gel Hold and Shine** *($10 for 8 ounces)* is a standard styling gel with medium hold. It leaves hair slightly stiff and sticky, but can be brushed through. The conditioning agents provide some protection during heat styling.

☺ **Quikk, Fast Dry Working Spray** *($13 for 10 ounces)* is a very good aerosol hairspray that does indeed dry quickly. It applies lightly, providing a light to medium hold that remains somewhat sticky but can be brushed through. The lanolin and silicone add shine. Note: This product is available in two formulas, an 80% VOC formula not for sale in California, and a 55% VOC formula for sale in California.

☺ **$$$ Texture Mud, Hard Hold Design Adhesive** *($16.95 for 3.5 ounces)* is a thick, slightly greasy pomade that contains film-forming/holding agents that work well to support more extreme styles but leave hair feeling sticky. This is a good option to smooth and tame unruly thick or coarse hair that is straight or curly.

☺ **Triple Play, Volumizing Mousse Strong Hold** *($12 for 7 ounces)* is a medium-hold styling mousse that goes on heavier than most, which makes it preferred for normal to slightly thick or coarse hair. This does leave hair feeling slightly sticky, but it can be brushed through.

☺ **$$$ Uncurl, Smoothing Glaze Keeps Hair Straight** *($16.95 for 8.4 ounces)* is a lightweight styling liquid that provides a soft hold and offers light conditioning for all hair types. This isn't as elegant as many of the silicone-based straightening balms, but it does provide a slight amount of protection from heat. Nothing in this product can keep hair straight unless it is first styled with heat and the appropriate styling tools.

☺ **Volume + Firm Texture Design Mist** *($10 for 8.4 ounces)* is a styling spray that is essentially a hairspray. It offers a medium hold that leaves hair slightly stiff and sticky, though hair can be brushed through.

☺ **Hi-Gloss** *($9.95 for 2 ounces)* is a standard, water-soluble pomade that contains several very good ingredients for dry to very dry hair. This non-sticky pomade works well to smooth the hair, add shine, and enhance curl, but use it sparingly to avoid a greasy look.

☺ $$$ **Hi-Shine Polishing Drops Protects and Shines** *($14.95 for 1.07 ounces)* is a standard silicone serum that would work as well as any. The tiny amount of alcohol present will evaporate before it can have a drying effect on the hair.

☺ **Mist n' Shine Ultra Fine Super Shine** *($10.50 for 2.2 ounces)* is a propellant-based silicone spray that works well as a lightweight option to add a glossy shine to all types of hair.

☺ $$$ **Spray and Shine Polishing Spray Seals and Shines** *($15.75 for 4 ounces)* is a slick, emollient shine spray that is a great finishing option for normal to very dry hair that is normal to thick or coarse. It adds shine and moisture without making hair feel too slick or heavy, although it could still be too much for those with fine or thin hair. The tiny amount of rosemary oil is unlikely to be a problem for the scalp.

HAYASHI SYSTEM HINOKI

Note: Hayashi claims the hinokitol (hinoki oil) in the products below can block the conversion of the hormone testosterone to dihydrotestosterone (DHT), a process that is one of the causes of male pattern baldness, and that this oil can therefore stimulate hair growth. However, there is no evidence or research to support this.

☺ **Shampoo Volumizing Cleanser for Fine and Thinning Hair** *($8 for 8.4 ounces)* is a very good shampoo for all hair types, and poses minimal to no risk of buildup.

☺ **Conditioner Texturizing Rinse for Fine and Thinning Hair** *($9 for 8.4 ounces)* is a fairly emollient conditioner that would work well for normal to dry hair of any thickness.

☺ $$$ **Hair Thickener Leave-In Body Booster for Fine and Thinning Hair** *($15 for 8.4 ounces)* is a very good leave-in conditioner for fine or thin hair.

☹ **Plus Hair and Scalp Revitalizer for Healthy Hair Growth, Fine and Thinning Hair** *($15 for 8.4 ounces)* contains alcohol as its main ingredient, and that won't help with healthy hair growth in the least. Ditto for the hinoki oil, which can be a scalp irritant. This scalp-specific product is more problematic than helpful.

HEAD GAMES

Here is yet another hair-care line aimed at teens and twenty-somethings looking to create modern hairstyles with edge and attitude. The marketing angle is all about providing unconventional, colorfully packaged products to help young adults discover themselves and the image they want to communicate (at least via their hair) to the world. Such deep sentiments go beyond what any hair-care product can provide, but I suppose the sense of empowerment these products try to convey is positive, and there's no doubt the product names and descriptions speak to most teens' sensibilities and spirit of fun, and the product's fragrances are kicky.

The Reviews H

Head GAMES is sold in salons and beauty supply stores. It is owned and distributed by Graham Webb International, itself a subsidiary of the Wella Corporation, which is owned by Procter & Gamble. Confused yet? For more information about head GAMES, call (800) 470-9909 or visit www.headgames.com.

What's Good About This Line: A varied group of styling products whose claims and level of hold should appeal to those looking to create trendy or extreme hairstyles.

What's Not So Good About It: A few of the styling products are either very difficult to work with, too sticky to tolerate, or poorly formulated.

☹ **Moisture Bliss, Hydrating Shampoo** *($8.50 for 12 ounces)* contains sodium C14-16 olefin sulfonate as one of its main detergent cleansing agents, which makes it too drying for both hair and scalp.

☺ **Thick Headed, Thickening Shampoo** *($8.50 for 12 ounces)* is a standard, but very good, shampoo that would work well for all hair types. Although there is some concern that the minerals in it can bond to the hair shaft and cause dryness with repeated use, they can also add a slightly thicker feel to hair.

☺ **Tangle Buster, Daily Detangling Conditioner** *($10 for 12 ounces)* is a standard lightweight conditioner that is a good option for normal to slightly dry hair that is normal to fine or thin.

☺ **All Whipped Up, Volumizing Mousse** *($10 for 10.5 ounces)* is a standard, propellant-based styling mousse that provides a light hold and is minimally stiff or sticky. It would work great for all hair types.

☺ $$$ **Attitude Adjustment, Reworkable Sculptor** *($15.50 for 2.5 ounces)* is a thick, water- and wax-based styling cream that can be difficult to work with because it is so gooey and stringy. This provides a medium, flexible hold that leaves hair coated and slightly sticky, but it can control unruly waves and curls for those with thick or coarse hair. It also comes in handy for creating exaggerated textures on shorter hairstyles. Removing this will take more than one application of shampoo.

☺ **Bizarre Twist, Molding Putty** *($14 for 4 ounces)* is an extraordinarily thick, lanolin wax–based styling putty that comes with a spatula so you can scoop it out (using your fingers would require digging into the product, which is messy). This is very difficult to apply as it does not distribute through wet hair evenly. It is also very sticky, and provides a matte finish. This is appropriate only for someone with thick or coarse hair who is up for the challenge of working with the product.

☺ **Gelous Rage, Hair Styling Gel** *($10 for 6 ounces)* is a standard styling gel capable of providing a medium to firm hold that leaves hair slightly stiff and sticky. The minerals in this product (particularly the copper, which can make hair look green) pose a small risk of binding to the hair and causing dryness, but the amounts included are likely too small to have this effect.

☺ **Green with Envy, Styling Pomade** *($10 for 2 ounces)* can be used by all hair types as a water-soluble pomade to add shine and smoothness to the hair. This feels thick initially, but ends up feeling lighter than most pomades once on the hair, and it provides a soft hold. Those with fine or thin hair should use it sparingly, while those with thicker hair can apply this liberally, especially if hair is dry.

☺ $$$ **Hard Ball, Hair Jam** *($15 for 1.9 ounces)* is a styling gel that has a jellylike texture and eschews conventional holding agents in favor of sucrose (sugar). This produces a lightweight gel that provides a medium to firm hold but, not surprisingly, leaves hair stiff and sticky. I suppose this could be useful for short, spiky hairstyles, but using this with a blow dryer can make hair feel fried and, for lack of a better word, crispy.

☺ **Messed-Up Madness, Molding Creme** *($14 for 4 ounces)* is an excellent hybrid styling cream/pomade product that works great to enhance hair texture and add definition to curls and waves without being stiff or sticky. This is fairly heavy and can become greasy if you use too much, but it remains a good option for normal to very dry hair that is coarse or thick.

☺ **Power Hungry, Maximum Hold Gel** *($10 for 6 ounces)* is a standard styling gel that provides a firm hold that leaves hair slightly stiff and sticky, though it can be brushed through.

☺ **Show Off, Texture Spray** *($14 for 6.8 ounces)* is a spray gel that contains mostly water, glucose (sugar), slip agent, preservative, film-forming/holding agents, thickeners, plant oil, anti-static agent, coloring agents, and fragrance. This is stiff stuff, and can definitely make hair stand on end, though not without a lot of stickiness. Contrary to claim, this product does not provide protection from heat. It is best for wet looks or when you intend to let your hairstyle dry naturally.

☹ **Split Personality, Dual-Purpose Smoothing Serum** *($12 for 8.2 ounces)* is a below-average smoothing gel that can ball up on the hair and flake during styling. There are much better options available for use when straightening hair with heat.

☺ **Stay Put, Firm Hold Hair Spray** *($10 for 10 ounces)* is a standard aerosol hairspray that distributes a fine, quick-drying mist capable of providing firm hold and long-lasting style support. It can be tricky to brush through, so it's best used as a final step to keep your hairstyle in place and add a touch of shine.

☺ **Thick Headed, Thickening Lotion** *($10 for 8.2 ounces)* is a gel, not a lotion, and one that's capable of providing a firm hold that leaves hair slightly stiff and very sticky. The conditioning agents provide some protection from heat, and hair can be brushed through, though not as easily as with most gels.

☺ **Wound Up, Elastic Styler** *($10 for 4 ounces)* is a watery, metallic blue styling gel (the blue color does not affect your hair color) that is designed for extreme hairstyles, meaning those that require a high degree of gravity-defying hold. This leaves hair uncomfortably stiff and sticky, but if your hair is resistant to most styling products and you want to spike, lift, or shape it, this works well.

HEAD & SHOULDERS

Head & Shoulders remains a mostly superior line to consider if you are struggling with dandruff. Their straightforward formulations (many of which have improved since I last reviewed this line) contain active ingredients that help mitigate the cause and flaky side effects of this common scalp condition. The main active ingredient used in the products below is zinc pyrithione. A potent anti-microbial agent, it is thought to act on the yeast believed to be responsible for causing dandruff. (It's not effective for dry scalp, which is a different condition that won't respond to treatment with zinc pyrithione.) As an over-the-counter drug, zinc pyrithione is allowed in concentrations up to 2% in rinse-off products, though concentrations below 0.5% in shampoos and conditioners tend to be less effective, especially for stubborn cases of dandruff. For leave-on products, the concentration of zinc pyrithione cannot exceed 0.25%. It is generally well tolerated and has a low incidence of side effects, the most common being skin irritation (Sources: www.nlm.nih.gov/medlineplus/druginfo/uspdi/202495.html; and *Journal of the American Academy of Dermatology*, December 2001, pages 897–903). For more information about Head & Shoulders, call (800) 723-9569 or visit www.headandshoulders.com.

What's Good About This Line: The active ingredients in these shampoos and conditioners can help control dandruff.

What's Not So Good About It: All of the shampoos contain ammonium xylenesulfonate, an ingredient that's counterproductive in products designed to help control flaking and itching; Head & Shoulders' leave-in anti-dandruff product is sullied by camphor.

Note: All of the shampoos below contain the solvent ammonium xylenesulfonate, which can cause scalp and hair dryness. I typically rate hair-care products that contain this ingredient poorly, but have made an exception in this case because the active ingredients in these shampoos are so effective. Also, while ammonium xylenesulfonate can be a problem in any amount, the amount used in the products below is only a small percentage of the total formula, which reduces the likelihood of problems for the hair.

☺ **Shampoo, Classic Clean** *($4.59 for 13.5 ounces)* is a standard, detergent-based shampoo that contains 1% zinc pyrithione to help control dandruff. This is otherwise an unremarkable formula, though the silicone can build up over time.

☺ **Shampoo, Dry Scalp Care** *($4.59 for 13.5 ounces)* is a standard, detergent-based shampoo that contains 1% zinc pyrithione as its anti-dandruff agent. This shampoo contains enough silicone to offer conditioning and detangling benefits, but it can quickly build up with repeated use, so alternate this with one that does not contain conditioning agents.

☺ **Shampoo, Extra Fullness** *($4.59 for 13.5 ounces)* is almost identical to the Shampoo, Classic Clean above, except this contains a tiny amount of film-forming agent, which poses a slight risk of buildup. Otherwise, the same basic comments apply.

☺ **Shampoo, Intensive Treatment** *($4.59 for 13.5 ounces)* is a standard detergent-based shampoo that contains 1% selenium sulfide as the active ingredient. Selenium sulfide is another anti-microbial/anti-fungal ingredient that is an option if your dandruff does not respond to treatment with zinc pyrithione. The downside of selenium sulfide is that it is particularly hard on hair and can strip hair color.

☺ **Shampoo, Refresh** *($4.59 for 13.5 ounces)* is nearly identical to the Shampoo, Dry Scalp Care above, and the same comments apply.

☺ **Shampoo, Ultimate Clean** *($4.59 for 13.5 ounces)* contains 1% zinc pyrithione as the active ingredient, and is a good conditioning shampoo for normal to dry hair of any thickness. The conditioning agents can build up with repeated use, so alternate this with a shampoo that does not contain them.

☺ **2-in-1 Shampoo Plus Conditioner, Classic Clean** *($4.59 for 13.5 ounces)* is identical to the Shampoo, Dry Scalp Care above, and the same comments apply. The high amount of silicone in this one is what makes it a two-in-one product, and it would be great for those with dry hair that is coarse or thick.

☺ **2-in-1 Shampoo Plus Conditioner, Smooth & Silky** *($4.59 for 13.5 ounces)* is identical to the Shampoo, Classic Clean above, and the same comments apply. This contains less silicone than the 2-in-1 Shampoo Plus Conditioner, Classic Clean above.

☺ **Conditioner, Dry Scalp Care** *($4.59 for 13.5 ounces)* contains 0.5% zinc pyrithione in a standard conditioner base of water, thickener, silicones, detangling agent, salt, fragrance, preservatives, and vitamins. This can be slightly helpful for a dry scalp, but the real reason to use this (and keep it on the scalp for several minutes while you shower) is the zinc pyrithione.

☺ **Conditioner, Extra Fullness** *($4.59 for 13.5 ounces)* contains 0.5% zinc pyrithione in a standard conditioner base of water, silicones, thickener, detangling agent, salt, fragrance, preservatives, and vitamins. The silicones present make hair feel silky smooth, but over time can build up on the hair, which won't help with its fullness.

☹ **Soothing Lotion for Dry Scalp Leave-In Treatment** *($4.99 for 6.8 ounces)* would have been a slam-dunk solution for all-day control of dandruff, but this product (which contains 0.1% zinc pyrithione as its active ingredient) contains camphor. Camphor does nothing to address the cause or symptoms of dandruff but will cause irritation and exacerbate an itchy scalp. If you're looking for an effective leave-on anti-dandruff product, consider Aveda's Scalp Remedy Anti-Dandruff Styling Tonic ($11 for 3.7 ounces) instead.

ICE

ICE is a strange name for a hair-care line. Is it supposed to mean the products are (or can make your hair) cold? And why would that be a good idea? If it's because of the connection to ice being a bright, reflective surface, as your shiny hair might be from using these products, then how do you explain the low luster many of the styling products have? Regardless of what the name means, ICE is a rather standard hair-care line, and its product names, claims, and packaging are the only truly unique characteristics it sports. Almost all of the products do perform well, and this Joico-owned line is clearly marketed toward young, hip urbanites who want their hairstyles to be more about shock value and high fashion than casual, traditional looks. That is a viable way to go if you're so inclined, and the ICE products can help you achieve styles that will definitely get you noticed, if for no other reason than curiosity about just how you got your hair to stay styled that way! For more information about ICE, call (800) 44-JOICO or visit www.icehair.com.

What's Good About This Line: Mostly excellent styling products, especially if you're looking for extreme hold or alternatives to standard products; good standard products.

What's Not So Good About It: A few of the styling products contain the sensitizing preservatives methylchloroisothiazolinone and methylisothiazolinone (Kathon CG); every ICE product contains irritating horseradish extract.

Note: There is less horseradish in the styling products than in the shampoos or conditioners, but use caution and try to keep the styling products off your scalp.

☺ **Washer Shampoo** ($8 for 10.1 ounces) is a standard shampoo that would work well for all hair types; it poses no risk of buildup.

☺ **Hydrater Conditioner** ($10 for 10.1 ounces) would work well for normal to slightly dry hair of any thickness.

☺ **Power Smoothie** ($10 for 6 ounces) is a very good conditioner for normal to dry hair that is normal to thick or coarse.

☺ **Amplifier Volumizing Mousse** ($12.50 for 8.8 ounces) is a standard, propellant-based mousse that offers a medium hold with a slight amount of stiffness and stickiness, though hair can be brushed through. This contains a nice array of conditioning agents to moisturize hair and provide some protection during heat styling.

☺ **Controller Firm Hold Gel** ($12.50 for 10.1 ounces) provides excellent control and offers one of the strongest holds I've found in a styling gel. The formula works well for slicked-back wet looks on hard-to-control hair. This is also a great taming product for unmanageable curly hair. The stiff, sticky finish may be off-putting, but this can be remedied by mixing this gel with a silicone serum or styling cream that does not contain holding agents.

☺ **Finisher Hair Spray** ($10 for 10.1 ounces) is an aerosol hairspray that provides a light, soft hold that allows hair to be reworked or brushed through as needed. Stickiness is present, but minimal, and this contains silicone for added shine.

☺ **Fixer Firm Hold Hair Spray** ($10 for 10.1 ounces) works well as a firm-hold hairspray, but it can leave hair feeling stiff and sticky. It can freeze styles in place, so it's great if you don't want your carefully constructed hairdo to be undone in the wind. This product advertises a sunscreen, and it does contain one, but there is no way to know how much UV protection you're getting. It could be an SPF 2 (which is no real protection at all) but even if it were higher, there are no standards to measure sunscreen in hair-care products.

☺ **Molder Matte Texture Cream** ($14.50 for 4.4 ounces) is a thick styling cream that provides a medium hold but contains conditioning agents to allow hair to remain flexible and moist. This begins slightly greasy but dries to a natural matte finish with some stickiness. It can work well to smooth stubborn frizzies or curls on thick or coarse hair, but it's too heavy for normal to fine or thin hair, unless used very sparingly.

☺ **Waxer Wax Pomade** *($12.50 for 3.8 ounces)* begins thick, but quickly emulsifies to a slick, greasy pomade that is best for smoothing frizzies or taming thick, coarse hair that is dry to very dry. The smooth texture makes this much easier to work with than traditional wax-based pomades, and it distributes well through the hair, but use it sparingly to avoid a greasy look.

☺ **Liquid ICE Spray Gel** *($10 for 10.1 ounces)* is a standard, alcohol-free spray gel that offers a light hold that remains soft and minimally sticky. The water-binding agent and vitamins provide no protection during heat styling, so this is best paired with a leave-in conditioner or silicone product prior to using a blow dryer or flat iron.

☺ **Slicker Defining Lotion** *($14.50 for 10.1 ounces)* is a very good styling lotion that provides a soft, non-sticky hold and would work brilliantly to straighten and smooth hair with heat.

☹ **Reactor Texture Transformer** *($14 for 1.7 ounces)* is a Jell-O-like pomade that looks solid but quickly liquefies once you emulsify it in your hands. It goes on fairly light, and works to add or enhance texture to hair, but not without a sticky, coated feel that is much more noticeable than standard pomades or styling waxes. This does have a tendency to ball up and flake if hair is manipulated too much after application, and that fact alone makes this difficult to enthusiastically recommend.

ICE SPIKER

☹ **Spiker Eraser Shampoo** *($9 for 8.45 ounces)* contains peppermint oil, which makes it too irritating for all scalp types. Further, this shampoo is sold as being adept at removing styling product buildup, yet it contains a high amount of film-forming agent, which will only create more buildup. What a misguided shampoo!

☺ **Spiker Blast Spray Adhesive, Extreme Hold** *($12 for 10 ounces)* is an aerosol hairspray that offers a light to medium hold with minimal stiff or sticky feel. This is easily brushed through and does not flake, but don't count on it for any sort of extreme hold.

☺ **Spiker Half Blast Spray, Flexible Hold** *($12 for 10 ounces)* is similar to the Spiker Blast Spray Adhesive, Extreme Hold above, except this offers more hold. Otherwise, the same comments apply.

☹ **Spiker Dis-Order Styling Gel** *($12.50 for 5.1 ounces)* contains the preservative Kathon CG, which is contraindicated for use in leave-on products if they come in contact with skin due to a risk of causing a sensitizing reaction.

☺ **Spiker Distortion Styling Gum** *($14 for 3.4 ounces)* is a water-based pomade in a tube. It has a slick, slightly greasy texture that works well to smooth frizzies or add shine and texture to dry hair that is thick or coarse. This does contain a film-forming/holding agent, but the mineral oil, lanolin, and silicones keep it from making hair stiff or sticky.

☹ **Spiker Erratic Molding Clay** *($15 for 3.4 ounces)* is a toothpaste-thick styling wax that contains the preservative Kathon CG, which is contraindicated for use in leave-on products due to a risk of causing a sensitizing reaction if they come in contact with skin.

☺ **Spiker Water-Resistant Styling Glue** *($12.50 for 6 ounces)* is not water-resistant, it's quite water-soluble, but that's great because it means this product is easy to shampoo out. This is an ideal choice for a very strong hold that can keep hair suspended straight up, slicked back, or molded into just about any style you can conjure up. The trade-off is the exceptionally sticky finish and the inability to comb through hair once it sets, though the hair is left with a slight amount of flexibility should you wish to reshape it.

INFUSIUM 23

The "23" in the name of this longstanding line represents the number of provitamin and treatment ingredients used in the products. Looking more closely, with the exception of panthenol and wheat protein, the remaining roster of special ingredients is just amino acids (as water-binding agents), none of which are capable of clinging to the hair because they are too fragile to withstand rinsing or styling. When used in leave-on products, amino acids theoretically can penetrate the cuticle layer and provide moisture to the hair shaft, but so can many other ingredients (such as glycerin or propylene glycol) that have a more dependable track record than amino acids. For more information about Infusium 23, call (800) DUART-33 or visit www.infusium.com.

What's Good About This Line: Most of the conditioners are very good; the prices for such generous sizes are a beauty bargain!

What's Not So Good About It: All of the leave-in treatments (which is what this line is known for) contain the sensitizing preservatives methylchloroisothiazolinone and methylisothiazolinone (Kathon CG); the styling products are an average lot, and several of them flake.

☹ **Colored/Permed Shampoo, for Chemically Treated and Over-Processed Hair** *($5.99 for 16 ounces)* contains sodium lauryl sulfate as one of its main detergent cleansing agents, which makes this shampoo too drying for all hair and scalp types.

☹ **Maximum Body Shampoo, for Fine/Thin Hair** *($5.99 for 16 ounces)* is nearly identical to the Colored/Permed Shampoo above, and the same comments apply.

☹ **Moisturizing Shampoo, for Normal to Dry Hair** *($5.99 for 16 ounces)* is nearly identical to the Colored/Permed Shampoo above, and the same comments apply.

☺ **Colored/Permed Revitalizing Conditioner, for Chemically Treated and Over-Processed Hair** *($5.99 for 16 ounces)* is an excellent conditioner for normal to dry hair of any thickness, though someone with overprocessed hair will need a richer, more emollient product to make their hair feel normal again.

☹ **Heat Activated/UV Protection Leave-In Treatment, for Damaged /Heat Styled Hair** *($5.99 for 16 ounces)* is a simple liquid leave-in conditioner that would be a problem for all scalp types because it contains the preservative Kathon CG, which is not recommended for use in leave-in products.

☹ **Maximum Body Leave-In Treatment, for Fine/Thin Hair** *($3.99 for 8 ounces)* has the same problem preservatives as the Heat Activated/UV Protection Leave-In Treatment above, and is also not recommended.

☺ **Maximum Body Revitalizing Conditioner, for Fine/Thin Hair** *($5.99 for 16 ounces)* is a standard, but good, conditioner for those with normal to slightly dry hair of any thickness, particularly those with normal hair.

☹ **Moisturizing Leave-In Treatment, for Normal to Dry Hair** *($5.99 for 16 ounces)* is nearly identical to the Heat Activated/UV Protection Leave-In Treatment above, and the same comments apply.

☺ **Moisturizing Revitalizing Conditioner, for Normal to Dry Hair** *($5.99 for 16 ounces)* is a very good moisturizing conditioner for normal to dry hair of any thickness.

☹ **Original Leave-In Treatment, for Damaged/Unmanageable Hair** *($5.99 for 16 ounces)* is nearly identical to the Heat Activated/UV Protection Leave-In Treatment above, and the same comments apply.

☺ **Power Pac Conditioner, 3-Minute Intensive Treatment** *($5.99 for 10.2 ounces)* is similar to the Moisturizing Revitalizing Conditioner above, except this contains a greater array of conditioning agents and fewer water-binding agents, which makes it preferred for dry hair of any thickness. This isn't all that intensive, and should be left on for longer than three minutes if your hair is dry (as in moisture-starved, not dry vs. wet application).

☹ **Shape & Hold Aerosol Hair Spray, Extra Firm** *($3.99 for 8 ounces)* is a very light-hold hairspray, but the film-forming/holding agents still tend to ball up and flake, especially when you brush through the hair.

☺ **Shape & Hold Non-Aerosol Hair Spray, Extra Firm** *($3.99 for 8 ounces)* is a standard hairspray that provides an incredibly soft hold that is not the least bit stiff or sticky. This is about as extra firm as cotton, and it's not recommended for any kind of structured hold. It works best for a natural, brushable hold.

☹ **Shaping Gel, Extra Firm** *($3.99 for 4 ounces)* is not extra firm in the least, and is actually a poorly formulated styling gel that tends to flake with little provocation.

☺ **Smoothing & Defining Lotion** *($3.99 for 6 ounces)* is a lightweight fluid styling lotion that provides a light hold that leaves hair minimally sticky and not stiff.

☺ **Styling Mousse, Extra Firm** *($3.99 for 6 ounces)* is a standard, propellant-based mousse that provides a light to medium hold with just a hint of stiffness and stickiness.

☺ **Volumizing Spray Gel, Extra Firm** *($3.99 for 8 ounces)* is a standard, but very good, spray gel for normal to fine or thin hair. It provides light to medium hold that is slightly sticky but does not make hair feel stiff. It is unlikely the sunscreen in this product can provide protection from UV rays. Not only do no standards exist to measure the amount of protection you would get, but heat styling and brushing the hair would negate any UV-protective benefit.

☺ **Split End Repair** *($5.99 for 3 ounces)* cannot repair split ends—no product can. This isn't a very impressive conditioner for dry or damaged hair. The film-forming agent can coat the hair and make it feel smoother, temporarily mending minor split ends, but the effect is gone as soon as you shampoo again.

INNER SCIENCE
(AVAILABLE IN CANADA ONLY)

For more information about Inner Science, owned by Procter & Gamble, call (800) 668-0150 or visit www.innerscience.com. **Note:** All prices are in Canadian dollars.

What's Good About This Line: Reliable conditioners for normal to dry hair of any thickness; reasonable prices.

What's Not So Good About It: Two of the three shampoos contain high levels of the solvent ammonium xylenesulfonate, which can cause dry hair and scalp, not to mention scalp irritation with continued use; the Strengthening and Rejuvenating mists are not capable of meeting any of their claims about making hair stronger.

☹ **Colour Care Shampoo** *($8 for 9 ounces)* is a standard shampoo that offers no special benefit for color-treated hair. This simple formulation can cleanse the hair and scalp, but the high amount of ammonium xylenesulfonate can cause unnecessary scalp dryness and irritation, and it is not recommended.

☹ **Extra Moisture Care Shampoo** *($8 for 9 ounces)* is nearly identical to the Colour Care Shampoo above, and the same comments apply. This does not provide moisture to the hair, but it will cause dryness.

☺ **Volume Care Shampoo** *($8 for 9 ounces)* is an OK, detergent-based shampoo for normal to fine or thin hair. The tiny amount of film-forming agent will not cause buildup. This does contain ammonium xylenesulfonate, but in a small amount that is unlikely to cause noticeable scalp dryness.

☺ **Colour Care Conditioner** *($8 for 6 ounces)* can be a good conditioner for normal to dry hair of any thickness, though the silicone can build up with repeated use. That means those with fine or thin hair should use this only on the ends of hair.

☺ **Colour Care Strengthening Mist** *($8 for 4.5 ounces)* is a liquid, leave-in conditioner that won't do much to strengthen hair, though it can help with combing and provide a feeling of thickness to fine or thin hair.

☺ **Extra Moisture Care Conditioner** *($8 for 6 ounces)* is a standard conditioner that would work well for normal to dry hair of any thickness.

☺ **Moisture Care Strengthening Mist** *($8 for 4.5 ounces)* is identical to the Colour Care Strengthening Mist above, and the same comments apply.

☺ **Volume Care Conditioner** *($8 for 6 ounces)* is similar to, but not as well formulated as, the Colour Care Conditioner above, primarily because many of the beneficial conditioning agents are listed after the fragrance on the ingredient list. This can still be a good, basic conditioner for normal to dry hair of any thickness, but those with fine or thin hair should apply it to the ends of the hair only.

☺ **Volume Care Rejuvenating Mist** *($8 for 4.5 ounces)* won't rejuvenate hair, but it can serve as a lightweight styling and combing spray for normal to fine or thin hair.

ION

Ion is an overwhelmingly large hair-care line with many formulas, but many of them are too similar to deserve their own category. Ion products are sold primarily through Sally Beauty stores nationwide. For more information about Ion, call (800) 777-5706 or visit www.sallybeauty.com.

What's Good About This Line: The prices are reasonable; many of the styling products are wonderful, especially for light, flexible hold; most of the shampoos and conditioners are worth considering by all hair types.

What's Not So Good About It: The line is much bigger than it needs to be; some of the styling products contain the problematic preservatives methylchloroisothiazolinone and methylisothiazolinone (Kathon CG); the anti-dandruff products are either too irritating or are ineffective; several Ion shampoos contain drying detergent cleansing agents; most of the "treatment" conditioners have completely uninspired formulas and are inferior to Ion's regular conditioners.

ION ANTI-FRIZZ SOLUTIONS

☺ **Anti-Frizz Solutions Smoothing Shampoo, Cleanser for Frizzy, Fly-Away Hair** *($4.99 for 12 ounces)* is an excellent shampoo for normal to dry hair that is normal to coarse or thick. The conditioning agents can build up with repeated use.

☺ **Anti-Frizz Solutions Straightening Shampoo, Cleanser for Curly, Wavy, Frizzy Hair** *($4.99 for 12 ounces)* is similar to the Anti-Frizz Solutions Smoothing Shampoo above, except this contains a larger amount of conditioning and film-forming agents. It is a very good option for someone with dry to very dry hair that is coarse or thick. The conditioning agents can build up with repeated use.

☺ **Anti-Frizz Solutions Leave-In Conditioner** *($4.99 for 12 ounces)* is a very standard leave-in conditioner that is an OK option for all hair types that need help with detangling.

☺ **Anti-Frizz Solutions Straightening Conditioner, Moisturizer for Curly, Wavy, Frizzy Hair** *($4.99 for 6 ounces)* works well to moisturize and help smooth curly or wavy hair that is normal to fine or thin; those with thick, curly hair will need something more emollient.

☺ **Anti-Frizz Solutions Liquid Mousse** *($4.99 for 12 ounces)* isn't a mousse; it's a standard styling spray that provides light hold with a minimal stiff or sticky feel. The conditioning agents are great for dry hair, and provide some protection during heat styling.

☹ **Anti-Frizz Solutions Lusterizing Cream** *($7.49 for 3.4 ounces)* contains the preservative Kathon CG, which is not recommended for use in leave-on products due to the high risk of causing a sensitizing reaction to skin (which includes the scalp). What a shame, because this is otherwise an excellent silicone-based smoothing cream for dry to very dry hair.

☺ **Anti-Frizz Solutions Straightener** *($5.99 for 8 ounces)* is a very good styling cream for smoothing stubborn frizzies or straightening hair with heat. It provides a light hold that is slightly sticky, and contains plant oil and silicones to make hair sleek and shiny. This is light enough for all hair types, though someone with fine or thin hair should use it sparingly.

☺ **Anti-Frizz Solutions Brilliance Shine Spray** *($5.99 for 6 ounces)* is an aerosol silicone spray that adds a glossy shine to all hair types. Those with fine or thin hair should use it sparingly to avoid a too-slick, greasy look.

☺ **Anti-Frizz Solutions Glossing Mist** *($6.99 for 4 ounces)* is a lightweight, alcohol-free silicone spray that is an excellent, affordable option for all hair types. Although this has a light texture and dry-down, it should still be used sparingly by those with normal to fine or thin hair.

☺ **Anti-Frizz Solutions Oil Free Glosser** *($7.99 for 4 ounces)* is a standard, simply formulated silicone serum that contains three types of silicone plus sunscreen (although that cannot be relied on to protect hair from sun damage). This works beautifully to smooth frizzies, provide heat protection, and add shine to hair. It is best for dry to very dry hair that is coarse or thick.

ION COLOR SOLUTIONS

☹ **Color Solutions Color Defense, Protective Shampoo** *($4.99 for 12 ounces)* contains sodium lauryl sulfate as its main detergent cleansing agent, which makes this too drying for all hair and scalp types, and negates any sort of protective benefits.

☺ **Color Solutions Color Defense Extra Control Styling Hair Spray** *($4.99 for 9.5 ounces)* is a standard, medium-hold aerosol hairspray that has a minimal stiff and sticky finish and is a good option for all hair types.

☺ **Color Solutions Color Defense After-Color Sealing Treatment** *($4.99 for 6 ounces)* is a standard conditioner that does not contain a single ingredient to help seal color in the hair. Still, it is a good conditioner for normal to slightly dry hair that is normal to fine or thin, but that's it.

☺ **Color Solutions Color Defense Leave-In Protector** *($4.99 for 8 ounces)* is an excellent spray-on, leave-in conditioner for all hair types. This cannot help preserve color, but it can help fortify and protect hair that has been damaged from chemical services.

ION DAILY SOLUTIONS

☹ **Daily Solutions Balanced Cleansing Shampoo, Gentle Cleanser for All Hair Types** *($4.99 for 16 ounces)* contains sodium C14-16 olefin sulfonate and TEA-dodecylbenzenesulfonate as its detergent cleansing agents, which is a doubly drying combination for all hair and scalp types. It is not recommended.

☺ **Daily Solutions Finishing Detangler, Conditioning After Shampoo Rinse** *($4.99 for 16 ounces)* is a very good conditioner for dry to very dry hair of any thickness.

ION DANDRUFF SOLUTIONS

☹ **Dandruff Solutions Clear-T Dual Action, Anti-Dandruff Shampoo** *($7.99 for 16 ounces)* is a standard anti-dandruff shampoo that contains 5% coal tar as its active ingredient. Coal tar can indeed help control dandruff, but it is more irritating and drying to the scalp and hair than the more commonly used anti-dandruff ingredients of zinc pyrithione or ketoconazole. The main problems with this shampoo are the inclusion of sulfur, which can strip hair color with repeated use, and menthol, which only exacerbates the irritation from coal tar. All in all, this formulation is less about dandruff and more about the treatment of psoriasis.

☹ **Dandruff Solutions Clear-T Dual Action Hair & Scalp Conditioner** *($6.99 for 8 ounces)* contains several mint extracts and oils along with menthol, and these are extremely irritating to the scalp, and that won't help dandruff in the least.

ION MOISTURE SOLUTIONS

☹ **Moisture Solutions Moisturizing Shampoo, Hydrating Cleanser for Color Treated, Relaxed or Permed Hair** *($4.99 for 16 ounces)* is identical to the Daily Solutions Balanced Cleansing Shampoo above, and the same comments apply.

☺ **Moisture Solutions Moisturizing Treatment, Hydrating Therapy Masque** *($4.99 for 4 ounces)* is a standard conditioner that isn't all that hydrating, at least not to the extent that it deserves consideration as a therapeutic treatment for hair. This is an OK option for normal to dry hair of any thickness.

ION PURIFYING SOLUTIONS

☹ **Purifying Solutions Clarifying Shampoo, for All Hair Types** *($4.99 for 16 ounces)* contains both sodium C14-16 olefin sulfonate and TEA-lauryl sulfate, which makes this shampoo too drying and irritating for all hair and scalp types.

☹ **Purifying Solutions Hard Water Shampoo** *($4.99 for 11.5 ounces)* is similar to the Purifying Solutions Clarifying Shampoo above, and the same comments apply.

☹ **Purifying Solutions Swimmer's Shampoo, Anti-Chlorine Cleanser** *($5.99 for 16 ounces)* contains sodium lauryl sulfate as one of its main detergent cleansing agents, which makes this too drying and irritating for hair and scalp. Further, this does not contain chelating agents, which are what's needed to remove minerals and chlorine from hair!

☺ **Purifying Solutions Hard Water Conditioner** *($4.99 for 11.5 ounces)* is a good, but boring, conditioner for normal to slightly dry hair of any thickness.

ION REPAIR SOLUTIONS

☺ **Repair Solutions Effective Care Intensive Therapy Treatment** *($3.99 for 4 ounces)* is nearly identical to the Moisture Solutions Moisturizing Treatment, Hydrating Therapy Masque above, and the same comments apply.

☺ **Repair Solutions Reconstructor Treatment** *($8.99 for 16 ounces)* is a poor formulation if you were hoping for any sort of hair conditioning. This is a very light formula that can minimally moisturize hair and would be an option only for someone with slightly dry fine or thin hair.

ION SALON SOLUTIONS

☺ **Salon Solutions Anti-Chlorine Swimmer's Dual Action Conditioner** *($3.99 for 8 ounces)* is a lightweight conditioner that can detangle normal to fine or thin hair, but provides nothing special for swimmers. It's actually a lackluster formula that pales in comparison to most other conditioners.

☺ **Salon Solutions Anti-Frizz Alcohol-Free Hair Spray** *($4.99 for 8 ounces)* is an alcohol-free hairspray that provides a medium hold that leaves hair feeling sticky and slightly difficult to brush through. The minimal amounts of silicone and conditioning agents have little effect on taming frizzies.

☺ **Salon Solutions Anti-Frizz Gel Styling Mist** *($4.99 for 11.5 ounces)* is a standard, alcohol-free styling spray that offers a light to medium hold. The film-forming/holding agent and glycerin combine to leave hair feeling sticky and moist, though it remains easy to brush through.

☺ **Salon Solutions Anti-Frizz Styling Gelle** *($4.99 for 6 ounces)* is a standard styling gel that provides a firm hold with a slightly stiff, sticky feel, though it does allow you to easily brush through hair. This can provide a minimal amount of protection during heat styling.

☺ **Salon Solutions Hard-To-Hold Hair Spray** *($2.99 for 11 ounces)* is an aerosol hairspray that offers such a light, soft hold that it is completely inappropriate for hard-to-hold hair. For a touchable hold that is easily brushed through, this is great.

☺ **Salon Solutions Styling Glaze** *($4.99 for 12 ounces)* is a light-hold, mildly conditioning styling gel that has a liquidy texture. It is a good option for all hair types, and can softly define curls and waves without stiffness or stickiness.

☺ **Salon Solutions Styling Spritz** *($4.49 for 8 ounces)* promises "super freeze" hold, and for the most part, this nonaerosol hairspray delivers just that, albeit with a considerable amount of stickiness. This is best for long-lasting hold on hairstyles you do not intend to brush through later.

☹ **Salon Solutions Conditioning Miracle Microwavable Treatment Pac** *($1.99 for 1 ounce)* is a mediocre conditioner that doesn't deserve to be sold as a special treatment for hair. This can be OK for normal to slightly dry hair that is fine or thin.

☺ **Salon Solutions Crystal Clarifying Treatment** *($2.29 for 0.18 ounce)* is a powder (so it must be mixed with water) clarifying treatment for hair that has been exposed to mineral buildup from hard water or swimming pools. It contains chelating agents to bind with and dislodge the mineral deposits from the hair shaft, but so do many shampoos, which makes this single-use product a somewhat expensive option.

☹ **Salon Solutions Hot 'n Moist Protective Hair and Scalp Treatment** *($1.99 for 1 ounce)* is too thin-textured to provide much moisture or smoothness to hair, and is easily replaced by an emollient conditioner with silicone or a silicone serum.

☺ **Salon Solutions Hot Oil Deep Penetrating Treatment** *($1.69 for 1 ounce)* is a boring conditioning "treatment" that lacks significant amounts of conditioning/moisturizing agents for hair. This can be an OK detangling solution for normal to fine or thin hair, but the price is high for such a small amount of product.

ION STYLING SOLUTIONS

☺ **Styling Solutions Flexible Hold Finishing Spray** *($4.49 for 8 ounces)* is a very good nonaerosol hairspray that does offer a flexible hold. Actually, the hold is so soft you may not believe this is hairspray! It is completely non-sticky and leaves hair very easy to brush through; just don't expect much hold, and you'll do well with this.

☺ **Styling Solutions Hydrolac Hair Spray** *($2.99 for 11 ounces)* is sold as "ultimate holding hair spray," but this aerosol hairspray provides quite a soft hold that is minimally sticky and does not leave hair feeling stiff. It's fine for casual hairstyles requiring light hold, but doesn't come close to approaching "ultimate."

☺ **Styling Solutions Shaping Plus Styling Spray** *($4.99 for 10.9 ounces)* works well as a medium-hold aerosol hairspray with added conditioning agents for smoothness and shine. This is a great finishing spray option for dry to very dry hair. It is slightly sticky, but can be easily brushed through.

☹ **Styling Solutions Styling Mousse** *($4.99 for 10 ounces)* contains the preservative Kathon CG, which is not recommended for use in leave-on products. This also contains peppermint, which can cause further scalp irritation.

☺ **Styling Solutions Texturizing Hair Wax** *($5.99 for 1.8 ounces)* is a thick, water-soluble pomade that has a creamy, slightly gummy texture that can be a bit tricky to work with. Still, it feels lighter than it appears, and can smooth dry ends and minimize frizzies without making hair look greasy.

ION VOLUMIZING SOLUTIONS

☺ **Volumizing Solutions Vitalizing Thickening Shampoo, for All Hair Types** *($4.99 for 16 ounces)* is similar to the Anti-Frizz Solutions Smoothing Shampoo above, and the same basic comments apply. The tiny amount of sodium lauryl sulfate present is unlikely to be a problem for hair or scalp.

☺ **Volumizing Solutions Vitalizing Thickening Conditioner, for All Hair Types** *($4.99 for 16 ounces)* is a standard, but good, conditioner that can work well for dry to very dry hair of any thickness. Just don't count on this making hair feel thicker.

☺ **Volumizing Solutions Vitalizing Hair Wax** *($5.99 for 1.8 ounces)* is a gel-type pomade that liquefies and spreads easily through the hair. This is water-soluble, and can be a very good finishing product to smooth dry ends or add shine (without greasiness) to all hair types. It does not contain wax, but does contain wax-like thickeners.

☺ **Volumizing Solutions Vitalizing Root Lift** *($4.99 for 10 ounces)* is a spray-on aerosol styling mousse that can be messy to use if you aim and shoot this product directly onto your hair. It is best applied to your hands, where you can work it into the hair one section at a time. This provides a firm hold that remains sticky, so it's best for stubborn hair that needs long-lasting support.

☺ **Volumizing Solutions Vitalizing Shaping Mist** *($4.99 for 11 ounces)* is similar to the Color Solutions Color Defense Extra Control Styling Hair Spray above, and the same comments apply.

☺ **Volumizing Solutions Vitalizing Thickening Styler** *($4.99 for 4 ounces)* is a light- to medium-hold styling gel whose film-forming/holding agents coat the hair shaft and provide a feeling of slight thickness with minimal stickiness. This gel does not contain any conditioning agents capable of protecting hair from the rigors of heat styling.

☹ **Volumizing Solutions Volume Builder** *($4.99 for 8 ounces)* contains the sensitizing preservative Kathon CG, which is not recommended for use in leave-on products, particularly spray products where scalp contact is guaranteed.

☺ **Volumizing Solutions Vitalizing Fortifying Treatment** *($4.99 for 8 ounces)* is an outstanding styling spray that contains a good amount of lightweight water-binding agents, panthenol, and chitosan (a substance from crab shells that can cling to hair and add a feeling of thickness). This provides a light, slightly sticky hold that can be easily brushed through, and it can provide some protection during heat styling.

ISO

All of the ISO products reviewed below contain vitamins, which the company maintains can do all sorts of wonderful things for the hair, from preserving color to protecting hair from sun damage. It isn't true. Vitamins are rather useless in hair-care products because they do not cling well to the hair, do not hold up under rinsing or styling, and cannot nourish something that is already dead—namely, hair! For more information about ISO (which stands for Innovative Styling Options), call 800-ISO-HAIR or visit www.isohair.com.

What's Good About This Line: For a salon-sold line, the shampoos and conditioners (almost all are worthwhile) have modest prices; the Multiplicity styling gels are outstanding options.

What's Not So Good About It: Some of the conditioners and several styling products contain the drying ingredient sodium polystyrene sulfonate; five of the styling products contain the sensitizing preservative Kathon CG.

☺ **Color Preserve Cleanse, Color Care Shampoo** *($7.25 for 13.5 ounces)* is a standard, but good, shampoo for normal to dry hair of any thickness, and the film-forming agents pose minimal risk of buildup. Despite the name, this cannot preserve color.

☺ **Daily Balancing Cleanse, Gentle Shampoo** *($7.25 for 13.5 ounces)* is a standard, but good, shampoo for all hair types. This poses minimal risk of buildup.

☺ **Purifying Cleanse, Deep Cleansing Shampoo** *($7.25 for 13.5 ounces)* is almost identical to the Daily Balancing Cleanse, Gentle Shampoo above, except this contains a larger amount of water-binding agents, making it slightly better for drier hair. Otherwise, the same comments apply.

☺ **Reviving Cleanse, Moisturizing Shampoo** *($7.25 for 13.5 ounces)* is a good shampoo for normal to dry hair. The tiny amount of the solvent ammonium xylenesulfonate is unlikely to cause hair or scalp dryness.

☺ **Color Preserve Condition, Color Care Conditioner** *($8.50 for 13.5 ounces)*. Nothing about this conditioner makes it preferred for color-treated hair, and it cannot make color last longer. It's just a good smoothing conditioner for normal to dry hair that is normal to coarse or thick.

☺ **Daily Nourishing Condition, Light Creme Conditioner** *($8.50 for 13.5 ounces)* is similar to the Color Preserve Condition, Color Care Conditioner above, except this contains less silicone, and that makes it preferred for normal to dry hair of any thickness. Otherwise, the same basic comments apply.

☺ **Recovery Condition, Intensive Treatment** *($8.50 for 5.1 ounces)* is nearly identical to the Daily Nourishing Condition, Light Creme Conditioner above, except this has a slightly thicker texture. Otherwise, the same comments apply. Price-wise, you're better off purchasing one of the other two conditioners above and leaving it on the hair as long as possible (if hair is dry, coarse, or thick).

☺ **Reviving Condition, Moisturizing Conditioner** *($8.50 for 13.5 ounces)* is nearly identical to the Color Preserve Condition, Color Care Conditioner above, and the same comments apply.

☺ **Stress Defense Condition, Leave-In Protection** *($8.50 for 8.5 ounces)* is a standard, very light conditioner that is best used to detangle normal to fine or thin hair. It affords a small amount of protection during heat styling.

☹ **Bouncy Creme Control, Texture Energizer** *($9 for 8.5 ounces)* contains the preservative Kathon CG, which is contraindicated for use in leave-on products due to its strong potential to cause a sensitizing reaction if it stays on the skin.

☹ **Bouncy Spray Control, Curl Activator** *($9 for 8.5 ounces)* contains a high amount of sodium polystyrene sulfonate, which can be drying to hair and can potentially strip dyed hair color with repeated use.

☺ **Creative Shaping Control, Flexible Spray** *($11 for 10.1 ounces)* is a standard aerosol hairspray whose fine mist provides a light hold that does indeed keep hair flexible (rather than stiff). This is minimally sticky and works well for all hair types seeking soft hold.

☹ **Intensifying Control, Shine Gel** *($9 for 5.1 ounces)* contains the preservative Kathon CG, and is not recommended due to the risk of causing a sensitizing reaction on the scalp.

☹ **Maximize Control, Extra-Firm Hold Gel** *($9 for 5.1 ounces)* contains the preservative Kathon CG, and is not recommended.

☺ **Tamer Control, Smoothing Foam Gel** *($10 for 6.7 ounces)* is a unique foaming gel whose texture is similar to that of a standard shaving cream. It feels creamy and spreads easily through the hair but provides minimal to no hold and offers insignificant protection from heat, so this is a poor choice to use alone when straightening wavy or curly hair. Combined with a silicone cream or serum, it can help smooth hair and keep it soft.

☺ **Thermal Set Control, Heat-Activated Styler** *($10 for 8.5 ounces)* is a standard, fast-drying, nonaerosol hairspray that provides a medium hold and leaves hair slightly stiff and sticky. The addition of a silicone thickener can add shine and make hair easier to comb through.

☹ **Transforming Control, Firm Hold Mousse** *($10 for 8.5 ounces)* contains the preservative Kathon CG, and is not recommended.

☺ **Ultimate Hold Control, Finishing Spray** *($11 for 10.1 ounces)* is a good, though standard, medium-hold aerosol hairspray. It leaves hair feeling slightly stiff and sticky, but contains silicone and conditioning agents to facilitate brushing and add shine. This is a good choice for dry hair.

☺ **$$$ Color Preserve Control, Protecting Serum** *($10 for 1.6 ounces)* is a standard silicone serum that can be a great option for dry to very dry hair that is normal to coarse or thick. It doesn't differ much from options sold at the drugstore for less money, and the drugstore silicone serums come in more generous sizes.

ISO MULTIPLICITY

☺ **Multiplicity Dimensions, Texture Shampoo** *($9.95 for 13.5 ounces)* is similar to the Daily Balancing Cleanse, Gentle Shampoo above, and the same comments apply.

☺ **Multiplicity Elevate, Volume Shampoo** *($9.95 for 13.5 ounces)* is a good shampoo for all hair types. The film-forming agents are present in amounts too small to impact hair, but that's OK because their negligible effect means there's no concern about buildup.

☺ **Multiplicity Moisture, Hydrating Shampoo** *($9.95 for 13.5 ounces)* is a standard, but good, detergent-based shampoo that poses minimal risk of buildup and is an option for all hair types. It is fairly similar to almost all of the ISO shampoos above. This shampoo is not particularly moisturizing, but it isn't drying either.

☺ **Multiplicity Reflect, Shine Shampoo** *($9.95 for 13.5 ounces)* is a good conditioning shampoo for normal to very dry hair, though the silicone can build up with repeated use.

☹ **Multiplicity Dimensions, Texture Conditioner** *($10.95 for 13.5 ounces)* is a basic conditioner that contains sodium polystyrene sulfonate, which can be drying to the hair and can potentially strip dyed hair color with repeated use.

☹ **Multiplicity Elevate, Volume Conditioner** *($10.95 for 13.5 ounces)* contains sodium polystyrene sulfonate, which can be drying to the hair and can potentially strip dyed hair color with repeated use.

☺ **Multiplicity Moisture, Hydrating Conditioner** *($10.95 for 13.5 ounces)* contains sodium polystyrene sulfonate, but a much lesser amount than the two Multiplicity conditioners above. This can be a very good smoothing conditioner for normal to very dry hair that is normal to coarse or thick. It contains mostly water, thickener, silicones, detangling agent, slip agent, plant oil, vitamins, glycerin, preservatives, and fragrance.

☹ **Multiplicity Reflect, Shine Conditioner** *($10.95 for 13.5 ounces)* contains sodium polystyrene sulfonate, which can be drying to the hair and can potentially strip dyed hair color with repeated use.

☹ **Multiplicity Disciplining, Smoothing Gel** *($11.75 for 7 ounces)* contains sodium polystyrene sulfonate, which can be drying to the hair and can potentially strip dyed hair color with repeated use, especially in leave-on products like this.

☹ **Multiplicity Escalate, Volume Whip** *($11.75 for 8.3 ounces)* is a styling mousse that contains sodium polystyrene sulfonate, which can be drying to the hair and can potentially strip dyed hair color with repeated use, especially in leave-on products. This also contains the skin-sensitizing preservative Kathon CG.

☺ **Multiplicity Finalize, Firm Hold Spray** *($11.75 for 10.1 ounces)* is a very good, firm-hold aerosol hairspray that leaves hair slightly stiff and sticky, though it remains relatively easy to brush through. This does contain a tiny amount of sodium polystyrene sulfonate, but probably not enough to cause noticeable dryness.

☺ **Multiplicity Luminate, Glossing Glaze** *($11.75 for 1.75 ounces)* is a thin, but still fairly greasy, pomade infused with mica for added shine. It can smooth dry ends and tame frizzies for all hair types, and the tiny amount of sodium polystyrene sulfonate (it's listed well after the fragrance and preservatives) is unlikely to cause dryness.

☹ **Multiplicity Mobilize, Working Spray** *($11.75 for 10.1 ounces)* contains a questionable amount of sodium polystyrene sulfonate, which can be drying to the hair and can potentially strip dyed hair color with repeated use, especially in leave-on products.

☹ **Multiplicity Multi-Texture, Styling Creme** *($11.75 for 7 ounces)* contains a high level of sodium polystyrene sulfonate as well as the preservative Kathon CG, and is absolutely not recommended.

☹ **Multiplicity Swax, Spray Wax** *($11.75 for 5.1 ounces)* contains too much sodium polystyrene sulfonate, which can be drying to the hair and can potentially strip dyed hair color with repeated use, especially in leave-on products.

☹ **Multiplicity Tactile, Texture Paste** *($11.75 for 1.75 ounces)* lists a lather agent/thickener as its second ingredient, and that can be drying for hair when used in this amount for leave-in products. This also contains sodium polystyrene sulfonate, which only adds to the potential for dryness.

☺ **Multiplicity Tousle, Cream n' Gel** *($14.50 for 5.1 ounces)* is a standard styling gel infused with a "strip" of emollients, so this makes for a visually appealing styling gel. It provides a light to medium hold that is easily brushed through, and the conditioning agents/emollients keep hair from being stiff and add some moisture. The tiny amount of sodium polystyrene sulfonate is very unlikely to cause dryness.

☺ **Multiplicity Twister, Firm Hold Gel** *($14.50 for 5.1 ounces)* is a very good medium- to firm-hold styling gel for all hair types except fine or thin. This contains an unusual (but excellent) blend of silicones, plant oil, and conditioning agents that can provide a significant amount of protection during heat styling. This gel does leave hair feeling slightly stiff and sticky, but that is the trade-off for so much hold. This is one of the few ISO styling products not plagued by problematic ingredients.

☹ **Multiplicity Upshoot, Styling Spritz** *($11.75 for 8.5 ounces)* contains a questionable amount of sodium polystyrene sulfonate, which can be drying to the hair and can potentially strip dyed hair color with repeated use, especially in leave-on products.

☺ **Multiplicity Whipped, Cream Wax** *($11.75 for 1.75 ounces)* is a creamy, reasonably water-soluble pomade that does not contain any waxes (though it does contain waxlike thickeners). It is surprisingly lightweight but does its job to smooth frizzies and add soft texture to hair with a low-wattage shine. It is one of the few pomades that are appropriate for all hair types (though someone with very thick or coarse hair would do better with a heavier product), and is minimally greasy. This does contain a tiny amount of sodium polystyrene sulfonate, but the amount is unlikely to cause dryness, especially in the presence of emollient ingredients.

☺ **Multiplicity Glosser, Shine Serum** *($12.75 for 1.7 ounces)* is a lighter-than-usual shine serum that contains a reduced amount of silicones, so it is thinner and less greasy and slick than most in this category. The slip agents and emollient also help smooth dry hair, with the silicones adding a silky softness and the light-reflecting shine that makes them such wonderful ingredients. This is a good silicone serum for all hair types, though someone with thick or coarse hair may desire a traditional (heavier) silicone product.

JASÖN NATURAL COSMETICS

This comprehensive skin-, body-, and hair-care line has been on health food and specialty market shelves since 1959. One of the original lines to tout natural ingredients, JASÖN deserves some credit for being at the forefront of the natural-ingredient trend that is still going strong today. The unfortunate issue with these elements, however, particularly plant and flower extracts, is that they are often the least effective part of a hair-care formulation. Extracts of lavender, goldenseal, sage, and horsetail sound appealing, but none of them can detangle, moisturize, smooth, or help style hair.

Where JASÖN differs from the competition is with the use of fairly gentle to very mild cleansing agents in all of its shampoos. As a refreshing bonus, many of the plant extracts in their hair-care products are innocuous, or—for a nice change of pace—really do have some benefit for the scalp, such as the anti-irritant properties of green tea or the soothing properties of chamomile. The catch is that these beneficial plant extracts are used in rinse-off products, and that means they have little time to exert their positive effect before they're washed away. Still, in many regards, JASÖN is among the gentlest of the so-called natural lines.

The only major issue I have with the JASÖN line is its contradictory nature. For example, a statement on their Web site reads, "We believe consumers must have a reliable natural alternative to chemically-synthesized, technical grade products, and to that end we are devoted to developing and manufacturing a wide range of personal care and beauty care products that are truly botanical in origin." Yet several of the JASÖN products contain disodium cocoamphodiacetate, cocamide DEA, cocamidopropyl betaine, and sodium myreth sulfate, among many others, none of which are the least bit natural! JASÖN's Web site also states that their products do not use lauryl or laureth sulfates, yet one of their shampoos contains sodium laureth sulfate. A similar inconsistency is found in their "How to Read a Label" Web article, where it's recommended that consumers avoid the synthetic ingredient sodium myreth sulfate. Didn't anyone at this company happen to notice that several of their shampoos do indeed contain this (gentle) detergent cleansing agent? The fact that JASÖN's hair-care products don't jibe with the anti-synthetic slant of their Web site should make any consumer question the company's commitment to creating natural products. They may be "natural in origin," but they are more hypocritical or just plain clueless than anything else. In the long run, botanicals won't clean, condition, or style the hair without essential help from decidedly unnatural ingredients. For more information on JASÖN Natural Cosmetics, call (877) JASON-01 or visit www.jason-natural.com.

What's Good About This Line: The shampoos and conditioners feature mostly excellent formulas at great prices; none of the dozens of shampoos contain drying detergent cleansing agents.

What's Not So Good About It: The anti-dandruff products contain hair-color-stripping sulfur; the styling products contain more plant extracts than they do beneficial ingredients that are necessary to hold hair in place and provide some heat protection.

☺ **Color Enhancing Shampoo for Black Hair** *($7.25 for 8 ounces)* is a very good conditioning shampoo for all normal to dry hair of any thickness.

☺ **Color Enhancing Shampoo for Blonde Hair** *($7.25 for 8 ounces)* is nearly identical to the Color Enhancing Shampoo for Black Hair above, except the decidedly unnatural dye agent in this one is preferred for blonde hair. The yellow tone of the dye is best for golden to dark blonde hair, though the color-depositing effect is minimal.

☺ **Color Enhancing Shampoo for Brown Hair** *($7.25 for 8 ounces)* is nearly identical to the Color Enhancing Shampoo for Black Hair above, except this contains basic unnatural dyes suitable for brown shades of hair. Otherwise, the same comments apply.

☺ **Color Enhancing Shampoo for Red Hair** *($7.25 for 8 ounces)* is nearly identical to the Color Enhancing Shampoo for Black Hair above, except this contains plant-based and synthetic dyes suitable for red shades of hair. The red henna can build up with repeated use and make hair feel dry, and the pomegranate poses a slight risk of leaving a red tinge on the scalp. This shampoo would be best for those with vivid, intensely red hair.

☺ **Color Enhancing Shampoo for Silver/Grey** *($7.25 for 8 ounces)* is nearly identical to the Color Enhancing Shampoo for Black Hair above, except this contains a blue dye agent that can minimally counteract brassy or yellow tones in gray, silver, and white hair. Otherwise, the same comments apply.

☹ **Dandruff Relief Shampoo** *($10 for 12 ounces)* can be an option for treating dandruff, but it contains 2% sulfur, which can be extremely drying to hair and irritating to the scalp. Sulfur can also strip dyed hair color, so this is not the dandruff shampoo to choose if you dye your hair. This is really too potentially problematic to consider, especially with the irritating wintergreen and rosemary oils it includes.

☺ **Damage Control Creme Shampoo, for Frizzy, Dry or Color-Treated Hair** *($12.50 for 16 ounces)* is a good conditioning shampoo for normal to dry hair of any thickness. This shampoo can moisturize hair but does not have a pronounced effect on frizzy hair.

☺ **Forest Essence Conditioning Shampoo** *($7.95 for 17.5 ounces)* contains a botanical garden full of plant extracts, none of which are all that helpful for hair or scalp. This is a very gentle shampoo whose detergent cleansing agents are too mild to handle oily hair and scalp, or remove multiple styling products. It can work well for normal to very dry hair of any thickness, provided your use of styling products is minimal.

☹ **For Kids Only! Extra Mild Shampoo** *($7.95 for 17.5 ounces)* is not as gentle or mild as the Forest Essence Conditioning Shampoo above, and the arnica, comfrey, and St. John's wort extracts it contains can be scalp irritants. Further, the essential oils can cause an itchy scalp, especially for children, whose immune defenses are still developing. This is an OK shampoo for adults with normal to dry hair of any thickness.

☺ **Hemp Enriched Shampoo for All Hair Types** *($7.95 for 17.5 ounces)* is an outstanding shampoo for dry to very dry hair of any thickness.

☺ **Natural Aloe Vera 84% Shampoo, Hair Nourishing Formula** *($6.55 for 16 ounces)* does contain aloe as its main ingredient, but aloe alone won't nourish the hair. It's just a decent water-binding agent with no real ability to cling to hair. This is a very gentle shampoo that is a significantly better option for kids (and babies) than the For Kids Only! Extra Mild Shampoo above. This shampoo is too mild to remove oil, dirt, and conditioner/styling product buildup from an adult's hair.

☺ **Natural Apricot Keratin Shampoo** *($6.50 for 16 ounces)* is similar to the For Kids Only! Extra Mild Shampoo above, except without the problematic plant extracts and essential oils. It is an excellent option for all hair types and poses minimal risk of buildup.

☹ **Natural Biotin Shampoo** *($6.50 for 16 ounces)* contains menthol and mint extracts, and is not recommended for any hair or scalp type.

☺ **Natural E.F.A. Shampoo, Extra Rich Hair Nourishing Formula for Normal to Dry Hair** *($6.50 for 16 ounces)* is a very good, extremely mild shampoo for normal to very dry hair of any thickness. The plant extracts in this product have soothing and/or anti-irritant properties—there's not a problematic one in the bunch—but this is too mild to cleanse adult hair of conditioner and styling product buildup. If you do not use styling products and do not have an oily scalp, this is worth considering.

☺ **Natural Henna Hi-Lights Shampoo** *($6.50 for 16 ounces)* is similar to the Natural Aloe 84% Shampoo above, except with henna extract instead of aloe. The high concentration of henna can build up on the hair and make it feel dry and slightly sticky, though initially this can be a great shampoo for fine or thin hair.

☺ **Natural Jojoba Shampoo, UV protection, Extra Body, Super Shine** *($6.50 for 16 ounces)* is nearly identical to the Natural Aloe 84% Shampoo above, and the same comments apply. This shampoo cannot provide UV protection.

☺ **Natural Sea Kelp Shampoo, Rich Concentrated Extra Gentle, Super Shine** *($6.50 for 16 ounces)* is similar to the Natural Apricot Keratin Shampoo above, and the same comments apply. This does contain fragrant plant extracts.

☺ **Natural Vitamin A, C & E Shampoo** *($6.50 for 16 ounces)* is nearly identical to the Natural Aloe Vera 84% Shampoo above, and the same comments apply.

☺ **Swimmers & Sports Hair and Scalp Reconditioning Shampoo** *($7.95 for 17.5 ounces)* is similar to the Natural Apricot Keratin Shampoo above, except this contains a chelating agent to help remove chlorine and mineral deposits from hair. Otherwise, the same basic comments apply.

☺ **Tall Grass Hi-Protein Shampoo** *($7.95 for 17.5 ounces)* is similar to the Natural Apricot Keratin Shampoo above, except this contains a tea of several grass extracts, which have no special benefit for hair or scalp, though they can aggravate allergies in susceptible persons. Otherwise, the same basic comments apply. The tiny amount of peppermint extract is unlikely to cause irritation.

☺ **Tea Tree Oil Hair and Scalp Therapy Shampoo** *($7.95 for 17.5 ounces)* contains witch hazel extract as its main ingredient, but in a shampoo it is rinsed out before it can dry the hair or scalp. Otherwise, this standard shampoo is a good option for someone with an oily scalp whose hair is normal to fine or thin.

☺ **Thin-to-Thick Hair and Scalp Therapy, Pro-Vitamin Hair Thickening Shampoo** *($8.89 for 8 ounces)* is similar to the Natural Apricot Keratin Shampoo above, except this contains minute amounts of problematic plant extracts. This shampoo does not contain film-forming agents, so is not adept at making hair feel thicker. It remains a good option for all hair types.

☺ **Color Sealant Conditioner, for All Shades of Hair** *($7 for 8 ounces)* can be a good, though standard, conditioner for normal to dry hair of any thickness.

☺ **Damage Control Creme Conditioner, for Frizzy, Dry or Color-Treated Hair** *($10 for 8 ounces)* is a lightweight conditioner that lists titanium dioxide as a UVA sunscreen. However, in this conditioner it is used strictly as an opacifying agent and cannot offer sun protection. This can be good option for normal to slightly dry hair that is normal to fine or thin, but it won't control or change the amount of damage your hair may have.

☺ **Forest Essence Vital Conditioner** *($7.35 for 8 ounces)* is an emollient conditioner that is excellent for normal to very dry hair that is normal to coarse or thick.

☺ **For Kids Only! Extra Gentle Conditioner** *($7.35 for 8 ounces)* is similar to the Forest Essence Vital Conditioner above, except this contains arnica, which can be a problem for the scalp. Kept on the hair, this can be a good conditioner for normal to very dry hair that is normal to coarse or thick.

☺ **Hemp Enriched Conditioner for All Hair Types, Especially Dry/Damaged Hair** (*$7.35 for 8 ounces*) can work well for normal to slightly dry hair that is fine or thin. It is too thin-textured and light for dry or damaged hair.

☺ **Natural Aloe Vera 84% Conditioner, Hair Nourishing Formula** (*$6.50 for 16 ounces*) is a standard, but good, conditioner that is an option for normal to dry hair of any thickness. The aloe vera at 84% is mostly water and not a helpful ingredient for hair.

☺ **Natural Apricot Keratin Conditioner** (*$6.50 for 16 ounces*) is similar to the Natural Aloe Vera 84% Conditioner above, except this contains a greater amount of detangling agent and more plant oil, which makes it preferred for normal to dry hair that is normal to coarse or thick.

☺ **Natural Biotin Conditioner** (*$6.50 for 16 ounces*) is similar to the Natural Aloe Vera 84% Conditioner above, and the same comments apply.

☺ **Natural E.F.A. Conditioner, Extra Rich Hair Nourishing Formula for Normal to Dry Hair** (*$6.50 for 16 ounces*) is similar to the Natural Aloe Vera 84% Conditioner above, except this contains a greater amount of detangling agents and fewer conditioning agents, and that makes it preferred for normal to dry hair that is normal to fine or thin.

☹ **Natural Henna Hi-Lights Conditioner** (*$6.50 for 16 ounces*) is similar to the Natural Aloe Vera 84% Conditioner above, except instead of aloe this contains henna extract, which can build up on the hair and cause dryness with repeated use. In a shampoo, henna extract is mostly rinsed away; but in conditioners, it tends to cling to the hair, where it lingers and can lead to problems.

☺ **Natural Jojoba Conditioner** (*$6.50 for 16 ounces*) is a very good option for normal to dry hair of any thickness. Despite the name, this contains only a tiny amount of jojoba.

☺ **Natural Sea Kelp Conditioner; Rich Concentrated Extra Gentle, Super Shine** (*$6.50 for 16 ounces*) is similar to the Hemp Enriched Conditioner for All Hair Types above, except this has a slightly thicker texture. Otherwise, the same comments apply.

☺ **Natural Vitamin A, C & E Conditioner** (*$6.50 for 16 ounces*) is similar to the Natural Sea Kelp Conditioner above, and the same comments apply.

☺ **Swimmers & Sports Hair and Scalp Reconditioning Conditioner** (*$7.35 for 8 ounces*) lists two sunscreens as active ingredients, but wisely does not list an SPF rating. That's because no such standards for figuring this number have been set for hair-care products, so even if the ingredients are present they can't be relied on for sun protection. This is otherwise a standard conditioner that can remove chlorine and mineral deposits from hair.

☺ **Tall Grass Hi-Protein Conditioner** (*$7.35 for 8 ounces*) is similar to the Hemp Enriched Conditioner for All Hair Types, Especially Dry/Damaged Hair above, minus the hemp oil and with the addition of grass juice, which has no significant effect on hair or scalp. Otherwise, the same basic comments apply.

☺ **Tea Tree Oil Hair and Scalp Therapy Conditioner** *($7.35 for 8 ounces)* is a lightweight conditioner that is an OK option for normal to slightly dry hair of any thickness. The AHAs present cannot exfoliate the scalp because this product's pH is too high. One more reason to keep this off the scalp is the inclusion of sage and rosemary oils. And the amount of tea tree oil is too small to have an effect on dandruff.

☺ **Thin-to-Thick Hair and Scalp Therapy, Pro-Vitamin Hair Thickening Conditioner** *($8 for 8 ounces)* is similar to the Natural Aloe Vera 84% Conditioner above, and the same basic comments apply. This does not contain ingredients that can make hair feel thicker, but it will make hair softer and smoother.

☺ **All Natural Hi-Shine Styling Gel, All Hair Types** *($7.50 for 6 ounces)* is a conditioning styling gel that provides a very soft hold that leaves hair feeling moist. This can be a great gel for enhancing curly or wavy hair without stiffness.

☹ **All Natural Mousse, Style & Shape All Hair Types** *($7.50 for 7 ounces)* is a liquid-to-foam mousse that offers a light, brushable hold but contains balsam, which adds an unpleasant stickiness and can eventually make hair feel brittle. There are better, less intensely fragranced styling mousses available. By the way, this formula is not "all natural"—when was the last time you saw a polyquaternium-11 tree?

☹ **Fresh Botanicals Hairspray Super Style Holding Mist** *($4.50 for 8 ounces)* is a light-hold, minimally sticky hairspray that is alcohol-free, so it takes much longer to dry than standard hairspray. This contains several plant extracts that can cause scalp irritation, but it is an OK option for normal to thick or coarse hair. It is too heavy for fine or thin hair, and can make it feel coated.

☺ **I'm Naturally Stuck-Up, a Stiff Hair Styling Wax** *($12.50 for 4 ounces)* is a thick, water-based, slightly greasy pomade that contains several heavy ingredients to smooth frizzies and the ends of dry to very dry hair that is normal to coarse or thick. Use this sparingly to avoid a coated feel on the hair. This product does not make hair feel the least bit stiff, so the name, while clever, is inaccurate.

☹ **Thin-to-Thick Hair & Scalp Therapy, Body Building Hair Spray (Non-Aerosol)** *($7 for 8 ounces)* is a styling spray that offers zero hold but can make hair feel slightly thicker, though not without some stickiness. It is an OK option for those whose hair needs minimal control, but this is mostly a prime example of how ineffective plant extracts are for styling hair.

☺ **All Natural Frizz Control, for Smooth, Soft Hair** *($7.50 for 2 ounces)* is an exceptional silicone serum for dry to very dry hair. It contains mostly silicone (a decidedly unnatural ingredient), emollient, plant extracts, conditioning agents, and vitamin A. The price for this product makes it a very good bargain.

☺ **All Natural Hi-Shine Plus, Instantly Tame and Control Fly-Aways** *($7.50 for 4 ounces)* is a lighter, spray-on version of the All Natural Frizz Control, for Smooth, Soft Hair above. It can add shine and smoothness to all hair types, though it should be used sparingly by those with fine or thin hair. Again, the price is excellent for what you get.

☹ **Dandruff Relief Aromatherapy Nourishing Spray Gel** *($7.50 for 2 ounces)* contains 2% sulfur, which can be extremely drying to hair and irritating to the scalp, especially in leave-on products like this.

☹ **Dandruff Relief Scalp Normalizing Tonic** *($7.50 for 2 ounces)* is even more problematic than the Dandruff Relief Aromatherapy Nourishing Spray Gel above. This leave-on product contains 2% sulfur along with the irritants camphor, wintergreen, lavender, cinnamon, and rosemary oils.

☺ **Hi-Shine Mends Ends** *($7.50 for 2 ounces)* is a lightweight, leave-in conditioner that can make split ends appear smoother and help make dry hair more manageable, but the only true solution for split ends is to cut them off.

☺ **Thin-to-Thick Hair & Scalp Therapy, Revitalizing Scalp Elixir** *($8.89 for 2 ounces)* contains mostly B vitamins, slip agents, vitamin C, amino acids, and proteins. In combination, these form a liquid solution of water-binding agents that can make hair feel smoother and more pliable but won't add thickness. Vitamins cannot perform on hair the way they do when they are taken orally or applied to the skin. With few exceptions (panthenol/vitamin B5 comes to mind), vitamins in hair-care products are ineffective. Contrary to claim, nothing in this product can dissolve "hair follicle debris."

JASÖN NATURAL COSMETICS SHAMAN

☹ **Shaman Light Hold Spray, with Panthenol & Orange** *($6.50 for 8 ounces)* is a light-hold, minimally sticky nonaerosol hairspray that contains several essential oils that can cause scalp irritation, including lavender and orange. This works for soft control, but why risk creating an itchy, irritated scalp when so many great hairsprays are available without the problematic essential oils?

☺ **Shaman Sculpting Gel, with Cucumber & Vitamin E** *($6.50 for 8 ounces)* is a light- to medium-hold styling gel with a slightly sticky finish. It can smooth and control hard-to-manage hair, but the witch hazel, lavender, and essential oil fragrance can be a problem if this gets on the scalp.

☺ **Shaman Smoothing Fixture, with Aloe & Orange** *($6.50 for 8 ounces)* is nearly identical to the Shaman Sculpting Gel above, except this has a thicker texture and provides a decidedly medium hold with a bit more stickiness. Otherwise, the same basic comments apply.

J.F. LAZARTIGUE

Jean Francois Lazartigue is a well-known (at least in Europe) French hairdresser who launched his own product line in 1977, supposedly because he found himself dealing with clients who presented "an overwhelming array of hair health problems." Believing that hair and scalp problems are symptoms of fatigue, anxiety, sickness, and pollution, he set out to create products to restore hair to a healthier state. However, what he created is an abundance of standard to poorly formulated products dressed up with prices that aren't justified by what they contain. The technology behind several of the products is dated, and larger lines, such as Pantene, L'Oreal, and Paul Mitchell, are a decade or two ahead of Lazartigue when it comes to modern hair-care products. That doesn't mean j.f. lazartigue products don't work or won't help you manage your hair, because they will; they just won't do it any better than products you would find for a fraction of the price at the drugstore. J.F. lazartigue may be a fantastic hairdresser and educator on such topics as performing relaxing salon treatments (such as scalp pressure-point massage), but his products are mostly disappointing and shockingly overpriced. For more information on j.f. lazartigue, call (800) 359-9345 or visit www.jflazartigue.com.

What's Good About This Line: Some very emollient products for those with dry to very dry hair; most of the styling products work well and are options if you have a limitless hair-care budget.

What's Not So Good About It: The claims for most of the products are borderline ludicrous; prices are astronomical for what amounts to either standard or below-average formulations; many of the shampoos contain drying detergent cleansing agents; and the hair-loss treatment products are useless and a complete waste of money.

☺ $$$ **Deep Action Treatment with Carrot Oil** (*$52 for 5.08 ounces*) is not a treatment in the least, it is just a conditioner. The claim is that it can repair the cortex within the hair shaft, but if it can do that (which it can't), then any other standard conditioner could make the same claim, because it contains standard conditioning ingredients that show up in lots and lots of products. The cortex layer of hair is essentially the heart of the hair shaft. In order for ingredients to affect it, they would have to break through seven to ten layers of cuticle, which would damage one part of hair to help another—a senseless endeavor to say the least. This conditioner contains mostly water, thickeners, carrot extract (which has no proven benefit for hair or scalp), plant oils, detangling agent, fragrance, slip agents, water-binding agents, preservatives, and coloring agents. It is a good, though wildly overpriced, conditioner for normal to dry hair of any thickness. Its function as a pre-wash conditioner is a foolish marketing ruse. Why condition the hair, then shampoo and wash out this expensive product, then have to condition again?

☹ **Marine Hair Care Mask** (*$28 for 3.5 ounces*) contains algae extracts with sea mud. Not only can the mud be very drying to the hair, it also completely negates the water-binding effect of the algae and glycerin.

☺ $$$ **Pre-Shampoo Cream with Shea Butter** (*$51 for 6.8 ounces*) is a very emollient conditioner for dry to very dry hair, but the price is outrageous for ingredients that show up in many other conditioners that cost much less. It contains mostly water, shea butter, plant oil, detangling agent, thickeners, glycerin, conditioning agents, Vaseline, fragrance, preservatives, and vitamin E. Using this as a pre-shampoo treatment is a waste of time (and money). If you're going to splurge on this product, use it after shampooing or as an overnight treatment.

☹ **Propolis Jelly for Oily Scalp** *($36 for 3.5 ounces)* is a useless product that contains mostly water, alcohol, propolis (a waxy substance gathered by bees), slip agent, thickener, pH adjuster, plant extracts, water-binding agents, preservatives, and fragrance. Nothing in this pre-shampoo product can regulate scalp oil, and the lactic and salicylic acids it contains cannot exfoliate because the product's pH is too high. Don't bother.

☺ **$$$ Salmon Protein Hair Restorer** *($28 for 2.54 ounces)* is another pre-shampoo product that claims to repair the hair's cortex. That's not possible given the ingredients— nor would you want your hair-care products to reach the cortex, because that would cause serious daily damage. For the money and the faulty claims, this is another "why bother?" product.

☹ **After Swimming Shampoo, Salt Neutralizer** *($20 for 5.07 ounces)* contains TEA-lauryl sulfate as one of the main detergent cleansing agents, which makes this too drying for all hair and scalp types. It does contain a chelating agent to remove minerals and chlorine from hair, but so do many other products that use gentler cleansing agents.

☺ **$$$ Anti-Dandruff Shampoo** *($26 for 8.4 ounces)* is a standard, rather gentle shampoo that contains a tiny amount of the antimicrobial agent piroctone olamine. As this book goes to print, the FDA is still evaluating that ingredient's efficacy against dandruff. In other words, piroctone olamine is not part of the FDA's over-the-counter monograph for dandruff products (Source: www.fda.gov). However, there is research showing that piroctone olamine is an effective ingredient in controlling dandruff, though it's no more effective than zinc pyrithione (found in Head & Shoulders) or ketoconazole (found in Nizoral A-D) (Source: *International Journal of Cosmetic Science*, October 2002, page 249) for far less money.

☹ **Body-Giving Shampoo** *($23 for 8.4 ounces)* contains TEA-lauryl sulfate as one of the main detergent cleansing agents, which makes this too drying for all hair and scalp types.

☺ **$$$ Cereal Shampoo** *($20 for 5.07 ounces)* is a standard shampoo that can be a good option for all hair types except oily. It contains mostly water, detergent cleansing agent, lather agent, water-binding agent, thickeners, detangling agent, film-forming agent, fragrance, plant extracts, and preservatives. This poses minimal risk of buildup.

☹ **Deep Cleansing Shampoo** *($25 for 8.4 ounces)* contains TEA-lauryl sulfate as the main detergent cleansing agent, which makes this too drying for all hair and scalp types. The camphor, phenol, and menthol in this product only make matters worse. Overall, this adds up to one of the most irritating shampoos reviewed in this book.

☺ **$$$ Marine Shampoo** *($22 for 8.4 ounces)* is a standard shampoo that is marred by a fairly stiff film-forming agent and clay, which can dry the hair. This is a decent option for someone with very oily hair or scalp, but should be alternated with a shampoo that does not contain the clay or film-forming agents.

☹ **Micro-Pearl Shampoo, for Dry Hair** *($32 for 6.8 ounces)* contains TEA-lauryl sulfate as the main detergent cleansing agent, which makes this too drying for all hair and scalp types.

☹ **Micro-Pearl Shampoo, for Oily Hair** *($32 for 6.8 ounces)* is similar to the Micro-Pearl Shampoo, for Dry Hair above, and the same comments apply.

☺ **$$$ Moisturizing Shampoo, for Colour Treated Hair** *($25 for 8.4 ounces)* is a standard, but good, shampoo that contains mostly water, detergent cleansing agent, lather agents, water-binding agent, waxlike emulsifier, thickeners, slip agent, film-forming agent, plant extracts, fragrance, chelating agent, and preservatives. This can work well for all hair types, and poses a slight risk of buildup with repeated use. However, the price does not jibe with the ingredients, and, for the money, almost any shampoo from L'Oreal would be every bit as effective.

☺ **$$$ Orchid Shampoo** *($24 for 8.4 ounces)* contains orchid extract, but that has no special benefit for hair or scalp; it's just a fragrant additive. This is similar to the Cereal Shampoo above, and the same basic comments apply, although this shampoo gives you more for your money (and with this line, every little bit helps!).

☺ **$$$ Shampoo for Frequent Use** *($25 for 8.4 ounces)* doesn't contain anything that makes it preferred for frequent use, though it is a fairly gentle shampoo. It is similar to the Moisturizing Shampoo, for Colour Treated Hair above, except it contains more detangling agent, which can make it preferred for longer hair.

☹ **Stymulactine 21 Shampoo, Hair Loss Specific Treatment** *($62 for 2 ounces)* has a preposterous price for what amounts to a tiny bottle of standard shampoo. This is almost identical to several other j.f. lazartigue shampoos above, including the Shampoo for Frequent Use. It does not contain a single ingredient that can change the loss of even one strand of hair. The "miraculous" ingredient is silanediol salicylate, which is nothing more than organic silicone, a conditioning agent for hair. Though I rarely rate products based on the claim a company makes about a product, the price and marketing angle for this product are just too over-the-top to warrant anything other than an unhappy face rating.

☺ **$$$ Treatment Cream Shampoo with Collagen** *($33 for 6.8 ounces)* is a good, though absurdly overpriced, standard shampoo for normal to very dry hair that is normal to coarse or thick.

☹ **Treatment Shampoo, Unstraightened** *($19.50 for 6.8 ounces)* contains TEA-lauryl sulfate as one of its main detergent cleansing agents, which makes it too potentially drying for all hair and scalp types. Nothing about this shampoo makes it preferred for curly or wavy hair.

☺ **$$$ Detangling & Nourishing Conditioner** *($19.50 for 6.8 ounces)* is a very standard conditioner that contains mostly water, thickener, detangling agents, conditioning agents, silicone, fragrance, water-binding agents, and preservatives. It can work well for normal to slightly dry hair of any thickness, and it's up to you if you want to pay significantly more than you have to for a conditioner.

☺ **$$$ Energizing Elixir, After Shampoo for All Hair Types** *($22 for 5.07 ounces)* is just a standard detangling conditioner that contains mostly slip agents, thickener, detangling/film-forming agents, fragrance, water-binding agents, and preservatives. It can make normal to fine or thin hair easier to comb, but that's about it.

☺ $$$ **Hair Body Emulsion, for Fine Hair** *($29 for 8.4 ounces)* is a standard conditioner for normal to slightly dry hair of any thickness, and the price is embarrassing for such a mundane formulation. There is more fragrance in this than "special" ingredients for hair.

☺ $$$ **Moisturizing Conditioner, for Colour Treated Hair** *($25 for 5.07 ounces)* contains mostly water, slip agent, thickener, detangling agents, more thickeners, silicone, plant oil, water-binding agents, fragrance, plant extracts, and preservatives. It is a good conditioner for normal to dry hair of any thickness.

☺ $$$ **Vita-Cream with Milk Proteins, After-Shampoo for Dry and Fine Hair** *($43 for 6.8 ounces)* is yet another standard conditioner that contains mostly water, thickener, detangling agents, water-binding agent, more thickeners, plant oils, silicone, fragrance, preservatives, and coloring agent. It's an OK (though absurdly priced) option for normal to slightly dry hair that is normal to fine or thin.

☺ $$$ **Vita-Cream with Milk Proteins, After-Shampoo for Normal Hair** *($43 for 6.8 ounces)* is nearly identical to the Vita-Cream with Milk Proteins product above, except this contains slightly more thickening agents, which makes it somewhat preferred for normal to dry hair of any thickness. Otherwise, the same review applies.

☺ $$$ **Disentangling Instant Silk Protein Spray** *($18 for 3.4 ounces)* is an effective spray-on detangler for fine or thin hair. It contains mostly water, amino acids (which serve as water-binding agents), film-forming/conditioning agent, silicone, emulsifier, slip agent, chelating agent, preservatives, and fragrance.

☺ $$$ **Especially for Curly or Frizzy Hair, Styling Gel to Straighten or Curl** *($17 for 3.4 ounces)* is a very standard styling gel that contains enough glycerin to add moisture to hair to aid with curl retention, although glycerin isn't preferred to silicones for straightening hair with heat. It provides a light hold with a moist, slightly sticky finish that is easily brushed through.

☹ $$$ **Hair Styling Gel** *($20 for 3.4 ounces)* is just a basic styling gel. It actually has a rather dated formula, offering not a single conditioning or shine-enhancing ingredient. It will provide medium hold that is slightly stiff and sticky, so it's best for normal to fine or thin hair.

☺ $$$ **Hair Volume Tonic** *($32 for 3.4 ounces)* is a non-sticky, spray-on product that contains mostly water, slip agent/thickener, film-forming agent, silicone, fragrance, more slip agent, and preservatives. It can add a feeling of thickness without stiffness or stickiness to normal to fine or thin hair, but the price is steep when you consider that much less expensive products can provide the same benefit.

☺ $$$ **Protective Hair Cream** *($21 for 2.54 ounces)* lists octyl dimethyl PABA as its second ingredient, a sunscreen that is rarely used anymore because it frequently causes a sensitizing reaction. It is rated as SPF 10, but that number is meaningless because there are no regulated standards for determining SPF numbers in hair-care products. That means this flies in the face of FDA cosmetic labeling regulations as well as cosmetics regulations for hair-care products worldwide. This is otherwise a thin-textured styling cream that can groom the hair without hold. It can work well for all hair types, but is absolutely not worth its price.

☺ $$$ **Protective Hair Milk** *($22 for 2.54 ounces)* is a fairly greasy styling cream that can be a decent option for dry to very dry hair that is coarse, curly, or thick. It contains mostly emollient thickener, water, mineral oil, PABA, slip agent, several more thickeners, fragrance, preservatives, and stabilizing agent.

☺ $$$ **Root Volumizer** *($18 for 2.54 ounces)* is a lightweight styling balm that contains mostly water, slip agent, silicone, film-forming agent, water-binding agent, thickener, preservatives, detangling agent, more water-binding agents, fragrance, and coloring agents. Whether applied at the roots or all over, this can add body or smooth hair during heat styling. It provides a soft hold with no stiffness and barely discernible stickiness.

☺ $$$ **Straightening Gel for Curly Hair** *($20 for 3.4 ounces)* is a standard styling gel that is similar to the Hair Styling Gel above, but this includes some water-binding agents that add softness and some smoothness to hair. Almost any styling gel at the drugstore can compete with or best this, but if you're inclined to overspend on hair care, this is a good gel.

☹ $$$ **Anti-Dandruff Cream** *($28 for 3.4 ounces)* makes confusing claims. The literature for the product says it contains a 2% concentration of zinc pyrithione, an anti-dandruff ingredient, but it doesn't appear on the ingredient list as an active ingredient. Without the percentage of zinc pyrithione appearing in the active ingredient list you're left to believe the claim, and this line doesn't have the best track record for reliable information. This rinse-out conditioner may have a positive effect on dandruff, but I wouldn't choose it over a Head & Shoulders product with the exact same active ingredient, a clearly listed concentration, a similar conditioner base, and a reasonable price.

☺ $$$ **Essentials for Curly or Frizzy Hair, Smoothing Shining Balm** *($17.50 for 3.4 ounces)* is simply Vaseline, coconut oil, fragrance, and carrot oil. It is a thick, greasy pomade that is an option only for very dry hair that is coarse or thick. Of course, plain Vaseline will have the same effect for mere pennies, but that choice is up to you.

☺ $$$ **Essentials for Curly or Frizzy Hair, Treatment Oil** *($39 for 3.4 ounces)* is a very emollient glossing and conditioning spray for dry to very dry hair that is coarse or thick with frizzies. It adds a glossy sheen to the hair, but can easily feel greasy and slick if not applied sparingly. This is the only j.f. lazartigue product whose formula somewhat justifies its high price by including more expensive and exotic plant oils, but that doesn't mean it's necessarily better for hair. Exotic plant oils do not have special restorative properties for the hair or scalp, but the sage and geranium oils can cause scalp irritation, so be careful to apply this only to the hair.

☹ $$$ **Intensive Scalp Revitalizer** *($36 for 10 ampoules)* cannot revitalize anything. It's a simple concoction of soy protein, water, preservative, fragrance, chelating agent, and more preservative. The soy protein can lightly moisturize the scalp, but for this amount of money and the elaborate presentation, you should expect (and receive) more.

☺ $$$ **Intensive Sebum Treatment, for Oily Roots** *($51 for 2.5 ounces)* is a spray-on product that contains mostly water, alcohol (which is too drying and irritating for the scalp and can't affect oil production), anti-inflammatory plant extract, anti-microbial plant extract, slip agents, conditioning agent, and preservatives. Nothing in this product can regulate oil or restore balance to your scalp. This product does not contain any sub-stantiated anti-dandruff agents.

☺ $$$ **Revitalizing Shining Blush for Hair** *($24 for 1.7 ounces)* is a standard sili-cone spray that contains an added emollient and conditioning agents that make it best for normal to very dry hair that is normal to coarse or thick. It is easily replaced by silicone sprays available at the drugstore for far less.

☹ **Stymulactine 21, Hair Loss Specific Treatment** *($62 for 2.5 ounces)* claims it can reduce hair loss by making hair healthier. Yet typical male and female pattern baldness (androgenetic alopecia) has nothing to do with how healthy your hair is, and everything to do with male hormones (testosterone), a specific enzyme (5 alpha-reductase or 5AR), and genetics. This is nothing more than a lightweight, leave-in conditioner that can hy-drate slightly dry hair. The price is insulting for what you get, and the claims are completely without substantiation.

JHERI REDDING

Jheri Redding was a hairstylist whose major claim to fame was developing pH-balanced shampoos. His namesake hair-care line was launched in the 1960s and has been owned for the past several years by Conair Corporation. Redding's family is responsible for creation of the Nexxus hair-care line, reviewed elsewhere in this book. For more infor-mation about Jheri Redding, call (800) 326-6247 or visit www.conairhaircare.com.

What's Good About This Line: Reasonable prices qualify the best of these products as bona fide beauty bargains; there are some excellent options for shampoos, condition-ers, and styling products, particularly silicone serums.

What's Not So Good About It: Several styling products contain the preservatives methylchloroisothiazolinone and methylisothiazolinone (Kathon CG), which are not rec-ommended for use in leave-on products; two of the three "Extra" shampoos contain drying detergent cleansing agents; a couple of the nonaerosol hairsprays flake.

☺ **Shine Shampoo with Vitamin C, for Dull, Dry Hair** *($2.49 for 16 ounces)* does contain vitamin C, but that won't do a thing for dull or dry hair (it won't help any hair type because vitamins cannot feed the hair). This standard, but good, shampoo is a great inexpensive option for all hair types, and poses no risk of buildup.

☺ **Mega-Vitamin Conditioner, for Dry, Damaged Hair** *($2.49 for 16 ounces)* is a standard, but good, conditioner that would work well for normal to slightly dry hair of any thickness. The vitamins it contains have no effect on hair or scalp.

☻ **Alcohol-Free Mousse, Volumizing Ultra Control** *($2.49 for 8 ounces)* is a standard mousse that contains the problematic preservative Kathon CG, which is not recommended for use in leave-on products due to the risk, when left on the skin, of causing a sensitizing reaction.

☹ **Alcohol-Free Mousse, Volumizing Ultra Control, Unscented** *($2.49 for 8 ounces)* is nearly identical to the Alcohol-Free Mousse, Volumizing Ultra Control above, and the same comments apply.

☹ **Curl Energizer, Frizz Control** *($2.49 for 14 ounces)* contains the preservative Kathon CG, and is not recommended.

☹ **Design Spritz, Super Hold (Non-Aerosol)** *($2.49 for 14 ounces)* is a terrible hairspray that takes too long to dry and then flakes easily.

☹ **Design Spritz, Unscented Super Hold (Non-Aerosol)** *($2.49 for 14 ounces)* is identical to the Design Spritz above, and the same comments apply.

☺ **Flexible Hold Hair Spray, Flexible Hold (Aerosol)** *($2.49 for 10 ounces)* is a standard, but very good, aerosol hairspray that provides a light to medium hold that allows hair to remain flexible. This can be a good finishing spray that allows you to play with your style before it sets and locks it into place.

☺ **Flexible Hold Hair Spray, Flexible Hold (Non-Aerosol)** *($2.49 for 12 ounces)* is a lightweight, light-hold hairspray that leaves hair flexible and slightly sticky. It's a great option for all hair types, and the price makes it almost a steal!

☺ **Flexible Hold Hair Spray, Unscented Flexible Hold (Non-Aerosol)** *($2.49 for 12 ounces)* is identical to the Flexible Hold Hair Spray, Flexible Hold (Non-Aerosol) above, except this contains less fragrance. Otherwise, the same comments apply.

☺ **Frizz Out Gel, Alcohol-Free** *($2.49 for 20 ounces)* is a standard, light- to medium-hold styling gel that can help smooth minor frizzies and leaves hair with a slightly sticky, stiff feel that can be easily brushed through.

☺ **Glossing Design Spritz, Super Hold (Aerosol)** *($2.49 for 10 ounces)* is a medium-hold aerosol hairspray that contains a small amount of silicone for shine.

☺ **Mega Hold Gel, Alcohol-Free** *($2.49 for 20 ounces)* is a very standard styling gel that provides a medium to firm hold with a stiff, sticky finish that can be brushed through.

☺ **Shine Hair Spray, Super Hold (Aerosol)** *($2.49 for 10 ounces)* is not super holding in the least. This is identical to the Flexible Hold Hair Spray, Flexible Hold (Aerosol) above, and the same comments apply.

☺ **Shine Hair Spray, Unscented Super Hold (Aerosol)** *($2.49 for 10 ounces)* is identical to the Shine Hair Spray Super Hold (Aerosol) above, and the same comments apply. This does contain fragrance, even though it is labeled as unscented.

☺ **Straightening Gel, Alcohol-Free** *($2.49 for 20 ounces)* is similar to the Frizz Out Gel, Alcohol-Free above, except this replaces the glycerin with collagen, another good water-binding agent for hair. Otherwise, the same comments apply. For straightening hair, pair it with a silicone serum or cream for best results.

☺ **Straightening Lotion, Blow-Dry Activated** *($2.49 for 6 ounces)* is a better solo choice to use before straightening hair with heat than the Straightening Gel above. This light-textured, slightly creamy styling lotion contains plant oil, panthenol, and several silicones to help shield hair from heat (though no product can offer complete protection from heat damage). It offers a silky-smooth, barely sticky finish that is easily brushed through, and this is light enough to use on all hair types.

☺ **Styling Gel, Alcohol-Free Salon Formula Firm Hold** *($2.49 for 8 ounces)* is similar to, but not as well-formulated as, the Mega Hold Gel, Alcohol-Free above. Given that the Mega Hold option gives you 20 ounces of product for the same price, there is no logical reason to consider this product.

☺ **Frizz Out Hair Serum** *($2.99 for 1.5 ounces)* is a standard silicone serum that contains a small amount of alcohol to help dilute the silicones, though this can still make hair look too slick and greasy if not used judiciously. For smoothing stubborn frizzies and making hair feel like silk, this inexpensive option is marvelous.

JHERI REDDING EXTRA

☹ **Extra Shiny Silver Conditioning Shampoo** *($7.95 for 13.5 ounces)* contains TEA-lauryl sulfate as its main detergent cleansing agent, which makes it too drying for all hair and scalp types.

☹ **Extra Theraplus Moisturizing Shampoo** *($6.95 for 13.5 ounces)* contains sodium lauryl sulfate as its main detergent cleansing agent, and that makes this nonmoisturizing shampoo too drying for all hair and scalp types.

☺ **Extra Therashine Smoothing Shampoo** *($6.95 for 13.5 ounces)* is a huge improvement over the two Extra shampoos above. This is a very good shampoo for all hair types and poses minimal risk of buildup.

☺ **Extra Humidicon Moisturizing Conditioner** *($8.95 for 13.5 ounces)* is a standard emollient conditioner for normal to very dry hair of any thickness.

☹ **Extra Natural Conditioner** *($7.95 for 16.5 ounces)* is an ultra-light conditioner that contains merely water, protein (which serves as a water-binding agent), salt, and vinegar. It can minimally assist with detangling fine or thin hair, but is basically a "why bother?" product.

☺ **Extra Straightening & Smoothing Lotion** *($10 for 13.5 ounces)* is nearly identical to the Straightening Lotion, Blow-Dry Activated above. This option costs more per ounce and has a slightly greater amount of silicone, but not enough additional silicone to choose this over the less expensive option above.

☹ **Extra Theramax Firm Control Styling Gel** *($6.95 for 13.5 ounces)* contains the preservative Kathon CG, and is not recommended.

☺ **Extra Protein Pac Vitamin Conditioning Treatment** *($6.95 for 8 ounces)* would be a great conditioner for normal to dry hair of any thickness, but the ingredients don't make it a special treatment for hair.

☺ **Extra Reflections Frizz Defense Serum** *($6.95 for 2 ounces)* is a standard, basic silicone serum that would work as well as any to smooth hair, add shine, and tame frizzies. It does contain fragrance.

☺ **Extra Reflections Polisher** *($8.95 for 4 ounces)* is nearly identical to the Extra Reflections Frizz Defense Serum above, except this option is fragrance-free, which is a definite plus!

☺ **Extra Reflections Spray-On Shine** *($5.95 for 4 ounces)* is a standard silicone spray that can be a good option for all hair types looking to boost shine and tame frizzies. Those with fine or thin hair, take care to apply this sparingly to avoid a greasy look.

JHERI REDDING RESQ

☹ **ResQ Polishing & Styling Gel** *($8.50 for 16 ounces)* contains the preservative Kathon CG, and is not recommended.

☺ **Extra ResQ Hair Polisher Daily Hair Treatment** *($13.98 for 6 ounces)* is a silicone serum with additional plant oils, both emollient (sweet almond, safflower) and fragrant (tea tree). This can work beautifully as a leave-in smoothing treatment for dry to very dry hair that is coarse, curly, or thick. It does contain fragrance.

☺ **Extra ResQ Hair Repair Conditioning Treatment** *($7.95 for 16 ounces)* can be a good conditioner for normal to dry hair, though the high amount of film-forming agent means it will build up with repeated use.

☺ **Extra ResQ Leave-In Hair, Shine & Scalp Treatment** *($6.95 for 15 ounces)* is a standard, but good, leave-in conditioner that can work well for slightly dry hair that is normal to fine or thin.

JOHN FRIEDA

What began as a small line of products aimed at turning dry, frizzy hair into the image of polished perfection has multiplied into an enormous assortment of products for a wide variety of hair types, styles, and colors. It is an understatement to say that Frieda's Frizz Ease products never worked remotely as well in real life as they seemed to in the astounding before-and-after pictures that graced the ads for those products, but they do make a significant difference in the feel of the hair and how it looks after styling. That's why, for its wide variety of choices in the category of silicone serums, sprays, and styling creams, this line is a frizzy-haired consumer's delight.

The Beach Blonde, Sheer Blonde, and Brilliant Brunette lines are add-ons that don't really bring anything new to the table, and regrettably they are all fraught with problematic formulations that make them poor choices for color-treated hair. In addition, the color-enhancing shampoos and conditioners do not use the basic dyes, like those selected by such other lines as ARTec and Aveda, to deposit a subtle amount of color on the hair. That means that these products won't do a thing for their targeted hair colors. This is disappointing because the marketing claims make these sound like products specially formulated for blonde and brunette hair, and that is absolutely not the case. Still, there is much to praise in this line; you just have to shop carefully and keep your expectations realistic (actually, that's good advice when considering any hair-care line). For more information about John Frieda, call (800) 521-3189 or visit www.johnfrieda.com.

What's Good About This Line: Frizz Ease products offer one-stop shopping for anyone battling frizzies; many conditioners have impressive formulations for normal to very dry hair; a few styling products are as unique as hair-care formulations can get, given the limited ingredients chemists have to work with; prices are more than reasonable.

What's Not So Good About It: Way too many Frieda shampoos are poorly formulated, with either drying detergent cleansing agents or other problematic ingredients such as sodium polystyrene sulfonate; a few styling products contain the sensitizing preservatives methylchloroisothiazolinone and methylisothiazolinone (Kathon CG).

JOHN FRIEDA BEACH BLONDE

☹ **Beach Blonde Cool Dip, Refreshing Shampoo** (*$6.49 for 10 ounces*) contains peppermint oil, which is irritating to the scalp, as well as sodium thiosulfate. Sodium thiosulfate is a reducing agent used to straighten or curl the hair, but it can swell the hair shaft, and that's not a great thing to do routinely.

☺ **Beach Blonde Life Preserver, Hair Conditioning Oil** (*$5.79 for 4 ounces*) contains mostly water, plant oil, fragrance, preservative, more plant oils, flower extract, and more preservatives. This is a very basic water-in-oil conditioner that isn't much different from using plain castor oil or canola oil on dry hair.

☹ **Beach Blonde Smooth Sailing, Detangling Conditioner** (*$6.49 for 10 ounces*) contains peppermint oil, and there are plenty of standard conditioners similar to this that do not contain this irritating ingredient.

☹ **Beach Blonde Ocean Waves, Sea Spray Texturizing Styler** (*$6.49 for 6 ounces*) contains the preservative Kathon CG, which is not recommended for use in leave-on products.

☺ **Beach Blonde Gold Rush, Shimmer Gel** (*$6.49 for 4 ounces*) is a basic styling gel that contains mostly water, slip agent, film-forming/holding agent, thickener, fragrance, silicone, preservatives, wax, and mineral pigments for shimmer. It offers a light hold that is minimally stiff and sticky, and is an option if you want to add subtle shimmer to your hair.

☺ **Beach Blonde Kelp Help, Deep Conditioning Masque** (*$6.49 for 8 ounces*) contains mostly water, thickeners, silicones, slip agent, film-forming/conditioning agent, detangling agent, glycerin, fragrance, preservatives, plant extracts, clay, water-binding agents, and coloring agents. It's a good emollient conditioner for normal to dry hair that is normal to thick or coarse. The tiny amount of clay will not cause dryness, though it is still an odd choice for use in a product that promises deep conditioning.

☹ **Beach Blonde Lemon Lights, Fresh Squeezed Highlighter** (*$6.49 for 6.2 ounces*) contains lemon juice, lemon peel, and grapefruit and pineapple juices, all of which are extremely irritating to the scalp and drying to the hair. And this is a spray-on product you're supposed to use with heat or in the sun to lighten hair (which it won't), which makes these ingredients even more problematic.

☺ **Beach Blonde Sun Streaks, Heat-Accelerated Highlighter** *($6.49 for 4.4 ounces)* contains hydrogen peroxide in a water-based spray, which can lighten hair in the sun or with the heat of a blow dryer. The amount of peroxide is not disclosed, but it is not enough to significantly blonde the hair. Products like this (think Sun-In®) typically can only lighten hair to a strawberry blonde or bronze tone, depending on your natural hair color, and have to be used repeatedly. It is far cheaper (though I don't recommend it) to just use an 89-cent bottle of 3% hydrogen peroxide daily during the summer and you will get the same, if not better, results.

JOHN FRIEDA FRIZZ EASE

☺ **Frizz Ease Smooth Start, Defrizzing Shampoo, Extra Strength Formula** *($5.29 for 12.7 ounces)* is a very good shampoo for normal to very dry hair that is normal to coarse or thick—frizzies or not. The film-forming agent agent poses a slight risk of buildup with repeated use.

☺ **Frizz Ease Smooth Start, Defrizzing Shampoo, Original Formula** *($5.29 for 12.7 ounces)* is a very good shampoo for normal to dry hair of any thickness. This can cause buildup with repeated use, so it is best alternated with a shampoo that does not contain conditioning or film-forming agents.

☺ **Frizz Ease Daily Nourishment, Leave-In Fortifying Spray** *($5.99 for 8 ounces)* is an excellent leave-in conditioner for normal to dry hair of any thickness. This can build up with repeated use, so it is slightly preferred for making normal to fine or thin hair more manageable. It can do a reasonably good job of taming frizzies.

☺ **Frizz Ease Emergency Treatment, Leave-In Conditioning Spray** *($4.29 for 3 ounces)* is similar to, but not as well formulated as, the Frizz Ease Daily Nourishment, Leave-In Fortifying Spray above. It contains fewer conditioning agents, and is still an option for normal to dry hair of any thickness (particularly normal to fine or thin-textured hair)—but for the money, the Leave-In Fortifying Spray is preferred.

☺ **Frizz Ease Glistening Creme, Defrizzing Conditioner, Extra Strength Formula** *($5.99 for 12.7 ounces)* is a standard, but good, conditioner. There is nothing extra strength about this product, but it can work well for smoothing normal to dry hair that is normal to thick or coarse.

☺ **Frizz Ease Glistening Creme, Defrizzing Conditioner, Original Formula** *($5.99 for 12.7 ounces)* can work well for normal to dry hair of any thickness except fine.

☺ **Frizz Ease Miraculous Recovery, Deep-Conditioning Treatment** *($6.99 for 4 ounces)* is a good conditioner for normal to very dry hair that is normal to coarse, curly, or thick. This more closely resembles a standard conditioner than a special treatment, and the only miracle you'll witness after using it is smoother, softer hair that is easier to comb through.

☹ **Frizz Ease 5-Minute Manager, Blow-Dry Styling Spray** *($5.29 for 6.7 ounces)* contains the preservatives methylchloroisothiazolinone and methylisothiazolinone (Kathon CG), which are not recommended for use in leave-on products due to the high risk of a sensitizing reaction.

☺ **Frizz Ease Corrective Styling Gel, with Encapsulated Silicone** *($4.29 for 4 ounces)* is a standard, medium-hold styling gel that leaves hair feeling slightly stiff and sticky. The silicone may be encapsulated, but there is such a tiny amount of it that your frizzies won't be improved very much.

☹ **Frizz Ease Corrective Styling Mousse, Curl Reviver** *($5.29 for 6 ounces)* contains the preservative Kathon CG, and is not recommended.

☹ **Frizz Ease Dream Curls, Curl Perfecter** *($5.99 for 6.7 ounces)* contains the preservative Kathon CG, and is not recommended.

☺ **Frizz Ease Moisture Barrier, Firm-Hold Hair Spray (Aerosol)** *($4.99 for 10 ounces)* is a standard (but very good) medium-hold aerosol hairspray. It leaves hair relatively flexible and easy to brush through, and provides a slightly glossy shine courtesy of silicones and lanolin.

☺ **Frizz Ease Secret Weapon, Flawless Finishing Creme** *($4.99 for 4 ounces)* would work beautifully as a lightweight smoothing cream for normal to dry hair that is normal to thick or coarse. It contains an impressive blend of water, plant oil, silicone, slip agents, emollients, and film-forming agents to give hair a sleek (but not greasy) appearance while helping to tame frizzies.

☺ **Frizz Ease Shape and Shine, Flexible-Hold Hair Spray (Non-Aerosol)** *($4.99 for 10 ounces)* is a great light- to medium-hold hairspray that holds hair in place with minimal stiffness or stickiness. This can be a good working spray for more detailed styles, and hair can be easily brushed through once this product dries.

☺ **Frizz Ease Wind-Down, Relaxing Creme, Extra Strength Formula** *($5.99 for 3.5 ounces)* is a commendable styling cream that has a cushiony, slightly emollient texture that is easy to distribute through hair. I don't agree with John Frieda that this product is "revolutionary," but it can (with heat, tension, and the right brush) help make hair straight.

☺ **Frizz Ease Wind-Down, Relaxing Creme, Original Formula** *($5.99 for 3.5 ounces)* is nearly identical to the Frizz Ease Wind-Down, Relaxing Creme, Extra Strength Formula above, and the same comments apply.

☺ **Frizz Ease 100% Shine, Glossing Mist** *($5.99 for 3 ounces)* is a very light silicone spray that can work well on all hair types. This does not leave hair as shiny as many silicone sprays, but it is also significantly less slick and potentially less greasy, which makes this an especially good choice for those with fine or thin hair. Use it sparingly until you are accustomed to this product's finish, and then use more if needed.

☺ **Frizz Ease Hair Serum, Extra Strength Formula** *($9.99 for 1.69 ounces)* is a standard silicone serum that has a slightly thicker texture and would work very well for smoothing and adding frizz-free shine to dry or very dry hair that is thick or coarse. This is too heavy (even when used sparingly) for fine or thin hair.

☺ **Frizz Ease Hair Serum, Lite Formula** *($9.99 for 1.69 ounces)* is a standard silicone serum made slightly lighter than usual by combining silicones with isododecane, a gel-based thickener with a matte feel. This can work well to smooth frizzies and add shine, but use it sparingly. Those with fine or thin hair should apply this only to the ends of hair.

☺ **Frizz Ease Hair Serum, Original Formula** *($9.99 for 1.69 ounces)* was one of the first mass-market silicone serums, one that started a trend that (for very good reasons) is still going strong today in almost every hair-care line. This contains merely silicones with a sunscreen (though it cannot significantly protect hair from UV damage or prevent color fading), and is an excellent choice to add shine and make hair feel silky smooth while taming frizzies. The Frizz Ease Hair Serum, Extra Strength Formula above adds aloe and vitamin E to the mix, but is otherwise identical to this product.

☺ **Frizz Ease Instant Touch-Up, Glossing Spray** *($5.99 for 3 ounces)* is a standard silicone spray that has a heavier texture than the Frizz Ease 100% Shine, Glossing Mist above, though it is still a good option for all hair types. Use this sparingly to avoid a slick, greasy look.

☺ **Frizz Ease Instant Mirror Image, Heat-Activated Laminator** *($13 for 1.69 ounces)*. The concept behind this product is to use it on dry, styled hair and then apply heat, which creates a super glossy, patent-leather shine. It can indeed do this (with or without heat, though heat "seals" this product faster than air drying does) and makes this an option for creating an ultra-shiny finish on all hair types, though someone with fine or thin hair should use just a few drops of it to avoid a greasy appearance. All in all, this is a nice twist on standard silicone serums.

JOHN FRIEDA FRIZZ EASE RELAX

☺ **Frizz Ease Relax Total Clarity, Moisturizing Shampoo** *($6.99 for 8.4 ounces)* is similar to the Frizz Ease Smooth Start, Defrizzing Shampoo, Original Formula above, except this contains a higher level of glycerin, which can provide more moisture for dry hair. Otherwise, the same comments apply.

☺ **Frizz Ease Relax Vital Strength, Fortifying + Moisturizing Conditioner** *($10.50 for 8 ounces)* is a very emollient conditioner appropriate for someone with dry to very dry hair of any thickness except fine or thin. This won't make hair stronger, but it can definitely condition and moisturize.

☺ **Frizz Ease Relax Revival, Re-Energizing Styling Mousse** *($10.50 for 8.6 ounces)* is a standard, propellant-based styling mousse that provides a light hold with minimal stickiness. Hair is easy to brush through, and the conditioning agents can smooth hair and provide a small amount of heat protection.

☺ **Frizz Ease Relax Ripple Effect, Wave-Maker Styling Spray** *($10.50 for 6 ounces)* is a dual-phase styling spray that must be shaken before each use. It is primarily water and silicones with two plant oils and lightweight holding agents. It works well to define curls and waves without stiffness or stickiness, and provides a good amount of heat protection. This unique product is well worth auditioning if you have normal to very dry hair that is normal to coarse, curly, or thick.

☺ **Frizz Ease Relax Straight Forward, Blow-Dry Straightening Creme** *($6.99 for 3.5 ounces)* is identical to the Frizz Ease Wind-Down, Relaxing Creme, Extra Strength Formula above, and the same review applies. Why this version costs $1 more is a mystery.

☺ **Frizz Ease Relax Daily Replenisher, Instant Surface Smoother** *($10.50 for 4.4 ounces)* is similar to the Frizz Ease Secret Weapon, Flawless Finishing Creme above, except this contains less plant oil and more glycerin and slip agent, which makes it preferred for normal to dry hair that is fine or thin. Otherwise, the same basic comments apply.

☺ **Frizz Ease Relax Moisture Remedy, Intensive Re-Hydrating Balm** *($10.50 for 2 ounces)* is an exceptionally emollient leave-in conditioner for dry to very dry hair and scalp. This is a heavy product, and absolutely not "ultra-light" and "non-greasy" as claimed. However, it can take very good care of dry, overprocessed hair.

☺ **Frizz Ease Relax Sheer Reflections, High-Gloss Finishing Spray** *($6.99 for 4.2 ounces)* is a standard silicone spray that contains a film-forming/holding agent for added control. It can work well for all hair types looking for a finishing touch of shine with a light, non-sticky hold—but use it sparingly.

☺ **Frizz Ease Relax Texture Correcting Serum** *($9.99 for 1.69 ounces)* is a water-based silicone serum that is much lighter than any of the Frizz Ease serums above. It is a good option for normal to fine or thin hair dealing with stubborn frizzies or flyaway strands. Use this sparingly until you are accustomed to how much product your hair can handle without looking slick or greasy.

JOHN FRIEDA SHEER BLONDE

☹ **Sheer Blonde Highlight Activating Shampoo, Formulated for Honey to Caramel Blondes** *($6.99 for 8.45 ounces)* contains sodium polystyrene sulfonate, which can be drying to hair and scalp and can potentially strip hair color. And this is supposed to be a highlight-enhancing shampoo!

☹ **Sheer Blonde Highlight Activating Shampoo, Formulated for Use on Platinum to Champagne Blondes** *($6.99 for 8.45 ounces)* contains TEA-lauryl sulfate as its sole detergent cleansing agent, along with a higher-than-usual amount of sodium polystyrene sulfonate. That makes this a poor choice for all hair types, but especially for color-treated hair.

☺ **Sheer Blonde Moisture Infusing Shampoo, Formulated for Use on Honey to Caramel Blondes** *($6.49 for 8.45 ounces)* is a very good shampoo for all hair types, and one that poses minimal risk of buildup.

☺ **Sheer Blonde Moisture Infusing Shampoo, Formulated for Use on Platinum to Champagne Blondes** *($6.49 for 8.45 ounces)* is nearly identical to the Sheer Blonde

Moisture Infusing Shampoo, Formulated for Use on Honey to Caramel Blondes above, and the same comments apply.

☹ **Sheer Blonde Volume Enhancing Shampoo with Highlight Activators, Formulated for Fine, Thin Honey to Caramel Blondes** *($6.49 for 8.45 ounces)* contains sodium polystyrene sulfonate, which makes this too drying for all hair and scalp types, and a definite problem for color-treated hair. The high amount of acrylate film-forming agent can immediately build up and make hair feel coated.

☹ **Sheer Blonde Volume Enhancing Shampoo with Highlight Activators, Formulated for Fine, Thin Platinum to Champagne Blondes** *($6.49 for 8.45 ounces)* is nearly identical to the Sheer Blonde Volume Enhancing Shampoo with Highlight Activators, Formulated for Fine, Thin Honey to Caramel Blondes above, and the same comments apply.

☺ **Sheer Blonde Blonde Hair Repair, Strengthening Conditioner** *($6.49 for 4.2 ounces)* is nearly identical to the Frizz Ease Miraculous Recovery, Deep-Conditioning Treatment above, and the same review applies. This one ends up costing less for slightly more product, and your hair won't notice the difference.

☺ **Sheer Blonde Instant Conditioner and Highlight Enhancer, Formulated for Use on Honey to Caramel Blondes** *($6.99 for 8.7 ounces)* is a very good conditioner for normal to dry hair of any thickness (and any hair color, for that matter).

☺ **Sheer Blonde Instant Conditioner and Highlight Enhancer, Formulated for Use on Platinum to Champagne Blondes** *($6.99 for 8.7 ounces)* is nearly identical to the Sheer Blonde Instant Conditioner and Highlight Enhancer, Formulated for Use on Honey to Caramel Blondes above, and the same review applies.

☺ **Sheer Blonde Instant Detangler with Weightless Conditioners, Formulated for All Shades of Fine, Thin Blondes** *($6.49 for 8.45 ounces)* is a very good leave-in conditioner for its intended hair type, and can provide some protection during heat styling.

☺ **Sheer Blonde Blonde Ambition, Dual Action Mousse** *($5.49 for 7.5 ounces)* is a standard, propellant-based mousse with a medium hold that leaves hair quite sticky. This does not have a good amount of conditioning agents, and the tiny amount of violet coloring has minimal effect on blonde hair. This is one of Frieda's weaker styling products.

☺ **Sheer Blonde Brand New Blonde, Revitalizing Styling Mousse** *($5.49 for 7.5 ounces)* is nearly identical to the Sheer Blonde Blonde Ambition, Dual Action Mousse above, except this does not contain coloring agents. Otherwise, the same review applies.

☺ **Sheer Blonde Crystal Clear, Shape, Shimmer & Hold Hairspray** *($4.99 for 8.5 ounces)* is a standard, light-hold aerosol hairspray that leaves a slightly sticky finish. Hair can be easily brushed through and the hairspray goes on very light, so there is little reason to be concerned about creating "helmet head."

☺ **Sheer Blonde Full-Blown Blonde, Volumizing Spray** *($5.49 for 6.7 ounces)* is a medium-hold, water- and alcohol-based styling spray that leaves hair feeling slightly stiff and sticky, though it can be easily brushed through without flaking.

☺ **Sheer Blonde Funky Chunky, Sheer Veneer Texturizer** *($5.49 for 4 ounces)* is a standard styling gel with an unusual name that has little to do with its formula. This provides a light to medium hold with some stickiness, though hair can be brushed through. The conditioning agents provide a slight amount of protection during heat styling.

☺ **Sheer Blonde Spun Gold, Shaping and Highlighting Balm** *($5.49 for 1.2 ounces)* is a thick, Vaseline- and mineral oil-based pomade (not a balm, which implies something much lighter) that is infused with shimmering gold particles that cling well to the hair. This is an option for smoothing dry to very dry hair that is thick or coarse, or use it sparingly to groom dry ends and calm frizzies.

☺ **Sheer Blonde Dream Creme, Instant Silkener** *($6.49 for 4.4 ounces)* is nearly identical to the Frizz Ease Secret Weapon Flawless Finishing Creme above, except this contains more slip agent than plant oil, which gives it a slightly lighter texture. Otherwise, the same comments apply.

☺ **Sheer Blonde Spotlight, Hi-Beam Glosser and Power Detangler** *($5.49 for 2.4 ounces)* contains mostly slip agent, silicone, water, film-forming agent, wax, and preservatives. This is fragrance-free, and can be an excellent lightweight detangling conditioner for all hair types.

JOHN FRIEDA BRILLIANT BRUNETTE

☹ **Brilliant Brunette Shine Release Moisturizing Shampoo, Amber to Maple** *($6.49 for 8.45 ounces)* contains sodium lauryl sulfate as one of its main detergent cleansing agents, which makes this too drying for both hair and scalp. The tea leaves and caramel coloring make the product look pleasingly brown in the bottle, but these ingredients cannot cling to the hair shaft, so this offers no color-enhancing benefits for brunettes.

☹ **Brilliant Brunette Shine Release Moisturizing Shampoo, Chestnut to Espresso** *($6.49 for 8.45 ounces)* is nearly identical to the Brilliant Brunette Shine Release Moisturizing Shampoo above, and the same basic comments apply.

☹ **Brilliant Brunette Shine Release Shampoo, Amber to Maple** *($6.49 for 8.45 ounces)* is nearly identical to the Brilliant Brunette Shine Release Moisturizing Shampoo above, and the same review applies.

☹ **Brilliant Brunette Shine Release Shampoo, Chestnut to Espresso** *($6.49 for 8.45 ounces)* is nearly identical to the Brilliant Brunette Shine Release Moisturizing Shampoo above, and the same basic comments apply.

☹ **Brilliant Brunette Shine Release Volumizing Shampoo, Amber to Maple** *($6.49 for 8.45 ounces)* is nearly identical to the Brilliant Brunette Shine Release Moisturizing Shampoo above, and the same review applies.

☹ **Brilliant Brunette Shine Release Volumizing Shampoo, Chestnut to Espresso** *($6.49 for 8.45 ounces)* is nearly identical to the Brilliant Brunette Shine Release Moisturizing Shampoo above, and the same basic comments apply.

☺ **Brilliant Brunette Light Reflecting Conditioner, Amber to Maple** *($6.49 for 8.45 ounces)* is a standard, though good, conditioner for normal to dry hair of any thickness, but the coloring agents have no effect on brunette hair.

☺ **Brilliant Brunette Light Reflecting Conditioner, Chestnut to Espresso** *($6.49 for 8.45 ounces)* is nearly identical to the Brilliant Brunette Light Reflecting Conditioner, Amber to Maple above, except this uses cocoa powder instead of tea leaves to add color (to the product, not to your hair). Otherwise, the same review applies.

☺ **Brilliant Brunette Simply Sleek Straightening Balm** *($5.49 for 3.8 ounces)* is nearly identical to the Sheer Blonde Dream Creme, Instant Silkener above, and the exact same comments apply. This product can straighten hair when used with heat and the proper brush.

☺ **Brilliant Brunette Satin Shine Finishing Creme** *($5.49 for 4.4 ounces)* is nearly identical to the Sheer Blonde Dream Creme, Instant Silkener above, and the same comments apply. Isn't it interesting how John Frieda has recycled this formula into so many different products? To his credit, though, if you are going to create several copycat products, this is a great formula to duplicate.

☺ **Brilliant Brunette Hold True Long-Lasting Finishing Spray** *($5.49 for 8.5 ounces)* is a light-hold, nonaerosol hairspray that has no special benefit for brunette hair, but can provide long-lasting style support without stiffness and with minimal stickiness.

☺ **Brilliant Brunette Shine Shock Leave On Perfecting Glosser** *($5.49 for 2.40 ounces)* is a thick silicone gel that can add dazzling shine to any shade of hair, not to mention smooth away frizzies. The texture of this product makes it best for dry to very dry hair that is normal to coarse or thick.

☺ **Brilliant Brunette Model Control Firm Hold Gel** *($5.49 for 6 ounces)* is a standard, but good, styling gel that provides medium hold with a slightly sticky/stiff finish. This gel contains nothing that makes it exclusive for use by brunettes.

JOHN MASTERS ORGANICS

John Masters is a New York City–based hairdresser who has formulated several hair-care products that contain primarily natural ingredients and essential oils (though the oils are basically just added fragrance). His unassuming approach, minimal packaging, and casual marketing angle (a prominent link on his Web site allows you to meet his dog, Amber) makes his small hair-care collection all the more appealing. His products are available online and in select department stores such as Barneys New York. For more information about john masters organics, call (800) 599-2450 or visit www.johnmasters.com.

What's Good About This Line: One of the few hair-care lines that lists the ingredients for each product on the company's Web site; this product line is a boon for fans of natural and organic ingredients, although the products are not even close to being all-natural.

What's Not So Good About It: Many of the essential oils offer no established benefit for hair or scalp, but they can cause scalp itching and irritation.

☺ $$$ **Evening Primrose Shampoo, for Dry Hair** *($16 for 8 ounces)* is an excellent shampoo for normal to very dry hair that is coarse or thick.

☺ $$$ **Lavender Rosemary Shampoo, for Normal Hair** *($16 for 8 ounces)* is nearly identical to the Evening Primrose Shampoo above, except this omits the plant oils and uses fewer essential oils for the fragrance. It is a good option for all hair types and poses no risk of buildup.

☺ $$$ **Lemongrass Shampoo, for Oily Hair** *($16 for 8 ounces)* is almost identical to the Lavender Rosemary Shampoo above, except this contains lemongrass instead. This can be a good, simple shampoo for all hair types.

☹ $$$ **Zinc & Sage Shampoo with Conditioner** *($20 for 8 ounces)* is, according to John Masters, his most popular shampoo. It is similar to all of his shampoos above, but adds an emollient thickener, which makes this more of a conditioning shampoo appropriate for normal to dry hair of any thickness. The zinc in it is said to regulate the scalp and put a stop to itching, but this is just plain zinc rather than the anti-dandruff ingredient zinc pyrithione or protective zinc oxide. Plain zinc is used as an astringent and a reducing agent (a substance that decreases the volume or concentration of another substance), and as such cannot regulate anything, though it may cause scalp dryness due to its astringent nature.

☺ $$$ **Citrus & Neroli Detangler** *($16 for 8 ounces)* is an emollient detangling conditioner, and would be best for someone with dry to very dry hair. The lemon, neroli, and grapefruit oils are a problem for the scalp, but if you apply this product on the hair only, that's a non-issue.

☹ $$$ **Herbal Cider Hair Rinse & Clarifier** *($17 for 8 ounces)* is an acidic finishing rinse for the hair that contains apple cider vinegar and lemon oil to help shut down (close) the hair's cuticle layer so hair is shinier. The lemon oil can be irritating to the scalp, and the cost of this product is high, considering you can try this yourself at home for pennies with vinegar (plain or apple cider) purchased at any supermarket.

☺ $$$ **Lavender & Avocado Intensive Conditioner** *($22 for 6.35 ounces)* can work well for dry hair of any thickness, but isn't intensive in the least, just overpriced for what is little more than a standard conditioner.

☺ $$$ **Personalized Color Conditioners** *($22 for 8 ounces)* is identical to the Citrus & Neroli Detangler above, but adds various basic dyes to create a color conditioner that can have a subtle impact on natural or dyed hair. It is available in ten shades, and the temporary dye agents shampoo out easily. But do keep in mind that even temporary dyes can cling strongly to highly processed or bleached hair because of its increased porosity.

☹ **Rosemary & Peppermint Detangler** *($16 for 8 ounces)* is almost identical to the Citrus & Neroli Detangler above, except this contains essential oils of peppermint, spearmint, and rosemary, which makes it too irritating and drying for all scalp types.

☺ $$$ **Bourbon Vanilla & Tangerine Hair Texturizer** *($21 for 2 ounces)* is a thick, but workable, plant oil–based pomade that can add soft texture and shine to all hair types while helping to control frizzies. It is moderately water-soluble and does not contain the typical waxes that can make hair feel heavy. This can still become greasy if not used sparingly, and is best for normal to very dry hair that is normal to coarse, curly, or thick.

☺ $$$ **Hair Pomade** (*$20 for 2 ounces*) is a very greasy pomade that contains olive oil, beeswax, mango butter, plant oils, essential oil fragrance, and vitamins. It is easy to work with, but can make hair feel slick and greasy unless used very sparingly. This is preferred for dry to very dry hair that is thick or coarse.

☹ **Sweet Orange & Silk Protein Styling Gel** (*$16 for 8 ounces*) is a light-hold styling gel that does not contain traditional film-forming/holding agents. That's to this gel's detriment because it can flake, especially when brushed through.

☹ **Deep Scalp Follicle Treatment & Volumizer for Thinning Hair** (*$21 for 2 ounces*) is a medicinal-smelling, spray-on, leave-in conditioner that contains some excellent (though standard) water-binding and conditioning agents. This goes astray and becomes a problem for the scalp and hair because it also contains arnica, sulfur, witch hazel, and essential oils of rosemary, thyme, and lavandin, among others. Considering this is meant to be applied to the scalp and left on, it is a significant problem for causing scalp itching and irritation and the sulfur is damaging to the hair shaft. None of these ingredients will affect hair growth in the least.

☺ $$$ **Dry Hair Nourishment & Defrizzer** (*$16 for 0.5 ounce*) is a wonderfully rich blend of plant oils along with squalene, an emollient. This is excellent for dry to very dry hair, and you need only a few drops to smooth the hair and control frizzies. This does contain essential oils for fragrance.

JOHNSON & JOHNSON HAIR CARE

For more information about Johnson & Johnson, call (800) 328-9033 or visit www.johnsonandjohnson.com.

What's Good About This Line: Johnson & Johnson is the originator of "no more tears" baby shampoos, and the majority of shampoos reviewed are suitable for use on babies and children; the prices are great, especially considering the generously large sizes of the shampoo containers.

What's Not So Good About It: All of the leave-on products contain sensitizing preservatives, which are of even greater concern for use on baby and children's scalps; it would have been nice for J&J to offer at least one fragrance-free shampoo for babies.

☺ **Baby Shampoo, Detangling Formula** (*$4.49 for 20 ounces*) is a very gentle shampoo that would be better if it did not contain fragrance, but it is still mild enough to clean the hair without dryness or irritation.

☺ **Baby Shampoo, Moisturizing Formula with Honey & Vitamin E** (*$4.49 for 20 ounces*) is nearly identical to the Baby Shampoo, Detangling Formula above, and the same comments apply. The addition of honey adds some water-binding properties, but vitamin E has no effect on hair or scalp.

☺ **Baby Shampoo, Natural Lavender** *($3.79 for 15 ounces)* is nearly identical to the Baby Shampoo, Detangling Formula above, and the same comments apply. This does not contain natural lavender; it just contains synthetic lavender fragrance.

☺ **Baby Shampoo, Original** *($4.49 for 20 ounces)* was Johnson & Johnson's first baby shampoo, the very one that ushered in the "no more tears" concept through J&J's patented use of extremely gentle detergent cleansing agents known as amphoteric surfactants. Amphoteric surfactants do not cleanse or foam as well as other surfactants, but their unique property is their very low irritation potential. Amphoterics (the one most commonly used is cocamidopropyl betaine) are so gentle that they can even reduce the irritation potential of other surfactants known for their sensitizing traits, such as sodium lauryl sulfate. This shampoo can work well to cleanse the hair of babies and children, but it is too mild to work effectively on adult hair, especially if you use styling products. Formula-wise, Baby Shampoo, Original is nearly identical to the Baby Shampoo, Detangling Formula above, and the same comments apply.

☺ **Head To Toe Baby Wash, Original** *($3.79 for 15 ounces)* is nearly identical to the Baby Shampoo, Detangling Formula above, except this does not contain coloring agents. Otherwise, the same review applies.

☹ **Softwash Baby Shampoo, Kissably Baby Soft** *($3.79 for 15 ounces)* is a stronger baby shampoo than all of the options above because it contains more standard detergent cleansing agents than cocamidopropyl betaine. This also contains an acrylate film-forming agent that can build up on a baby's hair with repeated use, so it is not as good a choice as any of the options above.

JOHNSON'S KIDS

☺ **Kids 2 in 1 Conditioning Shampoo, BlueBerry Bash** *($2.79 for 9 ounces)* is nearly identical to the Baby Shampoo, Detangling Formula above, except this contains silicone and additional conditioning agents, so it can be helpful for detangling children's hair while leaving it smooth and silky-soft.

☺ **Kids Arthur Conditioning Shampoo** *($3.49 for 11 ounces)* is nearly identical to the Softwash Baby Shampoo, Kissably Baby Soft above, except this omits the film-forming agent, which makes it a better choice if you want to avoid buildup.

☺ **Kids Blue's Clues Tickety Tock Strawberry Detangling Shampoo** *($3.49 for 11 ounces)* is nearly identical to the Kids 2 in 1 Conditioning Shampoo, BlueBerry Bash above, and the same comments apply.

☺ **Kids Head-to-Toe Body Wash, Berry Breeze** *($3.59 for 9 ounces)* is nearly identical to the Kids Arthur Conditioning Shampoo above, and the same review applies.

☺ **Kids Head-to-Toe Body Wash, Tropical Blast** *($3.59 for 9 ounces)* is nearly identical to the Kids Arthur Conditioning Shampoo above, and the same review applies.

☺ **Kids Head-to-Toe Body Wash, Watermelon Explosion** *($3.59 for 9 ounces)* is nearly identical to the Kids Arthur Conditioning Shampoo above, and the same review applies.

☺ **Kids Head-to-Toe Body Wash, Wild Orange Wave** *($3.59 for 9 ounces)* is nearly identical to the Kids Arthur Conditioning Shampoo above, but with a more intense fragrance. Otherwise, the same review applies.

☹ **Kids No More Bed-Head Spray, Watermelon Madness** *($3.59 for 10 ounces)* contains the preservatives methylchloroisothizolinone and methylisothiazolinone (Kathon CG), which are not recommended for use in leave-on products because they can cause sensitizing reactions on the scalp.

☺ **Kids No More Tangles Shampoo, StrawBerry Blast** *($2.79 for 9 ounces)* is, save for a change in fragrance, identical to the Kids 2 in 1 Conditioning Shampoo above, and the same comments apply.

☹ **Kids No More Tangles Spray Detangler, Jelly Bean Blast** *($3.49 for 10 ounces)* is identical to the Kids No More Bed-Head Spray, Watermelon Madness above, and the same comments apply.

☹ **Kids No More Tangles Spray Detangler, StrawBerry Blast** *($3.49 for 10 ounces)* contains the preservatives methylchloroisothizolinone and methylisothiazolinone (Kathon CG), which are not recommended for use in leave-on products because they can cause sensitizing reactions on the skin and scalp.

JOICO

Joico's claim to hair-care recognition over the years has been something called Triamine Complex. It is nothing more than hydrolyzed human hair keratin protein. Although it sounds like human hair protein should be able to bond better to hair and provide better conditioning, the reality is that after you take hair and get the protein molecules out, and then hydrolyze them, the hair is no longer hair, it's just another protein. That makes it a good conditioning agent, but no better than lots of other conditioning agents used in hair-care products. For more information about Joico, now owned by Shiseido, call 800-44-JOICO or visit www.joico.com.

What's Good About This Line: A nice variety of shampoos that are truly appropriate for their intended hair type; conditioners that run the gamut from light to substantial; some very good, silicone-based smoothing and straightening products.

What's Not So Good About It: A few of the styling products contain problematic ingredients such as sodium polystyrene sulfonate or the preservatives methylchloro-isothiazolinone and methylisothiazolinone (Kathon CG); there are no extra emollient conditioner options for very dry hair; claims for many products are way beyond what the ingredients they contain are really capable of doing.

☺ **Biojoba Treatment Shampoo, for Scalp and Chemically-Damaged Hair** *($10 for 10.1 ounces)* is a standard, but good, shampoo that contains very little of the bally-hooed hydrolyzed human hair keratin (Triamine Complex). This is a good option for all hair types and poses minimal risk of buildup. For some reason, Joico claims this shampoo "may help alleviate psoriasis," but there is nothing in it that can remotely help this stubborn skin and scalp condition.

The Reviews J

☺ **Kerapro Conditioning Shampoo, for Normal-to-Dry Hair** *($7 for 10.1 ounces)* is a standard, but very good, shampoo for all hair types, though it can cause slight buildup with repeated use.

☺ **Lavei Deep-Cleansing Shampoo, for Oily Hair** *($7 for 10.1 ounces)* is a good shampoo for all hair types, and poses minimal risk of buildup. The tiny amount of human hair keratin protein present won't have an impact on hair.

☺ **Resolve Chelating Shampoo, for Maximum Cleansing** *($8 for 10.1 ounces)* is a simple, but very good, chelating shampoo that can remove minerals, chlorine, and product buildup from all hair types. It does not contain conditioning or film-forming agents—just as it should be for a shampoo that promises to remove buildup!

☺ **Triage Moisture-Balancing Shampoo, for Normal Hair** *($7 for 10.1 ounces)* is an excellent conditioning shampoo for normal to very dry hair that is normal to coarse or thick.

☺ **Volissima Volumizing Shampoo, for Fine Hair** *($8 for 10.1 ounces)* can be a very good shampoo to make fine or thin hair feel thicker. This can build up with repeated use, but the film-forming agent and silicones are initially helpful for fine or thin hair. The tiny amount of witch hazel should not be a problem for the scalp or hair.

☺ **ALTima Daily Moisturizing Conditioner** *($10 for 10.5 ounces)* is a fairly light, standard conditioner that is a good option for normal to slightly dry hair of any thickness.

☺ **Integrity Leave-In Conditioning Detangler** *($10 for 10.1 ounces)* is a very good conditioning detangler for normal to slightly dry hair.

☺ **Lite Daily Conditioner, for All Hair Types** *($8 for 10.1 ounces)* is indeed light compared to most conditioners, and is a good option for slightly dry hair that is normal to fine or thin.

☺ $$$ **Moisturizer Intensive Moisture Treatment, Extra Conditioning** *($14 for 10.5 ounces)* is similar to the ALTima Daily Moisturizing Conditioner above, except this is slightly more emollient, which makes it slightly preferred for drier hair that is normal to fine or thin. The film-forming agent can build up with repeated use.

☺ **Phine Conditioning Chelating Treatment** *($8 for 5 ounces)* is a standard conditioner for normal to dry hair that is normal to fine or thin, though someone with moderately thick hair (not coarse) could also benefit.

☺ **Volissima Volumizing Conditioner, for Fine Hair** *($10 for 10.1 ounces)* is a standard, but very good, conditioner that is a good choice for normal to dry hair of any thickness, except coarse or very thick hair.

☺ **Brilliantine Shine and Defining Pomade** *($10 for 2 ounces)* is a very standard, Vaseline- and wax-based pomade that is best for dry to very dry hair that is thick or coarse. It can quickly feel heavy and look greasy unless used sparingly, but it can tame frizzies and smooth dry ends.

☺ $$$ **Hi-Rise Hair Volume Booster** *($14 for 10.5 ounces)* is a propellant-based mousse with a directional nozzle to focus application on the roots. The problem is that too much product is dispensed too forcefully, leaving you with an application that is too heavy in one area and not enough in another. It is best to dispense this into your hands, emulsify, and then apply to the hair. This provides a light to medium hold that is slightly sticky, but hair can be brushed through.

☹ **JoiGel Styling Gel, Medium Hold** *($10 for 10.5 ounces)* contains the preservative Kathon CG, which is contraindicated for use in leave-on products due to its high risk of causing a sensitizing reaction when left on skin.

☺ **JoiMist Firm Finishing Spray, Maximum Hold** *($11.50 for 11.2 ounces)* is a standard aerosol hairspray that provides a medium, brushable hold with a smooth, non-sticky finish. The conditioning agents and plant oil add shine and make this a preferred finishing spray for those with dry hair.

☺ **JoiMist Shaping and Finishing Spray, Medium Hold** *($11 for 11.2 ounces)* is nearly identical to the JoiMist Firm Finishing Spray, Maximum Hold above, although this provides a softer hold, but the difference is slight. Beyond this, the same comments apply.

☺ **$$$ Straight Edge Curl Straightener, Heat-Activated** *($14 for 10.1 ounces)* is a very good, light-textured styling cream that can work well to straighten hair with heat and the proper styling tool. The silicones add silky shine, and the film-forming agent provides a light, flexible hold that helps keep wavy or curly hair straight. This is not completely humidity-resistant—but then, no product is!

☺ **Travallo Design and Finishing Spray, Medium Hold** *($10 for 10.1 ounces)* is a standard hairspray that provides a light hold with minimal stiffness or stickiness. Hair is easy to brush through and restyle, which makes this a good working hairspray for more intricate styles you don't wish to instantly freeze in place.

☹ **Volissima Volumizing Gel, for Fine Hair** *($10 for 10.1 ounces)* contains film-forming agents whose seeming incompatibility with the base formula (or each other) causes this gel to ball up and eventually flake once dry. It is not recommended.

☺ **Volissima Volumizing Lotion, for Fine Hair** *($9 for 10.1 ounces)* isn't a lotion, it's a gel, and one that can provide a light, conditioned hold with minimal stickiness; it's incredibly easy to brush through. This is a much better formulation than the Volissima Volumizing Gel above.

☺ **Spray Glace Shine Enhancer** *($15 for 5 ounces)* is a standard silicone spray whose somewhat generous size helps offset its lofty price. As a spray, this goes on heavier than similar products, which means this can make fine or thin hair quickly look slick and greasy. It is best for dry to very dry hair that is normal to coarse or thick.

JOICO COLOR ENDURANCE

☺ **Color Endurance Color Lock Shampoo, for Color-Treated Hair** *($10 for 10.1 ounces)* contains not a single special (or proven) ingredient that can make color last longer, not to mention lock it into place. This shampoo is very similar to the Volissima Volumizing Shampoo, for Fine Hair above, and the same review applies.

☺ **Color Endurance Color Lock Conditioner, for Color Treated Hair** *($12 for 10.1 ounces)* is a very good, though surprisingly standard, conditioner for normal to dry hair of any thickness. It doesn't contain a single ingredient that can preserve even one molecule of color, especially when you consider that water alone (as when you rinse shampoo or conditioner) can also hasten the fading of dyed hair.

☹ **Color Endurance Color Lock Leave-In Protectant, for Color-Treated Hair** *($11 for 10.1 ounces)* is a standard styling spray masquerading as a specialty leave-on conditioner.

☺ **$$$ Color Endurance Thermal Styling Spray** *($16 for 8.5 ounces)* is a fairly sticky, alcohol- and water-based styling spray that provides a medium hold that can be brushed through. There is nothing in this product that can shield dyed hair from the inevitable fading. Ironically, this product contains a small amount of sodium polystyrene sulfonate, an ingredient that can potentially strip hair color (although for non-dyed hair, the tiny amount present is unlikely to cause problems).

☺ **$$$ Color Endurance Vibrant Shine Mist** *($14 for 3.4 ounces)* is a very standard silicone spray that can add a veil of glossy shine to all hair types, but the price is high considering you can achieve the same result with silicone sprays available at the drugstore.

JOICO CON_TEXT LINE

☺ **$$$ Con_text Assertion Finishing Spray** *($14 for 12 ounces)* is almost identical to the JoiMist Firm Finishing Spray, Maximum Hold above, and the same comments apply.

☺ **$$$ Con_text Conversion Texture Spray** *($12.50 for 6.5 ounces)* is a standard, alcohol-based, light- to medium-hold styling spray that has a slightly thick, sticky finish. The silicone and conditioning agents can provide a slight amount of heat protection during styling.

☺ **Con_text Organization Grooming Gel** *($12.50 for 6.8 ounces)* is a thick-textured styling gel that provides a medium to firm hold while leaving hair slightly stiff and moderately sticky, though this can be brushed through. It would work well for controlling detailed styles or for use on stubborn strands.

☺ **Con_text Orientation Light Wax** *($13 for 2 ounces)* is a fairly heavy pomade that can work well to add subtle texture and soft shine to all hair types, but those with fine or thin hair should apply this only to dry ends for on-the-spot smoothing. This is reasonably water-soluble.

☺ **$$$ Con_text Transformation Molding Putty** *($16 for 4.4 ounces)* is an impossibly thick, very heavy styling paste that can be difficult to distribute in your hands, let alone apply to the hair. It can add chunky texture with a low-wattage shine, but this remains sticky and does not shampoo out easily. If you're up for the challenge, this is an option for those with thick or coarse hair that is best described as "unruly" or "product-resistant."

☺ **Con_text Variation Pliable Paste** *($14 for 4.4 ounces)* is similar to, but much more workable than, the Con_text Transformation Molding Putty above. It has the same heaviness and stickiness issues, but is an option for stubborn hair that is thick or coarse.

JOICO I.C.E.

☺ **Forming I.C.E. Styling Creme** *($10.25 for 2 ounces)* is a light-hold, lightweight styling cream that can be a great product to "cocktail," or mix, with other styling products (such as gels or mousses) to create a softer hold, more shine, and additional heat protection. It is light enough to be used by those with fine or thin hair.

☹ **I.C.E. Gel Styling Gel, Maximum Hold** *($10 for 10.5 ounces)* contains the preservative Kathon CG, and is not recommended.

☺ **I.C.E. Mist Finishing Spray, Maximum Hold** *($10 for 10.1 ounces)* is a standard, medium-hold hairspray that leaves hair feeling minimally stiff and not at all sticky. The silicone adds a touch of shine and allows hair to be easily brushed through.

☹ **I.C.E. Sculpting Lotion** *($8 for 10.1 ounces)* contains the preservative Kathon CG, and is not recommended.

☺ **I.C.E. Whip Designing Foam, Firm Hold** *($14 for 10.5 ounces)* is a standard, propellant-based mousse that offers a light to medium hold with a non-sticky, minimally stiff finish that is easily brushed through. This would be a great option for normal to fine or thin hair, although it does not contain enough conditioning agents to provide decent protection during heat styling.

JOICO K-PAK

☺ **K-Pak Shampoo, for Damaged Hair** *($12 for 10.1 ounces)* is a standard, but very good, shampoo that is an option for normal to dry hair of any thickness, and poses minimal to no risk of buildup.

☺ **K-Pak Daily Conditioner, for Damaged Hair** *($12 for 10.5 ounces)* is nearly identical to the ALTima Daily Moisturizing Conditioner above, and the same review applies. The "extra" ingredients (alpha lipoic acid, vitamins) in this one have no effect on damaged (or any type of) hair, as those ingredients can't hold up under rinsing or styling tools.

☺ **$$$ K-Pak Deep-Penetrating Reconstructor, for Damaged Hair** *($18 for 5.2 ounces)* is nearly identical to the ALTima Daily Moisturizing Conditioner above, except this contains mineral oil, hardly an exciting or specialized hair-care ingredient. It simply makes this a more emollient option suitable for dry to very dry hair of any thickness. There is nothing in this product, or any hair-care product for that matter, that can reconstruct or repair hair. This product is overpriced for what you get, and you can achieve a similar effect by mixing a bit of plain mineral oil with your regular conditioner as a special treat for dry hair.

☺ **K-Pak Leave-In Protectant, for Damaged Hair** *($12 for 10.1 ounces)* is similar to, but not as elegant as, the Integrity Leave-In Conditioning Detangler above, except this contains more detangling agents and less silicone, which makes it not the best for those with damaged hair. This works well as a lightweight, leave-in detangler for all hair types, but the Integrity product is preferred.

☹ K-Pak Curl Revitalizer *($15.95 for 8.45 ounces)* contains a high amount of sodium polystyrene sulfonate, an ingredient that can be drying to hair and scalp and that can potentially strip hair color with repeated use.

☺ K-Pak Protective Hair Spray *($14 for 10 ounces)* is an aerosol hairspray that provides a light to medium hold that remains flexible and non-sticky. This contains added plant oils and conditioning agents, which does make it preferred for dry hair whose style needs the finishing touch a light mist of hairspray can provide.

☺ $$$ K-Pak Smoothing Balm *($16.95 for 6.8 ounces)* is a creamy, silky silicone lotion that would work great to smooth and add shine to dry hair, or it can work brilliantly to straighten curly or wavy hair when used with heat and a round brush. This does not contain any holding agents, so if your hair is on the stubborn side when it comes to straightening, consider Joico's Straight Edge Curl Straightener above.

☺ K-Pak Strengthening Tonic *($13.95 for 8.45 ounces)* is similar to the Color Endurance Color Lock Leave-In Protectant, for Color-Treated Hair above, except this adds silicone and some plant oil, which makes it better for drier hair. Otherwise, the same comments apply.

☺ K-Pak Styling Creme Elixir *($14.95 for 3.4 ounces)* is similar to the K-Pak Smoothing Balm above, only this contains more detangling/anti-static agent than silicone, which lends a lighter texture that is more appropriate for use on normal to fine or thin hair. Otherwise, the same basic comments apply.

☺ K-Pak Thermal Designing Foam, Medium Hold *($14.95 for 8.8 ounces)* is a very standard, light- to medium-hold propellant-based mousse that is slightly sticky but that does not leave hair stiff. The conditioning agents and plant oil provide a slight amount of heat protection, but this is a rather thin mousse from a product line designed for damaged hair.

☺ $$$ K-Pak Protect & Shine Serum *($15.50 for 2 ounces)* is an excellent emollient silicone serum that is a great (though pricey) choice for someone with dry to very dry hair that is coarse, curly, or thick. This is richer than most silicone serums, but you can still find similar products for less money, though you certainly won't be disappointed with this option.

KENRA

For more information about independently owned KENRA, call (800) 428-8073 or visit www.kenra.com.

What's Good About This Line: The styling products are mostly good options, though they're more standard than usual, especially for a salon line, where each product's bells and whistles tend to be the order of the day.

What's Not So Good About It: All but one of the shampoos is problematic; a few of the styling products are too lackluster to consider, especially given the salon prices.

☹ **Color Maintenance Shampoo, Gentle Formula to Help Preserve Color** (*$8 for 10.1 ounces*) contains sodium C14-16 olefin sulfonate as one of its main detergent cleansing agents, which makes this shampoo too drying for all hair and scalp types. This also contains irritating plant extracts and essential oils.

☺ **Dandruff Shampoo, Treatment for Dandruff and Other Scalp Conditions** (*$12 for 10.1 ounces*) lists zinc pyrithione as its active ingredient, but doesn't indicate the percentage used, so you're left to guess whether this shampoo will really be effective for dandruff. Chances are it will be, though this standard shampoo formulation holds no advantage over the zinc pyrithione–containing products from Head & Shoulders that cost far less.

☹ **Moisturizing Shampoo, Hydrating Formula for Added Moisture** (*$8 for 10.1 ounces*) is similar to the Color Maintenance Shampoo, Gentle Formula to Help Preserve Color above, and the same comments apply.

☹ **Volumizing Shampoo, Bodifying Formula for Volume and Fullness** (*$8 for 10.1 ounces*) is similar to the Color Maintenance Shampoo, Gentle Formula to Help Preserve Color above, and the same comments apply.

☺ **Color Maintenance Conditioner, Silk Protein Conditioner for Color-Treated Hair** (*$11 for 10.1 ounces*) contains essential oils of sage, peppermint, coltsfoot, rosemary, and horsetail, among others, which makes this conditioner an irritating proposition for the scalp. Used strictly on the hair, this can be a good emollient conditioner for dry hair of any thickness. Nothing in this conditioner can help make color last longer.

☺ **Daily Provision, Lightweight Leave-In Conditioner** (*$11 for 10.1 ounces*) is a good, though basic, leave-in conditioner for normal to fine or thin hair that is slightly dry and needs help with combing.

☺ **Moisturizing Conditioner, Deep Penetrating Formula for Maximum Hydration** (*$11 for 10.1 ounces*) is a very standard conditioner that is a good option for normal to slightly dry hair of any thickness, particularly if all that's needed is light moisture and detangling.

☺ **Volumizing Conditioner, Lightweight Formula for Volume and Fullness** (*$11 for 10.1 ounces*) is nearly identical to the Moisturizing Conditioner above, except this contains a greater amount of detangling agents. Otherwise, the same review applies. Does it make you wonder why this conditioner is sold as "lightweight" while the others above promise greater benefits, such as "deep penetrating"?

☺ **Artformation Spray, Firm Hold Styling and Finishing Spray 18** (*$13 for 12 ounces*) is a very standard, but good, firm-hold aerosol hairspray that leaves hair slightly sticky and a bit difficult to brush through. It is best for freezing styles in place and then letting them be.

☺ **Capture Glaze, Medium Hold Styling Fixative 14** (*$11 for 10.1 ounces*) is a standard styling gel that provides a light to medium hold with minimal stiffness or stickiness, allowing hair to be easily brushed through. This provides little protection during heat styling, so it's best combined with a product that contains more conditioning agents and/or silicone.

☺ **Design Spray, Light Hold Styling Spray 9** *($13 for 12 ounces)* is a very workable aerosol hairspray that provides a soft, flexible hold, perfect for natural styles where you want hair to have some movement. The conditioning agents make hair easy to comb through, and prevent it from getting stiff.

☹ **$$$ Molding Creme, Firm Hold Styling Fixative 18** *($15 for 6.95 ounces)* is more of a translucent gel than a cream. As a styling product, this takes longer than usual to dry and ends up providing a firm hold that is incredibly sticky, which can make hair difficult to brush through. There are hundreds of styling products with a more pleasant finish than this one, but it can work to create slicked-backed looks on hard-to-hold hair.

☹ **Root Volumizing Serum, Volumizer for Root Lift and Style Support 20** *($12 for 5.5 ounces)* is a fluid styling gel equipped with a special nozzle applicator for direct application to the roots. However, it can easily place too much product there, making hair too stiff and heavy in one place. This provides a medium to firm hold with a lot of stickiness.

☺ **Spray Gel, Firm Hold Styling Fixative 17** *($10 for 8 ounces)* is a standard spray gel that provides a medium hold with a moist finish that remains slightly sticky, though hair can be brushed through. It's not an exciting formula, but it does the job.

☺ **Straightening Serum, Softens, Smoothes and Controls Coarse, Curly Hair** *($14 for 8 ounces)* is a decent, serum-type styling gel that contains lightweight thickeners, detangling agents, and silicones for shine and for smoothing hair while straightening it with heat. This can work well for normal to fine or thin hair that is curly or wavy. It provides a soft hold without stiffness or stickiness.

☺ **Styling Gel, Firm Hold Styling Fixative 17** *($11 for 10.1 ounces)* is a standard styling gel that provides a firm hold that remains stiff and sticky, though it can help to style stubborn hair. The plant extracts and essential oil fragrance can cause scalp irritation and itching, so try to keep this on the hair only.

☺ **Thermal Styling Spray, Firm Hold Heat-Activated Styling Spray 19** *($12 for 10 ounces)* is a standard spray gel that provides a medium to firm hold that is slightly stiff and sticky. The tiny amount of silicones provides meager heat protection at best, so pair this with another product (such as a silicone styling cream) prior to using a blow dryer or flat iron.

☺ **Thickening Spray, Thickens Individual Strands for Increased Volume 4** *($13 for 8 ounces)* is one of the more impressive KENRA styling products, and can work well to thicken fine or thin hair while providing light conditioning with a soft, flexible hold that does not make hair feel stiff or sticky.

☺ **Volume Mousse, Medium Hold Fixative 12** *($11 for 8 ounces)* is a standard, but very good, mousse with a light to medium hold and a smooth, minimally sticky finish. It is a good option for normal to fine or thin hair, though it lacks a significant amount of heat-protecting ingredients.

☺ **Volume Mousse Extra, Firm Hold Fixative 17** *($11 for 8 ounces)* is almost identical to the Volume Mousse, Medium Hold Fixative 12 above, except this one provides a stronger hold with more apparent stickiness.

☺ **Volume Spray, Super Hold Finishing Spray 25 (Aerosol)** *($13 for 12 ounces)* is a standard, firm-hold hairspray that can leave hair feeling slightly sticky and stiff, though it can be brushed through.

☺ **Volume Spray, Super Hold Finishing Spray 25 (Non-Aerosol)** *($10 for 10 ounces)* is a standard hairspray with a medium hold and a minimally sticky finish. The plant extracts can be scalp irritants, so use caution during application.

☹ **Intensive Emollient Treatment, Advanced Moisturizing Formula for Dry and Chemically Stressed Hair** *($15 for 6 ounces)* contains balm mint as one of its main ingredients, which makes this too irritating for the scalp. Formula-wise, this is nearly identical to the Color Maintenance Conditioner above, except this contains plant oils.

KENRA PLATINUM

☺ **$$$ Platinum Freezing Gel, Lock & Hold 24** *($17.70 for 6 ounces)* is a somewhat fluid styling gel that provides an incredibly strong hold meant to create extreme hairstyles or to use on stubborn hair. A noticeably stiff, sticky feel accompanies all this hold, but (if your hair is in good condition) this can be brushed through with little effort, and it does not flake.

☺ **$$$ Platinum Grooming Pomade, Define & Control 4** *($17.70 for 2 ounces)* is a water-soluble, gel-type pomade that can add texture and shine while smoothing dry ends and frizzies without being overly greasy (if used sparingly). Platinum Grooming Pomade contains film-forming/holding agents, but the emollient and slip agents that precede them on the ingredient list are what prevent a stiff, sticky feel.

☺ **$$$ Platinum Shaping Cream, Smooth & Form 7** *($20 for 4 ounces)* is a true styling cream and one that, despite its steep price, is excellent for dry to very dry hair that is coarse, curly, or thick. It contains a blend of water with silicone, emollients, plant oil, and glycerin—just what dry hair needs to look and feel better. This provides a soft, flexible hold and unless hair is extremely thick or coarse, should be used sparingly.

☺ **$$$ Platinum Texturizing Taffy, Sculpt & Separate 13** *($20 for 2 ounces)* is a cross between a styling cream and a wax-based pomade, and does have a taffylike texture. Essentially, this is a very good smoothing product for dry hair that is thick or coarse, but the price is exorbitant for what you get (though the Lucite packaging is beautiful—too bad it can't help your hair). It provides moisture and can add texture and shine to the hair while being lighter than a traditional pomade. This should still be used sparingly and is preferred for use on dry (rather than damp) hair.

☺ **$$$ Platinum Silkening Gloss** *($17.70 for 2.26 ounces)* is a standard silicone serum that would work well for all hair types thanks to its thin, fluid texture, but those with fine or thin hair should still use it sparingly. As with all silicone serums, this will make hair incredibly shiny while working to tame frizzies. It's your call as to whether or not you should spend the extra money KENRA is charging, because formula-wise, this differs little from silicone serums available at the drugstore.

KÉRASTASE

Open up the brochure for this L'Oreal-owned, supposedly professional, salon-exclusive hair-care line and you are treated to such statements as "Relax your mind and place your trust in the only person who can heal your hair and lift your spirits … your Kérastase Certified Consultant." Sounds sort of like a salon witch doctor. I won't even get into the preposterous notion that hair can be healed, or why spirituality has nothing to do with how full or flat your hair looks. Only in the world of hair care could such an ordinary, unexceptional line gain such an aura of esteem and mystery. Kérastase is often featured in beauty and fashion magazines' "best of" lists, with celebrity stylists name-dropping left and right that their famous clients simply can't live without this or that Kérastase product. I don't know if it's ego at work here or just a resolute stubbornness to admit the obvious. Although Kérastase offers some very excellent products for taking good care of your hair, they're a far cry from special or unique, with similar versions for almost every one of them being available from L'Oreal's mass-market hair-care lines. Celebrity hairstylists have more talent going for them than anything in these pricey little bottles can possibly impart. The fact that there are so many comparable (sometimes even better) products available from L'Oreal at the drugstore makes it somewhat ridiculous to shop this line, although those with deep pockets won't be disappointed by most of what is available from the Kérastase product lineup. The rest of you can relax—you're not missing anything extraordinary if you skip this line altogether. For more information about Kérastase, call (877) 748-8357 or visit www.kerastase.com.

What's Good About This Line: Most of the shampoos, conditioners, and styling products work well, though often not for their intended hair type.

What's Not So Good About It: Often-outrageous prices for hair-care products that, for all their posturing, are incredibly standard, often boring formulations; none of the products come close to matching their unrealistic claims.

KÉRASTASE NUTRITIVE

The collection of Nutritive products is designed to tame and control dry, coarse hair. Although all of them have merit and are quite gentle, not a single one contains a unique list of ingredients to justify the cost. You will find that each of the products below has a similar L'Oreal counterpart at the drugstore, and that it's often available at one-half to one-third the price of the Kérastase product.

☺ $$$ **Nutritive Bain Elasto-Curl, Hydra-Toning Shampoo for Dry, Curly Hair** *($24 for 8.4 ounces)* is a very good, though extremely basic, shampoo. This will build up on hair with repeated use, but is a good alternate shampoo for all but very fine hair. Unless you have a penchant for overspending on shampoo, there is no reason to consider this over L'Oreal's Nutri Vive Shampoo ($3.99 for 13 ounces).

☺ $$$ **Nutritive Bain Oleo-Relax, Smoothing Shampoo for Dry Rebellious Hair** *($24 for 8.4 ounces)* is nearly identical to the Elasto-Curl, Hydra-Toning Shampoo for

Dry, Curly Hair above, only this contains less silicone, which means a lower rate of buildup. It would work well for normal to dry hair of any thickness.

☺ $$$ **Nutritive Bain Satin 1, Shampoo for Normal to Slightly Dry Hair** *($24 for 8.4 ounces)* is nearly identical to the Elasto-Curl, Hydra-Toning Shampoo for Dry, Curly Hair above, and the same comments apply.

☺ $$$ **Nutritive Bain Satin 2, Shampoo for Dry, Rebellious Hair** *($24 for 8.4 ounces)* is nearly identical to the Elasto-Curl, Hydra-Toning Shampoo for Dry, Curly Hair above, and the same comments apply.

☺ $$$ **Nutritive Bain Satin 3, Shampoo for Very Dry, Damaged Hair** *($24 for 8.4 ounces)* is essentially a differently packaged, renamed, and very expensive version of L'Oreal's Vive Color-Care Shampoo for Dry, Color-Treated, or Highlighted Hair ($4.49 for 13 ounces). Choosing this over the less expensive L'Oreal option only reinforces the mistaken belief that expensive hair-care products are better. If that were true, why would a company like L'Oreal model its Kérastase products so closely after their own drugstore product lines?

☺ $$$ **Nutritive Elasto-Curl, Hydra-Toning Core for Dry, Curly Hair** *($31 for 6.8 ounces)* is a very standard conditioner that can be a good (though absurdly priced) option for normal to slightly dry hair of any thickness.

☺ $$$ **Nutritive Lait Vital Proteine, Care for Dry and Sensitized Hair** *($31 for 6.8 ounces)* is such a basic, no-frills conditioner formulation that the price tag is truly embarrassing. Almost any conditioner from any other line will perform equally well (and many will surpass this) for a fraction of the cost. The L'Oreal main-line match to this would be their Vive Color-Care or Vive Nutri-Moisture Conditioners (each $4.49 for 13 ounces).

☺ $$$ **Nutritive Masquintense, Rich Nurturing Treatment for Thick Hair** *($36 for 5.1 ounces)* is a thick-textured conditioner marketed as a specialty treatment for the hair. It isn't—it is just a conditioner that would be appropriate for someone with normal to dry hair that is normal to thick or coarse.

☺ $$$ **Nutritive Nutri-Liss, Instant Smoothing Treatment for Dry and Unruly Hair** *($29 for 4.2 ounces)* is a lightweight, silicone-based, leave-in conditioner that is a good option for all hair types except very fine or thin. Leave-in conditioners such as this make hair feel very silky and aid in detangling.

☺ $$$ **Nutritive Lumi-Extract, Luminising Cream for Dry Hair** *($24 for 1.7 ounces)* is a water-based silicone serum for hair. It has a lotion-like appearance that quickly dissipates into a clear, slippery fluid that can easily make hair look limp or greasy if you use too much. Although this is a very good product, there is no logical reason to consider it over the silicone serums from John Frieda's Frizz Ease line or from other lines such as Citré Shine or Jheri Redding for a fraction of the price.

☺ $$$ **Nutritive Serum Nutri-Instant, Serum for Damaged Ends** *($29 for 1 ounce)* is a more traditional, waterless silicone serum that contains two forms of silicone, alcohol, and fragrance. This won't repair or heal damaged ends (if they're damaged or splitting, the only cure is to cut them off). Still, like all silicone serums in any price range, it can make hair look and feel smooth and silky, and appear incredibly shiny and radiant.

☺ $$$ **Nutritive Oleo-Relax, Smoothing Controlling Care for Dry and Rebellious Hair** *($29 for 4.2 ounces)* is a richer, waterless version of the Luminising Cream for Dry Hair above. This silicone- and oil-based product is an option for very dry, thick, or coarse hair, but I would recommend shopping John Frieda or Citré Shine before overspending here.

☺ $$$ **Nutritive Oleo-Relax, Relaxing Mask for Dry, Rebellious Hair** *($36 for 5.1 ounces)* is nothing more than a standard conditioner for the hair. Because it is a mask, the directions indicate that you should leave this on for longer than you would a "regular" conditioner—but the same effect can be achieved with any well-formulated conditioner, provided you leave it on the hair as long as possible.

☺ $$$ **Nutritive Masquintense, Rich Nurturing Treatment for Fine Hair** *($36 for 5.1 ounces)* is nothing more than a standard conditioner. Given the treatment positioning and imposing price, you would expect a few uniquely effective ingredients—but they are not present, and that makes this more a frivolous waste than a worthwhile product. That said, this could still be a good conditioner for normal to dry hair of any thickness.

☺ $$$ **Nutritive Emulsion Nutri-Instant, Enriching Conditioning Mousse for Dry and Sensitized Hair** *($29 for 5.1 ounces)* is a standard, propellant-based styling mousse that contains no holding agents and is mostly water, propellant, and silicone. This does contain a form of camphor that can be a significant scalp irritant, so avoid getting this near skin and apply it just to the hair.

☺ $$$ **Nutritive Elasto-Curl, Weightless Curl Defining Mousse for Fine, Curly Hair** *($29 for 5 ounces)* is an alcohol-based, standard styling mousse that provides a light hold with a slightly sticky finish that can be a bit tricky to brush through. The price for such a standard formulation is absurd.

☺ $$$ **Nutritive Elasto-Curl, Definition Forming Cream for Thick, Curly Hair** *($29 for 4.8 ounces)* is a leave-in conditioner that, despite its name, isn't all that creamy. This is fairly lightweight, and would not be emollient or moisturizing enough for thick or curly hair. It can work well to smooth normal to fine or thin hair and aid with combing. This product does not contain any holding agents, nor does it have anything "nutritive."

☺ $$$ **Nutritive Elasto-Curl, Weightless Curl Defining Mousse for Fine, Curly Hair** *($29 for 5 ounces)* is a liquid-to-foam mousse that provides a light hold while remaining moist and somewhat sticky in the hair. I wouldn't choose this over a L'Oreal mousse from the drugstore, but if you have money to burn, this is an option.

☺ $$$ **Nutritive Nutri-Build, Volumizing Treatment Mousse for Dry and Fine Hair** *($29 for 5.1 ounces)* is a standard, propellant-based mousse with an ultra-light texture and minimal to no hold. It can softly define curls or waves without a trace of stiffness or stickiness, but the basic formula doesn't jibe with the price.

☺ $$$ **Nutritive Oleo-Relax, Smoothing Holding Mist for Dry, Rebellious Hair** *($29 for 3.4 ounces)* is an alcohol-based silicone spray with a small amount of film-forming agent and plant oil mixed in. It goes on lightly (meaning without much weight) but adds a gleaming shine that is slightly greasy. This would work well as a finishing product for dry hair that is normal to coarse or thick.

KÉRASTASE RESISTANCE

The Resistance line is supposedly for weakened hair, and is meant to cure whatever is ailing the shafts of your hair. Claims run the gamut from "infuses body into fine hair" to "fortifies hair from within." It would be nice if standard hair-care products could really "feed" and "nourish" the hair, but that just isn't possible because, for one thing, hair is dead. The only living part of a hair is the part you can't see—because it's growing in the hair follicle under your scalp, where conditioners can't reach or stimulate growth in any way, shape, or form.

☺ $$$ Resistance Bain de Force, Fortifying Shampoo for Weakened Hair *($24 for 8.5 ounces)* is a very standard shampoo that contains minimal conditioning agents, so it should not be a problem for buildup. Not a single ingredient in this shampoo can fortify weakened hair, but it will cleanse it.

☺ $$$ Resistance Bain Volumactive, Bodifying Shampoo for Fine and Fly-Away Hair *($24 for 8.5 ounces)* is a very good, though exceptionally standard, shampoo that poses minimal risk of buildup and is suitable for all hair types. This claims to enhance volume and fullness, but that is what any good shampoo without conditioning agents and a little bit of film-forming ingredients can do, so what's the big deal?

☺ $$$ Resistance Ciment Anti-Usure, Fortifying Care for Worn Out Mid-Lengths and Ends *($31 for 6.8 ounces)* says it can "selectively treat, smooth, and fortify all sensitized areas from within," but notice that it does not actually say "within hair." That's actually good, because hair cannot be fortified or desensitized from within. The claims for this ordinary conditioner go way beyond what these standard ingredients can realistically accomplish.

☺ $$$ Resistance Expanseur Extra-Corps, Fortifying Care for Weakened Fine Hair *($29 for 3.4 ounces)* is about as fortifying as Twinkies snack cakes are nutritional. This is a very standard styling spray that goes on wetter than most styling sprays and provides a light hold with noticeable stickiness. It can work well for all hair types, but you should know that better products exist that cost a lot less than this.

☺ $$$ Resistance Volumactive, Bodifying Care for Fine Fly-Away Hair *($26 for 5.1 ounces)* is basically identical to the Nutritive Nutri-Build, Volumizing Treatment Mousse for Dry and Fine Hair above, only this alcohol-based formula has a slightly different holding agent and a bit more of the conditioning agents. However, these are not present in great enough concentrations that your hair will notice a difference. Otherwise, the same comments apply.

☺ $$$ Resistance Volumactive, Ultra-Light Vitalising Care for Fine Fly-Away Hair *($29 for 5.1 ounces)* claims it "adds substance to hair without heaviness," but the substance in this unnecessary product is simply a form of starch. It can coat and to some extent tame flyaway hair, but it doesn't have an elegant after-feel on the hair.

☺ **$$$ Resistance Age Recharge, Firming Masque** *($41 for 5 ounces)* is sold as a special treatment, chosen by your hairstylist based on your hair's "fiber condition" or "levels of sensitization." Regardless of either of those traits (and the fact that hair cannot become sensitive), this conditioner is so basic it is almost laughable. At best, this can lightly moisturize and help make normal to fine or thin hair feel slightly thicker while being easier to detangle.

☺ **$$$ Resistance Substance Constructive, Fortifying Treatment for Weakened Hair Coloured or Permed** *($26 for 2.5 ounces)* is a slick, water- and silicone-based styling cream that can work beautifully to smooth frizzies and add lots of shine to normal to very dry hair that is normal to coarse or thick. This product doesn't contain any ingredients that justify its price, but it is an undeniably good product.

KÉRASTASE SOLEIL PRODUCTS

Soleil translates to "sun," and that's the theme for this subcategory of Kérastase products, which is designed to treat hair that has been exposed to the damaging effects of not only the sun but also the ocean, wind, and chlorinated water (as in swimming pools). Perhaps no one in L'Oreal's marketing department noticed that these formulations are remarkably similar to every other Kérastase product. The "special" ingredients in this product category are ceramides and rice bran oil, which Kérastase claims combine to protect hair "from outside aggressions and repair damage from within." Ceramide can be a good hair-care ingredient, but not when present in the small amount in these products, and the benefits of rice bran oil are also found in many other oils and emollients in other hair-care products.

Please keep in mind that even if a hair-care product claims to contain a sunscreen, the FDA does not allow hair-care products of any kind to have an SPF rating due to the fact that sun-protecting ingredients can't cling reliably to the hair shaft, particularly not in a shampoo or conditioner that is rinsed off the hair. The same is true for styling products, where the sun-protecting ingredients would be brushed or combed away.

☺ **$$$ Soleil Bain Apres-Soleil, Repairing Shampoo Color Shine Treatment** *($24 for 8.5 ounces)* is nearly identical to the Nutritive Bain Satin 3, Shampoo for Very Dry, Damaged Hair above, and the same review applies.

☹ **$$$ Soleil Creme Richesse, Intensive Repair Treatment** *($36 for 5.1 ounces)*. If you want intensive conditioning, this is not the product. If you want a very standard, no-frills conditioner that outprices almost every other, here it is. There is nothing in this product, or any hair-care product for that matter, that can repair environmental damage or protect your hair from further UV assaults.

☺ **$$$ Soleil Aqua Protective, Anti-Drying Treatment UV, Sea, Pool** *($29 for 5 ounces)* is a lightweight, spray-on conditioner that claims to use nanotechnology to penetrate the hair shaft and protect it from environmental assaults. That sounds great, but even if this product could penetrate the hair shaft, none of the ingredients in here are capable of protecting hair from sun, salt water, or chlorinated swimming pools. This can work well for all hair types looking for a lightweight conditioner, provided you don't rely on it to protect your hair in the sun.

☺ $$$ **Soleil Creme Richesse, Intensive Repair Treatment** *($36 for 5.1 ounces)* is nearly identical to the Nutritive Masquintense, Rich Nurturing Treatment for Thick Hair above, and the same review applies.

☹ $$$ **Soleil Gelee Aqua-Proof, Wet Look Protective Care UV, Sea, Pool** *($29 for 4.8 ounces)* can indeed create a wet look, but this does not provide any degree of sun protection and can easily make hair feel too greasy. This is an OK option for dry to very dry hair that is coarse or thick and does not need hold.

☺ $$$ **Soleil Huile Genereuse, Smooth and Shiny Look UV, Sea, Pool** *($29 for 3.3 ounces)* is an emollient silicone spray that would be outstanding for dry to very dry hair that is coarse, curly, or thick—though the price is ridiculous when you consider the prices of identical products from drugstore lines.

☺ $$$ **Soleil Lait Apres-Soleil, Instant Hair Repair** *($29 for 5 ounces)* is primarily water, silicone, plant oil, more silicone, and preservatives. It can smooth hair and tame frizzies, but in no way, shape, or form can this repair the hair.

☺ $$$ **Soleil Voile Protecteur, Invisible Non-Oily Look UV, Sea, Pool** *($29 for 3.3 ounces)* is a standard silicone spray made richer by an additional emollient and plant oil, which can provide extra conditioning. Even so, this is primarily about the silky-feeling, smoothing, and shine-enhancing benefits of silicone, which can be had from many products that cost far less.

KIEHL'S

Though I wish the formulations were more exciting, Kiehl's is one of the few hair-care lines to feature product ingredient lists on its Web site (click on the "zoom the label" icon under the product's image), a welcome disclosure most other lines keep away from consumers. Even so, the price tags for many of the products are embarrassing for what amount to incredibly standard formulations whose unique or "buzz" ingredients are often a mere fraction of the product's contents. For more information about L'Oreal-owned Kiehl's, call (800) KIEHLS-2 or visit www.kiehls.com.

What's Good About This Line: Quite a few completely fragrance-free products; some great, reputation-worthy leave-in conditioning products for dry to very dry hair types; Kiehl's stores and department store counters always have samples of products, and actively encourage customers to try before they buy.

What's Not So Good About It: The high prices for mostly basic formulations and no-frills packaging; several shampoos contain drying detergent cleansing agents or irritating fragrant oils; conditioners tend to be either light or heavy, with no in-between options for normal to dry hair (though the creamier styling products make up for this).

☺ $$$ **Amino Acid Shampoo with Pure Coconut Oil** *($16.50 for 8.4 ounces)* contains a tiny amount of coconut oil and an even tinier amount of amino acids, certainly not enough to warrant naming this product after them. This is a very standard shampoo that contains primarily water, detergent cleansing agents, and fragrance. It would work well for all hair types and won't cause buildup, but the price is out of line for what you get.

☺ **Castille Shampoo, for Dry, Damaged, Thick or Coarse Hair** (*$13 for 8 ounces*) does not contain true castile soap, and that's a good thing, because it can be very drying to the hair and scalp. This is a very standard shampoo that contains tiny amounts of lanolin and olive oil, not enough to cause buildup. What's best about this gentle shampoo is that it is fragrance-free, which means it is excellent for someone with an easily irritated scalp.

☹ **Herbal Treatment Shampoo for Problem Hair and Scalp** (*$16 for 8 ounces*) lists sodium C14-16 olefin sulfonate as the first ingredient, which makes this a very drying shampoo for both hair and scalp. This also contains rosemary, wild mint, cedarwood, and lemon oils, which only increase the irritation.

☹ **Klaus Heidegger's All-Sport Every Day Shampoo** (*$12 for 8 ounces*) might work every day for Klaus (one of the founders of Kiehl's), but it's a problem shampoo for everyone else, thanks to the use of drying sodium C14-16 olefin sulfonate as its sole detergent cleansing agent.

☹ **Klaus Heidegger's All-Sport Every Day Shampoo, with Chamomile** (*$13.50 for 8 ounces*) is nearly identical to the Klaus Heidegger's All-Sport Every Day Shampoo above, and the same comments apply. The inclusion of chamomile doesn't offset the drying effect of the detergent cleansing agent.

☺ **Klaus Heidegger's All-Sport Swimmer's Cleansing Rinse for Hair and Body** (*$14 for 8 ounces*) is a very good, fragrance-free shampoo for all hair types, and it does not cause buildup.

☹ **Lecithin Conditioning Shampoo** (*$20 for 8 ounces*) contains sodium C14-16 olefin sulfonate as its sole detergent cleansing agent, and is not recommended. This also contains several irritating fragrant oils.

☺ **$$$ Mild, Gentle Shampoo for Babies** (*$15 for 8 ounces*) is a mild shampoo that is a good conditioning shampoo for babies as well as adults who do not use styling products and have dry hair.

☹ **Protein Concentrate Chamomile Shampoo** (*$14 for 8 ounces*) lists TEA-lauryl sulfate as the first ingredient, which makes this a very drying shampoo for all hair and scalp types. The rosemary, lavender, and sage oils only serve to add fragrance and more irritation.

☹ **Protein Concentrate Shampoo for Dry to Normal Hair** (*$13 for 8 ounces*) is nearly identical to the Protein Concentrate Chamomile Shampoo above, and the same review applies.

☹ **Protein Concentrate Shampoo for Oily Hair** (*$14 for 8 ounces*) is nearly identical to the Protein Concentrate Chamomile Shampoo above, and the same review applies.

☹ **Tea Tree Oil Shampoo** *($17 for 8 ounces)* contains several irritating fragrant oils, including lavender, coriander, sandalwood, patchouli, and rosemary oil, and not enough tea tree oil to have any effect on dandruff.

☺ **$$$ Extra-Strength Conditioning Rinse for Dry Hair** *($17.50 for 8 ounces)* isn't extra strength in the least. Who names these products? This is one of the lightest conditioners available that can work well to make fine or thin hair easier to comb, but it is too light for dry hair.

☺ **$$$ Extra-Strength Conditioning Rinse with Added Coconut** *($19 for 8 ounces)* is nearly identical to the Extra-Strength Conditioning Rinse for Dry Hair above, except this adds coconut oil, though in an amount too insignificant to make a noticeable difference for your hair. Otherwise, the same comments apply.

☺ **$$$ Hair Conditioning and Grooming Aid Formula 133** *($16.50 for 8 ounces)* is a lightweight, basic, leave-in conditioner that can make normal to slightly dry hair that is normal to fine or thin easier to manage.

☺ **$$$ Leave-In Hair Conditioner with Panthenol and Coconut Oil** *($16 for 4 ounces)* contains trivial amounts of plant oils, making this a very standard, overpriced conditioner for normal to slightly dry hair of any thickness. The best thing about this product is that it is fragrance-free.

☹ **$$$ Panthenol Protein Hair Conditioner Softener & Grooming Aid** *($14.50 for 6 ounces)* is a simple formulation of water, panthenol, preservative, detangling agent, alcohol, water-binding agent, slip agent, and emollient. This is fragrance-free, and can be of minimal benefit for fine or thin hair.

☺ **$$$ Creme with Silk Groom** *($17 for 4 ounces)* is the star of Kiehl's product lineup, in that this product is promoted most often in fashion magazines. In this case, its reputation as an excellent styling cream is well deserved. This is a wonderful product for normal to very dry hair that is normal to coarse or thick, and is a much better formulation than any of the Kiehl's conditioners above. Creme with Silk Groom contains no holding agents, and must be used sparingly to avoid weighing hair down or making it feel greasy. Those with thick or coarse hair can apply this more liberally, but should still use restraint.

☺ **$$$ Extra Strength Styling Gel** *($16 for 4 ounces)* is a thick styling gel that provides a medium hold with a slightly sticky finish. The conditioning agents provide some protection during heat styling. This fragrance-free gel can be too heavy for someone with fine or thin hair.

☺ **$$$ Hair Thickening Lotion, for Normal Hair Texture** *($12.50 for 4 ounces)* is a styling cream that is lighter than the Creme with Silk Groom above, but is still best for normal to very dry hair that is normal to coarse or thick. It does not contain ingredients to make fine or thin hair feel thicker, so don't let the name fool you. The tiny amount of film-forming/holding agent has no effect on hair.

☺ **$$$ Hair Thickening Spray, for Dry or Hard-to-Manage Hair** (**Non-Aerosol**) *($17 for 6 ounces)* is a very light styling spray that provides minimal to no hold, and contains primarily water and alcohols, which won't do much to make hair feel or look thicker. This is completely non-sticky, but is more of a do-nothing product than something to seriously consider if you have fine or thin hair.

☺ $$$ **Solid Grooming Aid** *($15.50 for 1.75 ounces)* is a water-based pomade that feels lighter than most pomades and offers a soft, groomed look that isn't greasy. This should still be used sparingly, and works best on hair that is normal to thick. Solid Grooming Aid shampoos easily from the hair, a trait many types of pomades and styling waxes lack.

☺ $$$ **Shine 'n Lite Groom for Dull or Thick Hair** *($12 for 4 ounces)* is similar to the Creme with Silk Groom above, except with a lighter texture, which makes it preferred for normal to dry hair of any thickness. Use this sparingly to avoid a heavy look, or mix it with a styling gel for a softer effect with conditioning benefits.

☺ $$$ **"Wet Look" Groom** *($13 for 4 ounces)* can work well as a lightweight, slightly slick grooming product for casual hairstyles requiring little to no hold. This can be a bit too heavy for fine or thin hair, but works well for all other hair types seeking a shiny, wet-looking finish. This product is fragrance-free.

☺ $$$ **Creme De La Creme Groom Repairateur with Silk** *($15 for 2 ounces)* is similar to the Creme with Silk Groom above, except this contains a greater amount of thickener to enhance the product's texture. Those with dry to very dry hair should stick with the original Creme above because this pricier formulation holds no special benefit other than its marketing claims.

☺ $$$ **Deep Conditioning Protein Pak** *($17.50 for 4 ounces)* is an excellent emollient conditioner for dry to very dry hair that is normal to coarse or thick.

☹ **Enriched Massage Oil for Scalp** *($15.50 for 4 ounces)* contains rosemary oil, which makes this a problem for direct use on the scalp. Those with a dry to very dry scalp should use plain oil, such as olive oil or canola oil, instead of this pricey concoction.

☹ **Herbal Toner for the Scalp** *($24 for 8 ounces)* is a basic liquid toner that contains several plant extracts that can be irritating to the scalp, causing dryness and itching. It is not recommended.

☺ $$$ **High-Gloss Conditioning and Styling Oil for Hair** *($20.50 for 1.5 ounces)* is mostly safflower oil along with an emollient thickener and several vitamins that have no effect on hair. Using plain safflower (or olive, almond, apricot, sunflower, or jojoba) oil not only would be less expensive, but also would be a way to moisturize very dry hair without adding fragrance (which this product contains).

☺ $$$ **Intensive Repairateur Deep Conditioning Pak** *($24.50 for 4 ounces)* is nearly identical to the Deep Conditioning Protein Pak above, and the same comments apply. Why this product costs several dollars more is a question worth asking, but don't expect a straight answer.

☺ $$$ **Lecithin and Coconut Enriched Hair Masque with Panthenol for Dry Hair** *($22.50 for 4.5 ounces)* is a good conditioner for normal to dry hair of any thickness.

KMS

KMS, which stands for "kinetic molecular systems," has changed its marketing method. Originally this line was showcased using a far more scientific approach, with the emphasis on "specialized" ingredients in the products and how they worked with your hair's chemistry. It was all very impressive sounding, even though their formulations weren't that different from what the rest of the hair-care industry was doing. Now the company emphasizes how their products can affect a consumer's lifestyle through the way they allow you to express yourself through the hairstyles you create using—what else?—the products KMS sells. This lifestyle-emphasizing approach to hair-care products is one many lines have been championing lately because consumers are highly motivated by brands they believe will help define who they are (or who they want to be or be seen as) and how they live.

Choosing to present this imposingly large hair-care line from the new go-with-the-flow angle that seeks to emulate the laid-back California lifestyle (which is more marketing finesse than reality, at least for those who live in California) may sound appealing. However, it doesn't help you determine which KMS products are best for your hair, and the choices in this line are numerous, to say the least. The good news is that if you gloss over the lifestyle positioning of this brand and focus on the reviews below, you can find some wonderful options for managing your hair, be it fine, normal, or thick. For more information about KMS, call (800) 342-5567 or visit www.kmshaircare.com.

What's Good About This Line: KMS is one of the few hair-care companies that list ingredients for each of their products on the company's Web site; the shampoos and conditioners are uniformly excellent; prices (for a salon line) are tolerable; the variety of styling products means there's something for everyone.

What's Not So Good About It: Several leave-in products (mostly for styling) contain the problematic preservatives methylchloroisothiazolinone and methylisothiazolinone (Kathon CG); their product selection is larger than it needs to be, which can create confusion while trying to decide what to buy.

KMS AMP VOLUME

☺ **AMP Volume Shampoo** (*$8.25 for 12 ounces*) is a standard shampoo that contains magnesium sulfate. This can swell the hair shaft, making fine or thin hair feel fuller, but it may also be drying when used routinely. The film-forming agent can build up with repeated use, but initially will also make fine, thin hair feel thicker.

☺ **AMP Volume 2-in-1 Thickening Creme** (*$5.75 for 4 ounces*) is a very good leave-in conditioner and a light-hold styling cream for normal to dry hair of any thickness. It leaves hair feeling soft and adds a natural shine without stiffness or stickiness. This can also provide protection during heat styling, and could work well as a mixer with other styling products.

☺ **AMP Volume Styling Foam** (*$10.75 for 8 ounces*) is an ultra-light, propellant-based mousse that offers soft hold with minimal stickiness. It can work well for fine or thin hair.

☺ **AMP Volume Reconstructor** *($8.95 for 8.1 ounces)* is nearly identical to the AMP Volume 2-in-1 Thickening Creme above, except this does not contain film-forming/holding agents. It can be a good lightweight conditioner for normal to slightly dry hair of any thickness, though it won't reconstruct one hair on your head.

KMS COLOR VITALITY

☺ **Color Vitality Blonde Shampoo** *($8.95 for 12 ounces)* is a good conditioning shampoo for normal to dry hair. This does contain a tiny amount of sulfur, but I suspect it's used to help pH-balance this product, though over the long term it may end up being somewhat drying to hair.

☺ **Color Vitality Shampoo** *($8.95 for 12 ounces)* is a standard shampoo that would work well for all hair types, but does pose a slight risk of buildup. This holds no special advantage for color-treated hair.

☺ **Color Vitality Blonde Treatment** *($8.50 for 5.1 ounces)* is a fairly heavy conditioner that could work well to smooth and form a protective seal over hair that is porous due to dyeing or bleaching. This ability to seal comes from the high amount of wax this conditioner contains, and it can build up with repeated use, especially on fine or thin hair. This conditioner cannot prevent premature color loss and fading, as claimed. It is best for normal to very dry hair that is normal to thick or coarse.

☺ **$$$ Color Vitality Intensive Treatment Leave-In** *($14.99 for six 0.34-ounce ampoules).* Despite the name, this product is basically just a standard silicone serum, so if you have one already, then this pricey product is unnecessary. KMS's claim that this will not build up with repeated use isn't true in the least because that is exactly what silicone does unless it is shampooed away.

☺ **Color Vitality Color Protectant** *($8.75 for 8.5 ounces)* is a lightweight, spray-on, leave-in conditioner that can detangle fine or thin hair, but contains nothing that will protect or preserve hair color.

☺ **Color Vitality Color Revitalizer** *($9.95 for 8.1 ounces)* is a standard conditioner that can be a good option for normal to slightly dry hair that is normal to fine or thin. This cannot, as claimed, prevent premature color loss or fading.

☹ **Color Vitality Solar Powered Highlighter** *($14.50 for 5 ounces)* is a water-based, spray-on lightening product that contains hydrogen peroxide, which can lighten hair in the sun or with heat, but this is no different than Sun-In® at the drugstore, which sells for less than half the price of this product. This contains the preservative Kathon CG, which poses a high risk of causing a sensitizing reaction on the scalp.

KMS CURL UP

☺ **Curl Up Shampoo** *($7.75 for 8.1 ounces)* is a good conditioning shampoo for normal to slightly dry hair, be it curly or straight.

☺ **Curl Up Bounce Back Spray** *($8.75 for 7 ounces)* is an alcohol- and water-based styling spray that provides a medium hold with a mildly sticky, stiff finish. It can work well to enhance curls and help them hold their shape, but curls aren't required to use it.

☺ **$$$ Curl Up Control Creme** *($15.95 for 5.1 ounces)* is a fairly thick, emollient styling cream that is a very good option for grooming and defining curls and waves on thick, coarse hair that's dry to very dry. It keeps hair pliable and adds shine without looking or feeling greasy, and does not get the least bit stiff or sticky. A few of the plant extracts can be scalp irritants, so use caution when applying this near the roots.

☺ **Curl Up Curl Gloss** *($12.95 for 6.8 ounces)* is an outstanding option for dry to very dry hair that is thick, curly, or coarse. This alcohol-free nonaerosol spray features an excellent blend of glycerin, silicones, wax, and emollients to moisturize and help define curly or wavy hair. It provides a light hold with a soft, moist finish, and a little goes a long way when it comes to adding gloss and smoothing frizzies. A few of the plant extracts (including arnica and sage) can be irritating if this gets on the scalp, so use caution during application.

☹ **Curl Up Curling Balm** *($13.50 for 6 ounces)* contains the preservative Kathon CG, which is contraindicated for use in leave-on products because it can cause a sensitizing reaction on skin and scalp. This product is not recommended.

☺ **Curl Up Curl Hydrator** *($9.75 for 8.1 ounces)* is a creamy conditioner for normal to dry hair of any thickness. It can be more helpful for curly hair that is normal to thin or fine in texture, but those with thick, dry curly hair will want something richer than this.

☺ **Curl Up Curl Prepare** *($9.75 for 8.28 ounces)* is similar to the Curl Up Curl Hydrator above, except it is slightly less emollient and contains a film-forming agent, which can be helpful for thin or fine hair that needs more manageability and weight to define or tame curls. The film-forming agent can build up with repeated use.

KMS DAILY FIXX

☺ **Daily Fixx Clarifying Shampoo** *($8.95 for 12 ounces)* is a very standard shampoo that is a great option for all hair types. The film-forming agent and silicone pose minimal risk of buildup.

☺ **Daily Fixx Dandruff Shampoo** *($8.95 for 12 ounces)* is a very good dandruff shampoo for normal to dry hair of any thickness. It contains 1.5% zinc pyrithione in a standard conditioning shampoo base that poses a slight risk of buildup with repeated use.

☺ **Daily Fixx Everyday Shampoo** *($8.95 for 12 ounces)* is an excellent shampoo for dry to very dry hair that is normal to coarse or thick.

☺ **Daily Fixx Moisture Shampoo** *($8.95 for 12 ounces)* is not as moisturizing as the Daily Fixx Everyday Shampoo above, but it is still a good option for normal to dry hair of any thickness. The film-forming agent poses a slight risk of building up on hair with repeated use.

☺ **Daily Fixx Totally Clean Shampoo** *($8.95 for 12 ounces)* is a very standard shampoo that does not contain conditioning or film-forming agents, so it will not cause buildup. The magnesium sulfate can swell the hair shaft and potentially cause dryness with routine use, but it can also temporarily make fine or thin hair feel fuller.

☺ **Daily Fixx Moisture Reconstructor** *($10.25 for 8.1 ounces)* is a great conditioner for dry to very dry hair that is normal to coarse or thick.

☺ **Daily Fixx Clarifying Treatment** *($10.25 for 8.1 ounces)* is a lightweight detangling conditioner that can work well for normal to slightly dry hair that is normal to fine or thin.

KMS DAILY REPAIR

☺ **Daily Repair Shampoo** *($8.25 for 12 ounces)* is nearly identical to the Daily Fixx Everyday Shampoo above, and the same review applies.

☹ **Daily Repair Leave-In Treatment** *($8.75 for 8.5 ounces)* would have been an excellent leave-in conditioner for hair, but it contains the preservative Kathon CG, and that makes this otherwise stellar product a sensitizing problem.

☺ $$$ **Daily Repair Pro-Gold Therapy** *($17.25 for 6.8 ounces)* is a good, though standard, conditioner for normal to dry hair that is normal to slightly thick or coarse.

☺ **Daily Repair Reconstructor** *($9.95 for 8.1 ounces)* is a good conditioner for dry hair that is normal to fine or thin, but don't expect any sort of hair reconstruction.

KMS FLAT OUT

☺ **Flat Out Shampoo***($7.75 for 8.5 ounces)* is similar to the Daily Fixx Moisture Shampoo above, and the same basic comments apply. This does contain a higher amount of film-forming agent and silicone, which increases the likelihood of buildup. This shampoo can have a minimal effect on smoothing coarse, textured hair.

☹ **Flat Out Hot Pressed Spray** *($8.75 for 7 ounces)* lists sodium polystyrene sulfonate as the second ingredient, which makes this product a good candidate for creating dry hair and potentially stripping hair color with repeated use.

☺ $$$ **Flat Out Lite Relaxing Creme** *($16.50 for 6 ounces)* is a very good styling cream to smooth dry, coarse hair and help tame frizzies. It provides a minimal hold without weight, and leaves hair feeling silky and looking sleek. The silicone blend can nicely protect hair during heat styling, which is exactly what you want if you plan to use this product to straighten curly or wavy hair with a blow dryer or flat iron.

☺ $$$ **Flat Out Relaxing Balm** *($18.95 for 6 ounces)* is more of a gel than a balm, and one that would be excellent for smoothing and straightening dry to very dry hair that is coarse or thick. This is water-based but contains several silicones, so it can feel greasy and should be used sparingly unless hair is extremely coarse or thick.

☺ **Flat Out Styling Shine Gel** *($9.75 for 7 ounces)* is a standard styling gel that offers little in the way of heat protection but much in the way of hold. This is a strong gel, and one that works well for stubborn hair, but not without noticeable stiffness and stickiness. It can be somewhat difficult to brush through, and would be best mixed with another product unless you're primarily concerned about hold.

☺ **Flat Out Hair Prepare** *($9.75 for 8.1 ounces)* claims to relax hair without creating buildup, but neither is true. It takes strong chemicals to relax curly or wavy hair, or at the very least, high heat, tension, and a round styling brush! This conditioner lists wax as its second ingredient, which can definitely build up on hair, as can the silicone. That doesn't mean this is a bad conditioner, because it isn't; it's just that the claim is misleading. This can be a very good conditioner for normal to dry hair that is normal to thick or coarse.

☺ $$$ **Flat Out Shine Serum** *($10.75 for 1.5 ounces)* is a very standard silicone serum that is more expensive than it needs to be, especially considering the inexpensive silicone serums available at the drugstore.

☺ **Flat Out Weightless Shine Spray** *($10.75 for 4 ounces)* is an emollient silicone spray that is a great option for adding a glossy shine and frizz control to dry or very dry hair that is coarse or thick.

KMS HAIR PLAY

☺ **Hair Play Configure Creme** *($13.50 for 4 ounces)* is a thick, slightly greasy molding cream that can work well to enhance texture on curly, wavy hair that is coarse or thick. It does not get stiff or sticky, and adds shine to hair while smoothing frizzies. It should be used sparingly unless your hair is extremely coarse.

☺ **Hair Play Defining Pomade** *($10.50 for 2 ounces)* is a water-soluble pomade that can still be greasy enough to deserve a recommendation only for those with coarse or thick hair. When used sparingly, this can smooth frizzies and add moisture to hair.

☺ **Hair Play Molding Paste** *($12.75 for 3.5 ounces)* does have a pastelike consistency, and works best on dry (not damp) hair to add strong texture and hold. Spiked or "bed head" hairstyles can be created easily with this paste, but the result can be quite sticky and this does not shampoo out easily.

☺ $$$ **Hair Play Paste Up Spray** *($15.95 for 7 ounces)* is essentially a spray-on styling wax that can be a lighter alternative to pomades for normal to slightly thick hair. It works well to create exaggerated texture and provides a flexible hold while not being too sticky, though the forceful aerosol application can take some getting used to!

☺ **Hair Play Stick-It Wax** *($12.75 for 2.3 ounces)* is a standard styling-wax stick that can work very well to smooth the hair and control stubborn frizzies when used sparingly. It contains mostly castor oil, waxes, thickener, preservative, and fragrance.

☺ **Hair Play Styling Grit** *($9.75 for 2 ounces)* is a thick, greasy pomade that has an initially gritty texture, though that can be blended away. This slightly water-soluble pomade is recommended only for dry to very dry hair that is coarse or thick.

☺ **Hair Play Tacky Gel** *($12.75 for 4 ounces)* is a silky-textured styling gel that dries to a tacky finish. It provides a firm hold that can be easily brushed through, and is a good option for creating slicked-back or more structured styles for all hair types.

☹ **Hair Play Texture Blast** *($12.75 for 6.8 ounces)* contains the preservative Kathon CG, and is not recommended.

KMS HAIR STAY

☺ **Hair Stay Max3 Gel Spray** *($10.50 for 8.5 ounces)* is a standard styling gel that offers a firm hold with a very sticky finish that can be a bit tricky to brush through. It would work well on short hair to add lots of hold and enhance texture.

☺ **Hair Stay Max Hold Spray (Aerosol)** *($10.75 for 9.5 ounces)* is a medium- to firm-hold hairspray that goes on light and can be easily brushed through. The silicones aid with comb-through and add an attractive sheen without looking greasy.

☺ **Hair Stay Max Hold Spray (Non-Aerosol)** *($8.75 for 8.5 ounces)* is a very good, firm-hold hairspray that can make hair feel slightly stiff and sticky, but can be easily brushed through without flaking.

☺ **Hair Stay Medium Hold Spray (Aerosol)** *($9.95 for 9.5 ounces)* is a light- to medium-hold hairspray that can be easily brushed through and is a good working hairspray for more involved hairstyles. The conditioning agents and silicone help prevent hair from getting stiff or sticky.

☹ **Hair Stay Sculpting Lotion** *($6.75 for 8.5 ounces)* contains the preservative Kathon CG, and is not recommended.

☺ **Hair Stay Styling Foam** *($10.75 for 8 ounces)* is a very standard, propellant-based mousse that provides a medium hold with a touch of stickiness, though hair is easily brushed through. This contains minimal conditioning agents to protect hair during heat styling.

☺ **Hair Stay Styling Gel, Maximum Hold, Natural Shine** *($7.50 for 8.1 ounces)* is a very standard, but good, firm-hold styling gel that has a sticky finish and can leave hair stiff, though it can be brushed through. This works best for shorter hairstyles where a strong or detailed hold is required.

KMS SILKER

☺ **Silker Shampoo** *($8.25 for 12 ounces)* is a standard conditioning shampoo that can work well for dry hair of any thickness. Silk amino acids can be good water-binding agents, but are not preferred over all the countless others, many of which are also used by KMS in this line and their other products.

☺ **Silker 2-in-1 Shaping Creme** *($10.75 for 4 ounces)* is an emollient, slightly greasy styling cream that is outstanding for dry to very dry hair that is normal to coarse or thick. This contains no holding agents, so hair does not become sticky or stiff.

☹ **Silker Leave-In Treatment** *($8.75 for 8.5 ounces)* contains the preservative Kathon CG, and is not recommended.

☺ **Silker Reconstructor** *($8.95 for 8.1 ounces)* is a good, though standard, conditioner for normal to slightly dry hair of any thickness.

KMS TURNSTYLE

☺ **Turnstyle Back to Life Revival Cream** *($11 for 4 ounces)* won't revive or resuscitate hair, but it is a very good leave-in conditioner that contains next to no holding agents. Back to Life Revival Cream would work well for all hair types except fine or thin.

☺ **Turnstyle Beach Head Sea Salt Spray** *($10 for 6.8 ounces)*. This non-sticky, water-based spray contains magnesium sulfate (commonly known as Epsom salts) along with slip agent, sea salt, film-forming agent, preservatives, and fragrance. The salt can help rough up the cuticle of the hair. You can enhance that further by hand or heat styling, as you're directed to do on the label, but that is not a great thing for hair in the long run.

☺ **Turnstyle Do-Over, Cleansing Spray** *($8.95 for 8.5 ounces)* is supposed to take the place of a full-on shampoo. You simply wet your hair with this spray-on product, towel dry, and restyle. This "quick shampoo alternative" contains mostly water, detergent cleansing agent, alcohol, slip agent, conditioning agents, preservatives, and fragrance. The inherent problem with regular use of this type of product is that you don't rinse out the detergent cleansing agent, and leaving these types of ingredients on the skin and hair can not only cause dryness of the scalp and hair but also irritate the scalp. The claim that it can remove smoke and other unwanted odors from the hair is based only on the intense fragrance of the product itself; it doesn't really remove anything—it simply covers odors up with a strong scent that many consumers rightly prefer over the smell of stale smoke. In the end, Turnstyle Do-Over, Cleansing Spray is more of an occasional-use product and, depending on your lifestyle and grooming habits, it may or may not be all that helpful to do-over more than once.

☺ **Turnstyle Head Wetter All Wet Spray** *($13 for 6.8 ounces)* is a new twist on standard spray gels. This formula is sort of like a silicone spray, styling gel, and pomade rolled into one. It provides a soft, flexible hold that is minimally sticky and stays moist. The only drawback is that it can have a somewhat heavy after-feel, which rules it out for anyone with fine or limp hair. Those with normal to thick hair that is normal to very dry would fare best with this wet-look spray.

L.A. LOOKS

Drugstore-sold L.A. LOOKS now has a new look plus a wider variety of styling products since I last reviewed the line. Unfortunately, most of what's new and what made the cut from the former lineup has one major problem: the use of preservatives methylchloroisothiazolinone and methylisothiazolinone (Kathon CG), which are not recommended for use in leave-in products due to the risk it poses for sensitizing skin reactions. That's not great news.

Despite the name, LA. LOOKS has little, if anything, to do with hair trends in Los Angeles, though the products are made there, but so are those from its sister company, Dep. Both lines have problematic products due to a poor choice of preservatives. For more information about L.A. LOOKS, call (800) 326-2855 or visit www.lalooks.com.

What's Good About This Line: The few styling products that don't contain problematic preservatives are definitely worth considering; prices are some of the best at the drugstore.

What's Not So Good About It: Over a dozen products with preservatives that pose sensitizing risks; no styling products for those who need only a light hold. For more details, see the reviews for the majority of L.A. LOOKS styling products below.

The Reviews L

☹ **Curl Look Curl Defining Spray, Mega Hold 8** *($2.99 for 10.5 ounces)*, **Curl Look Curl Enhancing Mousse, Extra Super Hold 7** *($2.99 for 7.4 ounces)*, **Curl Look Frizz Control Gel, Mega Hold 8** *($2.99 for 16 ounces)*, **Expressive Look Gel 2 Mousse, Mega Hold 8** *($2.99 for 7.5 ounces)*, **Expressive Look Spray Gel, Mega Mega Hold 9** *($2.99 for 12.2 ounces)*, **Expressive Look Styling Gel, Extra Super Hold 7** *($2.99 for 16 ounces)*, **Expressive Look Styling Gel, Mega Hold 8** *($2.99 for 16 ounces)*, **Expressive Look Styling Gel, Mega Mega Hold 9** *($2.99 for 16 ounces)*, **Mess It Up Look Fiber Creme Pomade, X-treme Hold 10** *($3.29 for 2.6 ounces)*, **Speed Dry Look Fast Drying Gel, X-treme Hold 10** *($2.99 for 8 ounces)*, **Spike It Look Styling Gel, X-treme Hold 10** *($2.99 for 7 ounces)*, **Sport Look Styling Gel, X-treme Hold 10** *($2.99 for 16 ounces)*, **Straight Look Styling Gel, Extra Super Hold 7** *($2.99 for 16 ounces)*, **Volume Look Mousse Spray, Mega Hold 8** *($2.99 for 8 ounces)*, and **Volume Look Styling Gel, Mega Hold 8** *($2.99 for 16 ounces)* would all be decent (and in the case of the styling gels, astonishingly similar) styling products, but they are not recommended because they all contain the problematic preservative Kathon CG, which is not recommended for use in leave-on products because it has a strong tendency to cause sensitizing reactions on the skin and scalp. What a shame, because the prices and generous sizes of these products are hard to resist.

☺ **Expressive Look Spritz-On Hair Spray, Mega Mega Hold 9** *($2.99 for 14 ounces)* is a standard nonaerosol hairspray that isn't "mega hold" in the least. It offers a very light hold without stiffness or stickiness, and allows hair to be easily brushed through.

☺ **Expressive Look Style & Lock Hair Spray, Mega Hold 8** *($2.99 for 10 ounces)* is identical to the Expressive Look Spritz-On Hair Spray, Mega Hold 9 above, except this uses an aerosol delivery method that can spray on unevenly, so it takes some patience during use.

☺ **Piece It Look Wax Stick** *($3.29 for 2.5 ounces)* is a very standard, but effective, wax stick packaged in a deodorant-style container. It contains little more than plant oils, waxes, fragrance, water, and preservative, but can work well to smooth frizzies or dry ends on dry hair that is also coarse or thick. It can be difficult to shampoo out, but that is typical of most wax-based products like this.

☺ **Straight Look Straightening Spray, Mega Hold 8** *($2.99 for 9 ounces)* is similar to the Expressive Look Style & Lock Hair Spray, Mega Hold 8 above, except this has a better aerosol dispersal nozzle and adds silicone to the mix for added shine and light conditioning. This can work well as a finishing spray after hair has been straightened, and provides a soft, minimally sticky hold that can tame flyaway strands.

☺ **Volume Look Volumizing Hair Spray, Mega Mega Hold 9** *($2.99 for 10 ounces)* is nearly identical to the Straight Look Straightening Spray, Mega Hold 8 above, except this provides a light to medium hold with slight stiffness and stickiness. It works fine as an all-purpose finishing spray for use once your hair is dry to set your style without adding weight.

LANCOME

Lancome's brochure for Hair Sensation makes it sound like they have saved the best for last when it comes to launching the ultimate in hair care. The sensuality angle is played up through each product's individual texture and scent. Although these two elements play an important role in consumer perception and preference, on their own they're not enough to constitute great hair-care products. Fortunately, Lancome's parent company L'Oreal does know a thing or two about creating excellent hair-care products—there is no question that the lineage behind Hair Sensation is solid. For those who know the association between L'Oreal and Lancome (L'Oreal owns Lancome), it won't come as a shock that Lancome's hair-care formulations are remarkably similar to, and in many cases almost identical to, what you find in L'Oreal's drugstore hair-care product selection. Of course, Lancome's hair products have sleeker, sexier packaging, but what's inside the bottles is what matters to your hair, and the fact remains that whether you spend $17 for a conditioner from Lancome or $4.49 on one from L'Oreal, your hair won't notice the difference. For more information about Lancome, call (800) LANCOME, or visit www.lancome.com.

What's Good About This Line: Almost all of the hair-care products reviewed will work beautifully and are definite options.

What's Not So Good About It: The prices! Spending the extra money to line your shower stall with Lancome hair-care products is completely about the prestige factor and not about superior hair care.

☺ $$$ **Intense Nutrition Nourishing Treatment Shampoo** *($16 for 8.4 ounces)* is a standard, but good, shampoo that contains gentle detergent cleansing agents and would work well for all but fine or thin hair. This also features conditioners that can build up on hair with repeated use, so alternate this shampoo with one that does not contain conditioners. A small amount of salicylic acid is present, but not enough to have an effect on hair one way or the other. Salicylic acid is included in hair-care products for its keratolytic (exfoliating) effect on the scalp, which can help with conditions like dandruff and psoriasis. However, in those specialty products it is an active ingredient, and is used in percentages (typically 3%) that have been proven effective at treating the intended condition (Source: *Journal of Dermatology Treatment,* June 2002, pages 51–60). This product does not share information about the percentage of salicylic acid, so there is no way to know if it is effective for anything relating to the hair or scalp. Intense Nutrition Nourishing Treatment Shampoo is similar to L'Oreal Vive Shampoo Color Care Regular ($4.49 for 13 ounces), only without the conditioning agents, so buildup with the latter product is not an issue.

☺ $$$ **Intense Nutrition Nourishing Daily Conditioner** *($17 for 6.7 ounces)* is an ordinary, lightweight, silicone-based conditioner that also contains enough film-forming agent to initially make hair feel smooth, though it can build up with repeated use and make hair feel coated and limp. This can be a good detangling conditioner for normal to dry hair, but it's best to alternate it with a second conditioner that does not contain as much (or any) film-forming agent.

☺ **$$$ Intense Nutrition Extra Rich Conditioning Mask** *($22 for 6.7 ounces)* is an extremely overpriced, very basic conditioner that contains standard conditioning agents along with isopropyl alcohol (what's that doing in a conditioning mask?) and some honey, which has water-binding properties but not in this small amount. The ballyhooed silk protein that supposedly "repairs and moisturizes instantly" is given short shrift compared to the coloring agents, which are there only to make the product look pretty on the shelf.

☺ **$$$ Intense Nutrition Damaged Tips Nutri-Serum** *($22 for 1.69 ounces)* is one of the most overpriced silicone serums sold today, and there isn't a drop of nutrition in it. This product consists solely of silicones, alcohol, and fragrance. Any (and I do mean any) silicone serum at the drugstore is a better choice than this product, unless you enjoy wasting money. Every line from Citré Shine to Jheri Redding or göt2b has excellent options for far less money, although Lancome's price doesn't change the fact that it is a good product.

☺ **$$$ Intense Nutrition Smooth and Shine Treatment** *($18 for 3.3 ounces)* is nearly identical to the Intense Nutrition Damaged Tips Nutri-Serum above, and the same comments apply. Given the similarities of the formulas, the price and size discrepancy makes no sense. Nothing in either product provides nutrition in any way, shape, or form to hair—not surprising, since that's not possible anyway.

☺ **$$$ Intense Volume Volumizing Gel Shampoo** *($16 for 8.4 ounces)* doesn't contain anything that will add volume to hair, but that also means it doesn't contain conditioning agents or film-forming agents that can build up on hair. That's good news for anyone who wants volume, because this shampoo will rinse cleanly—but so do many, many others that sell for much less than this standard shampoo, such as L'Oreal Vive Shampoo Color Care Regular ($4.49 for 13 ounces).

☹ **$$$ Intense Volume Extra-Body Non Rinse Conditioner** *($17 for 3.3 ounces)* is a spray-on, leave-in conditioner that contains mostly water, alcohol, thickener, plant oil, slip agents, silicone, and fragrance. The alcohol will prevent this product from weighing hair down, but some of the other ingredients can leave a slightly sticky feel to the hair that isn't as elegant as other leave-in conditioners such as Aveda Elixir ($9 for 8.5 ounces).

☺ **$$$ Intense Volume Extra-Volume Mousse** *($18 for 5 ounces)* is a traditional styling mousse that contains water, several propellants, film-forming agent, conditioning agents, preservatives, and fragrance. It offers a medium hold with a slightly stiff, sticky finish.

☺ **$$$ Radiant Color Reviving Treatment Shampoo** *($16 for 8.4 ounces)* features Lancome's patent-pending micro-emulsion gel technology, although what that has to do with preserving hair color is anyone's guess, because Lancome doesn't tell you how this technology works to keep hair color around. What this amounts to is another standard, but very good, shampoo that contains enough silicone conditioning agents to build up with repeated use.

☺ **$$$ Radiant Color Extra-Radiance Repairing Conditioner** *($17 for 6.7 ounces)* is nearly identical to the Intense Nutrition Nourishing Daily Conditioner above, and the same comments apply. If this one is formulated with the Sublime Color System (which Lancome refers to as an exclusive combination of repairing ingredients), then so is the Intense Nutrition Conditioner, despite the fact that it makes no such claims. Although this formula contains a good deal of silicone, it cannot repair hair, instantly or over the long term. It is a good option for someone with normal to dry hair of any thickness, but the silicone can build up with repeated use and make fine or thin hair limp.

☺ **$$$ Shine Vitality Gel Shampoo** *($16 for 8.4 ounces)* contains enough silicone to leave a smooth, shiny finish, and although you're bound to love the silky sheen, the silicone can cause buildup with repeated use, so it's best to alternate this with a shampoo that does not contain silicone or conditioning agents. This shampoo is remarkably similar to L'Oreal's Vive Shampoo Fresh Shine ($4.49 for 13 ounces).

☹ **$$$ Shine Vitality Express Shine Conditioner** *($17 for 6.7 ounces)* contains mostly water, emollient, thickener, and preservative. Actually, a preservative is the third listed ingredient, which is a bit startling—but then again, the conditioning agent that precedes it is enough for your hair to feel smoother and softer. What's almost insulting is the price for such an ordinary formulation. L'Oreal's Vive Conditioner Fresh Shine ($4.49 for 13 ounces) is nearly identical, although it contains more fragrance than preservative.

L'ANZA

L'ANZA's claim to fame is the "Keratin Bond System," featured in almost all of their products. The system was developed by chemist and company founder Robert De Lanza, who combined keratin protein and "select herbs" in a "unique hydrolization process" that is supposed to create a superb delivery system for the keratin, making it (at least according to L'ANZA) a superior conditioning agent. Is it? First, using keratin in hair-care products is not unique; and second, the herbs used in L'ANZA's products have no substantiated benefit for hair. Finally, to hydrolyze something simply means to decompose an ingredient by reacting it with water. Does that make for a conditioning agent superior to all others? Not at all. Despite the fact that hair is composed primarily of keratin, its function in hair-care products is primarily as a conditioning and water-binding agent. Because it does not cling well to the hair shaft, it tends to not be of much use when mixed into shampoos. In conditioners and styling products it can be more beneficial, but it offers no more advantages than many other conditioning agents, such as glycerin, ceramides, or panthenol. L'ANZA calls itself "The Company of Solutions," but the equations they've worked out (meaning the products they've formulated) are no different from those found in hundreds of other lines—and they still do not have a firm grasp on the shampoo category, where most of their options are disappointing. Still, many of their products are worth considering. For more information about L'ANZA, call (800) 341-2262 or visit www.lanza.com.

What's Good About This Line: For a salon line, the prices are mostly reasonable; the conditioners present some wonderful options for dry to very dry hair; the styling product lineup is comprehensive and quite versatile, with few negatives to worry about.

What's Not So Good About It: The majority of the shampoos contain drying detergent cleansing agents; the claims, particularly for the botanical ingredients in the Urban Elements line, are completely without support or substantiation.

L'ANZA BE LONG

☹ **Be Long, Long Hair Formula Cleanse** *($12 for 12 ounces)* contains TEA-lauryl sulfate as its main detergent cleansing agent, which makes this shampoo too drying for the hair while being drying and irritating to the scalp.

☹ **Be Long, Long Hair Formula Spray Cleanse** *($9.95 for 12.6 ounces)* is a spray-on cleanser that contains primarily water, alcohol, and the antiseptic ingredient benzalkonium chloride. None of these ingredients clean hair all that well, though they can help dissolve scalp oil in between shampoos. However, this product would be a problem for your scalp because it contains enough arnica extract to cause irritation, especially since this is not rinsed from the hair after application.

☺ $$$ **Be Long, Long Hair Formula Condition** *($14.25 for 12 ounces)* can detangle long hair that is normal to fine or thin, but so can many other conditioners that cost less than this. L'ANZA's Keratin Bond System is just a good conditioning/water-binding agent for hair that can make it smoother; it has no lasting effect on hair.

☺ $$$ **Be Long, Long Hair Formula Strengthen** *($14.25 for 5.07 ounces)* is a good basic conditioner for dry hair of any thickness, but does nothing lasting to make hair stronger.

☺ $$$ **Be Long, Long Hair Formula ProtecShine** *($11.95 for 1.7 ounces)* claims to provide "complete styling protection," which implies heat protection, something this silicone serum can provide only minimal help with. This product can nicely smooth frizzies and dry ends of normal to thick or coarse hair that is dry to very dry.

CTRL @ L'ANZA

☺ **Ctrl @ L'ANZA Modify Hair Molder <F5 Giga-Hold>** *($11 for 2.5 ounces)* is a thick, creamy concoction of water, Vaseline, mineral oil, wax, film-forming/holding agent, thickener, conditioning agent, silicone, preservatives, and fragrance. It is best for adding moisture, texture, and frizz control to dry or very dry hair that is coarse or thick, and should be used sparingly to avoid a heavy feel.

☺ **Ctrl @ L'ANZA Soft_Ware Soft Wax <F4 Giga-Hold>** *($11 for 2.5 ounces)* is a lightweight, water-soluble pomade that can smooth and groom dry hair while making it look shiny and slick. It is best for purposeful wet looks or for emphasizing curls for those with normal to slightly thick or coarse hair. If "Giga-Hold" means strong hold, you won't get it from this soft-finish pomade.

☺ **Ctrl @ L'ANZA Upgrade Hair Putty <F6 Giga-Hold>** *($11 for 2.5 ounces)* is a very thick pomade that works best when used on dry (rather than damp) hair for strong smoothing and control of stubborn frizzies. The heavy texture of this product makes it preferred for thick or coarse hair that needs groomed control or for emphasizing the texture of very short haircuts.

L'ANZA DRY HAIR FORMULA

☹ **Dry Hair Formula Moisturizing Shampoo** *($8.95 for 10.1 ounces)* contains TEA-lauryl sulfate as one of its main detergent cleansing agents, which is completely inappropriate for any hair type, but is especially a problem for dry hair.

☺ **Dry Hair Formula Detangler** *($10 for 10.1 ounces)* is similar to the Be Long, Long Hair Formula Condition above, and the same review applies.

☺ **Dry Hair Formula Moisture Treatment** *($8.90 for 4.2 ounces)* is a good lightweight conditioner for normal to slightly dry hair that is normal to fine or thin.

L'ANZA HAIR REPAIR FORMULA

☺ **Hair Repair Formula Protein Plus Shampoo** *($8.40 for 10.1 ounces)* is a standard, but very good, conditioning shampoo that contains less protein than the name implies. It does contain plant oil and conditioning agents that make it a good choice for dry to very dry hair that is normal to thick or coarse.

☺ **$$$ Hair Repair Formula Leave-In Protector** *($15.25 for 10.1 ounces)* is a very standard leave-in conditioner that is a good option for normal to dry hair of any thickness.

☺ **$$$ Hair Repair Formula Reconstructor** *($13.30 for 4.2 ounces)* is similar to the Be Long, Long Hair Formula Strengthen above, except this contains less plant oil, which makes it better for normal to dry hair of any thickness.

L'ANZA STRAIT-LINE TEMPORARY CURL RELAXING FORMULA

☺ **Strait-Line Temporary Curl Relaxing Formula Shampoo** *($10.95 for 8.5 ounces)* cannot relax curls in any way. This is just a standard, but very good, shampoo for dry to very dry hair that is normal to coarse or thick. It can cause buildup with repeated use.

☺ **Strait-Line Temporary Curl Relaxing Formula Conditioner** *($10.95 for 6.7 ounces)* is a very good moisturizing conditioner for dry to very dry hair that is normal to coarse or thick, but it cannot make curly hair straighter.

☺ **Strait-Line Temporary Curl Relaxing Formula Smoother** *($12.95 for 6.7 ounces)* is a slick, gel-based styling balm that contains a form of silicone to help create smooth, sleek hair while straightening it with heat. This product is light enough to be used by all hair types, and does a reasonably good job of keeping frizzies at bay. It does not provide hold and, therefore, is not sticky.

☺ **Strait-Line Temporary Curl Relaxing Formula Thermal Defense** *($10.95 for 8.5 ounces)* is basically a light- to medium-hold hairspray with added conditioning agent to help moisturize and make hair easier to comb through. The keratin does not offer much, if any, thermal defense from blow dryers or flat irons, and this remains slightly sticky once it dries.

☺ **$$$ Strait-Line Temporary Curl Relaxing Formula Shine Spray** *($14.25 for 3.5 ounces)* is a silicone-based spray that contains additional plant oils and conditioning agents that can benefit dry hair. It's pricey for what you get, but can work well to add a glossy sheen to hair. Use it sparingly to avoid a greasy appearance.

L'ANZA URBAN ELEMENTS

☹ **Urban Elements Deep Cleansing Shampoo** *($8.75 for 10.1 ounces)* has the same problem as most of the L'ANZA shampoos above, meaning it contains TEA-lauryl sulfate as its main detergent cleansing agent. As such, this is too drying to the hair and irritating to the scalp.

☺ **Urban Elements Remedy Shampoo** *($12 for 10.1 ounces)* is similar to the Hair Repair Formula Protein Plus Shampoo above, and the same basic comments apply. This shampoo eliminates the plant oil, which makes it preferred for normal to slightly dry hair. The salicylic acid can neither exfoliate the scalp nor damage the hair.

☹ **Urban Elements Shampoo Plus** *($7.90 for 10.1 ounces)* contains peppermint oil, which makes it too irritating for all scalp types. What a shame, because this is one of L'Anza's least expensive shampoos and the formulation is otherwise very good.

☹ **Urban Elements Daily Revitalizer** *($10.95 for 6.8 ounces)* is nearly identical to the Dry Hair Formula Moisture Treatment above, except this contains peppermint and clove oils, which makes it too irritating for the scalp.

☺ **$$$ Urban Elements Deep Conditioner** *($12.50 for 4.2 ounces)* omits the peppermint oil that's present in the Urban Elements conditioners above. It is similar to the Hair Repair Formula Reconstructor above, and the same review applies.

☺ **Urban Elements Leave-In Conditioner** *($10 for 10.1 ounces)* is similar to the Hair Repair Formula Leave-In Protector above, except this adds plant oil, which makes it preferred for dry hair. The peppermint and clove extracts are used in small amounts and as extracts, and therefore are less irritating than their oil forms. You should still be cautious and try not to apply this directly to the scalp.

☺ **Urban Elements Spray-In Conditioner** *($9.95 for 10.1 ounces)* is a boring spray-on, leave-in conditioner whose main benefit is detangling. It is an OK option for normal to fine or thin hair, but could be more exciting.

☺ **Urban Elements Bodifying Foam** *($10 for 7.1 ounces)* is a standard propellant-based mousse with light hold and a soft finish that is ideal for casual hairstyles or defining curls on fine or thin hair. It leaves hair minimally sticky and does not get stiff.

☺ **$$$ Urban Elements Design Wax** *($16.95 for 6.8 ounces)* isn't a wax of any kind and it doesn't contain any wax, so the name is misleading. This is a thick, clear gel that contains mostly water, slip agent, mineral oil, thickeners, panthenol, conditioning agents, aloe, preservatives, and fragrance. It is a versatile, water-soluble product that can smooth dry ends of all hair types while adding shine and moisture without noticeable heaviness.

It also works well mixed with other styling products to provide additional conditioning and a slight amount of heat protection.

☺ **Urban Elements Dramatic F/X Super Hold Finishing Spray** *($10.95 for 10.6 ounces)* is a standard aerosol hairspray with a medium hold that leaves hair slightly sticky, though it can be brushed through.

☺ **Urban Elements Finishing Freeze** *($11 for 10.1 ounces)* is a light-hold nonaerosol hairspray that leaves hair surprisingly soft and non-sticky. It is not a good choice if you're looking to freeze your style in place, but, for a touch of movable hold, this excels.

☺ **Urban Elements Hair Polish** *($12.10 for 4.2 ounces)* is a lightweight, but thick-textured, styling balm/pomade that can add soft shine and almost weightless moisture to all hair types. This offers no hold whatsoever, so think of it as an alternative leave-in conditioner for normal to slightly dry hair. Use it sparingly if your hair is fine or thin.

☺ **Urban Elements Liquid Texture** *($9.95 for 6.8 ounces)* is a standard styling gel with a very strong hold—stronger than many hairsprays, in fact. It can be a great ally to style stubborn hair, but the trade-off is the tacky, sticky after-feel that makes this somewhat difficult to brush through.

☺ **Urban Elements Mega Gel** *($9.85 for 6.8 ounces)* is similar to the Urban Elements Liquid Texture above, only with less hold and noticeably less stickiness. It is a standard, but good, option for all hair types.

☺ **Urban Elements Memory Hairspray** *($11.50 for 10.1 ounces)* is a very good, light-hold hairspray with a soft, non-sticky finish. It manages to keep hair in place while allowing some movement, and hair is easy to brush through and restyle, which makes this worthwhile for creating more complex hairstyles that require play time before the product dries and sets.

☺ $$$ **Urban Elements Molding Paste** *($16.95 for 6.8 ounces)* is a very thick, water- and wax-based paste that is best for someone smoothing dry to very dry hair or who is dealing with stubborn frizzies. It provides a natural shine rather than the slick, greasy shine associated with many pomades. The tube packaging is a mistake for this type of product because it is so dense that it's very difficult to squeeze out.

☺ **Urban Elements Spray Gel** *($10.50 for 10.1 ounces)* is a light- to medium-hold, light-textured spray gel that can work well for a variety of hairstyles from slicked-back to spiked—or for creating defined waves or curls—with minimal stiffness or stickiness. The conditioning agents make hair easy to brush through and help add smoothness.

☺ $$$ **Urban Elements Styling Cream** *($16.95 for 6.8 ounces)* is sold as being able to refine texture, add weight, and control frizz. It can do all of those things plus add a glossy shine. The emollient, slightly greasy texture of this product makes it well-suited for dry or very dry hair with stubborn curls or frizzies that need a heavier product to achieve smooth, defined styles.

☺ **Urban Elements Shine Gel, Oil-Free Weightless Glosser** *($13.60 for 3.5 ounces)* is a silicone-based gel that is quite slick and greasy, but it can add dazzling shine and expertly control frizzy hair, not to mention being of great help while straightening hair with heat. It is best for dry to very dry hair that is coarse or thick. This would quickly make normal to fine or thin hair limp and greasy.

L'ANZA VOLUME FORMULA

☺ **Volume Formula Bodifying Shampoo** *($8.40 for 12.6 ounces)* is a good shampoo for all hair types except oily, and the lack of film-forming agents means there is no risk of buildup.

☺ **Volume Formula Weightless Rinse** *($10 for 12.6 ounces)* is similar to the Dry Hair Formula Detangler above, except this replaces one of the thickeners with plant oil, and that makes it preferred for drier hair of any thickness. This is not really that weightless, and there are lighter options for fine or thin hair, but if dryness is a concern, this can help.

☹ **Volume Formula Body Styling Cream** *($9.40 for 8.5 ounces)* contains the preservative methylchloroisothiazolinone, which is not recommended for use in leave-on products due to its high risk of causing a sensitizing reaction on the scalp.

☺ **Volume Formula Final Effects, Maximum Hold Finishing Spray (Aerosol)** *($12.95 for 10.6 ounces)* is a standard, but good, hairspray that offers light hold with a minimal stiff or sticky feel. Hair can be easily brushed through, and you can reapply this while styling without making hair feel heavy or too coated.

☺ **Volume Formula Root Effects** *($13.60 for 7.1 ounces)* is an aerosol styling spray with a directional nozzle so you can apply product at the roots, but the forceful application tends to apply too much product at once, leading to coated, stiff, and sticky roots—probably not what you had in mind. This works best when it is dispensed into the palm of your hand and then applied to the hair in sections. It offers a medium hold that, when applied by hand, is slightly stiff and sticky. When used with heat, this can create long-lasting lift that can be brushed through.

☺ **Volume Formula Volumizing Dry Spray** *($10.50 for 8.5 ounces)* is a standard hairspray that provides a medium hold with some stickiness, so brushing through hair can be a challenge. Use this to set hairstyles you don't intend to brush through and it will work well to provide long-lasting control.

☺ **Volume Formula Zero Weight Gel** *($10.40 for 8.5 ounces)* is almost identical to the Urban Elements Liquid Texture above, and the same comments apply. It contains gold mica particles that add shimmer to hair, but they can easily flake off when hair is brushed through.

L'OREAL

For more information about L'Oreal, call 800-535-3457 or visit www.lorealparisusa.com.

What's Good About This Line: For the money, these are some of the best shampoos and conditioners available; the Studio and alt.Studio styling products have something for just about everyone; L'Oreal thinks highly enough of the formulations below that many of them were parlayed into their Lancome Hair Sensation line as well as their upscale (read: expensive) Kérastase hair-care products.

What's Not So Good About It: The shampoo formulas are fairly repetitive, despite claims for differing hair types and needs; the conditioners lack good leave-in options and rich, emollient options for dry to very dry or coarse hair; many of the styling gels tend to have a sticky after-feel not found in competing products, but they can certainly hold hair in place.

L'OREAL VIVE

L'Oreal's Vive products were renamed and updated in mid-2003 with what the company claims are more beneficial ingredients, better conditioning, new fragrances, and improved packaging. Visually, the face-lift is impressive, with brighter, bolder colors making each Vive category quite eye-catching as you peruse the selection of hair-care products at the drugstore. But how about what's inside these gleaming new bottles? For the most part, the formulas were barely altered and the differences between the Vive product categories are still strikingly minimal; some are almost identical. Still, for the money, these are some of the best shampoos and conditioners you're likely to find, and the prices are practically irresistible.

☺ **Vive Color-Care Shampoo, for Regular Color-Treated or Highlighted Hair** *($4.49 for 13 ounces)* is a standard shampoo that includes no special ingredients or benefits for dyed hair. It does contain a tiny amount of sunscreen, but that can't protect hair because it would be rinsed down the drain. This can be a very good shampoo for normal to slightly dry hair, and poses a slight risk of buildup.

☺ **Vive Color-Care Shampoo, for Dry Color-Treated or Highlighted Hair** *($4.49 for 13 ounces)* is nearly identical to the Vive Color-Care Shampoo, for Regular Color-Treated or Highlighted Hair above, and the same review applies. This contains nothing special for dry hair, and keep in mind that if your hair is color-treated, chances are it is indeed also dry.

☺ **Vive Curl-Moisture Shampoo, for Curly Hair** *($4.49 for 13 ounces)* is a great conditioning shampoo for dry to very dry hair that is normal to coarse or thick. The silicone can build up with repeated use, so alternate this with a shampoo that does not contain conditioning agents.

☺ **Vive Fresh-Shine Shampoo, for Frequent Use on All Hair Types** *($4.49 for 13 ounces)* is similar to the Vive Curl-Moisture Shampoo, for Curly Hair above, but this one contains slightly less silicone. Using this frequently will increase the rate at which the silicone builds up on hair, but it can help make it easier to comb and can help keep thin or fine hair from becoming too flyaway.

☺ **Vive Nutri-Moisture Shampoo, for Dry or Damaged Hair** *($4.49 for 13 ounces)* is nearly identical to the Vive Fresh-Shine Shampoo above, and the same review applies.

☺ **Vive Smooth-Intense Shampoo, for Dry, Frizzy or Rebellious Hair** *($3.99 for 13 ounces)* is yet another good shampoo for normal to dry hair of any thickness, and poses a slight risk of buildup with repeated use.

☺ **Vive Volume-Infusing Shampoo, for Fine Hair** *($4.49 for 13 ounces)* does not contain any silicone, and features a tiny amount of film-forming agent, so it ends up being a very good, basic shampoo for all hair types concerned about avoiding buildup.

☺ **Vive Fresh-Shine 2-in-1 Shampoo & Conditioner, for Frequent Use on All Hair Types** *($4.49 for 13 ounces)* is nearly identical to the Vive Color-Care Shampoo, for Regular Color-Treated or Highlighted Hair above, and the same review applies. Using this frequently will increase the rate at which the conditioning agents in this shampoo build up on the hair.

☺ **Vive Nutri-Moisture 2-in-1 Shampoo & Conditioner** *($4.49 for 13 ounces)* is similar to the Vive Fresh-Shine Shampoo, for Frequent Use on All Hair Types above, and the same review applies.

☺ **Vive Color-Care Conditioner, for Regular Hair** *($4.49 for 13 ounces)* is a basic, but effective, conditioner for normal to dry hair of any thickness. The sunscreen it contains cannot protect hair from UV damage because it does not cling well to hair nor does it hold up during rinsing. There are no standards for using sunscreens in hair-care products. Note that it carries no SPF rating (the FDA does not allow SPF ratings for hair-care products).

☺ **Vive Color-Care Conditioner, for Dry Hair** *($4.49 for 13 ounces)* is a good option for normal to dry hair of any thickness, and is basically similar to the Vive Color-Care Conditioner above.

☺ **Vive Curl-Moisture Conditioner, for Curly Hair** *($4.49 for 13 ounces)* contains some good conditioning agents for curly hair (and all dry hair of any texture, for that matter), including silicone and glycerin. It is lighter than the two Vive Color-Care conditioners above, and is an option for normal to slightly dry hair that is normal to fine or thin.

☺ **Vive Fresh-Shine Conditioner, for Frequent Use on All Hair Types** *($4.49 for 13 ounces)* is a very basic, but worthwhile, conditioner for normal to slightly dry hair that is normal to fine or thin.

☺ **Vive Nutri-Moisture Conditioner** *($4.49 for 13 ounces)* is identical to the Vive Color-Care Conditioner, for Regular Hair above, and the same review applies.

☺ **Vive Smooth-Intense Conditioner** *($3.99 for 13 ounces)* is nearly identical to the Vive Curl-Moisture Conditioner, for Curly Hair above, except that this product adds glycerin, even though it isn't an intense ingredient on hair. Otherwise, the same basic comments apply. The tiny amount of plant oil has little smoothing effect on hair.

☺ **Vive Volume-Infusing Conditioner** *($4.49 for 13 ounces)* is a good, basic conditioner for normal to slightly dry hair of any thickness.

☺ **Vive Color-Care Finishing Spray** *($4.49 for 8 ounces)* is a standard hairspray with a light hold and minimal stiff or sticky feel. It contains silicones to add shine and to make hair easy to brush through, but nothing in it can help protect hair color. The two sunscreen agents cannot prevent color loss from hair, and this product is not rated with an SPF number (in accordance with FDA regulations).

☺ **Vive Curl-Shaping Spray Gel** *($4.49 for 8 ounces)* is a very basic spray gel that offers a light to medium hold that remains sticky, which is not the best feel for curly hair, though this can help define stubborn curls.

☺ **Vive Color-Care Dry Defense 3-Minute Conditioning Treatment** *($5.99 for 6 ounces)* is nearly identical to the Vive Color-Care Conditioner, for Regular Hair above, and the same comments apply. Selling this formula as a special treatment is the epitome of hair-care product redundancy.

☺ **Vive Color-Care Masque, for Color Treated or Highlighted Hair** *($7.39 for 5 ounces)* is nearly identical in every respect to L'Oreal-owned Kérastase's Resistance Age Recharge, Firming Masque ($41 for 5 ounces), which further proves that expensive does not mean better when it comes to hair-care products. This "masque" can lightly moisturize and help make normal to fine or thin hair feel slightly thicker while being easier to detangle, but that's about it.

☺ **Vive Smooth-Intense Frizz Solution** *($5.99 for 3.4 ounces)* is a very good, attractively priced silicone serum that can work wonders (as most silicone serums can) for smoothing dry, frizzy hair and adding lustrous shine. Unless your hair is extraordinarily thick, use this sparingly to avoid a greasy, slick appearance.

L'OREAL VIVE FOR MEN

☺ **Vive for Men Daily Thickening 2-in-1 Shampoo & Conditioner, for Fine or Thinning Hair** *($3.69 for 13 ounces)* is more of a standard shampoo than a true two-in-one option because it contains small amounts of conditioning agents. This can work well for all hair types and poses no risk of buildup. The only thing that makes it preferred for men is the fragrance. Actually, the lack of film-forming agents means this shampoo won't be very effective at making fine or thin hair feel thicker.

☺ **Vive for Men Daily Thickening Anti-Dandruff Shampoo, for All Hair** *($3.69 for 13 ounces)* is a very good anti-dandruff shampoo that contains 1% zinc pyrithione as the active ingredient. This is appropriate for normal to dry hair of any thickness, and the silicone can cause buildup with repeated use (though it can also offset the drying effect of the anti-dandruff ingredient).

☺ **Vive for Men Daily Thickening Shampoo, for Fine or Thinning Hair** *($3.69 for 13 ounces)* is identical to the Vive for Men Daily Thickening 2-in-1 Shampoo & Conditioner, for Fine or Thinning Hair above, and the same review applies.

☺ **Vive for Men Thickening & Grooming Foam, for Fine or Thinning Hair** *($3.69 for 6 ounces)* is identical to the Studio Line Mega Mousse, Mega Hold Styling Mousse reviewed below, and the same review applies. This is indeed great for styling fine or thin hair.

☹ **Vive for Men Thickening & Grooming Gel, for Fine or Thinning Hair** *($3.69 for 6.8 ounces)* lists sodium polystyrene sulfonate as the second ingredient, which makes this drying for hair and irritating to the scalp, not to mention that it can potentially strip dyed hair color. This is a rare misstep for L'Oreal, but the good news for men is that any of the Studio Line or alt.Studio gels below are wonderful options to consider.

L'OREAL ALT.STUDIO

☺ **alt.Studio Crystal Wax, High Shine and Definition** *($5.99 for 1.7 ounces)* isn't a wax, nor does it contain any wax. It is a standard, water-soluble pomade with a thick texture that does spread easily through wet or dry hair. It can be heavy and slightly greasy, and is best for dry hair that is normal to coarse or thick. It adds a wet-look shine while allowing you to enhance hair's texture or define curls.

☺ **alt.Studio Freezer Gel, Hard Finish, Icy Shine** *($5.99 for 6.8 ounces)* is a standard styling gel that provides a firm hold with some stiffness and stickiness, though hair can be brushed through. This is best for slicked-back or spiked hairstyles, but it can also work well on hard-to-hold hair.

☺ **alt.Studio Iron-Tamer Spritz** *($5.99 for 5 ounces)* is a lightweight, slightly sticky, alcohol-based styling spray that offers a medium, flexible hold. This is sold as being able to protect hair from heat irons, but contains nothing to provide even a smidge of protection. Claim aside, this is a very good styling spray to use on wet hair you intend to let dry naturally.

☺ **alt.Studio Remix Paste, Extreme Texture, Reworkable Hold** *($5.99 for 3.1 ounces)* is less a paste and more a thick styling cream that is easy to work with and versatile enough to create smooth, sleek looks or exaggerated, highly textured styles. It is fairly water-soluble, which makes it easy to shampoo out, and provides a light to medium flexible hold that is slightly sticky but not stiff.

☺ **alt.Studio Up-Right Foam** *($5.99 for 7 ounces)* is a standard, propellant-based mousse that offers a medium to firm hold with enough stickiness to make this tricky to brush through. It is meant to be applied directly to the roots and then massaged into hair with fingers, and following these steps can indeed create long-lasting lift and, when used with heat, body. If you plan to use this with a heat-styling implement, it should be combined with a separate product that provides some heat protection, an area where this mousse falls short.

L'OREAL STUDIO LINE

☺ **Studio Line Anti-Frizz, Medium Hold Styling Gel** *($3.99 for 6 ounces)* is a simple, but excellent, anti-frizz styling gel for all hair types. It provides a light hold without stiffness but can be slightly tacky. It contains mostly water, glycerin, thickener, panthenol, silicone, and fragrance. This would work well to smooth hair or to shape and moisturize curly hair.

☺ **Studio Line Clean Gel, Strong Hold Styling Gel** *($3.99 for 6.8 ounces)* is a medium-hold, very standard styling gel that can feel a bit heavy on fine or thin hair. It is slightly sticky but can be easily brushed through. With the exception of the panthenol, the B vitamins have no effect on hair.

☺ **Studio Line Fast Forward, Strong Hold Finishing Spray** *($3.99 for 7 ounces)* is a standard aerosol hairspray that provides medium to firm hold with some stickiness but minimal stiffness.

☺ **Studio Line FX Aqua Gel, Strong Hold** *($3.99 for 5.1 ounces)* promises no stiffness or stickiness, but this is actually one of L'Oreal's stickiest styling gels. It provides a medium to firm hold that can be somewhat difficult to brush through. It is best for wet looks or more extreme hairstyles.

☺ **Studio Line Grab, Mega Hold Texture Gel** *($3.99 for 4 ounces)* is a thicker styling gel that contains an appreciable amount of plant oil, but this still ends up being fairly sticky. It offers a firm hold and is a good option for managing hard-to-hold hair that is coarse or thick.

☺ **Studio Line Invisi-Gel, Mega Hold Styling Gel** *($3.99 for 6.8 ounces)* is nearly identical to the Studio Line Clean Gel, Strong Hold Styling Gel above, and the same review applies. This isn't any more invisible on hair than L'Oreal's other gels.

☺ **Studio Line Invisi-Gel, Strong Hold Styling Gel** *($3.99 for 6.8 ounces)* is nearly identical to the Studio Line Clean Gel, Strong Hold Styling Gel above, except this has a softer hold. Otherwise, the same basic comments apply.

☺ **Studio Line Lasting Curls, Medium Hold Styling Gel** *($3.99 for 6 ounces)* is a standard styling gel that can work for all hair types requiring medium to firm hold. It leaves hair feeling slightly stiff and sticky, and is recommended only for curly hair that needs strong definition—there are softer options to groom curls without the residual stickiness.

☺ **Studio Line Liquid Gel, Strong Hold Styling Spray Gel** *($3.99 for 6 ounces)* is a standard, alcohol-free, light- to medium-hold spray gel. It leaves hair feeling slightly sticky, but is a better option for softly defining curls than the Studio Line Lasting Curls Medium Hold Styling Gel above. On non-curly hair, this gel is easily brushed through and the glycerin can add moisture.

☺ **Studio Line Mega Gel, Mega Hold Styling Gel** *($3.99 for 6.8 ounces)* is nearly identical to the Studio Line Lasting Curls, Medium Hold Styling Gel above, and the same comments apply.

☺ **Studio Line Mega Mousse, Mega Hold Styling Mousse** *($3.79 for 6.9 ounces)* is a propellant-delivered standard mousse. It provides a light hold with a minimal stiff or sticky feel, and allows hair to be easily brushed through. The tiny amount of conditioning agents makes this not the best choice for heat styling.

☺ **Studio Line Mega Spritz, Mega Hold Finishing Spritz** *($3.19 for ounces)* is a good, standard, light- to medium-hold nonaerosol hairspray that contains a fairly non-sticky film-forming/holding agent, which makes this a breeze to brush through as well as an effective working spray during styling.

☺ **Studio Line Melting Gel, Strong Hold Styling Gel** *($3.19 for 6.8 ounces)* does not offer strong hold. It actually does not contain any holding agents whatsoever! It can be an OK option for normal to fine or thin hair that needs light conditioning and some smoothing.

☺ **Studio Line Mighty Mist, Mega Hold Finishing Spray** *($3.79 for 8 ounces)* is nearly identical to the Studio Line Mega Spritz, Mega Hold Finishing Spritz above, and the same review applies.

☺ **Studio Line Pumping Curls, Medium Hold Finishing Spray** *($3.99 for 8 ounces)* is a lightweight, light-hold styling spray that can softly define curls without stiffness or stickiness. The texture of this product makes it best for normal to fine or thin curly hair, but there is no reason it cannot be used by those with non-curly hair.

☺ **Studio Line Springing Curls, Medium Hold Styling Mousse** *($3.79 for 6 ounces)* is a medium- to firm-hold, propellant-based mousse that contains glycerin to add moisture to hair. This can feel sticky, but it dissipates somewhat as it dries. Hair is easily brushed through, and this product can work well on curly hair of any thickness.

☺ **Studio Line Straight Up, Medium Hold Styling Gel** *($3.99 for 6.8 ounces)* isn't the best choice for straightening hair unless it is very stubborn. The stickiness can make this less than desirable as you're heat-styling your hair, but it can be a very good medium-hold styling gel for wet looks or textured hairstyles that don't need to be straightened.

☺ **Studio Line Volumatic, Strong Hold Styling Mousse** *($3.99 for 6 ounces)* is a light-hold, propellant-based styling mousse that can be a great option for normal to fine or thin hair needing body and lift. This can provide a slight amount of protection during heat styling, and allows hair to be easily brushed through.

☺ **Studio Line Volumatic, Strong Hold Styling Spray Gel** *($3.99 for 6 ounces)* contains mostly water, film-forming/holding agent, alcohol, silicone, preservative, fragrance, plant oil, and emulsifier. It is a good, light-hold, lightweight spray gel that works equally well for wet or dry hairstyling.

L'OREAL KIDS

☺ **Kids 2-in-1 Shampoo, Banana-Melon for Fine Hair** *($3.49 for 9 ounces)* is a standard conditioning shampoo whose only kid-like feature is the fruity fragrance. This can build up on hair with repeated use, but will make hair easier to comb. Those with fine hair may find this too conditioning; alternating it with a shampoo that does not contain conditioning agents will help eliminate that concern.

☺ **Kids 2-in-1 Shampoo, Cherry-Almond for Extra Conditioning** *($3.49 for 9 ounces)* is nearly identical to the Kids 2-in-1 Shampoo, Banana-Melon for Fine Hair above, and the same comments apply.

☺ **Kids 2-in-1 Shampoo, Fruity Apricot for Normal Hair** *($3.49 for 9 ounces)* is nearly identical to the Kids 2-in-1 Shampoo, Banana-Melon for Fine Hair above, and the same comments apply.

☺ **Kids 2-in-1 Shampoo, Tropical Punch for Extra Manageability** *($3.49 for 9 ounces)* is nearly identical to the Kids 2-in-1 Shampoo, Banana-Melon for Fine Hair above, and the same comments apply.

☺ **Kids 2-in-1 Shampoo, Watermelon for Thick, Curly or Wavy Hair** *($3.49 for 9 ounces)* is nearly identical to the Kids 2-in-1 Shampoo, Banana-Melon for Fine Hair above, and the same comments apply.

☺ **Kids 2-in-1 Swim Shampoo, Splash of Orange** *($3.49 for 9 ounces)* is nearly identical to the Kids 2-in-1 Shampoo, Banana-Melon for Fine Hair above, and the same comments apply.

☺ **Kids Fast Dry 2-in-1 Shampoo, Burst of Cool Melon for Thick, Curly or Wavy Hair** *($3.49 for 9 ounces)* doesn't contain anything that will make hair dry faster, and remains a good conditioning shampoo for normal to dry hair of any thickness.

☺ **Kids Fast Dry 2-in-1 Shampoo, Burst of Pineapple Flash for Normal to Fine Hair** *($3.49 for 9 ounces)* is, save for a change in fruity fragrance, identical to the Kids Fast Dry 2-in-1 Shampoo, Burst of Cool Melon for Thick, Curly or Wavy Hair above, and the same comments apply.

☺ **Kids Smoothie 2-in-1 Shampoo, Blueberry for All Hair Types** *($3.49 for 9 ounces)* is similar to the Kids 2-in-1 Shampoo, Banana-Melon for Fine Hair above, but contains a greater amount of conditioning agents, which makes it best for normal to very dry hair. This can be too conditioning for fine or thin hair, and will build up with repeated use.

☺ **Kids Smoothie 2-in-1 Shampoo, Orange Mango for Extra Shine** *($3.49 for 9 ounces)* is, save for a change in fruity fragrance, identical to the Kids Smoothie 2-in-1 Shampoo, Blueberry for All Hair Types above, and the same review applies.

☺ **Kids Smoothie 2-in-1 Shampoo, Strawberry** *($3.49 for 9 ounces)* is, save for a change in fruity fragrance, identical to the Kids Smoothie 2-in-1 Shampoo, Blueberry for All Hair Types above, and the same review applies.

☺ **Kids Conditioner, Burst of Juicy Grape for Normal to Fine Hair** *($3.49 for 9 ounces)* is a standard, but very good, smoothing conditioner that can work very well for normal to dry hair that is normal to fine or thin, and it does make hair easy to detangle.

☺ **Kids Tangle Tamer, Burst of Sweet Pear** *($3.49 for 9 ounces)* is an excellent spray-on detangler.

L'OREAL NATURE'S THERAPY

L'Oreal's Nature's Therapy line is probably their least-known collection of hair-care products. It is available primarily through beauty supply stores (Sally Beauty stocks it at most of their locations) and is sold under L'Oreal's Classic Salon banner. In a way, this sub-line is L'Oreal's attempt to join the natural craze because it is their only line of hair-care products that plays up the botanicals and plants in each product. However, the natural ingredients make up only a token amount of each product, and the formulations are (not surprisingly) similar to those of other L'Oreal hair-care products, notably those from their less expensive Vive line and the overpriced Kérastase brand.

☺ **Nature's Therapy Liquid Energy Fortifying Shampoo** *($7.49 for 12 ounces)* is a standard shampoo that is a good option for normal to dry hair of any thickness. This poses a slight risk of buildup.

☺ **Nature's Therapy Mega Moisture Nurturing Shampoo** *($4.99 for 12 ounces)* is similar to the Nature's Therapy Liquid Energy Fortifying Shampoo above, and the same

The Reviews L

basic comments apply. The tiny amount of film-forming agent in this product shouldn't pose a risk for buildup, but the conditioning agent can build up with repeated use.

☺ **Nature's Therapy Scalp Relief Treatment Shampoo** *($5.99 for 12 ounces)* is an excellent moisturizing shampoo for dry to very dry hair of any thickness. This can cause buildup with repeated use, but it can be helpful for a dry scalp.

☺ **Nature's Therapy Unfrizz Smoothing Shampoo** *($4.99 for 12 ounces)* is nearly identical to the Nature's Therapy Mega Moisture Nurturing Shampoo above, and the same review applies. The glycerin in this product can help smooth hair, but a shampoo cannot tackle frizzies as well as a conditioner or a styling product that contains silicone (or similar conditioning agents).

☺ **Nature's Therapy Liquid Energy Liquid Mousse Volumizer** *($6.99 for 5.5 ounces)* is a liquid-to-foam mousse that offers a very light hold without stiffness or stickiness. It is a good option for normal to fine or thin hair that needs an ultra-light styling product and just a hint of hold.

☺ **Nature's Therapy Mega Slick Moisturizing Pomade** *($5.99 for 2 ounces)* is fairly close to traditional pomade, containing primarily Vaseline, mineral oil, wax, silicone, thickeners, fragrance, and plant extracts. The plant extracts are present in token amounts— so much for this being from nature (though there is nothing unnatural about Vaseline or mineral oil). As with any emollient pomade, this should be used sparingly, and it's best for dry to very dry hair that needs help with frizzies and/or dry ends. This can be difficult to shampoo out, but it definitely adds shine and smoothes hair.

☺ **Nature's Therapy Unfrizz Taming Cream** *($7.49 for 4 ounces)* is a standard styling balm that can work well to straighten and smooth hair when used with heat and the proper styling tools. The paraffin, silicone, and glycerin that make up the backbone of this product are all worthwhile ingredients for dry to very dry hair.

☺ **Nature's Therapy Heat Control Leave-In Protection Creme** *($4.99 for 4 ounces)* is a great leave-in conditioner for normal to dry hair of any thickness except fine or thin.

☺ **Nature's Therapy Hot Oil Botanical Treatment** *($2.99 for 4 ounces)*, as is often the case with hair-care products claiming to be oil treatments, includes only a tiny amount of oil. This contains mostly water, conditioning agent, film-forming agent, thickener, fragrance, slip agent, water-binding agent, preservative, plant oils, and coloring agent. It is an OK option for normal to slightly dry hair, but is a far cry from being a botanical treatment.

☺ **Nature's Therapy Liquid Energy Fortifying Treatment** *($8.49 for 6 ounces)* is a basic, lightweight detangling spray that contains far more fragrance than fortifying ingredients, though it is still a decent option for fine or thin hair that is normal to slightly (very slightly) dry.

☺ **Nature's Therapy Mega Moisture Nurturing Creme** *($2.19 for 1 ounce)* is a very standard, but good, conditioner that would work well for normal to dry hair of any thickness.

☺ **Nature's Therapy Mega Repair Recovery Complex** *($5.99 for 6 ounces)* is similar to the Nature's Therapy Mega Moisture Nurturing Creme above, except this is a slightly more emollient option for dry hair of any thickness.

☹ **Nature's Therapy Scalp Relief Leave-In Treatment** *($6.99 for 4 ounces)* contains menthoxypropanediol, a combination of menthol and propylene glycol that can enhance the penetration of menthol into the skin. As a leave-in product, this is considerably irritating for the scalp, and is not recommended.

☺ **Nature's Therapy Unfrizz Smoothing Treatment** *($6.99 for 8 ounces)* is nearly identical to the Nature's Therapy Mega Moisture Nurturing Creme above, except this contains lanolin, though only a small amount. Still, it is enough to make this preferred for drier hair that is normal to slightly thick.

MASTEY

Henri Mastey's claim to fame is his refusal to use common detergent cleansing agents such as sodium and ammonium laureth sulfates in his products because he believes they are drying to the hair. Instead, the Mastey shampoos contain amphoteric surfactants (the gentlest category of surfactants, made famous by Johnson & Johnson's Baby Shampoo). In Mastey's case, the shampoos feature either sodium cocoyl isethionate or sodium cocoate or both. These cleansing agents are gentler to hair than the aforementioned laureth sulfates, but there is a downside—they do not cleanse hair and scalp as well. This means they often leave enough oil behind to make fine or thin hair feel limp, not to mention their limited ability to remove styling product and conditioner buildup. They are actually best used in conjunction with sodium or ammonium laureth sulfates, which themselves are not drying to the hair in the amounts used in most shampoos, so Mastey's cautions about avoiding these ingredients are unfounded. For more information about Mastey, call (800) 6-MASTEY or visit www.mastey.com.

What's Good About This Line: The shampoos are unusually gentle, and a few are superior options for dry to very dry hair types that do not use heavy styling products; some good detangling conditioners that can also remove mineral and chlorine buildup from hair.

What's Not So Good About It: Almost all the leave-on and styling products contain the problematic preservatives methylchloroisothiazolinone and methylisothiazolinone (Kathon CG); the shampoo and conditioner formulations are repetitive; some of the products recommended for fine hair are simply too heavy or emollient for fine hair.

☺ **Clarte Reconstructing Creme Shampoo, for Color Treated and Bleached Hair** *($11 for 12 ounces)* is a very good shampoo for all hair types except oily. Its cleansing ability is not strong enough to remove buildup from styling products, but it is a very gentle option for color-treated hair.

☺ **Color Refreshing Shampoo, Adds Color Highlights** *($10 for 8 ounces)* contains coloring agents, but not the type that can deposit color on the hair shaft. That means this shampoo, available in several different shades for various hair colors, is incapable of enhancing your hair color. However, it can work as a very gentle shampoo for all but oily hair. The conditioning agents can cause buildup with repeated use.

☺ **Enove Volumizing Creme Shampoo, for Fine Hair** *($11 for 12 ounces)* is similar to the Clarte Reconstructing Creme Shampoo above, except this contains emollient thickeners, which makes it preferred for dry to very dry hair of any thickness. This can cause buildup with repeated use, so those with fine or thin hair should alternate it with a shampoo that does not contain conditioning agents.

☺ **Le Remouver Hair Clarifier** *($11 for 12 ounces)* is a very standard, gentle shampoo that contains a chelating agent to help remove styling product and mineral or chlorine buildup from hair. It would be better if this contained stronger (but not drying) detergent cleansing agents because this shampoo's base is too mild to work for oily hair or heavy residue from styling products.

☺ **Traite Moisture Shampoo** *($15 for 16 ounces)* is nearly identical to the Enove Volumizing Creme Shampoo above, and the same comments apply.

☹ **HC Formula + B5 Leave-In Hair Mender** *($10 for 8 ounces)* contains the preservative Kathon CG, which is not recommended for use in leave-on products because it poses a high risk of causing a sensitizing reaction.

☺ **Liquid Pac** *($9 for 8.5 ounces)* is a bare-bones conditioner that would work best for fine or thin hair. This can remove mineral and chlorine buildup from the hair while helping make it easier to comb.

☹ **Activateur Curl Enhancer, Body & Shine Curl Builder** *($10 for 8 ounces)* contains the preservative Kathon CG, and is not recommended.

☹ **Designer Setting Spray, Flexible Hold Shaping Spray** *($10 for 8 ounces)* contains the preservative Kathon CG, and is not recommended.

☺ **Direction Shaping Hair Spray, Invisible Lift Style Support** *($10 for 8 ounces)* is a very standard, light-hold nonaerosol hairspray that dries to a minimally stiff and sticky finish. Hair is easily brushed through with no snags or snarls.

☺ **Fixe Super Hold Hairspray, Super Hold Shine & Support** *($10 for 8 ounces)* is almost identical to the Direction Shaping Hair Spray, Invisible Lift Style Support above, only with slightly more hold. The same basic comments apply.

☹ **Le Gel Super Hold, Super Hold Texture & Shine** *($10 for 8 ounces)* contains the preservative Kathon CG, and is not recommended.

☹ **Regide Mega Hold Spritz, Mega Hold Lift & Shine** *($10 for 8 ounces)* contains the preservative Kathon CG, and is not recommended.

☺ **Basic Superpac, Capillary Complex Reconstructor** *($10 for 6.8 ounces)* is a very standard conditioner that Mastey claims "drives deep into the cortex with the basic and vital nutrients to strengthen and revitalize damaged hair." The nutrients (vitamins) in this conditioner have no effect on hair because hair is dead and cannot be nourished from the outside in. This is a good conditioner for normal to dry hair of any thickness, but that's about it.

☺ **Moisturée Intensive Moisturizer** *($12 for 8 ounces)* is a good, though standard, conditioner for normal to slightly dry hair of any thickness.

MASTEY LUMINEUX

☹ **Lumineux Shine Gloss** *($15 for 5.1 ounces)* contains the preservative Kathon CG, and is not recommended.

☹ **Lumineux Super Body Shine Gel** *($15 for 5.1 ounces)* contains the preservative Kathon CG, and is not recommended.

☺ $$$ **Lumineux High Gloss Shine Mist** *($15 for 4 ounces)* is a standard silicone spray that can be a good option for adding a halo of shine to all hair types. This feels light but can make hair look greasy unless it is used sparingly.

MASTEY PURE COLORCARE

☺ $$$ **Pure Colorcare Moisture Sulfate-Free Shampoo** *($19.99 for 16 ounces)* is similar to the Enové Volumizing Creme Shampoo above, except this contains a greater amount of emollients and conditioning agents, which makes it a good choice for dry to very dry hair that is normal to coarse or thick. The sunscreen agents cannot protect hair from UV damage because they are rinsed away; also, no standards have been established to measure how much sun protection they would provide if they did cling to the hair shaft.

☺ $$$ **Pure Colorcare Volume Sulfate-Free Shampoo, for Fine Hair** *($19.99 for 16 ounces)* is nearly identical to the Pure Colorcare Moisture Sulfate-Free Shampoo, except this contains slightly fewer emollients, though it is still a rich shampoo. This is too heavy for fine hair, but otherwise the same basic comments apply.

☺ $$$ **Pure Colorcare Moisture Daily Conditioner** *($19.99 for 16 ounces)* is a good, though standard, conditioner for dry hair of any thickness, but the price is out of line for what you get.

☺ $$$ **Pure Colorcare Volume Daily Conditioner, for Fine Hair** *($19.99 for 16 ounces)* is nearly identical to the Pure Colorcare Moisture Daily Conditioner above, and the same comments apply. This is a bit too heavy for regular use by those with fine or thin hair.

☹ **Pure Colorcare Glaze Defining Creme, for Hold & Texture** *($14.99 for 8 ounces)* contains the preservative Kathon CG, and is not recommended.

☺ $$$ **Pure Colorcare Hold Super Hairspray, for Lasting Style Support** *($14.99 for 8 ounces)* is a very good, medium- to firm-hold nonaerosol hairspray that leaves hair feeling minimally stiff but slightly sticky, though it can be brushed through without incident.

☹ **Pure Colorcare Straight Styling Straightener, Controls Frizz** *($14.99 for 8 ounces)* contains the preservative Kathon CG, and is not recommended.

☹ **Pure Colorcare Lockdown Color Protector & Heat Shield, Leave-On Conditioner, Texturizer** *($14.99 for 8 ounces)* contains the preservative Kathon CG, and is not recommended.

☺ **$$$ Pure Colorcare Repair Intense Reconstructor, for Damaged Hair** *($19.99 for 8 ounces)* is similar to the Moisturée Intensive Moisturizer above, and the same basic comments apply. This formula is slightly better for drier hair, but is a very standard conditioner for the price, and it absolutely cannot reconstruct hair.

MASTEY SOLFILTRE

☺ **$$$ Solfiltre Swimmer's Shampoo** *($11 for 8.5 ounces)* doesn't contain any chelating agents, so it cannot remove mineral or chlorine buildup from hair. It is a standard, gentle shampoo that is similar to the Enové Volumizing Creme Shampoo above, only here you get less product for your money.

☺ **$$$ Solfiltre Protege Hair Sunscreen** *($11 for 8 ounces)* is nearly identical to the Liquid Pac above, and the same basic comments apply. The sunscreens it contains cannot protect hair from UV damage, and the preservative Kathon CG makes this a problem for the scalp if you leave it in the hair. The smiley face rating is for this lightweight conditioner's performance as a rinse-out product.

☺ **Solfiltre Swimmer's Shield** *($10 for 8 ounces)* would be a poor choice to use while swimming because the water-soluble ingredients cannot cling to hair when submerged in water, whether in a pool or the ocean. This can be a good rinse-out detangler to use after swimming, and the high amount of chelating agent can remove chlorine and minerals (such as those from salt water) buildup. For significant hair protection while swimming, either coat the hair from roots to tips with a silicone serum or wear a bathing cap.

MATRIX

Matrix is perhaps one of the best-known, most widely distributed, and heavily advertised salon hair-care lines. It is sold in over 80,000 salons in the United States, and rightly stakes its claim as the leading professional hair-care company. On the scene since 1980, Matrix began as an independent company and has had its share of owners over the past two decades, resulting in a huge assortment of products that could benefit from thoughtful streamlining. L'Oreal purchased Matrix from former owner Bristol Myers–Squibb in April 2000. Since then, Matrix has routinely launched new product lines, while doing little with the assemblage of products that have accumulated over the years. What's interesting to note is that since L'Oreal has been at the helm, Matrix products that have launched under their guidance are some of the best the company has produced in years. They are by no means groundbreaking or unique formulations, but they compete well with other salon lines such as Paul Mitchell, Joico, and Graham Webb.

Of course, the claims for these products run the gamut, with each sub-line touting its special benefits, whether it is creating measurably thicker hair, protecting color-treated hair from fading, or turning rebellious curls into humidity-resistant, well-mannered ringlets. To some extent, the ingredients in each respective line's products have capabilities that partially jibe with their claims, but to read the ad copy and the product descriptions, you would think every Matrix product was its own small miracle for whatever hair crisis it pledges to avert or remedy. When you sum up all the hype, it's clear that the majority of Matrix products cannot match their too-good-to-be-true claims. That's not to say that they aren't worth considering, because most of them will take care of your hair very nicely—just not to the extent stated in the claims.

Beneath the shiny veneer of attractive packaging and salon lineage, Matrix uses the same hair-care ingredients as countless other lines. That's primarily because the pool of ingredients from which to create hair-care products is quite limited, especially compared to the choices a cosmetics chemist has at his disposal for skin-care products. With hair-care products, it's essentially as if hundreds of chefs were preparing cuisine from the same cookbook, but serving each "new" dish on a different plate. For more information about Matrix, call (800) 6-MATRIX or visit www.matrix.com.

What's Good About This Line: A very good selection of conditioners, though those with very dry hair that is thick or coarse will want to look elsewhere; styling products feature a few unique options and almost all of them perform admirably for a wide variety of hair types and hairstyle preferences.

What's Not So Good About It: Matrix needs to overhaul many of its shampoos because too many contain drying detergent cleansing agents that harm the hair and scalp; a few random products contain the problematic preservatives methylchloroisothiazolinone and methylisothiazolinone (Kathon CG); Matrix Essentials contains a few dated products that the line could do without; formulations between lines tend to be repetitive.

MATRIX AMPLIFY VOLUMIZING SYSTEM

☹ **Amplify Volumizing System, Color XL Shampoo** *($11.95 for 13.5 ounces)* contains sodium lauryl sulfate as one of its main detergent cleansing agents, which makes it too drying for hair and too drying and irritating for the scalp.

☹ **Amplify Volumizing System, Volumizing Shampoo** *($11.95 for 13.5 ounces)* is similar to the Amplify Volumizing System, Color XL Shampoo above, and the same comments apply.

☺ **Amplify Volumizing System, Instant Conditioner** *($10.95 for 8 ounces)* is a good, fairly lightweight conditioner for normal to slightly dry hair that is normal to fine or thin.

☺ **Amplify Volumizing System, Volumizing Conditioner** *($12.95 for 13.5 ounces)* is a very standard, but good, conditioner that is best for normal to dry hair of any thickness.

☺ **Amplify Volumizing System, Foam Volumizer** *($11.95 for 9 ounces)* is a standard, propellant-based mousse that has a very light texture and provides minimal hold with not a trace of stiffness or stickiness. It can work well for normal to fine or thin hair that needs body.

☺ $$$ **Amplify Volumizing System, Gel-Wax** *($12.95 for 5.1 ounces)* is misnamed: There is no wax in this product, nor does it have a waxlike consistency. It's a jellylike styling gel that provides a light hold with a silky, almost weightless finish. It is ideal for smoothing normal to fine hair or creating softly defined curls or waves with no stiff or sticky feeling.

☺ **Amplify Volumizing System, Hair Spray** *($11.95 for 10 ounces)* is a great aerosol hairspray if you're looking for a weightless product that offers a light hold without stiffness or stickiness. Hair can be easily brushed through, and you can actually apply quite a bit of this before it starts to feel heavy, which makes this a smart choice for fine or thin hair.

☺ **Amplify Volumizing System, Liquid Gel** *($9.95 for 5.1 ounces)* is a standard styling gel capable of providing a light hold with minimal stiff or sticky feel, so hair is easy to brush through.

☺ **Amplify Volumizing System, Root Lifter** *($11.95 for 8.5 ounces)* is a standard, alcohol-free styling spray that offers a light, touchable hold without stickiness. This contains some good water-binding agents to moisturize dry hair and help it feel softer.

☺ **$$$ Amplify Volumizing System, Spray-Gel** *($12.95 for 5.1 ounces)* is a fairly basic, alcohol-free spray gel that contains mostly water, holding agent, plant oil, film-forming agent, fragrance, panthenol, and preservatives. It leaves hair feeling moist and flexible while providing a light hold with minimal stickiness.

☺ **Amplify Volumizing System, Spritz** *($9.95 for 8.5 ounces)* is a silky-feeling hairspray with a light hold and minimal stiff or sticky feel, and is easily brushed through.

MATRIX BIOLAGE

☹ **Biolage Color Care Shampoo** *($9.95 for 16 ounces)* contains sodium lauryl sulfate as one of its main detergent cleansing agents, and is not recommended.

☹ **Biolage Energizing Shampoo** *($9.95 for 16 ounces)* contains sodium lauryl sulfate, and can be drying to hair and drying and irritating to the scalp.

☹ **Biolage Fortifying Shampoo** *($9.95 for 16 ounces)* contains TEA-lauryl sulfate as its sole detergent cleansing agent, which isn't fortifying in the least. This shampoo is too drying for all hair and scalp types.

☹ **Biolage Hydrating Shampoo** *($9.95 for 16 ounces)* is almost identical to the Biolage Color Care Shampoo above, and the same comments apply.

☹ **Biolage Normalizing Shampoo** *($9.95 for 16 ounces)* is almost identical to the Biolage Color Care Shampoo above, and the same comments apply.

☺ **Biolage Ultra-Hydrating Shampoo** *($9.95 for 16.9 ounces)* is actually a very good conditioning shampoo for normal to dry hair.

☺ **Biolage Color Care Conditioner** *($10.95 for 13.5 ounces)* is a great conditioner for normal to dry hair of any thickness, color-treated or not. The sunscreen ingredient would be rinsed away and cannot provide any UV protection.

☺ **$$$ Biolage Conditioning Balm** *($14.95 for 8 ounces)* is a standard, rather boring, lightweight conditioner for normal to slightly dry hair that is normal to fine or thin.

☺ **Biolage Daily Leave-In Tonic** *($11.95 for 13.5 ounces)* is a lightweight, leave-in conditioner that can work well to smooth and detangle normal to fine or thin hair.

☺ **Biolage Detangling Solution** *($10.95 for 13.5 ounces)* is a very standard conditioner that is an option for normal to dry hair of any thickness.

☺ $$$ **Biolage Earth Tones Color Refreshing Conditioner** *($14.95 for 5.1 ounces)* is a standard, but good, conditioner for normal to slightly dry hair of any thickness. This is, of course, available in several shades to enhance hair color. The coloring agents are basic (not natural) dyes, and they can impart subtle color to hair, whether it is red, brunette, blonde, or silver/gray.

☺ $$$ **Biolage Fortifying Conditioner** *($14.95 for 8 ounces)* is about as fortifying for hair as dumping vitamins in the wastebasket would be for your body. This is a very standard conditioner that, for the money, can be easily replaced by any L'Oreal Vive conditioner. The plant and flower extracts have no effect on the hair, though they do contribute to this product's fragrance.

☺ $$$ **Biolage Fortifying Leave-In Treatment** *($12.95 for 8 ounces)* is a lightweight, leave-in conditioner that can work well for normal to slightly dry hair that is normal to fine or thin.

☺ $$$ **Biolage Ultra-Hydrating Balm** *($14.95 for 8.5 ounces)* is similar to the Biolage Fortifying Conditioner above, except this contains an increased level of emollients, and that makes it preferred for drier hair of any thickness, but especially coarse or thick.

☺ **Biolage Complete Control Hair Spray, Adjustable Hold** *($10.95 for 10 ounces)* is a weightless aerosol hairspray that can provide a light hold without stiffness or stickiness. It is an excellent option for those who need an extra touch of hold without any tackiness, and it allows hair to be easily brushed through.

☺ **Biolage Curl Defining Creme** *($12.95 for 8 ounces)* is a slightly creamy styling balm without hold that can work well to smooth slightly dry to dry hair that is normal to fine or thin. For curly hair, this can help define and shape curls while doing a reasonably good job of minimizing frizzies. The quantity of "special" milk proteins amounts to almost nothing.

☹ **Biolage Defining Elixir, Texturizing Jelly** *($10.95 for 3.5 ounces)* is a substandard styling gel that is prone to flaking and balling up in the hair, probably as a result of incompatibility between the film-forming/holding agent and the guar-based thickener.

☺ **Biolage Finishing Spritz, Firm Hold** *($9.95 for 13.5 ounces)* is a standard, medium-hold hairspray that leaves hair minimally stiff or sticky and can be easily brushed through.

☺ **Biolage Gelee, Firm Control** *($9.95 for 13.5 ounces)* is a standard styling gel that is capable of medium hold and leaves hair feeling slightly stiff and sticky, though it can be brushed through.

☺ **Biolage Glaze, Soft Control** *($10.95 for 13.5 ounces)* is a fluid styling gel with a light hold and a soft, minimally sticky finish. This can be a great option for creating softer styles or defining curls and waves without heaviness.

The Reviews M

☺ **Biolage Hydro-Foaming Styler, Firm Control** *($10.95 for 9 ounces)* is nearly identical to the Amplify Volumizing System, Foam Volumizer above, and the same review applies.

☺ **Biolage Shaping Creme-Wax** *($12.95 for 4.2 ounces)* is a lightweight, silky-feeling styling cream that is an option for straightening hair with heat- or diffuser-drying curly or wavy hair when soft texture and definition are preferred. Despite the holding agent, this does not get stiff or sticky.

☺ **Biolage Smoothing Shine Milk** *($12.95 for 8.5 ounces)* is a watery silicone spray that goes on light and not the least bit greasy. It is appropriate for all hair types that need minimal smoothing or a touch of extra conditioning with their styling products. This does not contain holding agents and dries to a silky-smooth finish.

☺ **Biolage Thermal-Active Setting Spray, Pre-Heat Styling Treatment** *($10.95 for 8 ounces)* contains little that makes it preferred to use prior to heat styling. This is just a standard styling spray with medium hold that remains slightly sticky, though it can be good for stubborn hair.

☹ **Biolage Hydro-Active Hair Masque** *($10.95 for 4 ounces)* contains the absorbent magnesium aluminum silicate as one of its main ingredients, which compromises this product's moisturizing abilities and makes it rather useless as a special treatment for hair. The water, slip agent, and thickener, which are listed before the absorbent, show up in almost every Biolage conditioner reviewed above, and you would be better off using any of those as a hair mask or overnight treatment.

☺ **Biolage Shine Renewal** *($13.95 for 3.9 ounces)* is a standard silicone serum with added plant oil and emollient. That makes it more conditioning, but this is not dramatically different from the silicone serums being sold at the drugstore for half the cost of this one. It can definitely help smooth frizzies and add shine.

MATRIX CURL.LIFE

☺ **curl.life shampoo** *($8.99 for 13.5 ounces)* is a great conditioning shampoo for normal to dry hair of any thickness, be it curly or straight.

☺ **curl.life conditioner** *($9.49 for 13.5 ounces)* is nearly identical to L'Oreal's Vive Curl-Moisture Conditioner, for Curly Hair ($4.49 for 13 ounces), and is a good conditioner for normal to slightly dry hair that is normal to fine or thin. As mentioned above, L'Oreal owns Matrix.

☺ $$$ **curl.life contouring cream, for thick/coarse hair** *($10.99 for 5.1 ounces)* is a thin-textured, well-formulated styling cream that is too light for thick or coarse hair but can be a great leave-in conditioner for normal to fine or thin hair, be it curly or straight. This can provide a slight amount of heat protection and help control frizzies.

☺ $$$ **curl.life contouring milk, for normal/fine hair** *($10.99 for 5.1 ounces)* is similar to, but slightly lighter than, the curl.life contouring cream, for thick/coarse hair above, and the same basic comments apply.

MATRIX ESSENTIALS

☹ **Matrix Essentials Actrol Dandruff Shampoo** *($12 for 16 ounces)* contains sodium lauryl sulfate as one of its main detergent cleansing agents, which makes this too drying for both hair and scalp. It also contains menthol, which increases the irritation factor even more.

☹ **Matrix Essentials Alternate Actions Clarifying Shampoo** *($11.45 for 16 ounces)* contains both sodium lauryl sulfate and TEA-lauryl sulfate, which makes this below-average shampoo doubly drying for hair and scalp.

☺ **Matrix Essentials Color Therapy Shampoo** *($10 for 16 ounces)* is a very good shampoo for all hair types and it poses no risk of buildup. This can remove mineral and styling product buildup from hair.

☺ **Matrix Essentials Nourishing Shampoo** *($10 for 16 ounces)* is a good, basic shampoo for all hair types that contains such a tiny amount of conditioning agents that buildup will not be a problem.

☺ **Matrix Essentials Perm Fresh Shampoo** *($9 for 16 ounces)* is a standard shampoo with light conditioning properties that can be helpful for normal to slightly dry hair that is normal to fine or thin. Nothing about this shampoo is particularly beneficial for permed hair.

☺ **Matrix Essentials Simply Clean Shampoo** *($10 for 16 ounces)* is nearly identical to the Matrix Essentials Nourishing Shampoo above, and the same review applies.

☺ **Matrix Essentials SoSilver Shampoo** *($9 for 16 ounces)* is nearly identical to the Matrix Essentials Nourishing Shampoo above, except this contains a violet coloring agent to help offset brassy or yellow tones. This type of coloring agent doesn't cling well to the hair, though, so you'll get little if any effect.

☹ **Matrix Essentials Color Therapy Leave-In Conditioner** *($9.25 for 12 ounces)* contains the preservative Kathon CG, and is not recommended. Even if it didn't contain this problematic ingredient, it would still be a below-average leave-in conditioner that pales in comparison to the other leave-in options by Matrix.

☺ **Matrix Essentials Color Therapy Revitalizing Conditioner** *($8 for 4 ounces)* is a good option for normal to dry hair of any thickness, but holds no special benefit for color-treated hair.

☺ **Matrix Essentials Nutrient-Rich Conditioner** *($9 for 4 ounces)* is similar to the Biolage Conditioning Balm above, except this is a more well-rounded formulation that can be better for dry (but not very dry or coarse) hair. Otherwise, the same basic comments apply.

☺ **Matrix Essentials Proforma Hair Spray** *($11.95 for 12 ounces)* is a standard aerosol hairspray with a light to medium hold and a slight stiff, sticky feel. It is basically interchangeable with the Matrix aerosol hairspray options above, though it's not quite as modern in feel and finish.

☺ **Matrix Essentials Sculpting Glaze** *($8 for 13.5 ounces)* is a lightweight, liquid styling gel that provides a light to medium hold with some residual stickiness, though hair is easy to brush through. The conditioning agents can have a slight impact on dry hair, but this product can work for any hair type, even if it is not much help for frizz control.

☺ **Matrix Essentials Vital Control Hair Spray** *($11.95 for 14.8 ounces)* is nearly identical to the Matrix Essentials Proforma Hair Spray above, and the same review applies.

☺ **Matrix Essentials 5+Protopak Restructurizing Treatment** *($3.25 for 1 ounce)* is a dated formulation that cannot restructure a single hair. It is an unexciting product that can be OK for creating a fuller appearance and thicker feel on fine or thin hair.

☺ **Matrix Essentials Body & Strength Reconstructor** *($11.50 for 8 ounces)* contains primarily shampoo-type ingredients as the backbone of a misguided formula, and it pales in comparison to almost all of the Matrix conditioners above. This provides little in the way of conditioning—and nothing in terms of reconstruction—for any hair type.

☺ **$$$ Matrix Essentials Instacure Leave-In Treatment** *($14.50 for 12 ounces)* is very similar to the Matrix Biolage Daily Leave-In Tonic above, and the same review applies.

☺ **Matrix Essentials Perm Fresh Leave-In Treatment** *($9.95 for 12 ounces)* is a very standard, leave-in conditioner that functions more as a setting lotion with light, flexible hold.

☹ **Matrix Essentials Perm Fresh Moisture Supply Hydrator** *($9 for 3.5 ounces)* contains several fragrant plant oils that can be irritating to the scalp, and the scalp of those with permed hair is likely already irritated from the chemical process.

☺ **Matrix Essentials Simply Silk Detangling Rinse** *($9 for 13.5 ounces)* is a good, basic conditioner for normal to dry hair that is normal to fine or thin.

MATRIX LOGICS

☹ **Logics Balancing Shampoo** *($9 for 13.5 ounces)* is similar to the Biolage Color Care Shampoo above, and the same review applies.

☹ **Logics Clarifying Shampoo** *($9.95 for 13.5 ounces)* is similar to the Biolage Color Care Shampoo above, and the same review applies.

☹ **Logics Remoisturizing Shampoo** *($9.95 for 13.5 ounces)* is similar to the Biolage Color Care Shampoo above, and the same review applies.

☺ **Logics Colorsure Conditioner** *($11 for 13.5 ounces)* is a very good conditioner for normal to dry hair of any thickness. The sunscreen ingredient cannot protect hair from sun damage.

☹ **Logics Leave-In Protector** *($11 for 13.5 ounces)* contains the preservative Kathon CG, which is contraindicated for use in leave-on products because of the risk of causing a sensitizing reaction on the skin and scalp.

☺ **Logics Forming Foam** *($11.95 for 10 ounces)* is nearly identical to the Amplify Volumizing System, Foam Volumizer above, and the same review applies.

☺ **Logics Performance Spray** *($11.95 for 10 ounces)* cannot protect color-treated hair from the damaging effects of the sun, even though it contains sunscreen, because without an SPF number you have no idea how much protection you're getting (for example, it could be an SPF 2). Moreover, the FDA has legitimate reasons for not allowing hair-care products to have an SPF rating. This is a good, standard aerosol hairspray capable of medium hold with a slightly sticky finish that can be brushed through.

☺ **Logics Thermal Fixative** *($11.95 for 13.5 ounces)* is nearly identical to the Biolage Thermal-Active Setting Spray, Pre-Heat Styling Treatment above, and the same review applies, though here you get more product for your money.

☺ **Logics Total Hold Spritz** *($8.95 for 13.5 ounces)* contains nothing that can revitalize color-treated hair, unless standard hairspray ingredients are your idea of a pick-me-up for dyed locks. This nonaerosol spray offers a light to medium hold with minimal stiff or sticky feel, and can be easily brushed through.

MATRIX SLEEK.LOOK

☺ **sleek.look Shampoo** *($10.95 for 13.5 ounces)* is a gentle conditioning shampoo that contains enough silicone to cause buildup with repeated use. This would work well for coarse, thick, or curly hair, but it should be alternated with a shampoo that does not contain conditioning agents. The small amount of salicylic acid will have no effect on hair, and that is a good thing, because there is no need to exfoliate the hair; doing so would only cause damage to the cuticle.

☺ **sleek.look Conditioner** *($12.95 for 13.5 ounces)* is a basic, though good, conditioner that is similar to L'Oreal's Vive Color- and Curl-Care conditioners. Remember, L'Oreal owns Matrix, and your hair won't notice a difference whether you choose their salon products or their drugstore products. This conditioner is best for all except fine or thin hair types, and, contrary to the claim, it cannot keep humidity off the hair. If that were the goal (and it's one that's nearly impossible to achieve), the ideal would be to use a leave-in anti-humidity product such as the Extreme Styling Cream below, or any silicone serum.

☺ $$$ **sleek.look Extreme Styling Cream** *($14.95 for 5.1 ounces)* is supposed to "transform curly, frizzy, dry, or coarse hair into a salon-smooth, sensuously sleek style." What Matrix leaves out is that it will take a good deal of time, tension, and heat styling to turn curly or frizzy hair into something resembling sleek (straight) hair. This very emollient cream can definitely help keep frizzies at bay, but it's best used by those with thick, coarse hair. Someone with fine to normal curly hair will find that it looks too greasy and feels heavy. Extreme Styling Cream contains mostly water, petrolatum (Vaseline), emollient, silicone, thickeners, preservative, fragrance, mineral oil, and water-binding agents. It does not offer any hold.

☺ $$$ **sleek.look Lite Styling Cream** *($14.95 for 5.1 ounces)* is similar to the Extreme Styling Cream above, only without the Vaseline and prominent silicone. This formula is ideal for normal to fine hair, whether curly or straight.

The Reviews M

☺ $$$ sleek.look Water-Free Lockdown Spray *($14.95 for 4.2 ounces)* doesn't contain any water, but that leaves alcohol as the carrier for this standard silicone spray. This also contains a film-forming agent that provides a light, non-stiff hold. There isn't anything about this formula that makes it worth considering over silicone sprays available at the drugstore, but it can help manage frizzies.

☺ $$$ sleek.look Deep Moisture Masque *($14.95 for 8.5 ounces)* is a great, though standard, conditioner for normal to dry hair of any thickness. It does not deserve consideration as a special treatment for hair because the formulation doesn't bear that out.

☺ $$$ sleek.look Sealing Serum *($12.95 for 1.7 ounces)* is a standard, but good, silicone serum that would work as well as any to tame frizzies and smooth dry ends while creating fantastic shine.

MATRIX TRIX

☺ BigTrix, Boost-It Mousse *($11.95 for 8.4 ounces)* is the only Matrix mousse that provides considerable hold, and that makes it a very good option for normal to fine or thin hair that needs body and fullness with strong style support. The only drawback is that this can leave hair feeling stiff and sticky, though it softens when the hair is brushed through.

☹ DirtyTrix Messy Matte Clay *($16.95 for 2.6 ounces)* is one of the newer breed of pomades that take traditional pomade ingredients like petrolatum, wax, and mineral oil and throw clay into the mix for a matte, pliable, moldable finish. This gives it an extremely thick, pastelike consistency that is difficult to work with and distribute evenly through hair, or even to control over individual sections. This particular product does feel like a dirty trick, because getting this stuff off your hands is difficult by itself, and then getting it out of your hair takes several attempts with shampoo, and even that doesn't remove all of it. I'm sure this might appeal to edgy, urban clients who wish to exaggerate the texture of their hair, and I wish them much luck in dealing with this product!

☺ $$$ FlikTrix, Piece-Out Wax *($16.95 for 2.6 ounces)* is a traditional styling wax, packaged in a decidedly untraditional roll-up, deodorant-style container. This castor oil–based wax is great for smoothing frizz or taming flyaway strands—but use it sparingly, or your hair will look too greasy or matted. This is much more water-soluble than the DirtyTrix Messy Matte Clay above, and you can achieve the same effect, albeit with shine.

☺ FreezeTrix, Fast Fix Spray *($11.95 for 12 ounces)* is a fast-drying aerosol hairspray meant to freeze hair in place within seconds, something it absolutely can do. This is Matrix's strongest-hold aerosol hairspray, but it still manages to be minimally sticky, although hair can be a bit difficult to brush through. This is best for hold you don't intend to disturb until your next shampoo.

☺ $$$ GlowTrix Luminous Creme Smoother *($16.95 for 3.4 ounces)* is a standard water- and silicone-based styling cream that contains additional emollients and plant oil for extra conditioning. This does not contain any holding agents, is excellent for smoothing the hair and adding shine when used sparingly, and does it without adding a stiff or sticky feel to hair. Those with thick or coarse hair will have the best results with this product, but normal hair can use it, too, though not with a heavy hand.

☺ $$$ **SwitchTrix, Wax-Gel Combo** *($15.95 for 3.4 ounces)* doesn't contain any wax, but it is a thick, heavy-duty gel that is best for creating sleek, frizz-free styles on thick or coarse hair that is straight or curly. It provides groomed control while maintaining a soft, pliable finish, works equally well on wet or dry hair, and is reasonably water-soluble.

☺ $$$ **TexTrix Texture Blast Spray** *($16.95 for 5.1 ounces)* is just a styling spray with a light to medium hold that allows hair to be easily brushed through. It is best used on damp hair, but also works on dry hair; just be aware that it has a longer drying time than traditional hairsprays.

☺ $$$ **TufTrix Strong Twisted Gel** *($16.95 for 5.1 ounces)* is a standard, firm-hold styling gel that can work well to create complex or detailed styles on all hair types. It is also a gel to consider if you have stubborn curls or waves, though it does leave hair feeling slightly sticky.

MATRIX VAVOOM

☹ **Vavoom Styling Shampoo** *($8 for 16 ounces)* contains sodium polystyrene sulfonate, which can be too drying for all hair and scalp types.

☺ **Vavoom Styling Conditioner** *($9 for 16 ounces)* is a very good moisturizing conditioner for normal to dry hair of any thickness, and can make unruly hair easy to comb through.

☺ $$$ **Vavoom Designing, Beam Shine Gloss** *($12 for 1.7 ounces)* is a standard, water-soluble, gel-based pomade that contains colored mica particles for shimmery shine. This can be a good smoothing pomade for all hair types, and can add a wet-look shine to hair while controlling frizzies. Use it sparingly on normal to fine or thin hair.

☺ **Vavoom Designing, Morph Cream Wax** *($10.50 for 3 ounces)* is a slightly thicker, more emollient version of the Vavoom Designing, Beam Shine Gloss above. It is preferred for grooming and curl/wave definition on dry to very dry hair that is thick or coarse. This is reasonably water-soluble, which makes it easier to shampoo out.

☺ **Vavoom Finishing, Freezing Spray** *($12.95 for 14.8 ounces)* is similar to the Amplify Volumizing System, Hair Spray above, and the same review applies.

☺ **Vavoom Finishing, Spritzing Spray Extra** *($8 for 13.5 ounces)* is nearly identical to the Biolage Finishing Spritz, Firm Hold above, and the same review applies.

☺ **Vavoom Styling, Forming Gel** *($10.30 for 13.5 ounces)* is a standard styling gel whose hold and finish are nearly identical to the TufTrix Strong Twisted Gel above, and the same comments apply.

☺ **Vavoom Styling, Glazing** *($10.30 for 13.5 ounces)* is a medium-hold styling gel with a liquidy texture that is easy to distribute through the hair. This is basically an all-purpose styling product for creating wet looks or adding body and brushable hold to uncomplicated hairstyles. If used to straighten hair, it should be mixed with a styling cream or silicone serum for frizz control and smoothness.

☺ **Vavoom Styling, Smoothing Gel** *($12.60 for 9.3 ounces)* is a silky, ultra-light smoothing gel that provides almost no hold but leaves hair feeling soft and lightly groomed. It is best for normal to fine or thin hair that does not require hold. Smoothing Gel does not leave a trace of stiffness or stickiness.

☺ **Vavoom Styling, Volumizing Foam** *($10.95 for 9 ounces)* is nearly identical to the BigTrix, Boost-It Mousse above, and the same review applies.

MICHAEL diCESARE

Celebrity hairstylist Michael diCesare began his career at age 18 under the tutelage of fellow hairstylist Paul Mitchell, and has been working steadily ever since, most frequently in the television industry where he has participated in many makeover shows and has attended to the coiffures of discerning famous women such as Martha Stewart and Oprah Winfrey. There is no doubt he can style hair, but what about the products that bear his name? Michael diCesare says he decided to create his own line of hair-care products because he wanted consumers to experience the same professional results at home that they receive in salons. That statement is a common hook to convince you that salon or "professional" lines are inherently better than "store-bought" or mass-market lines, but it's not true in the least. Research, professional industry journals, cosmetics chemists (and very likely your own experiences with hair-care products) have consistently demonstrated that this is just not the case.

What it boils down to is that the majority of hair-care products do their respective jobs very well, regardless of price or where they're retailed. What is left out of the whole "salon results at home" claim are the talented hairstylists themselves! There is no way any of the products below can help you experience the same results you get from your stylist unless you happen to be adept at styling your own hair. The stylist's skills (and his or her vantage point while heat-styling your hair) are what create the result you love when you look in the mirror, rather than the products themselves. The diCesare products include some great options, but nothing about the formulas is unique to this line, making it just one more hair-care line to consider. Michael diCesare products are sold primarily on the QVC shopping network. For more information about Michael diCesare, call (800) 367-9444 or visit www.michaeldicesare.com (**Note:** this Web site takes you to www.qvc.com).

What's Good About This Line: Some worthwhile conditioners for normal to fine or thin hair; a few of the styling products earn high marks for hold and smoothing ability.

What's Not So Good About It: Most of the shampoos use detergent cleansing agents that can be drying to hair as well as drying and irritating to the scalp; several of the spray-on styling products tend to ball up and flake after they are applied to hair, a rarity in today's hair-care market.

☺ **AquaBiotic Energizing Shampoo** *($12 for 8.75 ounces)* is a standard shampoo that is a good option for all hair types, and poses minimal to no risk of buildup.

☺ **Clarifying Oat Hair Wash** *($9.75 for 8.75 ounces)* is a standard shampoo that is an option for all hair types. It poses no risk of buildup.

☹ **For Blondes Shampoo** *($13.25 for 8.45 ounces)* contains sodium C14-16 olefin sulfonate as its main detergent cleansing agent, which makes this too drying and irritating for all hair and scalp types.

☹ **Purifying Oat Hair Wash, Daily Shampoo** *($9.75 for 8.75 ounces)* contains sodium lauryl and TEA-lauryl sulfates, and is not recommended for any hair or scalp type.

☹ **Sterling Silver Shampoo, Brightens Silver, White and Gray Hair** *($10.50 for 5.75 ounces)* contains a tiny amount of violet dye to help counteract yellow or brassy tones in silver hair, but the inclusion of sodium C14-16 sulfonate makes this shampoo too drying for this or any other hair color (or type). There are better, gentler color-enhancing shampoos available.

☺ **$$$ AquaBiotic Sea Rinse Daily Rinse Out Conditioner** *($13 for 8.75 ounces)* is an OK moisturizing and detangling option for normal to slightly thick hair that is dry.

☺ **$$$ Hydration Daily Conditioner** *($12.75 for 8.5 ounces)* is a silky-feeling conditioner that can be a very good option for normal to dry hair of any thickness, especially for those with hair that needs help with detangling and smoothing.

☺ **$$$ Amplifying Tonic Hair Thickener** *($16 for 8.75 ounces)* is a standard, water- and alcohol-based styling spray that goes on moist and slightly slippery, but dries to a light, minimally sticky hold that can help make fine or thin hair feel thicker. It contains conditioning agents that won't weigh hair down but can help smooth flyaways.

☺ **Defining Ice Humectant Frost Curl Enhancer** *($12 for 2 ounces)* is a standard, gel-type pomade that is fairly water-soluble. It works well to smooth frizzies while adding texture and shine on normal to very dry hair. This has a slightly greasy feel, so use it sparingly for best results.

☹ **LiquiFix BlowOut Blow Drying Lotion** *($12 for 8.75 ounces)* is a poorly formulated styling spray that tends to ball up and flake off hair before it dries. This is not what you want from any styling product, but especially not one you plan to use while heat-styling your hair.

☺ **LiquiFix LiquiCurl Curl Enhancing Spray** *($12 for 8.75 ounces)* is similar to the Amplifying Tonic Hair Thickener above, except this contains more detangling and conditioning agents, so it is slightly preferred for drier hair. This can make curls more manageable and shapely, but any hair type or texture could use this product.

☺ **LiquiFix Liquid Mousse** *($14.25 for 8.75 ounces)* is a very light styling spray (not a mousse) that provides minimal to no hold but can provide a slight smoothing benefit to flyaway or static-prone fine or thin hair.

☺ **LiquiFix LiquiThick Thickening Mousse** *($14.50 for 7 ounces)* is a liquid-to-foam mousse that provides a medium to firm hold with a slightly stiff, moderately sticky feeling. Hair can still be brushed through, but this product can be too heavy for very fine or thin hair. It is best for normal hair that is slightly dry and needs body or lift.

The Reviews M

☺ **Managel, Maximum Hold Styling Gel** *($13.75 for 4.75 ounces)* is a standard, ho-hum styling gel with a medium to firm hold that can be brushed through. It won't weigh hair down but can leave it feeling slightly stiff and sticky.

☹ **Preserving Spray, Super Hold** *($10.50 for 8.75 ounces)* is a nonaerosol hairspray that can ball up and flake on the hair, and is not recommended.

☹ **AquaBiotic Hair and Scalp Treatment** *($45 for 15 ampoules)* comes in tiny vials of liquid that contain mostly water, alcohol, glycerin, slip agent, sea salt, plant extracts, panthenol, water-binding agents, plant oil, fragrance, preservatives, and coloring agents. It is supposed to "remineralize" the scalp to restore moisture, but a dry scalp has nothing to do with loss or imbalance of minerals, and the skin's surface doesn't contain much in the way of minerals anyway. This formula is not very hydrating, and applying the alcohol directly to the scalp can cause it to become dry. Any lotion-type leave-in conditioner would be better than this gimmicky product.

☺ **Brilliance Serum** *($12 for 1 ounce)* is a standard silicone gel that would work as well as any to smooth dry, frizzy hair and add sleek shine.

☺ **$$$ Crystal Shine Lite** *($15 for 2 ounces)* is a very good, though standard, silicone spray that can be a good option for all hair types to add a veil of glossy shine to hair. This should be used sparingly to avoid a greasy appearance. It is fragrance-free.

☹ The **3-Piece Curly Hair Kit** *($21 for kit)* includes the ☹ **LiquiFix LiquiCurl Curl Enhancing Shampoo** *(2 ounces)*, which is not recommended due to the inclusion of drying TEA-lauryl sulfate, and 2-ounce and 8.75-ounce containers of the ☺ **LiquiFix LiquiCurl Curl Enhancing Spray** reviewed above. Skip this kit and go with the larger size of the LiquiCurl Curl Enhancing Spray above if that product sounds appealing to you.

☹ The **7-Piece "Instant Fix" Haircare Kit** *($45 for kit)* includes the following products that are reviewed above: ☺ **Clarifying Oat Hair Wash** *(two 0.2-ounce samples)*, ☹ **Purifying Oat Hair Wash, Daily Shampoo** *(8.75 ounces)*, ☹ **LiquiFix BlowOut Blow Drying Lotion** *(2 ounces)*, ☺ **LiquiFix Liquid Mousse** *(8.75 ounces)*, and ☺ **Brilliance Serum** *(1 ounce)*. The following items are also included in the kit: ☹ **Lift Style Lifter** *(5 ounces)*, another styling spray that is prone to balling up and flaking off the hair, and is not recommended; and ☺ **Climatize Climate Control for Hair Control** *(10 ampoules)*, a standard styling gel whose ampoule packaging is wasteful because once the product is opened it cannot be resealed and there is enough gel in each that someone with short to medium-length hair would consistently need less than what is provided per use. The gel itself offers a light, slightly sticky hold with a silicone-smooth shine, and the silicone does help keep humidity from making hair frizzy, but the presentation of this product needs to be improved. All told, this kit is a blend of good and bad products, and nothing in it really warrants the expense.

☺ **$$$ Colour Active 2-Piece Hair Care Kit** *($28.50 for kit)* includes the **Colour Active Shampoo-In Colour Treatment** *(5 ounces)*, a color-enhancing shampoo available in four shades. One of the better shampoos in the diCesare line, this contains basic dyes to deposit a small amount of color on hair. Don't expect dramatic color-enhancing benefits from these shampoos; at best, their effect will be subtle. The ☺ **Crystal Shine Lite** *(2 ounces)*, reviewed above, rounds out this kit.

☹ **FreezeFrame Finishing Hair Spray Duo** *($30 for kit)* includes two cans of Michael diCesare's aerosol **FreezeFrame Finishing Spray** *(10 ounces)*, which is another disappointing styling product that can easily flake, not to mention that the acetone in it can be a strong scalp irritant.

☹ **Thicker and Fuller 4-Piece Hair Care Kit** *($26.81 for kit)* includes the ☺ **Thicker Hair, Thickening Shampoo** *(8.75 ounces)*, a standard shampoo that contains conditioning and film-forming agents that make it preferred for dry hair that is normal to fine or thin, though it can cause buildup with repeated use. Also included is the ☺ **Restoring Emulsion Conditioner** *(2 ounces)*, which contains mostly water, film-forming/conditioning agent, slip agent, silicone, detangling agent, water-binding agents, fragrance, and preservatives. It would be a good detangling conditioner for normal to fine or thin hair, but it will build up on hair sooner than most conditioners. The ☺ **LiquiFix LiquiThick Thickening Mousse** *(7 ounces)*, reviewed above, is a good pairing with the shampoo and conditioner in this kit. Unfortunately, the kit also contains the flake-prone ☹ **FreezeFrame Finishing Spray** *(10 ounces)*, reviewed above, though it is the only disappointment in an otherwise well-assembled group of products.

MODERN ELIXIRS BY PAUL MITCHELL

It was no surprise that Paul Mitchell created a spin-off line of hair-care products whose title sounds new and familiar at the same time. I would love to say that these are the breakthrough, undeniably "modern" formulas that are truly a step above the rest, but as is so often the case when it comes to hair-care products, familiarity reigns.

Modern Elixirs does have its share of botanical cocktails, but it is the silicones in these products that impart shine and a silky feel to hair. Silicones are by far the unsung heroes in the world of hair care, rather than the more pleasant-sounding extracts of cherry bark, nettle, and watercress, to name a few. Beyond this, you'll find dozens of tried-and-true (and also decidedly "unnatural") ingredients that are doing all of the cleansing, conditioning, detangling, and holding hair in place. There are some winning products to consider in this line, as is true for most hair-care lines. If you don't mind the cost and can get past the notion that ingredients like poplar, carrot, and mallow are essential for healthy, shiny hair, you will find most of these products are effective and pleasant to use. For more information about Modern Elixirs, call (800) 793-8790 or visit www.paulmitchell.com.

What's Good About This Line: Most of the products are effective for basic cleansing, conditioning, and styling (once you get past the natural ingredient hoopla).

What's Not So Good About It: A couple of styling products contain problematic ingredients that can cause hair dryness or scalp irritation; Modern Elixirs is not as well-rounded a line as Paul Mitchell's namesake collection, but then again, it isn't as overwhelming either!

☺ **Bodifying Shampoo** *($9.99 for 8.5 ounces)* is a standard, detergent-based shampoo that lists a film former as the second ingredient, so this will easily build up on the hair with repeated use. It is an OK option for someone with normal hair that is fine or thin. Contrary to the claim, this will not strengthen hair or control split ends, though it will temporarily coat hair and hold split ends together (to some degree) and provide a feeling of fullness.

☺ **Color Therapy Shampoo** *($10.99 for 8.5 ounces)* is a good conditioning shampoo for someone with normal to dry hair of any thickness. It can cause buildup with repeated use. There is nothing in it that can lock in color any better than dozens of other shampoos, especially when the reality is that hair does not like holding onto dyes, making a certain amount of fading inevitable regardless of the shampoo you use (though using shampoos with problematic ingredients is rarely a good idea).

☺ **Refining Shampoo** *($9.99 for 8.5 ounces)* is a standard shampoo that would work well for normal to dry hair of any thickness except fine. The silicone and conditioning agents can contribute to product buildup when used repeatedly.

☺ **$$$ Bodifying Conditioner** *($12.49 for 8.5 ounces)* is a very standard conditioner for normal to slightly dry hair of any thickness. Although the claims make this sound like a superhero for hair, you won't find much difference between this and any conditioner from Pantene.

☺ **$$$ Color Therapy Conditioner** *($12.99 for 5.1 ounces)* is a very good, silky-feeling conditioner for someone with normal to dry hair that is normal to fine in texture. It cannot protect hair color from fading in the sun, so that claim is bogus.

☺ **$$$ Refining Conditioner** *($12.49 for 5.1 ounces)* is a fairly standard, leave-in conditioner that is an option for someone with normal to dry hair that is fine or thin. The claim that this keeps hair "soft and sane" all day is merely clever marketing copy.

☺ **Defining Pomade** *($13.99 for 1.8 ounces)* is a fairly standard pomade with a thick wax and mineral oil base that is about as modern as a typewriter. This does contain some film-forming agents that can help hold the hair along with the grease and wax, but they also lend a slightly sticky feel to this must-be-used-sparingly product.

☺ **Enhancing Foam** *($9.99 for 6.8 ounces)* is a very standard styling mousse that offers a light to medium hold with a slightly stiff, sticky feel. The silicones help keep the hair soft and brushable.

☺ **Finishing Spray** *($9.99 for 8.2 ounces)* and ☺ **$$$ Firm Finishing Spray** *($11.99 for 8.2 ounces)* are basically indistinguishable from each other. Both are standard, aerosol hairsprays that come in metal containers and offer a medium hold that can feel slightly stiff and sticky. The addition of silicones and conditioning agent allows hair to remain somewhat flexible and adds shine. The Firm Finishing Spray is rated lower because it contains an appreciable amount of acetone, which can be very irritating to the scalp and drying to hair.

☺ **Frizz Complex** *($12.49 for 5.1 ounces)* is a standard gel that has a minimal to light hold and a slightly greasy finish. It should work well for smoothing out coarse, thick hair, but use it sparingly to avoid a heavy look.

☹ **Styling Creme** *($13.99 for 5.1 ounces)* is a slippery gel-cream that contains a form of sulfonic acid that can be drying to the hair and can also potentially strip hair color. This would otherwise be a good, albeit basic, light-hold styling cream for normal to dry hair that is thick or coarse.

☺ **Style Serum** *($9.99 for 8.5 ounces)* is an intensely fragranced, soft-hold liquid gel with minimal stiff or sticky feel, and it can be easily brushed through. The claim that this offers protection from the heat of styling tools is not accurate, because no product can completely protect hair from the intense heat generated by most blow dryers and curling irons.

☺ **Illuminating Shine Spray** *($13.99 for 3.8 ounces)* is an aerosol silicone spray that provides a fine mist of shine to all hair types. This can be a great finishing touch for all hair types. It would take a lot of it to make hair feel heavy, though someone with fine or thin hair should apply this sparingly to keep hair from looking greasy rather than glossy.

MOP (MODERN ORGANIC PRODUCTS)

If it grows from the ground, and you put it in a cosmetic, they will come … and then they will buy. This must be the mantra of almost every hair-care, skin-care, and makeup line around the world. American Crew adds to this irksome, misleading trend with their mop line of hair-care products, all of which have a decidedly natural point of view. At least that's what they want you to think. Only the beauty industry can use ingredients like sodium laureth sulfate, cocamidopropyl betaine, and sodium cocoyl sarcosinate and tell you straight-faced that they are equal or similar to coconut oil. They aren't in the least—they're no more related to coconut oil than a tree is equal to or similar to a piece of paper.

A bit more perplexing is the claim that the ingredients in these products are "Certified Organic in accordance with the California Food [and Organic Food] Act of 1990." The California Organic Food Act of 1990 only regulates substances used in foods, not cosmetics (Source: www.fda.gov, Part 5 of Division 104 of the Health and Safety Code, which states that the Act is "applicable to producers of food sold as organic…"). Further, the Code states, "it is unlawful for any person to commingle nonorganic commodities with commodities sold as organic either in the same container…." So while sodium laureth sulfate (one of the cleansing agents in all the mop shampoos) is derived from coconut oil, it is processed either with sulfur trioxide or chlorosulfonic acid, both of which are decidedly inorganic. And that's not to mention that other ingredients in the product are strictly inorganic. This is only one small example, but it gives you an idea why it's just nonsense to refer to or claim compliance with any organic food code when all you're selling are hair-care products.

Nevertheless, to cultivate the impression that these products are loaded with plants, the labels list a cornucopia of botanical extracts. They're used only in trace amounts, but even if they were abundantly present in the formulations, there is no research showing that rosemary, ylang-ylang, sage, blackberry, hawthorn, calendula, or matricaria have any impact on hair other than to add fragrance or impress an unaware consumer. For more information about modern organic products, call (866) 699-4667 or visit www.mopproducts.com.

What's Good About This Line: Most of the styling products work beautifully, but not because of the plant extracts they contain; the conditioners offer a range of emolliency for all hair types.

What's Not So Good About It: Several plant extracts in these products, including peppermint, eucalyptus, sage, and others, cause scalp itching and irritation.

☹ **basil mint shampoo for normal to oily hair** *($10.99 for 10.15 ounces)* contains a slew of problematic plant extracts, as well as irritating eucalyptus oil and menthol, which makes it a problem for all scalp types.

☺ **lemongrass shampoo for fine hair** *($10.99 for 10.15 ounces)* is similar to the basil mint shampoo above, except this omits the menthol and eucalyptus in favor of lemongrass oil, which isn't great but it's less of a problem. It does contain a tiny amount of conditioning agents; these can cause buildup over time, but they also make this shampoo slightly better for dry hair of any thickness. The plant extracts, from calendula, matricaria, and *Ginkgo biloba,* have no effect on hair.

☹ **mixed greens shampoo for normal to dry hair** *($10.99 for 10.15 ounces)* is almost identical to the basil mint version above, and the same concerns apply.

☺ **pear shampoo for infants & toddlers** *($10.99 for 10.15 ounces).* Mop claims this shampoo is "The kindest way we know to cleanse the wee ones" and that it is supposed to "Contain no harsh lather additives or detergents to dry out skin and scalp." I agree that this is gentler than the shampoos above, as it leaves out the problematic plant extracts. Why they couldn't do that for the adult shampoos is disappointing. Other than that, there isn't much difference between the detergent cleansing agents in this shampoo and in the ones above, which makes this a far better choice for an adult's hair as well. Pear puree only adds fragrance and makes it necessary to increase the amount of preservatives so the pear doesn't turn brown or moldy.

☺ **burdock nourishing rinse, for all hair types** *($9.99 for 10.15 ounces)* is a standard emollient conditioner that is best for normal to dry hair of any thickness, so ignore the "all hair types" designation in the name.

☺ **daily rinse conditioner** *($9.99 for 10.15 ounces).* Although the plant extracts in this conditioner can be a problem for the scalp, if you can keep this away from the scalp it is a decent option for normal to dry hair of any thickness.

☺ **extreme moisture, treatment for dry hair** *($10.99 for 6.76 ounces)* isn't extreme in the least, but it is a good conditioner for normal to dry hair that has normal to dense thickness.

☺ **extreme protein treatment for damaged hair** *($10.99 for 6.76 ounces)* definitely contains a variety of proteins, and they can be decent conditioning agents—but they are not going to do anything to change or fix damaged hair. They work like any other conditioning agent to help hair feel temporarily smoother. This is another good conditioner for normal to dry hair that is normal to thick.

☺ **leave-in conditioner** *($9.99 for 10.5 ounces)* is a very good conditioner for normal to dry hair of any thickness, and it's great that this contains only a minimum of potentially irritating plant extracts.

☺ **lemongrass conditioner, for fine hair** *($11.99 for 10.15 ounces)* is a more emollient option than the burdock nourishing rinse above, and would be too heavy for someone with fine hair. Rather, this can be a great conditioner for dry to very dry hair that is coarse or thick.

☺ **mixed greens conditioner, for normal to dry hair** *($11.99 for 10.15 ounces)* is nearly identical to the burdock nourishing rinse above, except this contains slightly more plant oil, making it preferred for drier hair. The rosemary oil can be a scalp irritant, so be careful to apply this to the hair only.

☺ **pear detangler** *($10.99 for 8.45 ounces)* is a lightweight conditioner that can work decently to detangle normal to fine or thin hair, but is not the best if your hair is prone to snarls or is routinely difficult to comb through. The pear juice won't make hair easier to comb, but it can make it feel slightly sticky.

☹ **d-curl straightening balm** *($11.99 for 4.23 ounces)* is a decent balm to help style hair if you want minimal to light hold, no greasy feel, and don't need much control to get your hair to behave. But it assuredly doesn't work without the aid of a blow dryer or other heat-styling tool.

☺ **defining cream** *($11.99 for 4.23 ounces)* is a creamy pomade that has a medium hold and a slightly stiff feel. It does let you comb through hair easily, but it can leave a slightly greasy feel on hair, so use it sparingly.

☹ **form foaming gel, heavy hold** *($10.99 for 6.76 ounces)* lists sodium polystyrene sulfonate as the second ingredient, and that can be too drying for hair and irritating for the scalp, not to mention it can potentially strip dyed hair color.

☹ **form foaming gel, light hold** *($10.99 for 6.76 ounces)* is almost identical to the form foaming gel, heavy hold above, and the same comments apply.

☺ **lemongrass lift** *($13.99 for 8.45 ounces)* is a very standard styling spray whose fragrant plant extracts (which aren't helpful for hair) are its only unique feature. It provides a light to medium hold with a slightly stiff, sticky finish that can be easily brushed through. This would work best to define unruly curls or create smooth wet looks on normal to fine or thin hair.

☺ **orange peel molding cream** *($13.99 for 2.65 ounces)* is a very traditional, lanolin-based pomade that has a light to medium hold and can leave a greasy, sticky feel in hair. This provides a low-luster finish.

☺ **pomade** *($13.99 for 2.65 ounces)* is similar to the orange peel molding cream above, only with minimal hold and reduced stickiness.

☺ **styling tonic** *($11.99 for 8.45 ounces)* is a good leave-in conditioner that has some light hold, which means it would work as a styling spray as well. It is best for someone with normal to slightly dry hair that has normal to slight thickness.

MOP C-SYSTEM

☺ **$$$ C-system clean shampoo** *($14 for 10.15 ounces)* is a standard conditioning shampoo that is best for normal to dry hair of any thickness, though it can cause a slight buildup with repeated use.

☹ **C-system hydrating shampoo** *($14 for 10.15 ounces)* begins well but ends poorly thanks to the inclusion of several irritating fragrant oils, including spearmint, lemon, lime, and ginger. This shampoo is not recommended.

☹ **C-system moisture complex, for conditioning and detangling** *($14 for 6.76 ounces)* contains higher amounts of the same irritating fragrant plant oils as the C-system hydrating shampoo above, and is not recommended.

☺ **$$$ C-system conditioning mist, light hold styling spray** *($15 for 5.1 ounces)* is more like spraying orange-scented perfume on hair than styling it. This fragrant liquid provides minimal to no hold and minimal conditioning benefits, but it's an option for casual, unstructured hairstyles.

☹ **C-system C curl** *($15 for 5.1 ounces)* contains the same irritating fragrant plant oils as the C-system hydrating shampoo above, but can be even more problematic because this is a leave-on styling product. There is little doubt this product would eventually cause an itchy, irritated scalp.

☹ **C-system C straight** *($15 for 5.1 ounces)* is more a leave-in conditioner than a traditional straightening balm, and loses points for including the same irritating fragrant plant oils as the C-system hydrating shampoo above. This can smooth and straighten hair—with heat and the proper brush—but over time will cause an itchy, irritated scalp.

☺ **$$$ C-system finishing paste, pliable hold with light shine** *($15 for 2.65 ounces)* is closer to a thick cream than a paste, and it is quite easy to work with, though only if you're in need of a heavy product to smooth frizzies and create strong texture with a medium, slightly sticky hold. This does remain workable, so you can restyle your hair as needed, but use it sparingly.

☹ **C-system styling conditioner, water activated defining lotion** *($15 for 6.76 ounces)* contains the same irritating fragrant plant oils as the C-system hydrating shampoo above, but can be even more problematic because this is a leave-in product.

☺ **$$$ C-system texture lotion, light hold with a natural finish** *($15 for 6.76 ounces)* is a slightly thick styling lotion that can work well to provide light to medium hold and a moist finish that is minimally sticky. This can make curly or wavy hair look smooth and groomed while taming frizzies, or it can work (with heat) to straighten stubborn hair.

☹ **C-system reconstructing treatment, deep conditioning for dry hair** *($16 for 6.76 ounces)* contains higher amounts of the same irritating fragrant plant oils as the C-system hydrating shampoo above, and is not recommended.

MOP GLISTEN

☺ **glisten shampoo** *($11.50 for 8.45 ounces)* is a standard shampoo that can be a good option for normal to dry hair of any thickness.

☺ **glisten conditioner** *($12.50 for 8.45 ounces)* is a good conditioner for normal to dry hair of any thickness.

☺ **glisten eco-firm, firm hold hairspray** *($14 for 5.1 ounces)* is a standard hairspray that has a light to medium hold and lets you easily brush through hair.

☺ **glisten eco-light, variable hold hairspray** *($14 for 5.1 ounces)* is similar to the eco-firm hairspray above, except this has a softer, more flexible hold and is even easier to brush through because it contains silicone.

☺ **glisten light hold gel** *($11 for 8.45 ounces)* is a good gel that offers a light to medium hold with minimal to no stiff or sticky feel.

☺ **glisten heavy hold gel, for ultimate hold** *($12 for 8.45 ounces)* has a medium hold that leaves a slight stiff, sticky feel on hair, though it can easily be brushed through.

☺ $$$ **glisten high shine pomade** *($15 for 2.05 ounces)* is a thick, transparent gel-like pomade that has a light hold and a slightly sticky feel, though it can easily be brushed through. It will help to control hair without the heavy feel of most pomades, but use it sparingly. This is relatively easy to shampoo out.

☺ **glisten volumizing spray** *($12.50 for 8.45 ounces)* has a medium hold with a slightly stiff feel that does brush through, but use it sparingly if you have fine or thin hair to prevent weighing it down.

☺ **glisten shine drops** *($12.50 for 1.7 ounces)* is a standard silicone serum that would work as well as any to impart a silky feel and shine on hair. This does contain extra emollients and plant oil, which gives it a slight edge for very dry hair.

☺ **glisten weightless spray shine** *($12.50 for 4.23 ounces)* is similar to the glisten shine drops above, only this one is in spray form.

MOLTON BROWN LONDON

This English import began in 1973 when hairstylists at London's Mayfair Studio began creating products for their "discerning international clientele" (are clientele ever non-discerning? If so, whose products do they use?). Over the years this cosmetics line (they also sell skin-care and makeup) has evolved into somewhat of a cult favorite, though for the life of me I cannot figure out why. Especially for hair care, these formulations are as basic as tossing together a vinegar and oil salad dressing and leaving out any other seasoning. The showcased ingredients are present in meager amounts, unless they're used for fragrance, and while that may create a stress-relieving olfactory sensory experience it's rather useless for your hair or scalp. In the United States, you can find Molton Brown products at select highbrow department stores, such as Barneys New York and Neiman

Marcus, and at specialty cosmetics boutiques. It is not available in Canada, but to our neighbors up north let me say, don't worry, you're not missing a thing. For more information about Molton Brown London, visit www.moltonbrown.com.

What's Good About This Line: The shampoos are mostly gentle formulations suitable for most hair types, though the fragrance can be intense.

What's Not So Good About It: The prices are ridiculous for such standard formulations; you're paying for the prestige name and English pedigree, not the product.

☺ $$$ **Cassia Energy Hair & Body Wash** *($23 for 6.6 ounces)* is an exceptionally standard, ordinary shampoo. The real question is why this shampoo is so expensive, because it contains nothing spectacular or unique to justify the price. Aside from that, it can be a good shampoo for all hair types, and will not cause buildup.

☹ **Cool Mentha Hair & Body Sportswash** *($21 for 10 ounces)* contains essential oils of lemon and mint along with menthol, and these are irritating to the skin (if used as body wash) and scalp (when used as shampoo).

☺ $$$ **Healthy Hair Revitalising Shampoo** *($19 for 10 ounces)* is very similar to the Cassia Energy Hair & Body Wash above, except this adds a silicone conditioning agent and does not contain cassia bark. Instead, it adds a Chinese fruit extract that has no established benefit for hair or scalp. The same basic comments apply.

☺ $$$ **Travel Reviving Jinang Hair & Body Wash** *($23 for 6.6 ounces)* is nearly identical to the Cassia Hair & Body Wash above. The tiny amount of added conditioning agents has no effect on hair, which means this poses no risk of buildup.

☺ $$$ **Triple Action Biao Hairwash** *($23 for 10 ounces)* is sold as a special cleanser for men, said to reduce hair loss, fight dandruff, and reduce itchy scalp. It can do none of these things, so save your money (and your hopes). This is just another very standard, overpriced shampoo that works well for men or women with normal to dry hair of any thickness, and the conditioning agents can cause slight buildup with repeated use.

☺ $$$ **Wash Baby Wash** *($19 for 10 ounces)* is a surprisingly gentle shampoo. The absence of any preservatives is cause for concern, but I suspect the ingredient list for this product was incomplete, or this would quickly deteriorate and grow moldy once opened. This shampoo is OK for babies, but would also be good for adults with any hair type provided they use a minimal amount of styling products.

☺ $$$ **Indian Cress Instant Conditioner** *($21 for 10 ounces)* is a very standard conditioner that is a decent option for normal to slightly dry hair that is normal to fine or thin, but is absolutely not worth the money.

NEUTROGENA

For more information about Neutrogena, owned by Johnson & Johnson, call (800) 582-4048 or visit www.neutrogena.com.

What's Good About This Line: Some excellent shampoos and conditioners at prices you're bound to love; normal to dry hair types and most textures (from thin to thick) are well-served by the products reviewed; one of the few lines to offer effective shampoo treatments to combat seborrhea and psoriasis.

What's Not So Good About It: Some of the anti-dandruff shampoos contain drying detergent cleansing agents and/or unnecessary irritants such as menthol; the often-repetitive formulations are not radically different from those offered by countless other lines.

☺ **Clean Balance, Normalizing Shampoo** *($3.99 for 10.1 ounces)* is a standard, light-conditioning shampoo that can work great for all hair types. This does pose a slight risk of buildup with repeated use.

☺ **Clean for Color Color-Defending Shampoo** *($3.99 for 10.1 ounces)*. Although this is a gentle shampoo that avoids harsh cleansing agents, it is still just a standard shampoo. It contains enough film-forming agents to be a problem for buildup, despite the "no color-dulling residue" claim. There is no way this or any other shampoo can "lock in color," but this is a good shampoo for normal to dry hair that is normal to coarse or thick.

☺ **Clean Replenishing, Moisturizing Shampoo** *($3.99 for 10.1 ounces)* is identical to the Clean Balance, Normalizing Shampoo above, and the same review applies. This shampoo won't dry the hair, but it doesn't provide much in the way of moisture either.

☺ **Clean Volume, Body Volumizing Shampoo** *($3.99 for 10.1 ounces)* is identical to the Clean Balance, Normalizing Shampoo above, and the same review applies. The film-forming agents in this one are good for fine or thin hair, but have ability to increase the hair's volume over time.

☹ **Healthy Scalp, Anti-Dandruff Shampoo** *($5.99 for 6 ounces)* contains 1.8% salicylic acid, which can benefit those with dandruff. However, the inclusion of sodium C14-16 olefin sulfonate makes this too drying and irritating for hair and scalp. There are much better dandruff shampoos to consider.

☺ **Shampoo, Anti-Residue Formula** *($5.69 for 6 ounces)* is a very simple shampoo that can be excellent for all hair types. Because this contains no conditioning, detangling, or film-forming agents, it poses no risk of buildup, so it should be a good shampoo to alternate with your regular conditioning shampoo. By the way, Neutrogena has been selling this shampoo since 1980!

☺ **Shampoo, Moisturizing Formula for Permed/Color Treated Hair** *($4.99 for 6 ounces)* contains glycerin, which can be a great moisturizing ingredient for dry hair, but the amount is too small to have much impact. This is really just a standard shampoo that is fairly similar to the Shampoo, Anti-Residue Formula above, meaning it contains no conditioning or film-forming agents to cause buildup and it's an option for all hair types.

☺ **T/Gel Therapeutic Shampoo, Extra Strength** *($4.99 for 4.4 ounces)* is a 1% coal tar shampoo that can be very helpful for those suffering from psoriasis or seborrhea on the scalp. The shampoo base is very standard, but it's gentle and poses minimal risk of buildup. Coal tar shampoos can be drying for hair with repeated use, so use this as infrequently as you can and still control your symptoms or be sure to follow up with an emollient conditioner, keeping it off the scalp.

☹ **T/Gel Therapeutic Shampoo, for Fine/Oily Hair** *($4.99 for 4.4 ounces)* contains 0.5% coal tar, which is less drying to hair than higher amounts, but the shampoo base contains sodium lauryl sulfate, and that by itself can dry hair and the scalp, as well as cause scalp irritation.

☺ **T/Gel Therapeutic Shampoo, Intensive Anti-Flake Treatment** *($7.50 for 4.4 ounces)* is a very good 0.5% coal tar shampoo for battling psoriasis or seborrhea on the scalp. The shampoo base is gentle and does not contain conditioning or film-forming agents, so there is no concern about buildup. Actually, the chelating agent it contains can help remove buildup!

☺ **T/Gel Therapeutic Shampoo, Original Formula** *($4.99 for 4.4 ounces)* is nearly identical to the T/Gel Therapeutic Shampoo, Intensive Anti-Flake Treatment above, and the same review applies. Why this one costs less for the same amount of product is a mystery.

☹ **T/Gel Therapeutic Shampoo, Stubborn Itch Control** *($4.99 for 4.4 ounces)* is a 0.5% coal tar shampoo that contains menthol, a counter-irritant that just replaces one form of irritation (in this case, itching) with another, that being the stronger irritation caused by the menthol when it touches your scalp.

☹ **T/Sal, Maximum Strength Therapeutic Shampoo** *($5.99 for 4.5 ounces)* is similar to the Healthy Scalp, Anti-Dandruff Shampoo above, only with 3% salicylic acid. It still contains sodium C14-16 olefin sulfonate, and as such is not recommended.

☺ **Clean Balance, Normalizing Conditioner** *($3.99 for 10.1 ounces)* is a very good, though standard, conditioner for normal to slightly dry hair of any thickness.

☺ **Clean for Color Color-Defending Conditioner** *($3.99 for 10.1 ounces)* is a great inexpensive conditioner for normal to dry hair of any thickness, but the teeny amount of sunscreen agent in this product is lost when you rinse your hair.

☺ **Clean Replenishing, 60 Second Hair Repair** *($4.99 for 5.1 ounces)* The claim that this can repair hair in one minute is clearly ludicrous or the product description wouldn't include the claim that it can "be used every day." If it repaired hair, why would you need to reapply it? Wouldn't your hair be fixed and be normal without any dryness or damage? This ends up being a very good, fairly basic conditioner that would work well for someone with normal to dry hair that is thick or coarse.

☺ **Clean Replenishing, Instant Shine Detangler** *($3.99 for 6 ounces)* can work well for normal to fine or thin hair that needs help with combing and could benefit from light moisture. This does not contain the best detangling agents for hair that is damaged and/or difficult to comb through.

☺ **Clean Replenishing, Moisturizing Conditioner** *($3.99 for 10.1 ounces)* is identical to the Clean Balance, Normalizing Conditioner above, and the same review applies.

☺ **Clean Volume, Body Volumizing Conditioner** *($3.99 for 10.1 ounces)* is identical to the Clean Balance, Normalizing Conditioner above, and the same review applies.

☺ **Conditioner, Detangling Formula** *($4.69 for 6 ounces)* is a standard conditioner that can definitely detangle hair, but also provide moisture and smoothness. It is appropriate for those with normal to dry hair that is normal to slightly thick or coarse.

☺ **Conditioner, Revitalizing Formula for Permed/Color Treated Hair** *($4.69 for 6 ounces)* can be a very good, though standard, conditioner for normal to dry hair that is normal to thick or coarse. It can help smooth and soften dry, damaged hair.

☺ **T/Gel Therapeutic Conditioner, Treatment Conditioner** *($4.99 for 4.4 ounces)* is a lightweight detangling conditioner that contains 2% salicylic acid. There is research showing that salicylic acid can benefit those with dandruff, though the drawback is it can denature the hair shaft. As a conditioner, this can work well for normal to fine or thin hair that is slightly dry or needs help with combing. As an anti-dandruff product, it is best applied directly to the scalp and not distributed through the hair.

☺ **Overnight Therapy Replenishing Treatment** *($5.99 for 6 ounces)* is a very good, silicone-based conditioner that is an option for someone with normal to dry hair of any thickness. Any conditioner you leave on your hair for any length of time, day or night, ends up making hair feel better due to the enhanced penetration that can take place when it isn't rinsed away. This really is just a leave-in conditioner with an interesting marketing twist. It does contain fragrance.

☺ **T/Gel Overnight Dandruff Treatment** *($8.99 for 6 ounces)* is a spray-on treatment for fighting dandruff and its resulting flakes. Meant to be left on overnight (and to replace your regular dandruff shampoo), it contains 2% salicylic acid in a water and alcohol base with a pH of 4, which means enhanced exfoliation will occur. Although that can be beneficial for a flaky scalp (the salicylic acid can help dissolve dead skin cells, allowing them to be washed away), it can be a problem for the hair.

NEUTROGENA TRIPLE MOISTURE

☺ **Triple Moisture Cream Lather Shampoo** *($5.99 for 8.45 ounces)* is a standard, but good, mildly creamy conditioning shampoo that can be excellent for normal to dry hair that is normal to slightly thick or coarse. The plant oils can build up with repeated use, so this is best alternated with a shampoo that does not contain conditioning agents. Neutrogena claims the various oils it uses (meadowfoam, almond, and olive) can penetrate various layers of the hair strand. However, these (like all) oils do not penetrate the hair shaft. Rather, they coat it and help seal in moisture while adding shine and improving comb-ability.

☺ **Triple Moisture Daily Deep Conditioner** *($5.99 for 8.45 ounces)* claims to instantly detangle, add shine, improve manageability, and help tame frizzy hair—and it does deliver. This is an outstanding conditioner for dry or thick, coarse hair. Like any well-formulated conditioner, this can make hair feel smooth and soft all day.

☺ **Triple Moisture Healing Shine Serum** *($6.99 for 1.8 ounces)* is a silicone serum that is more fluid than most, but still does its job of smoothing frizzies, adding glossy shine, and leaving hair feeling like silk. It contains six forms of silicone (which can affect the product's texture but have little impact on performance), plant oils, preservative, sunscreens, and fragrance. The sunscreen cannot adequately shield hair from UV damage because there is no way to know whether sunscreens in hair-care products hold up on hair after it is brushed and styled, not to mention there are no standards for determining a hair-care product's SPF number, so how long your hair would be protected from sunlight is a mystery.

☺ **Triple Moisture Deep Recovery Hair Mask** (*$6.99 for 6 ounces*) contains ingredients that are found in hundreds of other conditioners, so why this is positioned as a mask is a marketing gimmick, nothing more. This standard formulation cannot rescue hair in need of "deep recovery" (meaning excessively damaged hair), but it is emollient enough to be a very good conditioner for dry hair of any thickness.

☺ **Triple Moisture Pure Strength Oil Therapy** (*$6.99 for two 0.68-ounce tubes*) contains little oil compared to the amount of water, glycerin, and other slip agents present. This is not as moisturizing or emollient for dry, damaged hair as the Triple Moisture Deep Recovery Hair Mask above, but it can benefit those with slightly dry hair that is normal to fine or thin and that needs help with smoothing and combing. It has a runny texture, and Neutrogena recommends applying this "therapy" prior to shampooing. That would be a mistake, because a shampoo would undo the benefits you just received from this lightweight conditioner! Instead, apply this to damp hair *after* shampooing, leave it in for the remainder of your shower, then rinse.

☺ **Triple Moisture Sheer Hydration Leave-in Foam** (*$6.99 for 6 ounces*) is one of the new leave-in conditioners that are brilliant options for fine or thin hair that is slightly dry. This water- and propellant-based foam has a weightless, non-sticky texture, yet does have smoothing and detangling properties courtesy of the silicone and plant oils it contains. The sunscreens cannot be relied on to protect hair from UV damage. Sheer Hydration Leave-In Foam is great for those whose hair could benefit from conditioning agents without added weight and not a hint of greasiness.

☺ **Triple Moisture Silk Touch Leave-in Cream** (*$6.99 for 6 ounces*) is a lotion-like leave-in conditioner that would work well for normal to dry hair that is normal to slightly thick but not coarse (which would need a heavier smoothing product than this). It contains mostly water, silicones, thickener, glycerin, film-forming/detangling agents, emollient, plant oils, sunscreens, preservatives, and fragrance.

NEXXUS

California-based Nexxus has been a salon staple for years, and has steadfastly stood by its "nature and earth united with science" tag line, despite the fact that uniting nature and science doesn't necessarily result in better hair-care products, at least not in this case. Still, it's the nature hook that pulls in many salon customers, and over the years Nexxus has gone from making questionable claims for many of its products to blatant dishonesty (see the Y Serum products below for a great example of how far this line will go to sell products).

Many of the products below have been completely reformulated since I last reviewed this line. What's interesting is not that the new formulations are good (many of them are), but that the various shampoos, conditioners, and hairsprays are more similar to each other than ever before. For example, a clarifying shampoo and a conditioning shampoo really should be completely distinct formulations, each with its own benefit for hair. That's not the case here, and the similarity makes for some very confusing products. These products can still be effective, but not necessarily in a manner that coincides with what each product claims, or for its intended hair type. For more information about Nexxus, owned and managed by founder Jheri Redding's family, call (800) 444-NEXXUS or visit www.nexxus.com.

What's Good About This Line: Some excellent shampoos and conditioners that can meet a variety of hair needs; most Nexxus hairsprays are very flexible and ideal for softer styles; the prices on many Nexxus items are on the low end considering its salon heritage.

What's Not So Good About It: The bad products here are *really* bad; the Phyto Organics line is considerably more problematic than helpful for hair and scalp; the Axios men's line is disappointing; Nexxus makes some of the poorest reconstructing products around (of course, no hair-care product can reconstruct damaged hair, but the term is used so often here that it is essentially its own category).

☺ **Aloe Rid Gentle Clarifying Shampoo** *($10 for 13.5 ounces)* is a standard, but good, shampoo. The chelating agent it contains can help remove mineral buildup. This excels as a shampoo for normal to dry hair of any thickness.

☺ **Assure Replenishing Nutrient Shampoo** *($8.50 for 13.5 ounces)* is quite similar to the Aloe Rid Gentle Clarifying Shampoo above, except this does not contain a chelating agent. It does use a film-forming agent that can help hair feel thicker, but it can also build up on hair with repeated use.

☺ **Botanoil Botanical Treatment Shampoo** *($8 for 13.5 ounces)* can be a good, basic shampoo for all hair types, and does pose a slight risk of buildup. The plant oils are present in amounts too small to be of much use for dry hair.

☺ **Dandarrest Dandruff Control Shampoo** *($8 for 10.1 ounces)* is a very good, simply formulated anti-dandruff shampoo that contains 1% zinc pyrithione as its active ingredient. Head & Shoulders shampoos cost less than this and contain the same active ingredient, but this is still an option.

☺ $$$ **Diametress Luscious Hair Thickening Shampoo** *($15 for 13.5 ounces)* isn't the best for helping hair feel thicker, though it is a better shampoo for dry to very dry hair that is normal to thick or coarse and needs smoothing.

☺ **Exoil Oily Hair Normalizing Shampoo** *($5.50 for 10.1 ounces)* cannot normalize an oily scalp and is actually a poor choice for that problem because it contains plant oil and conditioning agents that will only add to the problem of excess oil. This can be an excellent shampoo for normal to slightly dry hair of any thickness.

☹ **Pep 'R' Mint Herbal Energizing Shampoo** *($6 for 10.1 ounces)* contains, as the name indicates, peppermint. That makes this otherwise standard shampoo too irritating for all scalp types, and the lemon juice only makes matters worse.

☺ **Simply Silver Colour Toning Shampoo** *($8 for 10.1 ounces)* is an inky, blue-black-colored shampoo that can have a slight impact on toning down brassy or yellow/gold tones in silver or gray hair. This shampoo poses minimal risk of buildup, and is appropriate for all hair types.

☺ **Therappe Luxury Moisturizing Shampoo** *($8 for 13.5 ounces)* is fairly similar to the Aloe Rid Gentle Clarifying Shampoo above, and the same basic comments apply. This does not contain a chelating agent, but it does include a film former that can help make hair feel thicker but that will build up over time.

☺ **$$$ Aloxxi Conditioner, Color Infuser** *($12 for 6.8 ounces)* is a standard, color-depositing conditioner available in eight different shades, though half of them are vibrant purple, cherry red, copper, or mahogany, colors few consumers use to dye their hair. Still, these can work as well as any to deposit a subtle amount of color on the hair shaft. Nexxus uses the same basic dyes as other lines (such as ARTec and Aveda). The conditioner base is standard, but all hair types, save very dry or damaged hair, can use the Aloxxi conditioners.

☹ **Ensure Acidifying Conditioner & Detangler** *($14 for 13.5 ounces)* is an acidic conditioner (pH is 3) that can shut down the cuticle layers, making the hair appear smooth and light-reflective. However, the effect is temporary because hair's pH is fickle, and after this is rinsed out, the hair will quickly revert to its normal, higher pH. Plus, styling hair with heat roughs up the cuticle layer, so any smoothing you get from this conditioner will be all for naught once the blow dryer or flat iron touches the hair. Beyond this issue is the fact that Nexxus added an appreciable amount of grapefruit juice to this conditioner, which can be very irritating to the scalp and drying to hair.

☹ **Headress Volumizing Leave-In Conditioner** *($18 for 13.5 ounces)* could have been an excellent leave-in conditioner for all hair types, but it contains the preservatives methylchloroisothiazolinone and methylisothiazolinone (Kathon CG), which are not recommended for use in leave-in products due to their risk of causing a sensitizing reaction on the scalp.

☺ **$$$ Humectress Ultimate Moisturizing Conditioner** *($16 for 13.5 ounces)* is a very good conditioner for normal to very dry hair that is normal to thick or coarse. This isn't the "ultimate" moisturizing conditioner, but it is a thoughtful formulation that can make hair feel smooth and silky soft.

☺ **Comb Thru Natural Hold Design and Finishing Mist** *($9 for 10.6 ounces)* is an extremely light aerosol hairspray that provides minimal to no hold without a trace of stickiness or stiffness. It is a good option for uncomplicated styles that need the slightest hint of hold, and it contains conditioning agents that are helpful for dry hair. As the name implies, hair can be easily combed (or brushed) through.

☺ **Comb Thru Natural Hold Design and Finishing Sprae** *($11 for 13.5 ounces)* is the nonaerosol version of the Comb Thru Natural Hold Design and Finishing Mist above, and provides a bit more hold while maintaining the same qualities as its aerosol counterpart. This does contain sunscreens, but without an SPF rating (and no such standards exist anyway) it would be a mistake to rely on it for any amount of UV protection.

☹ **Designing Butter High Fashion Texture Creme** *($14 for 5 ounces)* contains a form of sulfonic acid that can be drying to hair and possibly strip hair color with repeated use. As one of the main ingredients in this styling product, it definitely poses a problem for all hair types.

☺ **Dzyn Maker Sheer Volume Design and Finishing Mist** *($11 for 14.1 ounces)* is an aerosol hairspray with properties that are identical to the Comb Thru Natural Hold Design and Finishing Mist above, and the same review applies.

☹ **Exxtra Gel Super Hold Styling Sculptor** *($15 for 13.5 ounces)* contains a form of sulfonic acid that can be drying to hair and possibly strip hair color with repeated use. There are too many styling gels that pose no such concern to make this one worth considering at all.

☺ **Maxximum Super Hold Styling and Finishing Mist** *($11 for 14.1 ounces)* is a very good, medium-hold aerosol hairspray with a slight stiff, sticky feel that can be brushed through. The silicone can add extra shine to hair, but the sunscreens cannot be relied on to protect hair from sun damage.

☺ **Maxximum Super Hold Styling and Finishing Spray** *($11 for 13.5 ounces)* is a good nonaerosol hairspray with a medium to firm hold that leaves hair feeling sticky and somewhat stiff, and brushing through hair can be a bit of a challenge. This would be best to set hairstyles you do not intend to brush through later, or to use on the roots for long-lasting lift without a coated, heavy feeling.

☺ **MaxxiStyler Sculpting Spray Gel (Pump)** *($13 for 13.5 ounces)* is a fairly sticky spray gel that provides a medium to firm hold and can be difficult to brush through. It works well for textured wet looks or can be used on dry hair to create gravity-defying lift with little movement. This formula contains no water; it is alcohol-based, but the alcohol will evaporate before it can dry the hair.

☺ **$$$ MaxxWax Creative Styling Stick** *($17 for 2.6 ounces)* is a standard wax stick packaged in a deodorant-style container that can be rolled up when more product is needed. This stiff, heavy wax is best for smoothing frizzies, stubborn curls, or dry ends of dry to very dry hair that is coarse or thick. It can be difficult to shampoo out.

☺ **Mousse Plus Alcohol Free Volumizing Foam Styler (Aerosol)** *($12 for 10.6 ounces)* is a very standard, propellant-based mousse that provides a light hold without stiffness or stickiness. Hair is easily brushed through, and this provides a slight amount of heat protection. It is a good, though overpriced, option for normal to fine or thin hair requiring body.

The Reviews N

☺ **NexxStyler Alcohol Free Sheer Volume Spray Gel (Pump)** *($13 for 13.5 ounces)* is a good, versatile styling spray that can provide a light, flexible hold with a soft, non-sticky finish. It works well when used on damp hair prior to heat styling or on dry hair to add soft control and texture. This can be easily brushed through and will not weigh down fine or thin hair.

☺ $$$ **Nexxtacy Alcohol Free Sustained Hold Styling and Finishing Spray** *($17 for 13.5 ounces)* is a standard styling spray that goes on slightly wet but dries quickly to a slightly sticky, stiff finish that can provide light to medium brushable hold. This is a great styling spray for normal to fine or thin hair.

☺ **Nexxtacy Sustained Hold Styling and Finishing Mist** *($11 for 14.1 ounces)* is a standard aerosol hairspray that offers a light to medium hold that keeps hair surprisingly pliable. That means this can come in handy as a working spray during styling, particularly for updos or for holding soft waves or curls. Hair can be easily brushed through and this remains minimally sticky and has an insignificant amount of stiffness.

☹ **Styling Gel Pure Control Stylizer** *($10.50 for 13.5 ounces)* contains a form of sulfonic acid that can be drying to hair and possibly strip hair color with repeated use. It is similar to the Exxtra Gel above, and neither is recommended.

☹ **VersaStyler Artistic Designing Lotion** *($10 for 13.5 ounces)* contains the preservative Kathon CG, and is not recommended.

☺ **Aloe Rid Treatment Deep Clarifying Solution** *($6 for 5 ounces)* is a very light conditioner that does contain a chelating agent, which can help remove mineral buildup from hair. This is a decent conditioner for fine or thin hair that is dry. Those with a sensitive scalp take note: This conditioner is fragrance-free.

☺ **Botanic Oil Essential Natural Oil Replenisher** *($10.25 for 10.1 ounces)* is nothing more than a mixture of plant oils with lecithin (a good conditioning agent) and vitamin E. Any oil from your kitchen cupboard would work as well as this for far less money. Still, this can be a rich conditioner for very dry hair of any thickness. Note that oil does not rinse well and, therefore, must be shampooed out.

☹ **Emergencee Strengthening Polymeric Reconstructor** *($14 for 3.3 ounces)* cannot reconstruct hair one bit. This contains a form of sulfonic acid as its main ingredient (it is listed before water), so the only emergency here is how dry this can make hair, not to mention the fact that this can potentially strip hair color.

☹ **Epitome Fortifying Botanical Reconstructor (Pump Spray)** *($15 for 10.1 ounces)* is a lightweight, but faulty, conditioner that contains minerals and enzymes that can chip away at and denature the hair shaft. This also contains sodium perborate, which can be drying to hair and have a bleaching action on hair.

☺ $$$ **KerapHix Restorative Protein Creme Reconstructor** *($18 for 13.5 ounces)* is nearly identical to the Humectress Ultimate Moisturizing Conditioner above, and the same review applies. The DNA and RNA in this product are there for show—these ingredients have no effect on hair.

☺ **Shinesque Dramatic Glistening Mist (Aerosol)** *($8.50 for 2.1 ounces)* is an aerosol glossing mist that contains a mineral oil derivative, along with silicones, so this can be quite greasy, though it will definitely add shine. It is best as a glossing spray for dry to very dry hair that is coarse, curly, or thick.

NEXXUS AXIOS MAN PRODUCTS

☺ **Axios Conditioning Shampoo and Body Wash** *($6 for 6 ounces)* is a standard shampoo that contains biotin, a B vitamin that Nexxus maintains is helpful against thinning hair, although it is not. It is a good shampoo for normal to dry hair that is normal to thick or coarse.

☺ $$$ **Axios Volumizing Shampoo and Scalp Clarifier** *($13 for 16 ounces)* is a standard shampoo that would work well for most hair types.

☺ $$$ **Axios Leave-In Conditioner and Volumizer** *($13 for 8 ounces)* is a lightweight conditioner with a small amount of film-forming agent that can help hair feel thicker. It is best for someone with normal to slightly dry hair that is fine or thin.

☹ **Axios Grooming Gel and Conditioner** *($8 for 4 ounces)* contains a form of sulfonic acid that can be drying to hair and possibly strip hair color with repeated use.

☹ **Axios Sculpting Pomade and Shine Glaze** *($14 for 4 ounces)* contains the preservative Kathon CG, and is not recommended.

☺ **Axios Styling Spray and Protectant (Pump Spray)** *($13 for 8 ounces)* is a light-hold hairspray that leaves a minimal stiff or sticky feel and can be easily brushed through. This contains potent fragrance, enough to serve as a man's cologne calling card. The sunscreen in here cannot protect hair from UV damage because it is not rated with an SPF number.

NEXXUS PHYTO ORGANICS

The Phyto Organics collection represents an attempt by Nexxus to get a foothold in the natural hair-care market. The "pure and natural" ingredients are strongly emphasized despite the fact that each product below contains the same standard hair-care ingredients as other Nexxus products. Sprinkled among these synthetic ingredients (which are responsible for almost all of the work in terms of cleansing, conditioning, and styling hair) are rare, exotic plant extracts "sourced from around the world." Nexxus thought of every angle with this line, from ingredients farmed organically by indigenous tribes to those used by ancient cultures whose mythology is steeped in folklore (rather than science), wrapping it up by using essential oils to add fragrance.

Perhaps the biggest boast made for this line is that the quinoa (pronounced "keen-wa") protein complex used in the Phyto Organics products can repair hair. Nexxus claims that this complex is the ideal combination of proteins of varying molecular weights, maintaining that high-, medium-, and low-weight segments can protect, repair, seal, strengthen, and penetrate the hair shaft. According to Nexxus literature, 12% of this protein complex can get through to the hair's medulla and cortex, the heart of each hair shaft that the cuticle layers are meant to protect. What is not mentioned (and why would it be, because it would refute the claim) is that protein molecules, regardless of the source, are too large to penetrate into the cortex or reach the medulla. Furthermore, although it sounds as if using hair-care products with specialized ingredients can replenish what hair has lost, it just isn't possible. Fancy charts and graphs showing how these ingredients supposedly work are interesting to look at, but the reality is that protein cannot repair hair. If it could, who would have damaged hair? We could all color-treat, perm, and heat-style the life out of our hair, and then just use the right hair-care products to bring everything back to normal. I wish that were true, but once healthy, intact hair is damaged, it is impossible to bring it back to its former glory. Using well-formulated hair-care products can provide some temporary fixes to make hair feel, look, and behave as if it were not damaged, but they are still just a Band-Aid over a wound that cannot be healed by products.

☺ **Phyto Organics Hydruss Moisturizing Shampoo** *($10 for 10.1 ounces)* is a good conditioning shampoo for normal to dry hair of any thickness. This can definitely cause buildup with repeated use.

☺ **Phyto Organics Inergy Nutrient Shampoo** *($10 for 10.1 ounces)* is nearly identical to the Phyto Organics Hydruss Moisturizing Shampoo above, except this contains a different blend of plant tea and essential oil fragrance.

☹ **Phyto Organics Kelate Purifying Shampoo** *($10 for 10.1 ounces)* contains essential oils of peppermint, cedarwood, and eucalyptus, which makes this shampoo too irritating for all scalp types. This also contains the decidedly unnatural ingredient sodium polystyrene sulfonate (doesn't that sound like something you would want on your vegetarian pizza?), which can make hair feel dry and stiff.

☺ **Phyto Organics Syntress Volumizing Lift Shampoo** *($10 for 10.1 ounces)* is a good shampoo for those with fine or thin hair because it contains a film-forming agent that can create a feeling of fullness, though over time it will build up and leave these hair types with hair that feels heavy and dry. It is best alternated with another shampoo that does not cause buildup.

☹ **Phyto Organics Luxxtress Leave In Hair Moisturizer** (**Pump Spray**) *($12.50 for 10.1 ounces)* contains the preservative Kathon CG, and is not recommended due to the high risk it poses of causing a sensitizing reaction on the scalp. This preservative could not be any more unnatural, and is a poor choice for a product line boasting of the miracles of plants.

☹ **Phyto Organics Nectaress Nourishing Conditioner** *($12 for 10.1 ounces)* contains a high amount of essential oil fragrance composed of grapefruit and orange oils, both of which can be exceedingly irritating to the scalp and drying to the hair.

☹ **Phyto Organics The Arts Absolute Finisher** (**Aerosol Spray**) *($11 for 10.6 ounces)* contains acetone, which can be very drying to hair and scalp, and this also includes irritating geranium, lemon, and lime oils to cause further scalp irritation.

☹ **Phyto Organics The Arts Brilliance Design Creme** *($22.50 for 10.1 ounces)* is problematic on several counts: It contains a form of sulfonic acid that can be drying to hair and possibly strip hair color, it uses the sensitizing preservative Kathon CG, and it contains tolu balsam, a tree-sap resin that can make hair feel dry and brittle. The price for such a poorly formulated product is insulting.

☹ **Phyto Organics The Arts Creative Sculpting Putty** *($11 for 10.1 ounces)* contains eucalyptus and rosemary essential oils in amounts that can be irritating to the scalp. This product is not recommended.

☺ **$$$ Phyto Organics The Arts Curl Relaxx Smoothing Gelee** *($23.50 for 10.1 ounces)* is a good, lightweight, thin-textured balm to smooth normal to fine or thin hair during heat styling. The price is out of line for what you get.

☺ **Phyto Organics The Arts Designing Spray Gel (Pump Spray)** *($13 for 10.1 ounces)* is a standard, lightweight styling gel with a light to medium hold and minimal to no stiff or sticky feel.

☺ **Phyto Organics The Arts Emphasis Redefining Gel** *($10 for 10.1 ounces)* is a very standard styling gel with a light hold and minimal to no stiff or sticky feel.

☺ **Phyto Organics The Arts Flexible Design Finisher (Aerosol Spray)** *($11 for 10.6 ounces)* is a standard aerosol hairspray with a decent flexible hold that can be brushed through.

☺ **Phyto Organics The Arts Resilient Hold Finishing Spray (Pump Spray)** *($11 for 10.1 ounces)* is a standard hairspray with a decent flexible hold that can be brushed through.

☹ **Phyto Organics The Arts Supple Hold Designing Spray (Pump Spray)** *($11 for 10.1 ounces)* contains essential oils of lemon, bergamot, and grapefruit, all of which can cause scalp irritation and cause further problems after application when the scalp is exposed to sunlight.

☹ **Phyto Organics Babassu Mud Revitalizing Hair Treatment** *($17 for 10.1 ounces)* lists kaolin (clay) as its second ingredient, which makes this a joke of a treatment because all it will do is cause dry hair. As the clay dries, it doesn't absorb impurities or toxins from hair, it just chips away at the cuticle, which results in more damage.

☺ **$$$ Phyto Organics Enphuse Intensive Reconstructor** *($22.50 for 10.1 ounces)* is, without question, the most intelligently formulated product in the Nexxus Phyto Organics range. This is a very good smoothing conditioner for normal to dry hair that is normal to thick or coarse.

NEXXUS RETEXXTUR

☺ **Retexxtur Curl Vitalizing Shampoo** *($8 for 10.1 ounces)* is a standard, but good, shampoo that can work well for normal to dry hair of any thickness, though it can cause buildup with repeated use. Nothing about this shampoo makes it particularly special for curly hair.

☺ **Retexxtur Curl Enhancing Styler (Pump Spray)** *($9 for 10.1 ounces)* is a very light, water- and alcohol-based styling spray that can provide a minimal hold without being stiff or sticky. It can softly enhance curls, but won't do much to change their texture or tame stubborn frizzies. There needs to be more to this to really benefit curly hair, which is why it does not earn a smiley face.

☹ **Retexxtur Texture Transforming Pomade** *($11.75 for 3.3 ounces)* contains the preservative Kathon CG, and is not recommended.

☹ **Retexxtur Curl Rejuvenating Treatment** *($7 for 3.3 ounces)* is similar to the Epitome Fortifying Botanical Reconstructor above, and the same review applies.

☺ $$$ **Retexxtur Hair Glow Anti Frizz Smoother (Pump Spray)** *($8.50 for 2 ounces)* is a standard silicone spray whose price for the amount you get is not too off-putting considering how well the product works to smooth frizzies and add a significant amount of shine to hair. This spray has a thicker texture and slightly greasier feel than most, which makes it preferred for dry hair that is normal to coarse or thick.

☺ $$$ **Retexxtur Smoothing Design Shine** *($14 for 1 ounce)* is an excellent silicone serum that contains additional conditioning agents to benefit dry to very dry hair. It is best for thick or coarse hair that needs additional smoothness, frizz control, and shine.

NEXXUS VITATRESSS

This sub-line is the Nexxus answer to the problem of fine, thinning hair for men or women. All of these products contain the B vitamin biotin along with several amino acids, which come with the claim that they can work on the scalp and inside the hair shaft to correct the causes of hair loss (one of which Nexxus incorrectly states is excess sebum production). There is no substantiated evidence anywhere that topical application of biotin or amino acids can slow hair loss and/or revive thinning hair to change it into a thicker, robust version of its formerly weak self. The amino acids (including cysteine) are indeed natural components of each hair's internal structure, but when they are depleted, whether because of hair damage, exposure to sun, or genetic influences, they cannot be replenished by hair-care products, mainly because they do not cling to the hair well. The VitaTress line has some good products, but the claims amount to hope and a prayer, not proven science. Besides, if boosting hair's nutrition could slow or stop hair loss, you would be better off taking oral nutritional supplements or adjusting the foods you eat to improve your hair's health, but it just doesn't work that way. See the section on hair loss in Chapter Three, "Hair Growth—Hair Loss" for a clear picture of why hair loss happens and what you can really do about it.

☺ **VitaTress Biotin Shampoo** *($9 for 10.1 ounces)* is a good shampoo for all hair types and poses minimal to no risk of buildup.

☺ **VitaTress Bodifying Mousse (Aerosol)** *($12 for 10.6 ounces)* is a very standard, propellant-based mousse that has a light hold with a slightly sticky feel that can be brushed through. This can work well to boost body in fine or thin hair, but the styling mousses recommended in these reviews and available at the drugstore can perform the same feat for less money.

☹ **VitaTress Conditioning Volumizer (Pump Spray)** *($10 for 10.1 ounces)* contains the preservative Kathon CG, and since this is a spray-on product it is guaranteed you will get this product on your scalp, and that is a problem.

☹ **VitaTress Liquid Gel** *($9.50 for 10.1 ounces)* contains the preservative Kathon CG, and is not recommended. Creating a sensitizing reaction on the scalp won't help thinning hair become stronger or slow hair loss.

☺ **VitaTress Styling Potion** *($9.50 for 10.1 ounces)* is a fluid styling gel that contains film-forming/holding agents typically found in hairsprays. This feels light in the hair but offers a medium to firm hold that remains slightly sticky. This can make fine or thin hair feel stiff and coated unless used sparingly, and there are better styling gels available for this hair type.

☺ **VitaTress Volume Hold Finisher** (**Aerosol Spray**) *($9 for 10.6 ounces)* is a standard hairspray that provides a light, touchable hold that can be easily brushed through and does not feel stiff or too sticky. The small amount of acetone can cause scalp irritation and be hard on hair with repeated use, making this tough to recommend wholeheartedly.

☹ **VitaTress Biotin Creme** *($11.50 for 2.1 ounces)* is a leave-in conditioner that contains wild mint oil, which serves no purpose other than to cause irritation while convincing the user that the product is "working."

☹ **VitaTress Cystine Treatment** *($7 for 3.3 ounces)* contains a form of sulfonic acid that can be drying to hair and potentially strip hair color with repeated use. Even though this is a rinse-out product, it is still not recommended. It isn't even a very good conditioner, and the vitamins do nothing for hair anyway.

NEXXUS Y SERUM

The Y Serum line is sold as the "anti-aging breakthrough for hair," with all manner of claims pertaining to bringing hair back to its youthful vitality. These products actually claim they can stop hair's aging process, which is completely untrue. Changes occurring in hair growth and color are biological processes influenced primarily by genetics and changing hormone levels, including the unknown cause of hair turning gray. Genetics and gray hair cannot be altered by hair-care products. Nexxus is still on the "amino acids as hair salvation" kick here, only this time they mix the water-binding agents with silicone. The silicone can attach to the hair shaft and help make hair smoother, feel silkier, and be easy to comb through, but it does not facilitate the penetration of amino acids into the inner portion of the hair shaft. The only thing that occurs is that these silicone-encased water-binding agents can cling to the hair longer, resulting in more manageable hair. The Y Serum products cannot repair damaged hair, promote color longevity, or reverse even one second of the hair's aging process. The three products below represent standard formulations that have merit for hair, just not in the manner in which they're presented.

☺ **Y Serum Younger Looking Hair Shampoo** *($11 for 10.1 ounces)* is a very good conditioning shampoo for normal to very dry hair that is normal to coarse or thick. It contains mostly water, detergent cleansing agents, thickener, plant extracts (Nexxus claims these have antioxidant benefits for hair, but that is not the case; even if they did, they wouldn't be effective because they would just be rinsed down the drain), several silicone conditioning agents, glycerin, more thickeners, detangling agents, pH adjuster, chelating agent, preservatives, and fragrance. This cannot permanently infuse ingredients into hair, nor can it stop hair's aging process. You've heard the expression "It's only a movie"? Well, this is only a shampoo.

☺ $$$ **Y Serum Younger Looking Hair Conditioner** *($16 for 10.1 ounces)* is a standard, but very good, conditioner for normal to very dry hair of any thickness.

☺ $$$ **Y Serum Younger Looking Hair Treatment** *($20 for 4.2 ounces)* is a water-based, ultra-light, leave-on spray that has mild conditioning properties suitable for detangling fine or thin hair. This cannot protect hair from UV damage, nor can it stop hair from aging.

NIOXIN

If there is a natural ingredient, herbal supplement, vitamin, enzyme, mineral, or amino acid out there that has ever been even remotely thought to have a hint of a chance to make thin hair look fuller, Nioxin probably uses it. This is the company whose entire existence hinges on its claim to be "the natural solution for fine and thinning hair." To that end, they have developed two dozen products (all with rather unnatural basic formulas) that they claim are capable of treating the various causes of thin hair, which, of course, includes hair loss. According to Nioxin's Web site, "Each product is designed to create and maintain an optimum scalp environment in order to address the problems associated with thin-looking hair, including hair loss through mechanical breakage, which leads to fine, fragile, thin-looking hair." Nioxin is quick to point out that their products cannot and do not regrow hair. Rather, they state that the products "help to create an optimum scalp environment for the body to perform its natural functions of hair growth." What isn't discussed is that when the biological process of hair loss begins, there is nothing in these products that can slow it down, and that simply improving the condition of the scalp is nowhere near enough.

Nioxin acknowledges that hormonal influences (in men and in women) are the major players when it comes to hair loss and baldness, but Nioxin literature also includes falsehoods that attribute hair loss and thinning to such elements as styling product buildup, environmental toxins, and a malnourished scalp. As causative factors, none of these affect hair growth, yet that's what Nioxin's claims depend on.

The only area where some truth comes into the picture is Nioxin's statement that chemical services and excessive hair manipulation (meaning rough brushing and heat styling) can cause hair loss and thinning. However, even this contention is not accurate, because what occurs after excessive chemical services (such as bleaching and perming hair within the same week) is hair *breakage*, not hair loss. Chemical treatments can indeed damage the hair shaft to the extent that hair that was once thick-feeling and healthy can turn to, for lack of a better word, mush. But once regrowth occurs (and chemical services are stopped) the hair will continue to grow and thrive as usual. In a nutshell, you don't need Nioxin products to bring thinning hair back to life. Nourishing the scalp with vitamins and amino acids sounds appealing, but you cannot feed the scalp from the outside in, and nothing in Nioxin's leave-on treatment products is capable of eliminating excess hormones and toxins. Unfortunately, Nioxin has built its success on such misinformation. They have toned down their claims quite a bit in the last few years, but falling for even these tamed versions will lead only to disappointment. For more information on Nioxin, call (800) 628-9890 or visit www.nioxin.com.

What's Good About This Line: Nioxin lists ingredients for all its products on the company's Web site; the aerosol hairsprays are all very good.

What's Not So Good About It: None of these products can stop hair loss or curb any part of the biological process that causes hair to thin; the products have incredibly long ingredient lists, but most of the them are window dressing to create treatments for thinning hair that offer false hope; the styling gels are below average.

NIOXIN BIONUTRIENT ACTIVES

☹ **Bionutrient Actives Cleanser** *($12.50 for 10.1 ounces)* contains TEA-lauryl sulfate as its main detergent cleansing agent, which makes it too drying for hair while also being drying and irritating for the scalp. This also contains rosemary, peppermint, and thyme, which create a tingle that may make you think this shampoo is working, when in fact it's just causing irritation. The enzyme-laced vitamins in this product cannot help thinning hair in the least.

☹ **Bionutrient Actives Cytonutrient Actives Treatment** *($24.99 for 3.4 ounces)* claims to provide scalp and hair protection from chemical residues, toxins, and buildup of DHT (dihydrotestosterone, the hormone responsible for male and female pattern baldness). It also promises to nourish the scalp so it can receive nutrients in an optimum condition, but the whole treatment is nothing but snake oil. There is no proof anywhere that the wild yam, ginkgo, milk thistle, and vitamins can reduce any sort of scalp buildup, and definitely nothing related to hormonal buildup. This is an overpriced product that isn't even a decent leave-in conditioner. Again, peppermint and rosemary are present for their tingling, bogus "it's working" effect.

☺ $$$ **Bionutrient Actives Scalp Therapy** *($15.99 for 10.1 ounces)* is a standard lightweight conditioner that contains mostly water, thickener, aloe, detangling agents, silicone, conditioning agent, vitamin E, water-binding agents, panthenol, film-forming agent, several plant extracts, vitamins, minerals, rosemary and peppermint extracts, and preservatives. It is an OK conditioner for normal to slightly dry hair that is fine or thin. The vitamins cannot nourish the scalp.

☹ **Bionutrient Actives Treatment** *($19.99 for 3.4 ounces)* is similar to the Bionutrient Actives Cytonutrient Actives Treatment above, and the same basic comments apply. Nothing in this product can "safeguard hair against the future buildup of toxins like DHT (dihydrotestosterone)." Here, it's important to mention that DHT isn't a toxin, it's a hormone created by the action of a naturally occurring enzyme that changes testosterone to DHT.

NIOXIN BIONUTRIENT CREATIVES

☺ **Bionutrient Creatives Lift Volumizing Mist** *($10.99 for 8 ounces)* is a very light, water-based, alcohol-free styling spray that provides minimal to no hold but can make hair feel coated. That can benefit fine or thin hair, but the film-forming agent will build up over time. This does have a non-sticky finish and is not stiff, which means hair stays touchable and is easily brushed through.

☹ **Bionutrient Creatives Liquid Foam** *($10.20 for 6.8 ounces)* is an average, liquid-to-foam styling mousse that provides a medium hold that can be brushed through. It leaves hair feeling somewhat sticky and stiff, and is overall not as elegant feeling as other mousses, many of which cost less than this.

☹ **Bionutrient Creatives Liquid Gel** *($9.99 for 5.1 ounces)* is a styling gel that offers a firm hold but with a very sticky finish that is difficult to brush through. Nioxin eschews the use of PVP (a standard film-forming/holding agent), maintaining that it can clog pores on the scalp and lead to hair loss. Yet the acrylate-based film former this does contain is virtually indistinguishable from PVP and it is just as likely to have the same effect. However, clogged pores do not cause hair loss and rarely amount to much of a problem if you shampoo regularly (and pay attention to massaging the scalp as you wash). This gel's feel and finish is a step below almost any styling gel at the drugstore; it just isn't pleasant to use and is not a necessity if your hair is thinning.

☹ **Bionutrient Creatives Niogel** *($7.99 for 5.1 ounces)* is a thicker, stickier version of the Bionutrient Creatives Liquid Gel above, and the same basic comments apply. This can easily make thin or fine hair feel glued together or look clumped.

☺ **Bionutrient Creatives Niospray, Extra Hold** *($10.99 for 8.8 ounces)* is a standard aerosol hairspray capable of a light to medium hold with a slightly stiff, sticky feel. This can be brushed through but it contains nothing special for fine or thin hair.

☺ **Bionutrient Creatives Niospray, Power Hold** *($10.99 for 8.8 ounces)* is a very good, though standard, firm-hold aerosol hairspray. It leaves hair feeling slightly stiff and sticky, though it can be brushed through. Nioxin actually states that this hairspray contains "no drying alcohol," yet denatured alcohol (which is a drying alcohol) is the first ingredient listed. It does evaporate before it can cause hair dryness, but the claim is still misleading.

☺ **Bionutrient Creatives Niospray, Regular Hold** *($10.99 for 8.8 ounces)* is another aerosol hairspray, this one similar to the Bionutrient Creatives Niospray, Power Hold above, and the same review applies.

☺ **Bionutrient Creatives Smoothly Defined** *($11.99 for 6.8 ounces)* is a liquid-to-foam mousse that is a very good option for fine or thin hair. It has light hold with a slight sticky feel but no stiffness, and it is easy to brush through. It would work particularly well on fine, curly hair that needs definition without weight.

☺ **Bionutrient Creatives Bliss** *($8.25 for 6.8 ounces)* is a spray-on, leave-in conditioner that contains mostly water, silicone detangling agent, conditioning agent, slip agent, film-forming agent, silicone, more conditioning agents, fragrance, and preservatives. This can be a good option for detangling fine or thin hair, but does feel slightly sticky. Contrary to Nioxin's claim, this product can cause buildup. It absolutely cannot remove DHT, excess hormones, or "pseudo-estrogens" from the scalp, so take that claim for what it is—nonsense. Even the notion that it could do these things flies in the face of human physiology and biology.

☹ **Follicle Booster** *($19.99 for 1 ounce)* is a scalp treatment that contains an ingredient that Nioxin refers to as Scalp Respiratory Complex, said to improve scalp cell activity and offer protection from free radicals. Does the activity of your scalp cells or free-radical damage have anything to do with hair loss? Not according to any published, peer-reviewed research. It would be nice if all it took to solve the problem of thinning hair was massaging this concoction of water, lecithin, algae, amino acids, coenzymes, vitamins, and minerals into the scalp, but it simply will not work. All this can really do is cause irritation, thanks to the peppermint and rosemary it contains. That probably makes hopeful consumers think this product is working, or that some sort of cellular respiration is occurring, but what's really going on is irritation.

NIOXIN BIONUTRIENT PROTECTIVES

☹ **Bionutrient Protectives Cleanser** *($12.50 for 10.1 ounces)* contains TEA-lauryl sulfate, which can be too drying for both hair and scalp and will not help "maintain an optimum scalp environment." This also contains wasabi (Japanese horseradish), peppermint, and rosemary to cause further scalp irritation.

☺ **Bionutrient Protectives Moisture & Strength** *($11.99 for 5.1 ounces)* is a standard conditioner that can work well to smooth and detangle normal to slightly dry hair that is fine or thin, but all other claims for this product are sheer fantasy.

☹ **Bionutrient Protectives Cytonutrient Protectives Treatment** *($24.99 for 3.4 ounces)* is similar to the Bionutrient Actives Cytonutrient Actives Treatment above, and the same review applies. This one adds a substantial amount of wasabi to the mix, and that can be a potent scalp irritant.

☹ **Bionutrient Protectives Scalp Therapy** *($15.99 for 10.1 ounces)* is similar to the Bionutrient Actives Scalp Therapy above, except this contains a different set of plant extracts. These add up to a blend of mostly irritating ingredients that have no effect on hair or scalp. In contrast to the Actives Scalp Therapy, this product contains a great deal of peppermint, which makes it too irritating to recommend, especially for massaging into the scalp.

☺ **Bionutrient Protectives Structure & Strength** *($11.99 for 5.1 ounces)* is a standard conditioner that has minimal to no impact on hair structure or strength. It contains mostly water, anti-static/detangling agent, thickener, water-binding agents, film-forming/conditioning agent, detangling agents, panthenol, more conditioning agents, plant extracts, fragrance, more water-binding agents, and preservatives. It is a good option for making fine or thin hair that is slightly dry easier to comb. This absolutely cannot rework the hair shaft to prevent damage or breakage.

☹ **Bionutrient Protectives Treatment** *($19.99 for 3.4 ounces)* is nearly identical to the Bionutrient Actives Treatment above, and the same review applies. This product has no effect on the buildup of environmental pollutants, nor does that type of buildup lead to thinning hair.

NIOXIN SEMODEX

Nioxin purports that thinning hair is caused by the presence of the *Demodex folliculorum* mite and that their Semodex products are designed to kill this mite, thus creating thicker hair and improving hair growth. The problem with this theory is that the *Demodex folliculorum* mite is present in the sebaceous glands, which are attached to the hair follicle, of lots and lots of people. In fact, up to 75% of the population—men, women, and children—have this mite, and clearly not all of them are balding (especially not kids), nor do they all have thin hair. Further, if the *Demodex folliculorum* mite was the reason for thinning hair or any kind of hair growth, then hair transplants wouldn't work because the mite, which is present in those hair follicles, would have the same effect; but that isn't the case. Hair transplants work exceedingly well; in fact, there has never been a case where transplanted hair follicles become thinner or fall out, though the *Demodex folliculorum* mite is still present (Source: www.keratin.com).

☹ **Semodex Sebolytic Cleanser, for Men** *($9.99 for 6 ounces)* contains TEA-lauryl sulfate, which makes this a poor shampoo for all hair types. This does not contain anything that can kill or control a mite infestation. This shampoo can dissolve and remove excess scalp oil, but so can countless other shampoos that contain detergent cleansing agents that won't dry out the hair and scalp.

☹ **Semodex Sebolytic Cleanser, for Women** *($9.99 for 6 ounces)* is slightly less drying than the Semodex Sebolytic Cleanser above, but the same review applies. The pumpkin seed oil, saw palmetto, and wild yam (among other plant extracts in this product) cannot treat *Demodex* mites and they do not make thin hair feel thicker. The balm mint in this product can cause scalp irritation.

☺ $$$ **Semodex Scalp Serum, for Men** *($30 for 2 ounces)* is sold as a product that can inhibit the buildup of lipase on a man's scalp. Lipase is an enzyme involved in hydrolyzing fats into fatty acids, which are a component of our scalp's (and our skin's) oil (sebum). Nothing in this product can control scalp oil or enzymes, especially not when the third ingredient in this product is, would you believe, another oil! The tiny amount of tea tree oil has no benefit for the scalp. Used in concentrations of 5% or more, tea tree oil can be a treatment for dandruff and have other anti-microbial properties, but the percentage in this product isn't even close to 5%. The numerous plant extracts in this product have no effect on mites, nor can they create a healthy scalp environment. At best, this pricey product can function as a light leave-in conditioner.

☺ $$$ **Semodex Scalp Serum, for Women** *($30 for 2 ounces)* is nearly identical to the Semodex Scalp Serum, for Men above, except this contains a slightly different mixture of plant extracts, none of which are effective against mites or in creating a healthy scalp. Otherwise, the same comments apply.

NIZORAL

The active ingredient in the Nizoral products is ketoconazole, an anti-fungal agent that debuted in 1981 as a prescription medicine for a variety of fungal and yeast-based infections, both topical and oral. Products containing 1% ketoconazole have been FDA-approved for over-the-counter use for dandruff since 1999, while 2% versions are still available by prescription only. The good news for those with mild to moderate dandruff is that research has shown 1% ketoconazole products to be as effective as the 2% prescription version (although the 2% version is preferred for severe dandruff, especially if it is accompanied by seborrheic dermatitis). There are conflicting studies on whether ketoconazole is more effective than products containing zinc pyrithione (found in shampoos in such hair-care lines as Head & Shoulders) as the active ingredient. However, the most current studies indicate that both of these active ingredients—ketoconazole and zinc pyrithione—are effective options in the battle against dandruff, and sufferers are urged to try each to see which medicine provides the best anti-dandruff effect for them. For some, a combination of both, alternated on different days in separate shampoos, may end up being an ideal solution (Sources: *Dermatology*, 2001, pages 171–176; *Skin Pharmacology and Physiology*, November-December 2002, pages 434–441; and *Journal of Dermatological Treatment*, June 2002, pages 51–60). For more information about Nizoral, call (800) 962-5357 or visit www.nizoral.com.

What's Good About This Line: Ketoconazole is an effective anti-dandruff agent, and Nizoral's shampoo base is non-drying; the conditioner, though nothing special, can detangle hair and make it feel softer.

What's Not So Good About It: The shampoo carries a considerably higher price compared to other anti-dandruff options.

☺ **$$$ Anti-Dandruff Shampoo** (*$15.39 for 7 ounces*) is a standard shampoo that contains 1% ketoconazole to help control dandruff. Besides this active ingredient, the shampoo contains mostly water, detergent cleansing agent, lather agent, thickener, film-forming agent, fragrance, chelating agent, preservatives, pH adjuster, and coloring agent. It can cause buildup with repeated use, though ketoconazole shampoos can still be effective against dandruff when used two or three times per week rather than daily.

☺ **Non-Medicated Daily Conditioner** (*$5.84 for 12 ounces*) is a very standard, but good, conditioner that contains mostly water, thickeners, anti-static agent, detangling agents, emollient, silicones, preservatives, and emulsifier. This would work well for normal to dry hair of any thickness, and it is fragrance-free!

NOLITA

For more information about Nolita, owned by Graham Webb, call (800) 470-9909 or visit www.nolitahair.com.

What's Good About This Line: Almost every product works well for its intended hair type and style; a couple styling products present unique twists on traditional options; none of the products contain unnecessary irritants.

What's Not So Good About It: The prices are rather high; the thymus extract in these products has no benefit for hair beyond that of a water-binding agent.

☺ **Moisturizing Shampoo** (*$12 for 8.5 ounces*) is a very standard shampoo that can be a great option for all hair types, and it poses minimal risk of buildup.

☺ $$$ **Moisturizing Conditioner** (*$14 for 8.5 ounces*) is a very basic, though effective, conditioner for normal to slightly dry hair that is normal to fine or thin.

☺ $$$ **Grit Gel, Beach Hair, City Style** (*$18 for 8 ounces*) is a medium- to firm-hold, fairly sticky styling gel that is meant for what Nolita describes as "that surf in the city look," and what they mean is that this gel contains sand-like particles meant to create a messy, "beachy" look. This is aptly named, because this gel does feel gritty, and remains so. Why anyone would want the feeling of sand in his or her hair all day is beyond me, but thanks to Nolita, it's an option, and it doesn't even require a trip to the beach.

☺ **Hair Spray** (*$12 for 10 ounces*) is a standard aerosol hairspray with a light to medium hold that's slightly stiff and sticky, though hair can be brushed through. It has a weightless feel and is a great option for keeping fine or thin hair in place, and the small amount of silicone can add a hint of shine.

☺ $$$ **Molding Clay, Uptown Hold, Downtown Style** (*$16 for 4 ounces*) is an impossibly thick, clay- and Vaseline-based pomade that can actually be quite drying to hair, not to mention extremely difficult to shampoo out. Really, this would work well only for short, spiked hairstyles that need strong texture and definition with a matte finish. If that describes your haircut and what you're looking for, proceed with caution—this is one of the trickiest pomades you're likely to come across.

☺ $$$ **Sheer Texturizer** (*$16 for 3.5 ounces*) is another thick pomade, but this one has a softer, creamier texture than the Molding Clay above that is much easier to work with on wet or dry hair. It adds a pliable, soft (but slightly sticky) hold with natural shine and a moist feel. This can still be too heavy for fine or thin hair, and should be used sparingly by normal to thick or coarse hair. It shampoos out fairly easily.

☺ $$$ **Straightening Spray, Chic Sleek, Smooth Sophisticate** (*$17 for 8 ounces*) is a water- and silicone-based straightening spray that goes on fairly greasy, though it can help make curly or wavy hair straight when used with heat. This is best for dry to very dry hair that is coarse or thick; all other hair types will find this liquid too greasy. It provides a soft hold without stickiness, and adds smooth shine plus a slight amount of heat protection.

☺ **Structure Gel, Vitamin Enriched Styling Gel** (*$14 for 5.1 ounces*) contains the tiniest amount of vitamins, and that's just fine, because vitamins are useless for hair. This is a very standard styling gel that provides a firm hold with considerable stiffness and stickiness, making hair somewhat difficult to brush through, especially if it is not in peak condition. If you're looking for a strong-hold gel, this is an option, but less expensive options are easy to find at the drugstore.

☺ **Styling Glue, Super Spiker, Hyper Hold** (*$14 for 6 ounces*) is a thick, slightly creamy styling gel that provides a firm yet flexible hold with some stickiness, though hair can still be brushed through. It is best for stubborn hair that needs hold with some smoothing and added shine. It can be used to slick back hair or exaggerate textured, choppy haircuts. This is relatively easy to shampoo out, but for the best results, I advise you to use it sparingly.

☺ $$$ **Thickening Serum, High Volume, Body Builder** *($16 for 8 ounces)* is a silky, lightweight styling gel that provides a light hold with a slight degree of stickiness but minimal to no stiffness. This doesn't contain any exciting conditioning agents, but it's a dependable gel for all but the most extreme, detailed hairstyles. Its light texture and finish makes it a good option for fine or thin hair, and the film-forming agents can make hair feel a bit thicker.

☺ $$$ **Whipped Wax, Lightweight Texture, Big City Shine** *($16 for 3.3 ounces)* is a styling cream that offers moisture without much heaviness. This lacks the conventional oils, emollients, and heavier waxes of most pomades, and can be a good smoothing, shine-enhancing option for normal to slightly thick, curly, or coarse hair. This can also smooth frizzies, though not to the same extent as silicone styling creams or serums. It provides a light, flexible, non-sticky hold.

ORIGINS

For more information about Origins, one of the many Estee Lauder Companies, call (800) ORIGINS or visit www.origins.com or www.gloss.com.

What's Good About This Line: Only one of the Origins hair-care products below is recommended, and that is only because it is the least problematic in terms of causing either hair dryness or scalp irritation.

What's Not So Good About It: Few product lines in this book offer such a disappointing, problematic selection of products filled with irritating essential oils. Based on the products reviewed below, it doesn't look like Origins can imagine creating a hair-care product without peppermint oil, which means they take the aromatic experience of using their products more seriously than they do what's good for your hair or scalp. Aveda, also a Lauder-owned company, uses far more restraint when it comes to irritating ingredients, often using the extract form in a dilute tea to minimize the irritation rather than using the potent essential oil.

☹ **Clear Head Mint Shampoo** *($11 for 8.5 ounces)* contains essential oils of peppermint along with several other types of mint, which makes this shampoo too irritating for all scalp types. It's enough mint to clear your sinuses, but that isn't helpful (or necessary) for hair and scalp.

☹ **Ginger Up Aromatic Shampoo** *($12.50 for 6.7 ounces)* contains essential oils of ginger, bergamot, clove, lime, eucalyptus, grapefruit, and several others, all extremely irritating to the scalp. This shampoo is not recommended.

☹ **Knot Free Shampoo** *($11 for 8.5 ounces)* contains TEA-lauryl sulfate as one of its main detergent cleansing agents, along with essential oils of peppermint and lemon, which makes this a drying, irritating problem shampoo for all hair and scalp types.

☺ $$$ **The Last Straw Conditioning Shampoo** *($12.50 for 7 ounces)* contains fewer essential oils (and none of the most irritating ones) than the Origins shampoos above. This is a good, mildly conditioning shampoo for normal to slightly dry hair of any thickness, and its creamy texture makes shampooing a bit more luxurious.

☹ **Clear Head Mint Conditioning Rinse** *($11 for 8.5 ounces)* contains a hefty amount of peppermint and several other mint oils, all of which are very irritating to the scalp.

☹ **Ginger Up Aromatic Conditioner** *($12.50 for 6.7 ounces)* contains a high amount of the same problematic essential oils described above for the Ginger Up Aromatic Shampoo. It is not recommended unless your goal is to cause significant scalp irritation. Actually, even without the essential oils, this is a very boring, standard conditioner.

☹ **Happy Endings Conditioner** *($12.50 for 5 ounces)* contains grapefruit, orange, and lemon essential oils (among others), which makes this too irritating and it isn't even a mediocre conditioner, especially since it features sodium lauryl sulfate as the third ingredient.

☹ **Knot Free Finishing Rinse** *($11 for 8.5 ounces)* is a decent conditioner that is ruined by the inclusion of a substantial amount of irritating essential oils, including peppermint, lemon, and wintergreen. It is not recommended for any hair or scalp type.

☹ **Rich Rewards** *($16.50 for 8.2 ounces)* is a standard emollient conditioner that contains a substantial amount of irritating peppermint, benzoin, and galbanum oils. This isn't a rich reward for the hair—it's punishment for the scalp.

OUIDAD

Ouidad is a New York City hair stylist on a mission to tame curly hair—not to straighten it, but to create soft coiled or loose cascading tendrils that bounce and feel soft to the touch. Aside from Ouidad's skill as a stylist and her bustling salon located in Manhattan, she created her own line of products sold with the tag line "a curl's best friend." Even though this is a small array of products, they are well-formulated and worth a look by any hair type. The claims for most of the products are refreshingly realistic rather than over-the-top, although the occasional "repairs hair" or "feeds your hair" does pop up.

For styling curly hair, no one seems to know more about the topic than Ouidad. But for factual information about hair, there is some irksome misinformation in Ouidad's book *Curl Talk* and on her Web site. For example she says, "The best treatment for split ends is to feed your hair, just like your skin. A nourished hair shaft will have enough internal weight to keep the cuticle closed so that each curl is smooth. Clearly, trimming split ends is not an option—you might as well shave your head. Split ends can appear anywhere so frequent deep conditioning is the only way to prevent them." Actually, the very definition of a split end is that it doesn't appear just anywhere; it appears only at the *ends* of hair. Hair can *break* anywhere, but that isn't the same as a frayed split end. And you can't feed hair, it's dead; when you cut it you don't say ouch or bleed, so the analogy to skin is bizarre. Moreover, it isn't the internal weight of the hair shaft that causes damage to the hair, it's the erosion of the external and internal structure of the hair from styling tools, sun damage, and chemical treatments such as perms and dyes.

Although this line fancies itself as the best solution for those with curly hair, the ingredients are not unique in the least, they're found in products throughout the hair-care industry. If Ouidad's products have any edge, it's for those with dry hair because several of these products work well to smooth and soften, whether hair is curly, wavy, or straight. For that alone, this line wins high marks. For more information about Ouidad, call (800) 677-HAIR or visit www.ouidad.com.

What's Good About This Line: Ouidad lists the ingredients for all its products on the company's Web site; it is one of the few lines reviewed in this book that managed to earn across-the-board smiling face ratings for every product.

What's Not So Good About It: The styling products, though all are great formulations, do not contain superior ingredients that justify their above-average prices.

☺ **Clear Shampoo** *($9 for 8 ounces)* is a thoughtfully formulated product that is a very good moisturizing shampoo for normal to dry hair that is normal to thick, curly, or coarse. It can cause buildup with repeated use, but it would take some time for that to occur.

☺ **Curl Quencher Shampoo** *($10 for 8 ounces)* is a creamier version of the Clear Shampoo above, although this contains less plant oil. This works well for normal to slightly dry hair of any thickness.

☺ **Water Works Shampoo** *($10 for 8 ounces)* contains several plant extracts that can be a problem for the scalp, though in a rinse-out product they aren't much cause for concern. This standard shampoo is a good option for all hair types, but is not recommended for someone with a sensitive scalp.

☺ **Balancing Rinse** *($10 for 8 ounces)* is an exceptionally standard, but good, conditioner for normal to dry hair of any thickness. Ouidad also recommends using this as a leave-in conditioner, and that would indeed be a good idea if you have dry hair that is normal to coarse, curly, or thick. This will not, as claimed, close the hair's cuticle layer. Once the cuticle layer is opened (several layers, actually), it can't be closed again like window blinds. Conditioners and styling products can smooth the layers, but once they're washed away, the cuticle remains damaged, especially if hair has been chemically treated or damaged from heat styling.

☺ **$$$ Botanical Boost** *($12 for 8 ounces)* is a very good, though basic, leave-in conditioning mist. Its ultra-light, non-sticky texture is ideal for fine or thin hair that is normal to slightly dry, curly, or straight.

☺ **$$$ Curl Quencher Conditioner** *($12 for 8 ounces)* is a good conditioner for normal to slightly dry hair of any thickness, and it definitely can detangle hair and help make curls more manageable, although it doesn't work as well on hair that is very thick or has tight, corkscrew curls.

☺ **$$$ Clear Control Pomade** *($25 for 4 ounces)* is a clear, gel-type pomade that is reasonably water soluble despite its slick, slightly greasy texture. This same basic formulation is seen in dozens of similar pomades that sell for much less than this overpriced option. It can smooth curls and tame frizzies while adding a glossy shine, but should be used sparingly unless hair is very dry and thick.

☺ $$$ **Climate Control Heat & Humidity Gel** *($16.20 for 8 ounces)* is a wonderfully silky styling gel that can provide a light hold with a soft, touchable finish and minimal stickiness. The conditioning agents and humectants can draw moisture to the hair, which in humid conditions is not what you want, because the added moisture (water) in the hair shaft can cause it to swell, which leads to big, frizzy hair. Sealing the hair shaft from moisture is one way to preserve a hair style and keep frizzies from leaving you frazzled. This product is an option for all hair types, but especially normal to fine or thin hair that needs soft hold with movement.

☺ **Styling Mist** *($10 for 8 ounces)* is a standard, light-hold, nonaerosol hairspray that has a minimal stiff or sticky feel and allows hair to be easily brushed through without flaking. The plant oil, silicone, and glycerin add a touch of conditioning and shine, and make this product preferred for those with drier hair of any thickness.

☺ **Tress F/X Styling Lotion** *($9 for 8 ounces)* is a liquid styling gel-lotion that is excellent for normal to dry hair of any thickness, curly or straight. It offers a light, flexible hold with a smooth, moist finish that's minimally sticky and not stiff. This can beautifully define curls, but is best used in climates where excess humidity is not a problem. For high-humidity climates, pair this with a silicone serum, hairspray, styling wax, or pomade to help repel moisture from hair and postpone the frizzies.

☺ $$$ **Deep Treatment** *($30 for 4 ounces)* is a well-formulated conditioner that is great on dry to very dry hair that is normal to coarse, curly, or thick. This was Ouidad's first product, the one that helped them build their reputation as *the* line for curly hair, but despite all of their exalted pronouncements, it really is just a very good conditioner. There are no unique ingredients present, but in combination they produce admirable results.

☺ $$$ **Shine Hair Glaze** *($25 for 4 ounces)* is a very standard, very overpriced silicone serum that can work as well as any to smooth hair, add shine, and make sure the frizzies don't come calling. If you're going to splurge on Ouidad products, save some money and purchase your silicone serum from Citré Shine, Jheri Redding, Avon, or Charles Worthington.

PANTENE PRO-V

Pantene has attained the status of a classic hair-care line. It's hard to miss this attractively packaged group of products in just about every mass-market outlet and drugstore worldwide. It is also one of the most heavily advertised hair-care lines, with print and television ads in constant rotation, each featuring actresses or models whose hair is so jaw-droppingly *perfect* you would be willing to drive uphill in a blizzard at 3 a.m. to get the same results. This is no doubt what makes Pantene one of the best selling hair-care lines around. Although Pantene likes to play up its "Pro-V" name, which refers to the conditioning agent panthenol, it turns out there is very little of this featured ingredient in most of their products. That's just fine, because panthenol is not the star ingredient for hair, it is just one of the more overly hyped (though still effective) ones.

The real star ingredient in Pantene's conditioners (which is really the main reason to shop this line) is not panthenol, but the unsung hero of hair-care, silicone. Combined with standard, hair-softening thickeners and detangling agents, Pantene has created an assortment of conditioners that leave all hair types feeling simply amazing. Of course, many other hair-care lines use silicone in their conditioners, but Pantene has proven to be a reliable choice that also happens to be more affordable than most. Pantene is owned by consumer product giant Procter & Gamble, which also owns Clairol, Head & Shoulders, and Wella hair-care brands, among others. For more information about Pantene, call (800) 945-7768 or visit www.pantene.com.

What's Good About This Line: Some of the best conditioners (that also happen to be some of the least expensive) can be found here; the styling products offer some pleasant-to-use, basic options as well as some more elegant choices for smoothing hair, including an excellent silicone serum.

What's Not So Good About It: Almost all Pantene shampoos need to be revamped on two counts: (1) the drying and irritating ammonium xylenesulfonate (present in all but one of them) should be removed and (2) Procter & Gamble needs to stop recycling the same shampoo, conditioner, and styling product formulations in product after product after product—you will not find another hair-care line where repetitiveness is so rampant. Pantene could be half the size it is now and still offer the same benefits to a wide variety of hair-care consumers.

☹ **Classically Clean Shampoo** *($4.99 for 13.5 ounces)* is a below-standard shampoo that contains the solvent ammonium xylenesulfonate, which can swell the hair shaft. This side effect can have short-term benefit for fine or thin hair, but it causes dryness for both hair and scalp.

☹ **Color Revival Shampoo** *($4.99 for 13.5 ounces)* is a conditioning shampoo that cannot revive color-treated hair. Rather, the ammonium xylenesulfonate it contains can cause dryness and irritation—not good news if you're trying to keep dyed hair in optimum condition.

☹ **Daily Moisture Renewal Moisturizing Shampoo** *($4.99 for 13.5 ounces)* is nearly identical to the Color Revival Shampoo above, and the same review applies.

☹ **Full & Thick 2 in 1 Shampoo + Conditioner** *($4.79 for 13.5 ounces)* is nearly identical to the Color Revival Shampoo above, and the same review applies.

☹ **Full & Thick Shampoo** *($4.79 for 13.5 ounces)* contains sodium lauryl sulfate as one of its main detergent cleansing agents, and that makes this shampoo too drying for all hair types as well as irritating to the scalp.

☹ **Hydrating Curls Shampoo** *($4.99 for 13.5 ounces)* is nearly identical to the Color Revival Shampoo above, and the same review applies. This is not hydrating, but it can be drying.

☹ **Purity Clarifying Shampoo** *($4.99 for 13.5 ounces)* contains an even greater amount of ammonium xylenesulfonate than the other Pantene shampoos above, and is not recommended.

☹ **Smooth & Sleek Shampoo** *($4.99 for 13.5 ounces)* is nearly identical to the Color Revival Shampoo above, and the same review applies.

☹ **Sheer Volume Shampoo** *($4.99 for 13.5 ounces)* is nearly identical to the Purity Clarifying Shampoo above, and the same review applies.

☹ **Classically Clean 2-in-1 Shampoo & Conditioner** *($4.99 for 13.5 ounces)* is nearly identical to the Color Revival Shampoo above, and the same comments apply.

☹ **Color Revival 2-in-1 Shampoo & Conditioner** *($4.99 for 13.5 ounces)* is nearly identical to the Color Revival Shampoo above, and the same comments apply.

☹ **Daily Moisture Renewal Moisturizing 2-in-1 Shampoo & Conditioner** *($4.99 for 13.5 ounces)* is nearly identical to the Color Revival Shampoo above, except this contains more conditioning agents. Otherwise, the same comments apply.

☹ **Hydrating Curls 2-in-1 Shampoo & Conditioner** *($4.99 for 13.5 ounces)* is nearly identical to the Color Revival Shampoo above, and the same review applies.

☹ **Pro-Vitamin Shampoo Plus Conditioner, Extra Body for Fine Hair** *($4.29 for 13 ounces)* is nearly identical to the Color Revival Shampoo above, and the same review applies. By now, after reading several of the reviews above, it has probably become clear to you that Pantene uses the same standard shampoo formula in various products meant for fine hair, curls, moisturization, classic cleansing, smoothness, and caring for color-treated hair. It makes you wonder why they don't release one "super shampoo" marketed to every hair type and condition imaginable. Of course if they did that, their shelf space at drug and mass-market stores would be greatly reduced, which would mean consumers might not notice them in the overwhelming sea of choices.

☹ **Pro-Vitamin Shampoo Plus Conditioner, for Permed/Color Treated Hair** *($4.29 for 13 ounces)* is nearly identical to the Color Revival Shampoo above, and the same review applies.

☹ **Sheer Volume 2-in-1 Shampoo & Conditioner** *($4.99 for 13.5 ounces)* is nearly identical to the Color Revival Shampoo above, and the same comments apply.

☹ **Smooth & Sleek 2-in-1 Shampoo & Conditioner** *($4.99 for 13.5 ounces)* is nearly identical to the Color Revival Shampoo above, and the same comments apply. By the way, the amount of panthenol (provitamin B5) in all of the Pantene shampoos is too minuscule to matter for any hair type.

☺ **True Confidence Anti-Dandruff 2-in-1 Shampoo & Conditioner** *($4.99 for 13.5 ounces)* is a very good anti-dandruff shampoo that contains 1% zinc pyrithione as its active ingredient. It is a good conditioning shampoo for those with dandruff and normal to slightly dry hair that is normal to fine or thin. It can cause buildup with repeated use. This is the only Pantene shampoo that does not contain ammonium xylenesulfonate.

☹ **Ultra Pro-Vitamin Shampoo Plus Conditioner, for Normal Hair** *($4.29 for 13 ounces)* is nearly identical to the Color Revival Shampoo above, except this contains an added conditioning agent. Otherwise, the same review applies.

☹ **Ultra Pro-Vitamin Shampoo Plus Conditioner, Moisturizing for Dry/Damaged Hair** *($4.29 for 13 ounces)* is nearly identical to the Color Revival Shampoo above, except this contains an added conditioning agent. Otherwise, the same review applies.

☺ **Classic Care Conditioner** *($4.99 for 13.5 ounces)* is a standard, but very good, conditioner that is a great option for dry hair that is normal to fine or thin.

☺ **Color Protect Conditioning Spray, with UV Filter** *($4.99 for 8.5 ounces)* is a lightweight, leave-in conditioner that also works as a lightweight styling spray. It can help make normal to fine or thin hair easy to comb through and provides a very light hold with a bit of stickiness but no stiffness. It is also useful for scrunching and shaping naturally curly, wavy, or permed hair. As for the UV filter, it is a bogus claim because there are no standards for measuring the amount of protection your hair would get from this product.

☺ **Color Revival Conditioner** *($4.99 for 13.5 ounces)* is similar to, but slightly more emollient than, the Classic Care Conditioner above, which makes it preferred for drier hair that is normal to slightly thick or coarse.

☺ **Daily Moisture Renewal Moisturizing Conditioner** *($4.99 for 13.5 ounces)* is a good, basic conditioner for normal to dry hair of any thickness.

☺ **Detangle Light Spray Conditioner** *($4.79 for 8.5 ounces)* is nearly identical to the Color Protect Conditioning Spray, with UV Filter above, and the same review applies.

☺ **Full & Thick Conditioner** *($4.79 for 13.5 ounces)* is similar to the Classic Care Conditioner above, except that this product contains a greater amount of panthenol, which makes this the preferred choice if hair has a normal to fine or thin texture and is also dry to very dry.

☺ **Hydrating Curls Conditioner** *($4.99 for 13.5 ounces)* is identical to the Daily Moisture Renewal Moisturizing Conditioner above, and the same review applies.

☺ **Sheer Volume Conditioner** *($4.99 for 13.5 ounces)* is identical to the Classic Care Conditioner above, and the same review applies.

☺ **Smooth & Sleek Conditioner** *($4.99 for 13.5 ounces)* is identical to the Daily Moisture Renewal Moisturizing Conditioner above, and the same review applies.

☺ **Body Builder Mousse** *($3.99 for 6.6 ounces)* is a standard, creamy-feeling mousse that provides a light hold with a minimal stiff or sticky feel, and allows hair to be easily brushed through. This is a good choice for fine or thin hair.

☺ **Body Builder Volume Gel** *($3.99 for 7.1 ounces)* is a standard, but good, styling gel with a light hold and a minimal stiff, sticky feel that allows hair to be easily brushed through. The conditioning agents can provide a slight amount of heat protection during styling.

☺ **Classic Hairspray, Flexible Hold** (Aerosol) *($3.79 for 8.25 ounces)* is a standard hairspray with a fine mist that provides a light, flexible hold without stiffness or stickiness. It can work well as a finishing touch for all hair types, and is easily brushed through.

☺ **Classic Hairspray, Flexible Hold** (Non-Aerosol) *($3.79 for 10.2 ounces)* offers a very light hold with just a trace of stickiness and no stiffness. It can work well on finished hairstyles that need just a bit more hold that can still be brushed through if desired.

☺ **Classic Hairspray, Ultra Firm Hold** (Aerosol) *($3.79 for 8.25 ounces)* is similar to the Classic Hairspray, Flexible Hold (Aerosol) above, except this offers a medium hold. Otherwise, the same comments apply.

☺ **Classic Hairspray, Ultra Firm Hold** (Non-Aerosol) *($3.79 for 10.2 ounces)* is similar to the Classic Hairspray, Flexible Hold (Non-Aerosol) above, except this offers slightly more hold. Otherwise, the same comments apply.

☺ **Classic Hairspray, Unscented** (Aerosol) *($3.79 for 8.25 ounces)* is similar to the Classic Hairspray, Flexible Hold (Aerosol) above, only with slightly more hold. Despite the name, this still contains fragrance, just a reduced amount for a subtle, but still detectable, scent.

☺ **Classic Hairspray, Unscented** (Non-Aerosol) *($3.79 for 10.2 ounces)* is identical to the Classic Hairspray, Flexible Hold (Non-Aerosol) above, except this contains a softer fragrance.

☺ **Curl Defining Mousse** *($3.99 for 6.6 ounces)* is identical in every respect, except for the name, to the Body Builder Mousse above, and the same review applies.

☺ **Curl Defining Scrunching Gel** *($3.99 for 7.1 ounces)* is a very standard, light- to medium-hold styling gel that can help scrunch curls or enhance wavy hair's texture, but not without some residual stickiness.

☺ **Curl Lock Hairspray, Flexible Hold** (Non-Aerosol) *($3.99 for 10.2 ounces)* is identical to the Classic Hairspray, Flexible Hold (Non-Aerosol) above, and the same comments apply.

☺ **Frizz Control Smoothing Creme** *($7.99 for 3.5 ounces)* is a very good water- and silicone-based styling cream that is a good choice to tame frizzies on dry to very dry hair that is normal to coarse or thick. It doesn't take much before this starts feeling greasy, so use it sparingly for best results. This also works well to straighten curly or wavy hair with heat and the proper styling tools.

☺ **Get It Straight Gel** *($3.99 for 7.1 ounces)* is identical to the Curl Defining Scrunching Gel above, and the same review applies. The tiny amount of conditioning agents make this inappropriate for use alone to heat-style hair, but it would be great on stubborn or unruly hair if mixed with the Frizz Control Smoothing Creme above.

☺ **In Control Mousse** *($4.79 for 6.6 ounces)* is identical to the Body Builder Mousse above, and the same review applies. Once again, Pantene has recycled the same mousse formula into four separate products (see the review for Radiant Response Mousse below). It isn't necessary, causes confusion, and yet it happens surprisingly often in the hair-care industry.

☺ **In Control Shaping Gel** *($3.99 for 7.1 ounces)* is identical to the Curl Defining Scrunching Gel above, and the same review applies.

☺ **Moisturizing Curls Shaper Anti-Frizz Creme** *($7.99 for 3.5 ounces)* is identical to the Frizz Control Smoothing Creme above, and the exact same review applies here, too.

☺ **Radiant Response Gel with Colorshine** *($3.99 for 5.1 ounces)* is a water-based, alcohol-free spray gel that offers a light to medium hold with a slightly sticky, stiff feel, though hair can still be brushed through. This is best for textured or slicked-back hairstyles that need hold with some pliability.

☺ **Radiant Response Mousse for Color-Treated Hair** *($3.99 for 6.6 ounces)* is identical to the Body Builder Mousse above, and the same review applies. Nothing in this mousse is particularly beneficial for color-treated hair.

☺ **Scrunching Curls Spray Gel** *($4.79 for 5.1 ounces)* is identical to the Radiant Response Gel with Colorshine above, and the same review applies. Why this one costs more is a mystery.

☺ **Stay Smooth Hairspray, Flexible Hold (Non-Aerosol)** *($3.99 for 10.2 ounces)* is identical to the Classic Hairspray, Flexible Hold (Non-Aerosol) above, and the same review applies.

☺ **Total Control Shaping Gel** *($4.79 for 7.1 ounces)* is identical to the Body Builder Volume Gel above, and the exact same comments apply.

☺ **Volumizing Hair Spray, Flexible Hold (Aerosol)** *($3.79 for 8.25 ounces)* is identical to the Classic Hairspray, Ultra Firm Hold (Aerosol) hairspray above, and the same comments apply.

☺ **Volumizing Hair Spray, Flexible Hold (Non-Aerosol)** *($3.79 for 10.2 ounces)* is identical to the Classic Hairspray, Flexible Hold (Non-Aerosol) hairspray above, and the same review applies.

☺ **Volumizing Hair Spray, Maximum Hold (Aerosol)** *($3.79 for 8.25 ounces)* is identical to the Classic Hairspray, Ultra Firm Hold (Aerosol) above, and the same comments apply. If you think this repetitiveness is tiresome to read, try writing about it!

☺ **Volumizing Hair Spray, Maximum Hold (Non-Aerosol)** *($3.79 for 10.2 ounces)* is identical to the Classic Hairspray, Ultra-Firm Hold (Non-Aerosol) above, and the same comments apply.

☺ **Volumizing Root Lifter Spray Gel** *($3.99 for 5.1 ounces)* is identical to the Radiant Response Gel with Colorshine above, and the same review applies.

☺ **Smooth & Shine Anti-Frizz Serum** *($5.89 for 1.7 ounces)* is a standard, but very good, silicone serum whose price makes it even more appealing. As with all silicone serums, it works beautifully to tame frizz, add brilliant shine, and make hair look sleek. Just use it sparingly to avoid a greasy appearance.

☺ **Curl Revive Frizz Control Treatment** *($4.79 for 8.5 ounces)* is nearly identical to the Color Protect Conditioning Spray, with UV Filter above, and the same comments apply. Neither this nor the Color Protect product above can protect hair from UV damage.

☺ **Deep Moisture Masque, for Color-Treated Hair** *($3.99 for 5.1 ounces)* is identical to the Daily Moisture Renewal Moisturizing Conditioner above, and there is no need to settle for this conditioner-masquerading-as-treatment when the same formula can be had in a much larger size for just one dollar more. The Daily Moisture Renewal product can be left on hair for as long as possible for maximum conditioning benefits.

☺ **Frizz Down Deep Moisturizing Treatment** *($4.79 for 6.8 ounces)* is identical to the Deep Moisture Masque, for Color-Treated Hair above, and the same comments apply.

☺ **Instant Defense Heat Protector Spray** *($4.79 for 8.5 ounces)* is nearly identical to the Color Protect Conditioning Spray, with UV Filter above, and the same review applies. Hair cannot be protected from the more than 300°F heat (water boils at 212°F) generated by curling irons, flat irons, and blow dryers. It is definitely better to have a styling product on the hair with smoothing ingredients than nothing at all, but that still doesn't stop the heat damage styling tools cause.

☺ **Pure Brilliance Deep Hydrating Treatment** *($3.99 for 6.8 ounces)* is identical to the Deep Moisture Masque, for Color-Treated Hair above, and the same comments apply.

☺ **Repair & Protect Intensive Restoration Treatment** *($4.79 for 6.8 ounces)* is identical to the Deep Moisture Masque, for Color-Treated Hair above, and the same comments apply.

☺ **Repair & Restructure Daily Strengthening Treatment** *($4.79 for 5.1 ounces)*. This spray-on product cannot strengthen hair, but it can make it easier to comb through while adding a slight feeling of thickness to fine or thin hair. As you may have guessed, nothing in this product can repair or restructure hair.

☺ **Restore & Renew Deep Fortifying Treatment** *($4.79 for 8.5 ounces)* is identical to the Deep Moisture Masque, for Color-Treated Hair above, and the same comments apply.

PANTENE PRO-V RELAXED & NATURAL

☺ **Relaxed & Natural Intensive Moisturizing Shampoo** *($3.99 for 13.5 ounces)* is a rich, conditioning shampoo suitable for dry to very dry hair that is coarse, curly, or thick. Pantene markets this line to women of color, but African-American consumers with thin, fragile hair may find this shampoo too emollient. It contains mostly water, Vaseline, detergent cleansing agents, lather agent, thickener, fragrance, salt, detangling agent, pH adjuster, preservatives, and panthenol.

☺ **Relaxed & Natural Daily Oil Cream Moisturizer** *($4.99 for 10.2 ounces)* is a heavy, greasy conditioner that is an option only for extremely dry, damaged, or overprocessed hair. It contains mostly water, mineral oil, Vaseline, thickener, silicone, emollient, preservative, pH adjuster, lanolin, alcohol, film-forming agent, plant oils, fragrance, preservatives, panthenol, and more thickeners. This is difficult to rinse from hair, but it definitely will make it smooth, soft, and easy to detangle.

☺ **Relaxed & Natural Intensive Moisturizing Conditioner** *($3.99 for 13.5 ounces)* is an excellent conditioner for normal to very dry hair that is normal to coarse, curly, or thick.

☺ **Relaxed & Natural Wrap & Set Lotion** *($4.99 for 10.2 ounces)* is similar to the Color Protect Conditioning Spray, with UV Filter above, except this adds two plant oils to the mix. They lend this product a slick but still light feel that can help set and condition braids or other textured hairstyles. This can work well as a leave-in detangling spray for dry hair of any texture.

☺ **Relaxed & Natural Intensive Oil Sheen Spray** *($4.99 for 10 ounces)* is a fairly greasy, slick aerosol glossing spray that is an OK option for dry to very dry hair that is thick, coarse, or highly textured. It adds lots of shine but can quickly become too heavy unless you use restraint as you apply it.

PAUL MITCHELL

This extensive product line has been a mainstay in salons for so long that it feels like an old, comfortable sweater that lasts season after season. Paul Mitchell was a hairstylist, and one of the first to launch his own line of products. The story of how this line came to be and how it grew into a company with sales of over $800 million per year is filled with classic American can-do attitude and more than a bit of risk-taking.

Mitchell and his business partner, John Paul DeJoria, devised the line in 1979, and spent all their savings to travel and promote the (then small) selection of products to salons across the country. Skeptical salon owners were offered a deal that was unheard of at the time: Buy Paul Mitchell products to use on your clients and if they (and the salon staff) were not happy with them, they could send them back for a full refund. The idea worked, and the seeds for what became one of the most distributed salon lines in the world were planted. If you are not familiar with this line, then you must not be frequenting one of the 90,000 U.S. salons where it is sold. There are many well-formulated products available from Paul Mitchell, but there are also enough missteps along the way that it's not a hair-care line to shop blindly. For more information about Paul Mitchell, call (800) 793-8790 or visit www.paulmitchell.com.

What's Good About This Line: Most of the shampoos and conditioners are highly effective options whose scope can meet the needs of every hair type and condition imaginable; one of the most reliable lines to shop for bountiful choices in styling products, again covering all the bases for every hair type and styling need, from minimal to cement-like hold; the color-enhancing shampoos are excellent; reasonable prices, for a salon-bred, salon-sold line.

What's Not So Good About It: The Tea Tree line is a collection that will only cause irritation thanks to the high amount of peppermint oil in all of the Tea Tree products; a few styling products contain drying sulfonic acid, film-forming agents, or sodium polystyrene sulfonate; a few shampoos contain drying detergent cleansing agents or other problematic ingredients that do more harm than good to hair.

☺ **Cleanse, Awapuhi Shampoo** *($5.99 for 8.5 ounces)* is a standard shampoo that can work well for normal to slightly dry hair that is normal to fine or thin. The awapuhi (white ginger) has no established benefit for hair, but it can impart a pleasant fragrance. This does pose a slight risk of buildup with repeated use.

☺ **Cleanse, Baby Don't Cry Shampoo** *($8.99 for 16.9 ounces)* is a very gentle shampoo that would be ideal for babies and children if it did not contain fragrance. For adults, this shampoo is an option for normal to slightly dry hair, but is not the best if you routinely use heavy styling products such as pomades or waxes.

☺ **Cleanse, Botanical Hydrating Shampoo** *($9.99 for 8.5 ounces)* isn't any more botanical than Paul Mitchell's other shampoos, which means almost not at all, and is fairly similar to (but more conditioning than) the Awapuhi Shampoo above. It is a very good option for normal to dry hair of any thickness. The conditioning agents can build up with repeated use.

☹ **Cleanse, Botanical Prep Shampoo** *($10.99 for 6.8 ounces)* contains sodium C14-16 olefin sulfonate as its main detergent cleansing agent, and also lists sodium polystyrene sulfonate, which makes this an incredibly drying shampoo that can potentially strip hair color with repeated use.

☺ **Cleanse, Shampoo One** *($6.49 for 8.5 ounces)* is a very standard, simple shampoo that is an option for all hair types, and poses minimal to no risk of buildup.

☺ **Cleanse, Shampoo Two** *($6.49 for 8.5 ounces)* is nearly identical to the Shampoo One above, except this contains a greater amount of film-forming agent, so it can definitely cause buildup with repeated use. It is preferred for normal to fine or thin hair that is normal to slightly dry.

☹ **Cleanse, Shampoo Three** *($8.99 for 8.5 ounces)* contains several problematic ingredients that can be irritating to the scalp, drying to hair, and potentially strip hair color. Sodium thiosulfate and sulfated castor oil are always a problem when used in shampoos. Paul Mitchell claims this shampoo can "increase hair's inner strength," when in reality the harsh ingredients in here will weaken it.

☹ **Cleanse, Tea Tree Special Shampoo** *($9.49 for 8.5 ounces)* contains tea tree oil, but not enough to help scalp problems such as dandruff, which would require a 5% concentration and this falls well under that. The problem ingredient in this product is peppermint oil—this shampoo contains quite a bit of it—which can cause pronounced scalp irritation. It also contains sodium lauryl sulfate as its main cleansing agent, which only makes matters worse.

☺ **Color Care, Color Shampoos** *($8.99 for 8.5 ounces)* is an excellent group of color-enhancing shampoos that present options for several shades of blonde, red/auburn, and brown hair, as well as an option for silver/gray hair. Their color-enhancing effect is subtle, but they are all recommended.

☺ **Color Care Shampoo, Color Protect Daily Shampoo** *($6.99 for 8.5 ounces)* is a standard, but very good, shampoo for normal to dry hair of any thickness. This can cause buildup with repeated use, but won't make thick or coarse hair feel stiff or wiry. Nothing in this shampoo can protect color better than any other standard shampoo.

☺ **Extra-Body Shampoo, Extra-Body Daily Shampoo** *($6.99 for 8.5 ounces)* is nearly identical to the Cleanse, Shampoo Two above, and the same review applies. The minor amount of conditioning agents does make this a clean-rinsing shampoo that can give fine or thin hair body.

☺ **Moisture Shampoo, Instant Moisture Daily Shampoo** *($5.99 for 8.5 ounces)* is nearly identical to the Cleanse, Shampoo Two above, and the same review applies. This is not a very moisturizing shampoo.

☺ **Moisture Shampoo, The Wash** *($10.99 for 16.9 ounces)* is similar to the Cleanse, Botanical Hydrating Shampoo above, and the same basic comments apply. This claims to supply the perfect balance of moisture, but there is no way for a shampoo to "detect" how dry your hair is, so that ends up being a bogus statement.

☺ **Smoothing Shampoo, Super Skinny Daily Shampoo** *($9.49 for 10.1 ounces)* is sold as a smoothing shampoo because "sleek and chic are in." That may be true, but there is nothing in this shampoo that is all that smoothing, nor is it all that different from most of the recommended Paul Mitchell shampoos above. This is a very good shampoo for normal to dry hair of any thickness, and poses just a moderate risk of buildup.

☺ **Color Care Condition, Color Protect Daily Conditioner** *($8.99 for 8.5 ounces)* is a standard, rather lightweight conditioner that is great for normal to slightly dry hair that is normal to fine or thin.

☺ **Condition, Botanical Body-Building Rinse** *($11.99 for 8.5 ounces)* is nearly identical to the Color Care Condition, Color Protect Daily Conditioner above, and the same review applies.

☹ **Condition, Tea Tree Special Conditioner** *($10.49 for 8.5 ounces)* contains peppermint and lavender oils, and neither is used in a token amount. Together, that greatly increases the potential for irritating the scalp, and the description for this conditioner clearly indicates it should be used on the scalp, which would be a mistake. The amount of tea tree oil in this product isn't enough to have any effect on scalp conditions such as dandruff.

☺ **$$$ Condition, The Conditioner** *($12.99 for 8.5 ounces)* is an exceptionally standard, but good, conditioner for normal to dry hair of any thickness.

☺ **$$$ Condition, The Cream, Leave-In Thickening Conditioner** *($14.49 for 6.8 ounces)* is a good conditioning balm for slightly dry hair. It contains a standard film-forming/holding agent to coat hair and make it feel thicker. This can leave hair feeling slightly sticky, but it is easy to brush through.

☺ **Condition, The Rinse** *($8.99 for 8.5 ounces)* is a lightweight detangling conditioner that is a good option for normal to fine or thin hair that is slightly dry.

☺ **Extra-Body Condition, Extra-Body Daily Rinse** *($8.99 for 8.5 ounces)* is identical to the Color Care Condition, Color Protect Daily Conditioner above, and the same review applies. This conditioner is not very heavy, which is why it can leave normal to fine or thin hair with some body, but over time it can make fine or thin hair feel limp unless it is washed out with a shampoo that doesn't cause buildup.

☺ **Extra-Body Style, Extra-Body Daily Boost, Root Lifter** *($10.95 for 8.5 ounces)* is a moist, slightly sticky, alcohol-free styling spray with a special directional nozzle to facilitate application at the roots. Applied on the roots, this can provide lift and volume with a light to medium hold that is easily brushed through.

☺ **Extra-Body Style, Extra-Body Finishing Spray, Firm-Hold, Volume and Shine** *($13.95 for 12 ounces)* is a standard aerosol hairspray that applies as a very fine mist that can keep fine or thin hair from becoming too coated. This provides a light, brushable hold that leaves hair feeling more silky than stiff or sticky. It is a great finishing product for those who normally avoid hairspray because they think it makes their hair too stiff and immovable.

☺ **Extra-Body Style, Extra-Body Sculpting Foam, Firm-Hold Thickening Foam** *($7.95 for 6 ounces)* is a standard, propellant-based mousse that offers a light hold with a soft, slightly sticky finish that is easily brushed through. The almost weightless texture and film-forming agents can make fine or thin hair feel slightly thicker, but they are not unique to this product.

☹ **Extra-Body Style, Extra-Body Sculpting Gel, Firm-Hold Thickening Gel** *($8.99 for 6.8 ounces)* contains a form of sulfonic acid that can be drying for hair and possibly strip hair color with repeated use.

☺ **Finish, Dry Wax, Clean Texture and Definition** *($12.95 for 1.8 ounces)* is an extremely thick styling wax with a natural matte finish. It is only for application on dry hair, and then is best used sparingly over stubborn frizzies, curls, or dry ends. It is difficult to shampoo out.

☺ **Finish, Foaming Pomade, Multi-Texture Smoothing Polish** *($10.95 for 5.1 ounces)* is a slick, greasy, liquid pomade that foams slightly as it is dispenses, similar to shaving cream. It is best for smoothing dry to very dry hair that is thick, coarse, and unmanageable. Unless used sparingly, it can make hair feel heavy and cause styles to fall flat.

☺ **$$$ Finish, Slick Works, Texture and Shine** *($16.95 for 6.8 ounces)* is a gel-type pomade packaged in a tube. It can indeed be slick, but it takes more than a little bit of this to make hair feel heavy. It is a good smoothing and shine-enhancing option for textured, curly, or wavy hair that is normal to fine, though it is still best used on the ends of hair rather than applied from root to tip. This does shampoo out easily.

☺ **Finish, Spray Wax, 3-D Texture and Flexible Hold** *($12.95 for 2.8 ounces)* is a unique, versatile, spray-on wax that works well to add instant texture and smoothness to dry, coarse hair, or it can be used for more extreme hairstyles where exaggerated texture is the goal. This is much lighter than a traditional wax, but can still make hair feel heavy and look greasy if it is not applied with restraint.

☺ **Finish, Super Clean Light, Soft-Hold Finishing Spray (Aerosol)** *($10.95 for 10 ounces)* contains more fragrance than conditioning agents, and it leaves hair feeling sticky and slightly stiff, though minimally so. This provides a light, flexible hold that is easily brushed through, making it a good working hairspray for casual hairstyles.

☺ **$$$ Finish, Wax Works, Extreme Texture and Shine** *($16.95 for 6.8 ounces)* is similar to the Slick Works product above, but with a thicker texture and more emolliency, which makes it preferred for drier hair that is thick or coarse. It has a light hold with no stiff or sticky feel.

☺ **Firm Hold Style, Freeze and Shine Super Spray, Firm-Hold Finishing Spray (Non-Aerosol)** *($10.95 for 8.5 ounces)* is a standard hairspray that has a medium to firm hold with a slightly stiff, sticky finish. It is difficult to brush through, so this is best used as a final finishing step when you are ready to hold hair in place while still allowing some movement.

☺ **Firm Hold Style, Super Clean Extra, Firm-Hold Finishing Spray (Aerosol)** *($10.95 for 10 ounces)* is similar to the Finish, Super Clean Light, Soft-Hold Finishing Spray (Aerosol) above, and the same basic comments apply. This does contain a greater amount of conditioning agents, which makes it easier to brush through and adds a touch more shine.

☺ **Firm Hold Style, Super Clean Sculpting Gel, Maximum Hold and Control** *($7.45 for 6.8 ounces)* is an excellent conditioning styling gel capable of a light to medium hold that is easily brushed through with minimal stiff or sticky feel. This is an excellent gel for enhancing curls and waves without feeling heavy.

☺ **Light Hold Style, Soft Sculpting Spray Gel, Flexible Styling Spray-On Gel** *($7.25 for 8.5 ounces)* is a water- and alcohol-based, light-hold spray gel that leaves hair feeling slightly stiff and sticky, though it is easily brushed through. This is a very good option for fine or thin hair that needs help with hold and could benefit from a slightly thicker feel.

☺ **Light Hold Style, Soft Spray, Light-Hold Finishing Spray (Non-Aerosol)** *($6.75 for 8.5 ounces)* is a standard, smooth-finish, light-hold hairspray that takes a bit longer than usual to dry, but leaves hair feeling minimally stiff and sticky. This is recommended for all hair types that need a shot of finishing-touch hold.

☺ **$$$ Medium Hold Style, Fast Drying Sculpting Spray, Medium-Hold Finishing Spray (Non-Aerosol)** *($16.95 for 16 ounces)* is almost identical to the Light Hold Style, Soft Spray, Light-Hold Finishing Spray above, except this offers more hold and more noticeable stickiness, though it can still be brushed through.

☺ **Medium Hold Style, Hair Sculpting Lotion, Versatile Styling Liquid** *($11.95 for 16.9 ounces)* is a watery styling product that works well on wet or dry hair to provide a light to medium hold. It isn't a heavy product, but can leave hair feeling slightly stiff and sticky, though it does brush through.

☺ **Medium Hold Style, Sculpting Foam, Conditioning Styling Foam** *($7.45 for 6 ounces)* is a creamy, but light-textured, propellant-based styling mousse. It provides a light, touchable hold that leaves hair smooth and soft, if just a bit sticky. Whereas most mousses feel like barely there fluff, this product has more "substance."

☺ **Medium Hold Style, Super Clean Spray, Medium-Hold Finishing Spray (Aerosol)** *($10.95 for 10 ounces)* is similar to the Finish, Super Clean Light, Soft-Hold Finishing

Spray (Aerosol) above, and the same basic comments apply. This does contain more conditioning agents, which makes it easier to brush through and adds a touch more shine to hair.

☺ **Medium Hold Style, Super Sculpt, Quick-Drying Styling Glaze** *($6.75 for 8.5 ounces)* has a slightly thicker texture than the Medium Hold Style, Hair Sculpting Lotion above, but otherwise offers the same amount of hold. The two products are basically interchangeable, though this one does have a slight apple scent that may or may not be to your liking.

☺ **Smoothing Style Straight Works, Straightens and Smoothes** *($14.95 for 6.8 ounces)* is a very good styling gel that contains enough silicone, film-forming agent, and wax to smooth wavy or curly hair and allow it to be straightened with heat and the proper brush. Those with fine or thin hair will likely find it too heavy, but it is excellent for coarse or thick hair that needs frizz control and lots of shine.

☹ **Style, Heat Seal, Multi-Purpose, Humidity Resistant Styling Spray** *($8.99 for 8.5 ounces)* contains sodium polystyrene sulfonate, which can be drying to hair and scalp while possibly stripping hair color with repeated use.

☺ **$$$ Style, Re-Works, Versatile Texture Cream** *($16.99 for 5.1 ounces)* is a thick, slightly creamy and quite sticky styling product. It offers a medium hold without any stiffness, and helps keep hair pliable. It is an excellent product for short, choppy haircuts where the emphasis is on defining texture and creating a purposefully messy, "bed head" look. Those with thick, coarse hair can also use this for extra manageability, shine, and structure. It is not recommended for fine or thin hair.

☺ **Style, Volumizing Spray, Root Lifter** *($9.99 for 8.5 ounces)* is nearly identical to the Extra-Body Style, Extra-Body Daily Boost, Root Lifter above, except this comes in a conventional spray-on applicator. Otherwise, the same basic comments apply.

☺ **Color Care, Color Protect Locking Spray** *($11.99 for 8.5 ounces)* won't protect hair color from fading, but is a very good spray-on, leave-in conditioner for normal to dry hair that is normal to fine or thin.

☺ **$$$ Condition, Botanical Body-Building Treatment** *($12.99 for 3.4 ounces)* does contain botanicals, but none of them are helpful for hair, though the licorice extract is a good anti-irritant for the scalp. (Still, the licorice extract will be rinsed out before it can have much of an effect.) Other than that, this is a rather boring conditioner that is mostly thickeners and fragrance. It is an OK option for normal to slightly dry hair of any thickness.

☺ **$$$ Condition, Hair Repair Treatment** *($12.49 for 6.8 ounces)* cannot repair hair, but is a very good conditioner for normal to dry hair that is normal to fine or thin.

☺ **Condition, Lite Detangler** *($8.99 for 8.5 ounces)* is a good, lightweight detangling solution for normal to fine or thin hair.

☹ **Condition, Seal and Shine** *($5.99 for 8.5 ounces)* contains a high amount of sodium polystyrene sulfonate, which can be drying to hair and scalp and has the potential to strip hair color.

☺ **Condition, Taming Spray** *($9.99 for 16.9 ounces)* can work well to detangle and lightly moisturize all hair types without adding a heavy, weighed-down feel to hair.

☺ **Condition, The Detangler** *($7.99 for 8.5 ounces)* can make all hair types easier to comb through while adding a silky smoothness.

☺ **Finish, The Shine** *($11.49 for 3.4 ounces)* is a standard, but effective, silicone spray that contains a small amount of alcohol to prevent the silicone from making hair feel too heavy, though this should still be used sparingly. It is a good shine-enhancing option for all hair types.

☺ **Moisture Condition, Awapuhi Moisture Mist** *($7.49 for 8.5 ounces)* can provide light moisture and moderate control of frizzies. It works great for normal to slightly dry hair that is fine or thin.

☺ **$$$ Moisture Condition, Instant Moisture Daily Treatment** *($18.99 for 16.9 ounces)* is a standard overpriced conditioner. It isn't any more intense than most of the Paul Mitchell conditioners above, but it is an option for all but fine or thin hair types.

☺ **$$$ Moisture Condition, Super-Charged Moisturizer** *($12.99 for 6.8 ounces)* is nearly identical to the Condition, The Conditioner above, and the same review applies.

☺ **Smoothing Condition, Super Skinny Daily Treatment** *($10.99 for 10.1 ounces)* is a very light conditioner that is an excellent option for normal to slightly dry hair that is normal to fine or thin.

☺ **$$$ Smoothing Condition Super Skinny Serum** *($16.99 for 5.1 ounces)* is a standard silicone serum whose texture is thinner than the Smoothing Style Gloss Drops below. It is a good option for all hair types that need help taming frizzies or restoring shine, but don't let its thinner texture fool you: this can still be too greasy if not used sparingly. It does have an intense fragrance, so be sure you like it before purchasing.

☺ **Smoothing Style Gloss Drops, Frizz-Free Defining Polish** *($14.95 for 3.4 ounces)* is a standard silicone serum that is pricier than similar options at the drugstore, though not outrageously so. It can work as well as any to smooth frizzies and add a lustrous shine to hair, and the thicker texture makes it preferred for coarse or thick hair.

PAUL MITCHELL LAB

☺ **$$$ Lab ESP, Elastic Shaping Paste** *($11.95 for 1.8 ounces)* is similar to the Finish, Dry Wax, Clean Texture and Definition above, except this is a water- and wax-based emulsion that has more pliability and is a bit easier to distribute through hair. It is still very heavy, and can make hair feel coated. However, it can be an amazing fix for stubborn frizzies and curls or it can be used to create extreme texture on short, choppy hairstyles. This is fairly difficult to shampoo out.

☺ **Lab XTG, Extreme Thickening Glue** *($10.95 for 3.4 ounces)* is Paul Mitchell's strongest-holding styling product, but if you want this much hold you'll have to tolerate a thick, gummy, glue-like texture that can be tricky to distribute through hair. It works best to emphasize short hairstyles that want a chunky, piece-y look with all-day styling support that remains pliable, but is uncomfortably sticky. Take the "glue" name seriously—they're not kidding about it.

PAUL MITCHELL TEA TREE

☹ Tea Tree Care, Tea Tree Special Shampoo, Invigorating Cleanser *($10.99 for 10.1 ounces)* is identical to the Cleanse, Tea Tree Special Shampoo above, save for a change in packaging. Both contain the exact same amount of tea tree oil, which is no more than a 1% concentration, and that's not enough to help scalp problems such as dandruff (that requires a 5% concentration). The problem ingredient in this product is peppermint oil—this shampoo contains quite a bit of it, and it can cause pronounced scalp irritation. It also contains sodium lauryl sulfate as its main cleansing agent, which only makes matters worse.

☹ Tea Tree Care, Tea Tree Hair and Body Moisturizer, Leave-In Conditioner *($11.99 for 10.1 ounces)* contains peppermint and lavender oils (and not in token amounts either), which will be especially irritating to the scalp when used in products such as this that are meant to be left on hair. In addition, it doesn't contain enough tea tree oil to be effective for any scalp problem.

☹ Tea Tree Care, Tea Tree Special Conditioner, Invigorating Conditioner *($11.99 for 10.1 ounces)* gets its invigoration from peppermint oil, which is too irritating for the scalp and makes this conditioner impossible to recommend.

☺ Tea Tree Groom, Tea Tree Grooming Pomade *($14.99 for 3.5 ounces)* is a standard, water-soluble pomade that is a decent option for smoothing ends and flyaways when used sparingly. The tea tree oil is a waste in here because using pomade on the scalp is a styling nightmare.

☺ $$$ Tea Tree Groom, Tea Tree Stick Wax *($17.49 for 2.6 ounces)* is a pomade in stick form and it works well to smooth hair. The tea tree oil is wasted, however, because you would not want to use this product on the scalp.

☹ Tea Tree Groom, Tea Tree Styling Gel *($10.95 for 6.8 ounces)* contains a form of sulfonic acid that can be drying to hair and potentially strip hair color with repeated use.

☺ $$$ Tea Tree Groom, Tea Tree Styling Wax, Definition and Control *($18.99 for 6.8 ounces)* is identical to the Finish, Wax Works, Extreme Texture and Shine above, and the same comments apply.

☹ Tea Tree Care, Tea Tree Hair and Scalp Treatment *($13.99 for 6.8 ounces)* contains a great deal of peppermint oil, and is not recommended for any scalp condition or skin type.

PAULA'S CHOICE

I developed and launched Paula's Choice skin care in 1995, and am proud of how the line has grown into an exciting array of effective yet affordable products. I originally had no intention of offering hair-care products (because the marketplace was already bursting at the seams with options), but it was a constant customer request, so I decided to offer a shampoo/body wash-in-one and a daily conditioner. A major point of difference for both of these products is that they are truly fragrance- and irritant-free. If you have ever tried to find fragrance-free hair-care products that work, you know what a daunting task it can be, since 99.9% of them either really do contain fragrance (sometimes listed as "perfume," "parfum," or just fragrance) or fragrant essential oils and plant extracts that are often, if not always, irritating to skin. I worked closely with the chemists involved in the creation of these products to be sure they met my strict performance standards and were every bit as elegant as the best hair-care products available.

Having analyzed and reported on the cosmetics industry for years, I am acutely aware that there are many products that perform as well as mine. I believe my products offer excellent value for their quality and performance. I leave them unrated because of my obvious bias, but as I have stated before, these products are just one set of great options among many—the final decision is yours. For more information about Paula's Choice, call (800) 831-4088 or visit www.paulaschoice.com.

All Over Hair & Body Shampoo *($12.95 for 16 ounces)* is a standard, detergent-based shampoo that is a very good option for all hair types, but particularly for those with a sensitive scalp. It poses minimal to no risk of buildup and is free of irritants, fragrance, and coloring agents. This is also an excellent shampoo for babies and children and, as the name states, as a body wash.

Smooth Finish Conditioner *($12.95 for 16 ounces)* is a moisturizing, daily-use conditioner with a slightly creamy texture that makes it appropriate for all hair types. It does not contain any needlessly irritating ingredients, and is completely fragrance- and colorant-free.

PERT PLUS

Procter & Gamble–owned Pert Plus was the first company to successfully develop and market the concept of a shampoo and conditioner in one product, otherwise known as "two-in-ones," back in 1985. This development changed the world of hair care forever. P&G used a form of silicone that had amazing properties for hair. Not only does silicone have an amazing silky texture, but its ability to cling to hair, even under water pressure and detergent cleansing agents, is astounding. Silicone's unique consistency can make hair feel satiny smooth with minimal to no greasy feel or weight. At the time Pert began incorporating silicones into shampoo, it was used in less than 5% of the hair-care industry. Today, silicone is found in more than 80% of the products being sold, and nowadays many shampoos, even those not labeled as two-in-ones, contain conditioning ingredients similar to Pert.

The only real downside to using a two-in-one is that the conditioners can build up on hair with repeated use. That's because every time you shampoo, the conditioning ingredients are being redeposited over what was already on the hair and not washed away. Over time, that can make hair feel heavy and weighed down. Washing with a "clarifying" shampoo (one that doesn't contain any conditioning or volumizing ingredients) every few times or every other time you shampoo will easily take care of that problem. Two-in-ones end up being best for those with normal to slightly dry hair that has normal thickness, though they're also excellent for those with short hair. Those with dry or damaged hair that is thick or coarse will not find two-in-ones emollient enough. For more information about Pert Plus, call (800) 543-1745 or visit www.pertplus.com.

What's Good About This Line: If you like two-in-ones, these are the products that started the trend.

What's Not So Good About It: The claim that each Pert Plus shampoo cleanses and conditions hair without any dulling residue or buildup is not true; conditioning agents in Pert Plus products cannot protect hair from the rigors of styling hair with heat; all but one of the shampoos below contain the solvent ammonium xylenesulfonate, which can cause scalp and hair dryness. I typically rate hair-care products that contain this ingredient poorly, but have made an exception in the case of the Pert Plus Dandruff Control Shampoo plus Conditioner because its active ingredient is so effective against dandruff. The other Pert Plus products were not rated highly because of their ammonium xylenesulfonate content.

☺ **2 in 1 Dandruff Control Shampoo plus Conditioner** *($3.99 for 13.5 ounces)* is a 1% zinc pyrithione anti-dandruff shampoo in a standard shampoo/conditioner base that works well for those with normal to dry hair that isn't thick or coarse.

☹ **2 in 1 Shampoo plus Deep Conditioner** *($3.49 for 13.5 ounces)* is a standard conditioning shampoo that can become drying for hair and scalp after repeated use due to the inclusion of ammonium xylenesulfonate (there is more ammonium xylenesulfonate in here than in the Dandruff Control Shampoo plus Conditioner above).

☹ **2 in 1 Shampoo plus Light Conditioner** *($3.49 for 13.5 ounces)* is, save for a lesser amount of silicone, nearly identical to the 2 in 1 Shampoo plus Deep Conditioner above, and the same comments apply.

☹ **2 in 1 Shampoo plus Medium Conditioner** *($3.49 for 13.5 ounces)* is, save for a lesser amount of silicone, nearly identical to the 2 in 1 Shampoo plus Deep Conditioner above, and the same comments apply.

☹ **Fresh 2 in 1 Refreshing Shampoo plus Conditioner** *($3.49 for 13.5 ounces)* is the lightest Pert Plus shampoo, but it's still not recommended because the ammonium xylenesulfonate can cause hair and scalp dryness with repeated use.

☺ **Kids 2 in 1 Shampoo plus Conditioner, Bananaberri** *($3.49 for 13.5 ounces)* is a very good conditioning shampoo for normal to dry hair that is normal to coarse or thick. However, the pervasive fruity scent is definitely more appealing to kids than adults. This is the only Pert Plus shampoo that does not contain ammonium xylenesulfonate.

PHILIP B. HAIR CARE

Philip B. is a successful hairstylist with salons in New York and Los Angeles, and his hair-care line includes some of the most expensive products around. Philip B. defends the expense as being related to the amount of plant extracts they contain. According to Philip B., "Extensive research with herbalists and chemists revealed a simple truth—few hair care formulations had more than 1% of the active ingredients that make them effective. In addition, many contained non-natural additives. Investigation and experimentation showed that by radically increasing the proportion of the effective ingredients, I could achieve this goal. Philip B. Hair Care is the only hair care line that contains ten to twenty times more natural elements that make them work better than any other hair care product."

I actually agree with part of his statement. It is absolutely true that when you add up all the plant extracts listed on most ingredient labels, almost all hair-care, skin-care, and cosmetic products contain far less of them relative to the amounts of the other ingredients. But the rest of what Philip B. is saying is little more than exaggeration designed to play on the consumer's obsession with natural ingredients.

Whether or not Philip B. products contain 10 to 20 times more of any plant extract than other products (a claim his own ingredient lists don't bear out), you are supposed to assume that there is research establishing that a greater amount of any plant has some enhanced benefit for hair. Herbalists or cosmetics chemists may believe these ingredients are good for the hair, but there is no data or research demonstrating that to be true. But don't worry, the Philip B. products also contain the same standard, synthetic, very effective ingredients that show up in all hair-care products. For more information about Philip B. Hair Care call (800) 643-5556 or visit www.philipb.com.

What's Good About This Line: Most of the shampoos, conditioners, and especially the styling products will nicely take care of hair, particularly hair that is dry to very dry.

What's Not So Good About It: The prices are astronomical for what you get because, regardless of how many plant extracts are in these products, almost all of them have minimal to no effect on hair or scalp; the few that do function as anti-irritants are coupled with potentially irritating plants, so the soothing benefit is lost.

☺ $$$ **Anti-Flake Relief Shampoo** *($32 for 8 ounces).* Other than the different name and price tag, this is essentially Head & Shoulders. Both contain zinc pyrithione as the main active ingredient (the label for this product uses the name zinc omadine, which is a trade name for zinc pyrithione). But this one also contains coal tar, an ingredient that is hard on hair and scalp, though it's an option for more serious scalp conditions such as psoriasis or seborrheic dermatitis. Before jumping into a coal-tar shampoo of any kind, start with the far less expensive Head & Shoulders or Nizoral (which contains the anti-dandruff ingredient ketoconazole) to see if those help control your dandruff.

☺ $$$ **African Shea Butter Shampoo for All Hair Types** *($21 for 8 ounces)* is a standard, detergent-based shampoo that also contains shea butter. That makes it best for someone with normal to very dry hair and scalp. The claim that this shampoo is fragrance-free is misleading, as several of the plant extracts it contains are extremely fragrant.

☹ **Peppermint and Avocado Shampoo Cool and Invigorating Clarifier** *($21 for 8 ounces)* is a standard, detergent-based shampoo that also contains a high level of peppermint oil, which is drying and unnecessarily irritating for the scalp. The plant oils are a problem for someone with an oily scalp.

☺ $$$ **Scent of Santa Fe Shampoo, Gentle Daily Cleansing for All Hair Types** *($29 for 8 ounces)* is a standard, detergent-based shampoo with plant extracts. It works well for all hair types, and without creating buildup. It does contain fragrance, and some of the plant extracts can be irritating to the scalp, but they will be washed away before they can cause much of a problem.

☻ $$$ **White Truffle Moisturizing Shampoo** *($45 for 8 ounces)* is a standard, detergent-based, lightly conditioning shampoo that works well for all but very fine or thin hair types—that is, if you aren't allergic to the cornucopia of plant extracts in here. The price tag is unwarranted, but then believing that the teeny amount of white truffle it contains can somehow help hair is as irrational as the price. It does contain fragrant plant extracts, as well as a small amount of lavender, lemon, and thyme oils—all potent scalp irritants that have no proven benefits for hair.

☺ $$$ **Deep-Conditioning Creme Rinse** *($23 for 6 ounces)* is a good standard conditioner for normal to dry hair, but it is absolutely overpriced, and the plant oils are not present in amounts that confer "deep conditioning" benefits to very dry, thick, or coarse hair.

☹ **Detangling Finishing Rinse for All Hair Types** *($19 for 6 ounces)* lists alcohol as its second ingredient, which can be drying for hair when used in a conditioner. It also contains silicone, detangling agent, vinegar, plant oils, fragrant oils, and preservative. The silicone and oils can make hair feel soft, but there are plenty of silicone serums and sprays on the market that don't use alcohol and therefore eliminate the risk of drying hair.

☺ $$$ **Creme of the Crop Hair Finishing Creme** *($25 for 2.5 ounces)* is a standard, pomade-style cream containing mostly water, Vaseline, wax, thickeners, lanolin oil, plant oils, fragrant plant oils (including rosemary oil, so keep this off the scalp), fragrance, and preservatives. Use it minimally, as it can leave a greasy buildup on hair. ($25 for Vaseline, wax, and lanolin. Is anyone else laughing besides me?)

☺ $$$ **Drop Dead Straight Hair Straightening Baume** *($19 for 6.5 ounces)* is a simple, lightweight styling balm with minimal hold and no stiff or sticky feel. It takes a lot of styling with a blow dryer or hair iron to get this product to help, and it does not work better than tons of other styling products that can help straighten hair. Actually, the lack of silicone and other anti-humidity ingredients makes this a subpar choice for making hair feel satiny smooth.

☺ $$$ **Self-Adjusting Hair Spray** *($18 for 8 ounces)* is a standard hairspray that doesn't self-adjust—you just use more if you want more hold. It has a light to medium hold and brushes through easily with minimal stiffness or sticky feel. It does contain fragrance.

☺ $$$ **Shin-Aid Matte Finish Pomade** *($24 for 2 ounces)* is a thick, slightly creamy pomade that does not leave a matte finish on hair. Rather, this leaves a natural shine that, while not as glossy or greasy as many pomades, is not anyone's definition of matte. This feels lighter in hair than it looks in the jar, and can do a very good job of smoothing frizz and enhancing texture without feeling heavy. It should still be used sparingly, but it's a somewhat unique alternative to traditional oil- and wax-based pomades.

☺ $$$ **Rejuvenating Oil for Dry to Damaged Hair** *($27 for 2 ounces)* contains olive, sesame, sweet almond, jojoba, and walnut oils, along with fragrant plant oils. You could create this concoction yourself for pennies. Only the hair-care industry can sell these everyday, easy-to-find oils for an absurd price accompanied by outlandish claims. Still, there is no denying that this product, though pricey, is helpful for dry to very dry hair that is thick or coarse.

☺ $$$ **Shin Shine** *($24 for 1.85 ounces)* contains liquid paraffin, silicones, fragrance, and plant extracts. It is a relatively standard silicone spray with a waxy base that is great for dry hair that needs help taming frizzies while adding a glossy shine. This can become greasy-feeling if not applied sparingly.

☺ $$$ **Styling Gel** *($16 for 4.25 ounces)* is a very standard gel with a light to medium hold and minimal to no stiff or sticky feel. The algae and seaweed extracts have a water-binding effect on hair, but nothing more.

PHYSIQUE

Procter & Gamble-owned physique claims that this line gives hair 20 full hours of hold, but even if you're awake for that long, these products don't contain anything different from what every other P&G hair-care line contains. Not to mention that 20 hours of hold doesn't tell you if your hairstyle will still be in place. The "hold" ingredients will indeed be there, but that doesn't mean that humidity, the weight of your own hair, or your styling technique won't have an effect in changing how your hair looks after one hour, five hours, or more.

According to the company's Web site, the science in each physique product "adjusts the spaces between your hair's strands ... and then holds for great style that lasts for 20 hours, guaranteed or your money back." But who's really going to ask for their money back on that claim? This all sounds convincing on the surface, until you ask yourself how creating separation space between each strand of hair can increase the amount of time your hair will hold its style, especially given the variables of weather, styling tools, and genetics that all affect how your hair looks. Besides, the silicones, serums, pomades, and waxes in this line smooth the hair together and reduce space, not increase it.

Most of the shampoo, conditioner, and styling-product formulas below are very similar, if not identical, to what Procter & Gamble offers in their Pantene and Pert Plus lines. physique's higher price point and reduced sizes are completely associated with marketing and not the result of some amazing formulary difference that makes these products worth considering over value-priced Pantene. For more information about physique, call (800) 214-8960 or visit www.physique.com.

What's Good About This Line: The styling products, though mostly standard, are worth auditioning; the conditioners, though mostly similar, work well for normal to dry hair of any thickness.

What's Not So Good About It: All the shampoos contain ammonium xylenesulfonate, which can swell the hair shaft and cause hair and scalp dryness with repeated use; the claim that physique products must be used together to obtain a long-lasting hairstyle—it just isn't true.

☹ **Clarifying Shampoo** *($6.99 for 10.2 ounces)* is a below-standard shampoo that contains the solvent ammonium xylenesulfonate, which can swell the hair shaft and result in dryness of the hair and scalp with repeated use.

☹ **Curl Defining Shampoo** *($6.99 for 10.2 ounces)* contains ammonium xylenesulfonate, and is not recommended. This shampoo will eventually make curly hair dry and frizzy.

☹ **Deep Hydrating Shampoo** *($6.99 for 10.2 ounces)*. Relative to the two physique shampoos above, this contains a reduced amount of ammonium xylenesulfonate, but so many shampoos omit this problematic ingredient that there is no logical reason to consider this option.

☹ **Straight & Control Shampoo** *($6.99 for 10.2 ounces)* is identical to the Curl Defining Shampoo above, and the same basic comments apply. Isn't it interesting that this shampoo is labeled for straight hair while the other is supposed to be the solution for defining curls?

☹ **Volumizing Shampoo** *($6.99 for 10.2 ounces)* contains ammonium xylenesulfonate in a base that is less conditioning than the Curl Defining Shampoo above, which will intensify this problematic ingredient's drying effect.

☹ **2-in-1 Shampoo + Conditioner** *($6.99 for 10.2 ounces)* contains ammonium xylenesulfonate, and is not recommended.

☺ **Curl Defining Conditioner** *($6.99 for 6.8 ounces)* is a standard, but very good, conditioner for normal to dry hair of any thickness. It is remarkably similar to most of Pantene's conditioners, all of which cost less and provide a greater amount of product.

☺ **Deep Hydrating Conditioner** *($6.99 for 6.8 ounces)* is slightly more emollient than the Curl Defining Conditioner above, and is an option for normal to dry hair of any thickness, though someone with very fine or thin hair should apply this only to the ends of hair.

☺ **Straight & Control Conditioner** *($6.99 for 6.8 ounces)* is nearly identical to the Deep Hydrating Conditioner above, and the same review applies. This won't make curly or wavy hair straight, but it can make it feel smoother.

☺ **Volumizing Conditioner** *($6.99 for 6.8 ounces)* is identical to the Curl Defining Conditioner above, and the same review applies.

☺ **Control + Freeze Hair Spray, Maximum Hold (Aerosol)** *($6.99 for 8.25 ounces)* is a standard hairspray that provides a light to medium, flexible hold with a minimal stiff or sticky feel. I strongly doubt this can provide 20-hour styling support (which the label claims) especially if you live in a humid climate. This brushes through easily and can be reapplied without making hair feel too heavy.

☺ **Curl Creating Gel** *($6.99 for 5.3 ounces)* is a very standard styling gel that offers no special benefit for curly hair. This provides a light to medium hold with a minimal stiff and sticky feel, allowing hair to be easily brushed through. This can't protect hair from styling stress, at least not if that stress is from high-heat sources such as blow dryers or curling irons.

☺ **Frizz Control Curl Cream** *($7.49 for 3.5 ounces)* is a very good, water- and silicone-based smoothing cream for dry, frizzy hair. It provides a light, pliable hold that can nicely define curls and waves without being sticky. It would also make a good finishing cream to add texture and smooth dry ends.

☺ **Keep It Flexible Hair Spray** *($8.99 for 8.25 ounces)* is nearly identical to the Control + Freeze Hair Spray, Maximum Hold (Aerosol) above, and the same comments apply. All of physique's hairsprays are adept at keeping hair flexible rather than stiff.

☺ **Keep It Straight Gel** *($6.99 for 5.1 ounces)* is nearly identical to the Curl Creating Gel above, and the same comments apply. Mixed with the Frizz Control Curl Cream above, this can work well to smooth and straighten hair with heat and the proper styling brush.

☺ **Keep It Straight Lotion** *($7.49 for 5 ounces)* is a great water- and silicone-based styling balm that can beautifully smooth frizzies and dry ends while adding shine to hair without excessive weight. It is an option for straightening hair with heat, but don't count on this (or any other styling product) to provide complete protection from the kind of heat required to make curly, wavy hair sleek and straight.

☺ **Keep Your Curls Hair Spray** *($6.99 for 5.9 ounces)* is a good nonaerosol hairspray that provides a silky-smooth, flexible hold that can help shape curls without making them sticky or stiff. This simple but effective formulation is a great hairspray for all hair types requiring an extra touch of hold that won't announce its presence in hair.

☺ **Precision Wax** *($7.49 for 1.7 ounces)* is a simple, Vaseline-based, waterless pomade that is an option for dry to very dry hair that is thick or coarse. It can nicely smooth frizzies and dry ends, but can quickly become heavy and greasy if not used sparingly.

☺ **Scrunching Foam** *($6.99 for 5 ounces)* is a standard, creamy-feeling mousse that provides a light hold with a minimal stiff or sticky feel, and allows hair to be easily brushed through. This is a good choice for fine or thin hair that is curly or straight.

☺ **Volume Boosting Foam** *($6.99 for 5 ounces)* is identical to the Scrunching Foam above, and the same review applies.

☺ **Volume Boosting Gel** *($6.99 for 5.1 ounces)* is a light-hold, standard styling gel with barely discernible stiffness and stickiness. It is light enough to help boost volume when fine or thin hair is heat-styled, but it lacks a sufficient amount of conditioning agents to provide heat protection. It is best to mix this gel with a dab of the Keep It Straight Lotion above prior to heat-styling your hair.

☺ **Volumizing Hair Spray (Aerosol)** *($6.99 for 5.5 ounces)* is similar to the Control + Freeze Hair Spray, Maximum Hold (Aerosol) above, and the same comments apply. This is so light it can keep fine or thin hair lifted, even if you apply too much.

☺ **Volumizing Hair Spray (Non-Aerosol)** *($6.99 for 5.9 ounces)* is identical to the Keep Your Curls Hair Spray above, and the same comments apply.

☺ **Volumizing Hair Spray, Unscented (Aerosol)** *($6.99 for 5.5 ounces)* is similar to the Control + Freeze Hair Spray, Maximum Hold (Aerosol) above, and the same comments apply. I would like to add that this option really *is* fragrance-free, which is great news for those with a sensitive scalp.

PHYTO

With plants aplenty and medicinal-looking packaging, the Phyto line is immersed in the (so-called) science of botanical extracts and how they affect our hair and scalp. Every Phyto product has at least a handful of plant extracts, but few of them have any effect when it comes to hair or scalp care. What Phyto doesn't discuss is the fact that although a certain plant extract may have beneficial active constituents, what the research has examined is the extract's pure, unadulterated form. Once extracts like this are commingled with standard ingredients such as sodium laureth sulfate, glyceryl stearate, and phenyl trimethicone (and these and all hair-care products do that), then mixed with water and processed for manufacturing, the extracts retain little, if any, of their original composition and benefit, assuming there was benefit originally.

Phyto also labels their detergent cleansing agents, thickeners, and several conditioning agents as being of "botanical origin." An ingredient such as disodium cocoamphodiacetate may sound less intimidating if you know it's from a plant, but you can't take coconut oil or milk or a tea or a palm leaf and use it to wash your hair, at least not if you want any sort of cleansing or lathering effect. Yes, many synthetic-sounding ingredients do have a botanical origin, but the process of creating a cleansing agent from a plant source involves many steps in the laboratory to chemically turn the natural source into an effective hair-care ingredient. For more information about Phyto, call (800) 55-PHYTO or visit www.phyto.com.

What's Good About This Line: Each category (shampoos, conditioners, and so on) has at least one good option for each hair type and condition.

What's Not So Good About It: Prices that are mostly out of line for what you get; many of the claims are ludicrous; many of the plant extracts and oils can be irritating for the scalp while having no established or proven benefit for hair; the shampoos are packaged in glass bottles, which makes them inconvenient for traveling or for use in the shower.

☺ **$$$ Phytoapaisant Soothing Shampoo, for Sensitive Scalp** *($20 for 6.7 ounces)* is a standard, but good, shampoo for normal to slightly dry hair of any thickness, although it has no special benefit for someone with a sensitive scalp. The *Piper mythisticum* (kava-kava) extract can have an analgesic (anti-inflammatory) effect, but it can also cause skin irritation and dermatitis (Sources: *Alternative Medicine Review*, December 1998, pages 458–460; and *Clinical Experimental Pharmacology and Physiology*, July 1990, pages 495–507). The extract would all be rinsed down the drain anyway, so it is more of a marketing gimmick than anything else. This shampoo poses a slight risk of buildup with repeated use.

☺ $$$ **Phytargent Whitening Shampoo, for Grey and White Hair** *($20 for 6.7 ounces)* is a standard, detergent-based shampoo that has light conditioning properties, which makes it suitable for normal to slightly dry hair that is normal to fine or thin. It poses a slight risk of buildup, and cannot whiten hair. Rather, the synthetic basic blue and red dyes it contains can help minimize yellow or brassy tones in white, silver, or gray hair. The effect will be subtle, but this is an option if your hair has unwanted yellow tones.

☹ $$$ **Phytoaxil Energizing Shampoo, for Thinning Hair** *($18 for 3.3 ounces)* doesn't contain any ingredients that are helpful for thinning hair. The extracts can cause irritation, but that doesn't help make hair thicker or regrow hair.

☺ $$$ **Phytobrush Special Smoothing Shampoo, for Blow-Drying** *($20 for 6.7 ounces)* is a standard shampoo that is an option for normal to slightly dry hair. The film-forming agents can initially make fine or thin hair feel thicker, but also can cause buildup with repeated use. If alternated with a shampoo that does not contain conditioners or volumizing ingredients, this is an option for all hair types except thick or coarse. There is nothing in this product that is helpful for blow drying or styling hair.

☹ **Phytocedrat Sebo-Regulating Shampoo, for Oily Scalp** *($20 for 6.7 ounces)* contains several irritating plant extracts rather high up on the ingredient list, and also adds lemon peel oil to the mix, which is very irritating to the scalp. Nothing in this product can reduce oil production.

☹ **Phytocitrus Shine Shampoo, for Colored or Permed Hair** *($20 for 6.7 ounces)* contains TEA-lauryl sulfate as one of its main detergent cleansing agents, and is not recommended for any hair or scalp type, especially not for permed or color-treated hair.

☺ $$$ **Phytocurl Curl Enhancing Shampoo, for Curly Hair** *($20 for 6.7 ounces)* is a great shampoo for normal to slightly dry hair of any thickness, but has no special benefit for curly hair, other than not being harsh or drying (and that can benefit all hair types).

☺ $$$ **Phytocyane Revitalizing Shampoo for Women, for Thinning Hair** *($20 for 6.7 ounces)* is a standard, rather boring, conditioning shampoo that is not exclusively for women, so ignore the label. The first plant extract listed is chinchona, a homeopathic remedy for tinnitus (ringing in the ears). Phyto appears to be the only company that holds this extract in high regard for thinning hair because there is no research demonstrating its benefit for that hair texture. This shampoo is a good option for normal to dry hair of any thickness, but differs little from what you'll find in L'Oreal's Vive line of shampoos, all of which cost a quarter of what this product does for twice the amount of product.

☺ $$$ **Phytojoba Hydrating Shampoo with Jojoba Oil, for Dry Hair** *($20 for 6.7 ounces)* contains a tiny amount of jojoba oil, and is a good shampoo for normal to slightly dry hair that is normal to fine or thin. It poses minimal risk of buildup.

☺ $$$ **Phytolactum Scalp-Regulating Shampoo with Phytolactine and Almond Milk Extract, for Frequent Use** *($20 for 3.3 ounces)* is just a standard, vastly overpriced shampoo. It is a good option for all hair types except thick or coarse. The film-forming agent will build up with repeated use. Nothing in it can regulate the condition of the scalp.

☺ $$$ **Phytomen Hair and Body Shampoo** *($18 for 5 ounces)* is a very standard shampoo for any gender that contains burdock extract, which has little effect on the scalp other than possibly being a mild anti-inflammatory, though in a shampoo it is just rinsed down the drain. The tiny amount of film-forming agent should not pose a risk of buildup.

☺ $$$ **Phytomousse Volume Foam Shampoo, for Fine and Limp Hair** *($20 for 5.07 ounces)* is a propellant-based mousse shampoo that has a foamy, light texture. The shampoo base is very standard, containing the same detergent cleansing agents found in countless other hair-care lines. This does include conditioning plant oil and shea butter, which can eventually make fine or limp hair feel too heavy. Still, it's a novel option for all hair types except thick or coarse.

☺ $$$ **Phytonectar Ultra Nourishing Shampoo, for Ultra-Dry Hair** *($20 for 6.7 ounces)* isn't ultra-nourishing in the least. Several of the Phyto shampoos above beat this for conditioning properties. It's a respectable shampoo for normal to slightly dry hair that is normal to fine or thin, and poses a slight risk of buildup with repeated use.

☹ **Phytoneutre Balancing Cream Shampoo, for All Hair Types** *($18 for 3.3 ounces)* contains eucalyptus oil, which makes this otherwise very standard shampoo too irritating to consider.

☺ $$$ **Phytopanama Mild Shampoo for Frequent Washing, for All Hair Types** *($20 for 6.7 ounces)* isn't really mild because it contains juniper oil, whose methanol content can be irritating to the scalp with repeated applications. For occasional use, this is a good shampoo for normal to dry hair of any thickness.

☺ $$$ **Phytorhum Fortifying Shampoo, for Lifeless Hair** *($20 for 6.7 ounces)* is a standard conditioning shampoo that doesn't contain any rum, but does contain sugarcane extract, which rum is made from. This also contains egg yolk extract, which makes this shampoo start to sound like a recipe for eggnog! Setting aside these strange additions, this shampoo can work well for normal to dry hair of any thickness and poses slight risk of buildup.

☹ **Phytosylic Shampoo with Salicylic Compound and Essential Oil of Cypress, for Dry Dandruff** *($20 for 6.7 ounces)* doesn't contain an active ingredient to fight dandruff. Although salicylic acid can help, it isn't as effective as zinc pyrithione or ketoconazole. The tea tree oil present could also have helped with dandruff if a greater amount was used, but instead this shampoo ends up being a problem for scalp irritation due to the inclusion of cypress and rosemary oils.

☺ **$$$ Phytovolume Volumizer Shampoo, for Fine and Limp Hair** *($20 for 6.7 ounces)* is similar to the Phytocurl Curl Enhancing Shampoo above, except this features different plant extracts; otherwise, the same comments apply.

☺ **$$$ Phyto 7 Daily Intense Hydrating Cream, for Dry Hair** *($22 for 1.7 ounces).* The only thing intense about this product is its price, which is sobering, considering that all you're getting is several plant extracts and preservatives. It isn't moisturizing (nor creamy), but it can make normal to fine or thin hair easier to comb without making it feel heavy or coated.

☺ **$$$ Phyto 9 Daily Ultra Nourishing Cream, for Ultra-Dry Hair** *($22 for 1.7 ounces)* is nearly identical to the Phyto 7 Daily Intense Hydrating Cream above, except this contains a small amount of nut oil, which makes it slightly better for dry hair that is normal to fine or thin. It is not preferred to the "natural" leave-in products from Aveda, such as their Elixir or Damage Control, both of which sell for less than this product and come in larger sizes.

☺ **$$$ Phytobaume Conditioner, for All Hair Types** *($18 for 6.7 ounces)* is a good, but standard, conditioner for normal to dry hair that is normal to fine or curly.

☺ **$$$ Phytokarite Ultra Nourishing Conditioner, for Ultra-Dry Hair** *($32 for 6.7 ounces)* is a very good, rich conditioner for dry to very dry hair that is normal to thick, coarse, or curly. It's way overpriced, but if you're going to splurge on this line, this is one of the top products to consider.

☺ **$$$ Phytomist Instant Hydrator with White Lotus Flowers** *($22 for 5 ounces)* is a lightweight, well-formulated, leave-in conditioning mist for normal to dry hair of any thickness.

☺ **$$$ Phytosesame Express Hydrating Conditioner, for Dry Hair** *($24 for 5 ounces)* is similar to, but less emollient than, the Phytokarite Ultra Nourishing Conditioner, for Ultra-Dry Hair above, and the same basic comments apply. This can be too heavy for those with fine or thin hair.

☹ **Phytodefrisant Botanical Hair Relaxing Balm, for Anti-Frizz** *($22 for 3.3 ounces)* contains the preservatives methylchloroisothiazolinone and methylisothiazolinone (Kathon CG), which are contraindicated for use in leave-on products due to their high risk of causing a sensitizing reaction on the scalp or skin. There are at least a dozen superior alternatives to this product available at the drugstore that don't contain these problematic preservatives.

☹ **Phytofix Setting Gel, for All Hair Types** *($18 for 3.3 ounces)* is an exceptionally standard styling gel that is not recommended because it contains enough rosemary oil to cause scalp itching and irritation.

☺ **$$$ Phytolaque Hair Spray with Vegetable Lacquer, for All Hair Types** *($18 for 3.3 ounces)* is a light- to medium-hold, nonaerosol hairspray whose formula is so basic the price is truly embarrassing. This dries to a smooth, minimally sticky and stiff finish, but so do innumerable hairsprays at the drugstore that carry much more realistic price tags.

☺ **$$$ Phytolaque Soie Hair Spray with Silk Proteins, for Sensitive Hair** *($18 for 3.3 ounces)* is almost identical to the Phytolaque Hair Spray above, except this adds a conditioning agent to improve hair's softness and comb-ability. Otherwise, the same review applies.

☺ **$$$ Phytovolume Actif Volumizer Spray Enriched with Keratin Amino Acids, for Fine and Limp Hair** *($22 for 3.3 ounces)* is more a hairspray than a styling spray, and is capable of a medium hold that leaves hair feeling slightly stiff and sticky. The film-forming agents can help make fine hair feel thicker, but they're not unique to this product. Again, for fans of "natural" hair-care products, I would consider Aveda's Flax Seed/Aloe Spray Gel or Volumizing Tonic before this pricier option.

☹ **$$$ Huile D'Ales Intensive Hydrating Oil Treatment, for Dry Hair** *($24 for five 0.33-ounce ampoules)* are capsules of castor oil (which isn't all that hydrating), along with several irritating plant extracts and rosemary oil. You can get the same, if not better results using oil from your kitchen cupboard, such as olive, almond, or safflower.

☹ **Phytoaxil Fortifying Intensive Care, for Thinning Hair** *($45 for 1.69 ounces)* leaves me speechless. Well, almost speechless. For $45, you get a liquid concoction of water, alcohol, plant extract, silicone, fragrance, fragrant flower oil, water-binding agent, more plant extracts, and preservatives. Not a single ingredient that can help thinning hair, and this product amounts to nothing more than a waste of money that completely dupes unsuspecting consumers.

☺ **$$$ Phytocitrus Vital Radiance Mask, for Color-Treated or Permed Hair** *($32 for 6.7 ounces)* is a standard conditioner that is an option for normal to dry hair of any thickness, but it is too ordinary to be considered a special treatment for hair, and the price is completely unrelated to what this product contains or can do for the hair.

☹ **Phytocyane Thinning Hair Revitalizing Lotion for Women, for Thinning Hair** *($45 for 12 0.25-ounce ampoules)* is almost as insufferable as the Phytoaxil Fortifying Intensive Care, for Thinning Hair above. It contains drying plant extracts along with soy protein, alcohol, and a form of sulfonic acid that can be drying to hair and scalp as well as having the potential to strip hair color. In addition, nothing in it can help stop hair from thinning in any way, shape, or form.

☺ **$$$ Phytodefrisant Relaxing Serum** *($24 for 1 ounce)* is as standard a silicone serum as they come, and although this can make dry, frizzy hair become smooth, sleek, and shiny, it is completely not worth the price. Identically effective options are available at the drugstore from such lines as Citré Shine and John Frieda.

☺ **$$$ Phytolisse Ultra Shine Smoothing Serum, for Anti-Frizz** *($24 for 1 ounce)* is similar to the Phytodefrisant Relaxing Serum above, and the same comments apply. The runny texture of this product makes it less substantial than many less expensive silicone serums.

☺ **$$$ Phytonectar Ultra Nourishing Oil Treatment, for Ultra-Dry Hair** *($26 for 2.5 ounces)* contains mostly corn, castor, and egg oils, along with plant extracts, sunflower seed oil, water-binding agents, fragrance, tea tree oil, slip agent, and preservatives. Save your money and moisturize dry hair with any oil from your kitchen.

☹ **Phytopolleine Botanical Scalp Stimulant, for Lifeless Hair** *($28 for 0.8 ounce)* contains corn oil along with a battery of very irritating fragrant oils, including rosemary, lemon, cypress, and eucalyptus. My scalp is itching just thinking about this problematic product.

PHYTO PHYTOSPECIFIC

☺ $$$ **Phytospecific Intense Nutrition Shampoo, with Kukui Oil** *($18 for 5.07 ounces)* is a conditioning shampoo that positions calendula and sage as nutrition for hair. The problem is that the hair is dead and cannot benefit from such ingredients, never mind the fact that these plants have no established benefit for hair anyway! This is a good option for normal to dry hair that is normal to slightly thick or coarse.

☺ $$$ **Phytospecific Hydra-Repairing Shampoo, with Shea Butter** *($18 for 5.07 ounces)* is similar to the Phytospecific Intense Nutrition Shampoo above, except this omits the plant extracts and nut oils and adds shea butter, making it better for dry to very dry hair that is normal to thick or coarse. This and the Phytospecific shampoo above will cause buildup with repeated use.

☺ $$$ **Phytospecific Vital Force Shampoo, with Illipe Butter and Barley Milk** *($18 for 5.07 ounces)* is nearly identical to the Phytospecific Intense Nutrition Shampoo above, and the same comments apply.

☺ $$$ **Phytospecific Restructuring Milk, with Canola Oil** *($20 for 5.07 ounces)* is an emollient, almost greasy conditioner for dry to very dry hair that is coarse, curly, or thick.

☺ $$$ **Phytospecific Shea Butter Beauty Styling Creme, for All Hair Types** *($18 for 3.38 ounces)* is a rich, greasy styling cream that consists primarily of Vaseline, mineral oil, and waxes. It can benefit very dry, thick, or coarse hair, but the price is ridiculous for what amounts to some very inexpensive ingredients. If you opt to try this, use it sparingly to avoid creating greasy-feeling hair.

☺ $$$ **Phytospecific Quinoa Oil Moisturizing Styling Balm, for All Hair Types** *($20 for 4.22 ounces)* does contain quinoa oil, but in a much smaller amount than the standard frontrunners on the ingredient list—mineral oil, Vaseline, and microcrystalline wax. This is a very standard, heavy styling balm that can be good for dry hair, but the price is laughable for what you get.

☺ $$$ **Phytospecific Intense Nutrition Mask, with Plant Marrow** *($22 for 6.75 ounces)* is a helpful conditioner for normal to dry hair of any thickness, but cannot supply nutrition to hair. Even if it did, hair is dead and cannot benefit from topically applied "nutritional" ingredients.

☺ $$$ **Phytospecific Revitalizing Treatment, with Vegetable Oils** *($24 for 3.35 ounces)* is nothing more than nut, plant, and mineral oil with thickeners and conditioning agents. It is effective for dry to very dry hair, but is absurdly overpriced for a treatment you can likely find in your kitchen pantry for pennies.

☺ $$$ **Phytospecific Multi-Regenerating Creme Bath, with Jojoba Oil** *($28 for 6.75 ounces)* is supposed to restore hair's bounce and vibrancy, something any good conditioner can do, and that's exactly what we have here, albeit for an absurd price. This is a standard, rank-and-file conditioner for normal to dry hair of almost any thickness; it is too emollient for thin hair.

PHYTO PLAGE

☺ $$$ **Phyto Plage Sun Shampoo** *($18 for 5 ounces)* is a standard, but good, shampoo that has no special benefit for hair that has been (or will be) exposed to the sun. It is an option for normal to slightly dry hair that is normal to fine or thin, but will cause buildup with repeated use.

☹ **Phyto Plage High-Protection Sun Oil, for Weakened Hair** *($20 for 3.3 ounces)* contains several oils, but none of them offer your hair sun protection, at least not in terms of protecting hair from UV-induced color fading. Any oil applied to hair can help counteract the sun's drying effect on hair, but still cannot offer complete protection. What is most troublesome about this product is the inclusion of lemon, rosemary, sage, and juniper oils, all of which are very irritating.

☺ $$$ **Phyto Plage Moisturizing Sun Gel** *($20 for 2.5 ounces)* is minimally moisturizing and certainly can't revive sun-damaged, dry hair. It is a decent, though unexciting, option for slightly dry hair.

☺ $$$ **Phyto Plage Protective Sun Veil** *($20 for 3.3 ounces)* is nothing more than plant extracts and a "UV filter," but it doesn't specify which UV filter. Nonetheless, without an SPF rating number, there is no way to know what you are really putting on your hair.

☺ $$$ **Phyto Plage Sun Protection Oil** *($18 for 3.3 ounces)* is nothing more than castor oil and some mostly irritating plant extracts. It can definitely moisturize dry hair and help keep it from becoming drier while exposed to sunlight, but so can plain plant oil (such as safflower or jojoba), and for far less money, too.

PHYTO PRO

☺ $$$ **Phyto Pro Extra Firm Holding Spray, Hold Factor 15** *($17 for 5 ounces)* is an incredibly standard hairspray with a light to medium hold and minimal stiff or sticky feel.

☺ $$$ **Phyto Pro Firm Holding Spray, Hold Factor 10** *($17 for 5 ounces)* is nearly identical to the Phyto Pro Extra Firm Holding Spray above, and the same review applies.

☺ $$$ **Phyto Pro Hard Spray, Hold Factor 20** *($17 for 4.2 ounces)* is nearly identical to the Phyto Pro Extra Firm Holding Spray above, and the same review applies.

☺ $$$ **Phyto Pro Intense Volume Mousse, Hold Factor 12** *($17 for 5 ounces)* is a standard, propellant-based mousse that offers a medium hold with a slightly stiff, sticky feel. Hair is easily brushed through, and this is a good, though pricey, mousse for normal to fine hair that is slightly dry.

☺ **$$$ Phyto Pro Sculpting Gel, Hold Factor 8** *($17 for 5 ounces)* is a standard, medium- to firm-hold styling gel that leaves hair feeling stiff and sticky, though it can be brushed through. L'Oreal's Studio Line or Garnier Fructis styling gels work as well as this option for a fraction of the price.

☹ **Phyto Pro Soft Setting Gel, Hold Factor 2** *($17 for 5 ounces)* is a below-standard styling gel because it is prone to flaking once dry. That side effect at this price is particularly embarrassing.

☺ **$$$ Phyto Pro Volumizing Mousse, Hold Factor 6** *($17 for 5 ounces)* is a weightless, propellant-based mousse with minimal to no hold and no stiff, sticky feel. It does have slight conditioning properties, but that's about all.

☺ **$$$ Phyto Pro Ultra-Brilliance Creme** *($17 for 2.5 ounces)* is a smooth, creamy styling balm that contains mostly water, Vaseline, silicones, plant extract, plant oil, thickener, wax, slip agent, film-forming agent, preservatives, and fragrance. It can smooth frizzies and moisturize dry to very dry hair without feeling overly greasy or slick. This can be too heavy for fine or thin hair; it's best for thick, coarse, or curly hair, and should be used sparingly until you're accustomed to how much your hair needs to stay smooth without becoming greasy.

PRELL

Ah, Prell. The shampoo brand that makes many hairstylists cringe with the myth that it could strip floor wax and remove hair color. Prell was originally launched by its then-owner Procter & Gamble in 1946. There never were any wax- or hair color-dissolving ingredients in this shampoo, but it was a rather harsh, drying shampoo that had a high alkaline pH. None of that was good for hair, but there wasn't much else around in those days that was very good for hair.

Procter & Gamble sold Prell to Prestige Brands International in late 1999. Since then, Prell's formulas and packaging have been revamped, though the original Prell Shampoo formula is still being sold, albeit with a lower pH value and kinder detergent cleansing agents. For more information about Prell, call (800) 33-PRELL or visit www.prellshampoo.com.

What's Good About This Line: Prell's latest formulations are a marked improvement and prove that its new owner intends to compete strongly with lines such as Suave, Clairol, and Finesse.

What's Not So Good About It: The original formulas have either stayed the same or been given a slight reworking that did not improve them to the standard of today's best shampoos.

☹ **Concentrate Shampoo, Rinse Clean Formula for All Hair Types** *($2.99 for 4 ounces)* contains sodium lauryl sulfate as one of its main detergent cleansing agents, along with SD-alcohol, and it is not recommended for any hair or scalp type.

☺ **Active Frequent Use Shampoo, Non-Drying Formula** *($3.19 for 11.25 ounces)* is a much gentler shampoo than the Concentrate Shampoo option above, and that makes it a good choice for normal to fine or thin hair. It poses a slight risk of buildup with repeated use.

☺ **Advanced Treatment Thickening Formula, Thickening Formula for Thin Hair** *($3.19 for 13.5 ounces)* is similar to the Active Frequent Use Shampoo, Non-Drying Formula above, except this contains a slew of plant extracts, including balm mint, which is irritating to the scalp. The amount used is probably too small to be a problem, but it is enough to keep this shampoo from earning a happy face rating.

☹ **Rinse Clean Shampoo, Original Formula for Normal/Oily Hair** *($3.19 for 13.5 ounces)* contains a high level of the solvent ammonium xylenesulfonate, which can swell the hair shaft and cause dry hair and scalp.

Prell Spa Formula

☺ **Hydra Care Rinse Clean Shampoo** *($3.19 for 13 ounces)* is a great shampoo for normal to dry hair of any thickness, and poses minimal to no risk of buildup.

☺ **Volume Care Rinse Clean Shampoo** *($3.19 for 13 ounces)* is nearly identical to the Hydra Care Rinse Clean Shampoo above, and the same basic comments apply, except that this one contains plant oil instead of a film-forming agent. However, the plant oil is present in an amount too small to be of benefit to dry hair.

☺ **Hydra Care Rinse Clean Conditioner** *($3.19 for 13 ounces)* is a standard conditioner and a very good option for normal to slightly dry hair that is normal to fine, thin, or slightly thick.

PROFESSIONAL

For more information about Professional, owned by Nature's Therapy, call (800) 382-3609 or visit www.customnails.com.

What's Good About This Line: Although I don't admire the business ethics of a company whose products try to capitalize on the success and reputation of an established brand, I have to concede that the products do work well and the prices are almost too good to resist.

What's Not So Good About It: Every product is compared to and attempts to copy another hair-care line's successful, well-known product.

☺ **Freezing Hair Spray, Extra Firm Hold (Aerosol)** *($3.86 for 10 ounces)* is a standard, firm-hold hairspray that, along with its strong hold, leaves hair feeling stiff and somewhat sticky. This can be tricky to brush through, and is best reserved as a final touch for freezing your style (or a section of hair) in place. The formula dries quickly, allowing little playtime.

☺ **Lift & Texture Root Boost** *($3.86 for 8 ounces)* is an aerosol styling spray with a directional nozzle designed to shoot a blast of foamy product at the roots of the hair. This has a medium hold and is sticky, but it definitely can provide lift and style support. On fine or thin hair, the force of the application means way too much product is dispersed at the roots, and that can weigh hair down and make it difficult to style. For best results, I suggest spraying this onto your hands and then working it through the hair.

☺ **Manipulator Styling Creme** *($3.64 for 2 ounces)* is a gel-based, water-soluble pomade with a stringy texture that can be tricky to work with, though it's easy to distribute through the hair. It offers a light to medium hold that keeps hair pliable without much stickiness and no stiffness. It is a versatile product for smoothing hair before heat styling, or can be used on dry hair to emphasize a textured, short haircut. It is effective, without being too heavy, for all but fine or thin hair types.

☺ **Shine Pomade Ultra-Hold** *($3.86 for 2 ounces)* is a thick, fairly greasy, but water-soluble, pomade that is excellent for smoothing hair or emphasizing waves and curls with a soft, frizz-free finish. It works best for normal to dry hair that is slightly thick to coarse. It adds a slick shine that can become too greasy unless used sparingly.

☺ **Ultra-Shaping Hair Spray (Aerosol)** *($3.86 for 10 ounces)* is nearly identical in feel and performance to the Freezing Hair Spray, Extra Firm Hold (Aerosol) product above, and the same review applies. The only difference between the two is that this one imparts some shine because of the silicone and conditioning agents it contains.

☺ **Ultra-Shaping Hair Spray Plus (Aerosol)** *($3.86 for 10 ounces)* is nearly identical in feel and performance to the Freezing Hair Spray, Extra Firm Hold (Aerosol) product above, except this offers slightly more hold and contains conditioning agents for shine. This is sticky enough to make it difficult to brush through, especially on drier hair.)

PROGAINE

If this product line reminds you of the hair-regrowth product Rogaine, it should—Progaine is made by the same pharmaceutical company that manufactures that over-the-counter topical drug. The rationale behind this line was that the scientists who spent years studying Rogaine learned a thing or two along the way about what fine, thin hair needs to look and feel its best. And because the majority of Rogaine users likely have fine or thin hair (or at least dwindling hair in some area), the Progaine line of shampoos and conditioners (which do not contain minoxidil, the active ingredient in Rogaine) was launched as an extension of the Rogaine products. Are they worth considering if you're using Rogaine? Not any more than countless other products available from other lines. The scientists behind Rogaine may know all about the FDA-approved ingredient minoxidil and its effect on hair loss, but their hair-care formulary knowledge isn't perfect, as evidenced by the individual product reviews below. For more information about Progaine, call (877) 776-4246 or visit www.progaine.com.

What's Good About This Line: One shampoo and one styling product are indeed great options for those with fine or thin hair.

What's Not So Good About It: One shampoo contains peppermint oil; the Volumizing Foam is below standard.

☹ **Deep Cleansing Shampoo** *($5.99 for 10 ounces)* is a standard shampoo that contains peppermint oil and balm mint, which may make those with fine or thin hair think it is stimulating hair growth, when in reality all that's occurring is irritation. There are better shampoos for fine or thin hair from L'Oreal, Neutrogena, and Aussie, to name just a few.

☺ **Volumizing Shampoo** *($5.99 for 12 ounces)* is an excellent shampoo for making fine or thin hair feel thicker, but that comes courtesy of the film-forming agent, which will cause buildup with repeated use. Ideally, this should be alternated with a shampoo that will not cause buildup to give fine or thin hair the best of both worlds.

☺ **2 in 1 Shampoo, Shampoo and Conditioner in One** *($5.99 for 12 ounces)* is a standard, but very good, conditioning shampoo that can be OK for alternate use on fine or thin hair. If used exclusively, the conditioning agents will quickly make fine or thin hair feel heavy and appear limp.

☺ **Weightless Conditioner** *($5.99 for 12 ounces)* isn't all that weightless, especially for someone with very fine or thin hair who is concerned about using anything too emollient. This is best for normal to slightly dry hair that is normal to slightly thick.

☹ **Volumizing Foam** *($5.99 for 6.7 ounces)* is a liquid-to-foam, medium-hold mousse that can make fine or thin hair feel thicker, but also sticky and slightly stiff. This can still be brushed through, but the sticky effect, while softened, is still apparent. This is not as elegant as many other mousses available from other equally inexpensive lines at the drugstore.

☺ **Volumizing Root Lifter** *($5.99 for 6 ounces)* is a root-lifting styling spray that does not leave hair feeling uncomfortably sticky. This water-based spray has a directional nozzle for direct application at the roots, and the amount sprayed as the pump is dispensed is a practical light mist rather than the overdose delivered by similar products. This offers a light, flexible hold without stiffness, is minimally sticky, and allows hair to be easily brushed through. It's an excellent option for building body and lift in fine or thin hair. It does contain fragrance.

PROVITAMIN

Since the last edition of this book, ProVitamin has made some major changes, eliminating almost all of its shampoos, conditioners, hot oils, and treatment products in favor of a seemingly endless procession of styling products. Many of their former products were poor formulations, so this change in marketing direction was a good one. As you will see from my reviews, this is not a hair-care line that should be overlooked even though the product names and packaging are clearly not designed to appeal to the sophisticated adult consumer. It is what's inside these funky-looking bottles and jars that counts and, for the most part, you will be impressed with what ProVitamin has to offer (hint: it's not vitamins). For more information on ProVitamin, call (813) 855-8035.

What's Good About This Line: Shopping for a silicone serum, spray, or gel? Look no further: this line has by far the most options, and at prices that are almost shockingly low compared to what you'll pay for similar (if not identical) products from salon lines; there's also a vast array of styling products that provide firm to bonded-like-glue hold.

What's Not So Good About It: A few styling gels contain the problematic preservatives methylchloroisothiazolinone and methylisothiazolinone (Kathon CG); the shampoo
and rinse-out conditioner are rather mundane compared to the styling products, which is
where this line really excels; the silicone products and a few styling sprays and gels suffer
from too much repetition, which makes shopping this line more confusing than it needs
to be.

☺ **ProVitamin Anti-Frizz Hair Serum** *($8.49 for 5.5 ounces)*, **ProVitamin Anti-Frizz
Hair Treatment Capsules** *($5.99 for 30 capsules)*, **ProVitamin Instant Repair Hair Serum**
($8.29 for 5.5 ounces), **ProVitamin Instant Repair Hair Treatment Capsules** *($5.99 for
30 capsules)*, **ProVitamin Maximum Body Hair Treatment Capsules** *($5.99 for 30 cap-
sules)*, **ProVitamin Mega Shine Hair Treatment Capsules** *($5.99 for 30 capsules)*, **ProVitamin
Perm/Color Hair Serum** *($8.29 for 5.5 ounces)*, **ProVitamin Perm/Color Repair Hair
Treatment Capsules** *($5.99 for 30 capsules)*, **ProVitamin Split Ends Mender Hair Serum**
($8.29 for 5.5 ounces), and **ProVitamin Split Ends Mender Hair Treatment Capsules** *($5.99
for 30 capsules)* are all nearly identical formulations that contain mostly vitamins, water-
binding agents, slip agent, silicones, film-forming agent, plant extract(s), fragrance, and,
for some of the products, coloring agents. All of these repetitive products are nothing more
than silicone serums, and they all can be excellent options for smoothing dry, frizzy hair
while making it feel silky-soft and radiant with shine. The Treatment Capsules contain the
most silicone, and are best for thick, coarse hair. The amount dispensed from each capsule
may be too much for shorter hair, so use only what you need. The multiple vitamins have
no effect on hair—it is the silicones and water-binding agents that are doing all the work.

PROVITAMIN SPECIAL EFFECTS

For a hair-care line so passionate about vitamins as hair's saving grace, you have to
wonder why so few of the products below contain them. True, they don't share the same
ProVitamin moniker, but they're from the same company. If this company thinks vitamins are so wonderful for hair, why not use them in every hair-care product they sell?
Wouldn't excluding them shortchange the consumer? Of course this is not the case, but it
should make you question this company's hype and claims.

☹ **Special Effects, Curls Up Shampoo** *($7.39 for 8.5 ounces)* is a below-average
shampoo whose vitamin content cannot save hair from the drying effects of the solvent
ammonium xylenesulfonate it contains. With repeated use, this can make hair and
scalp dry.

☺ **Special Effects, Curls Up Conditioner** *($7.39 for 8.5 ounces)* is a standard light-
weight smoothing conditioner that is a very good option for normal to slightly dry hair
that is normal to slightly thick or coarse.

☺ **Special Effects Moisture Junkie, Instant Leave-In Conditioner** *($7.29 for 6 ounces)*
is a very light, standard, leave-in conditioner that can work well for normal to fine or thin
hair that needs some help with combing and static.

☺ **Special Effects Chunky Ends, Instant Split Ends Mender** *($7.09 for 6 ounces)* cannot instantly mend split ends, at least not if you interpret "mend" to mean "fix" or "repair." This water-based, silicone-heavy conditioner can help make split ends look smoother, but, depending on how bad the damage is, the effect will be short-lived, and gone completely as soon as you shampoo again. The only way to fix split ends is to cut them off. This is still a very good leave-in conditioner for normal to slightly dry hair that is normal to thick or coarse.

☺ **Special Effects Curl Amplifier, Curl Reactivating Cream** *($7.39 for 4 ounces)* is a thick styling gel that is more for smoothing and adding frizz-free texture than for hold. This would work well for managing curly or wavy hair that is normal to slightly thick, and it is relatively water soluble.

☺ **Special Effects Curl Booster, Scrunching & Curling Spray** *($7.29 for 6 ounces)* is an alcohol-based styling spray that provides a firm hold with a noticeable stiff and sticky feel. I wouldn't recommend this for curls unless you want them to feel "crunchy," but it is a great styling spray for stubborn hair that is normal to fine.

☺ **Special Effects Curl Reaction, Curl Reactivating Texturizer** *($7.39 for 5.5 ounces)* is basically a water-based, lightweight silicone spray for hair. It can be used by all hair types to control frizz, and add smoothness and shine without weight or a greasy appearance. Those with fine or thin hair should still use this sparingly, perhaps mixing a couple pumps of this product with a styling gel for extra smoothing and a slight amount of heat protection. This does contain film-forming/holding agents, but remains pliable and non-sticky.

☺ **Special Effects Curls Up, Curl Reactivator & Defrizzant** *($5.99 for 6 ounces)* is a standard, silicone-based styling gel that can work beautifully to help straighten hair with heat and the proper brush, or to soften curls and reduce frizz.

☺ **Special Effects Fat Hair, Instant Thickening & Strengthening Serum** *($5.99 for 6 ounces)* is a lighter version of the Special Effects Curls Up, Curl Reactivator & Defrizzant above, and the same basic comments apply, except this is too light for someone with thick or coarse, curly hair. The ingredients can smooth hair and make it feel softer, but not thicker.

☺ **Special Effects Frizz Proof, Frizz Defiant Hair Pomade** *($7.39 for 2 ounces)* is not a pomade at all, though it is packaged like one. This is really just a nonaqueous silicone gel that does not offer any hold, but that can help smooth frizzies and add shine. It is relatively lightweight, and is appropriate for all hair types, though someone with fine, thin hair should use it sparingly.

☹ **Special Effects Hair Muscle, Hair Thickening Serum** *($7.39 for 4 ounces)* is a gel, not a serum, and it tends to flake even before it is dry. This product is not recommended.

☺ **Special Effects Hard Up, Extreme Hard Bodied Gel** *($7.29 for 6 ounces)* is a standard styling gel with a firm hold that leaves hair feeling stiff and sticky. It can be difficult to brush through if hair is dry, but is otherwise a perfectly workable gel for structured or wet-look hairstyles.

☺ **Special Effects Instant Straighten Out, Hair Straightener & Smoothing Treatment** *($7.09 for 6 ounces)* is nearly identical to the Special Effects Curls Up, Curl Reactivator and Defrizzant above, and the same review applies.

☺ **Special Effects Manipulative, Extreme Molding & Manipulating Cream** *($7.29 for 2 ounces)* is a smooth, creamy pomade that is excellent for adding a thicker feel to hair while emphasizing texture or adding smoothness with shine. This stays pliable in the hair yet works well to mold and shape it without feeling too greasy or heavy. It is best for normal to slightly thick hair that is straight, curly, or wavy. It does shampoo out fairly well.

☹ **Special Effects Mega Hold Curls Up Styling Gel** *($3.59 for 16 ounces)* contains the preservative Kathon CG, which is not recommended for use in leave-on products due to its risk of causing a sensitizing reaction on skin or scalp.

☹ **Special Effects Mega Hold Fat Hair Styling Gel** *($3.59 for 16 ounces)* contains the preservative Kathon CG, and is not recommended.

☹ **Special Effects Mega Hold Instant Straighten Out Styling Gel** *($3.59 for 16 ounces)* contains the preservative Kathon CG, and is not recommended.

☺ **Special Effects Molding Maniac, Extreme Texturizing & Molding Creme** *($7.09 for 6 ounces)* is nearly identical to the Special Effects Manipulative, Extreme Molding & Manipulating Cream above, except this has a slightly lighter, more lotion-like texture. The same comments still apply.

☺ **Special Effects Molding Wax, Pliable Hair Wax/Flexible Hold** *($7.29 for 2 ounces)* is a creamy, thick, but soft-textured styling wax that is much more versatile than traditional waxes. It is closer to a leave-in conditioner than a true wax, and as such can help groom and mold hair without making it feel too heavy or coated. It does not provide any hold, but can work well to shape and define curls or waves, or can be used to smooth dry ends while adding low-wattage shine.

☺ **Special Effects Polishing Serum, Smoothes, Seals & Shines Cuticle of Hair** *($7.09 for 6 ounces)* is a silicone-based gel that can work well to smooth frizzies and give hair a polished, glossy shine without a stiff, heavy feel. It can become greasy if not used sparingly.

☺ **Special Effects Power Pomade, Sculpts, Holds, Shines & Controls** *($7.29 for 2 ounces)* is a standard, gel-type pomade with a light hold that is slightly sticky. It's a good option to smooth and add moisture with control to stubborn curls or frizzies. It shampoos out easily and can work well for all but very fine or thin hair types.

☺ **Special Effects Root Booster, Root Lifting & Shaping Spray** *($7.29 for 6 ounces)* is a very standard styling spray with a firm hold that makes hair feel stiff and sticky, though it can still be brushed through if desired. It is best for hair that needs lots of control with little movement.

☺ **Special Effects Root Lifter, Volume Booster & Root Stimulating Serum** *($5.99 for 6 ounces)* doesn't contain anything to stimulate the roots. It's just a standard, medium-hold, slightly sticky styling gel that can be brushed through. This contains a tiny amount of conditioning agents, likely too small an amount to provide any heat protection.

☺ **Special Effects Spiked Out, A Water Resistant Hair Styling Glue** *($7.29 for 6 ounces)*. The name of this product is completely inaccurate because it is not water-resistant (it quickly rinses off with just water), it's not glue, and it does not have a glue-like hold. This is a silky-feeling styling gel with a light to medium hold that leaves hair slightly sticky but not stiff. It can be easily brushed through and is an excellent gel for normal to dry hair that is curly or wavy.

☺ **Special Effects Stay Straight, Humidity Resistant Straightening Spray** *($5.99 for 6 ounces)* is identical to the Special Effects Root Booster, Root Lifting & Shaping Spray above, and the same review applies.

☺ **Special Effects Ends Mender, Split-Ends Mender Serum** *($7.39 for 4 ounces)* is a very standard, but very good, silicone serum that would work as well as any to smooth frizzies and dry ends while adding a sleek, glasslike shine to hair. Use it sparingly or it can make hair look too slick and greasy. This is too heavy for fine or thin hair. Of course, this cannot mend or repair split ends or any amount of hair damage whatsoever.

☺ **Special Effects Extreme Shine, Weightless Shine & Anti-Frizz Treatment** *($7.29 for 6 ounces)* is a standard silicone spray that is a preferred option for taming frizzies and adding a glossy shine on normal to fine or thin hair. This product wins extra points because it is fragrance-free.

☺ **Special Effects Frizz Endz, Anti-Frizz Hair Serum** *($5.99 for 6 ounces)* is nearly identical to the Special Effects Curls Up, Curl Reactivator & Defrizzant above, except this contains slightly more silicone, which makes it preferred for drier hair. Otherwise, the same comments apply.

☺ **Special Effects Liquid Glass, Hair Polishing Serum** *($7.39 for 4 ounces)* is nearly identical to the Special Effects Ends Mender, Split-Ends Mender Serum above, and the same review applies. This does contain fragrance.

☺ **Special Effects Quick Fix, Instant Repair Serum** *($7.39 for 4 ounces)* is nearly identical to the Special Effects Ends Mender, Split-Ends Mender Serum above, and the same review applies. This does contain fragrance.

PROVITAMIN SPECIAL EFFECTS RAW TEXTURES

☺ **Special Effects Raw Textures Pliable Putty, Flexible, Moldable Hair Putty** *($5.99 for 2 ounces)* is a thick, fairly heavy pomade that is water-based and also contains plant oil, waxes, and film-forming/holding agent. It works well to smooth stubborn frizzies, dry ends, or unruly curls and waves while adding a soft shine. It is recommended for dry to very dry hair that is normal to coarse or thick.

☺ **Special Effects Raw Textures Raw Rubber, Rubberized Styling Sealant** *($9.79 for 4 ounces)* has a name that may make you think this offers heavy-duty, wind tunnel–tested hold, but that is not the case. This is a slightly thick smoothing balm that is a wonderful non-sticky option for dry to very dry hair that needs moisture, gloss, and frizz control. It is easy to distribute through the hair and contains some outstanding conditioning agents, including mineral oil, lanolin, and phospholipids. Unless your hair is extra thick or so coarse it's wiry, use this sparingly to avoid a greasy look.

☺ **Special Effects Raw Textures Rock Hard Epoxy, Rock-Hard Bonding Resin** *($5.99 for 2 ounces)* is like Crazy Glue for hair. This is an intensely strong-hold styling gel whose name is not a stretch of the truth. Use this only if you have impossibly stubborn hair or you want to create long-lasting, gravity-defying hold that you do not intend to brush through.

☺ **Special Effects Raw Textures Xtreme Spiking Blaster, Spray it! Spike it! Forget it!** *($9.79 for 4 ounces)* is an alcohol-based styling spray with very strong hold that can create long-lasting lift for extreme hairstyles. Spray it on wet or dry hair, style, and "fuggedaboutit."

☺ **Special Effects Raw Textures Xtreme Spiking Glue, Tell Your Hair Where to Stick It** *($9.79 for 4 ounces)* is indeed like glue—in appearance, texture, and amount of hold. This product is tricky to work with, especially on wet hair, but is an option for creating strong, exaggerated texture or to help keep stubborn, wayward strands in line. It can make hair feel quite coated and sticky, so use it sparingly and, preferably, only where needed.

PROXIPHEN & NANO

Nano Shampoo and Conditioner, Proxiphen, and Proxiphen-N are topical products for hair growth created and sold by a Dr. Peter Proctor, a physician with a Ph.D. in pharmacology. He is also the resident guru of an Internet hair-loss chat group. While the doctor's credentials are impressive, there are some serious questions regarding his hair-growth systems and claims. As is often the case with non-FDA-approved hair-regrowth products such as these (and because there are no studies supporting any of the claims), the authority of the endorsements is also questionable, because there is no research backing up what is being touted.

Nano shampoo and conditioner contains nicotinic acid N-Oxide (that's where the name Nano comes from) and superoxide dismutase (an antioxidant) for hair regrowth. None of these ingredients has any independent research showing it can grow hair. Actually, the claims made for these products are surprising because it is only supposed to be "as effective as minoxidil." You might wonder, if Nano is only as good as minoxidil, why not just use minoxidil, which does have extensive substantiated claims and is approved by the FDA for hair regrowth. The cost for a three-month supply of Nano Shampoo and Conditioner is $39.95, although the products rarely last three months.

Proxiphen, also developed by Proctor, is a topical prescription medication for hair regrowth, but it only takes a phone call to Proctor's office to obtain yours. Proxiphen contains a variety of ingredients, including minoxidil, retinoic acid (Retin-A), phenytoin (trade name Dilantin, an anticonvulsant and anti-seizure medication), spironolactone (a potent, topically effective anti-androgen), copper peptides (similar to those in Tricomin, reviewed later in this chapter), Nano (superoxide dismutase, an antioxidant, plus pyrmidine n-oxides, an amino acid), arginine (another amino acid), butylated hydroxytoluene (a preservative), and ascorbyl palmitate (a form of vitamin C). I've discussed some of these ingredients in the "Hair Growth—Scams or Solutions?" section in Chapter Three.

It is interesting to note that some people have reported loss of hair they gained with minoxidil when they began using Proxiphen, which has a lower concentration of commercial minoxidil. Others have reported that Proxiphen irritates the scalp, not surprising given the Retin-A and toluene it contains. Proctor says that Proxiphen stops hair loss, thickens hair, enlarges miniaturized hairs, and produces regrowth at the front of the hairline. And while the product has been prescribed by Proctor in various formulations for ten years, no independent, published clinical studies on its effectiveness are available. It costs $59.95 for a two-month supply.

There is also a nonprescription version of Proxiphen, called Proxiphen-N. The ingredients include superoxide dismutase, copper-binding peptides, and pyrmidine n-oxide, but there are none of the other more serious prescription-only ingredients that are found in the Proxiphen discussed above. Again, this product is promoted with no substantiating research or clinical data.

It is important to note also that Proctor does hold several patents for some of the ingredients in his products for hair regrowth. However, keep in mind that a patent doesn't have anything to do with efficacy; it simply establishes that Proctor is the one who can use these ingredients in hair-regrowth products. In other words, you could take a patent out establishing that you use tomatoes in your hair-regrowth products. The patent would then establish that you are the only one who can use tomatoes for that purpose—but it wouldn't in any way prove that tomatoes grow hair.

I would love to discuss the impact of these ingredients on the scalp in great detail, but the focus of this book isn't on balding, and it would take pages and pages. Proctor's Web site at www.drproctor.com is worth a visit. His information is based on some very interesting hypotheses that are worth looking at with an objective eye. The notion that his products are the answer for balding is, at best, questionable, but in the world of hair hope, that has never stopped an uninformed consumer from wasting his or her money.

PUREOLOGY

Pureology guarantees longer-lasting hair color thanks to its use of the trademarked ingredient Heliogenol, which is derived from sunflowers. Developed and sold by cosmetic ingredient supplier Croda, it is positioned as an herbal extract that can defend hair against ultraviolet (UV) and free-radical (oxidative) damage that can lead to color loss. Oxidation is definitely one of the causes of fading hair color, but Heliogenol is not the answer. The single study purporting to support its effectiveness was performed by Croda, and compared the effect of Heliogenol to vitamin E acetate, which does not have any research showing it can protect dyed hair from fading. Actually, no antioxidants have that ability because they do not cling well to hair and no one is sure how much of any antioxidant would be enough to prevent fading, or even how to keep it on the hair after shampooing, conditioning, or styling. The study results (with photographs) showed less fading on hair treated with Heliogenol than with vitamin E, but there is no independent research duplicating this proof. Besides, Croda recommends using Heliogenol at concentrations of at least 0.2%, and most of the Pureology products below use less than that. In short, there is no legitimate reason to hang your hope of color preservation on this one ingredient, or on this hair-care line. That doesn't mean Pureology lacks effective products—far from it. What they do lack is legitimate, substantiated proof that their products hold a singular advantage for consumers with color-treated hair. For more information about Pureology, call 800 331-1502 or visit www.pureology.com.

What's Good About This Line: Most of the shampoos and conditioners are effective, though overpriced, options for normal to dry hair; for a line that espouses plants and botanicals, each product does contain them, albeit as a plant tea or in amounts too small for hair to notice.

What's Not So Good About It: The prices are steep for what are mostly standard formulations; the fragrances are more potent than usual, which is bad news for those with sensitive, itchy scalps; a few products are exactly what you should avoid if you want to preserve your hair color as long as possible.

☺ $$$ **Hydrate Shampoo** *($19 for 10.1 ounces)* is a standard conditioning shampoo that is a very good option for normal to dry hair of any thickness. The conditioning agents can build up with repeated use. The botanical extracts and antioxidants absolutely cannot extend the life of dyed hair, as in a shampoo they are just rinsed down the drain.

☹ **Purify Shampoo** *($19 for 10.1 ounces)* contains sodium polystyrene sulfonate, an ingredient that can cause hair and scalp dryness as well as potentially strip hair color with repeated use. What is this ingredient doing in a hair-care line that pledges to be "the one and only for color-treated hair"?

☺ $$$ **SuperStraight Shampoo** *($19 for 10.1 ounces)* is similar to the Hydrate Shampoo above, except this contains several sunscreen agents, including avobenzone (listed by its technical name, butyl methoxydibenzoylmethane). Adding sunscreens to shampoo may look good on the label, but they cannot cling well to the hair or hold up under hairstyling and therefore end up being a useless inclusion. Furthermore, there are still no regulatory standards to determine how much, if any, UV protection sunscreens in hair-care products can provide. Hair-care products do not have SPF ratings. Given that, this is still an excellent shampoo for normal to dry hair of any thickness, though it has no special benefit for making curly hair straight. The silicones in it will build up with repeated use, so this should be alternated with a shampoo that does not cause buildup.

☺ $$$ **Volume Shampoo** *($19 for 10.1 ounces)* is, save for different botanicals used in the plant tea, nearly identical to the Hydrate Shampoo above, and the same comments apply. This shampoo is too conditioning to build volume in hair, especially if it is fine or thin.

☹ **Hydrate Conditioner** *($19 for 8.5 ounces)* contains peppermint oil, which is very irritating to the scalp. There are dozens of conditioners that improve on this formulation without the risk of scalp irritation, and most of them also cost less than this product.

☺ **$$$ SuperStraight Condition** *($22 for 10.1 ounces)* is a commendable, though pricey, conditioner for dry hair that is normal to thick, curly, or coarse. This is actually a somewhat original formula, and if you're prone to splurging on hair care this one won't disappoint if your goal is to create smooth, hydrated hair—just don't expect this to automatically make curly hair straight, because that isn't going to happen.

☺ **$$$ Volume Conditioner** *($19 for 8.5 ounces)* is a standard, but effective, light-weight conditioner for normal to slightly dry hair that is fine or thin and needs help with combing. The film-forming agents can make fine hair feel fuller and thicker, but they will build up with repeated use.

☺ **$$$ In Charge Plus, Finishing Spray, Super Firm Hold** *($16 for 9 ounces)* is a standard, light- to medium-hold aerosol hairspray that leaves hair feeling slightly sticky but not stiff, so it is easily brushed through. This is highly fragrant, so it's not the best choice if you have a sensitive, itch-prone scalp.

☺ **$$$ In Charge, Styling Spray, Firm Flexible Hold & Shine** *($17 for 9 ounces)* is a weightless aerosol hairspray with a light, flexible hold that leaves hair soft and minimally sticky. It would be a good working spray for more casual hairstyles that require movement.

☺ **$$$ Power Dressing, Body Hold Shine** *($17 for 5 ounces)* is a slightly creamy styling gel that provides a medium hold with a slightly sticky feel that can be easily brushed through. The conditioning agents and silicones make this a bit greasy, and it is best for drier hair that needs a smooth, conditioned hold with shine.

☺ **$$$ Pure Volume, Blowdry Amplifier** *($15 for 7 ounces)* is a standard styling gel that offers a medium to firm hold with a slightly sticky, stiff feel that is easily brushed through. The plant oil and conditioning agents provide a slight amount of protection during heat styling, but far from the "maximum thermal protection" highlighted on the label.

☺ **$$$ Root Lift, Spray Mousse** *($16 for 10 ounces)* is a standard, propellant-based mousse that offers a light, flexible hold with minimal to no stiffness and stickiness. The plant extracts and vitamins cannot protect color-treated hair from fading, nor do they provide any heat protection.

☺ **$$$ SuperStraight, Relaxing Serum** *($19 for 5.1 ounces)* is an excellent silicone-based straightening/styling serum with no stickiness for dry to very dry hair that is normal to coarse or thick.

☺ **$$$ Texture Twist, Styling Reshaper** *($19 for 3 ounces)* is a thick, standard styling balm whose wax content makes it good for smoothing stubborn frizzies or dry ends while adding shape and texture to hair. This is best for normal to thick or coarse hair that needs smoothing with a light hold and soft shine.

☺ $$$ **Colour Max, Seal & Detangle** *($16 for 8.5 ounces)* is a spray-on, leave-in detangling conditioner that is an option for normal to fine or thin hair that needs help with combing, and it won't add weight to hair. Contrary to claim, this product cannot "provide maximum protection against UVA and UVB sun fading, oxidation, and daily styling." How can a product claim to provide maximum UV protection when no such standard exists and the FDA does not even allow an SPF rating for hair-care products?

☺ $$$ **Reconstruct Repair, Rebuild & Minimize Breakage** *($20 for 8.5 ounces)* is a very standard, routine conditioner that cannot reconstruct or repair damaged hair, although it is a good conditioner for normal to slightly dry hair of any thickness.

☺ $$$ **Shine Max, Shining Smoother** *($17 for 2.5 ounces)* is an overpriced silicone serum that works as well as any to tame frizzies and add a brilliant shine to hair. The sunflower seed extract (Heliogenol) it contains cannot preserve hair color.

QUANTUM

For more information about Quantum, call (800) 621-3379 or, for Quantum Reds, call (800) 242-9283 or visit www.zotos.com.

What's Good About This Line: The prices match the simple, straightforward formulations; most of the shampoos are very good.

What's Not So Good About It: Some poor and dated formulations are present, including the Quantum Red Shampoo and Conditioner, because both contain drying red henna.

☺ **Clarifying Shampoo, for Deep Cleansing to Remove Build-Up** *($6.50 for 15 ounces)* is a very standard, simple shampoo that is an excellent option for all hair types, and can nicely remove product buildup.

☹ **Daily Cleansing Shampoo, for All Hair Types** *($6.50 for 15 ounces)* contains the ingredient diammonium dithioglycolate, a thioglycolic acid compound usually seen in perm and relaxing solutions. It can cause contact dermatitis and hair breakage with continued use, and is not recommended in a shampoo you're likely to use daily.

☺ **Moisturizing Shampoo, for Permed, Color-Treated & Dry Hair** *($6.50 for 15 ounces)* is a standard shampoo that is good for normal to dry hair of any thickness.

☺ **Volumizing Shampoo, for Fine, Limp, and Lazy Hair** *($6.50 for 15 ounces)* is a great shampoo for all hair types. The minuscule amounts of conditioning agents pose no risk of buildup.

☺ **Moisturizing Conditioner, for Permed, Color-Treated and Dry Hair** *($6.50 for 15 ounces)* is as basic as a conditioner gets, but this can still be an effective option for normal to dry hair that is normal to thick or coarse.

☹ **Daily Moisturizer, Leave-In Detangler and Conditioner** *($6.50 for 12 ounces)* contains the preservatives methylchloroisothiazolinone and methylisothiazolinone (Kathon

CG), which are contraindicated for use in leave-in products due to the probable risk of a sensitizing skin or scalp reaction.

☺ **Finishing Spray, for Firm, Flexible Hold** *($6.50 for 11 ounces)* is a standard, firm-hold aerosol hairspray with a slightly stiff, sticky feel that can be brushed through.

☺ **Spritz, for Firm Hold** *($6.50 for 8 ounces)* is a basic nonaerosol hairspray that provides a light to medium hold with a hint of stiffness and stickiness. It does not flake and the silicone helps you to brush through hair without snags along the way.

☺ **Styling Gel, Natural Hold for Sculpt, Style or Set** *($6.50 for 7 ounces)* is an average styling gel that can provide medium hold, but it remains uncomfortably sticky and stiff. It can work well for most hairstyles, but just isn't as modern or elegant as many other styling gels from other lines in all price ranges.

☺ **Volumizing Foam, for Instant Volume and Body** *($6.50 for 9 ounces)* is a standard, propellant-based mousse that has a light to medium hold and minimal stiff or sticky feel.

☺ **Perm Revitalizer, to Revive and Moisturize Curls** *($6.50 for 8 ounces)* is a standard water- and alcohol-based styling spray that has a light hold that remains slightly moist but minimally sticky. Hair can be easily brushed through, and nothing about this product makes it preferred for permed or curly hair.

QUANTUM REDS

☹ **Reds Daily Color Replenishing Shampoo, Deposits and Brightens All Shades of Red Hair** *($11 for 10.2 ounces)* contains a high amount of red henna extract, which tends to build up a sticky film over the hair that eventually makes hair feel dry and brittle—which is the main reason why you rarely see henna used in hair-care products. There are better color-enhancing shampoos available from Aveda, ARTec, and Paul Mitchell.

☹ **Reds Daily Color Refreshing Conditioner, Moisturizing & Protects All Shades of Red Hair** *($11 for 10.2 ounces)* contains a high amount of red henna extract, which tends to leave a sticky film over the hair that can dry out the hair shaft, making this a problem for most hair types.

☺ **Reds Daily 2-Phase Color Protector, Detangles, Brightens, & Protects All Shades of Red Hair** *($11 for 8 ounces)* is a lightweight, leave-in conditioner that works well to make normal to fine or thin hair feel smoother and be shinier.

QUEEN HELENE

Queen Helene is the great-grandmother of hair-care products, at least on the surface. Its parent company, Para Laboratories, has been in business for over 100 years, and Queen Helene is its longstanding brand, the source of hair-, skin-, and body-care products sold in drug and mass market stores nationwide. Sadly, it seems that somewhere in its history the Queen Helene hair-care line stopped innovating and simply rested on its now rather dated formulations. This is one of the few lines in this book that underutilizes one of the most modern and commonly seen hair-care ingredients, silicone. The products have their strong points, and that's good, particularly because this line is significantly less greasy than many others marketed toward African-American consumers, but the line still needs serious updating and a wider variety of products, particularly in the styling category. For more information about Queen Helene, call (800) 645-3752 or visit www.queenhelene.com.

What's Good About This Line: The prices and generous sizes are the main reason to pay attention to Queen Helene; there are some incredibly rich, emollient conditioners for dry to very dry hair; the silicone spray and serum are wonderful for performance and price.

What's Not So Good About It: Many of the shampoo formulas are either lackluster or dated; the styling gels are redundant, with the same basic formula recycled into *nine* different products, each with its own unique claims that turn out to be an amalgam of what all of the gels can do; the packaging for this line needs to be updated so it is more user-friendly.

☺ **Cholesterol & Tea Tree Shampoo** (*$5 for 12 ounces*) is a standard shampoo that is a good option for fine or thin hair that is slightly dry, but the film-forming agents can build up and make hair feel stiff.

☺ **Dandruff Shampoo, 6.5 pH Acid-Balanced** (*$3.50 for 16 ounces*) shares a pH typical of almost all shampoos, so singling this out and adding it to the name of the product is a bit strange. This shampoo has no effect on dandruff; it does contain a disinfectant, but not one that's known to help combat dandruff or a flaking scalp. It's just an average shampoo that won't do anything special for hair or scalp.

☺ **Ginseng & Tea Tree Shampoo, for All Types of Hair** (*$5.49 for 16 ounces*) is nearly identical to the Cholesterol & Tea Tree Shampoo above, except this contains a reduced amount of film-forming agent and replaces cholesterol with keratin amino acids. That makes it a better shampoo for normal to slightly dry hair of any thickness.

☺ **Mint Julep Shampoo with Protein, Concentrated with Protein** (*$3.50 for 16 ounces*) doesn't contain any mint, and that's a good thing for the scalp. It does contain a chlorophyll-derived coloring agent, but this product is minimally effective at cleansing the hair and scalp because it lacks detergent cleansing agents, instead relying on a lather agent. This will not remove styling product or conditioner buildup.

☺ **Natural Garlic Shampoo, Unscented** (*$3.75 for 21 ounces*) contains deodorized garlic, so no worries about your hair smelling offensive. The question is, why use garlic at all, since it has no established benefit for hair and scalp? It cannot stop excessive hair breakage, as claimed on the label. This is a very standard shampoo that is an option for all hair types and will not cause buildup.

☺ **Placenta Conditioning Shampoo, Acid-Balanced Concentrate with Panthenol** (*$4.50 for 16 ounces*) contains placental enzymes, and while the source is not identified it is likely they are derived from animals. Enzymes in hair-care products are notoriously unstable, and can actually have a detrimental effect on the cuticle if they remain active. That's not the case here though; this is just another standard shampoo that is an option for all hair types and poses minimal to no risk of buildup.

☺ **Cholesterol & Tea Tree Conditioner** *($5 for 12 ounces)* works well for slightly dry hair that is normal to fine or thin.

☺ **Ginseng & Tea Tree Conditioner, for All Types of Hair** *($5.49 for 16 ounces)* is a standard emollient conditioner that is an option for normal to dry hair of any thickness.

☺ **Placenta Cream Hair Conditioner, with Panthenol** *($4.25 for 15 ounces)* is a very emollient conditioner that is suitable for dry to very dry hair that is coarse or thick, but the tiny amount of placenta extract is a waste, offering no benefit for hair or scalp. For very dry hair, leaving a conditioner like this on hair overnight can make a noticeable difference.

☺ **Cholesterol Hair Conditioning Cream** *($3.50 for 15 ounces)* is similar to the Placenta Cream Hair Conditioner above, except this is less emollient and is preferred for dry hair of any thickness except fine or thin. The tiny amounts of cholesterol and lanolin don't have much impact on hair, but the mineral oil and emollient thickeners do.

☺ **Cholesterol Hot Oil Treatment** *($4.25 for 8 ounces)* is an OK moisturizing conditioner for normal to dry hair of any thickness.

☺ **Cholesterol with Ginseng Conditioning/Strengthening Cream** *($3.50 for 15 ounces)* is similar to the Placenta Cream Hair Conditioner above, except this is a less emollient option that is preferred for dry hair of any thickness except fine or thin. The ginseng component has no strengthening abilities for hair, so that claim is bogus.

☺ **Ginseng & Tea Tree Hot Oil Treatment, Dual Action** *($4.25 for 8 ounces)* is a slightly more emollient version of the Cholesterol Hot Oil Treatment above, except this one does not contain cholesterol. That's of little consequence, because the lanolin oil is an excellent (though heavy) emollient for dry hair.

☺ **Ginseng & Tea Tree Reconstructor, for Dry or Damaged Hair** *($1.99 for 1 ounce)* is similar to the Placenta Cream Hair Conditioner, with Panthenol above, and the same basic comments apply. Ginseng and tea tree may look enticing on the label, but they cannot reconstruct hair (nor can anything else in this product).

☺ **Jojoba Hot Oil Treatment** *($4.25 for 8 ounces)* is nearly identical to the Ginseng & Tea Tree Hot Oil Treatment, Dual Action above, except the plants are replaced by jojoba extract, which is not as effective as jojoba oil would be for hair. Otherwise, the same comments apply.

☺ **Placenta Hot Oil Treatment** *($4.25 for 8 ounces)* is nearly identical to the Cholesterol Hot Oil Treatment above, except that the placental enzymes, which have no effect on hair whatsoever, replace the cholesterol. Otherwise, the same comments apply.

☺ **Super Cholesterol Hair Conditioning Cream, for Extremely Damaged Hair** *($7 for 32 ounces)* is similar to most of the other conditioners from Queen Helene. It's an emollient formula that would be great for dry to very dry hair that is normal to thick or coarse, but it doesn't really deserve the "super" distinction because it isn't really distinctive.

☺ **Cholesterol Conditioning Styling Gel, Ultra Hold** *($3.50 for 16 ounces)*, **Crystalene Clear Moisturizing Styling Gel, Firm Hold** *($3.50 for 16 ounces)*, **Designing Gel, Alcohol Free for Maximum Hold and Extra Volume** *($3.75 for 16 ounces)*, **Pro-Rich, Protein Conditioning and Styling Gel** *($3.50 for 16 ounces)*, **Sculpturing Gel & Glaze** *($3.75 for 16 ounces)*, **Styling Gel, Hard to Hold** *($3.25 for 16 ounces)*, **Styling Gel, Mega Hold** *($3.50 for 16 ounces)*, **Styling Gel, Superhold** *($3.50 for 16 ounces)*, and **Super Protein 4 in 1, Hair Conditioner and Styling Gel** *($3.75 for 16 ounces)* all share the same basic styling-gel formula, with minor differences that have no discernible effect on hair. Each gel provides a medium hold that's slightly sticky but can be easily brushed through. The formulations make differing claims in terms of how fast each dries and the amount of conditioning they provide, but your hair will not notice a difference regardless of which one you choose. The jumbo jar packaging of each is a bit inelegant because you have to dig the gel out with your fingers. Only the Styling Gel, Mega Hold comes in a large, user-friendly squeeze bottle.

☺ **Shine Liquid, with Cholesterol** *($6.75 for 4 ounces)* is a standard, but very good and fairly priced, silicone serum that contains a tiny amount of cholesterol as added emollient for very dry hair. This is mostly silicone, and works as well as any serum at any price. The price tag should give you some idea of the markup for many salon-sold products.

☺ **Shine Spray, with Cholesterol** *($6.75 for 4 ounces)* is an excellent silicone spray for all hair types. It adds the requisite glossy shine and can help tame frizzies and smooth flyaway strands. Those with fine or thin hair should apply this product sparingly.

RALPH LAUREN

Ralph Lauren's small collection of hair-care products is known as Ralph Good Hair Day. Each of the six products reviewed below is fragranced with a floral scent marketed to a younger teen audience. The products are available in more than 2,000 department stores and the line will expand internationally in 2004. So does Ralph know hair care the way he knows polo and fashion? I'll let the reviews answer that question. For more information about Ralph Lauren hair care, owned by L'Oreal, call (888) 475-7674 or visit www.polo.com.

What's Good About This Line: For a designer line, prices are surprisingly realistic, though what you're paying for is the Ralph fragrance (and brand name) rather than superior hair care.

What's Not So Good About It: Nothing, unless you don't like the pervasive fragrance.

☺ **$$$ Balance Due Shampoo** *($12.50 for 8.4 ounces)* is a very standard shampoo that works well for all hair types and poses no risk of buildup.

☺ **$$$ Dish the Dirt, Clarifying Shampoo** *($12.50 for 8.4 ounces)* is a very standard, all-hair-types shampoo that poses no risk of buildup.

☺ $$$ **Flat-Free, Volumizing Shampoo** *($12.50 for 8.4 ounces)* is nearly identical to the Balance Due Shampoo above, and the same basic comments apply. This shampoo does not contain any volumizing agents.

☺ $$$ **Knot Now, Knot Ever, Conditioner** *($12.50 for 8.4 ounces)* is a simple conditioner that is primarily a way to add the teen-oriented Ralph scent to your hair. It is a decent option for normal hair of any thickness; but don't expect this to do wondrous things for dry, damaged hair.

☺ $$$ **Get Hold of Yourself Hair Spray** *($16.50 for 6.7 ounces)* has a great name, especially if styling your hair brings you to a panic! This is a non-aerosol hairspray that produces a fine, quick-drying mist and offers light, minimally sticky hold. It brushes through with ease and is excellent for all hair types, but be sure you like the perfume-y fragrance before purchasing.

☺ $$$ **Saved By the Gel Hair Gel** *($16.50 for 8.4 ounces)* is a liquidy gel that is easy to distribute through hair, and provides medium to firm hold. Due to this gel's sticky finish, it is somewhat difficult to brush through, and a little of this goes a long way, so the price isn't such a burn.

REDKEN

L'Oreal acquired Redken in 1995, and over the past few years their existing and new formulations have become increasingly standard and, in some cases, downright boring. When you're shopping a salon line, you should expect formulations that at least partially justify the higher prices compared to those of hair-care products sold in drug and mass market stores, though as it turns out that is rarely the case in the world of hair-care products. The number of Redken products whose special or "key benefit" ingredients are listed way after the preservatives and fragrance is staggering. Almost without exception, product after product is composed of four to six very standard ingredients, followed by preservatives and fragrance. That means the ingredients (such as the amino acid taurine) Redken touts as their unique selling point are barely present, and in all likelihood have no effect whatsoever on hair or scalp.

Under L'Oreal's ownership, the Redken line has expanded, offering several different categories, including options for dry, color-treated, long, curly, damaged, and sun-exposed hair, to name a few. All of the product categories make claims that make them sound like the ideal solution for their intended hair type or condition, but more often than not the formulas are interchangeable (particularly for shampoos and conditioners in the sub-lines). There are some very good products, but Redken just isn't as impressive as many other salon lines, including Paul Mitchell, Bumble and bumble, and Graham Webb. For more information about Redken, call (800) 423-5369 or visit www.redken.com.

What's Good About This Line: A few of the styling products are versatile, somewhat unique options well-suited for today's modern, textured yet casual hairstyles; the Color Extend color-enhancing conditioners are excellent; overall, the shampoos and conditioners are effective, though very standard, options.

What's Not So Good About It: Claims that are often unrealistic (though Redken is hardly the only company to cross that line); the numbered holding system for the main collection of styling products is more confusing than helpful, though the lower-numbered products do tend to have minimal to no hold as indicated; a few leave-on treatment products contain the drying sulfonic acid sodium polystyrene sulfonate; the styling gels are either problematic formulas or just not as elegant as many others.

☹ **Hair Cleansing Cream Shampoo** *($8.50 for 10.1 ounces)* contains sodium lauryl sulfate as its main detergent cleansing agent, and that makes this conditioning shampoo too drying for hair as well as drying and irritating for the scalp.

☺ **Airtight 12 Lock-Out Finishing Spray** *($11.95 for 11 ounces)* contains nothing that can "lock out environmental stress." Nature also has "keys" (such as high humidity and sunlight) to undermine whatever styling product you use. This is just a standard aerosol hairspray with a light, flexible hold that's neither stiff nor sticky. Hair is easily brushed through and maintains movement.

☹ **Clean Lift 07 Weightless Volume Gel** *($10.95 for 8.5 ounces)* is an ultra-light styling gel that would have been a great option for fine or thin hair, but it can ball up and flake off as it dries, making it more of a problem than a helpful body-boosting product.

☺ **Concrete 22 Cement Paste** *($13.95 for 5 ounces)* is a styling balm/gel hybrid that begins slick and slightly creamy but dries to a very strong, sticky hold that also makes hair stiff. That is great for creating extreme, gravity-defying hairstyles, but definitely not for softer styles you intend to brush through once they're dry. The name is almost self-explanatory, except this does not have a pastelike consistency.

☺ **Contour 08 Shaping Lotion** *($10.95 for 8.5 ounces)* is a standard styling gel with a basic, no-frills formula that provides medium hold with a slightly sticky, stiff feel that can be brushed through.

☺ **Framework 20 Workable Finishing Spray** *($11.95 for 11 ounces)* is a standard aerosol hairspray with a medium hold and a slightly stiff, sticky feel that can be brushed through. It dries too quickly to be considered a "working" hairspray.

☺ **Full Frame 07 Protective Volumizing Mousse** *($14.95 for 8.5 ounces)* is a propellant-based mousse with a medium to firm hold that leaves hair stiff and sticky, though it can be softened when hair is brushed through. This is a very good lightweight styling product for normal to fine or thin hair that is difficult to control.

☺ **Guts 10 Volume Spray Foam** *($12.95 for 10.58 ounces)* is, aside from a slightly different delivery system, identical to the Full Frame 07 Protective Volumizing Mousse above, and the same review applies.

☺ **Hardwear 16 Super Strong Gel** *($9.95 for 8.5 ounces)* is a standard gel with a medium hold and a slightly stiff feel that can be brushed through.

☺ **Hot Sets 22 Thermal Setting Mist** *($10.95 for 5 ounces)* is nothing more than a standard nonaerosol hairspray with a medium hold that's fairly sticky. It can indeed create long-lasting hot (roller) sets, but so can most other hairsprays, and using hairspray to heat-set hair can lead to excessive dryness and breakage. As a finishing spray, this works as well as any and it can be brushed through.

☺ **Inflate 14 Volumizing Finishing Spray** *($11.95 for 11 ounces)* is nearly identical to the Airtight 12 Lock-Out Finishing Spray above, and the same review applies.

☺ **In The Loop 02 Curl Booster** *($10.95 for 5 ounces)* credits the magnesium sulfate it contains as being able to fortify hair and eliminate frizzies, which is completely false. Magnesium sulfate is an alkaline ingredient that can raise the hair's cuticle layers to create a fuller, thicker appearance, but not without some dryness. It is the silicones in this light-weight, non-sticky spray that tame frizzies and help make curly hair more manageable, and that's about all this product has going for it.

☺ **Lift & Shine 15 Finishing Spritz** *($9.95 for 8.5 ounces)* is an ordinary, but good, nonaerosol hairspray that has a workable light hold that allows enough playtime to ar-range your hair before it sets. This can be easily brushed through and is great for all hair types. Considering the "shine" part of the name, this lacks shine-imparting ingredients.

☺ **Lush Whip 04 Styling Cream** *($14.95 for 4.2 ounces)* is a standard, water- and silicone-based styling cream with a light hold and minimal stickiness. This is a good grooming aid for use on wet or dry hair, and it can add moisture and shine while helping to shape hair. It is best for normal to dry hair that's normal to slightly thick.

☺ **Outshine 01 Anti-Frizz Polishing Milk** *($14.95 for 3.4 ounces)* is a slick, water-based styling balm that contains emollients, silicone, and detangling agents to help smooth and moisturize dry, frizzy hair of any texture. Those with fine or thin hair should use this very sparingly to avoid weighing hair down, but thick or coarse hair types can apply this liberally for moisture and shine.

☺ **Quick Dry 18 Instant Finishing Spray** *($11.95 for 11 ounces)* is nearly identical to the Airtight 12 Lock-Out Finishing Spray above, except this offers slightly more hold, though not enough to choose this option if you need extra hold. It does not contain shine-enhancing ingredients.

☺ **Rewind 06 Pliable Styling Paste** *($14.95 for 5 ounces)* is a gel-type, slightly creamy-feeling styling balm (not a paste) that can work well to shape and manage curly or wavy hair or add texture to straight hair. It offers a light hold with a moist, slightly sticky finish. True to its name, it leaves hair pliable, ready to be reshaped or coiffed into that perfectly disheveled "I just woke up" look. This also works reasonably well to control frizzies, but not in high humidity.

☺ **Rough Paste 12 Working Material** *($14.95 for 2.5 ounces)* is a thicker, heavier, version of the Rewind 06 Pliable Styling Paste above, and is well-suited for use on dry to very dry stubborn hair that is thick, curly, or coarse. This provides a medium, flexible hold with slight stickiness, and can be used on wet or dry hair, though it works best to shape and enhance texture when hair is dry.

☺ **Spray Starch 15 Heat Memory Styler** *($9.95 for 5 ounces)* contains potato starch, which Redken maintains can protect hair from heat. Even if that were true (it isn't), potato starch is the last ingredient listed, meaning there is only a trace amount, too little to affect hair. This is a standard styling spray with a medium hold and a slightly stiff, sticky feel. It does not contain a single ingredient to protect hair from heat, and is best used after heat-styling to hold hair in place.

☺ **Straight 05 Straightening Balm** *($12.95 for 5 ounces)* is a lackluster straightening balm that is an OK option for straightening fine or thin hair.

☹ **Thickening Lotion 06 Body Builder** *($10.95 for 5 ounces)* lists sodium polystyrene sulfonate as the third ingredient, so it poses a risk of dryness and even stripping hair color with repeated use. Even without this problematic ingredient, this is a rather unimpressive product.

☺ **Undone 02 Weightless Defining Cream** *($14.95 for 3.4 ounces)* is a very light styling cream that is ideal for smoothing normal to fine or thin hair without adding weight or a greasy feel. It offers no hold and thus is not stiff or sticky, and is a great mixer product to soften any gel, mousse, or styling spray.

☺ **Vinyl Glam 02 Mega Shine Spray** *($13.95 for 3.4 ounces)* is a standard, alcohol-based silicone spray that offers a tiny amount of hold along with a dazzling shine. It is a good frizz-fighting/glossing option for all hair types, though it should be used sparingly.

☺ **Water Wax 03 Shine Defining Pomade** *($13.95 for 1.7 ounces)* is a water-soluble, gel-type pomade that is quite thick and that lacks the elegant slip and shine of other pomades in this category. It is an OK option for smoothing frizz or shaping curls and waves on thick, coarse hair, but there are better options, many costing less than this product.

☺ **Willpower 26 Holding Spray** *($9.95 for 8.5 ounces)* is a standard, nonaerosol, medium-hold hairspray that makes hair feel quite stiff and sticky, though with some effort it can be brushed through. It is best for locking hairstyles in place with minimal movement. The sunscreens cannot be relied on for UV protection because this product is not rated with an SPF number, and no standards for protecting hair from the sun exist.

☺ **Glass 01 Smoothing Serum** *($13.95 for 2 ounces)* is a very standard silicone serum that works as well as any to turn dry, frizzy hair into sleek, shiny locks. It is best for thick or coarse hair.

REDKEN ACTIVE EXPRESS

☺ **Active Express Shampoo, Fast-Acting for All Hair Types** *($8.50 for 10.1 ounces)* used to be a unique shampoo that contained a high amount of witch hazel, whose alcohol content could help hair dry faster (if you used the entire Active Express system). It is now a standard conditioning shampoo that has no effect on how fast hair dries. It is a good option for normal to dry hair that is normal to thick or coarse.

☺ **Active Express Conditioner, Fast-Acting for All Hair Types** *($9.95 for 8.5 ounces)* is an exceptionally basic conditioner that isn't much faster acting than most others, though it does have a tiny amount of alcohol. This is a decent option for normal to dry hair of any thickness.

☺ **Active Express Quick Treat, Heat Styler for All Hair Types** *($12.95 for 8.5 ounces)* is primarily water, film-forming agent, detangling agent, preservative, and fragrance. Acrylates copolymer can provide a slight amount of heat protection, but the lack of moisturizing agents or proteins doesn't bode well for hair that's already dry or damaged.

☺ $$$ **Active Express Speed Control, Smoothing Treatment for All Hair Types** *($12.95 for 5 ounces)* is a very good styling cream for dry to very dry hair that is normal to thick or coarse. It does not provide any hold, but can help smooth hair and enhance its texture without looking or feeling overly greasy.

REDKEN ALL SOFT

☺ **All Soft Shampoo, Softness for Dry/Brittle Hair** *($8.50 for 10.1 ounces)* is, with a few inconsequential exceptions, nearly identical to the Active Express Shampoo above, and the same basic comments apply. The conditioning agents and silicone can make hair feel softer.

☺ **All Soft Conditioner, Softness for Dry/Brittle Hair** *($9.95 for 8.5 ounces)* is a standard, but good, option for normal to slightly dry hair of any thickness.

☺ $$$ **All Soft Addictive Hair Transformer, Softness for Dry Hair** *($14.95 for 3.4 ounces)* is a great spray-on conditioner for dry hair that is normal to coarse or thick, but it should be used sparingly or it will make hair look and feel greasy.

☺ $$$ **All Soft Heavy Cream, Super Treatment for Dry/Brittle Hair** *($12.95 for 8.5 ounces)* is an emollient, creamy conditioner for dry to very dry hair of any thickness.

REDKEN CLEAR MOISTURE

☺ **Clear Moisture Shampoo** *($8.50 for 10.1 ounces)* is a standard shampoo that contains a gentle detergent cleansing and lather agent combination with silicone added for conditioning (read: moisture). This shampoo is nearly identical in every respect to L'Oreal's Vive Curl-Moisture Shampoo, for Curly Hair ($4.49 for 13 ounces), and the amount of silicone makes it best for dry to very dry hair that is normal to coarse or thick.

☺ **Clear Moisture Conditioner** *($10.50 for 8.5 ounces)* is a very good conditioner that is an option for normal to slightly dry hair that is normal to fine or thin. For the cost-conscious, this is nearly identical to L'Oreal's Vive Curl-Moisture Conditioner, for Curly Hair ($4.49 for 13 ounces).

☺ $$$ **Clear Moisture Moist Ends Leave-In Treatment for Normal/Dry Hair** *($11.95 for 5 ounces)* is a basic, but good, leave-in conditioner for normal to slightly dry hair that is normal to fine or thin.

☺ $$$ **Clear Moisture Water Rush Moisturizing Treatment for Normal/Dry Hair** *($12.95 for 8.5 ounces)* is a lightweight conditioner that is appropriate for dry hair that is normal to fine or thin. It is similar to L'Oreal's Vive Color-Care Masque, for Color Treated or Highlighted Hair ($7.39 for 5 ounces), except Redken's option adds glycerin to the mix, and in an amount that can have a positive impact on dry hair, especially when left on for more than a few minutes. This conditioner does contain fragrance (in an amount greater than the "special" ingredients Redken included).

REDKEN COLOR EXTEND

☺ **Color Extend Shampoo, Protection for Color-Treated Hair** *($8.50 for 10.1 ounces)* contains nothing that can protect color-treated hair. If Redken believes their own claim, then they would have to concede that *every* standard shampoo available (and we're talking hundreds of products) can provide the same amount of protection their shampoo allegedly can. This is a good shampoo for all hair types, and poses no risk of buildup.

☺ **Color Extend Conditioner, Protection for Color-Treated Hair** *($9.95 for 8.5 ounces)* is a very basic conditioner for normal to dry hair of any thickness, but it cannot help preserve hair color.

☺ **$$$ Color Extend Injection, Color-Charged Conditioner** *($11.95 for 5 ounces)* is a collection of color-enhancing conditioners with options for blonde, auburn, red, burgundy, and silver or gray hair. The conditioner itself is excellent for dry hair of any thickness, and this does contain the requisite basic dyes that can deposit a subtle amount of color on the hair shaft.

☺ **$$$ Color Extend Total Recharge, Inner Hair Fuel for Color-Treated Hair** *($14.95 for 5 ounces)* claims to give color-treated hair a "shot of cuticle-reinforcing ceramide," but it does not contain this conditioning agent. This is a good detangling spray for normal to fine hair, although it can't recharge color-treated hair.

REDKEN EXTREME

☹ **Extreme Shampoo, Fortifier for Distressed Hair** *($8.50 for 10.1 ounces)* is extremely drying because it contains TEA-lauryl sulfate as its main detergent cleansing agent, which is too drying and irritating for all hair and scalp types.

☺ **Extreme Conditioner, Fortifier for Distressed Hair** *($9.95 for 8.5 ounces)* is similar to, but slightly more emollient than, the Color Extend Conditioner above, making it slightly preferred for drier hair of any thickness except very fine or thin.

☺ **$$$ Extreme Anti-Snap, Leave-In Treatment for Distressed Hair** *($13.95 for 8.5 ounces)* is little more than water, silicone, preservative, film-forming agent, fragrance, and wax—the other ingredients are present in amounts too small to matter for hair. This can help make hair smoother and temporarily improve the appearance of split ends, while also preventing damage to hair from combing or brushing. It doesn't take a special treatment product to do this—any silicone spray (or, if hair is very dry or coarse, a silicone serum) will do the same thing.

☹ **Extreme CAT, Protein Reconstructing Treatment for Distressed Hair** *($12.95 for 5 ounces)* contains only a tiny amount of protein (it's listed just before the preservative) and is primarily water, magnesium sulfate, surfactant, and taurine, the amino acid Redken likes to use in many of its products. The magnesium sulfate (Epsom salt) has an astringent effect on hair and scalp, and can lead to dryness and increased risk of hair breakage. This poorly formulated product is the wrong choice for hair in any state of distress.

☺ **$$$ Extreme Deep Fuel** *($14.95 for five 0.68-ounce tubes)* is packaged and marketed to appear as if it were intensive care for damaged hair. It turns out this is a fairly standard conditioner that cannot strengthen hair any better than most conditioners. It ends up being an expensive investment that is easily replaced by several other conditioners in this line.

REDKEN FRESH CURLS

☺ **Fresh Curls Shampoo, Moisture and Frizz Control for Curly Hair** *($8.50 for 10.1 ounces)* isn't as effective for curly, frizzy hair as the Active Express or All Soft shampoos above, but this is a good, standard shampoo for normal to slightly dry hair of any thickness. This poses a slight risk of buildup with repeated use.

☺ **Fresh Curls Conditioner, Moisture and Frizz Control for Curly Hair** *($9.95 for 8.5 ounces)* is a better product for curly hair, at least compared to the mismarketed Fresh Curls Shampoo above. This water- and silicone-based conditioner is an excellent smoothing, moisturizing option for dry, curly hair that is normal to thick or coarse.

☹ **Fresh Curls Curl Boost, Scrunching Spray Gel for Curly Hair** *($12.95 for 5 ounces)* lists sodium polystyrene sulfonate as its second ingredient, which makes this too drying for hair, not to mention that it can potentially strip hair color with repeated use.

☺ **$$$ Fresh Curls Spin Control, Curl Defining Leave-In Treatment** *($12.95 for 5 ounces)* is a very good leave-in smoothing conditioner for normal to dry hair of any thickness except very fine or thin. It can nicely smooth and help define curls and waves, as well as provide some protection during heat styling.

REDKEN HEADSTRONG

☺ **Headstrong Shampoo, Volume for Fine Hair** *($8.50 for 10.1 ounces)* is as standard as shampoos get. This is a good option for all hair types, and poses no risk of buildup.

☺ **Headstrong Conditioner, Volume for Fine Hair** *($9.95 for 8.5 ounces)* is yet another standard conditioner that is a good option for normal to dry hair of any thickness.

☹ **Headstrong Fine Shot, Root Boost Styling Treatment for Fine Hair** *($12.95 for 5 ounces)* contains sodium polystyrene sulfonate, which can be drying to hair and possibly strip hair color with repeated use. It is not recommended.

REDKEN SMOOTH DOWN

☺ **Smooth Down Shampoo, Anti-Frizz Smoothing for Very Dry/Unruly Hair** *($9.95 for 10.1 ounces)* is a standard, mildly conditioning shampoo that is a great option for all hair types. If you're looking for a shampoo to help combat frizzy hair, the Active Express or All Soft shampoos above are preferred over this one.

☺ **Smooth Down Conditioner, Anti-Frizz Smoothing for Very Dry/Unruly Hair** *($10.95 for 8.5 ounces)* is a standard conditioner that is similar to many in L'Oreal's Vive hair-care line that are available for a lot less money. This is a very good option for normal to slightly dry hair of any thickness.

☺ $$$ **Smooth Down Butter Treat, Smoothing Treatment for Very Dry/Unruly Hair** *($13.95 for 8.5 ounces)* is nearly identical to the Smooth Down Conditioner above, except this contains lanolin, which makes it preferred for dry hair that is normal to slightly coarse or thick.

☺ $$$ **Smooth Down Heat Glide, Protective Smoother for Very Dry/Unruly Hair** *($15.95 for 8.5 ounces)* is a standard silicone serum packaged in a generous-sized container. It is an outstanding frizz-smoothing option for dry to very dry hair that is coarse or thick.

REDKEN SO LONG

☺ **So Long Shampoo, Equalizing Strength for Long Hair** *($8.50 for 10.1 ounces)* is nearly identical to the Headstrong Shampoo above, and the same review applies. Nothing in this shampoo is special or preferred for cleansing long hair.

☺ **So Long Conditioner, Equalizing Strength for Long Hair** *($9.95 for 8.5 ounces)* is an excellent smoothing and detangling conditioner for normal to dry hair that is normal to fine or thin—and of any length.

☺ $$$ **So Long Heat Treat, Heat-Activated Leave-In Treatment for Long Hair** *($12.95 for 5 ounces)* is a spray-on, leave-in conditioner that works well to smooth and detangle normal to fine or thin hair while eliminating frizzies.

REDKEN SOLVE

☺ **Solve Dandruff Shampoo** *($9.95 for 10.1 ounces)* is a standard anti-dandruff shampoo that contains 1% zinc pyrithione, just like the Head & Shoulders shampoo that's available at the drugstore. It is an option for fighting dandruff, and although the conditioning agents can help offset the drying effect of the active ingredient, they also build up with repeated use.

☹ **Solve Purifying Shampoo, Purifying for Oily Hair and Scalp** *($9.95 for 8.5 ounces)* contains kaolin and montmorillonite as the main ingredients. As clays, both of these ingredients are too drying for any hair type.

REDKEN SUN SHAPE

☹ **Sun Shape Shampoo, After Sun & Sport Purifier** *($8.50 for 10.1 ounces)* is a chelating shampoo containing sodium lauryl sulfate as its main detergent cleansing agent, making it too drying for hair and too irritating for skin. There are much gentler shampoos available to remove mineral or chlorine buildup.

☺ $$$ **Sun Shape Sun Milk, Protective Leave-In Moisturizer** *($12.95 for 5 ounces)* is a very standard leave-in conditioner that is not as elegant as the silicone-based leave-in conditioners from Redken, but is nevertheless a good option for normal to dry hair that needs added moisture and help with combing. The buzz-worthy ingredients are listed well after the preservatives, so they don't amount to much when it comes to conditioning hair.

☺ $$$ **Sun Shape Swim Cream, Protective Hair Cream for Sun & Sport** *($12.95 for 5 ounces)* cannot shield hair from the damaging effects of the sun or water. Actually, a pure silicone serum would be a far better pre-swimming protective option than this water-based product. The key is to apply a generous amount of the silicone to dry hair before entering the pool.

RENE FURTERER

I suppose the interest and in and enthusiasm for this line has to do with its presence in upscale department stores and cosmetics boutiques such as Sephora. The made-in-France allure and the lofty prices surely must mean that you're buying something elite and special, right? Wrong, wrong, big time *wrong*. This line is one of the most disappointing around, full of products that are either so standard the prices are truly embarrassing, or so irritating and useless they would earn must-avoid status at any price.

One of the hooks of this line is, surprise, plant extracts and essential oils. All of the usual claims made for these ingredients are present, along with some new ones ranging from toning damaged hair (how is that even possible when hair is dead?) to controlling the amount of oil the sebaceous glands in your scalp secrete (not possible, oil production is controlled by hormones). Although some of the plant extracts used by Rene Furterer are harmless or even beneficial (most often for moisturizing dry hair), the ones used most frequently in these products tend to be skin irritants. Coincidentally, these same irritating essential oils and plant extracts have the least beneficial profiles for hair, with some, such as peppermint, serving only as a source of irritation.

All told, there is nothing in this line to get that excited about, unless you enjoy spending lots of money on very standard hair-care products. Even if you're someone who refuses to believe that drugstore hair-care products can be every bit as good (and often better) than salon or department store options, this is not one of the better lines to spend money on, or to take the time to shop, for that matter. For more information about Rene Furterer, call (800) 522-8285 or visit www.renefurterer.com.

What's Good About This Line: The rinse-out conditioners and a few of the leave-in conditioners have good moisturizing and smoothing formulas for dry hair; most of the styling products, though amazingly standard, do work well without being heavy, drying, or greasy.

What's Not So Good About It: Where to start! Each subcategory has its share of unimpressive products, ranging from those that contain irritating essential oils to hair-loss products that are useless for treating baldness, and the anti-dandruff and oily-scalp lines are entirely problematic, plus several hair masks contain drying clay. Prices are needlessly high, while the benefits are either negligble, nonexistent, or deliver the same result you can achieve from countless less expensive hair-care lines.

☹ **Astera Soothing Milk Shampoo** (*$20 for 5.07 ounces*) isn't soothing in the least. This detergent-based shampoo contains peppermint and rosemary oils, which make it too irritating for all scalp types. Even without the irritants, it is absurdly overpriced for what you get.

☺ **$$$ Karite Shampoo, for Extremely Dry Scalp and Hair** *($22 for 5.07 ounces)* is a very standard, but good, conditioning shampoo for dry hair of any thickness. For treating an extremely dry scalp, massaging on an emollient conditioner or nonfragrant oil is the preferred way to go.

☹ **Naturia RF6, Gentle, Balancing Shampoo** *($20 for 5.07 ounces)* contains peppermint and basil oils, which won't balance anything but can cause pronounced irritation and itching. The caraway oil (present in a high amount) can also cause irritation in the form of contact dermatitis.

☺ **$$$ Karite Nourishing Conditioning Cream** *($35 for 8.4 ounces)* is an extremely basic, drastically overpriced conditioner that is a mediocre option for slightly dry hair of any thickness.

☺ **$$$ Anti-Dehydrating Directional Treatment Spray, Firm Hold** *($18 for 6.7 ounces)* is a very standard nonaerosol hairspray with a medium to firm hold that leaves hair slightly stiff and sticky. Silicones are included to add shine and help make hair easier to comb through, but many inexpensive hairsprays use silicones too, so they're hardly unique to this pricey option.

☺ **$$$ Anti-Dehydrating Sculpting Gel, Strong Hold** *($18 for 4.3 ounces)* is an extremely standard, firm-hold styling gel that leaves hair feeling stiff and sticky, though it can be brushed through. Any of the L'Oreal Studio Line gels would perform as well as or better than this option.

☺ **$$$ Anti-Dehydrating Styling Gel, Soft Hold** *($18 for 4.3 ounces)* is nearly identical to the Anti-Dehydrating Sculpting Gel, Strong Hold above, except with a softer hold and less stickiness. Otherwise, the same comments apply.

☺ **$$$ Anti-Dehydrating Vegetal Styling Spritz, Soft Hold** *($18 for 6.7 ounces)* is as standard a styling spray as it gets, with light to medium hold and minimal stiff or sticky feel.

☺ **$$$ Anti-Dehydrating Volumizing Mousse, Soft Hold** *($18 for 6.7 ounces)* is a propellant-based mousse that provides very light, soft hold that is good for basic, low-maintenance hairstyles, especially on fine or thin hair. This weightless product is minimally sticky and easily brushed through.

☺ **$$$ Anti-Dehydrating Volumizing Mousse, Strong Hold** *($18 for 6.7 ounces)* is almost identical to the Anti-Dehydrating Volumizing Mousse, Soft Hold above, except this offers more hold and residual stickiness. It is still best for casual, unstructured hairstyles requiring weightless hold and body.

☺ **$$$ Anti-Dehydrating Volumizing Treatment Spray, Soft Hold** *($18 for 6.7 ounces)* is nearly identical to the Anti-Dehydrating Directional Treatment Spray, Firm Hold above, and the same comments apply.

☺ **$$$ Laque De Finition, Instant Hold Finishing Spray** *($26 for 6.9 ounces)* is a standard aerosol hairspray that is so basic its price is embarrassing. It distributes a fine mist capable of providing a light to medium, flexible hold with a minimal stiff or sticky feel. Choosing this hairspray over the myriad less expensive options is exclusively about the Furterer name, not the formulation.

☺ **$$$ Styling Wax, Sheer Shine** *($16 for 1.7 ounces)* is a standard, water-soluble, gel-type pomade that works as well as any to smooth dry ends and vanquish frizzies. It is light enough to be an option for all hair types, but persons with fine or thin hair should apply it only to the ends. This does shampoo out easily, and, despite the name, contains no wax.

☹ **Astera Soothing Fluid, for Sensitive, Irritated Scalp and Brittle Hair** *($36 for 1.69 ounces)* contains high amounts of peppermint, camphor, and eucalyptus oils, which is unbelievable in a product designed for an already irritated scalp. It also contains menthol, and is eligible for an award as one of the most needlessly irritating, insultingly priced hair-care products in this book.

☹ **Color Enhancing Mask, Auburn** *($22 for 5.5 ounces)* contains plant extracts to impart color to hair, but since these extracts don't cling as well to the hair as basic dyes do, they are only useful for coloring the product! Looking a little further, with kaolin (clay) as the third ingredient, this is too drying for all hair types. Clay can dry hair and scalp as well as chip away at the cuticle, leading to damaged, flyaway hair that won't take well to any color treatment.

☹ **Color Enhancing Mask, Blonde** *($22 for 5.5 ounces)* is, save for a change of plant extracts, identical to the Color Enhancing Mask, Auburn above, and the same review applies.

☹ **Color Enhancing Mask, Brunette** *($22 for 5.5 ounces)* is, save for a change of plant extracts, identical to the Color Enhancing Mask, Auburn above, and the same review applies.

☹ **Color Enhancing Mask, Silver** *($22 for 5.1 ounces)* is, save for a change of plant extracts and synthetic violet coloring, identical to the Color Enhancing Mask, Auburn above, and the same review applies.

☹ **Complex 5, Regenerating Extract with Stimulating Essential Oils** *($28 for 6 vials)* is sold as a specialty product for the scalp. It won't regenerate anything, but can cause irritation due to the orange and lavender oils it contains. This also uses a glycol carrier base, which helps enhance penetration of other ingredients into the skin, something you don't want when the other ingredients are unnecessary irritants.

☺ **$$$ High Control Emulsion Anti-Frizz, Radiance & Protection** *($18 for 8.5 ounces)* is a standard, but effective, leave-in conditioner/grooming cream for dry hair that is normal to coarse or thick.

☺ **$$$ Karite No Rinse Nutritive Concentrate, for Very Dry and Rebellious Hair** *($20 for 3.3 ounces)* is a lightweight, minimally creamy styling lotion that does a good job of adding moisture and smoothness to dry hair of any thickness except very fine or thin. Nothing in it is nutritive for the hair, but it definitely will condition it without being greasy or feeling heavy.

☺ **$$$ Spray Gloss** *($18 for 3.38 ounces)* is a standard, alcohol-based silicone spray that works as well as any to add shine and a silky feel to dry hair while helping to control frizzies. Less expensive options abound, but if you have to spend money on this line, this is a good bet.

RENE FURTERER ANTI-DANDRUFF TREATMENT

☺ $$$ Anti-Dandruff Shampoo, for Dry Scalp *($22 for 4.22 ounces)* contains salicylic acid as its active ingredient. That can be helpful for dandruff, but it would be better if it contained a more common anti-microbial agent such as zinc pyrithione (found in Head & Shoulders) or ketoconazole (found in Nizoral). This also contains thyme oil, which can be very irritating while offering little benefit other than itch relief.

☺ $$$ Anti-Dandruff Shampoo, for Oily Scalp *($22 for 4.22 ounces)* is a better anti-dandruff shampoo than the one above because it contains zinc pyrithione rather than salicylic acid. However, the orange and thyme oils it also contains are scalp irritants and make this overpriced dandruff shampoo difficult to recommend.

☹ Soothing Treatment Gel with Extract of Melaleuca *($20 for 2.5 ounces)* is a water- and alcohol-based gel that contains camphor, thyme, and orange—all of which are potent scalp irritants that have little to no benefit for a dandruff-prone scalp.

RENE FURTERER CARTHAME

☺ $$$ Carthame Cream Shampoo, for Thick Hair *($20 for 3.4 ounces)* is a rather standard shampoo that is an OK option for normal to dry hair that is normal to coarse or thick.

☺ $$$ Carthame Milk Shampoo, for Fine Hair *($22 for 5.07 ounces)* is a standard conditioning shampoo that can be a bit heavy for someone with fine hair. It is preferred for normal to slightly dry hair that is normal to slightly thick or curly.

☺ $$$ Carthame Intensive Oil Treatment *($30 for 1.98 ounces)* costs a lot of money for what amounts to soybean and safflower oils with thickeners and fragrant orange oil. Instead of getting taken by this product, take the plain soybean or olive oil from your kitchen cupboard and enjoy the same results, and without the potential irritation from the orange oil.

☺ $$$ Carthame No-Rinse Protective Cream *($22 for 2.6 ounces)* is an excellent, though simply formulated, leave-in smoothing conditioner for normal to dry hair that is normal to slightly thick, curly, or coarse.

RENE FURTERER CURBICIA

☹ Curbicia Cream Shampoo, for Oily Scalp and Oily Hair *($20 for 3.38 ounces)* contains camphor and juniper tar along with rosemary, thyme, and cypress oils, which makes this conditioning shampoo too irritating for all scalp types. Nothing about this product is beneficial for someone with an oily scalp.

☹ Curbicia Milk Shampoo, for Fine Hair *($22 for 5.07 ounces)* contains the same problematic ingredients as the Curbicia Cream Shampoo above, and the same review applies.

☹ **Curbicia Clay Mask Argilla, for Oily Scalp and Oily Hair** *($24 for 4.2 ounces)* lists kaolin (clay) as the second ingredient, which only serves to dry out hair and scalp while chipping away at the hair's cuticle layers. Making matters worse, it adds irritating pine oil, pine tar, and sage oil to the mix.

☹ **Curbicia Rebalancing Lotion, for Oily Hair and Scalp** *($22 for 3.4 ounces)* won't rebalance anything, but it will cause scalp irritation, as it contains rosemary and orange oils. At best, all this misguided product can do is make hair easier to comb, and there are plenty of other options to help with that task without subjecting your scalp to a dose of irritation with each use.

RENE FURTERER FIORAVANTI

☺ **$$$ Fioravanti Volumizing Shampoo** *($22 for 5.07 ounces)* is a standard shampoo that is a good, though overpriced, option for all hair types. This poses no risk of buildup.

☺ **$$$ Fioravanti Clarify and Shine Finishing Rinse, Super Shine** *($18 for 8.4 ounces)* is a standard conditioner that could be a decent option for very fine or thin hair that needs help with combing but cannot use leave-in detangling products because they make hair too heavy.

☺ **$$$ Fioravanti Lightweight Detangling Cream Rinse, Super Shine** *($22 for 5.07 ounces)* replaces the silicone in the Fioravanti Clarify and Shine Finishing Rinse above with standard thickeners, which makes it a more emollient option for normal to slightly dry hair that is fine or thin. The plant extract in it may be a good source of vitamin C, but topical application of that and most other vitamins is useless for hair and scalp.

☺ **$$$ Fioravanti No-Rinse Detangling Spray, Super Shine** *($18 for 5.07 ounces)* is a less interesting spray-on version of the Fioravanti Clarify and Shine Finishing Rinse above, and is an OK option for detangling fine or thin hair that would normally fall flat with more emollient products.

☹ **Fioravanti Straightening Gel** *($20 for 5.1 ounces)* is a basic, no-frills, water-based gel that can ball up and flake off hair during styling, and is not recommended.

RENE FURTERER OKARA

☺ **$$$ OKARA Re-Balancing Shampoo, for Colored Hair** *($22 for 5.07 ounces)* is a very standard shampoo with no special benefit for color-treated hair. This poses minimal risk of buildup and is an option for all hair types.

☺ **$$$ OKARA Repairing Shampoo, for Permed Hair** *($20 for 5.07 ounces)* is nearly identical to the OKARA Re-Balancing Shampoo above, and the same review applies.

☺ **$$$ OKARA 2 Phases No Rinse Conditioner** *($20 for 5 ounces)* is a basic, spray-on, leave-in conditioner that is a good option for normal to slightly dry hair that is normal to slightly thick or curly and needs help with combing.

☺ **$$$ OKARA Protective Mousse, for Color-Treated Hair** *($30 for 13.5 ounces)* isn't very protective, but it is a good, propellant-based mousse with minimal to no hold and no stiff or sticky feel. This can work well to lightly groom fine or thin hair that does not need control or shaping.

☺ **$$$ OKARA Repairing Treatment Mask, for Damaged Permed Hair** *($20 for 5.3 ounces)* is one of the few Rene Furterer hair masks that do not contain clay. This is a rather standard conditioner parading as a specialty treatment for hair. It is merely a good conditioner for normal to dry hair of any thickness.

☺ **$$$ OKARA Restructuring Mask, for Colored Hair** *($20 for 5.1 ounces)* is nearly identical to the OKARA Repairing Treatment Mask, for Damaged Permed Hair above, but adds silicones, which makes it preferred for normal to dry hair that is slightly thick, curly, or coarse and needs smoothing and some help with frizzies.

RENE FURTERER SUN PRODUCTS

☺ **$$$ Nourishing Sun Shampoo for Dry Hair—Frequent Use** *($22 for 5.3 ounces)* is similar to most of the Rene Furterer shampoos above and works well for most hair types, but it isn't nourishing in the least or helpful for sun exposure.

☹ **Refreshing Sun Shower Gel for Hair and Body** *($22 for 6.7 ounces)* contains peppermint and eucalyptus oils. They can feel refreshing, but the cooling, tingling sensation is your skin (and scalp's) way of communicating that it is being irritated.

☺ **$$$ Protective Sun-Moisturizing Mousse** *($18 for 2.9 ounces)* is a propellant-based conditioning mousse that does not offer any hold. As a leave-in conditioner, it is an option for fine or thin hair that is minimally dry. However, it cannot protect hair from the drying, color-fading effects of sun exposure. The KPS 30 statement is an unapproved, unregulated rating system that refers to this product's "keratin protection factor." It is a meaningless number and this product should not be relied on to protect hair from UV damage.

☺ **$$$ After-Sun Hair Balm, for Dry, Damaged Ends** *($22 for 2.5 ounces)* contains the tiniest amount of wax, and it's not enough to compete with the alcohol in here to really smooth and tame damaged ends. Any standard pomade at any price would do a better job than this to moisturize and help protect damaged ends. Of course, if your ends are that damaged, you really should cut them off— just a light trim can make an amazing difference in the hair's appearance and is well worth the added expense when compared to any hair-care product advertised as a treatment for damaged ends.

☺ **$$$ Repairing Sun Mask, for Damaged Hair** *($22 for 5.1 ounces)* is nearly identical to the OKARA Repairing Treatment Mask, for Damaged Permed Hair above, except this is slightly less emollient. Otherwise, the same basic comments apply.

☺ **$$$ Sun-Screen Nutrient Oil, Protects Against Sun, Seawater and Chlorine** *($18 for 2.2 ounces)* is an alcohol-based spray that also contains mineral oil, silicone, emollient, plant oils, sunscreens, preservative, and fragrance. This is fairly greasy, but is a good option for dry to very dry hair that is coarse or thick. The sunscreens cannot reliably protect hair from UV damage, because this is not rated with an SPF number. Moreover, no standards exist from which to figure the amount of sun protection sunscreens in hair-care products can provide.

RENE FURTERER THINNING HAIR TREATMENT FOR HAIR LOSS PREVENTION

☺ $$$ **Forticea Stimulating Shampoo** *($20 for 5.07 ounces)* is a detergent-based shampoo that contains a great deal of film-forming agent, which can make fine or thin hair feel thicker. However, those film-forming agents can quickly build up and make fine, thin hair feel heavy and limp, so this is not the best option for daily use.

☹ **RF 80** *($56 for 12 ampoules)* is sold as a special treatment to strengthen weak hair that has become thinner in appearance due to temporary hair loss. This concoction of water, slip agent, alcohols, plant oil, and water-binding agents cannot help thinning hair in the least, and is a problem to massage into the scalp because of the lemon and sage oils it contains. Consider this yet another product charade that will do nothing to restore thinning hair or stop hair loss, be it temporary or permanent.

☹ **Triphasic** *($56 for eight 0.18-ounce vials)* is another hair-loss "treatment," this one recommended for men suffering from male pattern baldness or any form of alopecia. The vials contain primarily water, alcohol, silicones, plant extract, whey, citrus oil, plant oil, coloring agent, lavender oil, preservatives, vitamins, and coloring agents. What each vial does not contain is anything that can have even a minor impact on hair loss or on encouraging hair to grow. It is a waste of time and money and is not recommended.

REVLON REALISTIC

For years, Revlon had a presence in the hair-care isles of drug and mass-market stores. Lines such as Flex, Outrageous, and ColorStay lined the shelves, offering mostly poor formulations rife with drying detergent cleansing agents, although the conditioners in each group had merit. These once-familiar hair-care products have all but vanished, and Revlon has wisely concentrated its efforts on what it does best: makeup. The Revlon Realistic line is sold in beauty supply stores and is marketed to African-American consumers. Although the line carries the familiar Revlon name, it is distributed by the Colomer Group, which purchased Revlon's Professional Products Worldwide division in 2000. The Colomer Group distributes many of the hair-care lines reviewed in this book, including American Crew, mop (Modern Organic Products) , and AFRiCAN PRIDE. For more information about Revlon Realistic, call (800) 223-2339 or visit www.thecolomergroup.com.

What's Good About This Line: Some extremely emollient, oil-rich products for very dry hair that is thick or coarse.

What's Not So Good About It: Shampoo is drying and styling products are all heavy, thick concoctions that leave hair looking and feeling greasy even when used sparingly— not good news from a line that boasts of anti-breakage formulas to deal specifically with the problems of chemically relaxed hair.

☹ **Moisturizing Shampoo** *($4.99 for 8.45 ounces)* contains sodium lauryl sulfate as its main cleansing agent, making this shampoo drying, not moisturizing, for all hair and scalp types.

☺ **Rinse Out Conditioner, with Cholesterol** *($4.99 for 8.8 ounces)* may include "Rinse Out" on the label, but this fairly greasy conditioner is difficult to rinse thanks to the mineral and plant oil. This is a very good option for dry to very dry hair that is normal to thick or coarse, but use it sparingly or your hair will likely end up feeling coated and heavy. The cholesterol is present in a very small amount, and is just a good conditioning agent for hair, no different from many others.

☹ **Dark Gel, Strong Hold** *($4.99 for 5.3 ounces)* is a mess of a gel that is mostly water and carbomers, which are gel-like thickeners that have a tendency to flake when used in higher-than-usual concentrations, and that's exactly what happens here. This gel is not recommended.

☺ **Finisheen Oil Sheen & Conditioning Spray, Aerosol** *($4.99 for 18 ounces)* is just wax, propellant, alcohol, emollients, and fragrance. It can work as a glossing spray for dry to very dry hair that needs shine, but the wax can make hair feel coated with repeated use. Silicone sprays with added emollients are the modern (and better) interpretation of products like this, and they are readily available.

☹ **Styling Gel, Strong Hold** *($4.99 for 5.3 ounces)* is similar to the Dark Gel, Strong Hold above, only with a slightly reduced tendency to flake. It's an antiquated formula that pales in comparison to almost every other standard styling gel you can buy at the drugstore.

☺ **Hairdress Hair & Scalp** *($4.99 for 5.3 ounces)* is a thick, greasy pomade that can smooth very dry, thick hair that is also frizzy, but even a tiny amount of this can leave hair looking overly slick and greased-up. This cannot restore the hair, but it will moisturize dry hair. Massaged into the scalp, it can clog the hair follicle and possibly stunt hair growth while preventing the dead skin cells on the scalp from being shed.

☺ **Hair Repair** *($4.99 for 8.8 ounces)* is a very standard conditioner that cannot repair one hair, but it is a decent option for normal to slightly dry hair of any thickness.

☺ **Moisturizing Hairdress, for Dry Hair & Scalp** *($4.99 for 5.3 ounces)* has a lighter texture than the Hairdress Hair & Scalp above, but is still incredibly greasy and slick. The Vaseline, mineral oil, silicone, and vegetable oil can all benefit very dry, thick, or coarse hair, but at the expense of making it look slick and greased-up, which may not be the look you're after. There are numerous more modern pomades and cream hairdressings available.

☺ **Oil Moisturizing Lotion** *($4.99 for 8.45 ounces)* is a very good conditioner for extremely dry hair that is normal to coarse or thick. The small amounts of oils will not make hair feel greasy, but this is still heavy-duty lotion, and would likely be best alternated with a lighter conditioner unless hair is unbearably dry.

ROGAINE

Minoxidil, the active ingredient in Rogaine, is still the only topical treatment for hair loss that has received FDA approval for that claim, and there is a plethora of independent research showing it is effective for regrowing hair, particularly for women. In-depth information regarding the science and statistics behind minoxidil is presented in Chapter Two, "To the Root of the Matter." For more information about Rogaine, call (800) 764-2463 or visit www.rogainedirect.com.

What's Good About This Line: Rogaine is available over-the-counter and is a viable option for treating male or female pattern baldness (androgenetic alopecia).

What's Not So Good About It: Rogaine does not work for everyone, and when it does work the results are not always spectacular. However, most users do notice some improvement in hair thinning and loss, provided they continue to use the treatment daily. To maintain results, Rogaine requires a lifetime commitment. If you stop using it, any new hair growth will soon be lost, and areas that were thinning will revert to the way they were before treatment with minoxidil began.

☺ $$$ **Men's Hair Regrowth Treatment, Extra Strength** *($29.99 for 2 ounces)* debuted in 1993 and contains 5% minoxidil in a base of 30% alcohol and 50% propylene glycol (which helps improve penetration of the active ingredient); the rest is water. It is certainly worth trying if your hair is thinning, although this combination of ingredients can cause scalp dryness and itching. Do keep in mind that Pfizer, the makers of Rogaine, does not hold a patent on minoxidil, and thus it is available for use by other companies. You can find store-brand "generic" versions with 5% minoxidil for half the price of Rogaine. Also note that, for men, Rogaine works best on hair loss at the crown area rather than thinning that begins at the temples and moves back.

☺ $$$ **Men's Hair Regrowth Treatment, Regular Strength** *($24.95 for 2 ounces)* is similar to the Men's Hair Regrowth Treatment, Extra Strength, above, except this contains 2% minoxidil, which is a good place to start to see if Rogaine will work for you. This also contains less alcohol than the Extra Strength version, which can make this slightly less irritating to the scalp.

☺ $$$ **Women's Hair Regrowth Treatment** *($24.95 for 2 ounces)* is identical to the Men's Hair Regrowth Treatment, Regular Strength above, and the same comments apply. Women who are pregnant or breast-feeding should not use Rogaine. As of this writing, the FDA has not approved products with 5% minoxidil for use by women. However, some dermatologists do prescribe a 5% concentration for female patients suffering from profuse hair loss or thinning, which can be an unwelcome side effect of menopause. One of the reasons stronger versions of minoxidil are not marketed (over-the-counter) to women is that, in studies, women who have used 5% concentrations noticed hair growth in areas they had not anticipated (nor desired), including the forehead, cheeks, upper lip, arms, and legs. Such side effects were reported far less frequently with 2% minoxidil preparations, so please don't let this dissuade you from considering Rogaine if you have thinning hair.

RUSK

For more information about salon-sold Rusk, owned by the Conair Corporation, call (800) 829-RUSK or visit www.rusk1.com.

What's Good About This Line: The selection of styling creams and balms is one of the most diverse, with options for every hair type except fine or thin (who shouldn't be using such products except sparingly anyway); some great light-hold hairsprays are present, as well as conditioners for normal to dry hair of any thickness.

What's Not So Good About It: A few of the shampoos contain drying detergent cleansing agents or other scalp irritants including the preservatives methylchloroisothiazolinone and methylisothiazolinone (Kathon CG); the color-protecting products are mostly disappointing.

RUSK BEING

☺ **Being Fresh Shampoo** *($11.90 for 13.5 ounces)* isn't any fresher than most shampoos, but it is a very good, mild conditioning shampoo for normal to slightly dry hair of any thickness. This does pose a slight risk of buildup.

☺ **Being Defensive Conditioner** *($11.90 for 13.5 ounces)* is an excellent, though standard, conditioner for normal to dry hair of any thickness.

☺ **Being Fierce Wax** *($11.90 for 1.8 ounces)* is a very thick, greasy pomade that contains primarily Vaseline and wax, along with a film-forming agent to help shape hair. It can add shine and texture to hair, but at the expense of feeling heavy. It is best for thick, coarse hair that is very dry, or used on very short hairstyles to exaggerate texture. This is difficult to shampoo out.

☺ **Being Flexible Hairspray** *($11.99 for 10.6 ounces)* is a standard aerosol hairspray with a very fine mist that provides a soft, flexible hold that can be brushed through with ease. It is a good finishing product when just a bit more hold is needed, either all over or in specific sections.

☺ **Being Gutsy Thickener** *($11.90 for 5.3 ounces)* is a thick-textured, but lightweight, styling cream that provides a light hold and a smooth finish that can tame minor frizzies and flyaway strands. It is minimally sticky and is a good choice to make normal to fine hair that is dry feel thicker. Don't let the initially creamy texture dissuade you—once dry, this is not an overly heavy product.

☺ $$$ **Being Primitive Clay** *($17 for 4.4 ounces)* doesn't contain any clay, and that's good, because it can be drying for hair. Rather, this is a standard, water- and beeswax-based pomade with additional thickeners and emollients that would be beneficial for dry to very dry hair that is thick or coarse. This feels heavy but does not look greasy. Instead, it has a soft matte finish and is minimally sticky. It works best used sparingly on dry (not damp) hair.

☺ $$$ **Being Rubber Gum** *($17 for 4.4 ounces)* is a standard, water-soluble pomade that, thankfully, is neither rubbery nor gummy. It does contain film-forming/holding agents to help shape and mold hair, but the mineral oil keeps it from getting stiff or sticky. This would be best for use on the ends of dry hair or for enhancing curls or waves in thick, coarse hair. It is relatively easy to shampoo out.

☹ **Being Shocked Adhesive** *($17 for 4.4 ounces)* is a cross between the Being Primitive Clay and Being Rubber Gum above, but it tends to ball up and flake on hair, not to mention being difficult to distribute evenly. This one needs to go back to the drawing board.

☺ **Being Slick Pomade** *($11.90 for 1.8 ounces)* is a lighter version of the Being Rubber Gum above. It omits the mineral oil, but the thickeners it contains can still make fine, thin hair feel greasy and limp. This is a very good smoothing, glossing pomade for normal to slightly thick hair that is normal to slightly dry. It is water soluble and shampoos out easily.

☺ **Being Smooth Creme** *($11.90 for 5.3 ounces)* is an emollient, oil-rich styling cream that is an excellent option for dry to very dry hair that is coarse, thick, or curly. It can add moisture, shine, and smoothness without feeling heavy, as long as it is used sparingly.

☺ **Being Strong Gel** *($11.90 for 5.3 ounces)* is a standard, water- and alcohol-based styling gel with a firm hold and a stiff, sticky finish. This can be brushed through, but is best for creating all manner of wet-look hairstyles or for spiking short hair.

☺ **Being Wild Paste** *($11.90 for 5.3 ounces)* is a creamy, thick styling balm that is a good option for thick, coarse hair that is stubborn and needs smoothing with hold. For some reason, this product has a much stronger, more masculine fragrance than all of the Rusk Being products above. The balm can be distributed throughout coarse or thick hair, but is best for just the ends of normal hair.

RUSK DEEPSHINE

☺ **$$$ Deepshine Sea Kelp Creme Shampoo** *($13 for 16 ounces)* is similar to the Being Fresh Shampoo above, and the same review applies. The sea kelp is not what makes hair shiny (that's what the silicone conditioning agent is for), but it can have water-binding properties for hair.

☺ **$$$ Deepshine Sea Kelp Conditioner** *($13 for 16 ounces)* is a very standard, but good, conditioner that can work well for normal to dry hair of any thickness.

☺ **$$$ Deepshine Sea Kelp Hold & Shine Hairspray** *($13 for 8 ounces)* is a nonaerosol hairspray with a heavier-than-normal application. It has a medium to firm hold and can leave hair feeling slightly stiff and sticky. This is not a breeze to brush through, but can work well to keep coarse, wiry hair in place.

☺ **Deepshine Sea Kelp Liquid Gel** *($10.99 for 16.2 ounces)* is a standard styling gel with a light to medium hold and minimal to no stiff or sticky feel.

☺ **Deepshine Sea Kelp Shining Gel** *($13 for 4.4 ounces)* is similar to the Sea Kelp Liquid Gel above except with more silicone, so it does add more shine.

☺ **$$$ Deepshine Anti-Frizz Serum** *($15 for 4.4 ounces)* is a standard silicone serum that contains an emollient for additional conditioning. It works as well as any to add shine and a silky feel to dry or very dry hair.

☺ $$$ **Deepshine Marine Nutrient Treatment** *($13 for 6 ounces)* contains more mica (a shiny, crystalline mineral pigment) than marine nutrients. This ends up being a very standard conditioner that is an OK option for normal to dry hair of any thickness, but is definitely not preferred to the Deepshine Sea Kelp Conditioner above.

☹ **Deepshine Phyto-Marine Lusterizer** *($13 for 4.4 ounces)* is a water- and silicone-based leave-in conditioning cream that contains the preservative Kathon CG, and as such is not recommended.

☺ $$$ **Deepshine Sea Kelp Shine Spray** *($15 for 8 ounces)* is a very good, alcohol-free silicone spray for dry hair that is normal to slightly thick or coarse. The combination of silicone and emollients produces a smooth, shiny finish while also moisturizing hair. The container size of this nonaqueous product makes it a bargain compared to many other silicone sprays. It does contain fragrance.

RUSK DESIGN SERIES

☺ **Design Series Blofoam, Root Lifter** *($11 for 10 ounces)* is a propellant-based mousse with a fine-point nozzle so you can apply it directly to the roots. This application method makes it all too easy to dispense more product in one area than you intended. It is best to dispense the foam into your hands, then apply it to the roots. This has a medium hold that is slightly stiff and sticky, but can be brushed through.

☺ **Design Series Cre8, Styling Creme** *($9.90 for 4 ounces)* is nearly identical to the Being Smooth Creme above, and the same review applies.

☹ **Design Series Jele Gloss, Bodifying Lotion** *($10 for 12 ounces)* contains the preservative Kathon CG, and is not recommended.

☺ **Design Series Jel FX, Forming Jel** *($7 for 5 ounces)* is a standard, lightweight styling gel that offers a light, flexible hold that is easy to brush through and leaves hair soft rather than sticky. It is a good option for all hair types.

☺ **Design Series Mousse, Volumizing Foam** *($11 for 8 ounces)* is a very standard, propellant-based mousse with a light hold and a minimal stiff, sticky feel. It is easy to brush through and works well to build volume in fine or thin hair when used with a blow dryer.

☺ **Design Series Radical Creme, Thickening/Texturizing Creme** *($10.95 for 4 ounces)* is nearly identical to the Being Gutsy Thickener above, except this has a slightly thinner texture. Otherwise, the same review applies.

☺ **Design Series Radical Sheen, Texturizing Polishing Gel** *($13.96 for 3 ounces)* is a standard gel that has light to medium hold with minimal to no stiff or sticky feel.

☺ **Design Series Worx, Working/Finishing Spray (Aerosol)** *($11 for 10 ounces)* is a standard, firm-hold hairspray that leaves hair feeling slightly stiff and sticky, though it can be brushed through.

☺ **Design Series Worx Atomizer, Fixing/Finishing Spray** *($11 for 10 ounces)* is nearly identical to the Design Series Worx, Working/Finishing Spray (Aerosol) above, except that this formula does not contain propellants and has a heavier application, which provides slightly more hold.

☺ **Design Series Sheer Brilliance, Polisher** *($13 for 4 ounces)* is a fluid silicone serum that can add a silky feel and glossy shine to hair, though it should be used sparingly to avoid a greasy look.

RUSK INTERNAL RESTRUCTURE

☹ **Internal Restructure Thickr, Thickening Shampoo** *($8 for 8.5 ounces)* contains sodium lauryl sulfate as its main detergent cleansing agent, which makes this too drying for all hair and scalp types.

☺ **Internal Restructure Thickr, Thickening Conditioner** *($8 for 8.5 ounces)* is similar to the Being Defensive Conditioner above, except this is a less interesting formula with more fragrance than water-binding agents. It can work for normal to dry hair, but won't make fine or thin hair feel thicker.

☺ **Internal Restructure Str8, Anti-Frizz/Anti-Curl Lotion** *($9.90 for 6 ounces)* is a very good conditioning styling lotion that can work well to smooth and straighten hair when used with heat and the proper styling brush. The film-forming/holding agent provides a flexible, minimally sticky hold, while the plant oil and silicones add shine and help prevent and control frizzies.

☹ **Internal Restructure Thick, Body & Texture Amplifier** *($9.90 for 6 ounces)* contains the preservative Kathon CG, and is not recommended.

☺ **Internal Restructure Thickr, Thickening Hair Spray** *($12 for 10.6 ounces)* is a standard aerosol hairspray whose film-forming/holding agents can make fine or thin hair feel thicker by virtue of their coating the hair shaft. Any hairspray can do this, but if you're looking for a light-hold, minimally stiff and sticky option, this is a good one.

☺ **Internal Restructure Thickr, Thickening Mousse** *($10.95 for 8.8 ounces)* is a standard, propellant-based mousse that provides medium hold but is slightly sticky. It can still be brushed through and can indeed make fine or thin hair feel thicker, but that benefit is not unique to this product.

☺ **Internal Restructure Thickr, Thickening Spray** *($7.50 for 4.2 ounces)* can't thicken hair, but it is a lightweight styling spray that has a light hold and does help fine or thin hair feel thicker.

☺ **Internal Restructure W8less, Shaping & Control Myst (Aerosol)** *($12.95 for 10 ounces)* is a very light hairspray that provides little to no hold and is neither stiff nor sticky. The lack of hold limits this product's versatility, but it's great for a soft finish on casual hairstyles.

☺ **Internal Restructure W8less, Shaping & Control Myst (Non-Aerosol)** *($11 for 10 ounces)* offers more hold than the Internal Restructure W8less, Shaping & Control Myst (Aerosol) above, and acquits itself nicely as a workable nonaerosol hairspray that can be easily brushed through.

☺ **Internal Restructure W8less Plus, Shaping & Control Myst** *($9.95 for 10 ounces)* is nearly identical to the Internal Restructure W8less, Shaping & Control Myst (Aerosol) above, but has a tangible hold that remains soft and flexible, which makes this a great working hairspray for all hair types.

☺ **Internal Restructure Wired, Multiple Personality Styling Cream** *($11 for 6 ounces)* is a very good water- and wax-based styling cream that provides a soft, groomed hold while keeping hair pliable and adding shine. It works well for thick, coarse, or curly hair that needs smoothing with support, and it can nicely tame frizzies and smooth dry ends. Those with normal hair can use this sparingly to smooth hair or add soft texture. The wax can make it difficult to shampoo out, and it will build up on hair with repeated use.

☺ **Internal Restructure Shine, Shine Spray** *($12 for 4.4 ounces)* is a standard aerosol silicone spray that goes on lighter than most and, as such, is a great shine-enhancing option for all hair types. Those with fine or thin hair should apply this sparingly.

☺ **Internal Restructure Shining, Sheen & Movement Myst** *($11 for 4 ounces)* is the nonaerosol counterpart to the Internal Structure Shine, Shine Spray above. It has a heavier application that can still be used by all hair types, though it can become greasy on fine or thin hair if not applied sparingly.

RUSK SENSORIES

☹ **Sensories Bright Chamomile & Lavender Color Brightening Shampoo** *($9.90 for 13 ounces)* contains TEA-lauryl sulfate as its main detergent cleansing agent, and that can be drying for hair while also being drying and irritating for the scalp. This also contains sulfated castor oil, which can strip (not brighten) hair color.

☹ **Sensories Brilliance Grapefruit & Honey Color Protect Shampoo** *($8 for 13.5 ounces)* contains sodium lauryl sulfate as its main detergent cleansing agent, and is not recommended for any hair or scalp type. The high amount of grapefruit can provoke further scalp irritation.

☹ **Sensories Calm Guarana & Ginger Nourishing Shampoo** *($8 for 13 ounces)* contains TEA-lauryl sulfate as one of its main detergent cleansing agents, and is not recommended for any hair or scalp type.

☺ **Sensories Clarify Rosemary & Quillaja Clarifying Detoxifying Shampoo** *($8 for 13.5 ounces)* does not contain any chelating agents, which are what is needed in a clarifying shampoo to remove the mineral deposits from hard water or the chlorine buildup from swimming pools. This is a standard shampoo whose conditioning agents pose no risk of buildup, but the TEA-lauryl sulfate (which is not present in a high amount) can still be drying for all but oily hair and scalp.

☺ **Sensories Full Green Tea & Alfalfa Shampoo** *($8.99 for 13 ounces)* is a very standard, but good, shampoo for all hair types and will not cause buildup.

☹ **Sensories Purify Cucurbita & Tea Tree Oil Deep Cleansing Shampoo** *($9.90 for 13 ounces)* is a standard shampoo marred by the inclusion of peppermint oil, which makes it too irritating for all scalp types.

☺ **Sensories Smoother Passionflower & Aloe Shampoo** *($8 for 13 ounces)* is, save for a change in fragrance and plant extracts that won't affect the hair, identical to the Sensories Full Green Tea & Alfalfa Shampoo above, and the same review applies.

☺ **Sensories Smoother Passionflower & Aloe Leave-In Texturizing Conditioner** *($9 for 8.5 ounces)* is a very good leave-in smoothing conditioner for all hair types except very fine or thin.

☺ **Sensories Brilliance Grapefruit & Honey Leave-In Color Protector** *($9 for 8 ounces)* is an excellent lightweight leave-in conditioner for normal to slightly dry hair that is normal to fine or thin.

☹ **Sensories Calm Detangler, Guarana & Ginger Leave-In Detangler** *($10 for 8.5 ounces)* contains the preservative Kathon CG, and is not recommended.

☺ **Sensories Calm Guarana & Ginger 60 Second Hair Revive** *($9 for 13 ounces)* is similar to the Being Defensive Conditioner above, and the same comments apply. This option ends up costing less per ounce, but its claim to revive hair in 60 seconds is a bit far-fetched. If all it took to revive hair was to use this product for one minute, why would you need to use it again?

☺ **Sensories Calm Guarana & Ginger Reconstructor** *($9.90 for 5.3 ounces)* is a standard, but good, conditioner for normal to dry hair of any thickness. If this can reconstruct hair (which it cannot) then every other Rusk conditioner should make the same claim because they contain similar, if not identical, ingredients.

☹ **Sensories Cure Vitamins & Protein Strengthening Treatment** *($9 for 8.5 ounces)* is a leave-in, spray-on detangling conditioner that contains the preservative Kathon CG, and is not recommended.

☹ **Sensories Invisible Hibiscus & Kukui Foaming Detangler** *($9 for 13 ounces)* is a leave-in conditioner that is a problem for the scalp because it contains the sensitizing preservative Kathon CG.

☺ **Sensories Moist Sunflower & Apricot Extract Moisturizing Creme Treatment** *($9 for 5.3 ounces)* is a standard conditioner that works well for normal to dry hair of any thickness.

Salon Grafix

For more information about Salon Grafix, call (248) 642-3041 or visit www.salon grafix.com.

What's Good About This Line: The prices—at any price, these are some of the best products in this book for cleansing, conditioning, and styling for those on a budget (or even those who are not, actually)! It is one of the few hair-care lines in this book to receive across-the-board smiling face ratings for every product.

What's Not So Good About It: My only nitpick is that a few of the styling products are copies of Paul Mitchell styling products, right down to the coconut fragrance and use of Mitchell's trademark ingredient, awapuhi extract. Imitation may be the sincerest form of flattery, but you shouldn't ride on the coattails of another company's successful marketing angle or product development (though Salon Grafix is hardly the only company to do this).

☺ **Moisture Balancing & Hydrating Shampoo** *($4.99 for 16 ounces)* is a very good shampoo for normal to dry hair that is normal to fine or thin. It can cause buildup with repeated use.

☺ **Shampoo for Color Treated Hair** *($4.99 for 16 ounces)* is nearly identical to the Moisture Balancing & Hydrating Shampoo above, except this contains fewer conditioning agents and poses minimal to no risk of buildup, which makes it a great option for all hair types, including color-treated hair.

☺ **Thickening & Volumizing Shampoo** *($4.99 for 16 ounces)* is nearly identical to the Moisture Balancing & Hydrating Shampoo above, except it does not contain film-forming agents so it won't have a thickening effect on hair. Otherwise, the same comments apply.

☺ **Daily Balancing Conditioner** *($4.99 for 16 ounces)* is a great conditioner for normal to dry hair of any thickness, though it won't balance anything.

☺ **Extra-Hold Sculpting Mousse** *($5.99 for 8 ounces)* is a standard, propellant-based mousse with a light to medium hold and a soft, minimally sticky finish. The conditioning agents and plant oil in it make it ideal for drier hair that is normal to fine and thin or curly.

☺ **Freezing Hair Spray, The Ultimate Mega Hold Styling Mist** *($5.99 for 10 ounces)* bills itself as "the absolute ultimate in hold and shine," but although it does offer some shine, the hold factor is medium at best, and just slightly stiff and sticky. It is easy to brush through, but doesn't distinguish itself as the "ultimate."

☺ **Freezing Hair Spray, The Ultimate Mega Hold Styling Mist, Unscented** *($5.99 for 10 ounces)* is identical to the Freezing Hair Spray above, and despite the name it does contain fragrance, though it is subtle. Otherwise, the same review applies.

☺ **Hair Pomade Styling Creme for Super Hold** *($5.99 for 8 ounces)* is a gel-type pomade with a slightly fluid texture, which does make it easier to work with than many of the thicker, paste-like pomades. This can work well to smooth and add moisture and definition to curly hair that is thick or coarse, but all hair types can use it sparingly to smooth dry ends and help control frizzies.

☺ **Mega-Hold Sculpting Mousse** *($5.99 for 8 ounces)* is nearly identical to the Extra-Hold Sculpting Mousse above, only this option has more hold and a stickier feel, but still with minimal stiffness. Otherwise, the same comments apply.

☺ **Micro-Fiber Extra Super Hold Hair Styling Gel** *($5.99 for 8 ounces)* really does offer extra-super hold, but not without the trade-off of considerable stickiness and a coated, thick feeling on hair. It is a great gel for managing and conditioning stubborn curls and waves, and is easily brushed through. This would also be excellent for use on short, textured styles that have not responded well (hold- and lift-wise) to other gels or styling sprays. It can be slightly heavy for fine or thin hair, so if that describes your hair, use this sparingly.

☺ **Non-Aerosol Freezing Hair Spray, The Ultimate Mega Hold Styling Mist** *($5.99 for 8 ounces)* works well for those who need a nonaerosol, firm-hold hairspray that can get stiff but is minimally sticky. It works best to freeze hair in place, or give long-lasting lift to roots.

☺ **Non-Aerosol Shaping Hair Spray, Extra Super Hold Styling Mist** *($5.99 for 8 ounces)* is identical to the Non-Aerosol Freezing Hair Spray above, and the same review applies.

☺ **Shaping Hair Spray, Extra Super Hold Styling Mist** *($5.99 for 10 ounces)* is a standard aerosol hairspray with a fine, almost weightless mist that can work well for a medium-hold finishing touch on fine or thin hair. It is minimally stiff, but stickier than the Salon Grafix aerosol and nonaerosol hairsprays above, though hair can be brushed through.

☺ **Shaping Hair Spray, Unscented** *($5.99 for 10 ounces)* is nearly identical to the Shaping Hair Spray, Extra Super Hold Styling Mist above, except this leaves hair feeling slightly more sticky, but only slightly. Despite the "unscented" in the name, this does contain a masking fragrance, although it's almost undetectable.

☺ **Shaping Hair Spray, Super Hold Styling Mist** *($5.99 for 10 ounces)* is nearly identical to the Shaping Hair Spray, Extra Super Hold Styling Mist above, except *this* is the option that is fragrance-free, which is good news for someone with a sensitive, itchy scalp. The film-forming/holding agents can still be a potential problem for a sensitive scalp, but there is no question that taking fragrance out of the equation helps.

☺ **Spiking & Freezing Styling Gel** *($5.99 for 8 ounces)* is only for those whose hairstyle demands an ultra-strong, cement-like hold. This is one strong gel that can achieve almost any extreme, gravity-defying look you care to try. The downside for all that hold is persistent stickiness—you will not be able to brush through your hair, but you'll get plenty of playtime to shape and mold hair into place before it dries.

SALON SELECTIVES

Over the years, Salon Selectives has had more revamping and repackaging than Madonna. Meanwhile, all this tinkering (mostly in the packaging department) still hasn't convinced me that this is a worthwhile line to consider over others. Although this line has an enticing name, that's about its only unique, interesting aspect. However, the line is not marketed to salons—it is a drugstore line that wants you to believe it is related to more pricey formulations. Despite its most recent visual and formulary tweakings, Salon Selectives still has a long way to go if it wishes to compete with more together and elegant lines such as, well, just about everyone else! For more information about Salon Selectives, owned by Unilever, call (866) 266-5367 or visit www.salonselectives.com.

What's Good About This Line: A few of the styling products feature fine formulations at fair prices.

What's Not So Good About It: The shampoos are repetitive formulations that are a notch below other options available at drugstores and salons; the conditioners are uninspired and also are repetitive formulas.

☺ **Clean Slate, Clarifying Shampoo** *($3.69 for 13 ounces)* is as standard as a shampoo gets, and this is an OK option for all hair types and won't cause buildup. However, the presence of a small amount of TEA-dodecylbenzenesulfonate is a potential problem for causing dry hair and scalp, and prevents this shampoo from getting a higher rating. By the way, it may look impressive to see vitamins listed so close to the beginning of the ingredient list, but they cannot affect hair or scalp, especially because in a shampoo they are just rinsed down the drain.

☺ **Completely Drenched, Moisturizing Shampoo** *($3.69 for 13 ounces)* is nearly identical to the Clean Slate, Clarifying Shampoo above, and is completely misnamed. This is an OK option for all hair types, but will likely leave those with dry hair wanting more.

☺ **Don't Fade On Me, Color Protecting Shampoo** *($3.69 for 13 ounces)* is nearly identical to the Clean Slate, Clarifying Shampoo above, and the same review applies. The TEA-dodecylbenzenesulfonate isn't what you want to see in a shampoo that purports to prevent hair-color fading (and even if it were a better formulation it couldn't do that).

☺ **Full of It, Bodifying Shampoo** *($3.69 for 13 ounces)* is nearly identical to the Clean Slate, Clarifying Shampoo above, and the same review applies.

☺ **Perfectly Normal, Balancing Shampoo** *($3.69 for 13 ounces)* is nearly identical to the Clean Slate, Clarifying Shampoo above, and the same review applies.

☺ **Completely Drenched, Moisturizing Conditioner** *($3.69 for 13 ounces)* is a boring, ultra-basic conditioner that is primarily water and cetearyl alcohol (a common thickening agent/emollient), along with several vitamins (which cannot nourish hair), plant extracts, fragrance, and preservatives. It's an OK option for normal to slightly dry hair, but the lack of detangling agents or other intriguing ingredients that would benefit hair doesn't make this worth considering strongly.

☺ **Don't Fade On Me, Color Protecting Conditioner** *($3.69 for 13 ounces)* is nearly identical to the Completely Drenched, Moisturizing Conditioner above, and the same review applies. There are much better conditioners available for color-treated (meaning damaged) hair.

☹ **Full of It Conditioner** *($3.79 for 13 ounces)* is similar to the Completely Drenched, Moisturizing Conditioner above, except this includes an appreciable amount of lemon and orange oils, which impart a fresh citrus fragrance but can be potent scalp irritants.

☺ **Perfectly Normal Balancing Conditioner** *($3.79 for 13 ounces)* is nearly identical to the Completely Drenched, Moisturizing Conditioner above, and the same review applies.

☺ **Control(d) Substance, Molding Putty for Short/Thick Hair** *($3.69 for 2.25 ounces)* is a styling gel/pomade hybrid that is more gooey than putty-like, and it can work well on wet or dry hair to create pliable shape and definition with a slight amount of stickiness but no stiffness. It is light enough for all hair types, but those with fine or thin hair should apply this sparingly and only to smooth out dry ends, and, as the name states, this also works well to add texture to short hair.

The Reviews S

☺ **Feel n' Control, Smoothing Gel for Flexible Control** *($3.69 for 13 ounces)* is a standard, alcohol-free gel without the usual holding/film-forming agents. It provides a light hold without stiffness and is minimally sticky, so hair is easy to brush through. This gel is best for creating softly defined curls or for smoothing and lightly shaping fine or thin hair.

☺ **Fully Pumped, Volume and Shine Styling Foam** *($3.69 for 7 ounces)* is a liquid-to-foam mousse with a light to medium hold that's slightly sticky but not stiff.

☺ **Get in Shape, Shaping Mousse for Thick/Curly/Wavy Hair** *($3.79 for 7 ounces)* is a standard, propellant-based mousse with medium hold and a slightly stiff, sticky feel, though hair is easily brushed through.

☺ **Hold Tight, Finishing Spray for Firm Hold (Aerosol)** *($3.99 for 7 ounces)* is a very standard hairspray with medium hold and a slightly stiff, sticky finish that is somewhat difficult to brush through due to the lack of silicone and conditioning agents.

☺ **Hold Tight, Finishing Spray for Firm Hold (Non-Aerosol)** *($3.79 for 8 ounces)* is a light- to medium-hold standard hairspray that feels quite light in hair and is minimally stiff or sticky. The tiny amount of silicone helps add a touch of shine and makes hair easier to comb through.

☺ **Hold Tight, Style Freeze Maximum Hold Finishing Spray (Aerosol)** *($3.79 for 7 ounces)* is almost identical to the Hold Tight, Finishing Spray for Firm Hold (Aerosol) above, except this offers slightly more hold (and resulting stickiness).

☹ **Rise Up, Volumizing Mousse for Thin/Straight Hair** *($3.69 for 7 ounces)* contains TEA-dodecylbenzenesulfonate, which serves no rational purpose in a styling product because it can be drying to the hair and it doesn't help with styling.

☺ **Sit Still, Finishing Spray for Medium Hold (Aerosol)** *($3.99 for 7 ounces)* is similar to, but has more hold than, the Hold Tight, Finishing Spray for Firm Hold (Aerosol) above, and the same basic comments apply.

☺ **Sit Still, Finishing Spray for Medium Hold (Non-Aerosol)** *($3.69 for 8.5 ounces)* is identical to the Hold Tight, Finishing Spray for Firm Hold (Non-Aerosol) above, and the same review applies.

☺ **Stay Flexible, Finishing Spray for Flexible Hold (Aerosol)** *($3.99 for 7 ounces)* is identical to the Hold Tight, Finishing Spray for Firm Hold (Aerosol) above, and the same review applies.

☺ **Stay Flexible, Finishing Spray for Flexible Hold (Non-Aerosol)** *($3.69 for 8.5 ounces)* is identical to the Hold Tight, Finishing Spray for Firm Hold (Non-Aerosol) above, and the same review applies.

☺ **Under Firm Control, Firm Hold Sculpting Gel** *($3.69 for 13 ounces)* is a relatively standard, light-hold styling gel that takes longer than usual to dry, but is minimally stiff or sticky. It is a good, basic option for all hair types whose hairstyle needs minimal control with slight smoothing and shine.

☹ **Air It Out, Odor Neutralizer for Hair** *($3.69 for 4 ounces)* is nothing more than cheap eau de cologne. This is just alcohol with water, fragrance, and coloring agents, and that doesn't neutralize odors, it just covers them up with a perfume-y scent. All of the Salon Selectives styling products reviewed above have rather potent scents, so adding this to the mix wasn't necessary, nor is it a must-have for you.

☺ **Lighten Up, Subtle Highlighting Foam Blonde** *($5.99 for 4 ounces)* is a liquid-to-foam, water-based mousse that contains no holding agents. What it does have is hydrogen peroxide to lighten hair in the sun or with heat from a blow dryer. More often than not, this is a tricky endeavor, because except for those with blonde hair the level of peroxide is too low to have a true blonding effect. Using this in the sun or even by itself can be drying and damaging to hair.

SCRUPLES

Many Scruples products contain what the company refers to as PBX, which is simply a complex of water-binding agents, silicone, wheat protein, and a sunscreen agent. These ingredients are beneficial for all hair types, though the sunscreen cannot be relied on to protect hair from UV damage (the FDA does not allow SPF ratings for hair-care products because of their inability to protect hair from sun damage). The main issue is that none of the ingredients in PBX are unique to Scruples, though the good news is that, for the most part, the claims made for this complex are in line with how each ingredient actually functions on the hair. The water-binding agents don't hold up well under heat-styling and brushing conditions, but they are still worthwhile ingredients to look for while shopping for hair-care products because they do help dry hair hold onto moisture. For more information about Scruples, call (800) 457-0016 or visit www.scrupleshaircare.com.

What's Good About This Line: The conditioners and most of the styling products are worth looking into if you don't mind the prices.

What's Not So Good About It: Several of the shampoos contain drying detergent cleansing agents; a few of the styling products contain problematic ingredients such as sodium polystyrene sulfonate; the prices for many of the products are out of line with the standard or (in some cases) boring formulations.

☹ **Hair Clearifier Purifying Shampoo** *($14.95 for 16 ounces)* can clarify hair. But this comes at the expense of causing unnecessary dryness and irritation because it contains sodium C14-16 olefin sulfonate as its main detergent cleansing agent.

☹ **Moisture Bath Moisture Replenishing Shampoo** *($14.95 for 16 ounces)* contains sodium C14-16 olefin sulfonate as its main detergent cleansing agent, which makes this shampoo too drying for hair, while also being drying and irritating to the scalp.

☺ **$$$ Renewal Color Retention Shampoo** *($14.95 for 16 ounces)* is a very standard shampoo that is a good option for all hair types and poses minimal risk of buildup. This cannot help hair retain color better than any other standard shampoo.

☹ **Smooth Out, Curl Control Shampoo** *($10.95 for 8.5 ounces)* is nearly identical to the Renewal Color Retention Shampoo above, except this contains balm mint, which can be a scalp irritant and makes this shampoo not worth considering.

☻ **Structure Bath Volumizing Shampoo** *($14.95 for 16 ounces)* contains sodium C14-16 olefin sulfonate and TEA-dodecylbenzenesulfonate, which can be doubly drying and irritating for all hair and scalp types.

☺ **$$$ Quickseal Fortifying Creme Conditioner** *($16.50 for 16 ounces)* is a very basic conditioner that is a good option for normal to dry hair of any thickness.

☺ **$$$ Reconstruct Leave-In Instant Repair** *($14.95 for 8.5 ounces)* is a lightweight, water-based, spray-on conditioner that works well for normal to fine or thin hair that is slightly dry and needs help with combing. It can build up on hair with repeated use, but will make fine, thin hair feel slightly thicker.

☺ **$$$ Renewal Color Retention Conditioner** *($22.50 for 16 ounces)* is a standard, but very good, conditioner for normal to dry hair of any thickness. This won't help you retain your color any longer or better than countless other conditioners.

☻ **Smooth Out, Curl Control Conditioner** *($14.95 for 8.5 ounces)* is similar to, but not as well formulated as, the Renewal Color Retention Conditioner above, and it loses points for including several irritating plant extracts, including balm mint and lemongrass.

☺ **$$$ Creme Parfait, Ultra Thick Styling Mousse** *($15.95 for 10.6 ounces)* is a thicker-than-usual, propellant-based mousse with a medium to firm hold and a stiff, sticky feel that can be brushed through. It is overpriced for what you get, but is a good option for fine or thin hair that needs volume with control.

☺ **Effects, Super Hold Finishing Spray** *($11.95 for 10.6 ounces)* doesn't offer super hold, if Scruples is using the word "super" to mean" "strong." This is a standard, light-hold aerosol hairspray with minimal stiff or sticky feel, so hair can be easily brushed through. This does contain added emollients, which make it preferred for use on drier hair.

☺ **Emphasis, Texturizing Styling Mousse** *($11.95 for 6 ounces)* is a very standard, propellant-based mousse that has a weightless texture and provides a light hold with a soft, non-sticky finish. This is a great option for fine or thin hair that is curly or straight.

☺ **Enforce, Fast Drying Styling Spray** *($12.50 for 8.5 ounces)* does dry fast, and works well as a light- to medium-hold styling spray for use on wet or dry hair. It is minimally stiff or sticky and easy to brush through—a versatile product to have on hand for simple or complex hairstyles.

☺ **Enforce, Sculpting Glaze Concentrate** *($12.95 for 8.5 ounces)* is a very standard, but good, medium- to firm-hold styling gel. It is sticky and can leave hair stiff, but is easy to brush through. The conditioning agents provide a slight amount of protection during heat styling.

☺ **High Definition, Extra Dry Hair Spray** *($13.95 for 10.6 ounces)* is a standard, quick-drying aerosol hairspray with a medium hold and some residual stickiness but little stiffness. For the money, it's nothing special, just a good hairspray for all hair types.

☺ **More Emphasis, Extra Body Styling Mousse** *($11.95 for 6 ounces)* is similar to the Emphasis, Texturizing Styling Mousse above, only with slightly more hold. Otherwise, the same comments apply.

☺ **Renewal, Forming Gel for Color Treated Hair** *($10.95 for 5 ounces)* holds no special benefit for color-treated hair. It's just a standard, water-based styling gel with medium hold and a sticky finish that is easily brushed through. This does contain mica, which imparts shimmery shine to hair, but the amount is so subtle you may not even notice.

☺ **Rock Hard, Extra Firm Finishing Spray** *($7.65 for 8.5 ounces)* is a standard nonaerosol hairspray with a medium hold and a minimal stiff, sticky feel. This does not dry immediately, and as such is a good working spray for finishing your hairstyle. The "Protective Barrier Complex" consists of water-binding agents, but the amounts here (as even greater amounts would be) are incapable of protecting hair or forming any type of barrier.

☺ $$$ **Smooth Out, Non-Chemical Straightening Gel** *($17.95 for 8.5 ounces)* is a slick, water-based gel that has a smooth texture and can work well to help straighten curly or wavy hair. However, it lacks silicones, which provide a sleeker finish and repel humidity. For use in non-humid climates, this is an option, though you do have to tolerate a large amount of shimmer particles from the mica in this. Although these don't flake excessively, they can stick to the scalp and to your brush.

☺ **Tea Tree, Sculpting Glaze Concentrate** *($12.95 for 8.5 ounces)* is nearly identical to the Enforce, Sculpting Glaze Concentrate above, except for the addition of tea tree oil and two other plant extracts that have no effect on hair but do impart fragrance. Otherwise, the same review applies.

☹ **Total Accents, Light Finishing Creme** *($15.95 for 4.2 ounces)* contains sodium polystyrene sulfonate, which can be drying for hair and scalp and possibly strip hair color with repeated use.

☹ **Total Accents, Precision Creme** *($15.95 for 5 ounces)* contains sodium polystyrene sulfonate, which can be drying for hair and scalp and possibly strip hair color with repeated use.

☺ $$$ **V² Double Volume for Hair** *($15.95 for 8.5 ounces)* is a standard alcohol- and water-based spray gel that offers a medium to firm hold that remains sticky, though this can be a good product to use on stubborn hair and it can make fine or thin hair feel thicker. It isn't easy to brush through, but excels for wet looks or finger-styled hair you allow to air dry.

☺ $$$ **ER Emergency Repair, for Damaged Hair** *($15.95 for 6 ounces)* has a thicker texture than other Scruples conditioners, but that doesn't mean this is what's needed for damaged hair. It's actually a rather standard, ho-hum conditioner.

☺ $$$ **Moisturex, Intensive Moisturizing Treatment** *($22.50 for 16 ounces)* is nearly identical to the ER Emergency Repair product above, and the exact same comments apply.

☺ $$$ **Renewal, Hair Therapy Polish** *($28.95 for 4.2 ounces)* is a standard, tremendously overpriced silicone serum that can work as well as any to smooth hair, add amazing shine, and tame frizzies. Citré Shine, Charles Worthington, L'Oreal, and Jheri Redding all have excellent and much less expensive options.

☺ **Spray Lites, Extreme Shine** *($12.95 for 4.2 ounces)* is an emollient spray for hair with added silicone for shine and a silky feel. This is great for dry hair that is normal to coarse, curly, or thick. This does contain mica, which imparts shimmer particles that tend to flake onto clothing.

SCRUPLES O_2 ORIGINALS

All but one of the products below contain "oxygen-energized water," which Scruples claims can become "hair's healthy solution" because oxygen-infused hair-care products are more effective and deeper penetrating than those without it. So that must mean that all of the Scruples products above, none of which contain this special water, aren't as good as the O_2 Originals products. Scruples doesn't explain this mystery, nor how their water is energized, but the whole claim is ludicrous because oxygen is already a major component of water, and energizing it (assuming the process keeps oxygen stable, which I strongly doubt) would theoretically just increase oxidative damage to hair, which would translate to color fading. That's probably not what you had in mind for your hair, but it's no cause for concern with these products because the claim is bogus.

☺ $$$ **O_2 Originals Hydrating Wash** *($12.95 for 12 ounces)* is a standard shampoo that is a good option for normal to slightly dry hair of any thickness. Nothing in it can penetrate to the hair's innermost structure, as claimed.

☺ $$$ **O_2 Originals Texturizing Wash** *($12.95 for 12 ounces)* is nearly identical to the Renewal Color Retention Shampoo above, and the same review applies. The oxygen-energized water has no special benefit for hair. After all, if the concept really worked, it would actually be detrimental.

☺ $$$ **O_2 Originals Hydrating Conditioner** *($16.95 for 8.5 ounces)* is similar to the ER Emergency Repair, for Damaged Hair above, and the same basic comments apply.

☺ $$$ **O_2 Originals Texturizing Conditioner** *($15.95 for 8.5 ounces)* is a basic and boring conditioner for normal to slightly dry hair that is fine or thin, but the price and silly oxygen marketing angle mean this is just not worth it.

☺ $$$ **O_2 Originals Designing Spray** *($15.95 for 8 ounces)* is nearly identical to the High Definition, Extra Dry Hair Spray above, and the same review applies.

☺ $$$ **O_2 Originals Direct Volume Spray Foam** *($15.95 for 10 ounces)* is a propellant-based, spray-on mousse with a light hold and a minimal stiff, sticky feel that is easily brushed through. Applied to the roots, it works well to add lift and volume without a trace of heaviness.

☺ $$$ **O_2 Originals Texturizing Gel** *($15.95 for 8.5 ounces)* is nearly identical to the Enforce, Sculpting Glaze Concentrate above, and the same review applies.

☺ **O_2 Originals Texturizing Styling Spray** *($12.95 for 8.5 ounces)* is more a hairspray than a styling spray, as the alcohol-based, fast-drying formula bears out. It provides a light hold with a minimally stiff, sticky feeling, and hair is easily brushed through.

☺ **O_2 Originals Soothing Polish** *($13.95 for 3.4 ounces)* is a water-based silicone lotion that doesn't contain much else that's especially advantageous for hair. It can smooth frizzies and add shine without significant weight, but those with fine, thin hair should use it sparingly.

SCRUPLES URBAN POTIONS

☺ **Urban Potions Cut & Style Foam** *($12.95 for 8.3 ounces)* is a propellant-based, medium-hold mousse that contains enough conditioning agent to leave hair feeling smooth and slightly moist, if a bit sticky. This is easy to brush through and is a great option for curly or wavy hair that is normal to fine or thin.

☺ **Urban Potions Snafu Styling Stick** *($14.95 for 3 ounces)* is primarily castor oil and several waxes, along with fragrance and fragrant plant extracts. It is an emollient, solid stick that can smooth stubborn curls, frizzies, or dry ends, but it should be used sparingly or hair can feel heavy and coated. This does not shampoo out easily. If you are interested in trying this type of product, L.A. LOOKS has a great option for far less money.

☹ **Urban Potions Texturizing Paste** *($14.95 for 3.5 ounces)* is a thick, stringy styling balm that is very messy to use and leaves hair feeling slick and sticky, not to mention heavy, even when used sparingly. This may work for thick, coarse hair that is unmanageable, but to use it requires patience and a willingness to tolerate your hair feeling goopy.

☹ **Urban Potions Texturizing Pomade** *($11.95 for 1.76 ounces)* is a standard, water-soluble, gel-like pomade that is a good option for all hair types except very fine or thin. As with all pomades of this ilk, it provides light smoothing and frizz control with a glossy, wet-look shine. Use it sparingly to avoid a greasy appearance.

☺ **Urban Potions Thermal Styling Spray** *($11.95 for 8.5 ounces)* is a standard nonaerosol hairspray with a medium to firm hold that leaves hair slightly stiff and sticky. Scruples claims this can protect hair from heat-styling implements, but the meager amount of conditioning agents will quickly be overcome by even a low heat setting, so the claim is erroneous. This is best used as a finishing product once hair has been heat-styled.

SEBASTIAN

This venerable, absolutely huge range of hair-care products has been lining salon shelves for over 30 years. Sebastian continues to offer an imposing selection of items that distinguish it from many other salon lines that don't have the scope or formulary variety it does. It is owned and distributed by the Wella Corporation professional division, and Procter & Gamble purchased a majority stake in Wella in late 2003. I hope that P&G doesn't overhaul this line and spin off more Pantene clones (which is what they have done and continue to do with the physique, Clairol, Aussie, and Infusium 23 lines they own) because there are some wonderful Sebastian products that shouldn't be altered. For more information about Sebastian, call (800) 829-7322 or visit www.sebastian-intl.com.

What's Good About This Line: If the prices don't bother you, this line can easily be one-stop shopping for all of your hair-care needs. The styling products really excel, with numerous options for every hair type, texture, and possible style. The Laminates line remains a top choice for those with thick, coarse, or frizzy hair and the Shaper line has some much-improved options for cleansing, conditioning, and styling. The lack of blatant repetition between formulas is refreshing, and really makes this line a winner for distinctive choices, though the label descriptions are not always accurate in terms of hold factor and recommended hair type.

What's Not So Good About It: A few products contain menthol, which is always a problem. Sebastian's choice of packaging for some of the gel-type products ends up being more frustrating than helpful; the Xtah line offers some intense styling products that are difficult to work with; a couple of the styling gels can become gummy and flake.

SEBASTIAN COLLECTION

☹ **Collection Mohair Shampoo** *($8.95 for 8.5 ounces)* contains menthol, which makes it too irritating for all scalp types. There are dozens and dozens of conditioning shampoos that are similar to this without the menthol or the strange 1960s throwback name.

☺ **Collection Spandex Shampoo** *($8.95 for 8.5 ounces)* is an excellent conditioning shampoo that is a very good option for normal to very dry hair that is normal to coarse or thick. It can cause buildup with repeated use and is best alternated with a shampoo that does not contain conditioning agents.

☹ **Collection Stark Naked Shampoo** *($8.95 for 8.5 ounces)* contains menthol, and is not recommended for any hair or scalp type.

☺ **Collection Slinky Conditioner** *($11.19 for 8.5 ounces)* is a standard conditioner that is a good option for dry hair that is normal to fine or thin.

☺ **Collection Titanium Protector, Leave-In Conditioner** *($9.95 for 8.5 ounces)* is a standard, but very good, leave-in conditioner for all hair types dealing with dryness. This can help protect hair from the rigors of brushing and heat styling, but don't be fooled by the titanium name—this is not a coat of armor for hair, and no leave-in conditioner can offer total protection from hair damage.

☺ **Collection Buff, Casual Waxless Pomade** *($13.95 for 4.4 ounces)* is an initially thick, creamy pomade that emulsifies into a smooth, rather lightweight styling balm that can work well to smooth and groom hair while providing a light hold that is not stiff or sticky. The silicones make this a good option for frizz control and adding soft shine to hair, though it can be slightly heavy for fine or thin hair.

☹ **Collection Control Top, Hardwear Gel for Extreme Hold** *($10.95 for 5.1 ounces)* is a below-standard styling gel that contains some good conditioning agents, but the film-forming/holding agent has a slight tendency to gum up on the hair and flake during brush-through, which makes it a poor option in light of the numerous styling gels that do not have this side effect.

☺ **Collection Fizz XL, Fashion Foam for Extra Hold** *($12.95 for 8.8 ounces)* is a standard, medium-hold, propellant-based mousse with a creamier texture than most. It leaves hair slightly stiff and sticky but does contain some very good conditioning agents, which can provide a slight amount of protection during heat styling. This mousse can be somewhat heavy for those with very fine or thin hair.

☺ **Collection Grease, Patent Leather Pomade for Flexible Hold** *($8.95 for 1.7 ounces)* is aptly named because greasy is how your hair will look and feel if you overuse this thick, heavy pomade. It can work well to smooth stubborn frizzies, but is best used on the ends of hair because it is difficult to shampoo out.

☺ **$$$ Collection Molding Mud, Street Chic Sculpting Bonder** *($16.95 for 4.4 ounces)* does allow you to mold hair into shape, and is a great option to define and smooth stubborn curls or waves in thick, coarse hair. Its waxlike base can be heavy and look greasy if not used sparingly. This keeps hair soft and pliable and is also an option for exaggerating texture on short or spiked hair. It is moderately difficult to shampoo out.

☺ **Collection Shpritz Forte, Glam Rock Finishing Spray for Strong Hold** *($9.95 for 8.5 ounces)* is a standard nonaerosol hairspray with a firm hold and a stiff, sticky finish that is somewhat difficult to brush through. This is a good finishing spray for updos or more complex styles where long-lasting hold is more important than flexibility and movement.

☺ **Collection Switch Craft, Changing Spray** *($12.95 for 8 ounces)* is an aerosol styling spray that keeps hair flexible during styling. It's essentially the antithesis of the Condition Shpritz Forte above, in that you can maintain a light degree of hold without stiffness, which is ideal for more casual hairstyles or for the finishing touch when you need hold with movement.

☹ **Collection Texturizer, Body Builder** *($16.50 for 8.5 ounces)* is a below-standard styling gel that becomes gummy as it dries, which leads to the product balling up and flaking. The problem isn't terrible, but with so many excellent styling gels available, you shouldn't have to tolerate it at all.

☺ **Collection Threads, Micro-Mesh Styler for Flexible Hold** *($13.95 for 3.4 ounces)* is similar to the Collection Molding Mud above, except this replaces the prominent wax with plant oil, so it has a softer, easier-to-work-with texture. This is a great option for adding smooth texture to all hair types, but especially thick, coarse, or curly hair that is stubborn. It is non-sticky and adds shine while providing soft control. Those with fine or thin hair need just a pea-sized dab for smoothing dry ends or frizzies.

☺ **Collection Volumizer, Working Spray** *($12.99 for 8.5 ounces)* is a nonaerosol hairspray with light to medium hold that is slightly stiff and sticky. The plant oil and emollients make this a better finishing-spray choice for dry or coarse hair and they lend this product a heavier, "wetter" texture that is not conducive to volumizing.

☺ **Collection Wet, Liquid Gel for Form Fitting Hold** *($7.50 for 8.5 ounces)* has been in the Sebastian lineup for years, and remains a standard, but very good, liquid gel that provides light hold and a soft, minimally sticky finish. It is a good option for all hair types, and works beautifully to shape and softly define curls and waves.

☺ **$$$ Collection Zero g, Runaway Finishing Spray for Dry Medium Hold** *($16.95 for 14.1 ounces)* is an aerosol hairspray that claims it "vaporizes in mid-air," and basically, it does. This dries very quickly and feels weightless, so it is a wonderful option for fine or thin hair that needs a light hold with minimal stickiness. It is easy to brush through and contains light conditioning agents for added shine.

☹ **Collection Dry Clean Only** *($9.95 for 8.5 ounces)* is a water- and alcohol-based product that's sold as a spray-on, quick-dry shampoo for people on the go. It doesn't have much cleansing ability and cannot absorb excess oils the way a dry, powder-based shampoo can. At best, it's a light mist of moisture for hair that doesn't come close to resembling what happens when you shampoo and rinse.

☺ **Collection Potion 9 Wearable Treatment to Restore and Restyle, Super Concentrated** *($13.99 for 5.1 ounces)* is a creamy, but light-textured, leave-in conditioner with a holding agent. Calling this a treatment is going a bit far, but it can moisturize slightly dry hair of any thickness and does help provide some protection during heat styling. It does not get stiff or sticky but can have a smoothing effect on frizzies, though not to the extent that a silicone serum would.

☺ **$$$ Collection Suedeluxe Reconstructor** *($17.95 for 8.5 ounces)* is a very standard, overpriced conditioner with no reconstructing ability. It's an option for normal to dry hair of any thickness.

SEBASTIAN COLLECTIVES

☺ **Collectives Cello Shampoo, for Normal to Oily Hair** *($8.50 for 10.2 ounces)* is a standard, but very good, shampoo for all hair types, and poses minimal risk of buildup.

☺ **Collectives Cello Shampoo, for Normal to Dry Hair** *($8.50 for 10.2 ounces)* is similar to the Collectives Cello Shampoo, for Normal to Oily Hair above, except with a greater amount of film-forming agent, enough to cause buildup with repeated use. However, this is a good shampoo for normal hair that is fine or thin.

☺ **Collectives Moisture Base, Moisturizing Conditioner** *($9.25 for 5.1 ounces)* is a very standard conditioner that works well for normal to dry hair of any thickness. It can cause buildup.

SEBASTIAN LAMINATES

☺ **Laminates Shampoo** *($9.99 for 8.5 ounces)* is very similar to the Collection Spandex Shampoo above, only with the addition of silicone and tiny amounts of plant oils, which makes this preferred for dry hair that is normal to thick or coarse. It can easily build up with repeated use, a characteristic of most conditioning shampoos.

☺ **$$$ Laminates Conditioner** *($13.19 for 8.5 ounces)* is an emollient conditioner that is well-suited for dry to very dry hair that is normal to coarse, curly, or thick.

☺ **Laminates Body, Thickening Polish** *($12.95 for 5.1 ounces)* is a standard styling gel whose water and alcohol base is augmented by silicones and several conditioning agents, all of which adds a smooth, shiny finish to hair. It provides a light to medium hold that is easily brushed through, is minimally stiff or sticky, and is an option for all hair types.

☺ **Laminates Crema Styler, Anti-Frizz Control** *($12.95 for 5.1 ounces)* is an emollient styling cream that is an outstanding option for dry to very dry hair that is thick or coarse. The water- and silicone-based formula contains an array of conditioning agents, including shea butter, and can beautifully smooth frizzies, add shine, and improve hair's texture without hold. It would also work well used with heat to straighten hair.

☺ **Laminates Curl, Curl Perfecting Polish** *($14.95 for 5.1 ounces)* is a thin-textured styling gel that offers minimal hold and almost no sticky after-feel. It is a very good option for fine or thin hair that needs styling support without weighing hair down. This is easily brushed through and can also be a boon for shaping fine, curly hair. This is the only Laminates product that does not contain any silicone.

☺ **$$$ Laminates Gel, Concentrated Smoothing Polish** *($17.95 for 5.1 ounces)* is one of the original silicone-based styling gels, and it remains one of the best. It is completely silicone-based (meaning no water), and as such is a concentrated formula that should be used sparingly by all hair types except very thick or coarse. It excels at smoothing and adding amazing shine, but offers little to no hold. It is a very good choice to straighten curly or wavy hair with heat.

☺ **Laminates Grip, Defining Polish** *($14.95 for 5.1 ounces)* is a very good styling gel that is similar to the Smoothing Polish above.

☺ **Laminates Hair Spray, Finishing Polish** *($10.95 for 8.5 ounces)* is a standard nonaerosol hairspray with a medium to firm hold that leaves hair quite sticky, though the silicone enhances brush-through. This is a fairly heavy finishing spray, and is best for use on normal to thick or coarse hair that needs extra styling support.

☺ **$$$ Laminates Straightening Spray, Transforming Gel Polish** *($17.95 for 8.5 ounces)* is a thinned-out, less greasy version of the Laminates Gel, Concentrated Smoothing Polish above. It is a more versatile option for all but fine or thin hair, and, like its counterpart, is better for smoothing/frizz control and shine enhancement than hold. It would indeed work well to straighten hair with heat. One other comment: The spray application method leaves much to be desired because this is too thick to be evenly (and consistently) dispensed through the tiny nozzle. You may want to just pour a small amount of it in your hands, and then apply it to the hair.

☺ **Laminates Detangling Milk, Leave-In Conditioner** *($9.95 for 8.5 ounces)* is an excellent leave-in conditioner for normal to fine or thin hair that is slightly dry and needs help with combing and static or flyaway hair.

☺ **Laminates Drops, Liquid Polish** *($14.95 for 1.7 ounces)* is a standard, but very good, silicone serum that works as well as any to smooth hair, add shine, and make frizzy hair a thing of the past. Use it sparingly to avoid a too slick, greasy look.

☺ **Laminates Hi Gloss Spray** *($9.99 for 1.7 ounces)* is a lighter, spray-on version of the Laminates Drops, Liquid Polish above, and is an option for all hair types that want a finishing touch of glossy shine. Use it sparingly or hair can become limp and greasy looking.

☺ **$$$ Laminates Masque Reconstructive Treatment** (*$14.95 for 8.5 ounces*) is nearly identical to the Laminates Conditioner above, except this includes more silicones, though not enough to make a noticeable difference between products. Either one would be great for normal to very dry hair that is normal to coarse or thick.

SEBASTIAN SHAPER

☺ **Shaper Color Survivor Daily Shampoo** (*$8.95 for 8.5 ounces*) is a very good, detergent-based shampoo for dry hair, but the film-forming agents and plant oil can build up and make hair feel coated and heavy. If you opt to use this, it is best to alternate it with a shampoo that does not cause buildup. Nothing in it can make color last any longer, but the film-forming agents can add an initial feeling of fullness.

☺ **Shaper Volume Boost Shampoo** (*$7.99 for 8.5 ounces*) is a conditioning shampoo that is not the best choice to build volume, but it's good for normal to dry hair of any thickness.

☺ **Shaper Color Survivor Daily Conditioner** (*$8.95 for 8.5 ounces*) is a very good smoothing conditioner for normal to dry hair of any thickness. The silicone can help smooth and add shine to color-treated hair, but cannot prevent color from fading.

☺ **Shaper Volume Boost Conditioner** (*$8.99 for 8.5 ounces*) is a good, basic conditioner for normal to slightly dry hair that is normal to fine or thin.

☺ **Shaper Blow Out Thermal Body Boost** (*$11.95 for 5.1 ounces*) is a slick, water- and plant oil-based gel that works well for smoothing hair without hold. The oil and conditioning agents can provide a slight amount of heat protection, and this is best for normal to dry hair that is slightly thick or coarse.

☺ **Shaper Full-On Body Mousse** (*$10.95 for 8.5 ounces*) is a standard, propellant-based mousse with a light hold and a moist finish courtesy of its high glycerin content. This is a very good product for normal to fine or thin hair that is dry and needs soft, conditioned control.

☺ **Shaper Hair Spray** (*$11.50 for 10 ounces*) is an aerosol hairspray with a light to medium, flexible hold that is minimally stiff or sticky. It can be a very good working spray for putting together complex hairstyles and is easily brushed through.

☺ **Shaper Hand Press Flattening Fluid** (*$13.95 for 5.1 ounces*) is a liquidy styling gel that is supposed to take the place of a flat iron to smooth hair. The idea is to spread this over your hands, then press hair flat, smoothing the product from roots to tip. Unless you have almost straight hair that is not stubborn, you will quickly find that you still need your flat iron to achieve a straight, smooth appearance. This is really just a light-hold, slightly sticky styling gel that has a relatively weightless feel in hair and is easily brushed through.

☺ **Shaper In Control Fiber Wax** (*$9.95 for 1.8 ounces*) doesn't contain any fibers. Rather, this is a water-based, emollient pomade/styling cream hybrid that is a good option for smoothing and frizz control on dry to very dry hair that is coarse or thick. It can quickly become greasy if not used sparingly.

☺ **Shaper Iron Works Hot Tools Protecting Spray** *($11.95 for 6.8 ounces)* is said to provide "direct" heat protection from all manner of heat-styling tools, but there is no way this water- and alcohol-based, light-hold styling spray can defend hair from heat damage, especially from direct-application sources such as flat or crimping irons. It is a good, lightweight, minimally sticky spray for normal to fine or thin hair.

☺ **Shaper Massive Texture Jel Mist** *($12.95 for 6.7 ounces)* is a gel packaged in a spray bottle. The packaging was a bad idea because it is difficult to spray this on evenly, and the pump clogs almost immediately. A tube or jar would have made this product much easier to use. That said, this is a basic, sticky styling gel that can add texture and a medium, slightly stiff hold to hair.

☺ **Shaper Mega Hold Hair Spray** *($13.95 for 10.6 ounces)* is a standard aerosol hairspray with medium to firm hold and a slightly stiff, sticky feel that can be brushed through.

☺ **Shaper Plus Hair Spray** *($12.50 for 10.6 ounces)* is similar to the Shaper Hair Spray above, except this offers more hold and has a stickier feel that can still be brushed through. Otherwise, the same comments apply.

☺ **Shaper Root Raise Lifting Spray** *($11.95 for 8.8 ounces)* is an aerosol hairspray with a directional nozzle for applying to the roots. It works well to provide long-lasting lift and a medium hold that is minimally stiff or sticky, though be careful applying this so you don't oversaturate the roots with too much product.

☺ **Shaper Sleek Hold Jel** *($9.95 for 8.5 ounces)* is a good basic styling gel with light hold that can impart shine to hair and has no stiff or sticky feel.

☺ **Shaper Smoothing Groomer** *($14.49 for 4.2 ounces)* is a water- and silicone-based styling cream that can feel fairly greasy even when used sparingly. It does not provide any hold, and is best for those with dry to very dry hair that is normal to coarse or thick.

☺ $$$ **Shaper Zero g Finishing Spray** *($15.95 for 14.1 ounces)* is a lighter-weight, faster-drying version of the Shaper Hair Spray above, and the same comments about hold and stickiness apply here, too. This would be preferred for fine or thin hair that needs added hold without weight.

SEBASTIAN XTAH

☺ **Xtah Raw Sensuality Hydration Shampoo** *($9.50 for 8.5 ounces)* is a creamy-feeling standard shampoo and there isn't anything raw or sensual about it. This is a good conditioning shampoo for dry hair of any thickness, though the film-forming and conditioning agents will build up with repeated use.

☺ **Xtah Raw Sensuality Hydration Conditioner** *($9.50 for 8.5 ounces)* is a very good conditioner for normal to dry hair that is normal to slightly thick or coarse. The amino acids it contains cannot fortify hair, though they can help as water-binding agents.

☺ $$$ **Xtah Raw Hair Bondage, Rock Hard Hold** *($19.50 for 4.4 ounces)* doesn't just provide rock-hard hold—it is like Crazy Glue for hair! Why anyone would need this much sticky hold is beyond me, but I suppose it can work for mohawks or other gravity-defying hairstyles you don't intend to brush through. This gel is difficult to shampoo out, and the high amount of film-forming agent will cause buildup almost immediately.

☺ $$$ **Xtah Raw Hair Crude Clay, Modeler** *($19.50 for 4.4 ounces)* is an impossibly thick, heavy Vaseline- and wax-based pomade that contains clay for a slight matte finish and a "chunky" look. The emollients keep the clay from being too drying for hair, but this product is very difficult to work with and its effects can be achieved with more user-friendly products.

☺ $$$ **Xtah Raw Hair Cy-Clone, Silkon Hair Cream** *($19.50 for 4.4 ounces)* is a thick, silicone- and wax-based pomade that contains so much menthol it can clear your sinuses. If the smell doesn't get you, it can work well (if used sparingly) to smooth frizzies and softly hold hair in place—but keep it away from the scalp to avoid irritation.

☺ $$$ **Xtah Raw Hair Dirty Workx, Rinse-Out Conditioner or Leave-In Styler** *($15 for 4.3 ounces)* fails as a rinse-out conditioner because the heavy wax and clay base is not water soluble, which means this will cause noticeable buildup with just one application. It is an OK option for making thick or coarse hair feel smoother, but there are much more elegant conditioners that do that without so much wax.

☺ **Xtah Raw Sensuality Loose Locks, Natural Styling Lotion** *($10.50 for 8.5 ounces)* is a lightly creamy, silky-feeling styling lotion that does not offer any hold, but can nicely smooth and groom hair that is dry, thick, or coarse.

☺ $$$ **Xtah Raw Hair Roxx, Rubber-Iced Gelatine** *($19.50 for 4.4 ounces)* is a thicker version of the Shaper Massive Texture Jel Mist above, but this option ends up feeling less sticky despite offering the same amount of hold. It is best for use on dry (not damp) hair to create exaggerated texture or spiked looks without a heavy after-feel.

☺ $$$ **Xtah Raw Hair Twisted Taffy, Free-Former** *($19.50 for 4.4 ounces)* has a creamy, gel-like texture that is reminiscent of the type of translucent icing usually seen on cinnamon rolls. It is a bit stringy at first, but emulsifies well and can add smooth texture and shine to hair without stiffness or a thick feel. It is best for dry to very dry hair that is normal to coarse or thick. This is relatively water-soluble despite its paraffin (wax) and plant-oil base.

SELSUN BLUE

This line offers a small group of products that contain selenium sulfide, an antimicrobial agent effective in the treatment of dandruff and seborrheic dermatitis. For more information about Selsun Blue, owned by Chattem, call (800) 366-6833 or visit www.chattem.com.

What's Good About This Line: The active ingredient, selenium sulfide, is an effective anti-dandruff option, though it's not without its drawbacks (Source: *Journal of the American Academy of Dermatology*, December 1993, pages 1008–1012).

What's Not So Good About It: Selenium sulfide can be drying for hair and strip hair color; it can also be extremely irritating if it gets in the eyes. If you decide to try one of the Selsun Blue shampoos, take special care during rinsing to avoid inadvertent eye exposure.

☺ **2-in-1 Treatment Dandruff Shampoo and Conditioner in One** *($7.89 for 11 ounces)* contains 1% selenium sulfide as its active ingredient. As an anti-microbial ingredient, it acts on the yeasts responsible for dandruff. Minimizing these yeasts will relieve the itching and flaking scalp associated with this common condition. However, the sulfur component of this ingredient can be very drying for hair and scalp while also stripping hair color. Therefore, this is best as a last resort when other over-the-counter anti-dandruff products have failed to produce positive results.

☺ **Balanced Treatment Dandruff Control for All Hair Types** *($7.89 for 11 ounces)* is nearly identical to the 2-in-1 Treatment Dandruff Shampoo and Conditioner in One above, except this option omits the conditioning agents, which means there's no risk of buildup. Otherwise, the same basic comments and concerns about selenium sulfide apply.

☹ **Medicated Treatment Dandruff Shampoo** *($7.89 for 11 ounces)* contains menthol, which makes it a problem for the scalp, and menthol has no effect on controlling dandruff or any other scalp problem. Combined with the selenium sulfide, this can be too irritating, and it is not recommended.

☺ **Moisturizing Treatment Dandruff Shampoo** *($7.89 for 11 ounces)* is nearly identical to the 2-in-1 Treatment Dandruff Shampoo and Conditioner in One above, and the same review applies. The conditioning agents are not present in high enough amounts to offset the drying effect of the selenium sulfide.

SENSCIENCE

For more information about Senscience, call (800) 242-9283 or visit www.isohair.com.

What's Good About This Line: This is a line of good, basic hair-care products.

What's Not So Good About It: There are only a few negative issues to point out, and other than that, these are mostly standard, sometimes boring formulations; the conditioner prices are on the steep side considering that most are similar to what you'll find from Pantene, L'Oreal, or Neutrogena's Triple Moisture line.

☺ **Energy Shampoo, for Dry Hair** *($9.50 for 16 ounces)* is a very standard shampoo that is a great option for all hair types, posing minimal to no risk of buildup with repeated use.

☺ **Energy Shampoo, for Normal Hair** *($9.50 for 16 ounces)* is identical to the Energy Shampoo, for Dry Hair above, and the same review applies.

☺ **$$$ Inner Conditioner, for Coarse Hair** *($13.15 for 16 ounces)* is a very good smoothing conditioner for normal to dry or slightly thick, coarse hair.

☺ **$$$ Inner Conditioner, for Fine Hair** *($13.15 for 16 ounces)* is a standard, but good, conditioner for normal to dry hair of any thickness.

☺ $$$ **Inner Conditioner, for Medium Hair** *($13.15 for 16 ounces)* is a very good, though standard, option for normal to slightly dry hair that is normal to slightly thick or coarse.

☺ **Inner Repair, Leave-In Conditioner** *($8.10 for 8 ounces)* is a very light, water- and alcohol-based, spray-on conditioner that can help detangle fine or thin hair and make it feel slightly thicker, though it offers little conditioning benefit. The film-forming/holding agents can leave hair feeling slightly stiff and sticky, and no part of this product can offer hair inner repair.

☺ **Maximum Memory, Firm Holding Spray** *($12.25 for 10.5 ounces)* is a very standard aerosol hairspray with a light hold and a slightly stiff, sticky feel that can still be brushed through. Senscience's Inner Cellular Membrane Complex is just a blend of silk and silicone—good conditioning agents for hair, but with no ability to penetrate that deeply or even mimic the hair's inner structure.

☺ **Memory Mist, Brushable Holding Spray** *($10.80 for 10.5 ounces)* is nearly identical to the Maximum Memory, Firm Holding Spray above, only with less hold and a softer, more flexible finish. It would be a great hairspray for those who have been disappointed in the past by heavy, sticky hairsprays.

☺ **Swing, Thermal Setting Spray** *($9.45 for 7.6 ounces)* is the nonaerosol counterpart to the Maximum Memory, Firm Holding Spray above, except this has a heavier application and is slightly more sticky. Which one you choose is a matter of personal preference.

☺ **Volumesse, Body Building Foam** *($9.50 for 7 ounces)* is a liquid-to-foam mousse with a medium to firm hold and a sticky, slightly stiff finish. This can be brushed through, and is a good choice for normal to fine, curly, or thin hair that is difficult to manage.

☺ **Hydrating Hair Masque** *($10.80 for 4 ounces)* is a conditioning mousse that is meant to replenish hair after chemical processing, but it is too light to make hair feel smooth and healthy. It is best for normal to fine or thin hair that needs light smoothing and minor frizz control.

☺ **True-Hue Color Treatment** *($10.80 for 18 0.58-ounce capsules)* is just plastic capsules filled with silicone, vitamins, sunscreens, and silk. This is akin to a standard silicone serum, and ends up being costly for what you get. The sunscreens cannot be relied on to protect color-treated hair from UV damage. As with all silicone serums, this can work well to smooth hair and tame frizzies.

☺ **VitalEsse, Repair and Shine** *($11.70 for 1.8 ounces)* is nearly identical to the True-Hue Color Treatment above, only this contains a small amount of alcohol to reduce the heavy effect of the silicones, and omits the sunscreens. Otherwise, the same comments apply.

SENSCIENCE BODY & SHINE

☺ **Body & Shine Bodifying Shampoo** *($7.65 for 12 ounces)* is a standard shampoo that is a good option for all hair types and poses no risk of buildup.

☺ **Body & Shine Daily Detangler** *($8.10 for 12 ounces)* is an ultra-light conditioner that is an OK option for normal to fine or thin hair that needs help with combing.

☺ **Body & Shine Glossifying Gel** *($8.10 for 6 ounces)* is a standard styling gel with a light hold and a minimal stiff, sticky finish that is easily brushed through. The vitamins it contains cannot add body or make hair glossy, though the small amount of silicone will add a bit of shine.

SENSCIENCE STRAIGHT SENSE

☺ **Straight Sense Shampoo** *($8.10 for 10.2 ounces)* is a very good conditioning shampoo for normal to slightly dry hair, but will not help make hair straighter.

☺ **Straight Sense Conditioner** *($8.10 for 10.2 ounces)* is a very good conditioner for normal to dry hair of any thickness. A conditioner with more silicone would be a more sensible choice if your goal is straight hair.

☺ **Straight Sense Smoothing Gel** *($9.90 for 6.8 ounces)* is a basic, rather boring smoothing gel, with minimal to no hold and a silky, slippery texture. It is somewhat effective for straightening hair with heat, but holds no advantage over more-elegant options with silicone. This is best for those with normal to fine or thin hair—it is too light for thick, coarse hair.

☺ **Straight Sense Defrizz Hairdress** *($7.60 for 3.4 ounces)* is a standard styling cream that contains enough silicone to provide a smoothing, frizz-taming benefit without making hair feel too heavy or greasy. It is a good finishing or mixing product for all but very thick or coarse hair.

SEXY HAIR CONCEPTS

What does it mean to have sexy hair? According to hairdresser Michael O'Rourke, who created this line, sexy hair is just about any hair that uses his products. So whether or not you have big, healthy, shiny, straight, curly, short, or wild hair, you can have sexy hair. There's little question that sex sells, and to date no one else has brought forth a hair-care line where sexiness is blatantly used as the major selling point for each shampoo, conditioner, and styling aid. The SEXY Hair Concepts products are loaded with names that conjure up double entendres, and the photographs of well-coiffed models on many of the products reinforce the company's message that, at least for younger generations, sex appeal has a lot to do with how your hair should look. But risqué names and flashy packaging mean little if the products themselves don't measure up. Unfortunately, that's all too often the case with SEXY Hair Concepts. There are some excellent products to consider, but to believe this line is the key to unlocking your hair's sex appeal would not only be faulty, but also downplay the real work of styling your hair into shape. For more information about SEXY Hair Concepts, call (800) 848-3383 or visit www.sexyhairconcepts.com.

What's Good About This Line: Conditioners with varied, mostly elegant formulas that are well-tailored to their intended hair type; prices that are on the low end for a salon-sold hair-care line; and a few novel products that take a standard concept (such as styling gel) and give it an unusual twist such as a metallic finish.

What's Not So Good About It: Irritating ingredients such as balm mint, lavender oil, and lemon show up in several products.

SEXY HAIR CONCEPTS BIG SEXY HAIR

☺ **Big Sexy Hair, Big Volume Shampoo** (*$6.95 for 8.5 ounces*) is a very good shampoo for all hair types and poses no risk of buildup, but it won't help create volume either.

☺ **Big Sexy Hair, Extra Big Volume Shampoo** (*$9.95 for 13.5 ounces*) is similar to the Big Sexy Hair, Big Volume Shampoo above, and the same comments apply.

☺ **Big Sexy Hair, Big Volume Conditioner** (*$6.95 for 8.5 ounces*) is an ultra-light conditioner that is suitable for fine or thin hair that is normal to slightly dry.

☺ **Big Sexy Hair Blow Dry, Volumizing Gel** (*$11 for 8.5 ounces*) is a standard gel with a light to medium hold that has minimal to no stiff or sticky feel.

☺ **Big Sexy Hair Dense, Thickening Spray** (*$11.95 for 8.5 ounces*) contains film-forming/holding agents that can make thin, fine hair feel thicker, and they do so with minimal stickiness or stiffness, making this an excellent light-hold styling spray. When used with heat and the proper styling techniques, this can indeed create big hair, but the sexy part has to come from you.

☹ **Big Sexy Hair Flip It Over, Full & Wild Spray** (*$13.95 for 4.4 ounces*) is an aerosol styling spray that offers a firm, bodifying hold but not without a great deal of stickiness that makes hair feel tacky to the touch. It is not a pleasant product to use unless you need strong hold and have no plans for that special someone to run their fingers through your hair (though it would be comical if they did and got stuck, which is possible given how sticky this product is).

☺ **Big Sexy Hair Root Pump, Volumizing Spray Mousse** (*$13 for 10.6 ounces*) is an aerosol spray mousse with a medium hold that remains slightly sticky but can be brushed through. It contains a minimal amount of conditioning agents, which makes this a poor choice to use by itself prior to heat-styling hair.

☺ **Big Sexy Hair Root Pump Plus, Humidity-Resistant Volumizing Spray Mousse** (*$14.50 for 10.6 ounces*) is nearly identical to the Big Sexy Hair Root Pump, Volumizing Spray Mousse above, except with slightly more hold. The tiny amount of silicone won't go far to keep humidity from getting to your hair.

☺ **Big Sexy Hair Spray & Play, Volumizing Hairspray** (*$13 for 10.6 ounces*) is a standard aerosol hairspray that could have been made even lighter if the goal was big volume, but it does work well for those who need light hold that is minimally stiff or sticky. The silicones add extra shine to hair.

☺ **Big Sexy Hair Spray & Play Harder, Firm Volumizing Hairspray** (*$14 for 10.6 ounces*) is almost identical to the Big Sexy Hair Spray & Play, Volumizing Hairspray above, only with slightly more hold. Otherwise, the same comments apply.

☺ **Big Sexy Hair Big Shine, Shine Spray** *($10.95 for 2.5 ounces)* is a standard silicone spray with a small amount of alcohol to help prevent it from getting too greasy.

☹ **Big Sexy Hair Volumizing Detangler** *($8.95 for 8.5 ounces)* contains the preservatives methylchloroisothiazolinone and methylisothiazolinone (Kathon CG), which are not recommended for use in leave-on products that come in contact with skin.

SEXY HAIR CONCEPTS CURLY SEXY HAIR

☺ **Curly Sexy Hair, Shampoo** *($6.95 for 8.5 ounces)* is a standard, but good, shampoo for normal to fine or thin hair that is curly or otherwise, though it can cause buildup with repeated use.

☺ **Curly Sexy Hair, Conditioner** *($6.95 for 8.5 ounces)* is very good for dry hair that is normal to thick or coarse, but keep in mind the plant oil will build up with repeated use and can make hair feel coated.

☺ **Curly Sexy Hair, Curl Power Curl Enhancer** *($11.95 for 8.5 ounces)* is a propellant-based, spray-on conditioner that has a silky, lightweight texture that can help softly define and shape curls without hold or a sticky feel. It is best for curly hair that is normal to fine or thin.

☺ **Curly Sexy Hair, Hot Curl Setting Lotion** *($9.95 for 8.5 ounces)* is a light-hold styling lotion that has no stiff or sticky feel. It works well for all hair types.

SEXY HAIR CONCEPTS HEALTHY SEXY HAIR

☺ **Healthy Sexy Hair, Soy Milk Moisture Shampoo** *($10.95 for 13.5 ounces)* is an excellent conditioning shampoo for dry hair of any thickness.

☺ **Healthy Sexy Hair, Soy Milk Shampoo** *($9.95 for 13.5 ounces)* is a less conditioning version of the Healthy Sexy Hair, Soy Milk Moisture Shampoo above, and the increased amount of film-forming agent makes this preferred for normal to fine or thin hair that is slightly dry.

☺ **Healthy Sexy Hair, Soy Milk Conditioner** *($9.95 for 8.5 ounces)* is a great conditioner for normal to dry hair of any thickness.

☹ **Healthy Sexy Hair, Soy Tri-Wheat Leave-In Conditioner** *($10.95 for 8.5 ounces)* contains the preservatives methylchloroisothiazolinone and methylisothiazolinone (Kathon CG), which is not recommended in a leave-in product like this.

☺ **Healthy Sexy Hair Soy Gelatine, Firm Holding Gel** *($12.95 for 4.4 ounces)* is a standard, medium-hold gel that has a slightly stiff feel, though it easily brushes through.

☺ **Healthy Sexy Hair Soy Paste, Texture Pomade** *($12.95 for 1.8 ounces)* is a thick, solid pomade that when used sparingly can help smooth flyaways and control frizzies.

☺ **Healthy Sexy Hair Soy Smoothie, Straightening Tonic** *($10.95 for 4.2 ounces)* is a light- to medium-hold, gel-like lotion that can work well for styling most hair types.

☺ **Healthy Sexy Hair Soya Want Flat Hair, Flat Iron Spray** *($11.95 for 5.3 ounces)* is a standard aerosol hairspray that contains conditioning agents and silicone to help offset its sticky feel and provide some moisture, but not enough to prevent hair from the heat damage that occurs when you use a flat iron. This can work well to help stubborn sections of hair respond better to flat ironing.

☺ **Healthy Sexy Hair Soya Want Full Hair, Firm Hairspray** *($13.50 for 10.6 ounces)* is identical in every respect to the Healthy Sexy Hair Soya Want Flat Hair, Flat Iron Spray above, and the same review applies. Notice the price and size difference? It doesn't make sense to me, either.

☹ **Healthy Sexy Hair Soy Sculpting & Braiding Clay** *($12.95 for 1.8 ounces).* The clay can dry the hair and slowly chip away at the cuticle layers, and isn't the best texture for styling hair.

☺ $$$ **Healthy Sexy Hair, Soy Fuel Power Conditioning Booster** *($14.95 for 1 ounce)* is a techno-blue fluid packaged in a science laboratory vial meant to convey that this is a serious treatment for distressed hair that has seen better days. You're supposed to mix a few drops of this with any conditioner to boost its power and provide "extreme protein" to hair. This water- and glycerin-based fluid does contain protein, but so do countless other products that cost much less. Proteins, like most conditioning agents, can form a temporary protective coating on the hair shaft, but in conditioners most of it is rinsed away since proteins don't hold up well under the pressure of water. This product is more gimmicky than effective, though it is still an option for all hair types, and the presentation is admittedly very cool.

☺ $$$ **Healthy Sexy Hair, Soy Potion Miraculous Leave-In Treatment** *($13.50 for 5.1 ounces)* is far and away the best product in the Healthy Sexy Hair lineup. This silky, gel-based, leave-in conditioner is an outstanding option for dry hair that is normal to slightly thick or coarse. If you're familiar with or use Sebastian's Potion 9 Leave-In Wearable Treatment, this is a similar but silkier formulation.

☺ $$$ **Healthy Sexy Hair, Soy Salvation Deep Treatment Hair Masque with Oatmeal** *($19.50 for six 1-ounce packets)* is a rather lackluster conditioner that, despite the name, does not contain any soy. I suppose "Oat Salvation" wouldn't be as trendy, because who wants to think of Wilford Brimley when they're going after healthy, sexy hair? Regrettably, this product isn't deep or much of a treatment, but it is OK for slightly dry hair of any thickness.

SEXY HAIR CONCEPTS HOT SEXY HIGHLIGHTS

☺ **Hot Sexy Highlights Color Stabilizing Shampoo** *($7.95 for 6.8 ounces)* is a standard shampoo that can work well for all hair types except dry, and poses a slight risk of buildup. It does contain henna.

☺ **Hot Sexy Highlights Highlighting Shampoo** *($7.95 for 6.8 ounces)* is nearly identical to the Hot Sexy Highlights Color Stabilizing Shampoo above, except this does not contain henna and has less film-forming agent, which makes it a very good option for all hair types. The coloring agents have minimal to no effect on reducing brassy or yellow tones in natural or dyed blonde hair.

☺ **Hot Sexy Highlights Color Conditioner** *($10.80 for 5.1 ounces)* is a color-enhancing conditioner available in five different shades to enhance blonde, red, brown, and black hair. The conditioner base contains mostly water, thickener, detangling agent, plant oil, panthenol, plant extracts, silicone, preservatives, and fragrance. Each conditioner contains basic dyes that do have some ability to cling to the hair shaft and impart a subtle color change.

☺ **Hot Sexy Highlights Whipped Up, Gel Foam** *($12.60 for 7 ounces)* is a foaming gel mousse with a light to medium hold and a slightly sticky feel that can easily be brushed through.

☻ **Hot Sexy Highlights High Drama, Glitter Spray Firm Hold** *($10.80 for 4.4 ounces)* is a light-hold aerosol hairspray infused with large flecks of glitter, available in gold, red, or blue hues. The glitter tends to flake off readily, which makes this more of a mess than a fun departure from standard hairspray.

☺ **Hot Sexy Highlights Aero Color, Poly-Ester Pink Color Spray** *($10.99 for 3.5 ounces)* is an aerosol hairspray with temporary dye to stain hair fluorescent pink. If you're looking for this type of product, you're probably not reading this book!

SEXY HAIR CONCEPTS SHORT SEXY HAIR

☺ **Short Sexy Hair Blow It Up, Gel Foam** *($11.50 for 5.3 ounces)* is almost identical to the Hot Sexy Highlights Whipped Up, Gel Foam above, and the same comments apply.

☺ **Short Sexy Hair Control Maniac, Wax** *($11.50 for 1.8 ounces)* is a thick, but workable, wax that contains more plant oil than actual wax, which means this leaves hair slightly greasy but shiny. A little of this goes a very long way, and it is best used to smooth stubborn curls or frizzies or on the ends of hair for added definition and texture.

☹ **Short Sexy Hair Fixed Up, Hard Hairspray** *($12.50 for 8.8 ounces)* is an aerosol hairspray that flakes before it has a chance to provide any sort of hold for hair, and flakes again as you try to brush through hair. It is not recommended.

☺ $$$ **Short Sexy Hair Frenzy, Bulked Up Texture** *($15.50 for 2.5 ounces)* is a thick, heavy-duty pomade that contains several emollients along with wax and film-forming agent. It can work well to create extreme textures on short hair, but should be used sparingly and not by those with fine or thin hair, unless it is buzz-cut short.

☺ **Short Sexy Hair Hard Up, Gel** *($10.50 for 4.2 ounces)* is a firm-hold gel that dries quickly and leaves hair feeling stiff and in place. It takes a bit of effort to brush through this.

☹ **Short Sexy Hair Play Dirty, Wax Master Dry Wax** *($11.95 for 4.4 ounces)* is an aerosol styling spray that has more glycerin, holding agent, and silicone than wax, and leaves hair feeling coated but not too heavy. Unfortunately, the lavender and rosewood oils can be irritating to the scalp, and this sprays on so forcefully you can't help but get it on your scalp, too. Paul Mitchell's Spray Wax, 3-D Texture and Flexible Hold ($12.95 for 2.8 ounces) is a much better option.

☺ **Short Sexy Hair Quick Change, Shaping Balm** *($11.50 for 1.7 ounces)* is a great emollient styling balm for dry to very dry hair that is normal to coarse or thick. Hair remains pliable with enhanced texture and shine, while stickiness is minimal. This works well to smooth stubborn frizzies and dry ends, or soften coarse curls and waves.

☺ **Short Sexy Hair Rough & Ready, Styling Gunk** *($13.95 for 4.4 ounces)* is a thick, jellylike styling balm that is meant to exaggerate or create a messy texture on dry (rather than damp) hair. It ends up being fairly easy to apply, but leaves hair very stiff and sticky, which isn't the best considering there are softer options that can also create the trendy bedhead look.

☹ **Short Sexy Hair Shatter, Separate & Hold Spray** *($11.95 for 4.2 ounces)* contains acetone as one of its main ingredients, which can be drying to the hair and, if it gets on skin, irritating. For a similar feel and hold without acetone, consider any of the Garnier Fructis Style hairsprays.

☺ **Short Sexy Hair Slept In, Texture Crème** *($11.50 for 4.2 ounces)* is basically a slightly creamy leave-in conditioner that can add soft texture and modest definition to hair while moisturizing it. The "special" ingredients are listed after the preservatives, and as such don't count for much.

☺ **Short Sexy Hair What a Body, Ultra Bodifying Blow Dry Gel** *($12.95 for 6.8 ounces)* is similar to many of the gels in the various product groups. It has a light to medium hold and minimal to no stiff or sticky feel.

SEXY HAIR CONCEPTS SILKY SEXY HAIR

☺ **Silky Sexy Hair, Silky Shampoo** *($8.95 for 8.5 ounces)* is a standard, but very good, conditioning shampoo that is ideal for normal to dry hair of any thickness, and will cause buildup with repeated use.

☺ **Silky Sexy Hair, Silky Conditioner** *($8.95 for 8.5 ounces)* is nearly identical to the Healthy Sexy Hair, Soy Milk Conditioner above, and the same review applies.

☺ $$$ **Silky Sexy Hair, Drench for Dry Hair** *($13.95 for 5.1 ounces)* is similar to the Healthy Sexy Hair, Soy Potion Miraculous Leave-In Treatment above, except this contains silicone, which makes it preferred for dry, frizzy hair that needs smoothing and added shine. It is too heavy for fine or thin hair, but all other hair types qualify for this very good leave-in conditioner.

☺ $$$ **Silky Sexy Hair, Frizz Eliminator** *($17.95 for 5.1 ounces)* is a standard silicone serum that works as well as any to smooth dry to very dry hair and ease away frizzies while adding brilliant shine. Use it sparingly to avoid a greasy, heavy feel.

☺ $$$ **Silky Sexy Hair, Remedy for Chemically Treated Hair** *($13.95 for 5.1 ounces)* is a leave-in conditioner that can work well for normal to dry hair that is normal to fine or thin. Although this can benefit chemically treated hair, it is not as elegant as the Silky Sexy Hair, Drench for Dry Hair above.

SEXY HAIR CONCEPTS STRAIGHT SEXY HAIR

☺ **Straight Sexy Hair Shampoo** *($6.95 for 8.5 ounces)* is a very good light-conditioning shampoo for normal to slightly dry hair of any thickness, but it won't help make hair straight.

☺ **Straight Sexy Hair Conditioner** *($6.95 for 8.5 ounces)* is a very standard conditioner that is an option for normal to slightly dry hair that is normal to fine or thin.

☺ **Straight Sexy Hair Power Straight! Straightening Balm** *($12.95 for 3.4 ounces)* is a very good, largely silicone-based straightening gel that works beautifully to turn curly or wavy hair into smooth, sleek locks (when used with heat and the proper styling brush, of course). This is an option for all but fine or thin hair.

☺ **Straight Sexy Hair Smooth & Seal, Aerated Anti-Frizz Spray** *($14.95 for 8.8 ounces)* is an aerosol silicone spray that produces a very fine mist. It is a great glossing option for all hair types, and has a silky-smooth finish that is minimally greasy or slick.

☺ **Straight Sexy Hair Straight Aero, Aerated Straightening Spray** *($14.95 for 8.8 ounces)* is a lightweight aerosol styling spray that has a smooth, light hold without being stiff or sticky. It is an option for straightening normal to fine or thin hair that is curly, but you will need to pair it with another product (such as a silicone serum or cream) to add extra smoothness and weight.

☺ **Straight Sexy Hair Shine On, Polishing Gloss** *($12.95 for 3.4 ounces)* is a very standard, but good, silicone serum that works as well as any to tame frizzies and add shine.

SEXY HAIR CONCEPTS WILD SEXY HAIR

☺ **Wild Sexy Hair Metal Head, Metallic Holding Gel** *($11.95 for 2.1 ounces)* is a firm-hold, liquidy styling gel that leaves hair stiff and slightly sticky. This is available in six colors, from copper to emerald green, and each shade tints hair with a metallic finish. This is for special-occasion use only, unless you're on a quest to become a rock star or just want to raise some eyebrows.

☺ **Wild Sexy Hair Unshakeable, Firm Holding Fixative** *($12.50 for 4.2 ounces)* is a nonaerosol, fast-drying hairspray with a rock-solid hold for extreme hairstyles. It remains very sticky, but will definitely come in handy for wind tunnel–proof styling support.

☺ **Wild Sexy Hair Untamed, Whipped Wax** *($14.95 for 3.5 ounces)* is an odd product that I am not sure how to classify. It's a propellant-based mousse/pomade/gel hybrid that is dispensed as foam, yet it has a gel-like texture with the greasy feel of a standard pomade. It provides a light to medium hold that leaves hair pliable but slightly sticky, and the overall weight and finish of this makes it preferred for dry hair that is coarse or thick.

☺ **Wild Sexy Hair Flashy, 3-D Shine Gloss** *($13 for 1.7 ounces)* has a tempting name that extroverts will gravitate toward, but they should know this is just a standard, gel-type, water-soluble pomade that works as well as any other to smooth frizzies and dry ends while imparting a glossy, wet-look shine. The only difference is the inclusion of

The Reviews S

sparkling blue particles, which does add a more dazzling shine, and the shiny particles tend not to flake.

SOFT & BEAUTIFUL

For more information about Soft & Beautiful, call (800) 527-5879 or visit www.proline-intl.com.

What's Good About This Line: You can tell that Soft & Beautiful has made an effort to offer lightweight products that are a refreshing departure from the typical oil- and Vaseline-laden products that make up most of every other ethnic hair-care line; there are numerous options for dry to very dry hair that is coarse or thick.

What's Not So Good About It: Even with the lighter options, the majority of styling and finishing products and many of the conditioners are examples of the way-too-famil-iar theme that runs through all African-American hair-care lines, namely grease, grease, and more grease. There are modern alternatives to such heavy products, something Soft & Beautiful clearly knows, as their glycerin-rich, low-oil products demonstrate; some leave-in products contain the skin-sensitizing preservatives methylchloroisothiazolinone and methylisothiazolinone (Kathon CG), which are not recommended for leave-in use.

☺ **Moisturizing Shampoo, Pro-Vitamin Formula** *($3.49 for 16 ounces)* is a very standard shampoo for all hair types, with minimal moisturizing properties. It will not cause buildup.

☺ **Conditioner, Hair Moisturizing Complex** *($7.99 for 6 ounces)* has a thin texture and is a good option for dry hair that is normal to slightly thick, curly, or coarse.

☺ **Holding Spray, Maximum Hold with Humidity Guard** *($2.29 for 12.5 ounces)* is a standard, weightless aerosol hairspray with a light hold and no stiff or sticky finish. The silicone makes the hair easier to comb through and adds a subtle amount of shine.

☺ **Extra Light Creme Moisturizer** *($3.59 for 4 ounces)* is about as extra light as a load of bricks! This conditioner is greasy but still a good choice for very dry hair that is coarse or thick. It doesn't rinse well and can make hair feel coated and heavy if not used sparingly.

☺ **Oil Moisturizing Lotion** *($6.69 for 16 ounces)* is a greasy, heavy-duty, leave-in conditioner that can make hair feel coated and slick if used as directed (meaning applying it generously to the scalp and throughout the hair). This is only for very dry hair that is extremely coarse, curly, or thick, and it should be used sparingly.

☺ **Oil Sheen** *($3.59 for 17.2 ounces)* is a glossing spray with a dry-feel finish, but it can still make hair look too slick and greasy if not used sparingly. The wax base can build up with repeated use and make hair look dull, so it is important to wash hair with a chelating shampoo to minimize buildup.

SOFT & BEAUTIFUL BOTANICALS

☹ **Botanicals Conditioning Shampoo** *($2.99 for 6 ounces)* contains sodium lauryl sulfate as its main detergent cleansing agent, which makes it too drying and irritating for all hair and scalp types. By the way, there are no botanical ingredients in this shampoo.

☹ **Botanicals Coco-Almond Moisturizing Shampoo** *($2.99 for 12 ounces)* is nearly identical to the Botanicals Conditioning Shampoo above, and the same review applies.

☺ **Botanicals Enriching Conditioner** *($2.99 for 6 ounces)* is similar to the Conditioner, Hair Moisturizing Complex above, and the same review applies. There is not a single botanical ingredient in this product, but that's OK, because they aren't of help to the hair or scalp anyway.

☺ **Botanicals Sculpting Foam** *($3.99 for 8 ounces)* is a standard, liquid-to-foam mousse with a light, soft hold and a slightly sticky feel that can still be brushed through. This contains conditioning agents that are beneficial to dry hair, and that lend this mousse a moist finish.

☺ **Botanicals Sculpting Gel** *($4.29 for 8 ounces)* does not contain any film-forming/holding agents, but it can be a good smoothing gel for dry hair. This can work well to soften and add shine to curly hair.

☺ **Botanicals Shining Gel** *($3.99 for 4 ounces)* is a heavier, greasier version of the Botanicals Sculpting Gel above. It's essentially a water-soluble, gel-type pomade that can work well to smooth coarse, dry strands while adding a glossy shine. It should be used sparingly to avoid making hair look too slick and greasy.

☺ **Botanicals Styling Creme, Firm Hold** *($4.49 for 3.4 ounces)* is too greasy and slick to offer anything resembling firm hold, but it is an option for smoothing very dry, coarse hair that's unruly or so wiry it does not respond well to traditional waxes and pomades. This does contain film-forming/holding agents, but they cannot firm up because of the slippery texture provided by the mineral oil.

☹ **Botanicals 3-in-1 Dry Scalp Treatment** *($5.19 for 4 ounces)* is an exceptionally greasy scalp treatment that contains menthol, which works to stop itching by virtue of producing a stronger irritant response than the itch itself. This also contains ground-up seeds that collect in the hair and can make the scalp feel grainy.

☺ **Botanicals Herbal Aloe Therapy Creme** *($4.29 for 3.4 ounces)* is a thick, emollient, leave-in conditioner whose Vaseline, mineral oil, and lanolin base can make even the driest hair feel exceptionally slick and greasy. This is an option for coarse, thick hair, but it's best used sparingly and only on the ends or to smooth stubborn frizzies.

☺ **Botanicals Lite Creme Moisturizer** *($3.99 for 6 ounces)* is indeed light, and is a very good leave-in conditioner for dry hair that is normal to fine, thin, or slightly thick.

☹ **Botanicals Moisturizing Braid Spray** *($5.19 for 12 ounces)* indicates that it should be sprayed directly on the scalp and then massaged in, but it contains the preservative Kathon CG, which is so sensitizing to skin (including the scalp) it is recommended for use only in rinse-out products, which this is not.

☺ **Botanicals Oil** *($4.29 for 4 ounces)* has an apt name because this is primarily oils—seven to be exact, although for dry to very dry hair just one oil will suffice. This is an option for overnight treatment of extremely dry hair that is also coarse or thick, but it should be shampooed out prior to styling to avoid limp, greasy hair.

SOFT & BEAUTIFUL JUST FOR ME

☺ **Just for Me Moisturizing Conditioning Shampoo** *($2.29 for 8 ounces)* is a very standard, but good, shampoo that's an option for normal to slightly dry hair that is normal to fine or thin, and it can cause buildup with repeated use.

☺ **Just for Me Creme Conditioner & Hairdress** *($2.99 for 3.4 ounces)* is an option for very dry hair that is coarse or thick, but use it sparingly to prevent hair from becoming greasy and heavy.

☹ **Just for Me Leave-In Conditioner** *($2.29 for 8 ounces)* contains the preservative Kathon CG, and is not recommended.

☺ **Just for Me Scalp Conditioner & Hairdress** *($2.99 for 3.4 ounces)* is similar to the Botanicals Herbal Aloe Therapy Creme above, and the same basic comments apply. This product is too greasy for daily use on the scalp. The oils it contains can clog the hair follicle and stop or inhibit the scalp's natural exfoliation process.

☺ **Just for Me Pressing Creme** *($4.09 for 3.4 ounces)* is another greasy pomade that is supposed to be used prior to pressing (straightening) curly hair. The emollients and oils it contains can provide some protection during heat styling, but nowhere near enough to avoid damage, and this can make all hair types feel extremely slick and oily. As a pomade for use on very dry ends, this is a decent option.

☺ **Just for Me Styling Creme** *($2.99 for 4 ounces)* is nearly identical to the Botanicals Styling Creme, Firm Hold above, and the same review applies.

☺ **Just for Me Detangler** *($2.99 for 8 ounces)* is a very good detangling conditioner for normal to dry hair that is normal to fine or thin. The film-forming agent can build up with repeated use, so be sure to wash with a chelating shampoo at least once per week.

☺ **Just for Me Oil Moisturizing Lotion** *($5.19 for 8 ounces)* is identical to the Oil Moisturizing Lotion above, and the same review applies.

SOFT & BEAUTIFUL PRO-LINE

☺ **Pro-Line Coconut Oil Conditioner** *($4.59 for 10 ounces)* is one of the greasiest, slickest products reviewed in this book. It has a heavy texture and can absolutely clog hair follicles when massaged into the scalp daily (as instructed). Even a tiny amount of this can instantly make hair feel greasy and heavy. For occasional use on very dry ends or stubborn frizzies, this is an OK option.

☺ **Pro-Line Comb-Thru Lite Creme Moisturizer, Hair & Scalp Conditioner** *($3.89 for 8 ounces)* really is a light conditioner that is an option for dry hair of any thickness.

☺ **Pro-Line Comb-Thru Greaseless Gel Pomade** *($3.75 for 2.99 ounces)* isn't completely greaseless (it contains mineral and sesame oils), but it is much lighter than most of the other pomades in this line, which makes it a better choice for dry to very dry hair that needs smoothing and frizz control but without a slick, heavy look. This should still be used sparingly for best results.

☹ **Pro-Line Perm Repair Setting Lotion for Wraps, Waves, Roller Sets** *($3.09 for 8 ounces)* contains the preservative Kathon CG, and is not recommended.

☺ **Pro-Line Comb-Thru Softener** (*$4.09 for 10 ounces*) is a creamy, leave-in conditioner that is a good option for normal to dry hair of any thickness except very fine or thin, but the fragrance is intense.

☺ **Pro-Line Comb-Thru Wave Keeper, Wave & Styling Gel** (*$3.09 for 8 ounces*) is a very good option for a non-sticky smoothing gel without hold. It works well for dry hair that is normal to fine or thin and could benefit from a moisturizing styling product.

☺ **Pro-Line Hair Food** (*$4.69 for 10 ounces*) is identical to the Pro-Line Coconut Oil Conditioner above, and the same comments apply.

☺ **Pro-Line Comb-Thru Oil Sheen** (*$2.99 for 11 ounces*) is nearly identical to the Oil Sheen above, except this has a slightly lighter texture and finish. Otherwise, the same basic comments apply.

☺ **Pro-Line Soft-n-Sheen for Extra-Dry Hair Oil Sheen and Comb Out Plus Moisturizers** (*$3.19 for 10 ounces*) doesn't contain any oils, but it is glycerin-rich, which makes it appropriate for dry hair of any thickness that needs moisture with some smoothing and slight frizz control.

SOFT SHEEN CARSON

This Chicago-based hair-care company is owned by L'Oreal, and is slowly coming around by offering a greater variety of lightweight, but still effective, products for African-American consumers. Their latest products feature some intriguing options, and show that Soft Sheen Carson is making a commitment (thanks to the cash flow from being owned by one of the largest cosmetics companies in the world) to offer the ethnic hair-care market some choices that have been sorely lacking. There are plenty of standard, overly greasy products still hanging on, but overall this is a worthwhile line to consider and it isn't just the same old, same old. For more information about Soft Sheen Carson, call (800) 442-4643 or visit www.softsheen-carson.com.

What's Good About This Line: A large variety of products that won't leave African-American hair looking like an oil slick; the prices are excellent, while the sizes are generous; the Care Free Curl line takes the lead by offering moisturizing options for curly hair that don't just load it up (and weigh it down) with grease and wax.

What's Not So Good About It: The "classic" products that have been around for years are some of the heaviest, greasiest products on the market; some products make completely unrealistic claims about stopping breakage and repairing hair, especially if your hair has been chemically treated or is routinely heat-styled; a few products contain problematic ingredients such as peppermint oil, balm mint, and the sensitizing preservatives methylchloroisothiazolinone and methylisothiazolinone (Kathon CG).

SOFT SHEEN CARSON ALTERNATIVES

☺ **Alternatives Conditioning Styling Gel** (*$2.99 for 6 ounces*) is a thick styling gel with a medium to firm hold that leaves a moist, slightly sticky finish. It can be brushed through easily, and the collagen base is a good water-binding agent for hair. The tiny amount of bergamot and peppermint extracts (not oils) is unlikely to be a problem for the scalp.

☹ **Alternatives Oil Moisturizer Lotion** *($3.10 for 16 ounces)* contains balm mint and peppermint oils, and that makes this mineral oil-based lotion too irritating for the scalp.

☺ **Alternatives Oil Sheen Spray** *($3.19 for 11.5 ounces)* is a fairly greasy aerosol glossing spray that is a good option for dry to very dry hair that is coarse and needs extra help to achieve a softer feel and smooth finish. Apply this sparingly to avoid a greasy appearance.

SOFT SHEEN CARSON BABY LOVE

☺ **Baby Love Conditioning Shampoo** *($3.55 for 12 ounces)* is a gentle shampoo that is an option for normal to dry hair of any thickness, though it is not capable of completely removing heavy styling products such as pomades or other styling product buildup. This would be a better option for babies if it did not contain fragrance.

☺ **Baby Love Conditioning Detangler** *($3.55 for 8 ounces)* is a very basic, spray-on detangling conditioner that is an option for normal to fine or thin hair that needs a slight amount of help with combing.

☺ **Baby Love Moisturizing Creme Hairdress** *($3.55 for 4 ounces)* is a water- and mineral oil-based styling balm that has a smooth, whipped-cream texture that is easy to distribute through wet or dry hair. It can still feel fairly greasy, so use it sparingly. The baby powder-like scent may not appeal to most adults, but this product is aimed at grooming children's hair anyway.

☹ **Baby Love Moisturizing Hairdress Lotion** *($3.95 for 8 ounces)* is similar to the Baby Love Moisturizing Creme Hairdress above, except with a more emollient, greasier texture. It contains balm mint, peppermint, and sage oils, which makes it an irritating problem for the scalp, especially for kids, and it is not recommended.

SOFT SHEEN CARSON BREAKTHRU

☺ **Breakthru Fortifying Moisturizing Shampoo** *($6.99 for 8.5 ounces)* is a standard, but very good, conditioning shampoo for normal to dry hair of any thickness. The tiny amount of balm mint extract is unlikely to be a problem for the scalp, but be sure to rinse this thoroughly. This can cause buildup with repeated use.

☺ **Breakthru Everyday Moisturizing Strength Lotion** *($5.99 for 8.5 ounces)* claims to help reduce hair breakage, but it's just another greasy styling lotion with a heavy, slick texture that can clog the hair follicles and potentially stunt healthy hair growth with long-term use. It is an option for smoothing frizzy areas or using on dry ends, but is just too greasy to apply all over. This product cannot stop or slow hair breakage because whether or not that happens depends on the chemical services you elect to have or on how much damage your hair incurs from heat-styling implements.

☺ **Breakthru Heat Strengthening Styling Cream** *($5.99 for 5 ounces)* cannot strengthen hair, but it is a very good styling and smoothing cream for normal to dry hair.

It has a light, but still creamy, texture that combines emollients with silicone and avoids the greasy ingredients characteristic of most ethnic hair-care products. This can groom the hair and add shine without pronounced heaviness or a slick finish.

☺ **Breakthru Heat-Style Protecting Foam** *($6.99 for 8.5 ounces)* is a liquid-to-foam mousse with minimal to no hold and a soft, moist finish. It is best for smoothing slightly dry hair that is normal to fine or thin, but should not be relied on to provide more than a slight amount of heat protection. Nothing in it can prevent or slow down hair breakage.

☺ **Breakthru Revitalizing Deep Conditioner** *($5.99 for 8.5 ounces)* is a very standard conditioner that isn't deep in the least, though it can still work well for normal to dry hair that is normal to fine or thin.

SOFT SHEEN CARSON CARE FREE CURL

☹ **Care Free Curl Conditioning Shampoo, with Protein** *($2.99 for 8 ounces)* contains sodium lauryl sulfate as its main detergent cleansing agent, and is not recommended for any hair or scalp type.

☺ **Care Free Curl Keratin Conditioner** *($3.99 for 8 ounces)* is an exceptionally standard conditioner that is a good option for normal to dry hair that is normal to fine or thin.

☺ **Care Free Curl Curl Activator** *($4.99 for 8 ounces)* is a creamy, leave-in conditioner that is somewhat greasy but not terribly so, and is an effective all-over option for very dry hair that is coarse, curly, or thick. Alternatively, it can be used by other hair types to smooth frizzies and dry ends, but it should be applied sparingly.

☺ **Care Free Curl Gold Hair and Scalp Spray** *($3.29 for 8 ounces)* is a moist, non-greasy, spray-on conditioner for dry hair that is normal to fine or thin. This works well to moisturize dry scalp and hair without severely weighing it down, though the moist finish can make hair feel somewhat coated.

☺ **Care Free Curl Gold Instant Activator, with Moisturizers** *($3.49 for 8 ounces)* is a water-based, leave-in conditioner that contains a good complement of lightweight moisturizing agents for dry hair, be it curly or straight. It offers a light, flexible hold and can work beautifully to shape and define curls without a greasy after-feel.

☺ **Care Free Curl Instant Moisturizer, with Glycerine & Protein** *($3.69 for 8 ounces)* is a lighter version of the Care Free Curl Gold Instant Activator above, and the same basic comments apply. Unless used sparingly, this can be a bit too heavy for fine or thin hair.

☺ **Care Free Curl Lite Gel Activator** *($3.49 for 11.5 ounces)* is a lightweight, water- and glycerin-based smoothing gel without any hold. It can leave a slightly sticky, moist feeling on hair, but is a good option for shaping curls or adding moisture without greasiness or a slick finish.

☺ **Care Free Curl Snap Back Curl Restorer** *($3.29 for 8 ounces)* says it can restore curls, but only if your hair is already curly. That's a bit confusing, but at least it's honest. This is a very basic, no-frills smoothing gel that replaces the glycerin in the Care Free Curl gels above with lanolin, so it is preferred for drier hair, but that also means it has a heavier texture that is best for normal to slightly thick or coarse hair. This does not contain any holding agents.

SOFT SHEEN CARSON DARK AND LOVELY

☺ **Dark and Lovely Moisture Seal 3-n-1 Conditioning Shampoo** *($3.49 for 13.5 ounces)* is a very good shampoo for all hair types, but the small amount of conditioning agents is of little help for dry hair. Buildup will be minimal and it will take several shampooings before that can occur.

☺ **Dark and Lovely Moisture Seal Deep Conditioner** *($3.49 for 8.5 ounces)* is a good emollient conditioner for dry hair that is normal to coarse or thick.

☺ **Dark and Lovely Moisture Seal Instant Conditioner** *($3.49 for 13.5 ounces)* is similar to, but slightly more emollient than, the Dark and Lovely Moisture Seal Deep Conditioner above, and the same basic comments apply.

☺ **Dark and Lovely Moisture Seal Daily Oil Moisturizer** *($3.49 for 8.5 ounces)* is a standard, greasy leave-in conditioner that is a good option for smoothing dry ends but can be too heavy for all-over use. The formula is primarily mineral oil, water, Vaseline, glycerin, and thickeners, and it does contain fragrance. This is difficult to shampoo out, and is best for very dry, coarse hair.

☺ **Dark and Lovely Moisture Seal Leave-In Styling Mist** *($3.49 for 8.5 ounces)* is a lightweight, water-based mist that provides a light hold with moderate stickiness. It can be brushed through and is an option for dry hair of any thickness thanks to the absence of heavy, greasy ingredients such as castor oil and Vaseline.

SOFT SHEEN CARSON MEGAHERTZ

☺ **Megahertz Gel>Wax** *($5.99 for 3.4 ounces)* is a thick gel that contains mineral oil to impart a flexible, slightly greasy texture and glossy finish. This offers a light hold that can feel moderately sticky, but leaves hair pliable. It is distinctly lighter than most pomades or styling lotions marketed in the ethnic hair-care market.

☺ **Megahertz Heat Smoothing>Balm** *($5.99 for 6.8 ounces)* is a silky, water- and alcohol-based styling balm that provides minimal to no hold with a slightly sticky finish. This is not the best choice for straightening hair with heat because it lacks a significant amount of conditioning agents and does not contain silicone, which is ideal for creating a straight, sleek look with a frizz-free finish. The packaging may look modern and the claims are enticing, but this is a lackluster entry in the overcrowded category of straightening balms.

☺ **Megahertz Heat>Styling Mist** *($5.99 for 8.5 ounces)* is a basic hairspray that offers a medium hold with a sticky finish, and can actually cause hair to stick *to* any heat-styling implement except a blow dryer. It is recommended only as a finishing spray to set your style when additional control is desired.

☺ **Megahertz Hi:Shine>Gel Pomade** *($5.99 for 2.5 ounces)* is a very standard, water-soluble, gel-type shimmer pomade that is a lighter alternative to the traditional

Vaseline- or lanolin-based pomades so often found in hair-care lines geared toward African-Americans. This can nicely smooth dry ends and frizzies while imparting a soft, wet-look shine. It shampoos out easily.

☺ **Megahertz Liquid>Gel Styler** *($5.99 for 8.5 ounces)* is a standard, lightweight liquid gel with a light hold and a minimally sticky finish that does not make hair feel dry or stiff. It brushes through easily, and is a good option for all hair types when the goal is a soft, casual style.

☺ **Megahertz Hi:Gloss>Serum** *($5.99 for 2.5 ounces)* is a standard, but very good, silicone serum with an attractive price. It is an excellent option for smoothing dry to very dry hair while controlling frizzies and imparting a silky feel and shiny finish.

SOFT SHEEN CARSON OPTIMUM CARE

☺ **Optimum Care Collagen Moisture Shampoo** *($2.29 for 8 ounces)* is a standard shampoo that is a very good option for all hair types, and it poses no risk of buildup.

☺ **Optimum Care Super Protecting Shampoo** *($3.59 for 16.9 ounces)* is a mild shampoo that is an option for any hair type that does not use heavy or emollient styling products.

☹ **Optimum Care Leave-In Conditioner** *($3.59 for 8 ounces)* contains bergamot, peppermint, and sage oils, and is not recommended because all of these ingredients can cause scalp itching and irritation.

☺ **Optimum Care Rich Conditioner** *($3.59 for 16.9 ounces)* works very well for normal to dry hair of any thickness, but for very dry, damaged hair, this is not a top choice for "optimum care."

☺ **Optimum Care Stay Strong Conditioner** *($3.59 for 16.9 ounces)* is nearly identical to the Optimum Care Rich Conditioner above, and the same comments apply.

☺ **Optimum Care Body & Shine Sheen Spray** *($3.59 for 9.5 ounces)* is a wax-based aerosol shine spray that can make hair feel slick and greasy even when used sparingly. It's an OK option if hair is very dry or coarse, but hold it at least 12 inches away from your hair and spray quickly to lightly coat hair without making it too heavy.

☺ **Optimum Care Soft Holding Spritz, with Panthenol** *($3.59 for 8 ounces)* is a very good nonaerosol hairspray that provides a medium hold with a slightly stiff, sticky finish that is easily brushed through. The small amount of conditioning agents can have a slight impact on drier hair.

☺ **Optimum Care Featherlight Hairdress** *($3.59 for 3.4 ounces)* isn't "featherlight" at all. This is one of the heaviest, greasiest pomades around, with a Vaseline, mineral oil, and lanolin base. It is recommended for use only on the ends of very dry, coarse hair; using it all over or massaging it into the scalp will only make hair feel slick and the scalp feel needlessly greasy.

☺ **Optimum Care Moisture Rich, with Vitamin E** *($3.59 for 4 ounces)* is another greasy pomade that can quickly make hair look and feel oily. It is too heavy to enhance texture, but is a decent option for smoothing very dry ends or stubborn frizzies. Use it only with the lightest touch to avoid an oily look and feel.

☺ **Optimum Care Nourishing Creme Hairdress** *($3.59 for 3.4 ounces)* is similar to the Optimum Care Featherlight Hairdress above, and the same review applies.

☹ **Optimum Care Nourishment, with Lanolin & Coconut Oil** *($3.59 for 3.5 ounces)* contains the preservative Kathon CG, which is not recommended for use in leave-on products due to the high risk of causing a sensitizing reaction.

SOFT SHEEN CARSON SPORTIN' WAVES

☺ **Sportin' Waves Gel Pomade, with Wavitrol III** *($2.59 for 3.5 ounces)* claims it is a gel formula that "goes on easy, rinses out clean," but that is absolutely not the case. This is a thick, greasy pomade whose Vaseline base is not easy to shampoo out. It can smooth dry ends and frizzies on very dry, coarse hair, but that's about all the grease your hair should take.

☺ **Sportin' Waves Maximum Hold Pomade** *($2.59 for 3.5 ounces)* is similar to the Sportin' Waves Gel Pomade above, except this is more emollient and greasier. The same basic comments apply. This contains no holding agents, so the "Maximum Hold" in the name is meaningless.

☺ **Sportin' Waves Oil Sheen Spray** *($2.99 for 16.8 ounces)* is an aerosol shine spray that is greasier than the others in the Soft Sheen Carson line. That is great for very dry, coarse hair, but it should be used sparingly to avoid a slick, oily look.

ST. IVES

For more information about St. Ives, whose specialty clearly does not appear to be creating superior hair-care products, call (800) 333-0005 or visit www.stives.com.

What's Good About This Line: The silicone serum is an inexpensive winner for very dry hair.

What's Not So Good About It: The shampoos all contain drying and irritating sodium lauryl sulfate; the conditioners are OK, but not as elegant as many other drug-store options; overall, too many products contain mint or menthol, making them poor choices.

☹ **Extra Body Shampoo Chamomile & Sunflower, for Fine or Thin Hair** *($2.99 for 20 ounces)* contains sodium lauryl sulfate as its main detergent cleansing agent, and that makes it too drying to the hair and also drying and irritating to the scalp.

☹ **Extra Shine Shampoo Raspberry & Jojoba, for Normal Hair** *($2.99 for 20 ounces)* is nearly identical to the Extra Body Shampoo Chamomile & Sunflower, for Fine or Thin Hair above, and is not recommended.

☹ **Revitalizing Shampoo Aloe and Echinacea, for Color Treated Hair** *($2.99 for 20 ounces)* is nearly identical to the Extra Body Shampoo Chamomile & Sunflower, for Fine or Thin Hair above, and is not recommended.

☺ **Extra Body Conditioner Chamomile & Sunflower Volumizing, for Fine or Thin Hair** *($2.99 for 20 ounces)* is a very standard conditioner for normal to slightly dry hair that is normal to fine or thin.

☺ **Extra Shine Conditioner Raspberry & Jojoba, for Normal Hair** *($2.99 for 20 ounces)* is nearly identical to the Extra Body Conditioner Chamomile & Sunflower version above, and the same comments apply. The tiny amount of plant oil it contains is not enough to sufficiently moisturize dry hair.

☺ **Revitalizing Conditioner Aloe and Echinacea, for Color Treated Hair** *($2.99 for 20 ounces)* is nearly identical to the Extra Body Conditioner Chamomile & Sunflower version above, and the same comments apply.

☹ **Hair Repair Hot Oil Moisturizing Treatment** *($3.99 for three 6.25-ounce treatments)* contains menthol, which makes this oil-free hot-oil treatment too irritating to consider unless you keep it completely off the scalp.

☹ **Hair Repair Intensive Conditioner Moisture Treatment** *($3.99 for 12 ounces)* contains mint oil and menthol rather high up on the ingredient list, which only serves to make this "treatment" intensely irritating.

☺ **Hair Repair Mud Miracle Deep Mineral Revitalizer** *($3.99 for 7 ounces)* is a surprisingly good conditioner for normal to slightly dry hair of any thickness. The tiny amount of mud has no negative impact on hair.

☺ **Hair Repair No Frizz Serum** *($7.50 for 1 ounce)* is a silicone serum that also contains several water-binding agents along with mineral and soybean oils, which makes it an especially good option for very dry hair that is coarse, curly, or thick. As with all silicone serums, it should be used sparingly to avoid a greasy appearance.

☺ **Hair Repair Strength & Shine Fortifying Reconstructor** *($3.99 for 10 ounces)* is similar to, but slightly more emollient than, the Extra Body Conditioner Chamomile & Sunflower Volumizing, for Fine or Thin Hair above, which makes it preferred for drier hair. The film-forming agent can build up with repeated use.

SUAVE

For more information about Suave, call (800) 782-8301 or visit www.suave.com or www.suaveformen.com.

What's Good About This Line: Don't let the rock bottom prices keep you from shopping this line—there are worthwhile options in each category, including some very good options for children and for most types of hairstyling.

What's Not So Good About It: Fragrance takes near-top billing in almost every shampoo and conditioner; Suave is a huge line where the majority of products have (for better or worse) nearly identical formulas, and that can make shopping this line cumbersome and confusing; the Performance Series and Professionals by Suave lines are terrible.

☺ **Balsam & Protein Shampoo, for All Hair Types** *($1.29 for 15 ounces)* is a very standard, but good, shampoo that poses no risk of buildup and is an option for all hair types. The tiny amount of balsam will not make hair feel dry or sticky.

☺ **Daily Clarifying Shampoo, for Normal to Oily Hair** *($1.29 for 15 ounces)* is a great inexpensive option for all hair types and will not cause buildup.

The Reviews S

☹ **Moisturizing Shampoo, for Dry or Damaged Hair** *($1.29 for 15 ounces)* contains ammonium xylenesulfonate, a solvent that can swell the hair shaft and cause both hair and scalp dryness.

☹ **Salon Formula Shampoo** *($1.29 for 15 ounces)* is nearly identical to the Moisturizing Shampoo, for Dry or Damaged Hair above, and the same review applies.

☺ **Balsam & Protein Conditioner** *($1.29 for 15 ounces)* is an exceptionally standard conditioner that is a decent option for normal to slightly dry hair that is normal to fine or thin. It does not contain a speck of protein, and the balsam is present in too small an amount to cause dryness or brittle-feeling hair.

☺ **Daily Clarifying Conditioner** *($1.29 for 15 ounces)* is similar to the Balsam & Protein Conditioner above, except that the balsam is replaced by PVP, a film-forming agent that can build up with repeated use, but that will initially make fine or thin hair feel thicker. Otherwise, the same basic comments apply.

☺ **Moisturizing Conditioner** *($1.29 for 15 ounces)* is a basic, no-frills conditioner for normal to slightly dry hair that is normal to fine or thin.

☺ **Salon Formula Conditioner** *($1.29 for 15 ounces)* is nearly identical to the Moisturizing Conditioner above, and the same comments apply.

☺ **Hairspray, Extra Hold (Aerosol)** *($1.29 for 6.5 ounces)* is a very standard, but completely worthwhile, hairspray that provides a light to medium hold with minimal stiff or sticky feel. It brushes through easily and doesn't dry instantly, so you have sufficient playtime to position hair in place before it sets.

☺ **Hairspray, Extra Hold (Non-Aerosol)** *($1.29 for 6.5 ounces)* is a standard, light-hold hairspray with a slightly stiff, sticky feel that can be brushed through easily. The lightweight finish makes it ideal for holding fine or thin hair, but all hair types can use this.

☺ **Hairspray, Extra Hold Unscented (Aerosol)** *($1.29 for 6.5 ounces)* is identical to the Hairspray, Extra Hold (Aerosol) above, except with a less obvious fragrance (meaning this is not fragrance-free).

☺ **Hairspray, Maximum Hold (Aerosol)** *($1.29 for 6.5 ounces)* offers a medium hold with a slightly stiff, sticky feel that can be brushed through with little effort. This contains conditioning agents and tiny amounts of silicone for added shine and a less dry feel.

☺ **Hairspray, Maximum Hold (Non-Aerosol)** *($1.29 for 6.5 ounces)* is a very standard, but good, hairspray with a medium hold and a slightly stiff, sticky feel that can be brushed through. The tiny amount of silicone can help make hair slightly shiny.

☺ **Hairspray, Maximum Hold Unscented (Aerosol)** *($1.29 for 6.5 ounces)* is identical to the Hairspray, Maximum Hold (Aerosol) above, except it contains a softer fragrance to mask the smell of the other ingredients.

☺ **Hairspray, Maximum Hold Unscented (Non-Aerosol)** *($1.29 for 6.5 ounces)* is identical to the Hairspray, Maximum Hold (Non-Aerosol) above, and the same comments apply. This contains a masking fragrance and as such is not technically fragrance-free.

☺ **Sculpting Gel, Maximum Hold** *($1.29 for 16 ounces)* doesn't provide maximum hold, but is a very good, medium-hold styling gel that allows you to create a wide variety of styles without getting too stiff or sticky. The price per ounce makes this one of the best hair-care bargains in this book!

☹ **Shaping Mousse, Extra Hold** *($1.29 for 5 ounces)* contains the problematic TEA-dodecyl-benzenesulfonate, which makes this otherwise standard mousse too drying for hair and irritating to the scalp.

☺ **Styling Gel, Extra Hold** *($1.29 for 16 ounces)* is nearly identical to the Sculpting Gel, Maximum Hold above, except this has slightly more hold and residual stickiness. It is a slightly better choice for styling unruly hair.

☺ **Volume & Control Mousse, Maximum Hold** *($1.29 for 5 ounces)* is a creamy, propellant-based mousse with light to medium hold and a slightly sticky, moist finish that is easily brushed through. This is an excellent mousse for fine or thin hair that is dry.

SUAVE AROMABENEFITS

☹ **AromaBenefits Citrus & Ginseng Energizing Shampoo** *($1.99 for 14.5 ounces)* contains lemon and orange oils along with a high amount of grapefruit extract. These oils and extract make this shampoo smell fresh and zesty, but can also cause scalp dryness and irritation, and that's not worth a pleasant aromatic experience.

☺ **AromaBenefits Cucumber & Melon Refreshing Shampoo** *($1.99 for 14.5 ounces)* is nearly identical to the Daily Clarifying Shampoo, for Normal to Oily Hair above, and the same review applies. The cucumber and melon are strictly for fragrance.

☺ **AromaBenefits Green Tea & Jasmine Soothing Shampoo** *($1.99 for 14.5 ounces)* is nearly identical to the Daily Clarifying Shampoo, for Normal to Oily Hair above, and the same review applies. The plant extracts have no beneficial impact on hair or scalp.

☹ **AromaBenefits Citrus & Ginseng Energizing Conditioner** *($1.99 for 14.5 ounces)* contains lemon and orange oils, making this otherwise very standard conditioner too irritating for the scalp, and the lemon oil is also too drying for hair.

☺ **AromaBenefits Cucumber & Melon Refreshing Conditioner** *($1.99 for 14.5 ounces)* is nearly identical to the Moisturizing Conditioner above, and the same review applies. The plant extracts may smell nice, but they won't help dry hair or add shine.

☺ **AromaBenefits Green Tea & Jasmine Soothing Conditioner** *($1.99 for 14.5 ounces)* is nearly identical to the Moisturizing Conditioner above, and the same review applies. Green tea can be soothing, but the amount in this conditioner is too small for the scalp to notice, and it would be rinsed away before it could have any effect anyway.

SUAVE FOR KIDS

☺ **Suave for Kids Cherry Blast 2-in-1 Shampoo Plus Conditioner** *($1.99 for 12 ounces)* is a standard, but very good, mild conditioning shampoo. It is a good option for shampooing a child's hair, but the fragrance is a bit much.

The Reviews S

☺ **Suave for Kids Orange Splash 2-in-1 Shampoo Plus Conditioner** *($1.99 for 12 ounces)* is, save for a change of fragrance, identical to the Suave for Kids Cherry Blast 2-in-1 Shampoo Plus Conditioner above, and the same review applies.

☺ **Suave for Kids Wild Watermelon 2-in-1 Shampoo Plus Conditioner** *($1.99 for 12 ounces)* is, save for a change of fragrance, identical to the Suave for Kids Cherry Blast 2-in-1 Shampoo Plus Conditioner above, and the same review applies.

☺ **Suave for Kids Go Go Grape Conditioner** *($1.99 for 12 ounces)* is actually a better conditioner formulation than most of the options Suave offers for adults! If you decide to try this, make sure you're OK with the sweet, candy-like grape scent.

☺ **Suave for Kids Awesome Apple Detangling Spray** *($1.99 for 10.5 ounces)* is a good, basic detangling spray for normal to fine or thin hair.

SUAVE HAIR VIBE

☺ **Hair Vibe Berry Shampoo** *($1.99 for 12 ounces)* is nearly identical to the Daily Clarifying Shampoo, for Normal to Oily Hair above, and the same comments apply.

☹ **Hair Vibe Melon 2-in-1 Shampoo** *($1.99 for 12 ounces)* contains TEA-dodecylbenzenesulfonate, which is irritating and drying to the scalp and drying for hair.

☺ **Hair Vibe Berry Conditioner** *($1.99 for 12 ounces)* is a very standard conditioner similar to most of the Suave conditioners above. It is a good, though very basic, option for normal to fine or thin hair that is slightly dry.

☺ **Hair Vibe Max Hold Gel, Apple** *($1.99 for 13 ounces)* is nearly identical to the Sculpting Gel, Maximum Hold above, and the same review applies. The apple fragrance is intense, so make sure you like it before buying.

☺ **Hair Vibe Shine & Shape Spray Gel, Melon** *($1.99 for 8.5 ounces)* is a more fluid version of the Sculpting Gel, Maximum Hold above, except with a melon fragrance and added mica for shimmery shine. The mica has a slight tendency to flake, but the gel itself does not.

SUAVE NATURALS

☺ **Naturals Aloe Vera Shampoo** *($1.29 for 15 ounces)* is nearly identical to the Daily Clarifying Shampoo, for Normal to Oily Hair above, and the same comments apply.

☺ **Naturals Chamomile Shampoo** *($1.29 for 15 ounces)* is nearly identical to the Daily Clarifying Shampoo, for Normal to Oily Hair above, but this contains a small amount of plant oil, which has a slight impact on drier hair. Otherwise, the same basic comments apply.

☺ **Naturals Freesia Shampoo** *($1.29 for 15 ounces)* is nearly identical to the Daily Clarifying Shampoo, for Normal to Oily Hair above, and the same comments apply.

☺ **Naturals Fresh Mountain Strawberry Shampoo** *($1.29 for 15 ounces)* is nearly identical to the Daily Clarifying Shampoo, for Normal to Oily Hair above, and the same comments apply. The strawberry juice only adds to the strong fragrance of this shampoo.

☺ **Naturals Juicy Green Apple Shampoo** *($1.29 for 15 ounces)* is nearly identical to the Daily Clarifying Shampoo, for Normal to Oily Hair above, and the same comments apply. This does have an intense apple fragrance, which may or may not be to your liking.

☹ **Naturals Lavender Shampoo** *($1.29 for 15 ounces)* contains peppermint, and that makes it a problem for all scalp types.

☺ **Naturals Ocean Breeze Shampoo** *($1.29 for 15 ounces)* is nearly identical to the Daily Clarifying Shampoo, for Normal to Oily Hair above, and the same review applies.

☹ **Naturals Passion Flower Shampoo** *($1.29 for 15 ounces)* is nearly identical to the Naturals Lavender Shampoo above, and the same review applies.

☺ **Naturals Sun-Ripened Raspberry Shampoo** *($1.29 for 15 ounces)* is nearly identical to the Daily Clarifying Shampoo, for Normal to Oily Hair above, and the same review applies.

☹ **Naturals Tropical Coconut Shampoo** *($1.29 for 15 ounces)* contains ammonium xylenesulfonate, a solvent that can swell the hair shaft and cause both hair and scalp dryness.

☺ **Naturals Vanilla Floral Shampoo** *($1.29 for 15 ounces)* is nearly identical to the Daily Clarifying Shampoo, for Normal to Oily Hair above, and the same review applies.

☺ **Naturals Aloe Vera Conditioner** *($1.29 for 15 ounces)* is nearly identical to the Hair Vibe Berry Conditioner above, and the same review applies.

☺ **Naturals Freesia Conditioner** *($1.29 for 15 ounces)* is nearly identical to the Hair Vibe Berry Conditioner above, and the same review applies.

☺ **Naturals Fresh Mountain Strawberry Conditioner** *($1.29 for 15 ounces)* is nearly identical to the Hair Vibe Berry Conditioner above, and the same review applies. The strawberry juice can make hair feel slightly sticky if this is not rinsed thoroughly.

☺ **Naturals Juicy Green Apple Conditioner** *($1.29 for 15 ounces)* is nearly identical to the Hair Vibe Berry Conditioner above, and the same review applies.

☹ **Naturals Lavender Conditioner** *($1.29 for 15 ounces)* contains peppermint, and is not recommended due to the potential risk of scalp irritation.

☺ **Naturals Ocean Breeze Conditioner** *($1.29 for 15 ounces)* is nearly identical to the Balsam & Protein Conditioner above, only without the balsam, and the same basic comments apply.

☹ **Naturals Passion Flower Conditioner** *($1.29 for 15 ounces)* contains peppermint, and is not recommended due to the potential risk of scalp irritation.

☺ **Naturals Sun-Ripened Raspberry Conditioner** *($1.29 for 15 ounces)* is nearly identical to the Balsam & Protein Conditioner above, only without the balsam, and the same basic comments apply.

☺ **Naturals Tropical Coconut Conditioner** *($1.29 for 15 ounces)* is nearly identical to the Hair Vibe Berry Conditioner above, and the same review applies.

☺ **Naturals Vanilla Floral Conditioner** *($1.29 for 15 ounces)* is nearly identical to the Hair Vibe Berry Conditioner above, and the same review applies.

☺ **Naturals Aloe Vera Extra Hold Frizz Control Gel** *($1.99 for 16 ounces)* is a very standard, medium-hold gel that leaves hair feeling minimally stiff but noticeably sticky. It's a decent option for most hair types; those with dry hair will likely want a product that will leave the hair feeling softer and conditioned.

☺ **Naturals Aloe Vera Extra Hold Hairspray (Aerosol)** *($1.79 for 8.5 ounces)* is a standard hairspray that provides a light hold with a minimal stiff, sticky feel that can be brushed through. The small amount of silicones can add a touch of shine to your finished style.

☹ **Naturals Aloe Vera Shaping Mousse** *($1.79 for 6 ounces)* is nearly identical to the Shaping Mousse, Extra Hold above, and the same review applies.

☺ **Naturals Freesia Flexible Hold Hairspray (Aerosol)** *($1.79 for 8.5 ounces)* is nearly identical to the Naturals Aloe Vera Extra Hold Hairspray above, and the same review applies.

☺ **Naturals Freesia Flexible Hold Non-Aerosol Hairspray** *($1.79 for 8.5 ounces)* is, with the exception of plant extracts that are present only for show, nearly identical to the Hairspray, Extra Hold (Non-Aerosol) above, and the same review applies.

☺ **Naturals Freesia Flexible Hold Shine & Shaping Gel** *($1.79 for 8.5 ounces)* is a water-based, alcohol-free gel that offers minimal to no hold with a barely sticky after-feel. This is a good option for smoothing hairstyles that don't demand hold, and its lightweight feel makes it appropriate for normal to fine or thin hair.

☺ **Naturals Ocean Breeze Extra Control Spray Gel** *($1.79 for 8.5 ounces)* is a medium- to firm-hold styling spray that is a great choice for styling stubborn, unruly hair. It has a slightly stiff, sticky finish, but can be brushed through. Used on dry (not damp) hair, this provides stronger hold and can nicely emphasize hair texture.

SUAVE PERFORMANCE SERIES

☹ **Performance Series Fruit Energy Fortifying Shampoo** *($1.99 for 14.5 ounces)* is a problem shampoo that contains TEA-dodecylbenzenesulfonate (which can strip hair color with repeated use) along with orange and lemon oils, which makes for one seriously drying and irritating shampoo for all hair and scalp types.

☹ **Performance Series 2-in-1 Shampoo Plus Conditioner** *($1.99 for 14.5 ounces)* contains TEA-dodecylbenzenesulfonate, and is not recommended.

☹ **Performance Series Cleansing Care 2-in-1 Shampoo Plus Conditioner** *($1.99 for 14.5 ounces)* contains TEA-dodecylbenzenesulfonate, and is not recommended.

☹ **Performance Series Smoothing 2-in-1 Shampoo Plus Conditioner, with Pro-Vitamin for Dry or Damaged** *($1.99 for 14.5 ounces)* contains TEA-dodecylbenzenesulfonate, and is not recommended.

☹ **Performance Series Fruit Energy Fortifying Conditioner** *($1.99 for 14.5 ounces)* contains TEA-dodecylbenzenesulfonate along with lemon and orange oils, and is absolutely not recommended.

☹ **Performance Series Smoothing Conditioner, with Pro-Vitamin for Dry or Damaged Hair** *($1.99 for 14.5 ounces)* contains TEA-dodecylbenzenesulfonate, and is not recommended.

☺ **Performance Series Vitamin Infusing Leave-In Conditioner** *($1.99 for 14.5 ounces)* is as standard as it gets for leave-in conditioners, but this is still a good option for fine or thin hair that needs help with combing and controlling static, flyaway strands.

☹ **Performance Series 2-Minute Recovery Deep Conditioner** *($1.99 for 8.5 ounces)* contains TEA-dodecylbenzenesulfonate, and is not recommended.

☺ **Performance Series Moisturizing Hot Oil** *($1.99 for three 0.5-ounce tubes)* is such a basic, do-nothing product it almost isn't even worth mentioning. This does not contain any oil; it's mostly water, film-forming/detangling agent, gel-based thickener, slip agent, preservatives, and fragrance. It can be minimally helpful for fine or thin hair that is difficult to comb through, but that's it.

☺ **Performance Series Strengthening Hot Oil** *($1.99 for three 0.5-ounce tubes)* is identical to the Performance Series Moisturizing Hot Oil above, and the same review applies.

SUAVE PROFESSIONALS

☹ **Professionals Amplifying Shampoo** *($1.99 for 14.5 ounces)* contains TEA-dodecylbenzenesulfonate, and is not recommended.

☹ **Professionals Awapuhi Shampoo** *($1.99 for 14.5 ounces)* contains ammonium xylenesulfonate, a solvent that can swell the hair shaft and lead to hair and scalp dryness, making this a poor choice for shampoo.

☹ **Professionals BioBasics Shampoo** *($1.99 for 14.5 ounces)* is similar to the Professionals Awapuhi Shampoo above, and the same comments apply.

☹ **Professionals Humectant Shampoo** *($1.99 for 14.5 ounces)* is similar to the Professionals Awapuhi Shampoo above, and the same comments apply.

☹ **Professionals Amplifying Conditioner** *($1.99 for 14.5 ounces)* contains TEA-dodecylbenzenesulfonate, and is not recommended.

☹ **Professionals Awapuhi Conditioner** *($1.99 for 14.5 ounces)* contains TEA-dodecylbenzenesulfonate, and is not recommended.

☹ **Professionals BioBasics Conditioner** *($1.99 for 14.5 ounces)* contains TEA-dodecylbenzenesulfonate, and is not recommended.

☹ **Professionals Humectant Conditioner** *($1.99 for 14.5 ounces)* contains TEA-dodecylbenzenesulfonate, and is not recommended.

SUAVE RAVE

☹ **Rave 2x Extra Bodifying Mousse** *($1.99 for 6 ounces)* is nearly identical to the Shaping Mousse, Extra Hold above, and the same review applies. In case you haven't noticed, Suave is adept at recycling the same basic formulas into all of their various hair-care sub-lines.

☺ **Rave 2x Extra Texture Creme** *($1.99 for 8 ounces)* is a very good, emollient styling cream that is a great option for dry hair that is coarse or thick. Its water and Vaseline base can leave hair feeling greasy if not used sparingly. It does provide a light, soft-touch hold that leaves hair smooth and pliable.

☺ **Rave 3x Ultra Holding Paste** *($1.99 for 2.25 ounces)* is the pomade version of the Rave 2x Extra Texture Creme above. It has a thick, creamy texture that can feel quite heavy, so it's best used sparingly on the ends of hair or to tame frizzies. It is an OK option to add extreme texture with hold to short, spiked hairstyles.

☺ **Rave 3x Ultra Scented Hairspray (Aerosol)** *($1.99 for 8.5 ounces)* is a standard, light hold hairspray with a minimal stiff, sticky feel that can be brushed through. It is very similar to most of the Suave aerosol hairsprays above.

☺ **Rave 3x Ultra Scented Hairspray (Non-Aerosol)** *($1.99 for 8.5 ounces)* is a standard, light-hold hairspray with a soft, minimally sticky finish that is a breeze to brush through. It is similar to most of the Suave nonaerosol hairsprays above.

☺ **Rave 3x Ultra Alcohol-Free Shaping Gel** *($1.99 for 13 ounces)* is a very standard gel that has a thick texture and provides a light to medium hold with a moist, sticky finish. For a wet-look gel, this isn't the best-feeling option available. However, once brushed through it softens and can be great for all but extreme or complex hairstyles.

☺ **Rave 3x Ultra Shaping Mousse** *($1.99 for 6 ounces)* is identical to the Volume & Control Mousse above, and the same review applies.

☺ **Rave 3x Ultra Styling Spray** *($1.99 for 8.5 ounces)* is nearly identical to the Hairspray, Extra Hold (Non-Aerosol) above, and the same review applies. This dries too quickly to be considered a styling spray, but as a hairspray, it's fine.

☺ **Rave 3x Ultra Unscented Hairspray (Aerosol)** *($1.99 for 8.5 ounces)* is not unscented because it contains masking fragrance to mask the smell of the other ingredients. Other than the reduced fragrance, this is identical to the Rave 3x Ultra Scented Hairspray (Aerosol) above, and the same review applies.

☺ **Rave 3x Ultra Unscented Hairspray (Non-Aerosol)** *($1.99 for 8.5 ounces)* is identical to the Rave 3X Ultra Scented Hairspray (Non-Aerosol) above, and the same review applies. Despite the name, this does contain fragrance, though it is subtle.

☺ **Rave 3x Ultra Volumizing Spray Gel** *($1.99 for 8.5 ounces)* is nearly identical to the Naturals Ocean Breeze Extra Control Spray Gel above, except this omits the plant extracts, which has no effect on its hold or finish.

☺ **Rave 4x Mega Scented Hairspray (Aerosol)** *($1.99 for 8.5 ounces)* is nearly identical to the Hairspray, Extra Hold (Aerosol) above, and the same review applies.

☺ **Rave 4x Mega Scented Hairspray (Non-Aerosol)** *($1.99 for 8.5 ounces)* doesn't offer any more hold than the 3x nonaerosol hairsprays above, and this is nearly identical to the Rave 3x Ultra Scented Hairspray (Aerosol) above, which means this collection of hairsprays is becoming awfully repetitive.

☺ **Rave 4x Mega Alcohol-Free Sculpting Gel** *($1.99 for 13 ounces)* is nearly identical to the Naturals Aloe Vera Extra Hold Frizz Control Gel above, and the same review applies.

☺ **Rave 4x Mega Unscented Hairspray (Aerosol)** *($1.99 for 8.5 ounces)* is, with the exception of reduced fragrance, identical to the Rave 4x Mega Scented Hairspray (Aerosol) above, and the same comments apply.

☺ **Rave 4x Mega Unscented Hairspray (Non-Aerosol)** *($1.99 for 8.5 ounces)* is identical to the Rave 3X Ultra Scented Hairspray (Non-Aerosol) above, and the same review applies. This does contain fragrance, though it is subtle.

☺ **Rave 6x Extreme Alcohol-Free Molding Gel** *($1.99 for 13 ounces)* is nearly identical to the Naturals Aloe Vera Extra Hold Frizz Control Gel above, except with slightly more hold and a stickier finish, but it can still be brushed through.

SUAVE FOR MEN

☹ **Suave for Men Deep Cleaning Shampoo** *($1.99 for 14.5 ounces)* contains orange and lemon oils, which makes this shampoo too irritating for the scalp, while the lemon oil can also be drying to hair.

☺ **Suave for Men Thickening Shampoo, for Thick Full Hair** *($1.99 for 14.5 ounces)* won't thicken hair in the least, so if the man you're shopping for has thinning hair, don't buy this and get his hopes up. On the other hand, it also won't build up on hair, which is good news for anyone with fine or thin hair, though film-forming agents in shampoos can initially make this hair type feel thicker. The small amount of wheat protein in this product is not enough to constitute a single breadcrumb, let alone offer benefit for the hair.

☹ **Suave for Men 2-in-1 Shampoo Plus Conditioner** *($1.99 for 14.5 ounces)* contains TEA-dodecylbenzenesulfonate, which can be drying to scalp and hair as well as potentially strip hair color with repeated use.

☹ **Suave for Men Dandruff 2-in-1 Shampoo Plus Conditioner, with Zinc Pyrithione** *($1.99 for 14.5 ounces)* contains both TEA-dodecylbenzenesulfonate and ammonium xylenesulfonate, which makes this shampoo a must to avoid, dandruff or not. (If you have dandruff, this product will make it worse.)

☺ **Suave for Men Holding Spray, Extreme Hold 10** *($1.99 for 8.5 ounces)* is a basic hairspray that does have a strong hold, meaning that once it's in place you won't be able to easily comb through your hair unless it's in optimum condition.

☺ **Suave for Men Style Gel, Max Hold 8** *($1.99 for 13 ounces)* is a very standard, but effective, styling gel that has a relatively firm hold and a minimally sticky finish that still brushes through easily. There are more exciting styling gels available, but for a man on a budget who just wants something to slick through his hair and go, this is a workable option—just make sure you like the potent scent before purchasing this for the man in your life.

☺ **Suave for Men Sport Gel, Extreme Hold 10** *($1.99 for 13 ounces)* is nearly identical to the Suave for Men Style Gel, Max Hold 8 above, and the same comments apply. The claim of extreme hold is not possible given the holding agent in this product. For very firm hold, combine this gel with the Suave for Men Holding Spray, Extreme Hold 10 above.

SUKESHA

For more information about Sukesha, call (800) 221-3496 or visit www.sukesha.com.

What's Good About This Line: The prices; there are some very good shampoos and hairsprays to consider.

What's Not So Good About It: Sukesha claims their products are made of all-natural ingredients, but when was the last time you saw a butyl ester of PVM/MA copolymer plant at your local greenhouse?

☺ **Extra Body Shampoo, Mild, Deep Cleansing for Added Texture** *($5.95 for 12 ounces)* is a very good shampoo for all hair types and it will not cause buildup.

☺ **Moisturizing Shampoo, Shampoo and Conditioner in One** *($5.95 for 12 ounces)* is similar to the Extra Body Shampoo, Mild, Deep Cleansing for Added Texture above, except this contains a film-forming agent and conditioning agents that can build up with repeated use. It is an option for normal to slightly dry hair that is normal to fine or thin to help make it feel thicker.

☺ **Natural Balance Shampoo, Pure and Gentle Shine and Volume** *($5.95 for 12 ounces)* is nearly identical to the Extra Body Shampoo, Mild, Deep Cleansing for Added Texture above, and the same review applies. The tiny amount of film-forming agent poses minimal to no risk of buildup.

☺ **Conditioning Rinse** *($5.95 for 8 ounces)* is a standard emollient conditioner that is good for normal to dry hair that is coarse or thick.

☹ **Shine and Body, Leave-In Conditioner** *($5.95 for 8 ounces)* contains the preservatives methylchloroisothiazolinone and methylisothiazolinone (Kathon CG), which are not recommended for use in leave-in products due to the risk of a sensitizing skin reaction.

☺ **Freeze Frame Super Spray, Superior Hold and Shine (Non-Aerosol)** *($6.95 for 8 ounces)* is a very light nonaerosol hairspray with a soft, flexible hold that is ideal for shaping hair while still allowing movement and easy comb-through. It does not leave hair stiff and is minimally sticky.

☺ **Glossing Gel, Brilliant Shine-Plus-Hold Formula** *($6.95 for 8 ounces)* is a well-named product. It is a light-hold styling gel with enough silicone and film-forming agent to impart shine and keep hair in place. This works well for all hair types, but should be used sparingly on fine or thin hair.

☺ **Maximum Hold Hair Spray, Ultimate Hold Formula (Aerosol)** *($8.95 for 10 ounces)* is a fairly sticky hairspray that provides a medium hold and is slightly difficult to brush through. It has a heavier finish that is inappropriate for fine or thin hair, but can work well to set normal to thick or coarse hair without getting stiff.

☺ **Sculpturing Lotion Extra Hold, Styling Formula for Extra Hold and Body** *($6.95 for 12 ounces)* is a medium- to firm-hold styling lotion that can have a somewhat stiff, sticky feel but can easily be brushed through.

☺ **Shaping & Styling Hair Spray, Firm Designing Formula (Aerosol)** *($8.95 for 10 ounces)* is the aerosol version of the Freeze Frame Super Spray, Superior Hold and Shine above, and the same review applies. Which hairspray to choose is a matter of preference, because both are excellent.

☺ **Styling Gel, Ultimate Body and Hold Formula** *($6.95 for 8 ounces)* is a standard gel that has a light to medium hold and minimal to no stiff or sticky feel.

☺ **Styling Hair Spray, Working Spray with Firm Control (Non-Aerosol)** *($6.95 for 8 ounces)* is a very standard hairspray that provides a firm hold with a stiff, sticky finish. It is best for hard-to-hold hair that needs long-lasting style support you don't intend to brush through later. This dries too fast and holds too strongly to be a good working spray.

☺ **Styling Mouse, for Extra Control and Volume** *($6.95 for 12 ounces)* is a standard, propellant-based mousse with a medium hold and a moist, sticky finish that can be brushed through. It is a good option for normal to fine or thin hair that is slightly dry.

☺ **Daily Hydrating Balm, Restores Vitality and Detangles** *($5.95 for 8 ounces)* is a lightweight detangling option for normal to fine or thin hair, but only goes so far to restore hair's vitality, especially if it is dry or damaged.

☺ **Hair Moisturizing Treatment, Intensive Formula for Elasticity & Strength** *($5.95 for 8 ounces)* is a standard, rank-and-file conditioner for normal to dry hair of any thickness. You can expect this to moisturize and soften hair, but not to restore strength to damaged hair, and it's not much of a treatment.

TCB

Owned by Alberto Culver and distributed by Proline International, tcb is an acronym for Taking Care of Beauty, a line of drugstore hair-care products marketed to the needs of African-American women. A couple of years ago, in an attempt to refresh the line's image, an updated logo and new packaging were created, and products were given more contemporary names, such as the Balancing Creme Conditioner and the Energizing Shampoo. The visual improvement is nice enough, but a bigger share of the budget might have been better spent improving the formulations because this line definitely has its share of dated ones. Ironically, the products offered in the Alberto VO5 and TRESemme lines have considerably better, state-of-the-art options than most of what is available here. African-American consumers would do well to venture beyond the ethnic hair-care section to see what's new in other recommended lines at the drugstore and in salons because these have wonderful properties for their hair-care needs, too. For more information about tcb, call (800) 333-6666 or visit www.proline-intl.com.

The Reviews T

What's Good About This Line; There are a few lighter, nongreasy textured products to consider.

What's Not So Good About It: The shampoos are drying to hair and scalp, and that's bad news for already dry, fragile African-American hair; several of the cream and leave-in conditioning hairdress products are moderately to intolerably greasy; tcb brags about their No Lye hair relaxer, but while the product doesn't contain lye, the pH is over 13 and that is what damages the hair and that *is* no lie.

☹ **Energizing Shampoo** *($2.49 for 6 ounces)* contains sodium lauryl sulfate as its main detergent cleansing agent, which isn't energizing, it's irritating to the scalp and drying to hair.

☹ **Maximum Moisture Shampoo** *($3.95 for 16 ounces)* is similar to the Energizing Shampoo above, and the same comments apply.

☺ **Balancing Creme Conditioner** *($1.99 for 6 ounces)* is an emollient conditioner that is an OK option for dry hair that is normal to thick or coarse.

☹ **Creme Protein Conditioner** *($3.95 for 16 ounces)* contains peppermint, which makes it too irritating to the scalp. The Balancing Creme Conditioner above is similar to this product, but without the potential scalp irritants.

☺ **Hair & Scalp Conditioner** *($4.35 for 10 ounces)* is mainly mineral oil, Vaseline, and lanolin, and is a very greasy, slick product that would be a problem for all-over scalp use because it can clog hair follicles, preventing natural exfoliation and stunting healthy hair growth. This liquefies to oil almost instantly, and is recommended (and receives a happy face rating) for use only on the ends of very dry, coarse hair.

☺ **Lite Hair & Scalp Conditioner** *($4.39 for 10 ounces)* is considerably lighter than the Hair & Scalp Conditioner above, and is on a par with, but slightly heavier than, a standard, water-soluble, gel-based pomade. This can work very well to smooth and soften coarse, unruly hair or to smooth very dry ends or frizzies. It can still be too greasy for daily use on the scalp.

☺ **Foaming Wrap-n-Set Lotion** *($3.79 for 6 ounces)* works well as a light-hold, moist-finish, liquid-to-foam mousse. It has a minimally sticky feel and does not stiffen on hair, and the conditioning agents provide a slight amount of protection from heat-styling implements.

☺ **Naturals Lite Gel Activator** *($3.69 for 10 ounces)* is a water- and glycerin-based smoothing gel with minimal to no hold. It is a good option for dry hair that is normal to fine and needs minimal shaping or control to maintain its style. This has a moist, slightly sticky finish that can be brushed through easily.

☺ **Thermal Pro, Blow Dry Lotion** *($3.79 for 6 ounces)* starts out creamy, but turns into a light styling cream with minimal to no hold. It's an option for slightly dry hair that is normal to slightly thick or coarse, but its basic formulation would have been much better had they included silicone, glycerin, or a small amount of plant oil. This can provide a very slight amount of protection during heat styling.

☺ **Creme Hairdress** (*$3.95 for 6 ounces*) is a water- and mineral oil-based styling cream that is a great choice for very dry hair that is extremely coarse or thick. Use it sparingly to avoid a heavy feel and greasy look, but it will make hair soft and shiny, and help keep frizzies at bay. It provides a soft hold and provides a slight amount of protection during heat styling.

☹ **Hair Food** (*$4.35 for 10 ounces*) isn't food for hair, it's more like grease for hair, plain and simple. It is a slick, emollient balm that is too oily for all but the select few whose hair is so coarse, dry, and wiry that they can almost break it by touching it. All others proceed with caution.

☹ **Hydrating Hot Oil Treatment** (*$2.89 for 2 ounces*) does not contain any oils, nor is it all that hydrating. It is of minimal benefit to slightly dry hair that is normal to fine or thin.

☹ **Oil Sheen and Conditioning Spray** (*$3.85 for 11 ounces*) is aerosol-propelled wax, along with small amounts of plant oils and plant extracts. This can add a smooth, shiny finish to the hair, but will quickly make it feel coated. Over time, repeated use of this product can make hair feel heavy and look dull.

TERAX

Terax is a line of Italian hair-care products marketed in the United States. It is available in some salons and at Sephora stores. For more information about terax, call (315) 458-2290 or visit www.teraxhaircare.com.

What's Good About This Line: Terax is one of the few cosmetics companies that provide complete product ingredient lists on their Web site; although the products are quite standard, there are some effective styling products.

What's Not So Good About It: All of the shampoos contain drying sodium lauryl sulfate as their main detergent cleansing agent; the prices are over-the-top, while the products are mostly below average.

☹ **Original Shamp Antiforfora** (*$16 for 8.4 ounces*) is a below-standard shampoo that contains sodium lauryl sulfate as its main detergent cleansing agent, which can make hair and scalp dry and irritate the scalp. This does contain anti-dandruff ingredients, but the percentages are not revealed (nor are they listed as active ingredients). Even if they had that part right, this would still be too drying, and there are gentler shampoos to help you battle dandruff.

☹ **Original Shamp Bambini** (*$12 for 8.4 ounces*) is as basic as shampoo gets, but this one contains sodium lauryl sulfate as its main detergent cleansing agent, which is too drying for hair and also drying and irritating for the scalp.

☹ **Original Shamp Bosco** (*$12 for 8.4 ounces*) contains sodium lauryl sulfate as its main detergent cleansing agent, and is not recommended for any hair or scalp type. This also contains peppermint, which only adds to the irritation from the detergent cleansing agent.

☹ **Original Shamp Collagene** *($12 for 8.4 ounces)* is nearly identical to the Original Shamp Bambini above, and the same review applies.

☹ **Original Shamp Delicato** *($12 for 8.4 ounces)* is nearly identical to the Original Shamp Bambini above, and the same review applies.

☹ **Original Shamp Fior Di Camomilla** *($12 for 8.4 ounces)* is nearly identical to the Original Shamp Bambini above, and the same review applies.

☹ **Original Shamp Latte** *($12 for 8.4 ounces)* is nearly identical to the Original Shamp Bambini above, and the same review applies.

☹ **Original Shamp Miele** *($12 for 8.4 ounces)* is nearly identical to the Original Shamp Bambini above, and the same review applies.

☹ **Original Lotion Hydrate** *($24 for 6.7 ounces)* is a basic, no-frills, leave-in conditioner that contains the preservatives methylchloroisothiazolinone and methylisothiazolinone (Kathon CG), which are not recommended for use in leave-on products due to the high risk of causing a skin-sensitizing reaction. Even without the preservative issue, this is one of the most boring leave-in conditioners around, and the price is ridiculous for what you get.

☹ **Original Lotion Life Drops** *($24 for 6.7 ounces)* lists two types of irritating alcohols high on the ingredient list, along with mostly wax, fragrance, and a minute amount of protein. This product is a mistake for any part of your life and a problem for your hair or scalp. It also contains the preservative Kathon CG, which adds injury to insult.

☺ **$$$ Original Lotion Rigene 8** *($20 for 6.7 ounces)* claims it is *the* conditioner for locking in hair color, but it contains nothing that can achieve that goal. This rinse-out formulation is nearly identical to the Original Lotion Hydrate above, so this is a very basic conditioner. It is an OK option for normal to slightly dry hair that needs help with combing and a dose of light moisture.

☹ **Original Lotion Shine** *($24 for 6.7 ounces)* is another leave-in conditioner that differs little from the Original Lotion Hydrate above, and it contains Kathon CG, which makes it a problem for the scalp.

☺ **$$$ Luxcent Hair Pomade** *($14 for 2.5 ounces)* contains merely polyethylene glycol (PEG) thickeners, sunscreen agent, preservatives, and fragrance. It has a thick texture but is easy to emulsify and distribute through hair. This can add texture and shine without being too heavy, but should be used sparingly to avoid a slick, greasy appearance. It is an option for all hair types except fine or thin.

☺ **$$$ Original Lotion Stirante, Leave-in Vegetable Straightening Lotion** *($18 for 5 ounces)* is an extremely ordinary, lightweight styling lotion that can add shine and smoothness, and will work for all hair types.

☺ **$$$ Original Lotion Volume, Leave-in Volumizing and Conditioning Spray** *($16 for 5 ounces)* is similar to the Stirante above, and the same basic comments apply. This version works better for those looking for minimal hold and more smoothness.

☺ **Original Spray Volumizing Hairspray, Forte** *($14 for 8.4 ounces)* is a standard, alcohol-based hairspray (don't worry, the alcohol evaporates before it can have a drying effect on the hair) with a light, touchable hold and a minimal sticky feel that can be brushed through easily.

☺ **Original Spray Volumizing Hairspray, Leggero** *($14 for 8.4 ounces)* is nearly identical to the Original Spray Volumizing Hairspray, Forte above, except this is slightly less sticky and has an even softer finish. Otherwise, the same review applies.

☺ **$$$ Original Volumizing Mousse** *($16 for 8.4 ounces)* is an exceptionally standard, propellant-based mousse with a light hold and a soft, non-sticky finish that is easily brushed through without flaking. The lightweight conditioning agents make this a good choice for fine or thin hair that is slightly dry.

☹ **Original Gel Styling Gel, for All Hair Types** *($8 for 5 ounces)* is an average styling gel that provides medium to firm hold with an intensely sticky finish that is moderately stiff, but it can still be brushed through. The high amount of glycerin makes this helpful for dry hair, but there are lighter, more elegant styling gels available.

☹ **$$$ Original Crema Hair Treatment** *($16 for 5 ounces)* is supposedly the hair-care product that gained this Italian hair-care line its reputation and instant cachet with the pop culture's beauty elite, but for the life of me I can't figure out why. Yes, this is a decent conditioner for slightly dry hair of any thickness except coarse, but it is so stunningly basic! It contains mostly water, thickener, pH adjuster, fragrance, more thickener, isopropyl alcohol, detangling agents, anti-static agent, and sodium lauryl sulfate (used in a tiny amount as an emulsifier, so it is not cause for concern). It's great that terax's press releases mention several celebrities who use this conditioner, but that doesn't automatically mean it's true (or that the products are good), and moreover celebrities can be just as fickle about products as any other consumer, or they may have moved on to better options which I recommend you do, too.

The big claim for this product's alleged superiority is that it has a slightly alkaline pH, which enhances the conditioner's penetration throughout the cuticle layers. It's all bogus. This conditioner actually has a pH similar to the pH of most conditioners, which is between 5.5 and 6.5 (which is acidic, not alkaline). If this were even slightly alkaline, it could cause the hair shaft to swell and actually damage the cuticle layers with repeated use. Opening up the cuticle layer only exposes it to damage, and that doesn't bode well for creating or maintaining healthy hair. Terax further claims that this conditioner contains natural proteins, but (at least according to the ingredient list, which I have to assume is accurate) proteins are nowhere to be found in this conditioner. Even if there were proteins, they are just one of many good conditioning/water-binding agents for the hair, and not in any way unique or worth the extra expense.

☺ **$$$ Original Gloss** *($16 for 1 ounce)* is a standard silicone serum, plain and simple. It works beautifully to smooth dry to very dry hair while adding lustrous shine and taming frizzies. Less expensive (and larger-sized) silicone serums abound at the drugstore, but if you're in the mood to splurge for no logical reason, this won't disappoint.

THERMASILK

Despite some excellent formulas, the claims made for these products about releasing moisturizing benefits under heat don't hold up, at least not all the way up, on high heat, which is the way most consumers use blow dryers, flat irons, or curling irons to style their hair. While it is indeed better to have styling products on the hair as a buffer to the rigors of styling tools, they can't keep the intense heat these implements generate from assaulting the hair.

You also have to wonder: What good are conditioning ingredients, even those supposedly meant to be activated by heat, when they're in a shampoo, which is mostly rinsed down the drain? Or what happens when they are added to finishing hairsprays, which are applied after the heat has been turned off? What's even more significant is that none of the conditioning agents thermaSilk uses are unique—they are the same ones that show up in countless other hair-care products, and include primarily silicone and silk amino acids.

What is true is that indirect or low heat can help all conditioning agents penetrate the hair cuticle. Both indirect heat and low heat are vastly better than high heat applied directly to the hair. Indirect heat is the type you get when you're sitting under a dryer bonnet at a salon and the heat source is at least six inches away from the hair. When a conditioner is left on your hair and the warmth circulates around it, the cuticle can open up and the conditioning agents can form a better bond with the hair shaft. However, that's not what happens with blow dryers and curling irons, which can heat up to over 300°F in direct contact with the hair! Think of it this way: If a flat iron or blow dryer can burn your skin, it can damage your hair. No matter how well formulated it is, no conditioner or styling product can protect hair from that kind of heat damage. In addition, when hair is wet (as it generally is before styling), heat can cause water inside the hair to literally boil (it only takes 212°F to get water to a rollicking boil), and even lower temperatures can cause water to agitate in the hair shaft. Bouts of high heat can burst the hair shaft and cause damage, and that's something no hair-care product in the world can address, regardless of the technology behind it.

Last, don't forget that heat is only one source of hair damage. The brushing and manipulation we do daily (sometimes several times per day) can be an even more significant source of damage, and conditioning agents of any kind can only protect so much. For more information about thermaSilk, owned by Helene Curtis, call (800) 621-2013 or visit www.thermasilkhair.com.

What's Good About This Line: Most thermaSilk styling products feature great formulations and even better prices; the conditioners rival drugstore competitor Pantene in terms of effective, silicone-based formulas.

What's Not So Good About It: All of the shampoos contain the problematic TEA-dodecylbenzene-sulfonate, and although it's only present in small amounts, repeated use could lead to unnecessary dryness and scalp irritation.

☺ **Clarifying Shampoo, for All Hair Types** *($3.99 for 13 ounces)* is a standard shampoo that is difficult to recommend wholeheartedly because it contains a small amount of TEA-dodecylbenzenesulfonate, which can lead to hair dryness and scalp irritation. This shampoo can remove minerals and styling-product buildup, but so can many others that don't include problematic ingredients.

☺ **Color Revitalizing Shampoo, for Colored or Permed Hair** *($3.99 for 13 ounces)* is a conditioning shampoo that contains a small amount of TEA-dodecylbenzenesulfonate, which can lead to hair dryness and scalp irritation with repeated use, though in the amount used here it would take awhile for that to occur. Nothing about this shampoo can revitalize colors or drooping curls.

☺ **Curl Defining Shampoo, for Naturally Curly or Wavy Hair** *($3.99 for 13 ounces)* is nearly identical to the Color Revitalizing Shampoo, for Colored or Permed Hair above, and the same comments apply.

☺ **Daily Balancing Shampoo** *($3.99 for 13 ounces)* is virtually identical to the Clarifying Shampoo, for All Hair Types above, and the same review applies.

☺ **Moisture Infusing Shampoo, for Dry or Damaged Hair** *($3.99 for 13 ounces)* is nearly identical to the Color Revitalizing Shampoo, for Colored or Permed Hair above, and the same comments apply. The only ingredient in this product that is helpful for dry, damaged hair is silicone, and for that hair type the benefits of silicone are better gained from a conditioner or styling product.

☺ **Volume Enhancing Shampoo, for Fine or Limp Hair** *($3.99 for 13 ounces)* is a standard, detergent-based shampoo that is similar to the Clarifying Shampoo above, but with a small amount of silicone that's not particularly helpful for fine or limp hair (though it is for dry hair). Unfortunately, this also contains a small amount of TEA-dodecylbenzenesulfonate, and that makes it less worthy of consideration than many other shampoos.

☺ **Moisture Infusing 2-in-1 Shampoo Plus Conditioner, for Dry or Damaged Hair** *($3.99 for 13 ounces)* is a decent conditioning shampoo, it but loses points for the needless inclusion of TEA-dodecylbenzenesulfonate.

☺ **Volume Enhancing 2-in-1 Shampoo Plus Conditioner, for Fine or Limp Hair** *($3.99 for 13 ounces)* is similar to the Moisture Infusing 2-in-1 Shampoo Plus Conditioner, for Dry or Damaged Hair above, except with a reduced amount of silicone and no glycerin, which makes it a lighter conditioning shampoo suitable for all hair types, though the TEA-dodecylbenzenesulfonate can be an eventual problem.

☺ **Clarifying Conditioner, for All Hair Types** *($3.99 for 13 ounces)* is a standard, but good, conditioner that is appropriate for normal to dry hair that is normal to slightly thick or coarse. Just to be clear, nothing in this can "clarify" the hair. If anything, the silicone will cling very well to the hair shaft and can build up with repeated use.

☺ **Color Revitalizing Conditioner, for Colored or Permed Hair** *($3.99 for 13 ounces)* is similar to the Clarifying Conditioner, for All Hair Types above, except this is a more impressive formula that contains higher amounts of water-binding agents, which makes it slightly preferred for drier hair. Otherwise, the same basic comments apply.

☺ **Curl Defining Conditioner, for Naturally Curly or Wavy Hair** *($3.99 for 13 ounces)* is an option for normal to slightly dry hair that is normal to fine or thin. For normal to fine curly hair, this can help moisturize without making curls feel heavy or go limp.

☺ **Intensive Daily Conditioner with Thermal Beads** *($4.99 for 6 ounces)* is nearly identical to the Clarifying Conditioner, for All Hair Types above, and the same review applies. The tiny amount of shea butter is not enough to make this conditioner an "intensive" option.

☺ **Light Detangling Mist, Leave-In Conditioner** *($3.99 for 10.5 ounces)* is indeed light, and is best for fine or thin hair that needs minimal moisture but could use some help with combing and static control.

☺ **Moisture Infusing Conditioner, for Dry or Damaged Hair** *($3.99 for 13 ounces)* is virtually identical to the Color Revitalizing Conditioner, for Colored or Permed Hair above, and the same review applies.

☺ **Volume Enhancing Conditioner, for Fine or Limp Hair** *($3.99 for 13 ounces)* is similar to, but not as elegant as, the Curl Defining Conditioner, for Naturally Curly or Wavy Hair above, and the same basic comments apply.

☺ **Control & Condition Cream** *($2.99 for 5.5 ounces)* is a creamy, water- and Vaseline-based styling cream that provides a soft, groomed hold and a smooth, frizz-free finish with shine. It is recommended for all hair types except fine or thin, and works especially well to enhance curls and waves without feeling too heavy or greasy.

☺ **Curl Perfecting Mousse** *($3.99 for 7 ounces)* is a standard mousse with a light hold and minimal to no stiff or sticky feel.

☺ **Firm Hold Hairspray (Aerosol)** *($3.99 for 7 ounces)* is a very good hairspray that provides a light mist application capable of providing a light (but not firm) hold with minimal stiff or sticky feel. It is easily brushed through and is an option for all hair types.

☺ **Firm Hold Hairspray (Non-Aerosol)** *($3.99 for 8.5 ounces)* is a standard, lightly conditioning hairspray capable of a light hold with absolutely no stiff or sticky feel. This is ideal for those who need a touch more hold but hate the stiff, tacky feel many hairsprays leave behind.

☺ **Flexible Hold Hairspray (Aerosol)** *($3.99 for 7 ounces)* is nearly identical to the Firm Hold Hairspray (Aerosol) above, except with slightly more hold and a bit more stickiness, though not enough to make it difficult to brush through hair.

☺ **Flexible Hold Hairspray (Non-Aerosol)** *($3.99 for 8.5 ounces)* is identical to the Firm Hold Hairspray (Non-Aerosol) above, and the same review applies.

☺ **Sculpting Gel** *($3.99 for 7 ounces)* is a very standard, but good, styling gel with a light hold and a smooth, non-sticky finish that can be brushed through easily. Because this offers such a light hold, it doesn't work as well for "sculpted" styles, but it's great for slicked-back or casual styles.

☺ **Shine & Shape Gel** *($3.99 for 8 ounces)* is a water-based gel with minimal to no hold, though it does contain a nice complement of lightweight water-binding agents for slightly dry hair. This would be best used to smooth normal to fine or thin hair or to enhance curls without a trace of stiffness or stickiness.

☺ **Ultra Hold Gel** *($3.99 for 7 ounces)* is nearly identical to the Sculpting Gel above, except this has slightly more hold, just not enough to earn an "ultra hold" designation. Otherwise, the same basic comments apply.

☺ **Ultra Hold Hairspray (Non-Aerosol)** *($3.99 for 8.5 ounces)* is similar to the Firm Hold Hairspray (Non-Aerosol) above, except it has slightly more hold (but definitely not ultra hold), and the same basic comments apply.

☺ **Volume & Shine Spray** *($3.99 for 7 ounces)* is a water- and silicone-based styling spray that is excellent for normal to thick or coarse hair. It provides a light hold that remains pliable, and adds soft shine with a minimal greasy, slick feel. It would also work well to enhance curls and waves on all but fine or thin hair.

☺ **Volume Infusing Mousse** *($3.99 for 7 ounces)* is a creamy-feeling, propellant-based mousse with a light hold and a minimally stiff, sticky finish that can be brushed through without incident. The water-binding agents can be helpful for slightly dry hair.

☺ **Frizz Fighter Weightless Hydrating Cream** *($3.99 for 4 ounces)* is a very good lightweight styling cream with minimal to no hold. Its primary benefits are smoothing frizzies and adding shine, and it does so without making hair heavy or greasy. Use this sparingly if you have fine or thin hair.

☺ **Moisture Recharging Thermal Wrap** *($6.99 for 1.5 ounces)* is nearly identical to the Color Revitalizing Conditioner, for Colored or Permed Hair above, except this comes with a thermal wrap. You apply the conditioner to hair, don the wrap, and then apply heat. This does allow the conditioning agents to better penetrate into and under the cuticle layers of the hair shaft, but you can achieve the same results with most of the thermaSilk conditioners above if you use them with a shower cap and a blow dryer. It is critical to keep the heat source at least six inches away from your head and to keep it moving because the ingredients in this conditioner cannot fully protect hair from heat damage.

THICKER FULLER HAIR

For more information about Thicker Fuller Hair, call (714) 556-1028 or visit www.advreslab.com.

What's Good About This Line: Nothing at all; for the reasons explained in the reviews below, it is actually the single most disappointing line in this book.

What's Not So Good About It: Each product is tainted by the inclusion of menthol and eucalyptus, whose chief function is not to help revitalize thinning hair, but to cause irritation and a false sense that the product is "working."

☹ **Moisturizing Shampoo, for Dry or Damaged Hair** *($3.99 for 12 ounces)* is a standard shampoo made irritating by the inclusion of menthol and eucalyptus, and it is not recommended. These common irritants may make you think the product is doing something special as your scalp tingles, but irritation is not the goal for hair care, and this has no positive effect on dry, damaged hair.

☹ **Revitalizing Shampoo, for All Hair Types** *($3.99 for 12 ounces)* is nearly identical to the Moisturizing Shampoo above, only with more menthol, and the same review applies.

☹ **Weightless Conditioner, for All Hair Types** *($3.99 for 12 ounces)* contains menthol and eucalyptus, which only cause scalp irritation and do nothing to make thin hair feel or appear thicker.

☹ **Full of Volume Thickening Mousse** *($3.99 for 6 ounces)*, **Instantly Thick Thickening Serum** *($6.49 for 4 ounces)*, **Volume Boost Volumizing Spray** *($3.99 for 8 ounces)*, and **Weightless Volumizing Hair Spray** *($3.99 for 8 ounces)* all contain high amounts of menthol and eucalyptus, along with other scalp irritants such as rosemary and thyme (which, contrary to claim, cannot control the scalp's output of oil). Each one of these can cause an itchy, irritated scalp, and that is not helpful for fine, thin hair. The Instantly Thick Thickening Serum above also contains sodium polystyrene sulfonate, which can dry the hair and scalp as well as potentially strip hair color with repeated use.

TIGI

If you like hair-care lines with kicky product names, colorful packaging, and a philosophy that all but demands its users have a sense of humor, welcome to TIGI. Founded over 30 years ago by the Italian brothers Toni and Guy Mascolo, it has grown into an international brand sold in dozens of countries. TIGI's educators (and the company's fervent belief in teaching all aspects of haircutting and styling to the salon owners and staff who sell their products) are admirable, and they have a well-earned reputation as trendsetters in the salon industry. Don't let the unconventional packaging and often risqué names fool you—this line really does take hair care and styling seriously, and has some outstanding products to prove it. For more information about independently owned and widely distributed TIGI, call (800) 256-9391 or visit www.tigihaircare.com.

What's Good About This Line: The shampoos are uniformly excellent, as are most of the conditioners, though there are no extremely emollient options for very dry or damaged hair; TIGI has some of the most creatively named and fun styling products around, and the really good news is that almost all of them perform well; the sheer extent and range of styling products means every hairstyle imaginable can be realized; best of all, this line does not suffer from blatant repetition in each product category as so many other lines do.

What's Not So Good About It: Although the styling product options are plentiful, enough of them have problematic ingredients to make it unwise to choose them at random or on a whim; the styling product prices are much higher than those of average salon lines, while the sizes for many of them may leave you and your hair feeling short-changed.

TIGI BED HEAD

☺ **Bed Head Control Freak Shampoo** *($7.95 for 12 ounces)* is a fairly standard shampoo that contains enough film-forming ingredients so that it is more of a volumizing shampoo for someone with fine or thin hair; however, that can cause buildup. It is best to alternate this with a shampoo that does not contain conditioners or volumizing ingredients.

☺ **Bed Head Dumb Blonde Shampoo, for After Highlights** *($9.95 for 12 ounces)* is a standard, rather than special, shampoo that carries no added benefit for use after your hair is highlighted. It is an excellent choice for all hair types (including color-treated), and poses a slight risk of buildup with repeated use.

☺ **Bed Head Manipulator, Daily Shampoo That Rocks!** *($8.95 for 12 ounces)* is similar to the Bed Head Dumb Blonde Shampoo, for After Highlights above, and the same basic comments apply. This does contain an increased amount of film-forming agent, which means buildup can happen sooner rather than later.

☺ **Bed Head Moisture Maniac Shampoo** *($7.95 for 12 ounces)* contains few moisturizing ingredients, and those that are included are present in such small amounts that it will not make a difference if your hair is dry. This is just another standard shampoo with a great name. It is an option for normal to slightly dry hair that is normal to fine or thin, and poses minimal risk of buildup.

☺ **Bed Head Self Absorbed, Mega Vitamin Shampoo** *($7.95 for 12 ounces)* is a very good, but standard, shampoo for all hair types, and it poses no risk of buildup.

☺ **Bed Head Control Freak Conditioner** *($11.95 for 8.5 ounces)* is a very light, rinse-out conditioner recommended for normal to fine or thin hair that needs help with combing, flyaway strands, and feeling thicker. It can cause buildup with repeated use.

☺ **Bed Head Dumb Blonde Conditioner, for After Highlights** *($9.95 for 12 ounces)* has no special benefit for blondes or color-treated hair, but it is a very good conditioner for dry hair of any thickness.

☺ **$$$ Bed Head Ego Boost, Split End Mender & Leave-In Conditioner** *($13.95 for 8 ounces)* can't repair a single split end, but it can make fine or thin hair that's slightly dry more manageable and easy to comb through, which may indeed boost your ego.

☺ **Bed Head Manipulator Conditioner** *($11.95 for 8.5 ounces)* is a standard, but good, conditioner for normal to dry hair of any thickness.

☺ **Bed Head Moisture Maniac Conditioner** *($11.95 for 8.5 ounces)* is nearly identical to the Bed Head Dumb Blonde Conditioner, for After Highlights above, and the same review applies.

☺ **Bed Head Self Absorbed Mega Vitamin Conditioner** *($11.95 for 8.5 ounces)* does contain vitamins, but all of them are present only in minute amounts. The amounts don't really matter, though, because they won't nutritionally boost hair in any way. This is a very good, though standard, conditioner for normal to dry hair of any thickness.

☺ **$$$ Bed Head, A Hair Stick for Cool People** *($17.95 for 2.7 ounces)* is a very standard castor oil- and wax-based styling stick that has a stiff texture that softens upon

The Reviews T

application. It can smooth sections of dry hair or tame frizzies, but must be used sparingly to avoid a coated, heavy feel and greasy appearance. Less expensive versions of this product are readily available at the drugstore.

☺ $$$ **Bed Head After-Party, Smoothing Cream for Silky, Shiny, Healthy Looking Hair!** *($17.95 for 3.4 ounces)* is an excellent pomade-style cream that, when used sparingly, can help smooth hair and provide a light hold that is neither stiff nor sticky.

☺ $$$ **Bed Head Boy Toys, Body Building Funkifier** *($17.95 for 3.4 ounces)* contains no holding agent, and its thick, gel-based texture is too heavy and moist to provide lift or fullness. What this can do is beautifully moisturize dry to very dry hair that is thick, curly, or coarse. It has high levels of glycerin and mineral oil, and is essentially a pomade in a can, dispensed like Cheez Whiz®. It is very easy to dispense more product than you'll need, and there's no putting it back, so use this carefully.

☹ $$$ **Bed Head Control Freak, Extra Extra Straight Hair Straightener** *($15.95 for 8 ounces)* claims to make hair straight without a flat iron and its resulting damage to hair, but there is nothing in this spray-on, pressurized foam that can turn curly or wavy hair into stick-straight hair. You still have to use this with a heat source and the proper styling tool to get any results. This ends up being a fairly unimpressive product that provides medium hold but leaves hair feeling stiff and sticky, rather than smooth and silky. It would be better to use this on dry hair as a finishing product than to straighten hair with heat.

☹ **Bed Head Control Freak, Serum Frizz Control & Straightener** *($15.95 for 9 ounces)* contains a form of sulfonic acid that can be drying to hair and scalp and also has the potential to strip hair color with repeated use.

☺ **Bed Head Creative Genius, Sculpting Liquid** *($13.95 for 8 ounces)* is a standard gel (with a fun name) that provides a medium to firm hold and a slightly stiff, sticky finish. It can still be brushed through, and is quite a versatile product, capable of creating numerous hairstyles—but the creativity has to come from you.

☺ **Bed Head Hard Head, Hard Hold Hairspray** (Aerosol) *($11.95 for 10.6 ounces)* is a standard hairspray that offers a firm hold with a slightly sticky finish and minimal stiffness. It contains conditioning agents and silicone to aid with brush-through and to add shine.

☺ $$$ **Bed Head Hard Head, Mohawk Gel for Spiking and Ultimate Hold** *($15.95 for 3.4 ounces)* is a creamy styling gel that provides very strong hold with a stiff, sticky finish. It is ideal for extreme, detailed hairstyles, and despite its strong hold this is not as rock-solid and glue-like as similar products. This option can actually be brushed through, but why would you want to do that and ruin your mohawk?

☺ $$$ **Bed Head Hard to Get, Texturizing Paste** *($17.95 for 1.5 ounces)* is a (surprise) unique styling product that combines elements of a pomade, leave-in conditioner, and styling cream into a workable paste that has a softer texture than most. It is excellent for adding non-sticky texture and piece-y definition to hair, especially if it is short or layered. It is reasonably water-soluble and can be used by all hair types, though someone with fine or thin hair should use it very sparingly to avoid weighing hair down.

☺ **Bed Head Head Shrink, Mega Firm Gel** *($11.95 for 8.5 ounces)* is as standard as styling gels get, and this medium-hold, slightly sticky option adds nothing new to the mix.

☺ $$$ **Bed Head Headbanger, Way-Out Wax for Rock Stars** *($18.95 for 4.5 ounces)* is an aerosol, spray-on wax with an intense citrus aroma that has nothing to do with rock stars. This is a very good option to add gloss and groomed control to coarse, frizzy hair. It sprays on much better than similar products, producing a fine mist rather than a concentrated blast. Hold it at least six inches from hair during application and use it sparingly, or it can make hair look greasy. This is too heavy for normal to fine or thin hair.

☺ $$$ **Bed Head Manipulator, A Funky Gunk That Rocks!** *($16.95 for 2 ounces)* is a creamy, slightly goopy pomade that is easy to emulsify and distribute through hair. It provides smooth, textured control with moderate shine, and is best for dry hair that is normal to coarse or thick. This works well to define thick, curly hair without being too heavy or greasy, but use it sparingly until you figure out how much of this product is best for your hair.

☺ $$$ **Bed Head Mastermind, Hair Candy for Separation and Texture!** *($16.95 for 2 ounces)* is a creamy, slightly stringy styling balm that can work well to smooth hair and add light hold with a soft, pliable finish. It is best for dry to very dry hair that is thick or coarse, but can be used sparingly to smooth dry ends or tame frizzies on normal to fine or thin hair.

☺ **Bed Head Maxxed-Out, Massive Hold Hairspray (Non-Aerosol)** *($12.95 for 8 ounces)* is a standard nonaerosol hairspray that provides medium to firm hold with a light finish that is minimally stiff and non-sticky. Hair can be brushed through, and this is a great, all-purpose hairspray—though the price is out of line for what you get.

☺ **Bed Head Power Trip, Hair Gel** *($11.95 for 7 ounces)* is a very standard, but effective, gel whose "Power Trip" name is related to the ironclad hold it provides. It does have a stiff, sticky finish, but will serve those looking to create detailed or gravity-defying hairstyles well. This can be slightly difficult to brush through, but it does not flake.

☺ $$$ **Bed Head Rubber Rage, Only for Cool People** *($17.95 for 1.25 ounces)* is a very expensive little product whose clever name and modern packaging don't mean as much as what's inside, and that is nothing more than a standard, gel-type pomade. Its water, castor oil, and mineral oil base is the same used in dozens of other pomades, most of which offer a greater amount of product for less money. As with all pomades of this type, it can smooth hair, reduce frizzies, and add shine. It should be used sparingly unless your goal is to create a greasy, slick look.

☺ **Bed Head Superstar, Thick Massive Hair** *($13.95 for 8.45 ounces)* is sold as a thermal-activated blow-dry lotion, and although it can work well with heat, you need to know how to position the heat and your brush to create thick, massive hair. This product has a thin, liquid-gel consistency and provides a light, minimally sticky hold with a smooth, shiny finish. It is ideal for all hair types except thick or coarse, and the silicone provides a slight amount of protection during heat styling.

☺ **Bed Head Uptight, Heat Activated Curl Maker** *($12.95 for 8 ounces)* is a light-weight, alcohol-free, water-based styling spray that contains an acrylate film-forming agent and silicone to define curls and enhance shine without weight. It is great for normal to fine or thin hair that is curly or straight, and provides light hold with a silky, completely non-sticky finish.

☹ **$$$ Bed Head Chocolate Head, Massive Hair Repair Treatment** *($15.95 for 3.7 ounces)* has an embarrassing formulation given its repair name and hair-saving claims. This does have some very good conditioning agents, but they are listed well after the fragrance, and as such don't count for much. It is an OK conditioner for normal to fine or thin hair that is minimally dry and needs help with combing. And you'll have to tolerate the intense chocolate fragrance that leaves hair smelling like a sundae or chocolate bar.

☺ **$$$ Bed Head Dumb Blonde Reconstructor, for After Highlights** *($15.95 for 6 ounces)* is nearly identical to the Bed Head Dumb Blonde Conditioner, for After Highlights above, and the same review applies. This product was an unnecessary addition, and its markup and reduced size (compared to the conditioner above) are completely unrelated to its formula and all about marketing this as a specialty product—when it is not.

☺ **$$$ Bed Head Girl Toys, Shine Serum** *($15.95 for 2 ounces)* is a standard silicone serum that works as well as any to tame frizz and add a silky feel with brilliant shine. The "Girl Toys" designation is strange because this can be used by either gender and contains nothing that would be off-putting to men. If anything, they might like the potent citrus fragrance more than women would.

☺ **$$$ Bed Head Headrush, Shine Adrenaline with a Superfine Mist** *($16.95 for 5.3 ounces)* is an aerosol silicone spray that does indeed have a superfine mist and as such is an outstanding (though pricey) glossing option for all hair types. It has an almost weightless, greaseless finish, but still adds an appreciable amount of shine. This is only a head rush if you apply it when you're hanging upside down!

☹ **Bed Head Health Goddess, A Vitamin Booster That Rehydrates & Detangles** *($14.95 for 6 ounces)* is supposed to revive your hair to its full, goddess-like potential, but don't count on anything close to that with this boring aerosol styling product. The bally-hooed vitamins (which cannot turn damaged hair into a vision of shining health) are present in the smallest amounts imaginable, and this is basically a minimal-hold spray that can provide minor control of static or flyaway hair.

☺ **$$$ Bed Head Shine Junkie, In a Can Outshine Everyone!** *($15.95 for 2 ounces)* is a silicone-based gel in an aerosol container, and dispensing it can be tricky because it tends to put out too much product and there is no way to put it back. As with all silicone gels, this can beautifully smooth dry to very dry, coarse hair and add radiant shine. This particular product is too heavy for normal to fine or thin hair.

☹ **Bed Head Treat Me Right, Peppermint Hair Mask** *($19.95 for 8 ounces)* is an emollient conditioner that would have been a good way to treat dry hair right, but it contains peppermint oil and menthol, and these can cause needless scalp irritation.

TIGI CATWALK

☺ **Catwalk Fashionista, Color Safe Shampoo** *($9.95 for 12 ounces)* is safe for color-treated hair, but so are all of the TIGI Bed Head shampoos above, so singling this out has more to do with marketing than any unique attribute. The risk of buildup is minimal.

☺ **Catwalk Oatmeal & Honey Treatment Shampoo** *($9.95 for 12 ounces)* doesn't contain oatmeal or honey, so the name is misleading. It is just a standard shampoo that offers no special treatment for hair. It can work well for any hair type.

☺ **Catwalk Sexed-Up, Body Building Shampoo** *($10.95 for 12 ounces)* is similar to the Bed Head Self Absorbed, Mega Vitamin Shampoo above, only without the vitamins (which were of little use to hair anyway) and plant oil. It is a very good shampoo for all hair types and poses minimal risk of buildup.

☺ **Catwalk Thickening Shampoo, for Fuller Hair** *($7.95 for 12 ounces)* is a good shampoo to make normal to fine or thin hair feel thicker. It can cause buildup, though, so it's best alternated with another shampoo.

☺ $$$ **Catwalk Fashionista, Color Safe Conditioner** *($12.95 for 8.5 ounces)* is TIGI's most basic conditioner, and is similar to, but less elegant than, the Bed Head Dumb Blonde Conditioner, for After Highlights above. Still, the same basic comments apply.

☺ **Catwalk Fast-Fixx, Lightweight Leave-In Conditioner** *($8.95 for 8 ounces)* is similar to the Bed Head Ego Boost, Split End Mender & Leave-In Conditioner above, and the same basic comments apply, though this one does have a lighter texture.

☺ $$$ **Catwalk Sexed-Up, Body Building Conditioner** *($12.95 for 8 ounces)* is similar to the Catwalk Fashionista, Color Safe Conditioner above, and the same basic comments apply, except this is actually a slightly better formulation that doesn't contain as much fragrance.

☺ $$$ **Catwalk Thickening Conditioner, for Fuller Hair** *($12.95 for 8 ounces)* won't thicken hair, but it is a good, though standard, conditioner for normal to slightly dry hair of any thickness.

☺ $$$ **Catwalk Catfight, Pliable Pudding** *($17.95 for 1.5 ounces)* is a standard, water-soluble pomade that promises, "it's so good, you'll fight over it!" I wouldn't take my admiration that far, but this can help smooth frizzies and create pliable texture while adding a soft shine and light hold. Whether or not you'll want to strut and pose after using this depends more on your attitude than anything else!

☺ **Catwalk Curls Rock, Curl Booster** *($13.95 for 7.7 ounces)* begs you to "blast in massive, flirty curls," and you can definitely use this aerosol styling spray for that purpose, but it's a rather boring formula. It does its job of providing a light, non-sticky hold and its weightless finish makes it preferred for fine or thin hair that's curly, but that's where the excitement stops.

☺ **Catwalk EnviroShape, Firm Hold Hairspray** *($12 for 8 ounces)* is a very good aerosol hairspray with a light hold and a completely non-sticky finish so hair can be brushed through easily. This won't hold up if you're under hot lights on the catwalk, but for creating soft hold on casual hairstyles, it's fine.

☺ **Catwalk Extra Strong Mousse, for Medium to Thick Hair** *($8.95 for 6.5 ounces)* is a very standard, propellant-based mousse that has a firm hold and a stiff, sticky finish. This can still be brushed through, and is a good option for hard-to-hold hair that is normal to fine or thin. The texture of this mousse is too light for thick hair.

☹ **Catwalk Fashionista, Smooth & Shine** *($13.95 for 8 ounces)* is a smoothing balm that is primarily water, fragrance, cellulose thickener, preservative, and wax. It can lightly smooth hair without any hold or heaviness, but that's about it. There are many more products to consider over this one-note option.

☺ **Catwalk Fashionista, Spritz & Shine** *($14.95 for 8 ounces)* is an alcohol-based styling spray whose slightly viscous texture is courtesy of the polyurethane this contains, which can make hair feel coated and slightly heavy. This is best for normal to slightly thick or coarse hair needing a medium hold that keeps hair flexible rather than stiff.

☺ **Catwalk Frisky, Scrunching Gel with Attitude** *($13 for 8 ounces)* is an excellent spray gel for all hair types, though it is best to spray this on your hands and then apply it to the hair where needed. This provides a light to medium hold without a stiff, sticky feel, though it can be used for more detailed styles if needed.

☺ **Catwalk Root Boost, Spray for Texture & Lift** *($11 for 8 ounces)* is one of the original, and still one of the best, root-boosting sprays. It has a directional nozzle for pinpoint application, and its spray, unlike many others of this ilk, is not intense or forceful. This provides a medium, movable hold with a slightly sticky feel and, when used correctly, can build incredible volume that lasts.

☹ **Catwalk Sexed-Up, Body Building Tonic** *($12.95 for 8 ounces)* lists sodium polystyrene sulfonate as its second ingredient, which can cause hair and scalp dryness and potentially strip hair color with repeated use.

☺ **Catwalk Strong Mousse, for Fine to Medium Hair** *($8.95 for 6.5 ounces)* is identical to the Catwalk Extra Strong Mousse, for Medium to Thick Hair above, and the same review applies.

☺ **Catwalk Texturizing Pomade** *($9.95 for 2 ounces)* is a very standard, water-soluble, gel-type pomade that is an option for smoothing frizzies and adding a wet-look shine. This can become greasy and slick if not used sparingly, and is best for normal to slightly thick, coarse, or curly hair. It contains several potentially problematic fragrant oils, so keep it away from the scalp.

☺ **$$$ Catwalk Thickening Cream, with Essential Oils** *($15.95 for 3.4 ounces)* is primarily water, slip agents, panthenol, and film-forming agent. It is a lotion-like gel that seems thick at first but ends up being a lightweight product suitable for all but very thick or coarse hair that needs a light, conditioned hold. It is slightly sticky, and the essential oils can be a problem if this gets on the scalp, but it is otherwise recommended.

☺ **Catwalk Work-It, Medium-Firm Hold Working Hairspray** *($12 for 8 ounces)* dries almost instantly, so it isn't a good choice if you need a working hairspray (meaning a slow drying time so hair stays pliable longer). It can, however, function beautifully as a firm-hold aerosol finishing spray for all hair types. It is relatively easy to brush through and doesn't make hair feel impossibly stiff.

☺ $$$ **Catwalk Oatmeal & Honey Treatment & Conditioner** *($13.95 for 8.5 ounces)* is more of a standard conditioner than special treatment, and is a good option for normal to dry hair of any thickness. It contains the tiniest amount of honey and not a single grain of oatmeal.

TRESEMME

For more information about TRESemme, owned by the Alberto Culver Corporation, call (800) 333-6666 or visit www.tresemme.com.

What's Good About This Line: The prices and generous sizes, not to mention that most of the products are effective for their intended purpose (barring any unrealistic claims such as repairing hair or preserving color); the styling products, though mostly standard fare, are worth a look, especially if you prefer medium- to firm-hold gels or mousses.

What's Not So Good About It: The line suffers from repetitive shampoo and conditioner formulations, particularly in the Total Solutions category; a few products contain problematic ingredients (luckily these are few and far between); the line lacks options for conditioning very dry, coarse hair, and its single leave-in conditioner is a problem.

☺ **European Deep Cleansing Shampoo** *($4.49 for 32 ounces)*. There is nothing European about this formula in the least, or in any of the European TRESemme products. This is just a very standard shampoo that works well for all hair types without causing buildup.

☺ **European Natural Shampoo** *($4.49 for 32 ounces)* is a very good shampoo for all hair types, and poses minimal risk of buildup.

☺ **European Revitalizing Colour Care Shampoo** *($3.69 for 32 ounces)* has no special benefit for color-treated hair, but is by no means detrimental either.

☺ **European Vitamin B12 & Gelatin Anti-Breakage Shampoo** *($4.79 for 32 ounces)* does contain vitamin B12 and gelatin, but neither of these can stop or correct hair breakage. The tiny amounts included in this product make them barely effective water-binding agents. This standard shampoo is similar to the European Revitalizing Colour Care Shampoo above, and the same comments apply.

☹ **European Vitamin E Moisture Rich Shampoo** *($4.49 for 32 ounces)* contains sodium lauryl sulfate as its main detergent cleansing agent, and that makes it too drying for the hair and too drying and irritating to the scalp.

☺ **European Natural Conditioner** *($3.69 for 32 ounces)* is a standard lightweight conditioner that is appropriate for someone with normal to slightly dry hair that is normal to fine or thin. The presence of plant extracts does not make this conditioner natural, and none of them have much conditioning benefit for hair—so that's where the synthetic ingredients come into play here.

☺ **European Remoisturizing Conditioner** *($4.49 for 32 ounces)* is similar to the European Natural Conditioner above, except with far fewer plant extracts. Otherwise, the same comments apply.

☺ **European Revitalizing Colour Care Conditioner** *($3.69 for 32 ounces)* is a good conditioner for normal to fine or thin hair that is slightly dry. The film-forming agents can build up and make hair feel heavy, so it is best to alternate this with a separate conditioner.

☺ **European Vitamin B12 & Gelatin Anti-Breakage Conditioner** *($4.79 for 32 ounces)* is nearly identical to the European Remoisturizing Conditioner above, except it includes vitamin B12 and gelatin in amounts great enough to serve as water-binding agents. However, that won't repair or prevent hair breakage. Otherwise, the same basic comments apply.

☺ **European Vitamin E Moisture Rich Conditioner** *($4.49 for 32 ounces)* is nearly identical to the European Remoisturizing Conditioner above, and the same comments apply. The vitamin E cannot make hair "moisture-rich."

☺ **Curl Care Curl Enhancing Mousse** *($4.29 for 10.5 ounces)* is a standard, propellant-based mousse whose airy foam offers a light to medium hold with minimal stiffness and a slightly sticky feel. It is easily brushed through, and works well for normal to fine hair, be it curly, wavy, or straight.

☺ **Curl Care Curl & Scrunch Hair Spray** *($4.29 for 10 ounces)* is a basic nonaerosol hairspray with added conditioning agents that make it suitable for dry hair of any thickness. This product has a medium hold that stays pliable, so it is indeed good for "scrunching" and shaping curly hair, but any hair type can use it, though it does dry slightly sticky.

☺ **European Mega Hold Sculpting Gel, Mega Hold** *($3.79 for 9 ounces)* doesn't provide mega hold, but it is a very good, medium-hold, alcohol-free gel that can be brushed through, and it's an option for all hair types except very fine or thin.

☺ **European Tres Gel Spray, Extra Hold** *($2.76 for 10 ounces)* is a slightly heavy spray gel that works well for normal to slightly thick or coarse hair that needs firm control. This alcohol-free formula leaves hair slightly stiff and moderately sticky, but it can be brushed through easily.

☺ **European Tres Mousse, Extra Hold** *($3.99 for 10.5 ounces)* is a standard, propellant-based mousse that offers medium hold with minimal stiffness or stickiness. This is great for normal to fine or thin hair that needs help taming unmanageable areas without adding weight or a greasy feel. It can be brushed through easily.

☺ **European Tres Spray, Super Hold** *($3.99 for 10 ounces)* is a nonaerosol hairspray that really does offer super (strong) hold. It dries quickly and can be tricky to brush through, but for long-lasting hold and support without heaviness, this wins high marks.

☺ **European Tres Two Hair Spray, Extra Hold** *($3.99 for 11 ounces)* is an aerosol hairspray with a medium to firm hold that leaves hair minimally stiff or sticky. It works well as an all-purpose finishing spray, though it does dry quickly, so be sure your hair is where you want it before applying this product.

☺ **European Tres Two Hair Spray, Ultra Fine Mist** *($3.99 for 11 ounces)* works well as a light-hold aerosol hairspray with a barely detectable stiff, sticky feel that can be brushed through easily. This has not only an ultra-fine mist, but also an ultra-light texture that won't weigh down or "coat" fine or thin hair.

☺ **European Volume & Body Styling Gel, Extra Hold** *($3.99 for 9 ounces)* is nearly identical to the European Mega Hold Sculpting Gel, Mega Hold above, except with slightly less hold, and the same basic comments apply.

☺ **Freeze Hold Freeze & Control Hair Spray** *($2.89 for 7 ounces)* is an aerosol hairspray with medium hold that is not stiff but is slightly sticky. It can be brushed through, and it dries quickly, so it's better as a finishing spray than a working spray.

☺ **Freeze Hold Shine Gel, Ultra Hold** *($4.29 for 9 ounces)* is nearly identical to the European Mega Hold Sculpting Gel, Mega Hold above, and the same comments apply. Despite the name, this does not freeze hair in place, nor is its hold close to being "ultra."

☺ **Hydrology Smoothing Moisture Pomade** *($4.99 for 3.5 ounces)* is a standard, gel-type pomade with a thick texture that goes on lighter than you might expect. It is a very good smoothing pomade that can help enhance texture and tame frizzies without making hair feel too greasy, though it should still be used sparingly on fine or thin hair. It is water soluble and shampoos out easily.

☺ **Smooth De-Frizzing Moisture Gel, Extra Hold** *($2.89 for 9 ounces)* is similar to the European Mega Hold Sculpting Gel, Mega Hold above, except that this option has a lighter hold and is less sticky. This is OK if frizzies are minor, but if not, it will need to be paired with a more potent frizz tamer, such as a silicone serum or styling cream.

☺ **Volume Volumizing Mousse, Mega Hold** *($2.89 for 10.5 ounces)* is nearly identical to the European Tres Mousse above, only this has a lighter hold and a softer finish. Otherwise, the same basic comments apply.

☹ **European Instant Self-Warming Hot Oil Treatment** *($2.99 for three 1-ounce tubes)* doesn't contain any oil and is a mediocre conditioner for slightly dry hair. This doesn't warm up on its own; you need to massage it into the hair and scalp to create friction, and that's where the warming comes from.

TRESEMME 4+4

☺ **4+4 Chamomile & Rosemary Infused Color Protecting Shampoo** *($5.49 for 16 ounces)* is a standard shampoo that is a good option for all hair types, and it poses minimal risk of buildup.

☺ **4+4 Guava & Keratin Infused Amplifying Shampoo** *($5.49 for 16 ounces)* is a very good, mildly conditioning shampoo for slightly dry hair of any thickness, and poses a slight risk of buildup with repeated use.

☹ **4+4 Green Tea & Ginger Infused Clarifying Shampoo** *($5.49 for 16 ounces)* is similar to the 4+4 Guava & Keratin Infused Amplifying Shampoo above, except this contains sodium polystyrene sulfonate, which can cause hair and scalp dryness and strip hair color with repeated use.

☺ **4+4 Marine Botanical & Cucumber Infused Hydrating Shampoo** *($5.49 for 16 ounces)* is nearly identical to the 4+4 Chamomile & Rosemary Infused Color Protecting Shampoo above, except this contains a different assortment of plant extracts (none of them particularly beneficial for hair or scalp). Otherwise, the same review applies.

☺ **4+4 Brushout Shaping Spray** *($4.69 for 10.5 ounces)* is nearly identical to the Freeze Hold Freeze & Control Hair Spray above, and the same review applies. Contrary to claim, the film-forming/holding agent in this product can indeed build up on hair, as it can with the use of any hairspray.

☺ **4+4 Extra Hold Hair Spray** *($4.69 for 12.2 ounces)* is a standard aerosol hairspray with a very light hold and a completely non-stiff, non-sticky finish. If you don't need much additional control or lift, this is an option, and it can be brushed through easily.

☺ **4+4 Extra Hold Styling Mousse** *($5.49 for 13.5 ounces)* performs nicely as a medium-hold, propellant-based mousse that has a slightly stiff, sticky finish but can still be brushed through without incident. It has a texture and finish that are slightly heavier than normal, and so it's best for normal hair that is curly, wavy, or straight and slightly dry.

☺ **4+4 Freezing Fixative Spray** *($4.69 for 10.5 ounces)* is nearly identical to the European Tres Two Hair Spray, Extra Hold above, and the same comments apply.

☺ **4+4 Intense Hold Super Mousse** *($5.49 for 13.5 ounces)* is identical in every respect to the 4+4 Extra Hold Styling Mousse above, and the same review applies.

☺ **4+4 Sculpting Gel** *($5.49 for 8.2 ounces)* is sold as a super-hold styling fixative, and that description is accurate. This water- and alcohol-based styling gel can provide a strong hold and leaves hair feeling stiff and sticky. It is recommended for slicking back stubborn hair or for creating more intricate styles that involve lift, definition, and long-lasting support. This can be slightly difficult to brush through, but it doesn't flake.

☺ **4+4 Spray F/X** *($5.49 for 8 ounces)* promises maximum hold, and it delivers, though not without residual stiffness and stickiness. This has an overall light feel in the hair, but is best used for areas that need extra hold or lift rather than used all over (whether hair is wet or dry). As expected, this is not the easiest product to brush through because it pretty much freezes hair in place.

☺ **4+4 Styling Glaze** *($5.49 for 19.2 ounces)* is a liquid styling gel that is easy to distribute through the hair. It provides a medium hold that leaves hair more sticky than stiff, but it can still be brushed through easily. The numerous film-forming and conditioning agents can make this a bit too heavy for very fine or thin hair, but all other hair types shouldn't find this too weighty, and it can nicely define curls or waves.

☺ **4+4 Ultra Fine Mist Hair Spray** *($3.69 for 12.2 ounces)* is identical to the European Tres Two Hair Spray, Ultra Fine Mist above, and the same review applies. This option does offer a bit more product for slightly less money.

☺ **4+4 Intensive Hair Balm** *($5.49 for 4 ounces)* isn't all that intensive. This is a rather standard conditioner with a texture that should be more emollient given the product's claims. Still, this is a very good option for normal to dry hair of any thickness.

☹ **4+4 Keratin Infused Hair Splash, Leave-In Treatment** *($5.49 for 8 ounces)* contains the preservatives methylisothiazolinone and methylchloroisothiazolinone (Kathon CG), which are not recommended for use in leave-on products due to the high likelihood of a sensitizing reaction on the scalp. In a spray-on product such as this, it is inevitable that some product will reach the scalp and cause irritation.

☺ **4+4 Marine Botanical & Mango Infused Hydrating Sealant** *($5.49 for 16 ounces)* is an excellent creamy conditioner that would be wonderful for dry hair of any thickness. The price and generous size makes this a near-bargain, and for those influenced by fragrance, the mango scent is soft rather than cloying.

TRESEMME TOTAL SOLUTIONS

☺ **Total Solutions Colour Care, Healthy Highlights Shampoo** *($3.79 for 14 ounces)* won't do a thing to enhance highlights, but this gentle shampoo won't wreck them either. It is a good option for slightly dry hair of any thickness, and poses a slight risk of buildup with repeated use.

☺ **Total Solutions Colour Care, Vibrant Colour Shampoo** *($3.99 for 14 ounces)* is nearly identical to the Total Solutions Colour Care, Healthy Highlights Shampoo above, and the same review applies.

☺ **Total Solutions Moisture, Gentle Moisture Shampoo** *($3.99 for 14 ounces)* is nearly identical to the Total Solutions Colour Care, Healthy Highlights Shampoo above, and the same review applies. This shampoo isn't much for moisture because the main conditioning agent won't cling well to hair or hold up during rinsing.

☺ **Total Solutions Moisture, Intense Moisture Shampoo** *($3.99 for 14 ounces)* is nearly identical to the Total Solutions Colour Care, Healthy Highlights Shampoo above, and the same review applies. The "Intense Moisture" in the name is nowhere to be found in the product, but this shampoo won't dry out hair.

☺ **Total Solutions Strength, Fortifying Shampoo** *($3.99 for 14 ounces)* is nearly identical to the Total Solutions Colour Care, Healthy Highlights Shampoo above, only without numerous plant extracts, and the same basic comments apply. Nothing in this shampoo can strengthen hair.

☺ **Total Solutions Strength, Replenishing Shampoo** *($3.79 for 14 ounces)* is nearly identical to the Total Solutions Strength, Fortifying Shampoo above, and the same comments apply.

☺ **Total Solutions Colour Care, Healthy Highlights Conditioner** *($3.79 for 14 ounces)* is nearly identical to the European Natural and European Remoisturizing conditioners above, and the same review applies. The citrus extracts in this product have no impact on highlights.

☺ **Total Solutions Colour Care, Vibrant Colour Conditioner** (*$3.99 for 14 ounces*) is a standard, but good, conditioner for normal to fine hair that is slightly dry.

☺ **Total Solutions Moisture, Smoothing Moisture Conditioner** (*$3.99 for 14 ounces*) is virtually identical to the Total Solutions Colour Care, Healthy Highlights Conditioner above, and the same comments apply.

☺ **Total Solutions Strength, Fortifying Conditioner** (*$3.99 for 14 ounces*) is very similar to the European Revitalizing Colour Care Conditioner above, except with a reduced amount of film-forming agent. Otherwise, the same basic comments apply.

☺ **Total Solutions Strength, Replenishing Conditioner** (*$3.79 for 14 ounces*) is nearly identical to the Total Solutions Strength, Fortifying Conditioner above, and the same comments apply. If your hair is very dry or damaged, this won't provide enough replenishment.

TRI

For more information about Tri, call (866) 644-7373 or visit www.trihaircare.com.

What's Good About This Line: Each category (shampoo, conditioner, styling product) has at least one very good option; for a salon-sold line, the prices are lower than average; there are some excellent emollient styling products for thick or coarse hair.

What's Not So Good About It: Tri has more than its fair share of problematic products, many rife with irritating ingredients that have no established benefit for hair or scalp; given the formulations, the price structure doesn't seem to follow any logical scheme.

☹ **Ecollogen Shampoo Treatment** (*$9.25 for 16 ounces*) contains TEA-lauryl sulfate as its main detergent cleansing agent, which makes this shampoo too drying for hair and also drying and irritating to the scalp.

☹ **Clarifying Shampoo, Build-Up/Mineral Remover** (*$9 for 10 ounces*) can remove buildup, but thanks to the sodium C14-16 olefin sulfonate this contains, it can also dry the hair and scalp. There are gentler options available that can remove mineral buildup just as well.

☺ **Jojoba Shampoo Treatment** (*$12 for 16 ounces*) is a very standard, but good, shampoo that is an option for normal to slightly dry hair of any thickness, and poses minimal to no risk of buildup.

☺ **Moisturizing Shampoo** (*$8 for 10 ounces*) is nearly identical to the Jojoba Shampoo Treatment above, minus the plant oil, and the same basic comments apply. The vitamins and antioxidants that are included have no effect on the hair beyond functioning as decent water-binding agents.

☹ **Whole Wheat Shampoo Treatment** (*$16.50 for 16 ounces*) contains sodium C14-16 olefin sulfonate as one of its main detergent cleansing agents, and that makes this shampoo a poor choice if you're trying to avoid dry hair and an irritated scalp.

☺ **Chamomile pH Rectifier, Leave-In Conditioner** *($6.50 for 8 ounces)* claims to adjust hair to its natural pH balance, but exactly what is it being balanced with? For example, dry hair actually has no pH. Only liquids or liquid solutions can have pH. When hair is dissolved in a liquid solution it has about the same pH as skin, about 4.5 to 5.5, which is somewhat acidic (water has a neutral pH of 7). Besides, it isn't the hair itself that has a pH; rather, there is an acid mantle made up of oil and sweat that covers the hair shaft, and it is this invisible layer that protects the hair. A pH over 7 (more alkaline) decomposes the hair's acid mantle and begins eating away at its outer layer, called the cuticle. So anything with a pH over 7 is bad for hair and anything with a pH of 4.5 to 7 works great for hair, either by complementing the hair's natural acid mantle or just leaving it alone and not disturbing it. The goal of any hair-care product should be to leave the pH of hair alone or to make it slightly more acidic (to help the cuticle shut down), and that's about it.

With that explanation in place, what we have here is nothing more than an ultralight, spray-on conditioner that is an OK, minimally effective option for fine or thin hair that needs help with combing. It has a pH of 6, which is a nice way to let hair do what it does naturally to establish its own pH.

☺ **Express Conditioning Detangler** *($8.25 for 8 ounces)* is a lightweight detangling conditioner suitable for normal to fine or thin hair that is minimally dry. The sunscreen it contains cannot protect hair from UV damage.

☹ **Jojoba Hair & Scalp Conditioner** *($12.25 for 8 ounces)* lists TEA-dodecylbenzenesulfonate as the second ingredient, and that makes this conditioner too drying for all hair types, and irritating if massaged onto the scalp as directed.

☺ **Moisturizing Conditioner** *($8 for 10 ounces)* is a standard, rank-and-file conditioner for normal to dry hair of any thickness. Although fragrance is not listed, the smell this product exudes is not one that would naturally emanate from the ingredients it contains.

☹ **Unific Energy Moisturizer** *($13.50 for 9 ounces)* contains a noticeable amount of peppermint oil, which makes this too potentially irritating for the scalp, and it would be painful if it accidentally got into your eyes as you're rinsing it off.

☺ **Whole Wheat Conditioning Rinse** *($10.50 for 8 ounces)* is an option for normal to slightly dry hair of any thickness.

☺ **AeroCurl Spray-In Curl Enhancer** *($12.95 for 7.6 ounces)* is an aerosol styling spray that has no special benefit for curly hair. It provides medium hold with a sticky finish that is difficult to brush through, yet the conditioning agents are helpful for dry hair. This would be best as a finishing spray on normal to thick or coarse hair, be it curly or straight.

☺ **Aerogel (Aerosol)** *($14.50 for 11 ounces)* is a fairly sticky aerosol hairspray that provides a firm hold with a slightly stiff finish. This has a heavier feel than most hairsprays (hence the "gel" portion of the product name) and can be too heavy for fine or thin hair. It is best as a finishing touch on thick, curly, or coarse hair that needs extra hold.

☺ **Aerogel-Light, Light Hold Hair Spray (Aerosol)** *($13.20 for 11 ounces)* is nearly identical to the Aerogel (Aerosol) above, except with slightly less hold and significantly less stickiness. Unlike the one above, however, this option is easy to brush through and is a more versatile option for all hair types.

☹ **AeroStraight Spray-In Straightener** *($12.95 for 8.5 ounces)* contains sodium polystyrene sulfonate as one of its main ingredients, and that makes this spray needlessly drying for hair and scalp, not to mention that repeated use can potentially strip hair color.

☺ **Body Infusion** *($9.75 for 9 ounces)* is nothing more than a standard aerosol hairspray, and when applied to the roots of damp or dry hair it can help build fullness and body, just like any hairspray. This offers a light to medium hold with a slightly stiff, sticky finish that can be brushed through.

☺ **Control and Finishing Mist** *($6.75 for 8 ounces)* is a standard, light-hold nonaerosol hairspray that dries to a minimally stiff, sticky finish. There isn't much else to say!

☺ **Covert Control Holding Spray** *($12 for 11 ounces)* is a standard aerosol hairspray with a light hold and a barely discernible stiff or sticky feel. It is easy to brush through, and light enough to use on fine or thin hair.

☺ **Fashion Styling Mousse** *($14 for 16 ounces)* is a standard, propellant-based mousse that provides a medium hold with a slightly stiff, sticky feel. If you prefer a mousse texture but need a stronger hold for more structured styles, this is a great option.

☺ **Gel Spray** *($7 for 8 ounces)* is a standard gel formula with clever packaging. This has a light to medium hold and minimal to no stiff or sticky feel.

☺ **Pom-Mousse, Hairstyle Forming Foam** *($14.25 for 3.75 ounces)* is a liquid-to-foam mousse with a heavier texture because of the plant oil it contains. This offers a medium hold with a slightly sticky, greasy finish. It is best for normal to thick or coarse hair that needs conditioned control.

☺ **Protein Bodifier, Spray In Body Builder** *($7.75 for 8 ounces)* is a standard water- and alcohol-based styling spray with light to medium hold that leaves hair slightly stiff and sticky. The collagen protein and panthenol do not become part of the hair structure (as Tri asserts on the label), but they are decent conditioning agents for all hair types. This is best for normal to fine or thin hair that needs hold and body.

☺ **Sculpture Styling Gel** *($6.50 for 5 ounces)* is the gel to choose if you need firm hold that you don't intend to brush through later. This water-based gel offers a glue-like hold and a very sticky finish. It is best for exaggerating texture or creating long-lasting hold on short or spiked hairstyles.

☺ **Shape and Shine** *($10.75 for 2 ounces)* is a water-soluble, gel-type pomade that works as well as any to add texture and shine to hair while smoothing frizzies. It can be used by all but very fine or thin hair types, and should be used sparingly for best results. This does shampoo out easily, and the mica it contains boosts shine without flaking.

☺ **Texture Styling Creme** *($9 for 4 ounces)* is a thick, fairly greasy styling cream that grooms and smoothes hair without any stiff or sticky feeling. It is ideal for dry to very dry hair that is thick or coarse. The mineral oil and Vaseline base can be difficult to remove with a single shampoo.

☺ **Bright Lites** *($9.75 for 3.5 ounces)* is a standard silicone spray dispensed via an aerosol container, and the fine mist it produces makes this an excellent glossing spray for all hair types. It adds brilliant shine without significant weight or greasiness, though it should still be used sparingly for best results.

☹ **Electri-Therm Control Treatment** *($5.35 for 8 ounces)* contains lime oil as one of its main ingredients, which makes this incredibly irritating to the scalp and also drying for hair. It also contains menthol, which only makes matters worse.

☹ **Unific Energy Protein Pac** *($3.85 for 1 ounce)* is sold to "reverse the effects of extremely damaged hair" and has an allegedly "miraculous" formula, but neither is true. With drying and irritating TEA-dodecylbenzenesulfonate listed as the third ingredient (after water and protein), this is much more problematic than helpful for damaged hair. There are some emollient ingredients in it, but countless other conditioners contain the same ones, so where is the miracle?

ULTRA SWIM

For more information about Ultra Swim, call (800) 421-1223 or visit www.chattem.com.

What's Good About This Line: The shampoo can remove chlorine and mineral buildup (such as those that can occur from hard water or pools that have copper pipes) from hair.

What's Not So Good About It: Ultra Swim's solution to removing chlorine includes adding two ingredients that can denature hair, making this a poor option for frequent use.

☺ **Shampoo Plus, Effectively Removes Chlorine and Chlorine Odor** *($4.69 for 7 ounces)* can indeed remove chlorine and its odor from hair thanks to the combination of chelating agents and other mineral-binding ingredients. However, both the urea and sodium thiosulfate it contains can denature the hair, leading to problems if you use this frequently. For occasional use (meaning no more than once per week) this is an OK option, but the potential risks don't make it worth choosing over many other chelating shampoos.

☺ **Ultra Repair Conditioner, Restores Protein & Moisture Lost Due to Chlorine Damage** *($4.69 for 7 ounces)* won't restore any more moisture to hair than any other standard conditioner, and it certainly cannot repair hair, but it is good for normal to dry hair of any thickness.

WASH & CURL

For more information about Wash & Curl, call (800) 595-6230 or visit www.wash ncurl.com.

What's Good About This Line: Two of the three shampoos are good (though not unique) options for normal to fine or thin hair.

What's Not So Good About It: The claims go too far by implying that straight hair will become curly after using Wash & Curl, while curly or wavy hair will be straight after shampooing with Wash & Straight, which contains a problematic detergent cleansing agent.

☺ **Extra Strength Wash & Curl Shampoo, for Dry, Damaged, Color-Treated Hair** *($4.20 for 8 ounces)* is a standard shampoo and, really, it doesn't get much more standard than this. The "Extra Strength Curl Enhancers" in this are actually just PVP, a film-forming/holding agent used in countless styling gels. This will build up on the hair with repeated use, but can make fine or thin hair feel thicker. It doesn't have much styling advantage when deposited during shampooing. Those with thick or coarse curly hair would do better without the PVP because it can make these hair textures feel heavier. It is best for normal to fine or thin hair, be it curly, wavy, or straight. Contrary to the directions, do not leave this shampoo on your hair for five minutes, especially if hair is dry or damaged or you have any scalp sensitivity, because that will only make matters worse.

☺ **Extra Strength Wash & Curl Shampoo, for Fine, Limp, Dry Hair** *($4.20 for 8 ounces)* is identical to the Extra Strength Wash & Curl Shampoo, for Dry, Damaged, Color-Treated Hair above, and the same review applies.

☹ **Wash 'n Straight Shampoo** *($5.95 for 10 ounces)* contains TEA-lauryl sulfate as its main detergent cleansing agent, which makes this too drying for all hair and scalp types. Furthermore, the film-forming agent in this product cannot discourage curly or wavy hair from "reverting to its natural state." It can coat the hair shaft and (until buildup becomes a problem) improve manageability, but that's it.

WELEDA

This Switzerland-based line has been in business since 1921, and made its U.S. debut in 1931 (its domestic office is now in New York State). How to explain this longevity is not easy because there isn't anything remotely exciting about these products, unless you put a high priority on choosing hair care that uses essential oils for fragrance. WELEDA (a name of Celtic origin) maintains that their products are "based upon the study of relationships between the processes of nature and the human being," which sounds very grounded and New Age–like, but philosophy won't clean or condition your hair. Nature (in the form of plant extracts and essential oils) is used in these products, but along with the plants are the same standard hair-care ingredients everyone else is using. And for good reason: plant and essential oils have little to no benefit when it comes to taking care of your hair. They are an enticing hook for many consumers, but if you tried to shampoo with calendula or condition your hair with rosemary essential oil, I can guarantee you would be disappointed. For more information about WELEDA, call (800) 265-2615 or visit www.usa.weleda.com.

What's Good About This Line: Shampoos that are all worth considering; if you are concerned about preservatives, this line uses a minimal amount of them.

What's Not So Good About It: The conditioners are lackluster in every respect but their scent, which has no effect on how smooth, soft, and easy to detangle your hair will be.

☺ **Calendula Phyto Shampoo** *($8.75 for 8 ounces)* is a standard, but very good, shampoo for all hair types, and it poses no risk of buildup. The fragrance is listed as "essential oils," but the specific oils are not identified, which can make this a risky proposition for someone with a sensitive, easily irritated scalp.

☺ **Chamomile Phyto Shampoo** *($8.75 for 8 ounces)* is nearly identical to the Calendula Phyto Shampoo above, except the calendula was replaced with soothing chamomile (and in a greater amount, too). Otherwise, the same basic comments apply.

☺ **Rosemary Phyto Shampoo** *($8.75 for 8 ounces)* is nearly identical to the Calendula Phyto Shampoo above, except the calendula was replaced with rosemary, which can be irritating to the scalp, though it does not appear that the product contains the potent oil form of rosemary. Otherwise, the same basic comments apply.

☺ **Aloe Phyto Conditioner** *($8.75 for 8 ounces)* is an extremely basic, rather light, conditioner that is an OK option for normal to slightly dry hair that is normal to fine or thin.

☺ **Chamomile Phyto Conditioner** *($8.75 for 8 ounces)* is even lighter than the Aloe Phyto Conditioner above, and contains merely water, anti-static agent, thickeners, aloe, essential oil fragrance, and calendula. The same basic comments apply.

☺ **Rosemary Phyto Conditioner** *($8.75 for 8 ounces)* is nearly identical to the Chamomile Phyto Conditioner above, except the soothing chamomile was replaced with potentially irritating rosemary. Otherwise, the same comments apply.

☺ **Rosemary Hair Oil** *($8.75 for 1.7 ounces)* is just almond oil with plant extract and fragrant plant oils. It is an option for dry to very dry hair if kept away from the scalp, but why use this when plain almond oil (or olive, canola, or safflower oil) works just as well without the potential for irritation?

WELLA

Internationally popular and trend-setting, Wella is a German-based company founded in 1880. Far less familiar in the United States, Wella made financial headlines in 2003 when consumer products giant Procter & Gamble acquired the brand in a two-part deal worth $5.7 billion. That's considerably more than the $4.95 billion P&G paid for Clairol in 2001, and it stands as the company's largest purchase to date (Source: *The Rose Sheet*, March 24, 2003, page 4). This purchase effectively makes P&G the largest hair-care company in the world. In buying Clairol, P&G also acquired their vast stable of products, and the purchase of Wella brings with that company Sebastian International, Graham Webb, and Back to BASICS. As this book goes to print, it was rumored that the Alberto-Culver Company may soon be added to the P&G ranks—unless competitor L'Oreal makes them an offer they can't refuse!

Wella's standing in the hair-care world is well established in salons, where their array of dye and perm products are considered some of the best in the business. For shampoos, conditioners, and styling products they fall far behind other lines, but now that P&G is in the picture I'm sure that will be changing over the next several years. For more information about Wella, call (800) 456-9322, extension 3, or visit www.wellausa.com.

What's Good About This Line: The prices are mostly reasonable. Wella makes some excellent styling products that cater to almost every styling taste and requirement; there are some wonderfully rich conditioners for thick, coarse hair that is dry to very dry; many of this line's claims are based more in reality than fantasy, which is refreshing.

What's Not So Good About It: Some Wella products are dated formulations containing mostly Vaseline and lanolin. There are far more hair-friendly ingredients and better products available from other lines (often less expensive) that could easily replace them.

☺ **Color Charm Care Rehydrating Shampoo, for Color Treated Hair** *($4.99 for 16 ounces)* is not hydrating in the least. The tiny amount of silk amino acids can't moisturize hair and has no benefit for color-treated hair. This is a basic, but good, shampoo for all hair types.

☹ **Color Charm Care Rehydrating Conditioner, for Color Treated Hair** *($4.99 for 16 ounces)* is an ordinary conditioner with minimal conditioning properties that would not be helpful for those with dry or damaged hair. This is an option only for someone with normal hair that needs help with comb-ability after hair is washed.

☺ **Kolestral Hot Oil Treatment** *($1.99 for 1 ounce)* does not contain any oil and remains another lackluster "treatment" product for hair. If you have fine or thin hair that is slightly dry, this is an OK, though unexciting, option.

☺ **Kolestral Concentrate, Intensive Conditioner** *($4.55 for 6 ounces)* is a thick, emollient conditioner that is an option for very dry hair that is coarse or thick. While it does contain lanolin and Vaseline, those ingredients are far less appealing for providing state-of-the-art benefits for hair in comparison to other ingredients.

☺ **In-Depth Treatment, for Problem Hair** *($7.95 for 16 ounces)* isn't more "in depth" than most other conditioners. This is a standard option for normal to dry hair of any thickness.

WELLA BONK

☺ **Bonk Amped, Long Hair Styler** *($9 for 5 ounces)* is a good option for all hair types looking for a styling spray that provides light hold and leaves hair flexible and minimally sticky. This is easy to brush through and adds soft shine to hair.

☺ **Bonk Crystal Dynamite, Iridescent Shine Gel** *($9 for 2.6 ounces)* is a water-soluble, gel-type pomade infused with tiny particles of mica for increased shine. It works very well to add texture to or to smooth hair (including frizzies) without being overly greasy. Despite this product's light attributes, it should still be used sparingly, especially if you have fine or thin hair.

☺ **Bonk Grounded, Frizz Eliminator** *($9 for 5.2 ounces)* is a very light water- and silicone-based styling cream that smoothes hair and calms frizzies without a heavy or greasy after-feel. This is ideal for use on normal to fine or thin hair; it is too light for thick or coarse hair. It would also be a good option to mix with gels or styling sprays to soften their effect while adding light conditioning hold to hair, as well as to provide a slight amount of heat protection.

☺ **Bonk Mega Spiker, Extreme Hold Styler** *($9 for 3.5 ounces)* does offer extreme hold, but not without lots of stickiness, which makes this tricky to brush through. It is best for detailed hairstyles that demand long-lasting hold and support.

☺ **Bonk Raw Hair Jam, Strong Hold Gel** *($9 for 5.5 ounces)* is a standard gel that provides medium hold with a moist, sticky finish that can still be brushed through. This does have a heavier texture, and is preferred for normal to slightly thick or coarse hair that is dry and needs extra styling support to make tresses manageable.

☺ **Bonk Warp Wax, Molding Agent** *($9 for 2.9 ounces)* is a fairly greasy pomade that is best for thick, coarse hair that needs smoothing and frizz control without the weight of Vaseline- or oil-based pomades. This is difficult to shampoo out.

WELLA COLOR PRESERVE

☺ **Color Preserve Daily Shampoo, for Color-Treated Hair** *($9.30 for 16 ounces)* is one of the most standard shampoos around, and has absolutely no benefit or edge for color-treated hair. All the claims about this shampoo's color-saving prowess are meaningless. It is an option for normal to fine or thin hair, but will cause buildup with repeated use.

☺ **Color Preserve Daily Conditioner, for Color-Treated Hair** *($10.30 for 16 ounces)* is a decent, though ordinary, conditioner for normal to slightly dry hair of any thickness.

☺ **Color Preserve Detangler and Leave-In Conditioner** *($10 for 8 ounces)* is a good leave-in conditioner for dry hair of any thickness, but it has no special advantage in terms of preserving hair color.

☺ **Color Preserve Deep Treatment** *($12.50 for 5.1 ounces)* is a basic emollient conditioner for dry hair that is normal to thick or coarse, but it cannot prolong hair color's depth and intensity.

☺ $$$ **Color Preserve Seal & Shine Drops** *($12.50 for 1.7 ounces)* is pricey for what you get, but it's worth checking out if you have dry to very dry hair and are battling frizzies.

WELLA ELAN PLUS

☺ **Elan Plus Conditioning Setting Lotion, Extra Hold** *($5.09 for 16 ounces)* is an old-fashioned setting lotion that has a liquidy texture and can provide light to medium hold with a slightly stiff, sticky feel. This is an OK option for setting or forming waves and curls, but lacks ingredients to help protect hair during heat-styling. It has an intense fragrance.

☺ **Elan Plus Conditioning Setting Lotion, Regular Hold** *($5.09 for 16 ounces)* is identical to the Elan Plus Conditioning Setting Lotion, Extra Hold above, only this offers slightly less hold, and the same basic comments apply.

WELLA LIFETEX WELLNESS

☺ **Lifetex Wellness Level Headed, Color Shine Shampoo** *($10 for 8.5 ounces)* is similar to the Color Charm Care Rehydrating Shampoo, for Color Treated Hair above, and the same review applies.

☺ **Lifetex Wellness Look Alive, Energizing Purity Wash** *($10 for 8.5 ounces)* is a standard shampoo that is a decent option for all hair types, though the lime, grapefruit, and orange extracts can be scalp irritants. This will not cause buildup.

☺ **Lifetex Wellness Wake-Up Call, Hydrating Purity Wash** *($10 for 8.5 ounces)* is nearly identical to the Lifetex Wellness Look Alive, Energizing Purity Wash above, and the same comments apply.

☺ **Lifetex Wellness Big Splash, Hydrating Purity Rinse** *($11 for 8.5 ounces)* is a very standard conditioner that is a good option for normal to slightly dry hair that is normal to fine or thin.

☺ $$$ **Lifetex Wellness Flash Flood, Hydrating Vitality Blast** *($16.50 for 5 ounces)* is an emollient, though standard, conditioner for dry to very dry hair that is coarse or thick. It is very similar to Wella's Kolestral Concentrate, Intensive Conditioner above, but costs almost four times as much.

☺ $$$ **Lifetex Wellness Power Plant, Energizing Vitality Blast** *($16.50 for 5 ounces)* is a stunningly basic conditioner that is an option for normal to fine or thin hair that is slightly dry, but the price is steep for what you get. Preservatives are not listed, but I suspect this was an oversight because this product would go rancid within weeks without a preservative system to keep it stable.

☺ **Lifetex Wellness Pumped Up, Energizing Purity Rinse** *($11 for 8.5 ounces)* is nearly identical to the Lifetex Wellness Power Plant, Energizing Vitality Blast above, save for a slightly different lineup of plant extracts, which won't impact hair in the least. Otherwise, the same review applies.

☺ **Lifetex Wellness Well Toned, Color Shine Purity Rinse** *($11 for 8.5 ounces)* is similar to, but not as well formulated as, the Lifetex Wellness Big Splash, Hydrating Purity Rinse above. The same basic comments apply, but I wouldn't choose this one over the Big Splash option.

☺ **Lifetex Wellness Well Defined, Sculpting Polisher** *($13.30 for 5 ounces)* is a thick, gel-type pomade that can be slightly heavy and greasy, but is still water-soluble. Those with normal to slightly thick, coarse, or curly hair would fare best with this, and it is infused with iridescent mica for increased shine. Note that the mica does not flake, which occurs more frequently when it is added to gels or mousses.

☹ **Lifetex Wellness Depth Charge, 60-Second Super Pak** *($17 for 5 ounces)* is similar to the Color Preserve Deep Treatment above, although that ends up being a much better product for dry hair because this option contains two forms of clay, which can damage the cuticle and make dry hair even drier. This is an overall poor choice and there is nothing "super" about it.

☺ $$$ **Lifetex Wellness Personal Trainer, Smooth and Defrizz Control** *($13 for 5 ounces)* is a lightweight, spray-on conditioner that has a lotion-like texture and can easily smooth flyaway strands and help manage frizzy hair. It has a silky finish and is not heavy or slick, which makes it a very good choice for normal or fine hair that is curly, wavy, or straight.

WELLA LIQUID HAIR

☺ **Liquid Hair Body Surf Beach Hair Styler, Strong Hold** *($11.30 for 4.2 ounces)* is a lightweight, minimal-hold styling spray that contains magnesium sulfate (an alkaline ingredient) and salt to rough up the hair's cuticle layer, which can add texture but can also cause damage when done repeatedly. This is OK for occasional use when creating highly textured hairstyles.

☺ **Liquid Hair Brilliant Spray Gel Volume & Texture, Strong Hold** *($10.30 for 6.8 ounces)* is an alcohol-free, water-based spray gel with a medium to firm hold that, thanks to glucose, leaves hair feeling stiff and sticky. It is slightly difficult to brush through, and is preferred for short, textured, or spiked hairstyles.

☺ **Liquid Hair Cross Trainer Straighten or Define Curl, Strong Hold** *($11.50 for 7 ounces)* is nearly identical to the Bonk Grounded, Frizz Eliminator above, except with slightly more hold. Otherwise, the same review applies.

☺ **Liquid Hair Crystal Styler Styling Gel, Extra Strong Hold** *($9.50 for 5 ounces)* is identical to the Bonk Mega Spiker, Extreme Hold Styler above, and the same review applies. Ounce for ounce, the Liquid Hair product is the better value.

☺ **Liquid Hair Energy Styler Volumizing Mousse, Strong Hold** *($11.50 for 10.6 ounces)* is a standard, propellant-based mousse that offers minimal hold with just a trace of stickiness. It is lighter than many mousses, and as such is a good option for fine hair that needs body and lift for casual hairstyles.

☺ **Liquid Hair Fast Finish Fixing Spritz** *($8.30 for 6.8 ounces)* is a very good styling spray that provides light hold and has a minimally stiff, sticky finish. It is easy to brush through and makes for a great working spray on wet or dry hair.

☺ **$$$ Liquid Hair Frozen Wax Sculpting Styler, Strong Hold** *($12.95 for 3.75 ounces)* is an aerosol spray-on wax that dispenses well, if a bit forcefully, and morphs into a thick, somewhat chunky wax that can be tricky to distribute through the hair. It has a heavy, greasy texture that is appropriate only for thick, coarse hair that is dry to very dry. It's better to apply this to your hands and then to your hair instead of spraying it directly on the hair.

☺ **Liquid Hair Gloss Jelly Finishing Polish, Soft Hold** *($10.99 for 1.7 ounces)* is a very standard gel-type pomade that can add texture and shine while smoothing dry ends or frizzies. It is reasonably water-soluble, but too greasy for use on fine or thin hair. All other hair types should use this sparingly for best results.

☺ **Liquid Hair Hair Putty Texturizer, Soft Hold** *($14 for 3.4 ounces)* is a thick styling lotion/pomade hybrid that is too thin to be considered a putty. It can help smooth coarse, frizzy hair while enhancing texture and adding shine, but can quickly become too heavy and greasy if not used sparingly.

☺ **Liquid Hair Kryptonite Acrylic Gel, Ultra Hold** *($11 for 3.5 ounces)* is a standard styling gel whose ultra hold description is entirely accurate. This is stiff, sticky stuff, but it can work wonders if you need gravity-defying lift and cement-like hold for extreme hairstyles. As you may have guessed, this cannot be brushed through without some snags along the way.

☺ **Liquid Hair Matte Finish Wax Hair Molder, Soft Hold** *($14 for 3.4 ounces)* is a standard styling wax with a soft texture, so it is easier to emulsify and apply to hair. It does have a matte finish and is heavy without feeling or looking greasy. This wax is recommended for coarse, thick hair that needs a substantial product to provide light grooming and control.

☺ **Liquid Hair Moonshine Foaming Pomade, Soft Hold** *($13 for 3.4 ounces)* is a liquid-to-foam mousse with the texture and feel of a water-soluble pomade. It is a unique product (well, as unique as hair-care products can get anyway) that would benefit dry to very dry hair that is coarse or thick. It offers no hold, and is best for enhancing hair's texture and adding a glossy shine with a moist finish. Curly, thick hair would also benefit from this product, but be sure to apply it sparingly.

☹ **Liquid Hair Power Shift Shaping Gel, Strong Hold** *($11.95 for 4.2 ounces)* is a styling gel/cream that ends up being problematic because it flakes terribly, and the mica particles will quickly fall from hair onto clothing, your car seat, bed sheets—everywhere.

☺ **$$$ Liquid Hair Restructurizer Leave-In Treatment, Soft Hold** *($16.50 for 6.8 ounces)* is a standard styling spray with light hold that keeps hair flexible and minimally stiff or sticky. The conditioning ingredients amount to lightweight anti-static and detangling agents, and offer little benefit for dry hair. This is good for use on normal to fine or thin hair that needs minor styling control, but needs help with combing.

☺ **Liquid Hair Structuring Mist Styling Hairspray, Strong Hold** *($9.50 for 8.4 ounces)* is a standard aerosol hairspray that can provide light to medium hold with a weightless feel that is slightly sticky. Less expensive versions of this product are available at the drugstore, but this remains a good "all hair types" hairspray.

WHITE RAIN

This venerable hair-care line has been repackaged and revived since severing ties with The Gillette Company in March 2000. The new look retains the classic appearance longtime users of this brand are familiar with, while the products themselves have improved formulas and less intense fragrances. As for a new name, the owners decided to stay with what has worked for several decades: The White Rain Company. For more information about White Rain, call (800) 575-7960 or visit www.whiterain.com.

What's Good About This Line: The prices! You're not likely to find a less expensive hair-care line that performs as well as this one does; there are excellent options in every category to meet most basic hair-care needs.

What's Not So Good About It: A few of the many shampoos contain problematic ingredients, and the conditioners offer options only for normal to slightly dry hair; the formulas are mostly repetitive, with the chief differences being fragrance and for-show-only additives such as plant extracts or vitamins; there are no styling creams, pomades, or silicone serums.

☹ **Daily Clarifying Shampoo, for Normal to Oily Hair** *($1.32 for 15 ounces)* is a below-standard shampoo that contains ammonium xylenesulfonate, a solvent that can swell the hair shaft and cause dryness with repeated use.

☺ **Extra Body Shampoo** *($1.32 for 15 ounces)* is a very good shampoo for all hair types and poses no risk of buildup. The chelating agent can remove chlorine, mineral, and styling product buildup.

☺ **Moisturizing Shampoo, for Normal to Dry Hair** *($1.32 for 15 ounces)* is nearly identical to the Extra Body Shampoo above, and the same review applies. This shampoo contains no conditioning agents, so the moisturizing claim isn't accurate, but this certainly won't strip color or make hair dry.

☺ **Regular Shampoo** *($1.32 for 15 ounces)* is nearly identical to the Extra Body Shampoo above, and the same review applies.

☺ **Salon Formula Shampoo, for Dull, Dry, Fly-Away Hair** *($1.32 for 15 ounces)* is nearly identical to the Extra Body Shampoo above, and the same review applies. The name may make you think this shampoo is different from the others, but it isn't, at least not in any way that's meaningful for your hair.

☺ **2 in 1 Shampoo Plus Conditioner, Extra Body** *($1.64 for 15 ounces)* is another very good shampoo that would serve normal to dry hair well. It contains mostly water, detergent cleansing agent, lather agent, thickener, emulsifier, pH adjusters, detangling agents, conditioning agents, fragrance, and preservatives. This is mildly conditioning and poses a slight risk of buildup with repeated use.

☺ **Extra Body Conditioner** *($1.49 for 15 ounces)* is an exceptionally basic conditioner that is an OK option for normal to slightly dry hair that is normal to fine or thin.

☺ **Moisturizing Conditioner** *($1.49 for 15 ounces)* is nearly identical to the Extra Body Conditioner above, and the same review applies.

☺ **Regular Conditioner** *($1.49 for 15 ounces)* is nearly identical to the Extra Body Conditioner above, and the same review applies.

☺ **Salon Formula Conditioner, for Dull, Dry, Fly-Away Hair** *($1.49 for 15 ounces)* is nearly identical to the Extra Body Conditioner above, and the same review applies. The only major difference between this conditioner and those above is that this one contains apple pectin fragrance, which doesn't affect hair's condition.

WHITE RAIN CLASSICS

☺ **Classics Color Nourish Mousse, Extra Body** *($1.32 for 5 ounces)* is a standard, propellant-based mousse that offers a light hold and a soft, non-sticky finish that can be brushed through with ease. It works great for soft, casual styles on normal to fine or thin hair.

☺ **Classics Hair Spray, Extra Hold (Aerosol)** *($1.59 for 7 ounces)* is a standard hairspray that, like many of its ilk, has a much softer hold than the name claims. This provides a light, minimally stiff hold with just a hint of stickiness. It is easy to brush through, and is a great option for all hair types.

☺ **Classics Hair Spray, Extra Hold (Non-Aerosol)** *($1.59 for 7 ounces)* is fine as a basic, no-frills hairspray for those who need medium hold. This remains sticky, and is not simple to brush through, but if you just need something to set and help maintain your style, it is a good option.

☺ **Classics Hair Spray, Extra Hold Unscented (Aerosol)** *($1.59 for 7 ounces)* is nearly identical to the Classics Hair Spray, Extra Hold (Aerosol) above, except this contains a softer fragrance (it is not unscented, however).

☺ **Classics Hair Spray, Extra Hold Unscented (Non-Aerosol)** *($1.59 for 7 ounces)* is identical to the Classics Hair Spray, Extra Hold (Non-Aerosol) above, and the same review applies.

☺ **Classics Hair Spray, Firm Hold (Aerosol)** *($1.59 for 7 ounces)* is identical to the Classics Hair Spray, Extra Hold (Aerosol) above, and the same review applies.

☺ **Classics Hair Spray, Maximum Hold (Aerosol)** *($1.59 for 7 ounces)* is similar to the Classics Hair Spray, Extra Hold (Aerosol) above, except this offers a medium hold with a stickier finish that makes it preferred for hard-to-hold hair.

☺ **Classics Hair Spray, Maximum Hold (Non-Aerosol)** *($1.59 for 7 ounces)* is similar to the Classics Hair Spray, Extra Hold (Non-Aerosol) above, except this offers slightly more hold and leaves a stickier finish. Otherwise, the same comments apply.

☺ **Classics Mousse, Extra Body** *($1.59 for 5 ounces)* is identical to the Classics Color Nourish Mousse, Extra Body above, and the same review applies.

☺ **Classics Spritz, Mega Hold (Non-Aerosol)** *($1.32 for 7 ounces)* is nearly identical to the Classics Hair Spray, Maximum Hold (Non-Aerosol) above, and the same review applies.

☺ **Classics Spritz, Super Hold (Non-Aerosol)** *($1.32 for 7 ounces)* is nearly identical to the Classics Hair Spray, Maximum Hold (Non-Aerosol) above, and the same review applies.

☺ **Classics Styling Gel, Extra Control** *($1.32 for 4 ounces)* is one of the most basic styling gels in this book, but for the money it does a good job providing a light to medium hold with a minimal stiff, sticky feel. The amount of panthenol (which is played up on the label) is too minuscule to matter for hair.

WHITE RAIN NATURALS

☺ **Naturals Shampoo Apple Blossom, for Dull, Limp Hair** *($1.32 for 15 ounces)* is nearly identical to the Extra Body Shampoo above, and the same review applies. This can indeed work well for limp hair because it can remove weighty buildup that results from use of conditioners and styling products.

☹ **Naturals Shampoo Energizing Citrus, for All Hair Types** *($1.32 for 15 ounces)* contains sodium lauryl sulfate as one of its main detergent cleansing agents, and that makes this shampoo too drying for the hair and scalp.

☹ **Naturals Shampoo Enriching Sunflower, for All Hair Types** *($1.32 for 15 ounces)* is similar to the Naturals Shampoo Energizing Citrus, for All Hair Types above, and the same review applies.

☺ **Naturals Shampoo Freesia Spirit, for Dull, Dry, Flyaway Hair** *($1.32 for 15 ounces)* is a much better option than the Naturals Citrus or Sunflower shampoos above. It works well for all hair types and poses minimal risk of buildup.

☺ **Naturals Shampoo Ginger Lily, for Normal to Dry Hair** *($1.32 for 15 ounces)* is nearly identical to the Extra Body Shampoo above, and the same review applies.

☺ **Naturals Shampoo Jasmine, for Flat, Fine, Thin Hair** *($1.32 for 15 ounces)* is nearly identical to the Extra Body Shampoo above, and the same review applies.

☺ **Naturals Shampoo Passion Flower, for Dry, Damaged, Overstressed Hair** *($1.32 for 15 ounces)* is nearly identical to the Extra Body Shampoo above, and the same review applies. This shampoo won't dry or strip the hair, but it isn't particularly helpful for damaged or overstressed hair.

☺ **Naturals Shampoo Pearberry Boost, for Permed/Color-Treated Hair** *($1.32 for 15 ounces)* is nearly identical to the Naturals Shampoo Freesia Spirit, for Dull, Dry, Flyaway Hair above, and the same review applies.

☹ **Naturals Shampoo Refreshing Lemongrass, for All Hair Types** *($1.32 for 15 ounces)* contains sodium lauryl sulfate as one of its main detergent cleansing agents, and that makes this shampoo too drying for the hair and scalp.

☹ **Naturals Shampoo Restoring Violet, for All Hair Types** *($1.32 for 15 ounces)* is nearly identical to the Naturals Shampoo Refreshing Lemongrass, for All Hair Types above, and the same review applies.

☺ **Naturals Shampoo Tropical Coconut, for Flat, Fine, Thin Hair** *($1.32 for 15 ounces)* is nearly identical to the Extra Body Shampoo above, and the same review applies.

☺ **Naturals Conditioner Apple Blossom, for Dull, Limp Hair** *($1.32 for 15 ounces)* is nearly identical to the Extra Body Conditioner above, and the same review applies.

☺ **Naturals Conditioner Energizing Citrus, for All Hair Types** *($1.32 for 15 ounces)* is a good, basic option for normal to slightly dry hair that is normal to fine, thin, or slightly thick.

☺ **Naturals Conditioner Enriching Sunflower, for All Hair Types** *($1.32 for 15 ounces)* is similar to the Naturals Conditioner Energizing Citrus, for All Hair Types above, except without the minerals or the citrus extracts. Otherwise, the same basic comments apply.

☺ **Naturals Conditioner Freesia Spirit, for Dull, Dry, Flyaway Hair** *($1.32 for 15 ounces)* is similar to the Naturals Conditioner Energizing Citrus, for All Hair Types above, except without the minerals or the citrus extracts. Otherwise, the same basic comments apply.

☺ **Naturals Conditioner Ginger Lily, for Normal to Dry Hair** *($1.32 for 15 ounces)* is nearly identical to the Extra Body Conditioner above, and the same review applies.

☺ **Naturals Conditioner Jasmine, for Flat, Fine, Thin Hair** *($1.32 for 15 ounces)* is nearly identical to the Extra Body Conditioner above, and the same review applies. The tiny amount of balm mint extract is unlikely to cause irritation, but it's still a good idea to keep this off the scalp.

☺ **Naturals Conditioner Passion Flower, for Dry, Damaged, Overstressed Hair** *($1.32 for 15 ounces)* is nearly identical to the Extra Body Conditioner above, but includes panthenol, which makes it slightly preferred. Panthenol actually works better in leave-in products because it doesn't hold up well during rinsing.

☺ **Naturals Conditioner Pearberry Boost, for Permed/Color-Treated Hair** *($1.32 for 15 ounces)* is nearly identical to the Extra Body Conditioner above, and the same review applies. The numerous plant extracts in this product have no effect on the hair's condition.

☺ **Naturals Conditioner Refreshing Lemongrass, for All Hair Types** *($1.32 for 15 ounces)* is similar to the Naturals Conditioner Energizing Citrus, for All Hair Types above, except without the minerals or the citrus extracts. Otherwise, the same basic comments apply.

☺ **Naturals Conditioner Restoring Violet, for All Hair Types** *($1.32 for 15 ounces)* is a good, though basic, conditioner for normal to slightly dry hair that is normal to fine or thin.

☺ **Naturals Conditioner Tropical Coconut, for Flat, Fine, Thin Hair** *($1.32 for 15 ounces)* is nearly identical to the Extra Body Conditioner above, and the same review applies. This does not contain coconut, but does have that familiar artificial coconut smell.

☺ **Naturals Anti-Frizz Gel Perfect Pearberry, Maximum Hold** *($1.59 for 8.25 ounces)* is a very standard, but good, styling gel that provides a firm hold with a stiff, sticky feel. This can still be brushed through and works well for unruly hair or intricate styles.

☺ **Naturals Hair Spray Angelica, Maximum Hold (Non-Aerosol)** *($1.32 for 7 ounces)* is, save for the addition of plant extracts (which have no benefit for hair), identical to the Classics Hair Spray, Extra Hold (Non-Aerosol) above, and the same review applies.

☺ **Naturals Hair Spray Chamomile, Extra Hold (Non-Aerosol)** *($1.32 for 7 ounces)* is, save for the addition of plant extracts (which have no benefit for hair), nearly identical to the Classics Hair Spray, Extra Hold (Non-Aerosol) above, except this is slightly less sticky. Otherwise, the same comments apply.

☺ **Naturals Hair Spray Enriching Sunflower, Extra Hold (Aerosol)** *($1.59 for 7 ounces)* is a standard hairspray with a light hold and no stiff or sticky finish, which means this can be brushed through easily. It is an excellent, inexpensive hairspray for those whose styles need a bit more structure and control.

☺ **Naturals Hair Spray Freesia Spirit, Extra Hold (Non-Aerosol)** *($1.59 for 7 ounces)* is a good option for a light-hold hairspray that is minimally stiff or sticky. The plant oil, silicone, and panthenol make this beneficial for dry hair and help add shine while allowing hair to be brushed through easily. This is the most elegant hairspray formula in the White Rain line.

☺ **Naturals Hair Spray Pearberry Boost, Maximum Hold (Aerosol)** *($1.59 for 7 ounces)* is similar to the Classics Hair Spray, Extra Hold (Aerosol) above, and the same basic comments apply.

☺ **Naturals Hair Spray Perfect Pearberry, Maximum Hold (Non-Aerosol)** *($1.59 for 7 ounces)* is, save for a change in plant extracts and fragrance, identical to the Naturals Hair Spray Freesia Spirit, Extra Hold (Non-Aerosol) above, and the same comments apply.

☺ **Naturals Nourishing Mousse Enriching Sunflower, Extra Body** *($1.59 for 5 ounces)* is a good, medium-hold, propellant-based mousse that has a slightly sticky finish that can be brushed through without flaking. It is an option for all hair types, but those with fine or thin hair will fare best with this lightweight product.

ZERO FRIZZ

For more information about Zero Frizz, call (800) 966-6960 or visit www.zerofrizz.com.

What's Good About This Line: Everything, from the products themselves to the prices, makes this line impressive for those with normal to dry hair of any texture; the silicone serum is one of the most affordable around, and performs every bit as well as serums sold in salons.

What's Not So Good About It: The name Zero Frizz sounds so definitive, yet even the best products cannot keep frizzies from coming back or showing themselves when the humidity rises; the products can go a long way to smooth frizzy hair, but the result depends on factors beyond your (or a hair-care product's) control—such as climate, genetics, and styling ability—so don't expect 100% frizz elimination.

☺ **Shampoo, Smoothing & Straightening** *($5.95 for 12 ounces)* is an excellent conditioning shampoo for normal to dry hair that is normal to coarse or thick, though it cannot automatically make curly hair straight. This will cause buildup with repeated use, so it would be best to alternate it with a shampoo that does not contain conditioning agents.

☺ **Daily Conditioner** *($5.95 for 12 ounces)* is a creamy, emollient conditioner that is a very good choice for dry to very dry hair that is coarse or thick.

☺ **Deep Conditioner** *($5.95 for 6 ounces)* is a more emollient, thicker version of the Daily Conditioner above, and the same basic comments apply.

☺ **Smooth Ends Leave-In Conditioning Treatment** *($3.99 for 6 ounces)* is a very good, leave-in conditioning fluid/lotion that can smooth hair while adding shine and taming frizzies. It cannot repair split ends, but can help them temporarily look smoother. As a leave-in conditioner, it is best for normal to dry hair that is normal to slightly thick or coarse.

☺ **Defining Touch, Anti-Frizz Styling Pomade** *($5.49 for 2 ounces)* isn't a true pomade. Rather, it is a whipped styling cream packaged in a jar. It has a smooth, moist texture that is easy to emulsify and distribute through the hair. Unless used sparingly, it can feel too heavy on all but thick or coarse hair. This works well to smooth frizzies without adding a glossy or greasy looking finish.

☺ **Hold It There, Anti-Frizz Treatment Styling Gel** *($3.99 for 6 ounces)* is a very good, silky-finish styling gel for all hair types. It provides a light to medium hold with a minimally stiff, sticky feel that is easily brushed through. This is not a good choice to use by itself if frizzies are a persistent problem (you would want to pair it with a silicone serum), but unless you aim to design an extreme hairstyle, this gel is a great option.

☺ **Smoothing + Styling Mousse** *($5.95 for 6 ounces)* is a propellant-based mousse with a light hold and a weightless, minimally sticky or stiff feel. It is a superb option for fine or thin hair that is slightly dry and needs mild conditioning without a trace of heaviness. If frizzies are a persistent problem, you will need to use this with a silicone serum to smooth them.

☺ **Straighten Out, Humidity Resistant Smoothing Cream** *($7.59 for 4.2 ounces)* is a thick, water- and silicone-based smoothing cream that works well to straighten hair—with heat and the proper styling tools. It offers a light hold with a trace of stickiness and leaves hair feeling silky but not greasy. It is an option for all hair types, though someone with curly hair that is fine or thin should use it sparingly.

☺ **Corrective Hair Serum** *($7.95 for 4 ounces)* is a standard silicone serum that works as well as any, but the price of this one makes it a genuine beauty steal! The sunscreen it contains cannot protect hair from UV damage, nor is this product rated with an SPF number, which is as it should be, since the FDA does not allow hair-care products to carry SPF ratings. This can work beautifully to tame frizzies and add shine, but, as with all silicone serums, it should be used sparingly.

☺ **Quick Fix Glistening Mist** *($7.95 for 4 ounces)* is a great silicone spray for all hair types. In addition to the silicone, this nonaqueous product contains water-binding agents and panthenol. Vitamins are present, too, but have no effect on hair.

ZIRH

For more information about Zirh, call (800) 295-8877 or visit www.zirh.com.

What's Good About This Line: This is a small line of men's products that is simple to figure out, which makes it even more appealing to men, who traditionally don't like too many choices when it comes to grooming products.

What's Not So Good About It: The prices are steep considering that the products are easily replaced with others available at the drugstore.

☺ **$$$ Shampoo, Premium Hair Shampoo** *($14.50 for 8.4 ounces)* claims that the alpha hydroxy acids in this are "hyper-effective cleansers" for all hair types, but the fact is that AHAs do not have any cleansing ability, and they can actually be detrimental for hair if the pH of the shampoo is acidic enough for them to exfoliate. However, that is definitely not the case here, and this ends up being a very standard, but good, shampoo for all hair types. It will not cause buildup.

☺ $$$ **Conditioner, Premium Hair Conditioner** *($14.50 for 8.4 ounces)* is too basic to be considered "premium," but it is a good option for normal to slightly dry hair that is normal to fine or thin. This cannot repair the hair's cuticle, as claimed.

☺ $$$ **Control, Lightweight Styling Wax** *($18.50 for 1.7 ounces)* is a clear, thick pomade that is fairly water-soluble. It is highly fragranced, but can indeed smooth dry sections of hair while adding a wet-look shine. It also works great (used in small amounts) to emphasize the texture of short hair, including flat tops and spiked dos.

☺ **Hold, Sculpting Hair Gel** *($14.50 for 3.4 ounces)* is a very basic, but effective, styling gel with a light hold and a smooth, non-sticky finish that is easily brushed through. This holds no advantage over any styling gel option from L'Oreal's Studio Line, but is an option nonetheless.

CHAPTER ELEVEN

The Best Products

SHOPPING MADE SIMPLE

Many readers of previous editions of this book have commented that my lists of best hair-care products were impossibly long. If the goal of this book is to make it easier for consumers to shop for effective hair-care products, they ask, then why are so many products recommended? Are they all *that* good? Good questions, and they can be answered with a simple yes—there are hundreds of excellent hair-care products available in all price ranges. However, for this third (and final) edition of *Don't Go Shopping for Hair-Care Products Without Me*, I decided, in response to my readers' requests, to offer streamlined lists in each product category (and subcategory, such as shampoos for specific hair and scalp types). All of the categories (and subcategories, where applicable) now feature lists of no more than 20 products within a range of prices. This will allow you to quickly find what you are looking for, rather than having to read through cumbersome lists. After analyzing thousands of products, these brief summaries list my favorites among the best of the best (of which there are many more), whether you want to spend realistically or extravagantly. My sincere hope is that this method helps direct you to the best products for your needs, and that shopping for hair-care products will become an empowering rather than intimidating or money-wasting experience.

Please note that there are fewer than 20 products listed in some hair-care categories due to the limited number of "best" options within those groups.

Because pricing in the different hair-care product categories varies widely, you will notice that each main category (such as shampoos, conditioners, styling products, and so on) has its own price dividing line to separate the inexpensive from the expensive options. These dividing lines between inexpensive and expensive products are based on the average price ranges observed while researching for this book. I may not agree with a company's prices, but that doesn't change the fact that the products it sells are worth considering.

One more thing: for more specific categories with limited options (such as color-enhancing or fragrance-free shampoos), the lists of best products are shorter by virtue of what's available and what was reviewed favorably.

DON'T JUDGE A PRODUCT BY ITS LABEL

Keep in mind that a hair-care company's name and/or claims for a product do not always correspond with my recommendations. Just because a product label says it "can repair hair" or a product is recommended for damaged hair or a sensitive, itchy scalp, or says it can "make hair feel fuller and thicker" doesn't mean the formulation itself supports that label or claim. Further, the hair-care industry's inane and meaningless terms like Mega,

Super, Firm, Super Firm, Flexible, Ultra Firm, Freeze, Soft, or Natural to describe hold are used randomly and vary wildly. It's not uncommon for there to be no difference between products with these arbitrary descriptive ratings, and I often found that the Mega-hold products had a softer hold than the Flexible-hold products. This was especially true for gels, mousses, and (more so than in the previous edition of this book) hairsprays. For this reason, while perusing the lists of best styling products you may see a firm-hold gel in the light-hold list.

Additionally, you will find many selections in the following lists of recommended products with names that make it sound as if they should be in the dry-hair group but that I have included in the normal or slightly dry hair group—and vice versa. What counts is the product formulation (meaning what each product contains), not what the companies want you to believe about their products. For example, there are many products labeled as good for one type of hair when they are really best suited for another type.

BEST SHAMPOOS

See Chapter Four for more information about shampoos.

BEST SHAMPOOS THAT WILL NOT CAUSE BUILDUP AND COST $8 OR LESS

Note: The hair-care lines marked with an asterisk feature one or more additional shampoos that are nearly identical to the recommended shampoo on the list.

Avon Advance Techniques Color-Protection Shampoo *($3.49 for 11 ounces)*

Bath & Body Works Bio Restorative Shampoo, Strengthens Damaged, Overstressed Hair *($7.50 for 12 ounces)*

Breck Beautiful Hair BRECK Shampoo for Normal Hair *($3.39 for 12 ounces)*

Charles Worthington Big Hair Body Beautiful Shampoo for Fine, Limp, and Flyaway Hair *($5.99 for 8.5 ounces)*

JASÖN Natural Cosmetics Swimmers & Sports Hair and Scalp Reconditioning Shampoo *($7.95 for 17.5 ounces)*

Jheri Redding Shine Shampoo with Vitamin C, for Dull, Dry Hair *($2.49 for 16 ounces)*

Joico Resolve Chelating Shampoo, for Maximum Cleansing *($8 for 10.1 ounces)*

*****Neutrogena** Shampoo, Anti-Residue Formula *($5.69 for 6 ounces)*

Prell Volume Care Rinse Clean Shampoo *($3.19 for 13 ounces)*

Quantum Clarifying Shampoo, for Deep Cleansing to Remove Build-Up *($6.50 for 15 ounces)*

Queen Helene Natural Garlic Shampoo, Unscented *($3.75 for 21 ounces)*

Salon Grafix Thickening & Volumizing Shampoo *($4.99 for 16 ounces)*

Senscience Body & Shine Bodifying Shampoo *($7.65 for 12 ounces)*

*****SEXY Hair Concepts** Big Sexy Hair, Big Volume Shampoo *($6.95 for 8.5 ounces)*

Soft & Beautiful Moisturizing Shampoo, Pro-Vitamin Formula *($3.49 for 16 ounces)*

Soft Sheen Carson Optimum Care Collagen Moisture Shampoo *($2.29 for 8 ounces)*

*****Suave** Daily Clarifying Shampoo, for Normal to Oily Hair *($1.29 for 15 ounces)*

*****Sukesha** Extra Body Shampoo, Mild, Deep Cleansing for Added Texture *($5.95 for 12 ounces)*

*TIGI Bed Head Self Absorbed, Mega Vitamin Shampoo *($7.95 for 12 ounces)*
*TRESemme European Deep Cleansing Shampoo *($4.49 for 32 ounces)*
*White Rain Extra Body Shampoo *($1.32 for 15 ounces)*

BEST SHAMPOOS THAT WILL NOT CAUSE BUILDUP AND COST MORE THAN $8

Note: *The hair-care line marked with an asterisk features one or more additional shampoos that are nearly identical to the recommended shampoo on the list.*

ABBA Complete, Shampoo for All Hair Types *($8.99 for 10 ounces)*
Alterna Life Volumizing Shampoo *($17 for 12 ounces)*
Aveda Brilliant Shampoo *($11 for 8.5 ounces)*
Aveda Hair Detoxifier *($9 for 8.5 ounces)*
Bumble and bumble Sunday Shampoo *($13 for 8 ounces)*
Framesi Biogenol Color Care System Clarifying Shampoo *($11 for 16 ounces)*
Frédéric Fekkai Technician Shampoo for Normal Hair *($18.50 for 8 ounces)*
Frédéric Fekkai Baby Blonde Color Enhancing Shampoo with Chamomile *($18.50 for 8 ounces)*
Goldwell Elumen Wash *($12 for 8.4 ounces)*
Graham Webb Classic Indulgence Pearl Enhanced Shampoo *($13.90 for 8.5 ounces)*
KMS Daily Fixx Totally Clean Shampoo *($8.95 for 12 ounces)*
Matrix Essentials Color Therapy Shampoo *($10 for 16 ounces)*
Michael diCesare Clarifying Oat Hair Wash *($9.75 for 8.75 ounces)*
NEXXUS VitaTress Biotin Shampoo *($9 for 10.1 ounces)*
Paula's Choice All Over Hair & Body Shampoo *($12.95 for 16 ounces)*
Philip B. Scent of Santa Fe Shampoo, Gentle Daily Cleansing for All Hair Types *($29 for 8 ounces)*
Redken Color Extend Shampoo, Protection for Color-Treated Hair *($8.50 for 10.1 ounces)*
Redken Headstrong Shampoo, Volume for Fine Hair *($8.50 for 10.1 ounces)*
*Rusk Sensories Full Green Tea & Alfalfa Shampoo *($8.99 for 13 ounces)*
Sebastian Collectives Cello Shampoo, for Normal to Oily Hair *($8.50 for 10.2 ounces)*

BEST SHAMPOOS FOR ADDING VOLUME OR CONDITIONING OR BOTH

BEST VOLUMIZING/CONDITIONING SHAMPOOS FOR HAIR THAT IS NORMAL TO FINE OR THIN THAT COST $8 OR LESS

Note: *The hair-care lines marked with an asterisk feature one or more additional shampoos that are nearly identical to the recommended shampoo on the list.*

*Charles Worthington Results Everyday Shine Shampoo, for Dull Lifeless Hair *($5.99 for 10.9 ounces)*
Citré Shine Color Brilliance Shampoo *($3.99 for 16 ounces)*
Citré Shine Moisture Burst Shampoo *($3.99 for 16 ounces)*
Garnier Fructis Fortifying Shampoo, for Fine Hair *($3.99 for 13 ounces)*
göt2b So Smooth Creme Shampoo *($5.99 for 8.5 ounces)*

ISO Daily Balancing Cleanse, Gentle Shampoo *($7.25 for 13.5 ounces)*
Jheri Redding Extra Therashine Smoothing Shampoo *($6.95 for 13.5 ounces)*
Joico Kerapro Conditioning Shampoo, for Normal-to-Dry Hair *($7 for 10.1 ounces)*
Joico Volissima Volumizing Shampoo, for Fine Hair *($8 for 10.1 ounces)*
L'Oreal Vive Fresh-Shine Shampoo, for Frequent Use on All Hair Types *($4.49 for 13 ounces)*
Paul Mitchell Cleanse, Awapuhi Shampoo *($5.99 for 8.5 ounces)*
*Paul Mitchell Cleanse, Shampoo Two *($6.49 for 8.5 ounces)*
Prell Active Frequent Use Shampoo, Non-Drying Formula *($3.19 for 11.25 ounces)*
Progaine Volumizing Shampoo *($5.99 for 12 ounces)*
Salon Grafix Moisture Balancing & Hydrating Shampoo *($4.99 for 16 ounces)*
*SEXY Hair Concepts Curly Sexy Hair, Shampoo *($6.95 for 8.5 ounces)*
Soft & Beautiful Just for Me Moisturizing Conditioning Shampoo *($2.29 for 8 ounces)*
Sukesha Moisturizing Shampoo, Shampoo and Conditioner in One *($5.95 for 12 ounces)*
TIGI Bed Head Control Freak Shampoo *($7.95 for 12 ounces)*
TIGI Bed Head Moisture Maniac Shampoo *($7.95 for 12 ounces)*

BEST VOLUMIZING/CONDITIONING SHAMPOOS FOR HAIR THAT IS NORMAL TO FINE OR THIN THAT COST MORE THAN $8

ARTec Textureline Smoothing Shampoo *($10.10 for 12 ounces)*
Bumble and bumble Thickening Shampoo *($16 for 8 ounces)*
Bumble and bumble Curl Conscious Shampoo, for Fine to Medium Hair *($18 for 8 ounces)*
Framesi Biogenol Color Care System Ultra Body Shampoo *($11 for 16 ounces)*
Garren New York Anyday Shampoo *($25 for 8 ounces)*
ISO Multiplicity Dimensions, Texture Shampoo *($9.95 for 13.5 ounces)*
ISO Multiplicity Moisture, Hydrating Shampoo *($9.95 for 13.5 ounces)*
j.f. lazartigue Orchid Shampoo *($24 for 8.4 ounces)*
Joico Biojoba Treatment Shampoo, for Scalp and Chemically-Damaged Hair *($10 for 10.1 ounces)*
KMS Color Vitality Shampoo *($8.95 for 12 ounces)*
KMS Daily Fixx Clarifying Shampoo *($8.95 for 12 ounces)*
Lancome Shine Vitality Gel Shampoo *($16 for 8.4 ounces)*
Matrix Essentials Perm Fresh Shampoo *($9 for 16 ounces)*
NEXXUS Assure Replenishing Nutrient Shampoo *($8.50 for 13.5 ounces)*
NEXXUS Phyto Organics Syntress Volumizing Lift Shampoo *($10 for 10.1 ounces)*
Phyto Phytojoba Hydrating Shampoo with Jojoba Oil, for Dry Hair *($20 for 6.7 ounces)*
Phyto Phyto Plage Sun Shampoo *($18 for 5 ounces)*
Redken Smooth Down Shampoo, Anti-Frizz Smoothing for Very Dry/Unruly Hair *($9.95 for 10.1 ounces)*
Sebastian Collectives Cello Shampoo, for Normal to Dry Hair *($8.50 for 10.2 ounces)*

BEST VOLUMIZING/CONDITIONING SHAMPOOS FOR HAIR THAT IS NORMAL TO DRY AND OF ANY THICKNESS THAT COST $8 OR LESS

Note: The hair-care lines marked with an asterisk feature one or more additional shampoos that are nearly identical to the recommended shampoo on the list.

Charles Worthington Results Moisture Seal Glossing Shampoo *($5.99 for 10.9 ounces)*

*Garnier Fructis Fortifying Shampoo + Conditioner, for Normal Hair *($3.99 for 13 ounces)*

ISO Color Preserve Cleanse, Color Care Shampoo *($7.25 for 13.5 ounces)*

JASÖN Natural Cosmetics Forest Essence Conditioning Shampoo *($7.95 for 17.5 ounces)*

JASÖN Natural Cosmetics Hemp Enriched Shampoo for All Hair Types *($7.95 for 17.5 ounces)*

JASÖN Natural Cosmetics Natural E.F.A. Shampoo, Extra Rich Hair Nourishing Formula for Normal to Dry Hair *($6.50 for 16 ounces)*

John Frieda Frizz Ease Smooth Start, Defrizzing Shampoo, Original Formula *($5.29 for 12.7 ounces)*

*KMS Curl Up Shampoo *($7.75 for 8.1 ounces)*

*L'Oreal Vive Color-Care Shampoo, for Regular Color-Treated or Highlighted Hair *($4.49 for 13 ounces)*

NEXXUS Exoil Oily Hair Normalizing Shampoo *($5.50 for 10.1 ounces)*

NEXXUS Retexxtur Curl Vitalizing Shampoo *($8 for 10.1 ounces)*

Prell Hydra Care Rinse Clean Shampoo *($3.19 for 13 ounces)*

Prell Volume Care Rinse Clean Shampoo *($3.19 for 13 ounces)*

Quantum Moisturizing Shampoo, for Permed, Color-Treated & Dry Hair *($6.50 for 15 ounces)*

Queen Helene Ginseng & Tea Tree Shampoo, for All Types of Hair *($5.49 for 16 ounces)*

Sebastian Shaper Volume Boost Shampoo *($7.99 for 8.5 ounces)*

SEXY Hair Concepts Straight Sexy Hair Shampoo *($6.95 for 8.5 ounces)*

*TRESemme Total Solutions Colour Care, Healthy Highlights Shampoo *($3.79 for 14 ounces)*

White Rain 2 in 1 Shampoo Plus Conditioner, Extra Body *($1.64 for 15 ounces)*

BEST VOLUMIZING/CONDITIONING SHAMPOOS FOR HAIR THAT IS NORMAL TO DRY AND OF ANY THICKNESS THAT COST MORE THAN $8

Note: The hair-care lines marked with an asterisk feature one or more additional shampoos that are nearly identical to the recommended shampoo on the list.

Aveda Shampure Shampoo *($9 for 8.5 ounces)*

Back to BASICS Pomegranate Peach Replenishing Shampoo *($8.95 for 12 ounces)*

*BioSilk Silk Therapy Smoothing Shampoo *($8.95 for 11.6 ounces)*

The Body Shop Olive Glossing Shampoo *($8.50 for 8 ounces)*

Bumble and bumble Alojoba Shampoo *($17 for 8 ounces)*

*Fudge Unleaded Shampoo 1, Mild Cleansing Shampoo for Everyday Use of Normal to Dry Hair *($13.55 for 16.8 ounces)*

*Graham Webb Making Waves Curl Defining Shampoo *($10.18 for 11 ounces)*

Hayashi System 911 Shampoo Emergency Repair for Dry Damaged Hair *($13 for 10.6 ounces)*

JASÖN Natural Cosmetics Damage Control Creme Shampoo, for Frizzy, Dry or Color-Treated Hair *($12.50 for 16 ounces)*

Joico K-Pak Shampoo, for Damaged Hair *($12 for 10.1 ounces)*

L'ANZA Urban Elements Remedy Shampoo *($12 for 10.1 ounces)*

*Matrix Biolage Ultra-Hydrating Shampoo *($9.95 for 16.9 ounces)*

Modern Elixirs by Paul Mitchell Color Therapy Shampoo *($10.99 for 8.5 ounces)*

mop (modern organic products) glisten shampoo *($11.50 for 8.45 ounces)*

*NEXXUS Phyto Organics Hydruss Moisturizing Shampoo *($10 for 10.1 ounces)*

Ouidad Curl Quencher Shampoo *($10 for 8 ounces)*

*Paul Mitchell Cleanse, Botanical Hydrating Shampoo *($9.99 for 8.5 ounces)*

*Phyto Phytocurl Curl Enhancing Shampoo, for Curly Hair *($20 for 6.7 ounces)*

*Pureology Hydrate Shampoo *($19 for 10.1 ounces)*

Senscience Straight Sense Shampoo *($8.10 for 10.2 ounces)*

SEXY Hair Concepts Silky Sexy Hair, Silky Shampoo *($8.95 for 8.5 ounces)*

BEST VOLUMIZING/CONDITIONING SHAMPOOS FOR DRY TO VERY DRY HAIR THAT IS NORMAL TO FINE OR THIN THAT COST $8 OR LESS

ISO Purifying Cleanse, Deep Cleansing Shampoo *($7.25 for 13.5 ounces)*

L'Oreal Nature's Therapy Unfrizz Smoothing Shampoo *($4.99 for 12 ounces)*

BEST VOLUMIZING/CONDITIONING SHAMPOOS FOR DRY TO VERY DRY HAIR THAT IS NORMAL TO FINE OR THIN THAT COST MORE THAN $8

Aveda Sap Moss Shampoo *($11 for 4.2 ounces)*

ISO Multiplicity Reflect, Shine Shampoo *($9.95 for 13.5 ounces)*

Kiehl's Mild, Gentle Shampoo for Babies *($15 for 8 ounces)*

Mastey Enove Volumizing Creme Shampoo, for Fine Hair *($11 for 12 ounces)*

Mastey Traite Moisture Shampoo *($15 for 16 ounces)*

Mastey Solfiltre Swimmer's Shampoo *($11 for 8.5 ounces)*

Rene Furterer Karite Shampoo, for Extremely Dry Scalp and Hair *($22 for 5.07 ounces)*

SEXY Hair Concepts Healthy Sexy Hair, Soy Milk Moisture Shampoo *($10.95 for 13.5 ounces)*

BEST VOLUMIZING/CONDITIONING SHAMPOOS FOR DRY TO VERY DRY HAIR THAT IS THICK OR COARSE THAT COST $8 OR LESS

Beauty Without Cruelty Moisture Plus Shampoo, Benefits Dry/Treated Hair *($6.95 for 16 ounces)*

ion Anti-Frizz Solutions Straightening Shampoo, Cleanser for Curly, Wavy, Frizzy Hair *($4.99 for 12 ounces)*

John Frieda Frizz Ease Relax Total Clarity, Moisturizing Shampoo *($6.99 for 8.4 ounces)*

L'Oreal Vive Curl-Moisture Shampoo, for Curly Hair *($4.49 for 13 ounces)*

Neutrogena Triple Moisture Cream Lather Shampoo *($5.99 for 8.45 ounces)*

Pantene Relaxed & Natural Intensive Moisturizing Shampoo *($3.99 for 13.5 ounces)*

BEST VOLUMIZING/CONDITIONING SHAMPOOS FOR DRY TO VERY DRY HAIR THAT IS THICK OR COARSE THAT COST MORE THAN $8

Aveda All-Sensitive Shampoo *($16 for 6.7 ounces)*
Back to BASICS Ginger Scalp Therapy Shampoo *($9.95 for 6 ounces)*
Back to BASICS Green Tea Ultra Hydrating Shampoo *($9.95 for 12 ounces)*
bain de terre Jasmine Moisturizing Shampoo *($10.49 for 13.5 ounces)*
BioSilk Silk Therapy Thickening Shampoo *($8.95 for 11.6 ounces)*
Garren New York Nourishing Creme Shampoo *($32 for 7 ounces)*
KMS Daily Fixx Everyday Shampoo *($8.95 for 12 ounces)*
KMS Daily Repair Shampoo *($8.25 for 12 ounces*
L'ANZA Hair Repair Formula Protein Plus Shampoo *($8.40 for 10.1 ounces)*
L'ANZA Strait-Line Temporary Curl Relaxing Formula Shampoo *($10.95 for 8.5 ounces)*
Mastey Pure Colorcare Moisture Sulfate-Free Shampoo *($19.99 for 16 ounces)*
Matrix sleek.look Shampoo *($10.95 for 13.5 ounces)*
NEXXUS Diametress Luscious Hair Thickening Shampoo *($15 for 13.5 ounces)*
NEXXUS Y Serum Younger Looking Hair Shampoo *($11 for 10.1 ounces)*
Ouidad Clear Shampoo *($9 for 8 ounces)*
Philip B. Hair Care African Shea Butter Shampoo for All Hair Types *($21 for 8 ounces)*
Phyto Phytospecific Hydra-Repairing Shampoo, with Shea Butter *($18 for 5.07 ounces)*
Redken Clear Moisture Shampoo *($8.50 for 10.1 ounces)*
Sebastian Laminates Shampoo *($9.99 for 8.5 ounces)*

BEST VOLUMIZING/CONDITIONING SHAMPOOS FOR NORMAL TO DRY HAIR THAT IS THICK OR COARSE THAT COST $8 OR LESS

Citré Shine Smooth Out Shampoo *($3.99 for 16 ounces)*
Goldwell Definition Dry & Porous Shampoo *($8 for 8.4 ounces)*
Goldwell Definition Permed & Curly Curl Care Shampoo *($8 for 8.4 ounces)*
ion Anti-Frizz Solutions Smoothing Shampoo, Cleanser for Frizzy, Fly-Away Hair *($4.99 for 12 ounces)*
ion Volumizing Solutions Vitalizing Thickening Shampoo, for All Hair Types *($4.99 for 16 ounces)*
John Frieda Frizz Ease Smooth Start, Defrizzing Shampoo, Extra Strength Formula *($5.29 for 12.7 ounces)*
Joico Triage Moisture-Balancing Shampoo, for Normal Hair *($7 for 10.1 ounces)*
Neutrogena Clean for Color Color-Defending Shampoo *($3.99 for 10.1 ounces)*
Neutrogena Triple Moisture Cream Lather Shampoo *($5.99 for 8.45 ounces)*
Pert Plus Kids 2 in 1 Shampoo plus Conditioner, Bananaberri *($3.49 for 13.5 ounces)*
Zero Frizz Shampoo, Smoothing & Straightening *($5.95 for 12 ounces)*

BEST VOLUMIZING/CONDITIONING SHAMPOOS FOR NORMAL TO DRY HAIR THAT IS THICK OR COARSE THAT COST MORE THAN $8

The Body Shop Honey Moisturizing Shampoo *($8.50 for 8 ounces)*
Darphin Gentle Shampoo with Calendula, for All Hair Types *($22 for 6.7 ounces)*
Darphin Shampoo with Gleditschia, for Thin and Dull Hair *($22 for 6.7 ounces)*

Frédéric Fekkai Glossing Shampoo *($20 for 8 ounces)*
Graham Webb Visibility Clarifying Shampoo *($9.25 for 11 ounces)*
j.f. lazartigue Treatment Cream Shampoo with Collagen *($33 for 6.8 ounces)*
John Masters Organics Evening Primrose Shampoo, for Dry Hair *($16 for 8 ounces)*
Lancome Radiant Color Reviving Treatment Shampoo *($16 for 8.4 ounces)*
Mastey Pure Colorcare Volume Sulfate-Free Shampoo, for Fine Hair *($19.99 for 16 ounces)*
Phyto Phytospecific Intense Nutrition Shampoo, with Kukui Oil *($18 for 5.07 ounces)*
Phyto Phytospecific Vital Force Shampoo, with Illipe Butter and Barley Milk *($18 for 5.07 ounces)*
Redken Active Express Shampoo, Fast-Acting for All Hair Types *($8.50 for 10.1 ounces)*
Redken All Soft Shampoo, Softness for Dry/Brittle Hair *($8.50 for 10.1 ounces)*
Rene Furterer Carthame Milk Shampoo, for Fine Hair *($22 for 5.07 ounces)*
Sebastian Collection Spandex Shampoo *($8.95 for 8.5 ounces)*

BEST DANDRUFF SHAMPOOS WITH ZINC PYRITHIONE, SELENIUM SULFIDE, OR KETOCONAZOLE (ALL PRICES)

Garnier Fructis Fortifying Anti-Dandruff Shampoo *($3.99 for 13 ounces)*
Head & Shoulders Shampoo, Classic Clean *($4.59 for 13.5 ounces)*
Head & Shoulders Shampoo, Dry Scalp Care *($4.59 for 13.5 ounces)*
Head & Shoulders Shampoo, Extra Fullness *($4.59 for 13.5 ounces)*
Head & Shoulders Shampoo, Intensive Treatment *($4.59 for 13.5 ounces)*
Head & Shoulders Shampoo, Refresh *($4.59 for 13.5 ounces)*
Head & Shoulders Shampoo, Ultimate Clean *($4.59 for 13.5 ounces)*
Head & Shoulders 2-in-1 Shampoo Plus Conditioner, Classic Clean *($4.59 for 13.5 ounces)*
Head & Shoulders 2-in-1 Shampoo Plus Conditioner, Smooth & Silky *($4.59 for 13.5 ounces)*
KENRA Dandruff Shampoo, Treatment for Dandruff and Other Scalp Conditions *($12 for 10.1 ounces)*
KMS Daily Fixx Dandruff Shampoo *($8.95 for 12 ounces)*
L'Oreal Vive for Men Daily Thickening Anti-Dandruff Shampoo, for All Hair *($3.69 for 13 ounces)*
NEXXUS Dandarrest Dandruff Control Shampoo *($8 for 10.1 ounces)*
Nizoral Anti-Dandruff Shampoo *($15.39 for 7 ounces)*
Pantene True Confidence Anti-Dandruff 2-in-1 Shampoo & Conditioner *($4.99 for 13.5 ounces)*
Pert Plus 2 in 1 Dandruff Control Shampoo plus Conditioner *($3.99 for 13.5 ounces)*
Redken Solve Dandruff Shampoo *($9.95 for 10.1 ounces)*
Selsun Blue 2-in-1 Treatment Dandruff Shampoo and Conditioner in One *($7.89 for 11 ounces)*
Selsun Blue Balanced Treatment Dandruff Control for All Hair Types *($7.89 for 11 ounces)*
Selsun Blue Moisturizing Treatment Dandruff Shampoo *($7.89 for 11 ounces)*

BEST LEAVE-IN DANDRUFF PRODUCTS (ALL PRICES)

Aveda Scalp Remedy Anti-Dandruff Styling Tonic *($11 for 3.7 ounces)*
Neutrogena T/Gel Overnight Dandruff Treatment *($8.99 for 6 ounces)*

BEST LINES WITH TEMPORARY COLOR-ENHANCING SHAMPOOS (ALL PRICES)

ARTec • Aveda • Bumble and bumble • Graham Webb • JASÖN Natural Cosmetics • Paul Mitchell

BEST LINES WITH TEMPORARY COLOR-ENHANCING CONDITIONERS (ALL PRICES)

ARTec • Aveda • BioSilk • Bumble and bumble • Graham Webb • John Masters Organics • Matrix (Biolage) • NEXXUS • Redken • SEXY Hair Concepts

BEST TEMPORARY COLOR-ENHANCING SHAMPOOS OR CONDITIONERS JUST FOR GRAY OR SILVER HAIR (ALL PRICES)

American Crew Classic Gray Shampoo *($9.99 for 8.45 ounces)* and Classic Gray Conditioner *($9.99 for 8.45 ounces)*

BioSilk Silver Lights Conditioning Shampoo *($9 for 11.6 ounces)*

JASÖN Natural Cosmetics Color Enhancing Shampoo for Silver/Grey *($7.25 for 8 ounces)*

NEXXUS Simply Silver Colour Toning Shampoo *($8 for 10.1 ounces)*

Phyto Phytargent Whitening Shampoo, for Grey and White Hair *($20 for 6.7 ounces)*

BEST CONDITIONERS

See Chapter Four for more information about conditioners.

BEST CONDITIONERS FOR NORMAL OR NORMAL TO DRY HAIR OF ANY THICKNESS THAT COST $8 OR LESS

Note: *The hair-care lines marked with an asterisk feature one or more additional conditioners that are nearly identical to the recommended conditioner on the list.*

Avon Advance Techniques Color-Protection Conditioner *($3.49 for 11 ounces)*

*****Bath & Body Works** Bio Color Protect Conditioner, Helps Protect Color and Revitalizes Its Shine *($7.50 for 12 ounces)*

Citré Shine Color Brilliance Conditioner *($3.99 for 16 ounces)*

*****Clairol** Daily Renewal 5x Replenishing Conditioner, for Dry/Damaged Hair *($4.99 for 13.5 ounces)*

Garnier Fructis Fortifying Deep Conditioner 3 Minute Masque *($3.99 for 5 ounces)*

Goldwell Definition Dry & Porous Intensive Treatment, for Dry/Coarse Hair *($8 for 5 ounces)*

*****göt2b** Instantly Gratified Instant Conditioner *($5.99 for 8.5 ounces)*

*****Infusium 23** Colored/Permed Revitalizing Conditioner, for Chemically Treated and Over-Processed Hair *($5.99 for 16 ounces)*

*****Inner Science** Colour Care Conditioner *($8 for 6 ounces)*

*****JASÖN Natural Cosmetics** Color Sealant Conditioner, for All Shades of Hair *($7 for 8 ounces)*

Jheri Redding Mega-Vitamin Conditioner, for Dry, Damaged Hair *($2.49 for 16 ounces)*

*****L'Oreal** Vive Color-Care Conditioner, for Dry Hair *($4.49 for 13 ounces)*

Neutrogena Clean for Color Color-Defending Conditioner *($3.99 for 10.1 ounces)*

*Pantene Daily Moisture Renewal Moisturizing Conditioner *($4.99 for 13.5 ounces)*
Prell Spa Formula Hydra Care Rinse Clean Conditioner *($3.19 for 13 ounces)*
Salon Grafix Daily Balancing Conditioner *($4.99 for 16 ounces)*
*Soft Sheen Carson Optimum Care Rich Conditioner *($3.59 for 16.9 ounces)*
St. Ives Hair Repair Mud Miracle Deep Mineral Revitalizer *($3.99 for 7 ounces)*
TRESemme 4+4 Intensive Hair Balm *($5.49 for 4 ounces)*

BEST CONDITIONERS FOR NORMAL OR NORMAL TO DRY HAIR OF ANY THICKNESS THAT COST MORE THAN $8

Note: *The hair-care lines marked with an asterisk feature one or more additional conditioners that are nearly identical to the recommended conditioner on the list.*

Alterna Hemp Seed Deep Conditioner *($23.75 for 8.3 ounces)*
*Aveda Shampure Conditioner *($9 for 8.5 ounces)*
*Back to BASICS Tangerine Twist Daily Radiance Conditioner *($9.95 for 12 ounces)*
Bath & Body Works Botanical Nutrients Wheat Germ Almond Hair Reconstructor, for All Hair Types *($10 for 5 ounces)*
*The Body Shop Honey Moisturizing Conditioner *($8.50 for 8 ounces)*
*Bumble & bumble Super Rich Conditioner *($17 for 8 ounces)*
*Framesi Biogenol Color Care System Moisture-Rinse *($10 for 10.1 ounces)*
*Frédéric Fekkai Glossing Conditioner *($20 for 8 ounces)*
Fudge The Conditioner, Conditioner for Normal to Dry Hair *($10.20 for 10.1 ounces)*
Hayashi System Hinoki Conditioner Texturizing Rinse for Fine and Thinning Hair *($9 for 8.4 ounces)*
ICE Hydrater Conditioner *($10 for 10.1 ounces)*
*ISO Daily Nourishing Condition, Light Creme Conditioner *($8.50 for 13.5 ounces)*
Joico Volissima Volumizing Conditioner, for Fine Hair *($10 for 10.1 ounces)*
KMS Silker Reconstructor *($8.95 for 8.1 ounces)*
*Mastey Basic Superpac, Capillary Complex Reconstructor *($10 for 6.8 ounces)*
*Matrix Biolage Color Care Conditioner *($10.95 for 13.5 ounces)*
Michael diCesare Hydration Daily Conditioner *($12.75 for 8.5 ounces)*
*Rusk Being Defensive Conditioner *($11.90 for 13.5 ounces)*
Sebastian Shaper Color Survivor Daily Conditioner *($8.95 for 8.5 ounces)*
Senscience Straight Sense Conditioner *($8.10 for 10.2 ounces)*
*SEXY Hair Concepts Healthy Sexy Hair, Soy Milk Conditioner *($9.95 for 8.5 ounces)*

BEST LEAVE-IN CONDITIONERS FOR NORMAL TO FINE OR THIN HAIR THAT COST $8 OR LESS

Note: *The hair-care lines marked with an asterisk feature one or more additional conditioners that are nearly identical to the recommended conditioner on the list.*

AFRiCAN PRIDE Leave-In Conditioner *($3.99 for 12 ounces)*
*AFRICAN ROYALE Daily Doctor Maximum Strength Leave-In Conditioner *($4.49 for 12 ounces)*
Aussie Hair Insurance Leave-In Conditioner for Weak, Distressed Hair *($3.99 for 8 ounces)*

The Body Shop Amlika Leave-In Conditioner, for All Hair Types *($6 for 3.4 ounces)*
*Clairol Daily Renewal 5x Daily Nourishment Creme, Leave-In *($4.99 for 4.2 ounces)*
Jheri Redding Extra ResQ Leave-In Hair, Shine & Scalp Treatment *($6.95 for 15 ounces)*
John Frieda Frizz Ease Daily Nourishment, Leave-In Fortifying Spray *($5.99 for 8 ounces)*
Neutrogena Triple Moisture Sheer Hydration Leave-in Foam *($6.99 for 6 ounces)*
Pantene Repair & Restructure Daily Strengthening Treatment *($4.79 for 5.1 ounces)*
Soft & Beautiful Botanicals Lite Creme Moisturizer *($3.99 for 6 ounces)*
Soft Sheen Carson Care Free Curl Gold Instant Activator, with Moisturizers *($3.49 for 8 ounces)*

BEST LEAVE-IN CONDITIONERS FOR NORMAL TO FINE OR THIN HAIR THAT COST MORE THAN $8

Note: The hair-care lines marked with an asterisk feature one or more additional conditioners that are nearly identical to the recommended conditioner on the list.

Alterna Volumizing Spray Leave-In Conditioner *($16.50 for 8.5 ounces)*
*Aveda Elixir Daily Leave-On Hair Conditioner *($9 for 8.5 ounces)*
bain de terre Herbal Sea Mist Leave-In Detangler *($9.19 for 6.7 ounces)*
Bumble and bumble Prep *($13 for 8 ounces)*
Framesi Biogenol Color Care System Leave-In Conditioner *($10 for 10.1 ounces)*
*Hayashi System 911 Protein Mist Leave-In Conditioner Detangler Body Builder *($11 for 8.4 ounces)*
j.f. lazartigue Disentangling Instant Silk Protein Spray *($18 for 3.4 ounces)*
Joico Integrity Leave-In Conditioning Detangler *($10 for 10.1 ounces)*
Matrix Biolage Fortifying Leave-In Treatment *($12.95 for 8 ounces)*
mop (modern organic products) leave-in conditioner *($9.99 for 10.5 ounces)*
Ouidad Botanical Boost *($12 for 8 ounces)*
Paul Mitchell Color Care, Color Protect Locking Spray *($11.99 for 8.5 ounces)*
Phyto Phytomist Instant Hydrator with White Lotus Flowers *($22 for 5 ounces)*
Pureology Colour Max, Seal & Detangle *($16 for 8.5 ounces)*
Quantum Reds Daily 2-Phase Color Protector, Detangles, Brightens, & Protects All Shades of Red Hair *($11 for 8 ounces)*
Redken So Long Heat Treat, Heat-Activated Leave-In Treatment for Long Hair *($12.95 for 5 ounces)*
Rusk Sensories Brilliance Grapefruit & Honey Leave-In Color Protector *($9 for 8 ounces)*
*Sebastian Laminates Detangling Milk, Leave-In Conditioner *($9.95 for 8.5 ounces)*
SEXY Hair Concepts Curly Sexy Hair, Curl Power Curl Enhancer *($11.95 for 8.5 ounces)*
Wella Color Preserve Detangler and Leave-In Conditioner *($10 for 8 ounces)*

BEST LEAVE-IN CONDITIONERS FOR DRY TO VERY DRY OR COARSE HAIR THAT COST $8 OR LESS

Bath & Body Works Botanical Nutrients Leave-In Creme Conditioner, for Damaged or Color-Treated Hair *($7.50 for 6 ounces)*
ion Color Solutions Color Defense Leave-In Protector *($4.99 for 8 ounces)*

John Frieda Sheer Blonde Instant Detangler with Weightless Conditioners, Formulated for All Shades of Fine, Thin Blondes *($6.49 for 8.45 ounces)*

L'Oreal Nature's Therapy Heat Control Leave-In Protection Creme *($4.99 for 4 ounces)*

Neutrogena Overnight Therapy Replenishing Treatment *($5.99 for 6 ounces)*

Neutrogena Triple Moisture Silk Touch Leave-in Cream *($6.99 for 6 ounces)*

ProVitamin Special Effects Chunky Ends, Instant Split Ends Mender *($7.09 for 6 ounces)*

Soft & Beautiful Oil Moisturizing Lotion *($6.69 for 16 ounces)*

Soft Sheen Carson Care Free Curl Curl Activator *($4.99 for 8 ounces)*

Zero Frizz Smooth Ends Leave-In Conditioning Treatment *($3.99 for 6 ounces)*

BEST LEAVE-IN CONDITIONERS FOR DRY TO VERY DRY OR COARSE HAIR THAT COST MORE THAN $8

Goldwell Kerasilk Rich Care Leave-In Silk Fluid *($16 for 4.2 ounces)*

Kérastase Nutritive Nutri-Liss, Instant Smoothing Treatment for Dry and Unruly Hair *($29 for 4.2 ounces)*

Ouidad Balancing Rinse *($10 for 8 ounces)*

Redken All Soft Addictive Hair Transformer, Softness for Dry Hair *($14.95 for 3.4 ounces)*

Redken Fresh Curls Spin Control, Curl Defining Leave-In Treatment *($12.95 for 5 ounces)*

Rene Furterer Carthame No-Rinse Protective Cream *($22 for 2.6 ounces)*

Rusk Sensories Smoother Passionflower & Aloe Leave-In Texturizing Conditioner *($9 for 8.5 ounces)*

Sebastian Collection Titanium Protector, Leave-In Conditioner *($9.95 for 8.5 ounces)*

SEXY Hair Concepts Healthy Sexy Hair, Soy Potion Miraculous Leave-In Treatment *($13.50 for 5.1 ounces)*

SEXY Hair Concepts Silky Sexy Hair, Drench for Dry Hair *($13.95 for 5.1 ounces)*

BEST CONDITIONERS FOR NORMAL TO DRY HAIR THAT IS NORMAL TO FINE OR THIN THAT COST $8 OR LESS

Note: *The hair-care lines marked with an asterisk feature one or more additional conditioners that are nearly identical to the recommended conditioner on the list.*

*****Alberto VO5** Balsam & Protein Conditioner *($1.29 for 15 ounces)*

Aussie Slip Detangler for Tangly Hair *($3.99 for 12 ounces)*

*****Avon** Advance Techniques Curly & Chic Conditioner *($3.49 for 11 ounces)*

Charles Worthington Results Superconditioner *($5.99 for 10.9 ounces)*

Citré Shine Moisture Burst Conditioner *($3.99 for 16 ounces)*

*****Dove** Foam Conditioner, Extra Volume *($3.99 for 9 ounces)*

*****finesse** Color Care Conditioner *($3.79 for 15 ounces)*

ion Anti-Frizz Solutions Straightening Conditioner, Moisturizer for Curly, Wavy, Frizzy Hair *($4.99 for 6 ounces)*

Joico Lite Daily Conditioner, for All Hair Types *($8 for 10.1 ounces)*

*****L'Oreal** Vive Curl-Moisture Conditioner, for Curly Hair *($4.49 for 13 ounces)*

SEXY Hair Concepts Big Sexy Hair, Big Volume Conditioner *($6.95 for 8.5 ounces)*

TRESemme European Revitalizing Colour Care Conditioner *($3.69 for 32 ounces)*

BEST CONDITIONERS FOR NORMAL TO DRY HAIR THAT IS NORMAL TO FINE OR THIN THAT COST MORE THAN $8

Note: The hair-care lines marked with an asterisk feature one or more additional conditioners that are nearly identical to the recommended conditioner on the list.

*Alterna Caviar Treatment Conditioner with Age-Control Complex *($24 for 8.5 ounces)*
ARTec Textureline Volume Conditioner *($9.50 for 8 ounces)*
*Back to BASICS Marine Color Protection Conditioner *($9.95 for 12 ounces)*
BioSilk Silk Filler *($12 for 11.6 ounces)*
The Body Shop Nettle Oil Balance Conditioner *($8.50 for 8 ounces)*
*Frédéric Fekkai Apple Cider Clean Conditioner *($18.50 for 8 ounces)*
*Graham Webb Condition 30 Second Sheer Conditioner *($11.11 for 11 ounces)*
*Hayashi System 911 Daily Remedy Conditioner for Damaged Hair *($13 for 10.6 ounces)*
head GAMES Tangle Buster, Daily Detangling Conditioner *($10 for 12 ounces)*
*JASÖN Natural Cosmetics Damage Control Creme Conditioner, for Frizzy, Dry or Color Treated Hair *($10 for 8 ounces)*
*Kiehl's Extra-Strength Conditioning Rinse for Dry Hair *($17.50 for 8 ounces)*
*KMS Color Vitality Color Revitalizer *($9.95 for 8.1 ounces)*
L'ANZA Dry Hair Formula Moisture Treatment *($8.90 for 4.2 ounces)*
*Matrix Amplify Volumizing System, Instant Conditioner *($10.95 for 8 ounces)*
Modern Elixirs by Paul Mitchell Color Therapy Conditioner *($12.99 for 5.1 ounces)*
Nioxin Bionutrient Protectives Moisture & Strength *($11.99 for 5.1 ounces)*
*Paul Mitchell Smoothing Condition, Super Skinny Daily Treatment *($10.99 for 10.1 ounces)*
Redken So Long Conditioner, Equalizing Strength for Long Hair *($9.95 for 8.5 ounces)*
Senscience Hydrating Hair Masque *($10.80 for 4 ounces)*
TIGI Bed Head Control Freak Conditioner *($11.95 for 8.5 ounces)*

BEST CONDITIONERS FOR DRY TO VERY DRY HAIR THAT IS NORMAL TO FINE OR THIN THAT COST $8 OR LESS

Note: The hair-care lines marked with an asterisk feature one or more additional conditioners that are nearly identical to the recommended conditioner on the list.

*Charles Worthington Results Daily Treat Conditioner, Normal Hair *($5.99 for 10.9 ounces)*
Garnier Fructis Fortifying Cream Conditioner, for Fine Hair *($3.99 for 13 ounces)*
Infusium 23 Power Pac Conditioner, 3-Minute Intensive Treatment *($5.99 for 10.2 ounces)*
ion Daily Solutions Finishing Detangler, Conditioning After Shampoo Rinse *($4.99 for 16 ounces)*
ion Volumizing Solutions Vitalizing Thickening Conditioner, for All Hair Types *($4.99 for 16 ounces)*
L'Oreal Nature's Therapy Mega Repair Recovery Complex *($5.99 for 6 ounces)*
Neutrogena Triple Moisture Deep Recovery Hair Mask *($6.99 for 6 ounces)*
Pantene Full & Thick Conditioner *($4.79 for 13.5 ounces)*
*Pantene Classic Care Conditioner *($4.99 for 13.5 ounces)*
St. Ives Hair Repair Strength & Shine Fortifying Reconstructor *($3.99 for 10 ounces)*
TRESemme 4+4 Marine Botanical & Mango Infused Hydrating Sealant *($5.49 for 16 ounces)*

BEST CONDITIONERS FOR DRY TO VERY DRY HAIR THAT IS NORMAL TO FINE OR THIN THAT COST MORE THAN $8

Note: The hair-care line marked with an asterisk features one or more additional conditioners that are nearly identical to the recommended conditioner on the list.

ARTec Textureline Smoothing Conditioner *($9.99 for 8 ounces)*

fresh Meadowfoam Cream Treatment Conditioner *($32 for 5.1 ounces)*

Fudge 1 Shot Hair Reconstructing Clinic in a Bottle *($12.35 for 4.2 ounces)*

H₂O+ Sea Plankton Restructuring Conditioner *($16 for 8 ounces)*

Jheri Redding Extra Humidicon Moisturizing Conditioner *($8.95 for 13.5 ounces)*

John Masters Organics Citrus & Neroli Detangler *($16 for 8 ounces)*

Joico Moisturizer Intensive Moisture Treatment, Extra Conditioning *($14 for 10.5 ounces)*

KMS Daily Repair Reconstructor *($9.95 for 8.1 ounces)*

L'ANZA Be Long, Long Hair Formula Strengthen *($14.25 for 5.07 ounces)*

L'ANZA Volume Formula Weightless Rinse *($10 for 12.6 ounces)*

NEXXUS Y Serum Younger Looking Hair Conditioner *($16 for 10.1 ounces)*

Redken All Soft Heavy Cream, Super Treatment for Dry/Brittle Hair *($12.95 for 8.5 ounces)*

Redken Water Rush Moisturizing Treatment for Normal/Dry Hair *($12.95 for 8.5 ounces)*

Sebastian Collection Slinky Conditioner *($11.19 for 8.5 ounces)*

*TIGI Bed Head Dumb Blonde Conditioner, for After Highlights *($9.95 for 12 ounces)*

Wella Lifetex Wellness Personal Trainer, Smooth and Defrizz Control *($13 for 5 ounces)*

BEST CONDITIONERS FOR DRY TO VERY DRY HAIR THAT IS NORMAL TO THICK OR COARSE THAT COST $8 OR LESS

Note: The hair-care lines marked with an asterisk feature one or more additional conditioners that are nearly identical to the recommended conditioner on the list.

AFRiCAN PRIDE Instant Oil Moisturizing Hair Lotion *($3.99 for 12 ounces)*

bain de terre Cucumber Moisturizing Conditioner *($11.89 for 13.5 ounces)*

*Bath & Body Works Bio Straight & Sleek Conditioner, Relaxes Curls and Fights Frizz for a Smooth, Shiny Finish *($7.50 for 12 ounces)*

binge 2,500 Calorie, Intensive Conditioner *($5.99 for 8.5 ounces)*

The Body Shop Brazil Nut Deep Conditioning Hair Treatment for, Dry, Damaged & Chemically Treated Hair *($8 for 8.4 ounces)*

Clairol Herbal Essences Intensive Blends Restoring Conditioning Balm *($3.99 for 12 ounces)*

*Goldwell Definition Dry & Porous Strengthening Treatment, for Fine & Stressed Hair *($8 for 5 ounces)*

*göt2b So Blonde Blonde Aid Intensive Hair Repair *($5.99 for 6 ounces)*

JASÖN Natural Cosmetics Forest Essence Vital Conditioner *($7.35 for 8 ounces)*

*John Frieda Frizz Ease Glistening Creme, Defrizzing Conditioner, Extra Strength Formula *($5.99 for 12.7 ounces)*

*Neutrogena Triple Moisture Daily Deep Conditioner *($5.99 for 8.45 ounces)*

*Pantene Relaxed & Natural Intensive Moisturizing Conditioner *($3.99 for 13.5 ounces)*

ProVitamin Special Effects, Curls Up Conditioner *($7.39 for 8.5 ounces)*

*Queen Helene Placenta Cream Hair Conditioner, with Panthenol *($4.25 for 15 ounces)*

Revlon Realistic Rinse Out Conditioner, with Cholesterol *($4.99 for 8.8 ounces)*

SEXY Hair Concepts Curly Sexy Hair, Conditioner *($6.95 for 8.5 ounces)*

*****Soft Sheen Carson** Dark and Lovely Moisture Seal Instant Conditioner *($3.49 for 13.5 ounces)*

Sukesha Conditioning Rinse *($5.95 for 8 ounces)*

*****thermaSilk** Color Revitalizing Conditioner, for Colored or Permed Hair *($3.99 for 13 ounces)*

*****Zero Frizz** Daily Conditioner *($5.95 for 12 ounces)*

BEST CONDITIONERS FOR DRY TO VERY DRY HAIR THAT IS NORMAL TO THICK OR COARSE THAT COST MORE THAN $8

Note: *The hair-care lines marked with an asterisk feature one or more additional conditioners that are nearly identical to the recommended conditioner on the list.*

*****Aveda** Scalp Benefits Balancing Conditioner *($12 for 6.7 ounces)*

Back to BASICS Vanilla Plum Fortifying Conditioner *($8.95 for 12 ounces)*

bain de terre Lavender Color Protecting Conditioner *($10 for 13.5 ounces)*

*****BioSilk** Fruit Cocktail *($12 for 11.6 ounces)*

Burt's Bees Avocado Butter Hair Treatment with Nettles and Rosemary *($9 for 4 ounces)*

Charles Worthington Dream Hair Stay True Moisture Surge Conditioner, for Color-Treated and Dehydrated Hair *($14 for 8.7 ounces)*

*****Frédéric Fekkai** Moisturizing Conditioner with Shea Butter *($22.50 for 6 ounces)*

Fudge Oomf Conditioner, Extra Gutz for Fine Limp Hair *($10.20 for 10.1 ounces)*

*****Graham Webb** Making Waves Curl Defining Conditioner *($11.11 for 11 ounces)*

*****H$_2$O+** Milk Conditioner *($16 for 12 ounces)*

ICE Power Smoothie *($10 for 6 ounces)*

ISO Color Preserve Condition, Color Care Conditioner *($8.50 for 13.5 ounces)*

KMS Daily Fixx Moisture Reconstructor *($10.25 for 8.1 ounces)*

L'ANZA Strait-Line Temporary Curl Relaxing Formula Conditioner *($10.95 for 6.7 ounces)*

Matrix Biolage Ultra-Hydrating Balm *($14.95 for 8.5 ounces)*

mop (modern organic products) lemongrass conditioner, for fine hair *($11.99 for 10.15 ounces)*

*****NEXXUS** Humectress Ultimate Moisturizing Conditioner *($16 for 13.5 ounces)*

Pureology SuperStraight Condition *($22 for 10.1 ounces)*

Redken Fresh Curls Conditioner, Moisture and Frizz Control for Curly Hair *($9.95 for 8.5 ounces)*

*****Sebastian** Laminates Conditioner *($13.19 for 8.5 ounces)*

BEST STYLING PRODUCTS

See Chapter Four for more information about styling products.

BEST SILICONE SPRAYS & SERUMS

BEST SILICONE SPRAYS FOR ALL HAIR TYPES (PARTICULARLY NORMAL TO FINE OR THIN HAIR) THAT COST $12 OR LESS

Note: The hair-care lines marked with an asterisk feature at least one additional product that is nearly identical to the product listed.

Avon Advance Techniques Straight & Sleek Shine Spray *($4.99 for 3.4 ounces)*

Charles Worthington Shine, Shine, Shine Gloss and Refresh Spray, All Hair Types *($5.99 for 5.9 ounces)*

göt2b Dazzling Shine Spray *($5.99 for 6 ounces)*

Graham Webb Brit Style Shine Spray *($12.04 for 4 ounces)*

Hayashi System Design Mist n' Shine Ultra Fine Super Shine *($10.50 for 2.2 ounces)*

*****ion** Anti-Frizz Solutions Brilliance Shine Spray *($5.99 for 6 ounces)*

JASÖN Natural Cosmetics All Natural Hi-Shine Plus, Instantly Tame and Control Fly-Aways *($7.50 for 4 ounces)*

Jheri Redding Extra Reflections Spray-On Shine *($5.95 for 4 ounces)*

*****John Frieda** Frizz Ease 100% Shine, Glossing Mist *($5.99 for 3 ounces)*

Paul Mitchell Finish, The Shine *($11.49 for 3.4 ounces)*

*****ProVitamin** Special Effects Curl Reaction, Curl Reactivating Texturizer *($7.39 for 5.5 ounces)*

Queen Helene Shine Spray, with Cholesterol *($6.75 for 4 ounces)*

*****Rusk** Internal Restructure Shine, Shine Spray *($12 for 4.4 ounces)*

Sebastian Laminates Hi Gloss Spray *($9.99 for 1.7 ounces)*

SEXY Hair Concepts Big Sexy Hair Big Shine, Shine Spray *($10.95 for 2.5 ounces)*

Tri Bright Lites *($9.75 for 3.5 ounces)*

Zero Frizz Quick Fix Glistening Mist *($7.95 for 4 ounces)*

BEST SILICONE SPRAYS FOR ALL HAIR TYPES (PARTICULARLY NORMAL TO FINE OR THIN HAIR) THAT COST MORE THAN $12

Alterna Hemp Seed Spray Shine *($18.60 for 4 ounces)*

ARTec Pure Hair Neroli Reflecting Sprayshine *($12.99 for 4 ounces)*

Aveda Brilliant Spray-On Shine *($18 for 3.4 ounces)*

BioSilk Silk Therapy Shine On *($12.50 for 5.3 ounces)*

Curl Friends Anti-Frenzy Smootherator *($21 for 2 ounces)*

Goldwell Trendline Shine Spray *($12.50 for 3.7 ounces)*

Joico Color Endurance Vibrant Shine Mist *($14 for 3.4 ounces)*

Mastey Lumineux High Gloss Shine Mist *($15 for 4 ounces)*

Matrix Biolage Smoothing Shine Milk *($12.95 for 8.5 ounces)*

Modern Elixirs by Paul Mitchell Illuminating Shine Spray *($13.99 for 3.8 ounces)*

Redken Vinyl Glam 02 Mega Shine Spray *($13.95 for 3.4 ounces)*

Rene Furterer Spray Gloss *($18 for 3.38 ounces)*

SEXY Hair Concepts Straight Sexy Hair Smooth & Seal, Aerated Anti-Frizz Spray *($14.95 for 8.8 ounces)*

TIGI Bed Head Headrush, Shine Adrenaline with a Superfine Mist *($16.95 for 5.3 ounces)*

BEST SILICONE SPRAYS FOR DRY TO VERY DRY HAIR THAT IS NORMAL TO COARSE OR THICK THAT COST $12 OR LESS

Note: The hair-care lines marked with an asterisk feature at least one additional product that is nearly identical to the recommended product on the list.

Citré Shine Shine Mist Anti-Frizz Spray Laminator *($4.99 for 3 ounces)*

*Conair Headcase Bee Good, Shape & Define Spray Wax *($3.99 for 4.5 ounces)*

*göt2b Roughed Up Spray Wax Pomade *($5.99 for 3.3 ounces)*

ion Anti-Frizz Solutions Oil Free Glosser *($7.99 for 4 ounces)*

KMS Flat Out Weightless Shine Spray *($10.75 for 4 ounces)*

*NEXXUS Retexxtur Hair Glow Anti Frizz Smoother (Pump Spray) *($8.50 for 2 ounces)*

BEST SILICONE SPRAYS FOR DRY TO VERY DRY HAIR THAT IS NORMAL TO COARSE OR THICK THAT COST MORE THAN $12

Bumble and bumble Gloss *($13 for 4 ounces)*

Framesi Shine In Polishing Spray *($17 for 8 ounces)*

Frédéric Fekkai Protein Rx Reparative Spray *($18.50 for 4 ounces)*

Hayashi System Design Spray and Shine Polishing Spray Seals and Shines *($15.75 for 4 ounces)*

j.f. lazartigue Revitalizing Shining Blush for Hair *($24 for 1.7 ounces)*

Joico Spray Glace Shine Enhancer *($15 for 5 ounces)*

mop (modern organic products) glisten weightless spray shine *($12.50 for 4.23 ounces)*

Philip B. Hair Care Shine *($24 for 1.85 ounces)*

Rusk Deepshine Sea Kelp Shine Spray *($15 for 8 ounces)*

BEST SILICONE SERUMS FOR ALL HAIR TYPES (PARTICULARLY NORMAL TO FINE OR THIN HAIR) THAT COST $12 OR LESS

Note: The hair-care lines marked with an asterisk feature at least one additional product that is nearly identical to the recommended product on the list.

Alterna Hemp Seed Shine & Texturizing Catalyst *($10.75 for 3.4 ounces)*

Avon Advance Techniques Straight & Sleek Dry Ends Serum *($3.49 for 1 ounce)*

Bath & Body Works Bio Curl on Cue Shine Serum *($10 for 3.4 ounces)*

BioSilk Silk Therapy *($12 for 2.26 ounces)*

*Charles Worthington Shine Silkening Serum *($5.99 for 1.7 ounces)*

*Citré Shine Color Miracle Color Protecting Polishing Serum *($6.99 for 4 ounces)*

Fudge Head Polish Hair Shiner *($9.25 for 1.6 ounces)*

*göt2b Glossy Anti-Frizz Shine Serum *($5.99 for 4 ounces)*

*Jheri Redding Frizz Out Hair Serum *($2.99 for 1.5 ounces)*

John Frieda Frizz Ease Hair Serum, Lite Formula *($9.99 for 1.69 ounces)*

Neutrogena Triple Moisture Healing Shine Serum *($6.99 for 1.8 ounces)*

Pantene Smooth & Shine Anti-Frizz Serum *($5.89 for 1.7 ounces)*

*ProVitamin Anti-Frizz Hair Serum *($8.49 for 5.5 ounces)*
Queen Helene Shine Liquid, with Cholesterol *($6.75 for 4 ounces)*
Zero Frizz Corrective Hair Serum *($7.95 for 4 ounces)*

BEST SILICONE SERUMS FOR ALL HAIR TYPES (PARTICULARLY NORMAL TO FINE OR THIN HAIR) THAT COST MORE THAN $12

Note: The hair-care lines marked with an asterisk feature at least one additional product that is nearly identical to the recommended product on the list.
Aveda Light Elements Smoothing Fluid *($23 for 3.4 ounces)*
*Fudge De Frizz Polish and Control for All Types of Hair *($16.96 for 1.69 ounces)*
Goldwell Kerasilk Rich Care Leave-In Silk Fluid *($16 for 4.2 ounces)*
ISO Multiplicity Glosser, Shine Serum *($12.75 for 1.7 ounces)*
KENRA Platinum Silkening Gloss *($17.70 for 2.26 ounces)*
*Matrix Biolage Shine Renewal *($13.95 for 3.9 ounces)*
Paul Mitchell Smoothing Condition Super Skinny Serum *($16.99 for 5.1 ounces)*
Rusk Design Series Sheer Brilliance, Polisher *($13 for 4 ounces)*
Sebastian Laminates Drops, Liquid Polish *($14.95 for 1.7 ounces)*
*SEXY Hair Concepts Silky Sexy Hair, Frizz Eliminator *($17.95 for 5.1 ounces)*
TIGI Bed Head Girl Toys, Shine Serum *($15.95 for 2 ounces)*

BEST SILICONE SERUMS FOR DRY TO VERY DRY HAIR THAT IS NORMAL TO COARSE OR THICK AND THAT COST $12 OR LESS

Note: The hair-care line marked with an asterisk features at least one additional product that is nearly identical to the recommended product on the list.
AFRICAN ROYALE Diamond Drops *($4.99 for 2 ounces)*
American Crew Shine Tonic *($11.99 for 1.7 ounces)*
ARTec Kiwi Coloreflector Blow Silk, Silk Shine for Dry and Wet Styling *($11 for 2 ounces)*
Bath & Body Works Bio High Shine Gloss *($12 for 2 ounces)*
ISO Color Preserve Control, Protecting Serum *($10 for 1.6 ounces)*
JASÖN Natural Cosmetics All Natural Frizz Control, for Smooth, Soft Hair *($7.50 for 2 ounces)*
*John Frieda Frizz Ease Hair Serum, Extra Strength Formula *($9.99 for 1.69 ounces)*
L'Oreal Vive Smooth-Intense Frizz Solution *($5.99 for 3.4 ounces)*
Soft Sheen Carson Megahertz Hi:Gloss>Serum *($5.99 for 2.5 ounces)*
St. Ives Hair Repair No Frizz Serum *($7.50 for 1 ounce)*

BEST SILICONE SERUMS FOR DRY TO VERY DRY HAIR THAT IS NORMAL TO COARSE OR THICK AND THAT COST MORE THAN $12

Note: The hair-care line marked with an asterisk features at least one additional product that is nearly identical to the recommended product on the list.
Alterna Hemp Seed Polishing Gloss *($14.10 for 2.5 ounces)*
Frédéric Fekkai Finishing Polish *($20 for 1.7 ounces)*
Jheri Redding Extra ResQ Hair Polisher Daily Hair Treatment *($13.98 for 6 ounces)*
mop (modern organic products) glisten shine drops *($12.50 for 1.7 ounces)*
NEXXUS Retexxtur Smoothing Design Shine *($14 for 1 ounce)*

Paul Mitchell Smoothing Style Gloss Drops, Frizz-Free Defining Polish *($14.95 for 3.4 ounces)*
Pureology SuperStraight, Relaxing Serum *($19 for 5.1 ounces)*
***Redken** Smooth Down Heat Glide, Protective Smoother for Very Dry/Unruly Hair *($15.95 for 8.5 ounces)*
Rusk Deepshine Anti-Frizz Serum *($15 for 4.4 ounces)*
Wella Bonk Amped, Long Hair Styler *($9 for 5 ounces)*

BEST STYLING SPRAYS (INCLUDING SPRAY GELS)

BEST STYLING SPRAYS WITH LIGHT HOLD THAT COST $12 OR LESS

Note: The hair-care lines marked with an asterisk feature at least one additional product that is nearly identical to the recommended product on the list.
Beauty Without Cruelty Volume Plus Spray Gel *($6.95 for 8.5 ounces)*
binge Give It a Swirl, Curl Enhancer *($5.99 for 8.5 ounces)*
Charles Worthington Hair Makeover Blow-Drying Spray, Medium Hold for All Hair Types *($5.99 for 9 ounces)*
Clairol Herbal Essences Natural Volume Root Volumizer *($3.49 for 6 ounces)*
Framesi Biogenol Color Care System Snapp, Curl Rejuvenator *($10 for 10.1 ounces)*
Garnier Fructis Curl Shaping Spray Gel Curl Defining, Strong *($2.64 for 8.5 ounces)*
Graham Webb Brit Style Volumizing & Thickening Spray *($10.18 for 8.5 ounces)*
***ion** Anti-Frizz Solutions Liquid Mousse *($4.99 for 12 ounces)*
***L'Oreal** Studio Line Pumping Curls, Medium Hold Finishing Spray *($3.99 for 8 ounces)*
Paul Mitchell Light Hold Style, Soft Sculpting Spray Gel, Flexible Styling Spray-On Gel *($7.25 for 8.5 ounces)*
Progaine Volumizing Root Lifter *($5.99 for 6 ounces)*
Rusk Internal Restructure Thickr, Thickening Spray *($7.50 for 4.2 ounces)*
Sebastian Shaper Iron Works Hot Tools Protecting Spray *($11.95 for 6.8 ounces)*
SEXY Hair Concepts Big Sexy Hair Dense, Thickening Spray *($11.95 for 8.5 ounces)*
Soft Sheen Carson Dark and Lovely Moisture Seal Leave-In Styling Mist *($3.49 for 8.5 ounces)*
thermaSilk Volume & Shine Spray *($3.99 for 7 ounces)*
***Wella** Bonk Amped, Long Hair Styler *($9 for 5 ounces)*

BEST STYLING SPRAYS WITH LIGHT HOLD THAT COST MORE THAN $12

Note: The hair-care line marked with an asterisk features at least one additional product that is nearly identical to the recommended product on the list.
ABBA Sets Spray Gel *($12.75 for 10.1 ounces)*
***Frédéric Fekkai** Instant Volume Root Lifting Spray *($17.50 for 8 ounces)*
Garren New York Designing Spray Tonic *($26 for 6 ounces)*
KENRA Thickening Spray, Thickens Individual Strands for Increased Volume 4 *($13 for 8 ounces)*
KMS Curl Up Curl Gloss *($12.95 for 6.8 ounces)*
NEXXUS NexxStyler Alcohol Free Sheer Volume Spray Gel (Pump) *($13 for 13.5 ounces)*
TIGI Bed Head Uptight, Heat Activated Curl Maker *($12.95 for 8 ounces)*

BEST STYLING SPRAYS WITH LIGHT TO MEDIUM HOLD THAT COST $12 OR LESS

Note: *The hair-care line marked with an asterisk features at least one additional product that is nearly identical to the recommended product on the list.*

Framesi Biogenol Color Care System Spray Gel, Firm Hold *($10 for 10.1 ounces)*
Infusium 23 Volumizing Spray Gel, Extra Firm *($3.99 for 8 ounces)*
L'ANZA Urban Elements Spray Gel *($10.50 for 10.1 ounces)*
***Pantene** Radiant Response Gel with Colorshine *($3.99 for 5.1 ounces)*

BEST STYLING SPRAYS WITH LIGHT TO MEDIUM HOLD THAT COST MORE THAN $12

Note: *The hair-care lines marked with an asterisk feature at least one additional product that is nearly identical to the recommended product on the list.*

***Matrix** Logics Thermal Fixative *($11.95 for 13.5 ounces)*
***Michael diCesare** Amplifying Tonic Hair Thickener *($16 for 8.75 ounces)*
Scruples Enforce, Fast Drying Styling Spray *($12.50 for 8.5 ounces)*
TIGI Catwalk Frisky, Scrunching Gel with Attitude *($13 for 8 ounces)*

BEST STYLING SPRAYS WITH MEDIUM TO FIRM HOLD THAT COST $12 OR LESS

***Aveda** Flax Seed/Aloe Strong Hold Spray-On Styling Gel *($11 for 8.5 ounces)*
ProVitamin Special Effects Curl Booster, Scrunching & Curling Spray *($7.29 for 6 ounces)*
ProVitamin Special Effects Raw Textures Xtreme Spiking Blaster, Spray it! Spike it! Forget it! *($9.79 for 4 ounces)*
Suave Naturals Ocean Breeze Extra Control Spray Gel *($1.79 for 8.5 ounces)*
TIGI Catwalk Root Boost, Spray for Texture & Lift *($11 for 8 ounces)*
TRESemme European Tres Gel Spray, Extra Hold *($2.76 for 10 ounces)*

BEST STYLING SPRAYS WITH MEDIUM TO FIRM HOLD THAT COST MORE THAN $12

Note: *The hair-care line marked with an asterisk features at least one additional product that is nearly identical to the recommended product on the list.*

ARTec Pure Hair Borage Supporting Liquidgel *($14.30 for 9 ounces)*
NEXXUS Nexxtacy Alcohol Free Sustained Hold Styling and Finishing Spray *($17 for 13.5 ounces)*
Scruples V² Double Volume for Hair *($15.95 for 8.5 ounces)*

BEST STYLING CREAMS AND LOTIONS

BEST STYLING CREAMS AND LOTIONS FOR NORMAL TO FINE OR THIN HAIR THAT COST $10 OR LESS

Note: *The hair-care line marked with an asterisk features at least one additional product that is nearly identical to the recommended product on the list.*

BioSilk Silk Therapy Smoothing Balm *($8.95 for 6 ounces)*
The Body Shop Define & No Frizz Styling Cream *($10 for 3.4 ounces)*

Garnier Fructis Smoothing Milk Instant Smoothing & Frizz Control, Strong ($2.64 for 5.1 ounces)

Infusium 23 Smoothing & Defining Lotion ($3.99 for 6 ounces)

Ouidad Tress F/X Styling Lotion ($9 for 8 ounces)

Senscience Straight Sense Defrizz Hairdress ($7.60 for 3.4 ounces)

SEXY Hair Concepts Curly Sexy Hair, Hot Curl Setting Lotion ($9.95 for 8.5 ounces)

Soft & Beautiful Pro-Line Soft-n-Sheen for Extra-Dry Hair Oil Sheen and Comb Out Plus Moisturizers ($3.19 for 10 ounces)

thermaSilk Frizz Fighter Weightless Hydrating Cream ($3.99 for 4 ounces)

*****Wella** Bonk Grounded, Frizz Eliminator ($9 for 5.2 ounces)

BEST STYLING CREAMS AND LOTIONS FOR NORMAL TO FINE OR THIN HAIR THAT COST MORE THAN $10

Note: *The hair-care lines marked with an asterisk feature at least one additional product that is nearly identical to the recommended product on the list.*

*****American Crew** Texture Creme ($18.99 for 8.45 ounces)

Bumble and bumble Brilliantine ($15 for 2 ounces)

Framesi Biogenol Color Care System Stop-Frizz, Anti-Humectant ($12.50 for 2 ounces)

Frédéric Fekkai Luscious Curls ($18.50 for 4 ounces)

Garren New York Styling Creme ($25 for 4 ounces)

j.f. lazartigue Root Volumizer ($18 for 2.54 ounces)

Joico Forming I.C.E. Styling Creme ($10.25 for 2 ounces)

*****Matrix** Biolage Curl Defining Creme ($12.95 for 8 ounces)

mop (modern organic products) C-system texture lotion, light hold with a natural finish ($15 for 6.76 ounces)

*****Redken** Lush Whip 04 Styling Cream ($14.95 for 4.2 ounces)

*****Rusk** Being Gutsy Thickener ($11.90 for 5.3 ounces)

BEST STYLING CREAMS AND LOTIONS FOR THICK OR COARSE HAIR THAT COST $10 OR LESS

Note: *The hair-care line marked with an asterisk features at least one additional product that is nearly identical to the recommended product on the list.*

Alberto VO5 Sheer Hairdressing, Lightweight Leave-In Anti-Frizz & Shine Creme ($5.99 for 4 ounces)

Back to BASICS Green Tea Texturizing Lotion ($8.95 for 6.8 ounces)

binge Hair Pudding, Texturizing Cream ($5.99 for 5.1 ounces)

Citré Shine Taking Hold Styling Glue ($4.99 for 6 ounces)

göt2b Glued Styling Spiking Glue ($5.99 for 6 ounces)

John Frieda Frizz Ease Secret Weapon, Flawless Finishing Creme ($4.99 for 4 ounces)

*****Pantene** Frizz Control Smoothing Creme ($7.99 for 3.5 ounces)

physique Frizz Control Curl Cream ($7.49 for 3.5 ounces)

Soft Sheen Carson Breakthru Heat Strengthening Styling Cream ($5.99 for 5 ounces)

Suave Rave 2x Extra Texture Creme ($1.99 for 8 ounces)

tcb Creme Hairdress ($3.95 for 6 ounces)

thermaSilk Control & Condition Cream *($2.99 for 5.5 ounces)*
Tri Texture Styling Creme *($9 for 4 ounces)*
Zero Frizz Defining Touch, Anti-Frizz Styling Pomade *($5.49 for 2 ounces)*

BEST STYLING CREAMS AND LOTIONS FOR THICK OR COARSE HAIR THAT COST MORE THAN $10

Note: The hair-care lines marked with an asterisk feature at least one additional product that is nearly identical to the recommended product on the list.

Alterna Caviar Age-Free Protectant Smoothing Creme *($18.90 for 8.5 ounces)*
American Crew Liquid Line Structure, Firm Hold Styling Lotion *($12.99 for 6.76 ounces)*
*****ARTec** Textureline Texture Creme, Weightless Volume for Moisture Deprived Hair *($15.70 for 8.4 ounces)*
*****Aveda** Brilliant Universal Styling Creme *($15 for 5 ounces)*
Back to BASICS Holding Paste, for Men *($12.95 for 4 ounces)*
Framesi Shine In Polishing Cream *($16 for 5 ounces)*
head GAMES Messed-Up Madness, Molding Creme *($14 for 4 ounces)*
KENRA Platinum Shaping Cream, Smooth & Form 7 *($20 for 4 ounces)*
*****Kiehl's** Creme with Silk Groom *($17 for 4 ounces)*
KMS Curl Up Control Creme *($15.95 for 5.1 ounces)*
L'ANZA Urban Elements Styling Cream *($16.95 for 6.8 ounces)*
Matrix sleek.look Extreme Styling Cream *($14.95 for 5.1 ounces)*
Nolita Whipped Wax, Lightweight Texture, Big City Shine *($16 for 3.3 ounces)*
Paul Mitchell Style, Re-Works, Versatile Texture Cream *($16.99 for 5.1 ounces)*
*****Phyto** Pro Ultra-Brilliance Creme *($17 for 2.5 ounces)*
*****Redken** Outshine 01 Anti-Frizz Polishing Milk *($14.95 for 3.4 ounces)*
*****Rusk** Being Smooth Creme *($11.90 for 5.3 ounces)*
*****Sebastian** Collection Buff, Casual Waxless Pomade *($13.95 for 4.4 ounces)*
SEXY Hair Concepts Short Sexy Hair Quick Change, Shaping Balm *($11.50 for 1.7 ounces)*
TIGI Bed Head After-Party, Smoothing Cream for Silky, Shiny, Healthy Looking Hair! *($17.95 for 3.4 ounces)*

BEST STYLING GELS (INCLUDING LIQUID GELS)

BEST STYLING GELS WITH LIGHT HOLD THAT COST $10 OR LESS

Note: The hair-care lines marked with an asterisk feature at least one additional product that is nearly identical to the recommended product on the list.

AFRiCAN PRIDE Wonder Weave Moisturizing Styling Gel *($3.99 for 8.5 ounces)*
Aussie Natural Gel *($3.99 for 7 ounces)*
Back to BASICS Basic Style Curl Catalyst, Curl Activating Gel *($9.95 for 6 ounces)*
The Body Shop Hold Still Styling Gel *($8 for 3.4 ounces)*
Garnier Fructis Wet Shine Gel All Day Wet Look & Hold, Strong *($2.64 for 6.8 ounces)*
ion Salon Solutions Styling Glaze *($4.99 for 12 ounces)*
JASÖN Natural Cosmetics All Natural Hi-Shine Styling Gel, All Hair Types *($7.50 for 6 ounces)*

Joico Volissima Volumizing Lotion, for Fine Hair *($9 for 10.1 ounces)*
L'Oreal Studio Line Anti-Frizz, Medium Hold Styling Gel *($3.99 for 6 ounces)*
*Pantene Body Builder Volume Gel *($3.99 for 7.1 ounces)*
Rusk Design Series Jel FX, Forming Jel *($7 for 5 ounces)*
Salon Selectives Feel n' Control, Smoothing Gel for Flexible Control *($3.69 for 13 ounces)*
Sebastian Collection Wet, Liquid Gel for Form Fitting Hold *($7.50 for 8.5 ounces)*
*Soft & Beautiful Botanicals Sculpting Gel *($4.29 for 8 ounces)*
Soft Sheen Carson Megahertz Liquid>Gel Styler *($5.99 for 8.5 ounces)*
Suave Naturals Freesia Flexible Hold Shine & Shaping Gel *($1.79 for 8.5 ounces)*
Sukesha Glossing Gel, Brilliant Shine-Plus-Hold Formula *($6.95 for 8 ounces)*
tcb Naturals Lite Gel Activator *($3.69 for 10 ounces)*

BEST STYLING GELS WITH LIGHT HOLD THAT COST MORE THAN $10

Note: The hair-care lines marked with an asterisk feature at least one additional product that is nearly identical to the recommended product on the list.
ABBA Botz *($12.25 for 5.5 ounces)*
*Aubrey Organics B-5 Design Gel *($10.75 for 8 ounces)*
*Aveda Confixor Conditioning Fixative *($15 for 8.5 ounces)*
Frédéric Fekkai Straight Away Straightening Balm *($16.50 for 4 ounces)*
Fudge Oomf Booster, Styling Muscle for Fine Limp Hair *($10.20 for 10.1 ounces)*
*Garren New York Holding & Molding Gel *($20 for 4 ounces)*
Goldwell for Men Power Gel, Extreme Wet Look *($12 for 5 ounces)*
*Matrix Amplify Volumizing System, Gel-Wax *($12.95 for 5.1 ounces)*
Nolita Thickening Serum, High Volume, Body Builder *($16 for 8 ounces)*
Ouidad Climate Control Heat & Humidity Gel *($16.20 for 8 ounces)*
*Sebastian Laminates Curl, Curl Perfecting Polish *($14.95 for 5.1 ounces)*
TIGI Bed Head Superstar, Thick Massive Hair *($13.95 for 8.45 ounces)*

BEST STYLING GELS WITH LIGHT TO MEDIUM HOLD THAT COST $10 OR LESS

Conair Headcase Out There, Beads-of-Shine Defining Gel *($3.99 for 8 ounces)*
John Frieda Brilliant Brunette Model Control Firm Hold Gel *($5.49 for 6 ounces)*
Paul Mitchell Firm Hold Style, Super Clean Sculpting Gel, Maximum Hold and Control *($7.45 for 6.8 ounces)*
ProVitamin Special Effects Spiked Out, A Water Resistant Hair Styling Glue *($7.29 for 6 ounces)*
Zero Frizz Hold It There, Anti-Frizz Treatment Styling Gel *($3.99 for 6 ounces)*

BEST STYLING GELS WITH LIGHT TO MEDIUM HOLD THAT COST MORE THAN $10

Note: The hair-care line marked with an asterisk features at least one additional product that is nearly identical to the recommended product on the list.
*Aveda Custom Control Styling/Finishing Emulsion *($16.50 for 2.6 ounces)*
Frédéric Fekkai Texturizing Balm *($16.50 for 4 ounces)*

Graham Webb Brit Style Exothermic Styling Gel *($10.18 for 8.5 ounces)*
Graham Webb Making Waves Curl Defining Gel *($15.60 for 8.5 ounces)*
mop (**modern organic products**) glisten light hold gel *($11 for 8.45 ounces)*
Sebastian Laminates Body, Thickening Polish *($12.95 for 5.1 ounces)*

BEST STYLING GELS WITH MEDIUM TO FIRM HOLD THAT COST $10 OR LESS

Note: The hair-care lines marked with an asterisk feature at least one additional product that is nearly identical to the recommended product on the list.

ARTec Textureline Control Gel, Exceptionally Strong All Day Hold for Curly and Wavy Hair *($10 for 8 ounces)*
Conair Headcase Mind Bender, Ruthless Hold Gel *($3.99 for 5 ounces)*
*d:fi Hi:fi Firm Hold Gel *($7.95 for 8.45 ounces)*
L'Oreal Studio Line FX Aqua Gel, Strong Hold *($3.99 for 5.1 ounces)*
L'Oreal Studio Line Grab, Mega Hold Texture Gel *($3.99 for 4 ounces)*
ProVitamin Special Effects Hard Up, Extreme Hard Bodied Gel *($7.29 for 6 ounces)*
Soft Sheen Carson Alternatives Conditioning Styling Gel *($2.99 for 6 ounces)*
*Suave Sculpting Gel, Maximum Hold *($1.29 for 16 ounces)*
*TRESemme European Mega Hold Sculpting Gel, Mega Hold *($3.79 for 9 ounces)*
White Rain Naturals Anti-Frizz Gel Perfect Pearberry, Maximum Hold *($1.59 for 8.25 ounces)*

BEST STYLING GELS WITH MEDIUM TO FIRM HOLD THAT COST MORE THAN $10

Note: The hair-care lines marked with an asterisk feature at least one additional product that is nearly identical to the recommended product on the list.

Alterna Styling & Nutritive Creme Gel *($15.30 for 8.5 ounces)*
Goldwell Trendline Lagoom, Strong *($12.50 for 5.7 ounces)*
ISO Multiplicity Twister, Firm Hold Gel *($14.50 for 5.1 ounces)*
Joico Con_text Organization Grooming Gel *($12.50 for 6.8 ounces)*
*Matrix TufTrix Strong Twisted Gel *($16.95 for 5.1 ounces)*
mop (**modern organic products**) glisten heavy hold gel, for ultimate hold *($12 for 8.45 ounces)*
Nolita Styling Glue, Super Spiker, Hyper Hold *($14 for 6 ounces)*
*Pureology Power Dressing, Body Hold Shine *($17 for 5 ounces)*
Ralph Lauren Saved by the Gel Hair Gel *($16.50 for 8.4 ounces)*
Sebastian Xtah Raw Hair Roxx, Rubber-Iced Gelatine *($19.50 for 4.4 ounces)*

BEST STYLING GELS WITH EXTREMELY STRONG HOLD THAT COST $10 OR LESS

Note: The hair-care lines marked with an asterisk feature at least one additional product that is nearly identical to the recommended product on the list.

Aussie Smoothy Gel, Medium Hold *($3.99 for 8 ounces)*
Conair Headcase Act Up, Gravity-Defying Spiking Glue *($3.99 for 4 ounces)*
Garnier Fructis Fiber Gum Putty Pliable Molding, Extra Strong *($2.64 for 5 ounces)*
*Giga.Hold by Salon Grafix Freeze Hair Putty *($5.99 for 2 ounces)*

L'ANZA Urban Elements Liquid Texture *($9.95 for 6.8 ounces)*
*ProVitamin Special Effects Raw Textures Rock Hard Epoxy, Rock-Hard Bonding Resin
($5.99 for 2 ounces)
Salon Grafix Micro-Fiber Extra Super Hold Hair Styling Gel *($5.99 for 8 ounces)*
Salon Grafix Spiking & Freezing Styling Gel *($5.99 for 8 ounces)*
TRESemme 4+4 Sculpting Gel *($5.49 for 8.2 ounces)*
Tri Sculpture Styling Gel *($6.50 for 5 ounces)*

BEST STYLING GELS WITH EXTREMELY STRONG HOLD THAT COST MORE THAN $10

Note: *The hair-care line marked with an asterisk features at least one additional product that is nearly identical to the recommended product on the list.*

ABBA Gelsential Maximum Support Styling Gel *($11 for 10.1 ounces)*
ARTec Textureline Adhesive, Radical Hair Glue *($15.95 for 5.75 ounces)*
BioSilk Rock Hard Gelee Hard Hold Gel *($11 for 6 ounces)*
*ICE Controller Firm Hold Gel *($12.50 for 10.1 ounces)*
KENRA Platinum Freezing Gel, Lock & Hold 24 *($17.70 for 6 ounces)*
Redken Concrete 22 Cement Paste *($13.95 for 5 ounces)*
TIGI Bed Head Hard Head, Mohawk Gel for Spiking and Ultimate Hold *($15.95 for 3.4 ounces)*
Wella Liquid Hair Kryptonite Acrylic Gel, Ultra Hold *($11 for 3.5 ounces)*

BEST MOUSSES (LIQUID-TO-FOAM AND PROPELLANT-BASED)

BEST MOUSSES WITH MINIMAL TO LIGHT HOLD THAT COST $8 OR LESS

Note: *The hair-care lines marked with an asterisk feature at least one additional product that is nearly identical to the recommended product on the list.*

*Aussie Mega Hold Mousse, Extra Hold & Control *($3.99 for 6 ounces)*
*Clairol Herbal Essences Natural Volume Bodifying Foam *($3.79 for 7 ounces)*
*finesse Touchables Mousse, Curl Defining *($3.79 for 7 ounces)*
L'Oreal Studio Line Volumatic, Strong Hold Styling Mousse *($3.99 for 6 ounces)*
L'Oreal Nature's Therapy Liquid Energy Liquid Mousse Volumizer *($6.99 for 5.5 ounces)*
*Pantene Body Builder Mousse *($3.99 for 6.6 ounces)*
*Paul Mitchell Extra-Body Style, Extra-Body Sculpting Foam, Firm-Hold Thickening Foam *($7.95 for 6 ounces)*
*physique Scrunching Foam *($6.99 for 5 ounces)*
Soft & Beautiful Botanicals Sculpting Foam *($3.99 for 8 ounces)*
tcb Foaming Wrap-n-Set Lotion *($3.79 for 6 ounces)*
thermaSilk Volume Infusing Mousse *($3.99 for 7 ounces)*
*White Rain Classics Color Nourish Mousse, Extra Body *($1.32 for 5 ounces)*
Zero Frizz Smoothing + Styling Mousse *($5.95 for 6 ounces)*

BEST MOUSSES WITH MINIMAL TO LIGHT HOLD THAT COST MORE THAN $8

Note: The hair-care lines marked with an asterisk feature at least one additional product that is nearly identical to the recommended product on the list.

Alterna Caviar Mousse with Age-Control Complex *($19 for 14.1 ounces)*

Aveda Phomollient Styling Foam *($12 for 6.7 ounces)*

Bath & Body Works Botanical Nutrients Neroli Flaxseed Styling Foam *($9.50 for 6.7 ounces)*

The Body Shop Wheat Protein Volumizing Mousse *($10 for 6.75 ounces)*

Charles Worthington Dream Hair Feels Fabulous Supercontrol Mousse, Light for All Hair Types *($10 for 5.25 ounces)*

Goldwell Definition Permed & Curly Curl Care Foam, Leave-In *($14 for 6.7 ounces)*

head GAMES All Whipped Up, Volumizing Mousse *($10 for 10.5 ounces)*

KMS AMP Volume Styling Foam *($10.75 for 8 ounces)*

L'ANZA Urban Elements Bodifying Foam *($10 for 7.1 ounces)*

*Matrix Amplify Volumizing System, Foam Volumizer *($11.95 for 9 ounces)*

Nioxin Bionutrient Creatives Smoothly Defined *($11.99 for 6.8 ounces)*

Rene Furterer Anti-Dehydrating Volumizing Mousse, Soft Hold *($18 for 6.7 ounces)*

Rusk Design Series Mousse, Volumizing Foam *($11 for 8 ounces)*

*Scruples Emphasis, Texturizing Styling Mousse *($11.95 for 6 ounces)*

Sebastian Shaper Full-On Body Mousse *($10.95 for 8.5 ounces)*

Wella Liquid Hair Energy Styler Volumizing Mousse, Strong Hold *($11.50 for 10.6 ounces)*

BEST MOUSSES WITH LIGHT TO MEDIUM HOLD THAT COST $8 OR LESS

*Note: The hair-care lines marked with an asterisk feature at least one additional product that is nearly identical to the recommended product on the list.

Citré Shine Big Volume Styling Foam *($4.99 for 8.5 ounces)*

L'Oreal Studio Line Springing Curls, Medium Hold Styling Mousse *($3.79 for 6 ounces)*

Salon Grafix Extra-Hold Sculpting Mousse *($5.99 for 8 ounces)*

Salon Selectives Get in Shape, Shaping Mousse for Thick/Curly/Wavy Hair *($3.79 for 7 ounces)*

*Suave Volume & Control Mousse, Maximum Hold *($1.29 for 5 ounces)*

*TRESemme European Tres Mousse, Extra Hold *($3.99 for 10.5 ounces)*

White Rain Naturals Nourishing Mousse Enriching Sunflower, Extra Body *($1.59 for 5 ounces)*

BEST MOUSSES WITH LIGHT TO MEDIUM HOLD THAT COST MORE THAN $8

*Note: The hair-care lines marked with an asterisk feature at least one additional product that is nearly identical to the recommended product on the list.

Charles Worthington Dream Hair Feels Fabulous Supercontrol Mousse, Firm Hold for All Hair Types *($10 for 5.25 ounces)*

Frédéric Fekkai Full Volume Mousse *($18.50 for 5 ounces)*
ICE Amplifier Volumizing Mousse *($12.50 for 8.8 ounces)*
*Joico I.C.E. Whip Designing Foam, Firm Hold *($14 for 10.5 ounces)*
KENRA Volume Mousse, Medium Hold Fixative 12 *($11 for 8 ounces)*
Rene Furterer Anti-Dehydrating Volumizing Mousse, Strong Hold *($18 for 6.7 ounces)*
Scruples O₂ Originals Direct Volume Spray Foam *($15.95 for 10 ounces)*
*SEXY Hair Concepts Hot Sexy Highlights Whipped Up, Gel Foam *($12.60 for 7 ounces)*

BEST MOUSSE WITH MEDIUM TO FIRM HOLD THAT COSTS $8 OR LESS

Salon Grafix Mega-Hold Sculpting Mousse *($5.99 for 8 ounces)*

BEST MOUSSES WITH MEDIUM TO FIRM HOLD THAT COST MORE THAN $8

Note: The hair-care lines marked with an asterisk feature at least one additional product that is nearly identical to the recommended product on the list.
ARTec Kiwi Coloreflector Shaping Foam, Shapes and Conditions Hair *($8.50 for 7 ounces)*
Goldwell Trendline Volume Mousse, Extreme *($14.50 for 10.2 ounces)*
KENRA Volume Mousse Extra, Firm Hold Fixative 17 *($11 for 8 ounces)*
*Matrix BigTrix, Boost-It Mousse *($11.95 for 8.4 ounces)*
Michael diCesare LiquiFix LiquiThick Thickening Mousse *($14.50 for 7 ounces)*
*Redken Full Frame 07 Protective Volumizing Mousse *($14.95 for 8.5 ounces)*
Scruples Creme Parfait, Ultra Thick Styling Mousse *($15.95 for 10.6 ounces)*
Scruples Urban Potions Cut & Style Foam *($12.95 for 8.3 ounces)*
Sebastian Collection Fizz XL, Fashion Foam for Extra Hold *($12.95 for 8.8 ounces)*
Senscience Volumesse, Body Building Foam *($9.50 for 7 ounces)*
Tri Fashion Styling Mousse *($14 for 16 ounces)*
Tri Pom-Mousse, Hairstyle Forming Foam *($14.25 for 3.75 ounces)*

BEST POMADES, PASTES, AND STYLING WAXES

BEST WATER-SOLUBLE POMADES WITH MINIMAL TO LIGHT HOLD THAT COST $12 OR LESS

Note: The hair-care lines marked with an asterisk feature at least one additional product that is nearly identical to the recommended product on the list.
Citré Shine Texture Play Chunking Creme *($4.99 for 2 ounces)*
Conair Headcase Motivator, Style Defining Pomade *($3.99 for 2 ounces)*
d:fi d:tails Pomade for Hold and Shine *($9.95 for 2.6 ounces)*
*göt2b Defiant Define & Shine Pomade *($5.99 for 2 ounces)*
Hayashi System Design Hi-Gloss *($9.95 for 2 ounces)*
head GAMES Green with Envy, Styling Pomade *($10 for 2 ounces)*
ion Volumizing Solutions Vitalizing Hair Wax *($5.99 for 1.8 ounces)*
ISO Multiplicity Whipped, Cream Wax *($11.75 for 1.75 ounces)*
*Matrix Vavoom Designing, Beam Shine Gloss *($12 for 1.7 ounces)*
Professional Shine Pomade Ultra-Hold *($3.86 for 2 ounces)*

ProVitamin Special Effects Power Pomade, Sculpts, Holds, Shines & Controls *($7.29 for 2 ounces)*
Salon Grafix Hair Pomade Styling Creme for Super Hold *($5.99 for 8 ounces)*
*****Soft Sheen Carson** Megahertz Gel>Wax *($5.99 for 3.4 ounces)*
TRESemme Hydrology Smoothing Moisture Pomade *($4.99 for 3.5 ounces)*
Tri Shape and Shine *($10.75 for 2 ounces)*
*****Wella** Bonk Crystal Dynamite, Iridescent Shine Gel *($9 for 2.6 ounces)*

BEST WATER-SOLUBLE POMADES WITH MINIMAL TO LIGHT HOLD THAT COST MORE THAN $12

Note: The hair-care lines marked with an asterisk feature at least one additional product that is nearly identical to the recommended product on the list.
American Crew Pomade *($15.99 for 3.53 ounces)*
ARTec Textureline Texture Shine *($12.75 for 2.64 ounces)*
Aveda Brilliant Humectant Pomade *($18 for 2.6 ounces)*
Bumble and bumble Styling Wax *($15 for 1.5 ounces)*
Frédéric Fekkai Pomade Cristal *($18.50 for 2.6 ounces)*
Goldwell Trendline Gel Wax, Normal *($14.50 for 3.3 ounces)*
Graham Webb Brit Style Wax Pomade *($17 for 1.7 ounces)*
ICE Spiker Distortion Styling Gum *($14 for 3.4 ounces)*
KENRA Platinum Grooming Pomade, Define & Control 4 *($17.70 for 2 ounces)*
L'ANZA Urban Elements Design Wax *($16.95 for 6.8 ounces)*
mop (modern organic products) glisten high shine pomade *($15 for 2.05 ounces)*
*****Paul Mitchell** Finish, Slick Works, Texture and Shine *($16.95 for 6.8 ounces)*
Philip B. Hair Care Shin-Aid Matte Finish Pomade *($24 for 2 ounces)*
*****Rusk** Being Rubber Gum *($17 for 4.4 ounces)*
*****SEXY Hair Concepts** Healthy Sexy Hair Soy Paste, Texture Pomade *($12.95 for 1.8 ounces)*
TIGI Bed Head Boy Toys, Body Building Funkifier *($17.95 for 3.4 ounces)*
Wella Lifetex Wellness Well Defined, Sculpting Polisher *($13.30 for 5 ounces)*
Zirh Control, Lightweight Styling Wax *($18.50 for 1.7 ounces)*

BEST WATER-SOLUBLE POMADES WITH MEDIUM TO FIRM HOLD THAT COST $12 OR LESS

Note: The hair-care line marked with an asterisk features at least one additional product that is nearly identical to the recommended product on the list.
BioSilk Silk Pomade Designing Finish *($11 for 4 ounces)*
L'Oreal alt.Studio Remix Paste, Extreme Texture, Reworkable Hold *($5.99 for 3.1 ounces)*
*****ProVitamin** Special Effects Manipulative, Extreme Molding & Manipulating Cream *($7.29 for 2 ounces)*
Salon Selectives Control(d) Substance, Molding Putty for Short/Thick Hair *($3.69 for 2.25 ounces)*
Sebastian Shaper In Control Fiber Wax *($9.95 for 1.8 ounces)*

BEST WATER-SOLUBLE POMADES WITH MEDIUM TO FIRM HOLD THAT COST MORE THAN $12

Alterna Life Pliable Molding Paste *($14.10 for 3 ounces)*
ICE Waxer Wax Pomade *($12.50 for 3.8 ounces)*
Kiehl's Solid Grooming Aid *($15.50 for 1.75 ounces)*

BEST TRADITIONAL (MEANING OIL- OR WAX-BASED) POMADES THAT COST $12 OR LESS

Note: The hair-care lines marked with an asterisk feature at least one additional product that is nearly identical to the recommended product on the list.
Charles Worthington Lasting Impression Defining Wax *($5.99 for 1.7 ounces)*
*Fudge Hair Shaper, Firm Hold Factor 2 *($11.75 for 3.5 ounces)*
John Frieda Sheer Blonde Spun Gold, Shaping and Highlighting Balm *($5.49 for 1.2 ounces)*
Joico Brilliantine Shine and Defining Pomade *($10 for 2 ounces)*
*L'ANZA Ctrl @ L'ANZA Modify Hair Molder <F5 Giga-Hold> *($11 for 2.5 ounces)*
L'Oreal Nature's Therapy Mega Slick Moisturizing Pomade *($5.99 for 2 ounces)*
physique Precision Wax *($7.49 for 1.7 ounces)*
Sebastian Collection Grease, Patent Leather Pomade for Flexible Hold *($8.95 for 1.7 ounces)*
Soft & Beautiful Pro-Line Comb-Thru Greaseless Gel Pomade *($3.75 for 2.99 ounces)*

BEST TRADITIONAL (MEANING OIL- OR WAX-BASED) POMADES THAT COST MORE THAN $12

Note: The hair-care line marked with an asterisk features at least one additional product that is nearly identical to the recommended product on the list.
Alterna Hemp Seed Hair Concrete *($18 for 2 ounces)*
*ARTec Pure Hair Watercress Finishing Purehold *($14.85 for 2 ounces)*
Aveda Brilliant Anti-Humectant Pomade *($18 for 2.6 ounces)*
Bumble and bumble Sumotech *($19 for 1.5 ounces)*
Frédéric Fekkai Fekkai for Men Grooming Clay *($18.50 for ounces)*
JASÖN Natural Cosmetics I'm Naturally Stuck-Up, A Stiff Hair Styling Wax *($12.50 for 4 ounces)*
John Masters Organics Hair Pomade *($20 for 2 ounces)*
Joico Con_text Orientation Light Wax *($13 for 2 ounces)*
Modern Elixirs by Paul Mitchell Defining Pomade *($13.99 for 1.8 ounces)*
mop (modern organic products) orange peel molding cream *($13.99 for 2.65 ounces)*
Nolita Sheer Texturizer *($16 for 3.5 ounces)*
Rusk Being Primitive Clay *($17 for 4.4 ounces)*
SEXY Hair Concepts Short Sexy Hair Frenzy, Bulked Up Texture *($15.50 for 2.5 ounces)*
TIGI Bed Head Manipulator, A Funky Gunk That Rocks! *($16.95 for 2 ounces)*

BEST STYLING WAXES AND PASTES WITH MINIMAL TO LIGHT HOLD THAT COST $12 OR LESS

L.A. Looks Piece It Look Wax Stick *($3.29 for 2.5 ounces)*
ProVitamin Special Effects Molding Wax, Pliable Hair Wax/Flexible Hold *($7.29 for 2 ounces)*

SEXY Hair Concepts Short Sexy Hair Control Maniac, Wax *($11.50 for 1.8 ounces)*
Soft Sheen Carson Optimum Care Body & Shine Sheen Spray *($3.59 for 9.5 ounces)*

BEST STYLING WAXES AND PASTES WITH MINIMAL TO LIGHT HOLD THAT COST MORE THAN $12

Note: The hair-care line marked with an asterisk features at least one additional product that is nearly identical to the recommended product on the list.

*****American Crew** Classic Wax, Pliable Styling Wax *($14.95 for 3.53 ounces)*
ARTec Kiwi Coloreflector Manipulating Wax *($12.50 for 3 ounces)*
Aveda Light Elements Detailing Mist-Wax *($21 for 6.7 ounces)*
Bumble and bumble Sumowax *($19 for 1.5 ounces)*
KMS Hair Play Paste Up Spray *($15.95 for 7 ounces)*
KMS Hair Play Stick-It Wax *($12.75 for 2.3 ounces)*
Matrix FlikTrix, Piece-Out Wax *($16.95 for 2.6 ounces)*
Paul Mitchell Finish, Spray Wax, 3-D Texture and Flexible Hold *($12.95 for 2.8 ounces)*
Pureology Texture Twist, Styling Reshaper *($19 for 3 ounces)*
TIGI Bed Head, A Hair Stick for Cool People *($17.95 for 2.7 ounces)*
TIGI Bed Head Hard to Get, Texturizing Paste *($17.95 for 1.5 ounces)*
TIGI Bed Head Headbanger, Way-Out Wax for Rock Stars *($18.95 for 4.5 ounces)*
Wella Liquid Hair Matte Finish Wax Hair Molder, Soft Hold *($14 for 3.4 ounces)*

BEST STYLING WAX AND PASTE WITH MEDIUM TO FIRM HOLD THAT COSTS $12 OR LESS

Paul Mitchell Lab ESP, Elastic Shaping Paste *($11.95 for 1.8 ounces)*

BEST STYLING WAXES AND PASTES WITH MEDIUM TO FIRM HOLD THAT COST MORE THAN $12

KMS Hair Play Molding Paste *($12.75 for 3.5 ounces)*
L'ANZA Urban Elements Molding Paste *($16.95 for 6.8 ounces)*
NEXXUS MaxxWax Creative Styling Stick *($17 for 2.6 ounces)*
Paul Mitchell Finish, Dry Wax, Clean Texture and Definition *($12.95 for 1.8 ounces)*
Redken Rough Paste 12 Working Material *($14.95 for 2.5 ounces)*
Sebastian Collection Molding Mud, Street Chic Sculpting Bonder *($16.95 for 4.4 ounces)*

BEST STRAIGHTENING BALMS, LOTIONS, CREAMS, & GELS

BEST STRAIGHTENING BALMS, LOTIONS, CREAMS AND GELS WITH MINIMAL TO LIGHT HOLD THAT COST $12 OR LESS

Note: The hair-care lines marked with an asterisk feature at least one additional product that is nearly identical to the recommended product on the list.

Alberto VO5 Straight Hair, Straightens, Smoothes and Shines *($5.99 for 4 ounces)*
Avon Advance Techniques Straight & Sleek Smoothing Balm *($3.99 for 5.1 ounces)*
Back to BASICS Basic Style Sleek Creme, Anti-Frizz Straightening Balm *($9.95 for 5.5 ounces)*

Bath & Body Works Bio Straight & Sleek Extreme Smoothing Creme (*$9 for 3.4 ounces*)
BioSilk Silk Strate (*$11 for 11.6 ounces*)
Charles Worthington Relax and Unwind Blow-Dry Straightening Balm for Curly, Frizzy, and Unruly Hair (*$5.99 for 9 ounces*)
Citré Shine Get Smooth Straightening Balm ($4.99 for 3.3 ounces*)
göt2b Smoothed Over Straightening Balm (*$5.99 for 4.2 ounces*)
ion Anti-Frizz Solutions Straightener (*$5.99 for 8 ounces*)
Jheri Redding Straightening Lotion, Blow-Dry Activated ($2.49 for 6 ounces*)
John Frieda Frizz Ease Wind-Down, Relaxing Creme, Extra Strength Formula ($5.99 for 3.5 ounces*)
physique Keep It Straight Lotion (*$7.49 for 5 ounces*)
ProVitamin Special Effects Curl Amplifier, Curl Reactivating Cream ($7.39 for 4 ounces*)
Rusk Internal Restructure Str8, Anti-Frizz/Anti-Curl Lotion (*$9.90 for 6 ounces*)
Zero Frizz Straighten Out, Humidity Resistant Smoothing Cream (*$7.59 for 4.2 ounces*)

BEST STRAIGHTENING BALMS, LOTIONS, CREAMS & GELS WITH MINIMAL TO LIGHT HOLD THAT COST MORE THAN $12

Note: *The hair-care lines marked with an asterisk feature at least one additional product that is nearly identical to the recommended product on the list.*
Alterna Hemp Seed Straightening Balm ($15.30 for 8.3 ounces*)
Aveda Hang Straight (*$16 for 6.7 ounces*)
Bumble and bumble Straight (*$20 for 5 ounces*)
Fudge Erekt, Non Chemical Hair Straightener Heat Sensitive (*$13.05 for 4.2 ounces*)
Graham Webb Stick Straight Super Strength Smoothing Gel (*$16.69 for 6 ounces*)
ICE Slicker Defining Lotion (*$14.50 for 10.1 ounces*)
Joico Straight Edge Curl Straightener, Heat-Activated ($14 for 10.1 ounces*)
KENRA Straightening Serum, Softens, Smoothes and Controls Coarse, Curly Hair (*$14 for 8 ounces*)
KMS Flat Out Lite Relaxing Creme ($16.50 for 6 ounces*)
Matrix SwitchTrix, Wax-Gel Combo (*$15.95 for 3.4 ounces*)
Nolita Straightening Spray, Chic Sleek, Smooth Sophisticate (*$17 for 8 ounces*)
Paul Mitchell Smoothing Style Straight Works, Straightens and Smoothes (*$14.95 for 6.8 ounces*)
Sebastian Laminates Crema Styler, Anti-Frizz Control (*$12.95 for 5.1 ounces*)
Sebastian Laminates Gel, Concentrated Smoothing Polish ($17.95 for 5.1 ounces*)
SEXY Hair Concepts Straight Sexy Hair Power Straight! Straightening Balm (*$12.95 for 3.4 ounces*)

BEST HAIRSPRAYS (AEROSOL & NON-AEROSOL)

BEST NON-AEROSOL HAIRSPRAYS WITH MINIMAL TO LIGHT HOLD THAT COST $10 OR LESS

Note: The hair-care lines marked with an asterisk feature at least one additional product that is nearly identical to the recommended product on the list.

American Crew Grooming Spray *($9.75 for 8.45 ounces)*

ARTec Textureline Texture Freeze, Super Fast Drying Hair Spray with Shine (Non-Aerosol) *($8.20 for 8 ounces)*

Avon Advance Techniques Daily Results Flexible Hold Hair Spray *($3.99 for 6.7 ounces)*

BioSilk Spray Spritz Firm Hold Styling Spray (Non-Aerosol) *($10 for 11.6 ounces)*

Clairol Herbal Essences Styling Spritz, Maximum Hold *($3.99 for 8.5 ounces)*

*finesse Touchables Hair Spray, Extra Hold, Scented (Non-Aerosol) *($3.89 for 8.5 ounces)*

Infusium 23 Shape & Hold Non-Aerosol Hair Spray, Extra Firm *($3.99 for 8 ounces)*

ion Styling Solutions Flexible Hold Finishing Spray *($4.49 for 8 ounces)*

*Jheri Redding Flexible Hold Hair Spray, Flexible Hold (Non-Aerosol) *($2.49 for 12 ounces)*

Matrix Amplify Volumizing System, Spritz *($9.95 for 8.5 ounces)*

Ouidad Styling Mist *($10 for 8 ounces)*

*Pantene Classic Hairspray, Flexible Hold (Non-Aerosol) *($3.79 for 10.2 ounces)*

Paul Mitchell Light Hold Style, Soft Spray, Light-Hold Finishing Spray (Non-Aerosol) *($6.75 for 8.5 ounces)*

*physique Keep Your Curls Hair Spray *($6.99 for 5.9 ounces)*

Redken Lift & Shine 15 Finishing Spritz *($9.95 for 8.5 ounces)*

Sukesha Freeze Frame Super Spray, Superior Hold and Shine (Non-Aerosol) *($6.95 for 8 ounces)*

*thermaSilk Firm Hold Hairspray (Non-Aerosol) *($3.99 for 8.5 ounces)*

BEST NON-AEROSOL HAIRSPRAYS WITH MINIMAL TO LIGHT HOLD THAT COST MORE THAN $10

Note: The hair-care line marked with an asterisk features at least one additional product that is nearly identical to the recommended product on the list.

Aveda Brilliant Hair Spray *($13 for 8 ounces)*

Back to BASICS Basic Style Final Fix, Firm Hold Hair Spray *($10.95 for 10 ounces)*

Bumble and bumble Holding Spray *($13 for 8 ounces)*

*L'ANZA Urban Elements Finishing Freeze *($11 for 10.1 ounces)*

NEXXUS Comb Thru Natural Hold Design and Finishing Sprae *($11 for 13.5 ounces)*

Ralph Lauren Get Hold of Yourself Hair Spray *($16.50 for 6.7 ounces)*

Rusk Internal Restructure W8less, Shaping & Control Myst (Non-Aerosol) *($11 for 10 ounces)*

Scruples O$_2$ Originals Texturizing Styling Spray *($12.95 for 8.5 ounces)*

BEST NON-AEROSOL HAIRSPRAYS WITH LIGHT TO MEDIUM HOLD THAT COST $10 OR LESS

Note: The hair-care lines marked with an asterisk feature at least one additional product that is nearly identical to the recommended product on the list.

Beauty Without Cruelty Natural Hold Hair Spray *($6.95 for 8.5 ounces)*
***Clairol** Restyle Extra Hold Extra Control Hairspray, 7 *($2.99 for 9 ounces)*
***John Frieda** Frizz Ease Shape and Shine, Flexible-Hold Hair Spray (Non-Aerosol) *($4.99 for 10 ounces)*
Joico Travallo Design and Finishing Spray, Medium Hold *($10 for 10.1 ounces)*
***L'Oreal** Studio Line Mega Spritz, Mega Hold Finishing Spritz *($3.19 for ounces)*
Quantum Spritz, for Firm Hold *($6.50 for 8 ounces)*
***Salon Selectives** Hold Tight, Finishing Spray for Firm Hold (Non-Aerosol) *($3.79 for 8 ounces)*
Scruples Rock Hard, Extra Firm Finishing Spray *($7.65 for 8.5 ounces)*
Soft Sheen Carson Optimum Care Soft Holding Spritz, with Panthenol *($3.59 for 8 ounces)*
***White Rain** Naturals Hair Spray Freesia Spirit, Extra Hold (Non-Aerosol) *($1.59 for 7 ounces)*

BEST NON-AEROSOL HAIRSPRAYS WITH LIGHT TO MEDIUM HOLD THAT COST MORE THAN $10

Paul Mitchell Medium Hold Style, Fast Drying Sculpting Spray, Medium-Hold Finishing Spray (Non-Aerosol) *($16.95 for 16 ounces)*
Sebastian Collection Volumizer, Working Spray *($12.99 for 8.5 ounces)*

BEST NON-AEROSOL HAIRSPRAYS WITH MEDIUM TO FIRM HOLD THAT COST $10 OR LESS

Note: The hair-care lines marked with an asterisk feature at least one additional product that is nearly identical to the recommended product on the list.

ARTec Pure Hair Sandalwood Finishing Spray *($10 for 12 ounces)*
***Aussie** Sprunch Spray, Non-Aerosol *($3.99 for 16 ounces)*
Garnier Fructis Full Control Non-Aerosol Hairspray All Day Hold, Ultra Strong *($2.64 for 8.5 ounces)*
ICE Fixer Firm Hold Hair Spray *($10 for 10.1 ounces)*
KMS Hair Stay Max Hold Spray (Non-Aerosol) *($8.75 for 8.5 ounces)*
***Salon Grafix** Non-Aerosol Freezing Hair Spray, The Ultimate Mega Hold Styling Mist *($5.99 for 8 ounces)*
Salon Selectives Sit Still, Finishing Spray for Medium Hold (Non-Aerosol) *($3.69 for 8.5 ounces)*
TRESemme Curl Care Curl & Scrunch Hair Spray *($4.29 for 10 ounces)*

BEST NON-AEROSOL HAIRSPRAYS WITH MEDIUM TO FIRM HOLD THAT COST MORE THAN $10

Aveda Firmata Hair Spray *($11 for 8.5 ounces)*
Bath & Body Works Botanical Nutrients Willow Bark Firm Hold Hair Spray *($10.50 for 7.5 ounces)*

Goldwell Trendline Finish Spray, Strong (Non-Aerosol) *($12.50 for 6.7 ounces)*
Graham Webb Brit Style Finishing Spray *($10.18 for 8.5 ounces)*
Mastey Pure Colorcare Hold Super Hairspray, for Lasting Style Support *($14.99 for 8 ounces)*
NEXXUS Maxximum Super Hold Styling and Finishing Spray *($11 for 13.5 ounces)*
TIGI Bed Head Maxxed-Out, Massive Hold Hairspray (Non-Aerosol) *($12.95 for 8 ounces)*

BEST NON-AEROSOL HAIRSPRAYS WITH EXTREMELY STRONG HOLD THAT COST $10 OR LESS

Aussie Instant Freeze Super-Hold Hairspray, Non-Aerosol *($3.99 for 8 ounces)*
Clairol Herbal Essences Non-Aerosol Hairspray, Maximum Hold *($3.79 for 8.5 ounces)*
Giga.Hold by Salon Grafix Freeze Hair Spray Non-Aerosol Styling Mist *($5.99 for 8 ounces)*
ion Salon Solutions Styling Spritz *($4.49 for 8 ounces)*
TRESemme European Tres Spray, Super Hold *($3.99 for 10 ounces)*
TRESemme 4+4 Spray F/X *($5.49 for 8 ounces)*

BEST NON-AEROSOL HAIRSPRAYS WITH EXTREMELY STRONG HOLD THAT COST MORE THAN $10

Note: *The hair-care line marked with an asterisk features at least one additional product that is nearly identical to the recommended product on the list.*
*****ABBA** Exacting Medium-Hold Working Hair Spray *($11.50 for 10.1 ounces)*
Fudge Creative Hair Cement, Very Strong Styling Mist *($10.25 for 10.1 ounces)*
SEXY Hair Concepts Wild Sexy Hair Unshakeable, Firm Holding Fixative *($12.50 for 4.2 ounces)*

BEST AEROSOL HAIRSPRAYS WITH MINIMAL TO LIGHT HOLD THAT COST $10 OR LESS

Note: *The hair-care lines marked with an asterisk feature at least one additional product that is nearly identical to the recommended product on the list.*
*****Aussie** AirDo Flexible Hold Styling Mist, Aerosol *($3.99 for 7 ounces)*
Bath & Body Works Bio Max Volume Finishing Spray *($9 for 8 ounces)*
*****Garnier Fructis** Full Control Aerosol Hairspray All Day Firm Hold, Ultra Strong *($2.64 for 8.25 ounces)*
ICE Finisher Hair Spray *($10 for 10.1 ounces)*
ion Salon Solutions Hard-to-Hold Hair Spray *($2.99 for 11 ounces)*
*****NEXXUS** Comb Thru Natural Hold Design and Finishing Mist *($9 for 10.6 ounces)*
Soft & Beautiful Holding Spray, Maximum Hold with Humidity Guard *($2.29 for 12.5 ounces)*
Sukesha Shaping & Styling Hair Spray, Firm Designing Formula (Aerosol) *($8.95 for 10 ounces)*
*****thermaSilk** Firm Hold Hairspray (Aerosol) *($3.99 for 7 ounces)*
*****TRESemme** European Tres Two Hair Spray, Ultra Fine Mist *($3.99 for 11 ounces)*
*****White Rain** Classics Hair Spray, Extra Hold (Aerosol) *($1.59 for 7 ounces)*

BEST AEROSOL HAIRSPRAYS WITH MINIMAL TO LIGHT HOLD THAT COST MORE THAN $10

Note: The hair-care lines marked with an asterisk feature at least one additional product that is nearly identical to the recommended product on the list.

Bumble and bumble Does It All Styling Spray *($19 for 10 ounces)*

ISO Creative Shaping Control, Flexible Spray *($11 for 10.1 ounces)*

KENRA Design Spray, Light Hold Styling Spray 9 *($13 for 12 ounces)*

Matrix Amplify Volumizing System, Hair Spray *($11.95 for 10 ounces)*

Pureology In Charge, Styling Spray, Firm Flexible Hold & Shine *($17 for 9 ounces)*

Redken Airtight 12 Lock-Out Finishing Spray *($11.95 for 11 ounces)

Rusk Being Flexible Hairspray *($11.99 for 10.6 ounces)

Scruples Effects, Super Hold Finishing Spray *($11.95 for 10.6 ounces)*

Sebastian Collection Switch Craft, Changing Spray *($12.95 for 8 ounces)

SEXY Hair Concepts Big Sexy Hair Spray & Play, Volumizing Hairspray *($13 for 10.6 ounces)

TIGI Catwalk EnviroShape, Firm Hold Hairspray *($12 for 8 ounces)*

BEST AEROSOL HAIRSPRAYS WITH LIGHT TO MEDIUM HOLD THAT COST $10 OR LESS

Note: The hair-care lines marked with an asterisk feature at least one additional product that is nearly identical to the recommended product on the list.

finesse Touchables Hair Spray, Extra Hold, Scented (Aerosol) *($3.89 for 7 ounces)

Framesi Shine In Take Hold (Aerosol) *($10 for 10 ounces)*

ion Styling Solutions Shaping Plus Styling Spray *($4.99 for 10.9 ounces)*

Jheri Redding Flexible Hold Hair Spray, Flexible Hold (Aerosol) *($2.49 for 10 ounces)

John Frieda Frizz Ease Moisture Barrier, Firm-Hold Hair Spray (Aerosol) *($4.99 for 10 ounces)*

KMS Hair Stay Medium Hold Spray (Aerosol) *($9.95 for 9.5 ounces)*

physique Control + Freeze Hair Spray, Maximum Hold (Aerosol) *($6.99 for 8.25 ounces)

Salon Grafix Shaping Hair Spray, Extra Super Hold Styling Mist *($5.99 for 10 ounces)

Suave Hairspray, Extra Hold (Aerosol) *($1.29 for 6.5 ounces)

Wella Liquid Hair Structuring Mist Styling Hairspray, Strong Hold *($9.50 for 8.4 ounces)*

White Rain Classics Hair Spray, Maximum Hold (Aerosol) *($1.59 for 7 ounces)*

BEST AEROSOL HAIRSPRAYS WITH LIGHT TO MEDIUM HOLD THAT COST MORE THAN $10

Note: The hair-care lines marked with an asterisk feature at least one additional product that is nearly identical to the recommended product on the list.

ARTec Kiwi Coloreflector Blaster Spray, Fast Drying Super Hold Hairspray *($12 for 10 ounces)

Frédéric Fekkai Sheer Hold Hairspray *($22.50 for 5.8 ounces)*

Fudge Skyscraper, Firm Hold Hairspray *($14.95 for 21.5 ounces)*

Graham Webb Vivid Color Color Locking Hair Spray *($11.16 for 10 ounces)*

Hayashi System Design Quikk, Fast Dry Working Spray *($13 for 10 ounces)*
ISO Ultimate Hold Control, Finishing Spray *($11 for 10.1 ounces)*
Joico K-Pak Protective Hair Spray *($14 for 10 ounces)*
NEXXUS Nexxtacy Sustained Hold Styling and Finishing Mist *($11 for 14.1 ounces)*
Nolita Hair Spray *($12 for 10 ounces)*
*Sebastian Shaper Hair Spray *($11.50 for 10 ounces)*
Tri Covert Control Holding Spray *($12 for 11 ounces)*

BEST AEROSOL HAIRSPRAYS WITH MEDIUM TO FIRM HOLD THAT COST $10 OR LESS

Note: The hair-care line marked with an asterisk features at least one additional product that is nearly identical to the recommended product on the list.
finesse Touchables Hair Spray, Maximum Hold (Aerosol) *($3.89 for 7 ounces)*
göt2b Glued Spiking Freeze Spray *($5.99 for 12 ounces)*
Salon Selectives Sit Still, Finishing Spray for Medium Hold (Aerosol) *($3.99 for 7 ounces)*
*Suave Hairspray, Maximum Hold (Aerosol) *($1.29 for 6.5 ounces)*

BEST AEROSOL HAIRSPRAYS WITH MEDIUM TO FIRM HOLD THAT COST MORE THAN $10

Note: The hair-care lines marked with an asterisk feature at least one additional product that is nearly identical to the recommended product on the list.
*Goldwell Trendline Finish Spray, Extreme (Aerosol) *($14.50 for 8.6 ounces)*
ISO Multiplicity Finalize, Firm Hold Spray *($11.75 for 10.1 ounces)*
*Joico JoiMist Firm Finishing Spray, Maximum Hold *($11.50 for 11.2 ounces)*
KENRA Artformation Spray, Firm Hold Styling and Finishing Spray 18 *($13 for 12 ounces)*
KMS Hair Stay Max Hold Spray (Aerosol) *($10.75 for 9.5 ounces)*
NEXXUS Maxximum Super Hold Styling and Finishing Mist *($11 for 14.1 ounces)*
*Nioxin Bionutrient Creatives Niospray, Power Hold *($10.99 for 8.8 ounces)*
*Sebastian Shaper Plus Hair Spray *($12.50 for 10.6 ounces)*
TIGI Catwalk Work-It, Medium-Firm Hold Working Hairspray *($12 for 8 ounces)*

BEST AEROSOL HAIRSPRAYS WITH EXTREMELY STRONG HOLD THAT COST $10 OR LESS

Note: The hair-care line marked with an asterisk features at least one additional product that is nearly identical to the recommended product on the list.
*Aqua Net 2 Super Hold All Day All Over Hold, Fresh Fragrance *($2.59 for 14 ounces)*
Aussie Instant Freeze Super-Hold Hairspray, Aerosol *($3.99 for 7 ounces)*
Giga.Hold by Salon Grafix Freeze Hair Spray Ultra Intense, Aerosol *($5.99 for 10 ounces)*

BEST AEROSOL HAIRSPRAYS WITH EXTREMELY STRONG HOLD THAT COST MORE THAN $10

Alterna Hemp Seed Maximum Hold Volume Lock *($21.60 for 14.1 ounces)*
Matrix FreezeTrix, Fast Fix Spray *($11.95 for 12 ounces)*

BEST SPECIALTY PRODUCTS
(ALL PRICES)

Note: The products in the following list are unusual options that can be effective for their intended hair type, condition, or purpose—but that were difficult to classify within the other Best Product groups. Please refer to each product's specific review in Chapter Ten for details and recommended hair type/condition.

AFRiCAN PRIDE Spray On Braid Shampoo *($3.99 for 8 ounces)*
AFRICAN ROYALE Hot Six Oil *($4.79 for 8 ounces)*
Charles Worthington Perfect Reflection Wax, for Dark Hair Shades and Perfect Reflection Wax, for Blonde Hair Shades *(both $12 for 1.7 ounces)*
Clairol Metalex Hair Conditioner 511 *($12.99 for 4 ounces)*
Curl Friends Gooey-Goo Wonder Wax *($18 for 2 ounces)*
Darphin Protective Shining Oil, for All Hair Types *($25 for 1.6 ounces)*
fresh Sugar Shea Butter *($38 for 3.5 ounces)*
Goldwell Colorance Color Soft Color Foam Colorant *($11.12 for 4.2 ounces)*
Goldwell Colorance Color Styling Mousse *($7.97 for 2.4 ounces)*
Graham Webb Brit Style Sculptor *($14.83 for 3.4 ounces)*
Graham Webb Color Care Blonde Shimmer Cream *($12.95 for 1.7 ounces)*
John Frieda Beach Blonde Gold Rush, Shimmer Gel *($6.49 for 4 ounces)*
John Frieda Frizz Ease Instant Mirror Image, Heat-Activated Laminator *($13 for 1.69 ounces)*
John Frieda Frizz Ease Relax Ripple Effect, Wave-Maker Styling Spray *($10.50 for 6 ounces)*
John Masters Organics Dry Hair Nourishment & Defrizzer *($16 for 0.5 ounce)*
KMS Turnstyle Head Wetter All Wet Spray *($13 for 6.8 ounces)*
Nolita Grit Gel, Beach Hair, City Style *($18 for 8 ounces)*
Sebastian Xtah Raw Hair Twisted Taffy, Free-Former *($19.50 for 4.4 ounces)*
SEXY Hair Concepts Wild Sexy Hair Metal Head, Metallic Holding Gel *($11.95 for 2.1 ounces)*
SEXY Hair Concepts Wild Sexy Hair Untamed, Whipped Wax *($14.95 for 3.5 ounces)*
Soft & Beautiful Botanicals Oil *($4.29 for 4 ounces)*
Wella Liquid Hair Moonshine Foaming Pomade, Soft Hold *($13 for 3.4 ounces)*

BEST FRAGRANCE-FREE PRODUCTS
(ALL PRICES)

Note: All of the products listed below deserve special recognition because they are completely fragrance-free and, therefore, are excellent for anyone with a sensitive, easily irritated, or itchy scalp.

BEST FRAGRANCE-FREE SHAMPOOS

Aveda Personal Blends Shampoo Formula *($10.50 for 7 ounces)*
DHC Baby Hair Shampoo *($6 for 3.3 ounces)*
Framesi Shine In Shampoo *($11 for 10 ounces)*
Free & Clear Shampoo, for Sensitive Skin & Scalp *($7.80 for 8 ounces)*

Kiehl's Castille Shampoo, for Dry, Damaged, Thick or Coarse Hair *($13 for 8 ounces)*

Kiehl's Klaus Heidegger's All-Sport Swimmer's Cleansing Rinse for Hair and Body *($14 for 8 ounces)*

Paula's Choice All Over Hair & Body Shampoo *($12.95 for 16 ounces)*

BEST FRAGRANCE-FREE CONDITIONERS

DHC Head Conditioner *($16 for 6.7 ounces)*

Framesi Shine In Conditioner *($10 for 10 ounces)*

Free & Clear Hair Conditioner, for Normal & Sensitive Skin *($7.80 for 8 ounces)*

John Frieda Sheer Blonde Spotlight, Hi-Beam Glosser and Power Detangler *($5.49 for 2.4 ounces)*

Kiehl's Leave-In Hair Conditioner with Panthenol and Coconut Oil *($16 for 4 ounces)*

Kiehl's Panthenol Protein Hair Conditioner Softener & Grooming Aid *($14.50 for 6 ounces)*

NEXXUS Aloe Rid Treatment Deep Clarifying Solution *($6 for 5 ounces)*

Nizoral Non-Medicated Daily Conditioner *($5.84 for 12 ounces)*

Paula's Choice Smooth Finish Conditioner *($12.95 for 16 ounces)*

BEST FRAGRANCE-FREE STYLING PRODUCTS

Bumble and bumble Straight *($20 for 5 ounces)*

Free & Clear Hair Spray for Sensitive Skin, Soft Hold *($10.95 for 8 ounces)*

Free & Clear Hair Spray for Sensitive Skin, Firm Hold *($10.95 for 8 ounces)*

Jheri Redding Extra Reflections Polisher *($8.95 for 4 ounces)*

Kiehl's Extra Strength Styling Gel *($16 for 4 ounces)*

Kiehl's "Wet Look" Groom *($13 for 4 ounces)*

Michael diCesare Crystal Shine Lite *($15 for 2 ounces)*

physique Volumizing Hair Spray, Unscented (Aerosol) *($6.99 for 5.5 ounces)*

ProVitamin Volumizing Hair Spray, Unscented (Aerosol) *($6.99 for 5.5 ounces)*

Salon Grafix Shaping Hair Spray, Super Hold Styling Mist *($5.99 for 10 ounces)*

APPENDIX

Animal Testing

COMPANIES THAT *DO NOT* TEST ON ANIMALS:

ABBA
AFRICAN ROYALE
...rto VO5
...na
...ony Logistics
...ec
...ey Organics
...e

...o BASICS
Bath & Body Works
Beauty Without Cruelty
    (BWC)
BioSilk
The Body Shop
Bumble and bumble
Burt's Bees
Citré Shine
Clairol
Clinique
Curl Friends
Dep
Framesi
Fudge
Garnier Fructis
Goldwell
göt2b
Graham Webb
H₂O+

head GAMES
ICE
ion
Jheri Redding
John Masters Organics
Joico
KENRA
Kiehl's
KMS
L.A. LOOKS
Lancome
L'ANZA
L'Oreal
Mastey
Matrix
NEXXUS
NIOXIN
Nolita
Origins
Ouidad
Paul Mitchell
Paula's Choice
Philip B. Hair Care
Prell
Professional
Pureology
Queen Helene
Ralph Lauren
Redken
Salon Grafix

Scruples
SEXY Hair Concepts
Soft & Beautiful
Soft Sheen Carson
St. Ives
Sukesha
tcb
Thicker Fuller Hair
TRESemme
Tri
WELEDA
Zero Frizz
Zirh

COMPANIES THAT *DO* TEST ON ANIMALS:

Aqua Net
Breck
Dove
finesse
Head & Shoulders
Infusium 23
Johnson & Johnson
Pantene PRO-V
Pert Plus
physique
Salon Selectives
Suave
thermaSilk

COMPANIES THAT HAVE AN UNKNOWN STATUS:

Adorn
AFRiCAN PRIDE
American Crew
Avacor
bain de terre
binge
Charles Worthington
Conair
d:fi
Darphin
Denorex
Folligen
Frédéric Fekkai
fresh
Garren New York
Hayashi
Inner Science
    (Canada Only)
ISO
j. f. lazartigue
JASÖN Natural Cosmetics

John Frieda
Kerastase
Michael diCesare
Molton Brown
mop (modern organic
    products)
Neutrogena
Nizoral
Phyto
ProVitamin
Progaine
Proxiphen & Nano
Quantum
Rene Furterer
Revlon Realistic
Rogaine
Rusk
Sebastian
Selsun Blue
Senscience
terax

TIGI
Ultra Swim
Wash & Curl
Wella
White Rain

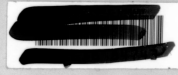
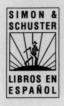

SIMON &
SCHUSTER

LIBROS EN
ESPAÑOL

Fairb

CRIANDO A

Educando a niños

NUESTROS

latinos en

NIÑOS

un mundo bicultural

GLORIA G. RODRIGUEZ, PH.D.

TRADUCIDO POR CAMI J. LICEA

LIBROS EN ESPAÑOL

SIMON & SCHUSTER
LIBROS EN ESPAÑOL
Rockefeller Center
1230 Avenue of the Americas
New York, NY 10020

Copyright © 1999 por Gloria G. Rodriguez, Ph.D.

DISEÑADO POR PATRICE SHERIDAN
PRODUCIDO POR K&N BOOKWORKS INC.

Hecho en los Estados Unidos de América

10 9 8 7 6 5 4 3 2 1

Datos de catalogación de la Biblioteca del Congreso puede
solicitarse información.

ISBN 0-684-84126-6

Dedicatoria

Le dedico este libro a mi madrecita, Lucy Villegas Salazar, a quien quiero con toda mi alma y corazón. Mi madre me hizo comprender que ningún otro papel en la vida es más importante que aquél de padre o madre, y así se convirtió en mi inspiración para comenzar AVANCE en 1973.

Este libro también se lo dedico a mi familia querida: mi esposo maravilloso y media naranja, Salvador C. Rodríguez, y nuestros niños, Salvador Julián, Steven René, y Gloria Vanessa, a quienes amamos mucho y a Sonya Yvonne, nuestro ángel en el cielo. Que este libro les ayude a nuestros niños con sus futuros papeles de padres y también a conservar nuestra bella y rica cultura hispana. Lo que deseamos para nuestros niños, deseamos para todos los niños latinos.

Prólogo

Hace más de veinte años fui invitada a ser testigo de un tesoro nacional floreciente. En 1973, Gloria Rodríguez, una joven e inteligente mujer México-americana, recién graduada de la universidad y con todas las oportunidades del éxito material por delante, decidió renunciar a su empleo como maestra para comenzar a trabajar en el complejo de viviendas subvencionadas más carenciado del lado oeste de San Antonio. Recuerdo vívidamente el entorno tan deprimente y amenazador al caminar ese día gris de febrero, a través del laberinto desconocido de edificios que conducía al primer Centro de AVANCE. Aun más imponente era la tarea que tenía ante mí: ayudar a desarrollar unas estrategias para utilizar el subsidio inicial, el cual se estaba acabando rápidamente. Adentro, el cuarto estaba calientito, lleno de los aromas de café y tacos y el parloteo de alrededor de una docena de muchachas, algunas con bebés en los brazos y otras con bebés todavía dentro de sus vientres jóvenes. Estaban cosiendo unos títeres hechos de calcetín, mientras Carmen Cortez, la nueva socia de Gloria, les hablaba sobre el desarrollo de lenguaje en los niños muy pequeños. Cuando Gloria Rodríguez se acercó a la mesa, le enseñaron orgullosamente sus trabajos manuales y el parloteo llegó a un punto culminante al comprometerse cada una a volver para la siguiente sesión. El programa llenó mi corazón y lo envolvió con tanta fuerza que nunca lo ha soltado. Yo supe en ese momento que ninguna persona de consciencia, que viera lo que AVANCE significaba en la vida de estas jóvenes, pudiera dejar de apoyar su trabajo.

A través del cuarto de siglo subsiguiente, eruditos, encargados de la formulación de políticas, directores generales de la Salud Pública, numerosas primeras damas y aun el príncipe de Gales atravesarían el camino a ese departamento transformado en ese complejo de viviendas públicas. Lo que fue creado en ese lugar empobrecido se duplicaría en sitios a través de dos estados y en once programas afiliados. La filosofía y metodología de AVANCE se ha extendido a través de los Estados Unidos y Latinoamérica debido a la influencia del Centro de Entrenamiento de AVANCE. El programa de estudios de AVANCE, escrito a mano, progresaría de una serie de gastados blocs estilo legal de papel amarillo, a un sistema sofisticado y completo que permite la reproducción. Eventualmente, a las primeras 35 madres jóvenes, se les unirían más de 80,000 madres y padres. El personal ha ascendido a cientos. AVANCE transformaría muchas vidas—las vidas de madres (y ahora

padres) jóvenes, cuyos futuros antes se definían con un sentido de desesperanza. Ahora se les ayuda a lograr el poder de tomar control de sus
vidas por medio de terminar sus estudios de preparatoria (high school),
asistir a la universidad, recibir entrenamiento y preparación para trabajos específicos—y ante todo, a llegar a ser unos padres competentes, con
confianza, optimistas y capaces de transformar la vida de sus propios
hijos. Muy pronto el éxito de AVANCE se hizo indisputable. Sin embargo, lo que persistía como una pregunta en la mente de los eruditos, de
aquellos encargados de la formulación de políticas, y de otros escépticos
de tales programas sociales era: "¿Por qué funciona y cómo?" Los científicos sociales examinarían minuciosamente el programa, componente
por componente, sólo para descubrir que era imposible establecer con
exactitud por qué es tan exitoso el programa.

Este libro, desde su enfoque en la Virgen de Guadalupe a su o-
rientación sobre los principios de Piaget sobre el desarrollo de los niños,
provee algunas respuestas a aquellas preguntas. Y aun más importante es
el hecho de que amplía y extiende el poder de AVANCE para llegarles a
todas las familias latinas, ya sean encabezadas por muchachas adolescentes que están luchando por completar su educación preparatoria, o
bien parejas profesionales que están ascendiendo dentro de sus carreras,
o personas con doctorados en el estudio del desarrollo de los niños.
AVANCE funciona porque está cimentado en la aceptación incondicional de jóvenes latinos, madres y padres, que llegan a sus centros,
además de una creencia y fe rotunda en su potencial y en la creación de
unas duraderas y estrechas relaciones de apoyo al dedicarse los padres al
trabajo más exigente de la vida. AVANCE funciona porque los padres
jóvenes y vulnerables se dan cuenta que pueden confiar en sus enseñanzas. Este libro es una invitación a esas enseñanzas, una celebración a
ellas, y una bienvenida a las alegrías, las luchas, y los triunfos de carácter íntimo y privado de las familias latinas.

Este libro, tal como el programa construido por la autora, es impulsado con la energía de su creadora, una energía que contagia a la mayoría
que llega a tener contacto con AVANCE y con Gloria Rodríguez. Es una
energía que no aceptará restricciones ni limitaciones de parte de estructuras tradicionales y la cual insiste que todo es posible, para todos. Es una
energía que es una amalgama de las creencias arraigadas y la sabiduría
tradicional de la crianza de las familias latinas, el poder inherente de
nuestros conocimientos científicos y comprensión actual de cómo se
desarrollan los niños físicamente, intelectualmente, emocionalmente, y
socialmente, además de las lecciones sobre sentido común que se
adquieren a través de la lucha por la dignidad y plena participación de

una comunidad que históricamente ha sido excluida. Aun más valiosa es la rica amalgama de historia, tradiciones y experiencias de la propia familia de Gloria—una riqueza con la cual se identificarán todos los latinos.

En muchos sentidos este libro es parecido a la comunidad a la cual está diseñado a informar y a servir. La comunidad latina representa la erupción de energía nueva en este país. Esta fuerza poderosa de demografía y de energía espiritual y cultural definirá, en muchos sentidos, el siglo veintiuno de los Estados Unidos, de una manera muy similar a como lo hicieron los "baby boomers" (personas nacidas inmediatamente después de la segunda guerra mundial) en el siglo veinte. Con la anticipación de llegar a formar el veinticinco por ciento de la población de los Estados Unidos durante los próximos cincuenta años, los latinos tendrán un impacto sobre todas las instituciones y la vida de casi todos los demás americanos. La naturaleza de ese impacto depende enormemente de nuestra capacidad para desarrollar en nuestros niños la capacidad para contribuir y participar en las instituciones de los Estados Unidos, y al mismo tiempo fortalecer, en lugar de destruir, los atributos familiares, éticos, y espirituales que componen el sello distintivo de nuestra cultura tradicional y profunda, en toda su diversidad.

Los profesionales de educación, del desarrollo de los niños, y de los servicios sociales y de salud que trabajan con familias latinas pueden encontrar en este libro no sólo una perspicacia profunda sobre la interacción de la cultura, la mente, y el espíritu de esta comunidad, sino también innumerables herramientas para ayudarles a llegar y alcanzar a las familias latinas. Yo recomendaría que los lectores utilicen este libro como un recurso para sus niños y familias, una fuente de canciones, recetas, y dichos, los cuales forman una parte tan importante de la cultura latina y deben ser atesorados y pasados de generación a generación.

Los padres latinos se encontrarán a sí mismos y a sus padres y abuelos reflejados y celebrados en estas páginas. Ya sean de descendencia mexicana, puertorriqueña, dominicana, centroamericana, cubana, o sudamericana, o bien india, negra, blanca o mestiza, los latinos en los Estados Unidos se enfrentarán al reto y se sentirán emocionados por las posibilidades de criar unos niños fuertes que no le piden nada a nadie— que saben quiénes son y los dones y talentos maravillosos que traen a este amado país en el emocionante siglo al cual ellos darán forma.

—Blandina Cárdenas
Professora adjunta, La Universidad de Texas en San Antonio;
Antigua comisionada de la Administración
de Niños, Jóvenes, y Familias

Reconocimiento

Ante todo, quiero reconocer y agradecer a mi familia más cercana por su gran paciencia y apoyo mientras escribía este libro. También quiero agradecer a mi familia nuclear, a mi familia extensa, a la familia extensa de mi esposo, y a mi familia de AVANCE por darme recuerdos tan bellos y por hacer posible este libro. He intentado compartir las experiencias de mi vida, mi orgullo cultural latino, además de mi entrenamiento y mis conocimientos profesionales con el fin de ayudar a todos los padres actuales y futuros que lean este libro.

Quiero ofrecer un agradecimiento especial a Elena Cabral y a Rebecca T. Cabaza, dos grandes escritoras hispanas, por compartir conmigo sus extraordinarios talentos literarios y editoriales. También quiero agradecerle a Cami Licea por traducir a español este libro, a Blandina Cárdenas por escribir el prólogo, y a las muchas personas que compartieron sus recetas, dichos, juegos, canciones, y canciones de cuna.

Sobre todo, quiero reconocer, agradecer, alabar, y honrar a Dios Todopoderoso, por brindarme Su amor, bendiciones, orientación, y fortaleza. Él es quien me sostiene. No hubiera podido completar este libro sin Su presencia en mi vida, porque cuando me encontraba a la mitad de escribirlo, perdí a mi queridísima amiga, Carmen P. Cortez, cuya amistad y bella sonrisa verdaderamente echo de menos.

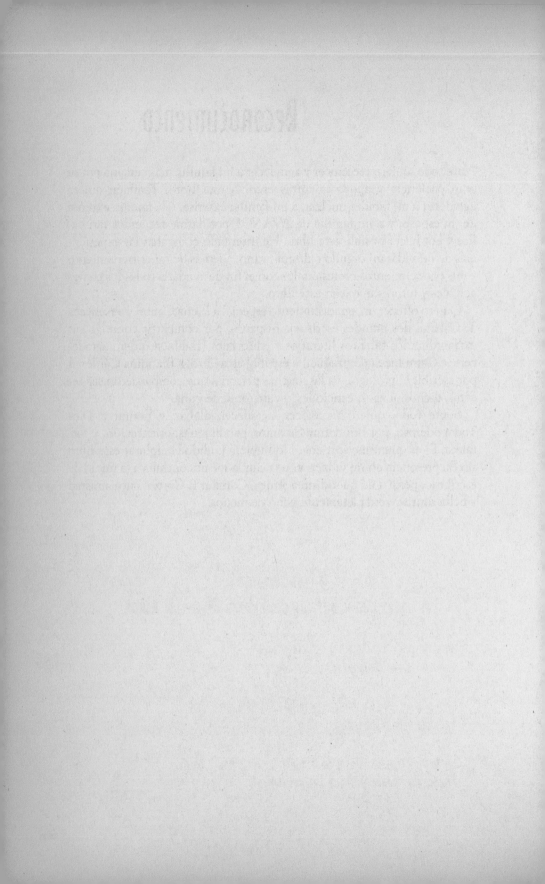

Contenido

Tercera parte
Los tres pilares de una crianza efectiva:
El matrimonio, la familia, y la comunidad

Introducción

En 1970, cuando era una estudiante de primer año de universidad, con asignaturas principales de sociología y educación, me enteré de que yo era una niña a riesgo. Por ser hija de una madre que estaba criando a sus hijos sin pareja, quien me crió a mí y a siete otros niños en los barrios de San Antonio, yo, según algunos expertos, no debí haber llegado a mi graduación de preparatoria. En una época cuando las estadísticas comenzaban a pintar un cuadro muy desolado de jóvenes hispanos en crisis, con índices alarmantes de abandono de estudios, bajos logros académicos, y delincuencia juvenil, yo me maravillaba ante el hecho de que según las normas de la sociedad, yo era un misterio.

Cuando yo leí esos números de malos presagios, yo comencé a recordar el pasado—recordé el complejo de viviendas subvencionadas, llamado Alazán, y nuestra pequeña casita de madera en la calle Colima, en el lado oeste de la ciudad, donde mi madre, una viuda con una educación de solamente tercer año de primaria, crió exitosamente a sus hijos a pesar de las drogas, la violencia, y el crimen que amenazaba las calles. Yo me pregunté, ¿qué era lo que esta mujer hizo, qué secreto o qué magia extraña poesía que la ayudó a criar exitosamente a sus niños a pesar de las probabilidades en su contra?

Después de varios años de estudios, un doctorado, y tres hijos propios, yo me enteré que no fue ni un secreto ni un hechizo. En el caso de mi madre, Lucy Salazar, fue una combinación de su fe inalterable, su profundo sentido de compromiso a la familia, además del apoyo que recibió de su extensa familia y de sus vecinos en el barrio, una combinación exclusiva a ella. El apoyo principal provenía de mi abuelo Lázaro "Papayo" Villegas, quien llegó a ser para mí, a la edad de dos años, una amorosa figura paterna, después del fallecimiento de mi padre. Como valores centrales y fundamentales en mi familia, se encontraban un amor incondicional, una dedicación, y altas expectativas para los niños. También existía un profundo sentido de compromiso a la cultura que se nos obsequiaba tal como un regalo especial, el cual necesitaba ser conservado y apreciado.

A pesar de que éramos pobres, yo recuerdo siempre volver al hogar para encontrar a una madre amorosa quien había preparado una mesa llena de comida, con todo y una pila de tortillas calientitas. Aunque teníamos un patio pequeño donde vivíamos, mi madre siempre se las arreglaba para llenarlo con aromáticas flores perennes y hermosos rosales, que juntos con los árboles de nuez, sirvieron para darle a nuestro patio una apariencia más bella y más grande de lo real. Aunque mi madre nos enseñó la importancia de la humildad, también puso énfasis en el orgullo, recalcando que siempre debíamos mantener las cabezas bien erguidas. A mis hermanas y a mí, nos vestía como muñecas, con guantes y lindos sombreros para hacer resaltar los vestidos de colores vibrantes, con enaguas, que nos cosía para la Navidad y para Domingo de Pascua. A todos, sin falta, nos hicieron sentir importantes y especiales. Un intenso sentido de obligación a la familia se formó durante estos primeros años, ya que como hermanos, se esperaba que nos cuidáramos unos a otros. Cuando éramos niños, se esperaba que mostráramos respeto a la gente mayor. Como latinos, se nos infundía un sentido de orgullo y dignidad porque formábamos parte de *nuestra gente*.

El dicho favorito de mi madre, *no hay mal que por bien no venga*, se convirtió en un credo familiar en nuestra casa. Aunque contaba con mi abuelo para brindarle apoyo, mi madre funcionó como ambos madre y padre para mí. Ella era, tal como también lo era mi suegra, la Doña, siempre dejando muy en claro, sin ninguna duda, lo que ella esperaba de sus niños, y nunca se desviaba de las reglas que ella misma imponía. Tal como es el caso de muchos padres hispanos, entre aquellas cosas que ella consideraba más importantes figuraba nuestra educación, un aprendizaje que incluía no solamente lo que leíamos en libros, sino también nuestro comportamiento, nuestras actitudes, nuestros principios, y nuestras creencias. Ser bien educados significaba no solamente que sabíamos leer y escribir, sino que también poseíamos ciertas virtudes tales como el respeto, la lealtad, la compasión, la dedicación al trabajo, y la capacidad de distinguir entre el bien y el mal.

Uno de los recuerdos más vívidos de mi niñez ocurrió cuando yo contaba con sólo cuatro años de edad. Yo estaba parada en la acera enfrente de mi edificio en el complejo de viviendas subvencionadas cuando una niña mayor me embistió con su bicicleta, estrellándome de cara contra el cemento, dándole a los pedales para alejarse con una total indiferencia a mis heridas. Mi madre, quien observó el incidente desde una ventana del segundo piso de nuestro edificio, estaba tan enfurecida y alterada que llamó a la policía, y el incidente, muy para la sorpresa de mis vecinos, aun salió luego como reporte en el periódico local. Lo que quedó grabado en mi memoria por mucho tiempo después de ese día fue la manera en que mi madre, siempre vigilante, valiente, y tenaz, nunca dejó de utilizar cada uno de sus recursos y toda gota de energía para mantener erguidos a sus hijos. Mientras hubiera aliento en su cuerpo, ella estaba resuelta a asegurarse de que nadie nos iba a tumbar ni a impedir que llegáramos a ser lo que era la intención de Dios.

Esta mujer que poseía tan poco, se las arreglaba para llenarnos de tanto amor, esperanza, y orgullo que nunca hubiéramos podido imaginar no cumplir con sus expectativas de mantenernos lejos de los problemas y de luchar por alcanzar nuestras metas. Ambos, ella y mi abuelo, se aseguraron que nosotros supiéramos y sintiéramos que éramos especiales. Yo recuerdo que mi abuelo nos decía: "Dios cuida a los huérfanos y a las viudas. Él tiene una meta especial para cada uno de ustedes".

Mi meta en la vida durante los últimos veinticinco años, además de mi familia, ha sido AVANCE, una organización sin fines de lucro que ha sido mundialmente reconocida como una organización líder en la educación a los padres sobre la crianza de sus niños y el apoyo familiar, y se ha hecho merecedora de recibir elogios de medios de comunicación ambos hispanos y convencionales además de políticos de todo el espectro político. Muchos dignatarios, incluyendo al príncipe Carlos, Barbara Bush, Jesse Jackson, la gobernadora Ann Richards, el director de la Salud Pública, David Satcher, y el senador de los Estados Unidos Bill Bradley, han visitado los programas de AVANCE. AVANCE ha sido reconocido en los libros escritos por tres primeras damas de los Estados Unidos: *First Teachers (Los primeros maestros)* de Barbara Bush, *It Takes a Village (Se necesita a todo el pueblo)* de Hillary Clinton, y *Helping Someone with Mental Illness (Ayudar a alguien con una enfermedad mental)* de Rosalynn Carter. En 1997, a una familia participante de AVANCE y a mí nos invitaron el presidente Bill Clinton y la primera dama Hillary Rodham Clinton a la Casa Blanca para representar a AVANCE como un programa modelo en la Conferencia de la Casa Blanca sobre el Desarrollo y Aprendizaje de los Niños Pequeños. AVANCE pudo ampliar sus servicios en los campos de educación a los padres sobre la crianza de sus niños y el apoyo familiar gracias al apoyo de algunas de las más grandes fundaciones y corporaciones en los Estados Unidos, incluyendo a Carnegie, Ford, Kellogg, Rockefeller, Hilton, Mott, Hasbro, y Kraft/General Foods.

Este libro les lleva a todos los padres hispanos las estrategias y los principios que han ayudado a tantos padres de AVANCE, provenientes del barrio donde yo crecí y más allá. El modelo que ha cultivado AVANCE, con más de veinticinco años de investigación y experiencia, tiene como base la satisfacción de las cuatro necesidades básicas de los niños: las físicas, las cognoscitivas, las sociales, y las emocionales. En adición a éstas, para el propósito de este libro, yo he añadido una quinta necesidad, la cual está inextricablemente unida a todo elemento de la cultura hispana: nuestra fe y espiritualidad. Utilizando actividades que abrazan y celebran las tradiciones de nuestra raza, yo les muestro a los padres cómo su cultura puede realzar la experiencia de la crianza de los niños. Yo refuerzo y fortalezco nuestros puntos fuertes, como latinos, concretamente nuestro idioma y nuestros valores culturales, al ayudar a los padres a adquirir los conocimientos y las habilidades esenciales para llegar a ser mejores padres. Estos valores incluyen la devoción a los niños, al matrimonio, a la familia, a la fe, y a la comunidad. Nuestras costumbres son fuerzas poderosas que pueden moldear las mentes y los corazones de los niños, creando unos individuos orgullosos y seguros quienes tienen algo muy especial que ofrecerle a la sociedad.

Todos nosotros queremos ver a nuestros niños llegar a ser seres humanos sanos, felices, competentes, y exitosos. Queremos que sobresalgan en la escuela y crezcan para ser personas honestas, compasivas, trabajadoras, y responsables. Claro que los niños no vienen automáticamente empaquetados con estas maravillosas virtudes, ni tampoco vienen con un librito de instrucciones. De la misma manera, una efectiva crianza a los niños no es algo natural para los padres; es un arte e incluye habilidades que deben ser aprendidas tal como las de cualquier otro papel en la sociedad. Usted ya posee muchos de los ingredientes que son esenciales para una crianza efectiva, incluyendo el amor, las esperanzas, y los sueños que tiene para sus niños. Con las herramientas apropiadas, la crianza de los niños puede ser la experiencia que le proporciona más satisfacción y gratificación que ninguna otra en su vida.

Los hispanoamericanos, ya casi llegando a componer quienes ya casi componen el grupo étnico más grande de los Estados Unidos, encaran grandes oportunidades y desafíos. En su papel de madres y padres, muchos se encuentran luchando por orientar y conducir a sus niños a través de una sociedad cada vez más urbana, móvil, impersonal, y competitiva, donde las influencias negativas parecen acechar a la vuelta de cada esquina. Los sistemas naturales de apoyo asociados con la familia, o sea, un matrimonio firme y un sistema de tíos, primos, amigos, y vecinos, aún son muy fuertes entre muchos hispanos, sin embargo, deben reforzarse al volverse más móviles y más americanizadas las familias. Mi esposo y yo somos iguales a muchos padres hispanos que trabajan, y quieren mantener las antiguas tradiciones en este mundo de constantes cambios, al mismo tiempo de hacerles frente a las demandas de dos carreras profesionales. Yo conozco los obstáculos que muchos de ustedes tienen que encarar. Sin embargo, también sé que existen maneras de unir lo mejor de ambos mundos, la cultura latina y la americana, para ayudar a mantener la solidez del matrimonio y de la familia y para ayudar a sus niños a tener éxito en un mundo bilingüe, de dos culturas.

A través de mi entrenamiento en los campos de la educación y el crecimiento y desarrollo de los niños, yo puedo proporcionarle la información y las investigaciones más actualizadas para ayudarle a orientar a sus niños. Ciertamente, los niños alrededor del mundo tienen las mismas necesidades básicas. Sin embargo, como latina que ha estado criando a tres niños y que ha trabajado con innumerables otros padres hispanos, yo quiero discutir estos principios, con una voz que le habla a nuestra comunidad. Al hacer esto, yo recurriré a las experiencias de mi propia crianza, de mi entrenamiento y desarrollo profesionales, de mi experiencia como maestra, y de ejemplos derivados de AVANCE y de la familia Rodríguez. También aplicaré conocimientos que he obtenido por medio de mis propios hijos varones, Salvador y Steven, y de mi hija, Vanessa, al aprender ellos de su mundo y de su rico patrimonio hispano y al desarrollar su enorme potencial. Mis niños han servido como mi laboratorio al intentar aplicar las teorías que yo aprendí sobre el desarrollo y crecimiento de los niños, a cada uno de ellos, a través de cada etapa de desarrollo. La crianza de los niños puede ser un verdadero desafío cuando nuestros niños ponen a prueba los límites impuestos y luchan por conseguir autonomía e independencia. A veces cómicas, con frecuencia angustiosas, las anécdotas que compartiré, las ofrezco, por encima de todo, de todo corazón, ya que le harán comprender que usted no está solo al sufrir frustraciones y temores, ni tampoco al gozar de esperanzas y sueños para sus niños.

Por medio de anécdotas, dichos, canciones, y juegos, este libro le ofrecerá un rico marco cultural para absorber la información que necesita para criar a sus niños. Estos elementos quizá le enseñen, le entretengan, le provoquen gracia, y tal vez aun le sorprendan. Pero más que todo, le recordarán lo singular e importante que es su cultura y cómo puede enriquecer a su familia y a su comunidad y ayudarle a usted a cumplir con su papel y con sus responsabilidades de padre o madre. En una época cuando las familias y las comunidades en todas partes están buscando nuevas barreras contra las fuerzas que las destruyen o dividen, usted encontrará que los consejos en este libro todavía guardan un mensaje que les habla a todos en éste, el siglo veintiuno. Lo sagrado de los vínculos de la familia extensa, la fe en la comunidad, y nuestro sentido único del compadrazgo, reflejan nuestra devoción a las relaciones. Por generaciones, estos lazos han mantenido a las familias hispanas juntas y unidas. Igual como los innumerables ancianos que aconsejaron a mi madre y cuyas palabras de sabiduría se nos pasaron a mí y a mis propios hijos, este libro también ofrecerá algunos consejos acerca de cómo criar a un niño bien educado y bien equilibrado.

Este libro cubre los primeros doce años de la vida de un niño. Con el último de mis tres niños, mi hija, Vanessa, quien acababa de cumplir trece años cuando comencé a escribir este libro, yo me maravillo ante todo lo que ella y mis dos hijos varones, Sal y Steven, aprendieron durante sus primeros doce años de vida. Muchos logros importantes se forman durante este período crítico, desde su capacidad para aprender conceptos básicos y absorber diferentes idiomas, hasta adquirir sus valores, su amor propio, y su personalidad. Éstos son los años importantes cuando establecen su carácter y sus valores, y cuando sus intereses y talentos emergen. La mitad de lo que aprenden los niños entre el tiempo cuando están dentro de la matriz y la edad de diecisiete años se ha aprendido ya para la edad de cuatro años. Por lo mismo, el mensaje crítico de este libro, es que nunca habrá otra persona que tendrá mayor influencia en el desarrollo de sus niños que usted mismo. Si usted construye unos cimientos fuertes y sólidos, y establece una buena relación entre padre e hijo durante estos años importantes de la vida, se aumentarán aun más las probabilidades de éxito escolar y de la vida que tendrán sus niños.

Este libro es para personas quienes ya son padres, o bien, están planeando serlo. Yo quiero ayudarles a aprender qué es lo que se espera y se necesita durante estos años, para que pueda crear un medio ambiente apropiado para sus niños. El ser un padre efectivo requiere una gran cantidad de tiempo, energía, paciencia, y compromiso. Requiere una enorme cantidad de conocimientos y habilidades. Yo espero que este libro le ayude a conseguir esa información y a adquirir las habilidades necesarias para ayudarle a mejorar su interacción y su relación con sus niños. Tal como fue cierto para mi madre, una combinación de fe, un profundo sentido de compromiso a su cultura y a sus niños, además del apoyo que recibirá de su pareja, su familia, sus vecinos, sus amigos, y su comunidad, le ayudarán enormemente para cumplir su papel de padre y para posibilitar a sus niños a alcanzar su potencial.

Cuando lo lea, deseo que este libro le atraiga intelectualmente, como a un adulto racional que quiere proveerle la mejor crianza a sus niños. Pero también quiero que le llegue al alma, como a un latino o latina que reconoce y se enorgullece de sus raíces culturales. Es claro que tenemos mucho de qué enorgullecernos. Yo quiero que los padres hispanos o aquellas personas casadas con hispanos puedan ayudarles a sus niños a encontrar un lugar en el mundo donde puedan brillar. Al aprender nuestros niños acerca de su rico patrimonio cultural latino, su historia, y su idioma, al mismo tiempo de estar absorbiendo la cultura americana y el idioma inglés, ellos estarán preparados para asumir sus papeles de liderazgo en este país, y en el mundo entero.

A través de los años, he recibido muchos premios y reconocimientos por mi trabajo en la educación a los padres sobre la crianza de sus niños, desde revistas hispanas tales como *Hispanic*, *Hispanic Business*, y *Latina*, hasta las de los medios de comunicación convencionales, incluyendo a *New York Times*, ABC *World News Tonight*, Lifetime Television, *Parent's* magazine, y *Working Mother* magazine. Al mismo tiempo que algunos otros quizá me consideren una experta en el campo de la crianza de los niños y la educación temprana de los niños, no profeso ser yo una madre perfecta, ni mis hijos, unos niños modelos. Yo realmente dudo que existan tales personas. Ciertamente he cometido errores al criar a mis niños, y en retrospectiva, pude haber hecho algunas cosas de manera diferente. Sin embargo, sí sé, por experiencia, que una crianza efectiva, con algo de entrenamiento y orientación y apoyo, se puede lograr a alto grado. Tal como ocurre con todo en la vida, usted también se desviará de su camino, pero con unos fuertes cimientos, encontrará que puede sobrevivir a los obstáculos y se dará cuenta que su experiencia será tan repleta de alegría y satisfacción como la mía.

Tal vez recuerde que le haya dicho las siguientes palabras su padre o su abuelo: *Hijo eres, padre serás, según lo hiciste, así lo verás*. Como yo era una niña tenaz, mi madre me decía, *"Vas a pagar todas las que debes"*. Ésta era una advertencia, la cual recordaba con una extraña mezcla de entusiasmo y temor con el nacimiento de cada uno de mis hijos. Yo me preguntaba, ¿estaba yo preparada, de la misma forma que mi madre lo había estado, para cumplir los enormes desafíos que conllevaba criar a estos pequeñísimos seres humanos, quienes seguramente crecerían para ser tan tenaces y obstinados como su madre? ¿Cómo podría yo tomar las lecciones derivadas de sus experiencias y aplicarlas a mi propia realidad?

Éstos son los tipos de preguntas que usted también quizá se esté haciendo, al comenzar la odisea más grande de su vida, al preparar a la próxima generación de líderes, ciudadanos, trabajadores, y padres. Yo espero que las siguientes páginas le proporcionen algunas respuestas, mientras usted proceda, paso por glorioso paso.

Nuestros niños

Nuestros niños son como unas rosas deliciosamente aromáticas
que en una fresca mañana primaveral de mayo, se ponen a florar.

Nuestros niños son como unas gloriosas y vívidas puestas de sol,
grabadas en nuestras mentes, para siempre perdurar.

Nuestros niños son como los vientos relajantes y a la vez rugientes,
con lo que hacen y dicen, logran un revuelo de emociones provocar.

Nuestros niños son como los radiantes y cálidos rayos del sol,
dolor y gran alegría nos pueden causar.

Nuestros niños son como los pájaros de dulce cantar,
llenan el aire con risa y alegría al jugar.

Nuestros niños son como las mariposas que se transforman,
y cada día sus talentos únicos vuelven a desplegar.

Nuestros niños poseen, igual como los arroyos serpenteantes,
un rico patrimonio en sus venas, que del ayer viene a resaltar.

Nuestros niños poseen, igual como las maravillas asombrosas del mundo,
una belleza y un resplandor sin iguales para mostrar.

Nuestros niños son los regalos más grandes de Dios,
creados para amar, para cuidar, y por su camino orientar.

—Gloria G. Rodríguez

Primera parte

Destinados a la grandeza:

Enseñando a niños hispanos

quiénes son, de dónde vienen,

y hacia dónde van

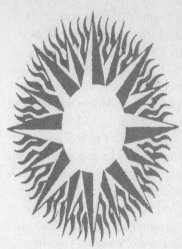

Capítulo I

Destinados a la grandeza: La demografía y la historia hispanas

¿Quiénes somos?

NUESTROS NIÑOS: EL TESORO MÁS GRANDE DE LA CULTURA HISPANA

En virtud de nuestro pasado, los padres hispanos ya poseemos mucho para poder ayudar a preparar a nuestros niños para el futuro. En esencia, el ser hispano significa valorar a los niños. Amamos y atesoramos a nuestros niños, y mucho de lo que hacemos, lo hacemos para ellos y con ellos. Para ser testigo de esto, tan sólo hay que asistir a una boda o quinceañera hispana, donde generalmente se pueden observar a los niños, jugando a mitad de la pista de baile, bailando orgullosamente al son de cumbias, polkas, salsas, o merengues. Durante estos acontecimientos, los niños son mostrados y presentados a los amigos y parientes como nuestras más preciadas posesiones. Rara vez son los niños tan bienvenidos y tan visibles con los adultos como en la cultura latina. Ciertamente, *los hijos son la riqueza de los padres, son nuestro gran tesoro.* Ellos enriquecen y dan valor a nuestras vidas. Mientras que nuestros niños, como todos los niños, pueden producir tensión y ansiedad al explorar su mundo y probar sus límites, también nos pueden proporcionar un enorme placer y gratificación. Son nuestras vidas, los núcleos de nuestras existencias.

Los padres tienen la esperanza y el deseo de que sus niños tengan éxito y sienten un gran orgullo cuando lo logran. Este gran sentido de esperanza y orgullo de los padres se convierte en una tremenda fuerza impulsora para los padres latinos. El saber esto fue lo que me ayudó a llegarles, exitosamente, a las familias hispanas pobres hace veinticinco años cuando comencé AVANCE. Yo sabía que los padres latinos, sin importar su posición en la vida, tenían esperanzas y sueños para sus niños, especialmente cuando eran pequeños. Yo pensaba que aun si los padres perdieran las esperanzas para ellos mismos, o se habían resignado a su posición en la vida, aún perduraría un destello de esperanza para sus niños. Cuando yo tocaba las puertas de los padres en un esfuerzo para reclutarlos al programa de AVANCE, yo les preguntaba: "¿Aman a sus niños? ¿Desean lo mejor para ellos?" Cada vez la respuesta era una rotunda: "¡Sí, cómo no!" Yo aprendí que los hispanos harán cualquier cosa necesaria para ayudar a sus niños a desarrollarse bien, tener éxito en la vida, y obtener sus derechos básicos de dignidad y respeto.

Para poder ayudar a nuestros niños, necesitamos recurrir a su rico patrimonio cultural e historia para inculcarles fortaleza y un sentido de identidad. Si nosotros queremos que nuestros niños tengan confianza en sí mismos y un amor propio sano, ellos deben extraer esta fuerza del conocimiento y la comprensión de qué es lo que significa ser latino. Vamos a tomar un momento para considerar quiénes son nuestros niños, de dónde se remontan sus orígenes, y cómo su destino está ligado a su espiritualidad.

Como padre, es crítico que se dé cuenta de los cambios ocurriendo en los demográficos de este país. La cara de América no será la de un blanco anglosajón por mucho tiempo más. Pronto será hispana, y eso traerá un gran destino para nuestros niños. Cosas maravillosas y extraordinarias les esperan a nuestros niños. Bendecidos con un legado de logros y un rico patrimonio de sus ancestros además de un despliegue de talentos y habilidades, nuestros niños tienen mucho sobre el cual construir, ya que algún día serán el grupo étnico más grande de los Estados Unidos. Igual a cualquier planta que necesita haber echado bien sus raíces para poder crecer sana y fuerte, también nuestros niños necesitan comprender sus raíces para poder alcanzar su destino. Necesitan entender quiénes son, de dónde vienen, y hacia dónde van. Necesitan apreciar las esperanzas, las luchas, y los triunfos de nuestros antepasados. Usted debe ayudarles a reconocer que ellos forman parte de un eslabón de una larga cadena, y que son los beneficiarios de la búsqueda de nuestros antepasados de una mejor vida. Ellos se paran en los hombros de personas que vinieron antes que ellos para que ellos pudieran subir la escala social al éxito y alcanzar sus metas y su potencial. No estarán solamente en una posición de ayudarse ellos mismos y ayudar a sus familias, sino que también podrán brindar sus talentos, sus habilidades, y sus posiciones de influencia para mejorar la calidad de vida de muchos latinos que los seguirán.

Para poder dar fruto, toda planta necesita más que simplemente haber echado buenas raíces. También debe estar arraigado en unos cimientos sólidos y ricos. Al ayudar a sus niños a comprender la fuerza de nuestra cultura y su relación a la historia del pasado, usted está preparando el rico suelo de donde ellos podrán orgullosa y lentamente salir al mundo. De esos cimientos, usted también podrá extraer la fuerza y la energía que le ayudarán a ser el jardinero competente que le posibilitará producir la fruta que llegará a ser su más preciado tesoro.

¿QUIÉNES SOMOS?

Según los demógrafos, en 1997, los hispanos constaban de casi 30 millones de personas, o sea 11 por ciento de la población de los Estados Unidos, mientras que los blancos no hispanos, constaban del 73 por ciento. Para el año 2000, los hispanos constarán del 15 por ciento de la población, o sea 39 millones. Para el año 2010, los hispanos habrán sobrepasado a la población afroamericana, con una población proyectada de 41 millones, comparada con la suya proyectada de 37.5 millones. Si usted tiene un niño que nace hoy, al llegar al año 2010, su niño será menor de doce años de edad y no solamente formará parte del grupo más grande de minorías en los Estados Unidos, pero, en combinación con las otras minorías, compondrán la mayoría. Para el año 2050, la población hispana, proyectada para llegar casi al triple en cantidad, con un total de 87.4 millones, entonces compondrá alrededor de un cuarto de la población total de 392 millones de personas. A causa del alto índice de fertilidad e inmigración entre los hispanos, y por el pronóstico que la población de blancos va a disminuir alrededor del año 2030, se proyecta que los hispanos algún día compondrán el grupo de mayoría en los Estados Unidos.

Los hispanos, como grupo, son jóvenes. La edad promedia para los hispanos es de veinticinco años, comparada con treinta y cuatro para la población en general. Alrededor de un tercio son niños menores de quince años, lo cual refleja la juventud de nuestra población, comparada con 20.4 años para los blancos no hispanos. El tamaño promedio de un hogar es de 3.6 personas para los hispanos, y 2.6 para los no hispanos. De acuerdo al *National Center for Health Statistics* (Centro Nacional para Estadísticas de la Salud), en 1992, el índice de fertilidad para los blancos era de 1.8 niños, comparado con 3.0 para los hispanos, y 2.5 para los negros. Los México-americanos tienen un índice más alto de fertilidad cuando se comparan con otros grupos hispanos; tienen un promedio de 3.78 niños por familia, seguidos por 2.85 para los puertorriqueños, y los cubanoamericanos son más comparables a los blancos.

Desde los salones de clase hasta el mercado, nuestra influencia ya se siente en casi todos los sectores de la sociedad. En muchas escuelas de hoy en día, especialmente aquellas ubicadas en estados con gran número de hispanos tales como Texas y California, los niños hispanos ya componen la mayoría. Nuestro poder de compras de $350 billones ha estimulado nuevas pautas en las industrias de modas, publicaciones, y cinematografía, y nuestra fuerza se ha hecho sentir en varias de las últimas elecciones presidenciales y para gobernador, debido a la alta concentración de hispanos en claves estados políticos como California (35 por ciento), Texas (20 por ciento), Nueva York (10 por ciento), y Florida (7 por ciento). Estas influencias económicas y políticas se hicieron sentir a pesar de que el presupuesto anual promedio de una familia hispana es de $25,561, a comparación con $33,864 para todas las familias.

LAS RAÍCES HISTÓRICAS HISPANAS

A nosotros como pueblo se nos conoce por diferentes nombres: latinos, hispanos, chicanos, o latinoamericanos, todos los cuales utilizaré de manera intercambiable a través del libro. El 64 por ciento de los hispanos son México-americanos, 11 por ciento son puertorriqueños, 13 por ciento son del Caribe y Centro- y Sudamérica, casi 5 por ciento son cubanoamericanos, y 7 por ciento son de otro origen hispano. Dentro de esos nombres que catalogan y son tan amplios, se encuentra una gama de experiencias que distinguen a los mexicanos, cubanos, puertorriqueños, dominicanos, nicaragüenses, venezolanos, y peruanos. Los hispanos tienen distintos antecedentes, historias, educación, y afiliaciones socioeconómicas y políticas. Los orígenes de la población latina han sido ya por mucho tiempo un motivo de intensa investigación y debate. Algunos han establecido una conexión entre los latinos y la gente nómada que cruzó el estrecho de Bering, originarios de Asia, hace entre 11,000 y 20,000 años, formando así la base de nuestra herencia indígena

("Paleo-Indian"), o de primeros americanos, cuyos descendientes emigraron más tarde a través de las Américas: América Central y las Américas del Sur y del Norte además de las islas del Caribe. La más antigua presencia humana en las Américas se ha remontado a Monte Verde, Chile, hace 12,500 años y también a Clovis, Nuevo México, hace 11,200 años. Muchos de nuestros niños son descendientes de las grandes naciones indígenas incluyendo los olmecas, los mayas, los toltecas, los aztecas, los incas, los taínos, los quechuas, y los anasazis.

De acuerdo a las leyendas, los aztecas hablaron de haber salido de cuevas en un mítico lugar llamado Aztlán, el cual se dice estar localizado en alguna parte del sector sudoeste de los Estados Unidos. De allí, guiados por *Huitzilopochtli*, su dios del sol, anduvieron por zonas inexploradas en busca de una señal profética, un águila con una serpiente en su pico parado encima de un nopal. La encontraron en 1323 en *Tenochtitlán*, el sitio donde construyeron su imperio, y donde ahora se encuentra la Ciudad de México.

Hoy en día, los hispanos hacen sus búsquedas genealógicas por otros rumbos. Una puertorriqueña de piel blanca y cabello rizado a quien yo conozco es orgullosa de sus raíces africanas, y también pudo descubrir que algunos de sus antepasados eran los vikingos, originarios de Suecia y Noruega que habitaron las islas del Caribe y Latinoamérica muchos años antes de la llegada de Cristóbal Colón. Aquellos recién llegados se casaron con los indios, después con los españoles, y más adelante, con los africanos que habían sido traídos al área como esclavos.

Otros hispanos también establecen una conexión con África, lugar donde se originó toda la civilización humana hace más de tres millones de años. Tal como dice un dicho hispano, *todos tenemos negro detrás de las orejas*. Sin embargo, algunos hispanos miran hacia el viaje de Cristóbal Colón en 1492 a Mesoamérica, la cual incluye a México, América Central, y las Indias del Oeste, como el nacimiento de la gente latina, el cual fue el resultado del mestizaje, la mezcla de las sangres española e india y de sus culturas.

El cuadro de razas y culturas divergentes uniéndose en el mundo hispano con frecuencia ha conllevado nombres especiales. Los descendientes de los primeros colonizadores españoles fueron conocidos como *criollos*. Los *mestizos* eran el producto de sangres españolas e indias, tal como los *mulatos* eran el producto de la mezcla de negros y españoles. Los negros que se casaban con indios tenían niños llamados *cambujos,* y a los niños productos de la mezcla de *mulatos* y *criollos* les llamaron *chinos*. Aun los indios americanos nativos quienes se adaptaron a la cultura española recibieron un nombre; se les llamaron *jenízaros*.

LA VENIDA A AMÉRICA

Es importante que usted les provee a sus niños una perspectiva latina de la historia, la cual generalmente falta en los libros escolares. Llévelos a la biblioteca para investigar si tienen una colección latina de libros. Con estos libros, usted y sus niños se podrán enterar de que la migración de los hispanos a América tiene orígenes múltiples. Como hispanos, nos podemos enorgullecer del hecho de que el explorador español Pedro Menéndez de Avilés estableció el primer asentamiento permanente en St. Augustine, Florida, en 1565, cuarenta y dos años antes de que los primeros colonizadores llegaran a Plymouth Rock en 1607. Aun el poblado de Santa Fe, Nuevo México, fue establecido antes, en 1598.

Muchos de los primeros colonizadores y sus descendientes eventualmente se emigraron a lo que ahora es el sudoeste de los Estados Unidos. El 2 de febrero de 1848 es considerado por algunos como el nacimiento oficial de hispanoamericanos en los Estados Unidos. Ésta es la fecha en que se firmó el Tratado de Guadalupe Hidalgo, después de la victoria americana en la guerra entre México y los Estados Unidos. Bajo las condiciones del Tratado de Guadalupe Hidalgo, México vendió a Estados Unidos los estados de California, Texas, Nevada, Utah, y porciones de Arizona, Colorado, Kansas, Nuevo México, Oklahoma, y Wyoming por quince millones de dólares, y después reajustaron las líneas divisoras en 1853 con la Adquisición de Gadsden. Todas las personas que vivían dentro de estas regiones automáticamente se convirtieron en ciudadanos de los Estados Unidos. Así, muchas familias que vivían como mexicanos antes de esta guerra ahora eran americanos, o en otras palabras, México-americanos. Ellos se convirtieron, tal como ha sido el caso de tantos latinoamericanos, en unas personas de dos mundos y dos culturas.

Como resultado de la guerra, a los puertorriqueños les tocó una suerte parecida a la de los mexicanos en lo referente a convertirse en ciudadanos. Con la victoria de la guerra entre España y los Estados Unidos en 1898 y la consecuente firma del Tratado de París en 1899, Puerto Rico se convirtió en un territorio de los Estados Unidos. Más tarde, la aprobación de la Ley de Jones de 1917 les otorgó a los residentes puertorriqueños la ciudadanía de los Estados Unidos y les confirió el derecho de viajar libremente entre los Estados Unidos continentales y la isla. Grupos grandes de puertorriqueños se establecieron principalmente en Nueva York, Nueva Jersey, y hasta fechas recientes, en Florida. Entre los años de 1940 y 1960, más de 545,000 puertorriqueños vinieron a este país en busca de trabajo a causa de las malas condiciones económicas en la isla. En la mayoría de los casos, los hombres vinieron a este país primero, se mudaron con unos parientes, y más tarde trajeron al resto de la familia.

Otros hispanos vinieron a América impulsados por guerras y condiciones económicas que cada vez se empeoraban en sus propios países, y alentados por la promesa implícita de una mejor vida en los Estados Unidos. Hasta el año de 1924, la gente podía viajar libremente entre México y los Estados Unidos. Sin embargo, cuando se vio afectada la economía de los Estados Unidos y hubo una escasez de trabajo, se estableció el Departamento de Inmigración de los Estados Unidos para controlar la inmigración, sólo para volver a abrir convenientemente las puertas de la frontera cuando se mejoró la economía. En 1900 había entre 380,000 y 560,000 México-americanos que vivían en los Estados Unidos y aproximadamente tres millones en 1930. Entre 1900 y 1940 hubo una gran demanda de mano de obra barata para construir ferrocarriles, y para trabajar en las minas y fábricas. También se necesitaban a peones en los ranchos de ganado ovino y de reses, y en las granjas para hacer trabajo agrícola, pizca de algodón, y cosechar frutas y verduras. Muchos hispanos vinieron a este país a través de permisos de trabajo o contratos laborales. Su ética firme de trabajo los llevó a las plantas de laminación de acero, a las fábricas de automóviles y conservas, y las empacadoras de carne, dispersando a mexicanos a través de los Estados Unidos, especialmente en Texas, California, Arizona, Nuevo México, Colorado, Washington, Montana, Idaho, y otros partes del país, específicamente Chicago, y la Ciudad de Kansas.

Cuando se terminaron los trabajos, muchas familias hispanas se quedaron en aquellas ciudades y se convirtieron en ciudadanos a través del matrimonio y sus hijos se convirtieron en ciudadanos de los Estados Unidos. Muchos de mis amigos hispanos del sudoeste tienen un padre o una madre que es mexicano(a) o México-americano(a) y otro(a) que es americano(a) nativo(a), descendiente de naciones como los navajos o los pueblos. Con el Programa de Repatriación de 1939 se deportó alrededor de 500,000 personas de descendencia mexicana. Este programa les provocó mucho resentimiento, humillación, e ira a los hispanos que habían estado viviendo en este país por más de una década, aun si bien no eran ciudadanos. Sin embargo, de nuevo hubo una gran demanda de latinos para suplir la enorme falta laboral durante la Segunda Guerra Mundial. El Programa de Braceros, patrocinado por el gobierno, el cual comenzó en 1943, animó a muchos mexicanos a aceptar trabajos de baja categoría y de bajo pago. Igual que anteriormente ocurrió, muchas de estas personas se casaron y se establecieron en este país y se convirtieron en ciudadanos de los Estados Unidos. Los hispanos que fueron a la guerra tuvieron mejores oportunidades para mejorar su educación y su calidad de vida a través del proyecto de la ley para soldados (*G.I. Bill*). Muchos llegaron a ser líderes de su comunidad y lucharon incansablemente por conseguir igualdad y derechos civiles para hispanos, a través de organizaciones como *Lulac* (*The League of United Latin American Citizens*) y *G.I. Forum*.

Otros hispanos vinieron a este país, igual como lo hicieron mis propios antepasados de México, para escaparse de la persecución y la guerra. Mi abuelo Lázaro Villegas, orgulloso de su patrimonio indio y mexicano, trajo a su esposa, Rosario, y su hijo, Pascual, a América, impulsado por la época turbulenta causada por la Revolución Mexicana de 1910. Mi abuelo paterno, Julián Garza, conocido como "el general", fue un *Carrancista* que luchó en la revolución contra Pancho Villa. Él murió en la lucha, en un intento por proteger su tierra y el honor de su familia en la época cuando las fuerzas de Villa asaltaban los pueblos y violaban a mujeres mestizas y criollas, incluyendo a una de mis parientes. Fue durante una de estas épocas tumultuosas que mi abuela enviudada, María de Jesús "Chita" Lombraña Garza, principalmente de sangre española, emigró a los Estados Unidos con sus hijos.

La más reciente oleada de latinos a los Estados Unidos ha sido de países hispanohablantes de América Central, el Caribe, y Cuba. Aproximadamente 200,000 cubanos vinieron a los Estados Unidos entre 1959 y 1962 para escaparse de la Revolución Cubana. Otros 50,000 llegaron entre 1962 y 1965, y 250,000 más vinieron por vía aérea entre 1966 y 1973. En 1980, hubo un gran éxodo de 125,000 "marielitos", quienes fueron mandados por el gobierno cubano por barco a Miami, del Puerto de Mariel, y en 1994, arribaron miles cubanos más, huyendo de la pobreza y la opresión política—muchos de ellos hicieron el viaje en pequeñas embarcaciones construidas a mano.

Los dominicanos, quienes inmigraron a los Estados Unidos entre 1945 y 1959, eran semejantes a los cubanos en que abandonaron su país por razones políticas, muchos de ellos de similar opulencia y educación. La mayoría de los latinos de América Central vinieron a través de México, buscando asilo de los estragos de una guerra civil, cuando estuvo su país bajo gobierno militar. Éstos incluían a escuadrones de la muerte y atrocidades contra los derechos civiles cometidas en contra de las guerrillas que rebelaban y luchaban por la igualdad y por una más justa distribución de los recursos nacionales. Miles de personas, principalmente de Guatemala, Nicaragua, y El Salvador, fueron forzados a salir de sus países. Con fuertes cicatrices emocionales, viajaron a través de condiciones peligrosas en busca de asilo en América. Sin embargo, la mayoría de ellos fueron rechazados por el gobierno debido a la política de los Estados Unidos con estos países, lo cual obligó a muchos a entrar ilegalmente al país. Muchos de los sudamericanos vinieron a los Estados Unidos a trabajar y a estudiar. Sin importar de cuál país vinieron, muchos latinos eventualmente se casaron con estadounidenses y se convirtieron en ciudadanos legales, mientras que otros se quedaron ilegalmente.

La Ley de Reforma y Control de Inmigración de 1986 les otorgó la amnistía a todos los inmigrantes ilegales que habían estado en este país desde el 1 de enero de 1982. Como resultado de esta ley, 2.3 millones de mexicanos y 100,000 sudamericanos se convirtieron en residentes permanentes legales.

AYUDAR A NUESTROS NIÑOS A DESCUBRIR SUS RAÍCES

Al ayudar a nuestros niños a estudiar sus raíces en un mundo multicultural, muchos descubrimos que nuestros valientes antepasados vinieron a este país en busca de asilo, libertad, y una mejor vida, igual a los inmigrantes europeos que llegaron a la Isla Ellis. Los ancestros que dejaron sus queridas patrias, ya sean cubanos, mexicanos, salvadoreños, o dominicanos, lo hicieron motivados por la seguridad y el bienestar de sus niños. Yo he leído historias sobre los viajes valientes realizados por muchas mujeres solas, incluyendo a mi propia abuela, quien cruzó la frontera de los Estados Unidos con sus niños para comenzar una vida nueva de esperanza y oportunidad. Igual como en muchas otras familias hispanas, esto señaló el comienzo de un nuevo capítulo en la historia de nuestra familia.

Mi abuelita María de Jesús Garza y sus niños se establecieron en Zuehl, Texas, como aparceros. Muchos años después, mi padre y abuelo se mudaron a la "gran ciudad" de San Antonio donde mi padre trabajó como carnicero, para su tío que vivía en el barrio. Mi madre, que nació en Laredo, Texas, en 1920, al poco tiempo de haber cruzado la frontera sus padres, se estableció con ellos a unas cuantas cuadras de donde vivía y trabajaba mi padre en los barrios de San Antonio. Ella trabajó pelando nueces, junta con su madre, hasta que se casó con mi padre, y se mudaron al lado de la casa de la madre de ella. Fue para ellos una época de gran determinación y sacrificios, de recuerdos dejados atrás, y de nuevos comienzos en la pequeña casa de madera en la calle Colima.

Con un padre mexicano con raíces españolas, y una madre de primera generación, nacida en los Estados Unidos, con antecedentes principalmente indígenas, yo estoy orgullosa de mi patrimonio mixto. Igual a otros hispanos, probablemente tenga raíces africanas, dicho por mi cabello tan rizado, o un linaje chino, por los ojos que se miran un poco orientales, o aun algo de patrimonio judío, ya que los Garza que originalmente se asentaron en México, se me dijo, eran judíos sefarditas de España. Yo comparto todo esto con ustedes con el propósito de establecer el hecho de que por ser latinos, cada uno de nosotros tiene una historia y un viaje genealógico, ambos de los cuales son ricos y únicos.

¿Usted sabe cuáles son sus raíces genealógicas? ¿Hasta qué fecha se remonta su linaje familiar? Sería un proyecto familiar muy interesante e importante investigar y anotar su ascendencia familiar, o sea, hacer un árbol genealógico. Yo quisiera haber grabado en vídeo a mi abuelo y a mis tíos antes de su fallecimiento. Pongan a sus niños a entrevistar y grabar en vídeo a sus abuelitos, a sus tíos mayores, o a cualquier otra persona que conoció a su familia antes de venir a este país. Visite el lugar de origen de sus familiares, tal como lo hice yo al ir a Nava, México, para ver el lugar donde nació mi padre. Para mi sorpresa, yo hablé con personas que habían conocido muy bien a mi padre y a su familia. Reúna un álbum de recortes, o libro de recuerdos, que consista de antiguas fotografías familiares que se remontan a los años 30 y 40. Prepare un árbol genealógico con los nombres de todos sus parientes, comenzando por su familia inmediata. Mi esposo talló unos pequeños árboles de madera, y los puso en unos marcos para fotos, con los nombres de su familia inmediata, y obsequió uno a cada uno de sus hermanos como regalo de Navidad.

Entreviste a otras personas y pregúnteles de dónde vinieron, cuándo, cómo, y por qué vinieron a este país. ¿Estuvieron sus antepasados en este país antes del Tratado de Guadalupe Hidalgo? Algunos hispanos se enorgullecen mucho de ser hispanoamericanos de quinta generación. Pídales que cierren los ojos. ¿Qué recuerdan acerca de su niñez? Dígales que piensen en todas las imágenes, los sonidos, los aromas, al contestar algunas de las siguientes preguntas.

1. Describa su casa, su vecindario. ¿Adónde iba de compras?
2. ¿Cuáles son algunos de los juegos, canciones, dichos, celebraciones, cuentos tradicionales, canciones de cuna, que usted recuerda?
3. ¿Qué instrumento musical tocó usted o escuchó tocarse en su comunidad?

4. ¿Qué tipo de alimentos comía? (Consiga recetas favoritas.)

5. Describa las flores, los árboles, y el paisaje de su país.

6. Describa sus escuelas. ¿Qué estudió? ¿Y sus hermanos? ¿Qué habilidades aprendió?

7. ¿Cómo pasaba los fines de semana?

8. ¿Cómo iba de un lugar a otro? ¿Qué tipo de transportación usaba?

9. Describa su educación religiosa.

10. ¿Qué tipo de trabajo tenía?

11. ¿Qué fueron sus momentos más tristes y más alegres, y por qué?

12. Describa su personalidad. ¿Qué le gusta hacer?

13. ¿A cuáles parientes le tiene parecido físico?

14. ¿Qué tipo de ropa usaba?

15. ¿Cuántos idiomas habla?

16. Describa su viaje a los Estados Unidos.

17. Nombre a cuantos familiares pueda.

18. ¿Hay alguna historia interesante o emocionante que le gustaría compartir conmigo acerca de su lugar de origen?

UN LEGADO DE LOGROS Y RICO PATRIMONIO

Como miembros de lo que algún día será el grupo étnico más grande de la diversa sociedad multicultural de nuestra nación, nuestros niños necesitan estar confiados y orgullosos de que son los herederos de cuando menos dos grandes culturas, dos idiomas, y siglos de historia. Queremos que sepan el idioma inglés y que estén cómodos con la cultura y tradiciones americanas, pero también queremos que hablen el idioma español, y que conserven su identidad hispana. Queremos que conozcan sus raíces históricas y que se sientan orgullosos de su legado y de su rico patrimonio.

Los libros de historia en las escuelas americanas no ponen suficiente énfasis en nuestros antepasados y nuestra historia. Nuestros niños no reciben suficiente información acerca de los maravillosos logros de los aztecas, olmecas, toltecas, e incas. Estos grandes imperios, construidos alrededor de los años 200 a. de C. y 400 d. de C., tuvieron poblaciones de hasta treinta millones de personas, mayores que las de cualquier otro imperio de esa época. Construyeron enormes pirámides y palacios hechos de piedra, con cientos de cuartos. Es asombroso preguntarse cómo lograron esto. Tenían templos religiosos, centros recreativos, escuelas, plazas, prisiones, barberías, jardines, y zoológicos, tal como una principal ciudad metropolitana de la actualidad. Los arquitectos y los ingenieros también construyeron avenidas, canales, puentes, represas, y sistemas de irrigación. Astrónomos inquisitivos analizaban los cielos a través de observatorios e inventaron el más preciso calendario hasta la fecha, el cual se utilizaba para planear las ceremonias religiosas y también las temporadas de siembra y de cosecha. El pueblo hispano ha producido relucientes creaciones a través de treinta siglos espectaculares de arte, desde la joyería fina y elaboradas cerámicas hasta detalladas tapices y magníficas estatuas expuestas en museos a través del mundo entero. En estos imperios, los hispanos reunieron fuerzas militares, establecieron comercio, y celebraron acontecimientos religiosos, sociales, artísticos y recreativos. Yo les digo a mis hijos que son hábiles en matemáticas, ciencia, y arte gracias al rico patrimonio hispano que fluye por sus venas. Para mantener esta compleja orden social se requerían buenas habilidades para dirigir, elaboradas formas de gobierno, además de una fuerza laboral enorme, hábil, e inteligente.

Existen muchas maneras en que usted les puede proporcionar esta rica historia cultural a sus niños. Llévelos a la biblioteca y saque libros sobre los mayas, los aztecas, y los incas. Llévelos a los museos para aprender acerca de la época precolombina. Si tiene la oportunidad de viajar, llévelos a visitar la Pirámide del Sol que está cerca de la Ciudad de México, o las ruinas mayas que se encuentran en Chichén Itzá, Uxmal, o Palenque en la península de Yucatán, o Tikal en Guatemala, o las magníficas ruinas incas en Machu Picchu en Perú, o el antiguo fuerte español llamado El Morro y La Fortaleza, el palacio del gobernador, en Puerto Rico. Sus niños seguramente estarán orgullosos de estar vinculados a estos maravillosos descubrimientos arqueológicos, y sitios históricos que son admirados por millones de personas a través del mundo. El Canal de Descubrimiento (*Discovery Channel*), en la televisión por cable, y la revista *National Geographic* en ocasiones destacan artículos con información sobre nuestros ancestros. Ya que las escuelas presentan más la perspectiva europea occidental de América, nos toca a nosotros, como padres, proporcionarles a nuestros niños los capítulos de historia que faltan para brindarles una fuente de orgullo y un sentido de identidad con relación a sus raíces latinas.

LA RAZA CÓSMICA Y EL DESTINO DE NUESTROS NIÑOS

La llegada de los españoles al Caribe en 1492, a México en 1519, y a Perú en 1532, cambiaría el curso de la historia y la cultura para nuestra gente. José Vasconcelos, el antiguo ministro de educación de México, se refirió a este fenómeno como *la raza cósmica*, una mezcla variada de todas las razas y grupos étnicos. El 12 de octubre, el día en que se celebra el descubrimiento de América por Cristóbal Colón, es conmemorado por muchos hispanos como el Día de la Raza. Los niños latinos de hoy en día son el producto de muchos matrimonios mixtos y la mezcla de muchas razas. La mezcla de las razas ha creado una gama tan amplia como la de un arco iris en lo que se refiere a la cantidad de hermosos tonos de color de piel. Los hispanos difieren en el color y la forma de los ojos, la piel, y el cabello. Sin tomar en cuenta nuestras diferencias físicas, históricas, y aun sutiles diferencias lingüísticas, estamos unidos, conectados por una rica y variada cultura que incluye tradiciones duraderas y valores fundamentales básicos, tales como creer en lo sagrado de los niños, la familia, la comunidad, y la espiritualidad.

EL ORIGEN Y LA ESPIRITUALIDAD DE LOS HISPANOS

En adición a las ruinas antiguas, el calendario azteca, y el bello arte popular, nuestros ancestros nos dejaron una fuerte espiritualidad que ha orientado nuestros pensamientos y acciones. Yo veo a nuestros niños, quienes representan la mezcla de muchos grupos étnicos y diferentes creencias religiosas, como haberse levantado, en cierto sentido, de las cenizas de grandes civilizaciones y poderosos imperios para asumir los destacados papeles a los cuales están destinados.

Hay muchos relatos documentados acerca de los acontecimientos misteriosos que ocurrieron antes de la ascensión y subsecuente destrucción de las magníficas civilizaciones de los aztecas en México y de los incas en Perú, y de la aparición de la Virgen de Guadalupe. Estos increíbles acontecimientos están relatados en numerosos libros, incluyendo el libro de Richard E. W. Adams titulado *Prehistoric MesoAmerica* y el libro de Earl Shorris titulado *Latinos*. Parece ser que todos los incidentes, por más incredulidad que esto pueda provocar, fueron Divinamente creados y orquestados.

Entre los primeros de los misterios, fue la señal profética que los aztecas buscaban por lugares inexplorados que les avisaría dónde construir su imperio. Ciento cincuenta años más tarde, encontraron un magnífico águila encima de un nopal, con una serpiente en su pico, en una isla en medio de un lago en Tenochtitlán, donde ahora está la Ciudad de México.

Luego hubo una profecía que se predijo y se anotó antes de la llegada de Cristóbal Colón al Caribe, concerniente a la destrucción de los indios taínos. Earl Shorris cita una porción del libro de Fray Ramón Pane titulado *Account of the Customs of the Indians*, donde menciona que los taínos vieron en su país "una gente ataviada quien los gobernarían, y darían muerte, y ellos morirían de hambre". Los indios taínos en Puerto Rico y Cuba en verdad fueron destruidos y los arawaks también fueron completamente aniquilados por los españoles.

En su libro titulado *Kingdom of the Sun*, Ruth Karen ilustra la sincronización coincidente de la llegada de los españoles. El imperio inca cayó en treinta y tres minutos, debido en gran parte al hecho de que dos hermanos de la realeza inca habían estado envueltos en una guerra, uno contra el otro, y estaban agotados. Antes de la guerra, el moribundo padre real fue recipiente de la siguiente profecía de parte de su profeta: "La luna, tu madre, te dice que Pachacuti, el creador y dador de la vida, amenaza a tu familia, a tu reino, y a tus súbditos. Tus hijos se harán una guerra cruel, aquéllos de sangre real morirán, y el imperio desaparecerá". Su profecía fue acertada; sin embargo, desdichadamente, el profeta fue ejecutado por haberla revelado.

Los incas creían que Pizarro, el explorador español, era el héroe y dios de piel blanca y barba, quien, de acuerdo a la leyenda inca, había venido a enseñarles acerca de "importantes artes de la vida" y después partió por el este, con la promesa de volver por el mar. Los aztecas tenían una leyenda similar. Ellos creían que Hernán Cortés era Quetzalcoatl, el dios de la luz, la verdad, y la bondad, quien partió de Tenochtitlán y prometió regresar del este. Los aztecas tenían muchos otros dioses, incluyendo a Huitzilopochtli, el dios de la guerra, quien exigía periódicos sacrificios humanos para poder hacer que el sol subiera cada día. Quetzalcoatl partió de México en el año de 895 porque estaba muy en contra de estos sacrificios humanos.

Este folklore preparó el escenario para el drama de la conquista española, cuyo desarrollo ya se había predicho. El drama de la vida real tenía suspenso, drama humano, y mucho derramamiento de sangre. Justo antes de la llegada de los españoles, los aztecas anotaron varios acontecimientos y presagios poco usuales. Primero, un cometa de tres cabezas apareció durante el día sobre Tenochtitlán. Segundo, el templo de Huitzilopochtli quedó reducido a cenizas en un incendio sin explicación, y un relámpago producido por una gran tormenta dañó otro templo de Huitzilopochtli. Además, Nezahualpilli, el rey texcoco de la nación azteca náhuatl, predijo que en 1519 su dios Quetzalcoatl volvería del este en la forma de un hombre alto de ojos azules y cabello rubio y que toda la civilización azteca llegaría a su fin. En 1519, de acuerdo a la profecía, un español blanco de ojos azules, Hernán Cortés, arribó del este. En adición, fue anotado que algunos pescadores recibieron una profecía de "gente de apariencia extraña siendo llevada a Moctezuma, el rey azteca".

Esas personas de extraña apariencia que solicitaron una entrevista con Moctezuma, resultaron ser los españoles, quienes más tarde tomaron prisionero al rey azteca. Hernán Cortés aprovechó el hecho de que los aztecas creían que él era un dios y que los estados sometidos aztecas no eran leales a Moctezuma. A pesar de que las fuerzas aztecas tuvieron una gran victoria en 1520, conocida en la historia española como "la noche triste", un año después de esta batalla, novecientos soldados y miles de indios de los estados sometidos aztecas conquistaron la dinastía azteca.

Después de la conquista, los españoles infligieron gran dolor y sufrimiento a los aztecas, incluyendo a aquéllos que se alinearon a su favor, en contra de Moctezuma. Las familias fueron destrozadas. Todos fueron privados de comida, torturados, forzados a esclavitud; y su cultura, religión, y percepción del mundo cambiaron abruptamente. Una de las más grandes civilizaciones de todos los tiempos fue destruida.

La heroína principal, quien eventualmente llevó a entre ocho y nueve millones de aztecas a cambiar al cristianismo en un período de diez años, y a la pacífica y gradual mezcla de dos culturas, fue la Virgen de Guadalupe. Ella fue el puente cultural y espiritual entre los aztecas y los españoles. La aparición de la Virgen María ante un pobre indio azteca náhuatl llamado Juan Diego en 1531 fue el punto culminante de este increíble drama. Por el hecho de aparecer como una mestiza morena que hablaba el idioma náhuatl, la gente mexicana podía identificarse con ella.

De acuerdo al libro de Jeanette Rodríguez titulado *Our Lady of Guadalupe: Faith and Empowerment Among Mexican-American Women*, Juan Diego declaró que la Virgen de Guadalupe le dijo: "...a todos los habitantes de esta tierra y a todos que me aman, apelan a mí, y confían en mí. Yo escucharé sus lamentos y remediaré todas sus miserias, sus dolores, y sus sufrimientos". Cuando la Virgen de Guadalupe apareció ante el tío enfermo de Juan Diego y lo sanó, ella le dijo que su nombre era Tlecauhtlacupeuh. El nombre sonaba como Guadalupe, el nombre de la virgen que los españoles trajeron de Extremadura, España. Pero en náhuatl significa "la que viene volando de la luz como el águila de fuego".

Los aztecas tenían su propia diosa que era una madre virgen, llamada Tonantzín, quien era la madre de Huitzilopochtli. Era adorada por los aztecas cada 12 de diciembre. La Virgen de Guadalupe milagrosamente apareció ante Juan Diego en ese mismo día, el 12 de diciembre, en el cerro de Tepeyac, el lugar donde se adoraba a Tonantzín. La Virgen de Guadalupe eventualmente reemplazó a Tonantzín, y el dios Huitzilopochtli fue reemplazado por el Dios cristiano que los españoles trajeron de España.

La milagrosa aparición de Nuestra Señora de Guadalupe ante Juan Diego ocurrió durante una época cuando la gente náhuatl estaba muy confundida y sufría enormemente. Nuestra Señora quería que se construyera una iglesia en Tepeyac para mostrarles a todos su amor y para reconfortar a los necesitados. Ella les trajo esperanza y les dio fortaleza.

LA VIRGEN DE GUADALUPE: NUESTRO SÍMBOLO CULTURAL DE ESPERANZA Y FORTALEZA

Esa misma esperanza y esa misma fortaleza que le fueron otorgadas a la gente náhuatl, nos ha otorgado a los hispanos a través de Latinoamérica y Estados Unidos. Esto es especialmente cierto para los muchos hispanos que emigraron a los Estados Unidos sin un sistema social de apoyo, sin saber el idioma y las costumbres y lo que se esperaba de ellos en esta nueva tierra. Por su milagrosa aparición y el importante papel que ha jugado para tantos latinos a través de las Américas, la Virgen de Guadalupe fue oficialmente reconocida por el Papa Pius XII como la Patrona de las Américas. Ella aun se considera una protectora contra fuerzas malévolas, las cuales a veces son simbolizadas por serpientes y dragones.

Una vez, en el Complejo de Viviendas Subvencionadas de Mirasol en San Antonio, donde estaba ubicado el primer centro de AVANCE, un horroroso dibujo de un dragón con fuego brotando de su hocico y los números 666 escritos junto a él, cubría una pared cerca de la oficina de AVANCE. Éste era más o menos la época cuando los narcotraficantes y los adolescentes delincuentes estaban causando una gran cantidad de dolor y sufrimiento a los residentes. Un miembro de la mesa directiva de AVANCE, quien es hispano y un católico devoto, estuvo tan horrorizado cuando vio este dibujo que aportó los fondos necesarios para reemplazarlo con un mural de la Virgen en el cual ella abraza a una madre y a un niño hispanos. Este mural se mantuvo intacto, sin estropearse con graffiti, debido al respeto y la devoción que la gente le tiene. En esa comunidad hispana y en muchas otras, Ella aparece como una fuerza invencible que vela por las familias. Ella proveyó una fuente de fortaleza y valentía a esas familias, capacitándolas a desafiar a los narcotraficantes que estaban destruyendo a los jóvenes y empujándolos hacia una vida de drogas y crimen. A través de su unión y su fortaleza, los padres expulsaron a los narcotraficantes de su comunidad.

Nuestra Señora de Guadalupe nos ha dejado su increíble milagro, la fenomenal tilma que Juan Diego vestía el día en que Ella apareció ante él. Cuando Juan Diego dejó caer las rosas de su tilma como prueba al obispo de su autenticidad, la imagen de la Virgen milagrosamente apareció en el manto. A pesar de la textura áspera de la tela, la increíble imagen de la Virgen María ha permanecido en el manto de Juan Diego desde 1531 y aún existe hoy en la Basílica de Nuestra Señora de Guadalupe en la Ciudad de México.

Hay muchos sitios interesantes en la internet incluyendo (http://ng.netgate:net/~norberto/eye.html) donde se encuentran cosas como "The Mystery in the Eyes of Our Lady of Guadalupe" (El misterio en los ojos de Nuestra Señora de Guadalupe). También usted se dará cuenta de varios descubrimientos de la existencia de siluetas en las pupilas de ambos ojos de la imagen de la Virgen María que apareció en el manto original. En el centro de una de las pupilas de la Virgen de Guadalupe se encuentra la imagen de una familia con varios niños, uno de los cuales es un bebé cargado dentro en un rebozo, en la espalda de su madre. Yo creo que Nuestra Señora de Guadalupe nos continúa hablando hoy a los latinos con una voz que cura, tal como lo hizo en la época de los aztecas.

La revelación me llevó a pensar que quizá Nuestra Madre, conocida por muchos nombres, está tratando de decirnos algo sobre la familia. Tal vez sepa que la familia está bajo un serio ataque en nuestro mundo moderno tal como lo estuvo la gente náhuatl hace tantos siglos. Posiblemente, está tratando de decirnos que ella escucha los lamentos de muchas familias hispanas que están sufriendo porque sus niños son víctimas de las drogas, el alcohol, y el crimen. Los adultos se enfrentan a demasiado analfabetismo, desempleo, y discriminación. Entre los niños, un 15 por ciento se acuestan en la noche con hambre, casi el 50 por ciento abandonan sus estudios, y cerca del 40 por ciento viven en la pobreza. El amor al dinero y a las cosas materiales también puede destruir a los niños y a las familias. La Virgen María tal vez está mandando un mensaje que dice que debemos buscar la fortaleza y una orientación en ella y en Dios, su hijo.

Yo creo que para mantener la solidez de las familias, debemos comenzar por volver a construir los cimientos, con nuestras virtudes culturales: nuestra espiritualidad, además del valor que les conferimos a los niños, al matrimonio, a la familia, y a la comunidad. La familia, aun con todas las fuerzas adversas que la amenazan, puede sobrevivir si nosotros abrazamos la riqueza cultural que hemos heredado.

Las rosas que saltaron milagrosamente del manto de Juan Diego son una metáfora del renacimiento de una nueva raza latina en una época y en un lugar donde nadie esperaba que aparecieran. Igual como las innumerables variedades de rosas, los latinos reflejan un bello surtido de colores y variedades. Tal como aquellas delicadas flores crecen con fuerza con los nutrientes apropiados, con amor, y con persistencia, también así se desarrollarán nuestros niños latinos y llegarán a ser unas promesas para un futuro mejor. Nuestros niños han sido destinados a orientar y a crear una mejor nación y un mejor mundo para toda la gente.

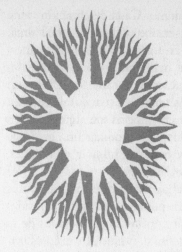

Capítulo II

La cultura hispana

La cultura es un modo de vivir que abarca todo, desde nuestras creencias y formas de celebración, hasta nuestros alimentos y nuestra ropa. Incluye a nuestro idioma, alimentos, religión, música, tradiciones, y valores. La cultura consiste en cómo nos relacionamos unos con otros, cómo pensamos, cómo nos comportamos, y qué percepción tenemos del mundo. La cultura es la manera en que un niño es socializado desde su nacimiento, comenzando con su familia, y más tarde con instituciones tales como la iglesia y las escuelas en la comunidad y el medio ambiente a su alrededor. La que tiene más influencia es la cultura del hogar, la cual se pasa de generación en generación y se aprende durante el período más critico de la vida. La cultura hispana es rica y vibrante, llena de tradiciones, celebraciones, y relaciones sólidas. Nuestra cultura incluye canciones alegres, alimentos deliciosos, creencias religiosas firmes y sólidas, y el idioma español. Es nuestro modo de vivir, es quienes somos como latinos.

Del bautismo hasta la quinceañera, una celebración que conmemora el rito de paso a la edad adulta de una joven, los padres hispanos han celebrado acontecimientos que unen a la familia y los amigos para proclamar la importancia del niño, con plenitud de comida, música, alegría, y significado espiritual. Los hispanos creen que se debe celebrar la vida. Nuestra cultura está imbuida de música estimulante y animadora que restaura y llena de energía al espíritu humano. Cada celebración tiene sus propias canciones que elevan nuestras sensibilidades y llegan al alma, como cuando se cantan "Las Mañanitas" en los cumpleaños mexicanos, cuando se canta "Madre Querida" a las madrecitas en el día de las Madres, o cuando las Posadas son representadas con canción y drama en la Navidad. Las guitarras, las marimbas, los tambores (conga), las claves, los güiros, las maracas, los acordeones, y las trompetas son algunos de los instrumentos musicales típicamente usados para producir una gama de optimista música latina, desde cumbias y polkas a salsas y merengues, todos los cuales son apreciados a través del mundo.

El día de los Muertos, una de las muchas tradiciones hispanas, nos ayuda a encarar la muerte de una manera positiva. Nuestras coloridas fiestas, llenas de vida, nos ayudan a lidiar con las cargas pesadas de la vida. En el mundo hispano, la vida se celebra con música y colores brillantes. Igual como las flores de papel de colores fuertes y los listones coloridos de nuestras celebraciones, la imaginación y la creatividad de un niño se vuelven abundantes a través de nuestros ritos y folklore. Las actividades como el cantar, bailar, dar palmadas, y dar gritos como "ajúa" nos llenan de energía y nos mantienen felices y sanos. Los ritos ceremoniales nos unen a Dios, a la familia, y a los amigos. Aunque sea un hecho reconocido que los hispanos tienen una sólida ética de trabajo, también creemos en disfrutar de la vida. Este concepto es el énfasis del dicho *come, bebe, que la vida es breve*, y del popular brindis latino *salud, amor, pesetas, y tiempo para disfrutarlos*.

Nuestra cultura ha jugado un importante papel en mantener a la familia unida y fuerte, a través de tradiciones y ritos. Ha hecho posible que las familias celebren la vida y ha ayudado a construir relaciones sólidas y duraderas. Estos vínculos con nuestros niños y con la familia extensa, los vecinos, y los amigos, son evidentes al unirnos en momentos felices para celebrar la Navidad, el día de la Acción de Gracias, Pascua, el día de la Madre, cumpleaños, bautismos, quinceañeras, y bodas, además de también unirnos en momentos tristes al compartir la profunda pena con nuestros seres queridos en los velorios.

Los hispanos a través de los Estados Unidos están recobrando su rico patrimonio a través de innumerables maneras. Quizá les enseñen a sus niños a apreciar su folklore, por ejemplo los mariachis o la música jíbara o los cuentos tradicionales. Quizá también animen a sus niños a estudiar el baile folclórico. Si no ponemos a nuestros niños en contacto con estas tradiciones culturales, seguramente éstas morirán, junto con los beneficios que producen. Los padres deben hacer todo el esfuerzo posible por enseñarles a sus niños el idioma español, orientar su conducta con dichos perspicaces, y ayudarles a enorgullecerse de los exquisitos platillos tradicionales de nuestra gente. Aun se ha comprobado que algunos de nuestros tradicionales remedios caseros y hierbas, tales como el té de manzanilla, de canela, y de hierbabuena, poseen un valor medicinal valioso.

Los padres hispanos, al igual que sus niños, necesitan celebrar el hecho de que son únicos y especiales porque son latinos. Por muchas generaciones en los Estados Unidos, nunca existieron muchos premios por ser hispano. Cuando yo estaba en la escuela, por ejemplo, si se pescaba a alguien hablando español, se le daba un golpe veloz en la mano con una regla, o se le forzaba a soportar la humillación de tener que estar parado con la nariz vuelta hacia el centro de un círculo en el pizarrón. Yo pasé muchas tardes con la nariz pegada al pizarrón porque entré a la escuela hablando principalmente español. Igual a muchos hispanos, algunos de mis amigos también escondían sus taquitos que les hacían sus mamás, dentro de las bolsas de papel que les servían de loncheras, como si les causara vergüenza el no tener un emparedado de jamón y queso. Nadie quiere que nuestros niños se avergüencen de quiénes son. Yo quiero que ni mis niños ni ningún otro niño hispano tenga que pasar por lo que muchos de nosotros pasamos durante nuestra niñez y juventud. Aquéllos que logramos éxito tuvimos padres que nos alentaron a descubrir quiénes somos y a estar orgullosos de nuestra identidad. En una época cuando nuestra música y nuestro arte son valorados y apreciados por millones de personas, y nuestra cocina, incluyendo los tacos, los burritos, y la salsa picante, son tan populares como las hamburguesas, la pizza, y la salsa catsup, puede que sea más fácil para los niños hispanos celebrar su patrimonio cultural con gusto, confianza, y orgullo.

NUESTROS NOMBRES

Los nombres hispanos hablan volúmenes sobre nuestra historia y cultura y nos recuerdan quiénes somos. Muchos nombres hispanos tienen significado religioso, incluyendo el nombre de Guadalupe o Lupe, en honor a Nuestra Señora de Guadalupe. Uno de mis primos varones y mi cuñada se llaman Guadalupe, y a ambos les decimos Lupe por corto. Casi no puede uno entrar a un vecindario hispano sin encontrar un tesoro, una cantidad asombrosa, de niñas y mujeres llamadas Mary, o María, en alguna combinación como María Elena, María Antonieta, María Luisa, Ana María, o Mary Ann, Mary Lou, o Mary Helen. Yo recuerdo que siendo adolescente, cuandoquiera que yo iba al autocine con mis amigos, los muchachos inevitablemente nos llamarían diciendo: "Eh, María". Ellos sabían que había una gran probabilidad de que alguna de nosotras se llamara María. Los nombres hispanos reflejan la alegría y la espiritualidad de nuestra cultura, desde Luz, hasta Esperanza.

Y, claro, otro nombre religioso que se encuentra comúnmente entre familias hispanas es el nombre de Jesús, en inglés y en español. El nombre de nacimiento de mi hermana Susie es Jesusita, llamada así por mi abuela. Otros nombres tradicionales hispanos que tienen un significado religioso incluyen los nombres de los discípulos: Juan, Lucas, Pablo, o Pedro. Se les recuerda a los santos y otras figuras bíblicas con nombres tales como Lourdes, Teresita, Ana, y Tomás, José, Moisés, e Israel, Lázaro, Ester, Magdalena, Marta, Rebeca, Raquel, Mercedes, Ángel, Angélica, Santos, Gloria, y Luz.

Mi hijo, Salvador Julián, volvió muy disgustado de la escuela un día porque uno de los niños de su clase de primer año de primaria le dijo que su nombre era tan largo como una culebra. Ya no quería llamarse Salvador. Él quería un nombre corto como Tom o Bill. Mi esposo y yo nos sentamos con él y le explicamos qué especial era llevar los nombres de su padre y de dos abuelos, y el nombre de nuestro Salvador. "No hay nombre más grande que ese", le dijimos. "Yo sé que mi nombre es especial. No me molesta tener un nombre largo en la casa, pero en la escuela, ¿está bien si me llaman Sal, por corto?" Salvador respondió. Le dije: "Claro que sí. A Papi también le llaman Sal sus amigos. Pero él sabe que su verdadero nombre es Salvador, y está orgulloso de él, tal como nosotros queremos que tú lo estés".

Si usted vive en una comunidad de diversidad étnica o sus niños asisten a una escuela con variados orígenes étnicos, quizá se entere de que las personas que no están acostumbradas a escuchar nombres españoles tal vez traten a su niño de manera distinta, y quizá aun le hagan broma o burla. Como padres, nosotros necesitamos ayudar a nuestros niños a encarar los comentarios negativos y a sensibilizar a los maestros para que hagan lo mismo. Hágale saber a la maestra que usted no quiere que se cambie ni se anglicanice el nombre de su niño por conveniencia, tal como si llamaran a Rafael "Ralph". Cuando habla con la maestra, pronuncie el nombre de la manera que usted quiere que sea pronunciado. Tal vez algunas personas no puedan hacer vibrar las erres tan bien como usted, pero comprenderán que el nombre de su niño es importante y significativo.

Si usted cree que los nombres tienen significado, debe enorgullecerse de aquellos nombres que les proporcionan a sus niños un sentido de su historia. Cada vez más escuchamos a nombres como Valerie, Crystal,

Brian, o Jeffrey juntos a apellidos como García o Hernández. Estas combinaciones sugieren que estamos en una encrucijada entre dos culturas y que tenemos la capacidad de abrazar a ambas. En algunos casos, como los de mi hija, Gloria Vanessa, y mi hijo Steven René, los niños hispanos tal vez lleven un nombre de un mundo y un nombre del otro. Muchos nombres como Ana o Benjamín pueden complacer a ambos mundos.

¿Tiene usted un nombre especial para sus niños? Entre los amigos hispanos, a veces son más conocidos los sobrenombres que los nombres. A una persona se le puede llamar *Araña* si tiene piernas muy largas, *Güera* si tiene el cabello rubio o piel blanca, o *Chino* si tiene el cabello rizado. A mí me llamaban *GoGi*; a Yolanda, la más chica de los hermanos en mi familia, le llamábamos *Baby*; Susi era *Tuti*; Rosa Linda era *Chata*; y a la mayor generalmente se le llama *Mami*. A mi esposo le llamaban *Nuni*, porque era un "Junior", y a uno de sus hermanos le llamaban *Mito* por "hermanito". A muchos nombres hispanos los acortan, para convertirlos en sobrenombres. Por ejemplo, Enrique muchas veces se cambia a Quique; Antonio a Tone; Isabel(a) a Chabela; Gregorio a Goyo; José a Pepe; Guillermo a Memo; Ignacio a Nacho; Alberto, Gilberto, y Roberto a Beto; Elena a Nena; Jesús a Chuy; Consuelo a Chelo; Luciano a Chano; y Rosalía a Chayo. Al añadir *ita* o *ito* a algunos nombres se convierten en "nombres de cariño", tales como Juanito, Rosita, y Panchito. Otras palabras de cariño son *mi hijita, mi amor, mi cielo, mi corazón,* o *mi luna de miel.*

A veces, las palabras como *gorda(ita), negra(ita), ruquita, viejito* son tan sólo una expresión de cariño. A menos que uno esté metido a fondo en la cultura, le puede parecer difícil comprender las matices culturales, tal como cuando yo le llamo a mi hija "mi mamita", "mi princesita", "mi hijita", y "mi chulita". Puede que sea mi princesa, mi hija, mi niña linda, pero de ninguna manera es mi madre.

¿Tenía usted un sobrenombre especial cuando estaba creciendo? ¿Utiliza algunas palabras hispanas de cariño con sus niños? Hacer esto es una maravillosa manera de celebrar nuestra cultura y de crear una cálida relación duradera con sus niños.

NUESTRA RELIGIÓN

Un examen de los aspectos más atrayentes de nuestra cultura quizá comenzaría con lo que yo considero ser uno de nuestros más sólidos valores—nuestra fe. Los hispanos representan a una gran cantidad de denominaciones, incluyendo a las de los bautistas, los metodistas, los testigos de

Jehová, los adventistas del Séptimo Día, y los judíos. Pero por lo mismo de que muchos siguen siendo un producto de nuestra historia, el 75 por ciento de los hispanos son católicos. Cada religión organizada tiene sus doctrinas, tradiciones, y prácticas valiosas, y la mayoría de los hispanos son profundamente espirituales, sin importar su ideología. Mi esposo y yo fuimos bautizados en la religión católica y estamos criando a nuestros niños como católicos. Como católica, quisiera compartir con ustedes qué tan integrada está la religión católica a la cultura hispana. Algunas personas tal vez hayan hecho la conversión a otra religión, pero han conservado muchas de las prácticas que han llegado a ser conocidas como hispanas, porque han permanecido con nosotros a través de los siglos.

Por ejemplo, nuestra sólida tradición religiosa se refleja en los objetos sagrados que adornan muchos hogares hispanos y que traen bendiciones, paz, y harmonía a nuestras vidas. Comenzando por los móviles de "ojos de Dios" que se sostienen encima de la cuna de un bebé latino, los rosarios que cuelgan orgullosamente de los espejos retrovisores, y las veladoras religiosas, los crucifijos, las virgencitas en los altares, éstos son algunos símbolos que reflejan la conexión de la familia hispana al mundo espiritual. Se puede observar en las medallas y los angelitos que las personas lucen y en los santitos, retablos, bultos, y nichos que se usan para decir oraciones o para exponerse. Muchos hispanos van de peregrinaje a santuarios o capillas tal como el de San Juan de los Lagos en el Valle del Río Grande en Texas, para rezarle a la Virgen María y pedirle milagros o para hacerle promesas. En muchas iglesias latinas, se puede rezar por un milagro para su niño al dejar su retrato en un salón especial en la iglesia y prenderle una veladora, o al sujetarle un brochecito en la forma del parte de cuerpo que quiere que se cure, a la estatua de cierto santo. Muletas, vestidos de novia, y aun medallas militares que se encuentran en estos lugares sirven de testimonio a las muchas oraciones que fueron contestadas.

Muchos hispanos les entregan su fe, sus esperanzas, y sus peticiones a santitos tales como Santa Ana. Hay canciones que le piden a Santa Ana, a la Virgen, o a Jesús, que acallen y arrullen a sus bebés hasta dormirlos mientras ellos los cuiden y protejan. Como madre de la Virgen María, Santa Ana es la patrona de las madres y las abuelas, y ella recalca a los hispanos la importancia de las relaciones entre madres e hijos y de la familia extensa. Algunos otros santos que quizá jueguen un papel en la vida de una familia hispana incluyen a San Antonio de Padua, quien cuida a parientes enfermos o ayuda a encontrar a animales extraviados. Otros santos populares incluyen a San Judas Tadeo, santo patrón de las causas perdidas; Santa Rita de Casia, para las mujeres que están buscando marido; Santa Inés, conocida por proteger la pureza de las jovencitas;

y Santa Bárbara, quien protege contra los relámpagos y contra el maltrato a los niños. Un santo favorito de muchos hispanos en México y Nuevo México es el Santo Niño de Atocha, el santo patrón de los niños, los prisioneros, y las enfermedades. Este santo también se conoce como protector de los viajeros, por lo cual también se conoce a San Cristóbal. Usted puede utilizar las historias de los santos para enseñarles a sus niños conducta y características positivas, tales como la bondad, y al mismo tiempo desalentar otras, como el egoísmo. Para muchas generaciones de latinos, los santitos han servido como modelos de moralidad.

Los *retablos* son piezas de dos dimensiones de arte popular hispano, hechos de hojalata, cobre, lona, o madera, que ilustran las caras o las obras de los santos o de acontecimientos bíblicos. Los *nichos*, pequeñas cajas que sirven como capilla a los bultos, los cuales son esculturas de tres dimensiones, labradas de madera, de Jesús, la Virgen María, o un santo, se están volviendo tan populares hoy en día como lo fueron en el siglo doce. Hay nichos de todos tamaños, colores, y diseños. Puede familiarizar a sus niños con estas bellas obras de arte en los museos y las tiendas de arte popular.

En momentos de pesar, los católicos también encuentran gran paz y fortaleza al buscar a Nuestra Santa Madre por medio del rosario. A través de Latinoamérica, se le conoce por muchos nombres incluyendo a María, la Madre Dolorosa, la Madre de Socorros, la Virgen de Caridad del Cabre, la Virgen de San Juan de los Lagos, Nuestra Señora de Alta Gracia, y Nuestra Señora del Rosario. También es conocida como Nuestra Señora del Carmen y Nuestra Señora de la Luz. Nuestra Señora de los Ángeles y la Inmaculada Concepción se ven como protectoras contra los monstruos o la maldad. La mejor conocida es Nuestra Señora de Guadalupe. Junta con la Santa Trinidad y los Ángeles, a ella se le ve como alguien que protege, que cura, que consuela, que intercede, y que es una fuente de poder para los latinos. Como figura cultural y religiosa, Ella nos proporciona un sentido de identidad, propósito, y valor.

HONRAR A LA VIRGEN DE GUADALUPE

Al llevar a sus niños de paseo por las comunidades hispanas, muéstreles los muchos altares construidos en honor a la Virgen en los patios y sitios prominentes de los hogares. Algunas personas, como mi suegra, tienen altares de la Virgencita que están adornados con velas y flores. Yo tengo un cuadro de Ella encima de la repisa de la chimenea. Mi vecina, quien le reza a la Virgen todos los días, tiene un altar rodeado de una nube de algodón y una lámpara de techo alumbrándola. Algunos altares llegan a ser el foco central de un cuarto donde los cuadros o iconos de la Virgen María, arreglados en un collage, comparten el espacio con imágenes de Jesús, los santos, y miembros de la familia. Estos altares unen los mundos divinos y terrenales. Hoy en día, aún se pueden observar altares de patio en honor a la Virgen, que se conocen como grutas y están hechas de piedra, losas, conchas, y flores. Su imagen está ilustrada en velas, medallas, murales, y aun en tatuajes en los pechos, las espaldas, y los brazos de hombres musculosos.

Los católicos devotos honran a Nuestra Señora de Guadalupe el 12 de diciembre. Pero a través de todo el año, las Guadalupanas y los Guadalupanos, un grupo de mujeres y hombres hispanos cuya misión exclusiva es servirla y honrarla, colocan rosas frescas y velas enfrente de la estatua de la Virgen. Ellos también son los responsables de organizar la celebración llevada a cabo en su día. Por toda la semana, hay varios rosarios, misas, velorios, festivales, y bailarines. En México, hay un peregrinaje a Tepeyac, el lugar donde primero se le apareció a Juan Diego. Miles de personas del mundo entero vienen a pagarle homenaje. Sería una asombrosa experiencia cultural y religiosa llevarles a sus niños a ser testigos de tal acontecimiento, además de observar la tilma original, la cual se encuentra dentro de la Basílica de Guadalupe.

Cada año, mi esposo fielmente se une a otros miembros del coro, comenzando a las cinco de la mañana, para llevarle serenata a la Virgen en Su día especial. Cada vez que yo asisto a estas reuniones, me conmuevo al ver la devoción de la gran cantidad de personas que se levantan tan temprano para cantar las bellas canciones escritas especialmente para Ella. Éstas incluyen "Buenos días"; "Paloma blanca"; "Adiós, O Virgen de Guadalupe;" "La virgen ranchera", como también aquellas que se cantan a todas las madres, "Madre querida," "Canto a la madre," y "Las mañanitas". Hay cancioneros en español que contienen las melodías de estas canciones, en las librerías católicas, especialmente en las ciudades donde hay grandes poblaciones hispanas.

Buenos días, Paloma Blanca

Buenos días, Paloma Blanca,
hoy te vengo a saludar,
saludando tu belleza
en tu trono celestial.

Eres Madre del Creador,
y a mi corazón encantas;
gracias te doy con amor.
Buenos días, Paloma Blanca.

Niña linda, niña santa,
tu dulce nombre alabar;
porque eres tan sacrosanta,
hoy te vengo a saludar.

Reluciente como el alba,
pura, sencilla, y sin mancha;
¡Qué gusto recibe mi alma!
Buenos días, Paloma Blanca.

Qué linda está la mañana,
el aroma de las flores
despiden suaves olores
antes de romper el alba.

Mi pecho con voz ufana,
gracias te da, Madre mía;
en este dichoso día
antes de romper el alba.

Cielo azul yo te convido
en este dichoso día
a que prestes tu hermosura
a las flores de María.

Madre mía de Guadalupe,
dame ya tu bendición;
recibe estas mañanitas
de un humilde corazón.

Adiós, O Virgen de Guadalupe

Adiós, O Virgen de Guadalupe,
Adiós, O Virgen del Salvador,
Desde que niño nombrarte supe
Eres mi vida, eres mi vida, mi solo amor.

Adiós, O Virgen, Madre querida;
Adiós refugio del pecador.
Eres mi encanto, eres mi vida,
Dulce esperanza en mi dolor.

Adiós, O Virgen de Guadalupe,
Adiós, O Madre del Redentor,
Ante tu trono siempre se agrupe
Todo tu pueblo lleno de amor.

Adiós, O Madre la más amable,
Aquí te dejo mi corazón;
Adiós, O Virgen incomparable,
Dame, Señora, tu bendición.

La virgen ranchera

A ti, Virgencita, mi Guadalupana
Yo quiero ofrecerte un canto valiente
Que Méjico entero te diga sonriente.

Yo quiero decirte lo que tú ya sabes
Que Méjico te ama, que nunca está triste
Porque de nombrarte el alma se inflama.

Tu nombre es arrullo y el mundo lo sabe
Eres nuestro orgullo, mi Méjico es tuyo,
Tú guardas la llave.

Que viva la Reina de los Mejicanos
La que con sus manos sembró rosas bellas
Y puso en el cielo millares de estrellas.

Yo sé que en el cielo escuchas mi canto
Y sé que con celo nos cubre tu manto
Virgencita chula eres un encanto.

Por patria nos diste este lindo suelo
Y lo bendijiste porque era tu anhelo
Tener un santuario cerquita del cielo.

Mi virgen ranchera, mi virgen morena,
Eres nuestra dueña, Méjico es tu tierra
Y tú su bandera.

Que viva la Reina de los Mejicanos
La que con sus manos sembró rosas bellas
Y puso en el cielo millares de estrellas.

En muchas comunidades hispanas, las extravagantes festividades del 12 de diciembre incluyen a bailarines especiales llamados *concheros* y *matachines*, quienes crean música con cascabeles, conchas amarradas a tiras en los tobillos, flautas, y conchas de armadillos. Están ataviados con brillantes disfraces llenos de lentejuelas, listones, plumas, cuentas, espejos, y bellos tocados que representan su ancestral cultura azteca. Los matachines bailan hasta doce danzas diferentes, incluyendo "La batalla", "La cruz", "La procesión", "El abuelo", "The Maypole", y "El toro".

Esta danza ritual de las espadas originalmente se bailó en épocas medievales para representar el conflicto entre los moros y los cristianos. Se trajo a México y al sudoeste de los Estados Unidos para simbolizar la resistencia de los indios a la conquista española, y la subyugación posterior que sufrieron. En el 12 de diciembre, se representa el drama de la aparición de la Virgen de Guadalupe ante Juan Diego, con el contexto del choque de religiones y culturas que fue el resultado de la entrevista entre Cortés y Moctezuma. También se representa para mofarse o burlarse del papel que hizo la *Malinche* en la conquista, por medio de presentaciones durante las cuales unos jovencitos se visten como jovencitas con máscaras cómicas o grotescas, pelucas, y disfraces para representarla a ella. Por medio de drama, humor, y simbolismo, representan la transformación de un pueblo.

Adquiera para su niño el libro de Sylvia Rodríguez titulado *The Matachines Dance* para aprender más sobre estas danzas rituales y sus significados. Si usted vive en una comunidad donde se celebra el Día de la Virgen de Guadalupe, lleve a sus niños para que conozcan este rico aspecto de nuestra cultura. Puede que su hijo o hija se interese por representar uno de los papeles de la ceremonia, por el cual quizá tendría que confeccionar elaborados disfraces, como aquéllos lucidos actualmente por los indios pueblos e hispanos de Nuevo México. Yo estoy segura que su niño nunca olvidaría el día que representara uno de estos papeles, si acaso tuviera la suerte de ser escogido. Los adultos también representan los papeles y se divierten aun más que sus niños. Se dice que la participación voluntaria trae honor y bendiciones a la familia del actor, y a la comunidad en general. Si no existen estas ceremonias en su comunidad, quizá usted las pueda iniciar.

NUESTRAS CELEBRACIONES RELIGIOSAS

Muchas de nuestras tradiciones, creencias, prácticas, y ritos giran alrededor de la religión. Están centradas en ceremonias religiosas que reúnen a familias y amigos para bautismos, primeras comuniones, confirmaciones, quinceañeras, y bodas, además de los días festivos religiosos incluyendo a Navidad, la noche de Fin de Año, Domingo de Pascua, y el Día de los Muertos. También hay muchas fiestas y festivales religiosos que se celebran con mucha comida deliciosa, flores de papel de colores vívidos, y entrenamiento alegre, que, juntos con el significado espiritual, hacen que nuestras vidas sean más excitantes y alegres.

Celebrar la Nochebuena

Al atardecer de Nochebuena, las familias hispanas a través de las Américas se preparan para las Posadas. La tradicional representación del viaje que hicieron María y José para encontrar alojamiento en Belén, se celebra por nueve días en México y otros países latinoamericanos, comenzando el 16 de diciembre. Cada noche un grupo de vecinos llevando farolitos con velas camina a varias casas en el barrio con estatuas de María y José encima de un burro. Unas luminarias, bolsas de papel hechas pesadas con arena y un votivo, iluminan la oscuridad de la noche y guían a los viajeros, o peregrinos, por su camino. Quizá su familia pueda participar en una Posada patrocinada por su iglesia o iniciada por usted o algún vecino de su comunidad. Improvise con la hechura de los disfraces de los pastores y los instrumentos, o bien, verdaderamente planee y organice el acontecimiento con toda la pompa y esplendor y gala de una escena navideña.

Sigue la tradicional canción que se utiliza para esta representación. Los peregrinos tocan la puerta de la casa de un vecino y solicitan alojamiento, cantando la canción que está a continuación (afuera de la casa). Los familiares de esa casa responden de manera similar con canción (adentro de la casa):

Las Posadas

EL CORO:

(José y María y el grupo
de viajeros cantan esto)

EL JEFE DE LA FAMILIA:

(La familia abre la puerta y el
jefe de la familia responde)

AFUERA

1. En nombre del Cielo,
Os pido posada,
Pues no puede andar
Mi esposa amada.

3. No seas inhumano,
Tennos caridad.
Que el Dios de los Cielos
Te lo premiará.

5. Venimos rendidos
Desde Nazaret.
Yo soy carpintero
De nombre José.

7. Posada te pide,
Amado casero,
Por sólo una noche
La Reina del Cielo.

9. Mi esposa es María,
Es Reina del Cielo
Y madre va a ser
Del Divino Verbo.

11. Dios pague, señores
Vuestra caridad,
Y así os colme el Cielo
De felicidad.

ADENTRO

2. Aquí no es mesón.
Sigan adelante.
Yo no puedo abrir.
No sea algún tunante.

4. Ya se pueden ir
Y no molestar,
Porque si me enfado
Los voy a apalear.

6. No me importa el nombre.
Déjenme dormir.
Pues ya se los digo
Que no hemos de abrir.

8. Pues si es una Reina
Quien lo solicita,
¿Cómo es que de noche
Anda tan solita?

10. ¿Eres tú José?
¿Tu esposa es María?
Entren, peregrinos,
No los conocía.

12. Dichosa la casa
Que abriga este día
A la Virgen pura
La hermosa María.

TODA LA FAMILIA: (Cuando se abre la puerta, la familia anfitriona
responde)

Ábranse las puertas, rómpanse los velos,
Que viene a posar el Rey de los Cielos.

Entren, santos peregrinos, peregrinos.
Reciban este rincón,
No de mi pobre morada, mi morada,
Sino de mi corazón.

Al entrar la gente a la casa, se arrodillan ante el pesebre del nacimiento, en recuerdo al nacimiento de Cristo, y el verdadero significado de la Navidad. En Nochebuena, las familias sacan un muñeco que representa al niño Jesús y la dueña de la casa escoge a una mujer que le cae bien y que será su comadre por tres años. Como madrina del niño Jesús, ella arrullará al Santo Niño antes de ponerlo en el pesebre. Todos cantan la siguiente canción de cuna, la cual es seguida por el rompimiento de la piñata y su canción correspondiente.

El rorro

A la rururu, niño chiquito.
Duérmase ya mi Jesusito.
Los animales grandes y chiquitos,
guarden silencio, no le hagan ruido.

Noche venturosa, noche de alegría.
Bendita la dulce, divina María.

Coros celestiales, con su dulce acento,
Canten la ventura de este nacimiento.

La canción para la piñata de las Posadas

En las noches de Posada, la piñata es lo mejor
Aun las niñas remilgadas, se animan con gran fervor.

Con los ojitos vendados, y en las manos un bastón
La olla rómpela a pedazos, no le tengas compasión.

Dale, dale, dale
no pierdas el tino

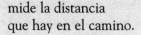

mide la distancia
que hay en el camino.

Que si no le das
de un palo te tiro.
Que si no le das
de un palo te tiro.
Dale, dale, dale

Muchos van a misa para colocar un regalo enfrente del nacimiento. El regalo, u ofrenda, puede ser una flor de Nochebuena, comida para los pobres, o una promesa, una piadosa ofrenda de portarse mejor. Los vecinos preparan alimentos especiales tales como pan dulce, bizcochitos, chocolate mexicano, o ponche, y dulces. Cada uno de los nueve días incluye cosas festivas y brillantes, sonidos alegres, y aromas deliciosos. Uno puede encontrar golosinas dulces, una colorida piñata, música, y canto, todo lo cual produce una impresión duradera a cualquier niño.

Como parte de la celebración de las Posadas, haga los siguientes alimentos tradicionales con sus niños. Solicite la ayuda de un miembro mayor de la familia si nunca antes ha intentado hacer estos por su propia cuenta. Lo más probable es que las generaciones actuales y pasadas encontrarán muchos puntos en común al confeccionar las más deliciosas golosinas y reposterías hispanas. Quizá sus niños puedan ayudarles a cortar las galletas, estirar las bolitas, o cubrir las galletas con la mezcla de canela y azúcar.

Bizcochitos

1   libra de manteca de puerco (2 tazas)
1   taza de azúcar
2   huevos batidos
1   cucharadita de vinagre (solamente si usa jugo de naranja)
2   cucharadas soperas de semillas de anís
6   tazas de harina
3   cucharaditas de polvo de hornear
1   cucharadita de sal
⅓   taza de jugo de naranja, ¼ taza de brandy, coñac, jerez, borbón (depende del gusto)
⅔   taza de azúcar y 1 cucharadita de canela, para cubrir las galletas

Precaliente el horno a 350 grados. Bata la manteca y el azúcar hasta hacer una mezcla ligera y esponjosa. Ponga los huevos, el vinagre, y el anís en un tazón; bata hasta que esté cremosa la mezcla. En otro tazón, combine la harina, el polvo de hornear, y la sal. Añada a la mezcla de manteca, alternando la harina con el licor o jugo de naranja, mezclando hasta que tenga una consistencia firme la masa. Estire la masa con un palote de amasar, en una superficie enharinada, hasta que tenga ½ pulgada de grosor. Corte la masa con un pequeño cortador de galletas de la forma que usted prefiera (yo prefiero las de una pulgada de ancho), y métalas en la mezcla de azúcar y canela, dándoles vuelta hasta cubrirlas. Colóquelas en una bandeja de horno sin engrasar y hornéelas por 10 a 20 minutos o hasta que se doren ligeramente. La receta rinde entre cuatro y doce docenas de galletas, dependiendo del tamaño.

Pan de polvo

1   paquete de semillas de anís (2½ onzas) ó ¾ taza
1   paquete pequeño de canela entera ó 5 trozos de canela de 3 pulgadas cada uno
1   libra de manteca de puerco (2 tazas)
1   libra de manteca vegetal (2 tazas)
1   paquete de levadura (¼ onza)
1   taza de azúcar
12   tazas de harina
⅔   taza de azúcar y 1 cucharadita de canela (para la mezcla de azúcar y canela)

Precaliente el horno a 350 grados. En una olla de un litro de capacidad, ponga a hervir las semillas de anís y la canela en agua; deje hervir por varios minutos. Quite la olla del fuego y aparte hasta que se enfríe a temperatura ambiental. Disuelva la levadura y el azúcar en este "té" de canela y anís. Mezcle las mantecas de puerco y vegetal hasta que queden cremosas. Comience a mezclar la harina con la mezcla de manteca, y añada el té poco a poco, amasando hasta lograr una masa firme. Estire la masa con el palote para amasar hasta que tenga un grosor de ¼ pulgada. Corte la masa con un pequeño cortador de galletas de la forma que usted prefiera (yo prefiero las redondas de una pulgada de ancho o las de forma de corazón). Colóquelas en una bandeja de horno sin engrasar y hornéelas por 15 a 20 minutos o hasta que se doren ligeramente. Meta las galletas, mientras estén calientes, en la mezcla de azúcar y canela, dándoles vuelta hasta cubrirlas. La receta rinde de seis a ocho docenas, dependiendo del tamaño. Pueden ser almacenadas en un recipiente cerrado herméticamente, por hasta cuatro semanas. Se sirven estas galletas en las bodas y quinceañeras.

Polvorones de canela

      1   taza de mantequilla o margarina
    ½   taza de azúcar glas (azúcar en polvo)
      1   cucharadita de extracto de vainilla
    2½ tazas de harina
      1   cucharadita de canela molida
    ¼   cucharadita de sal
      1   taza de nueces finamente picadas
      1   taza de azúcar glas y 1 cucharadita de canela (para la mezcla de
           azúcar con canela)

Precaliente el horno a 350 grados. Utilizando una batidora eléctrica, bata la mantequilla o margarina hasta que esté cremosa, y después añada el azúcar y la vainilla. Poco a poco, añada 2 tazas de harina, la canela, y la sal. Junto con la última tanda de harina (cuando menos ½ taza), añada las nueces. Mezcle y luego añada a la masa. Cubra y ponga a enfriar en el refrigerador por dos horas. Separe y forme bolitas de masa de una pulgada cada una. Coloque en una bandeja de horno sin engrasar y hornéelas por 15 minutos. Meta las galletas, mientras estén calientes, en la mezcla de azúcar y canela, dándoles vuelta hasta cubrirlas. La receta rinde de cuatro a cinco docenas de galletas.

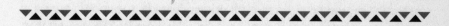

Pasteles de boda

      1   taza de mantequilla
      1   cucharadita de vainilla
    ½   taza de azúcar glas
      2   tazas de harina

¼ cucharadita de sal
1 taza de nueces finamente picadas
azúcar glas (para cubrir las galletas)

Precaliente el horno a 350 grados. Utilizando una batidora eléctrica, bata la mantequilla y la vainilla hasta quedar esponjosa la mezcla. Añada el azúcar y mezcle hasta que se quede cremosa. En otro recipiente, mezcle la harina con la sal y luego añada la mezcla cremosa. Añada las nueces. Mezcle. Forme la masa en pequeñas bolitas de alrededor de una pulgada de ancho, y aplane ligeramente cada una con la mano. Haga una forma de un cilindro con la masa, con un diámetro de más o menos 1¼ pulgadas, envuelva en papel encerado, y refrigere por dos horas, hasta que esté firme. Corte la masa cilíndrica en rodajas con ½ pulgada de grosor. Coloque en una bandeja de horno sin engrasar y hornéelas por 15 a 20 minutos. Meta las galletas, mientras estén calientes, en el azúcar glas, dándoles vuelta hasta cubrirlas. La receta rinde dos docenas de galletas.

A pesar de que algunos hispanos en América todavía celebran las Posadas por nueve días, la mayoría llevan a cabo una versión condensada de las mismas en Nochebuena. En mi familia, los niños se visten de pastores y ángeles. En una celebración verdaderamente de dos culturas, el varón más joven generalmente hace el papel del niño del tambor, una tradición de Norteamérica.

En mi antiguo barrio, los peregrinos caminaban a alojamientos construidos en nuestro patio grande enfrente de la casa, para simbolizar el viaje de María y José a las diferentes posadas. Cuando nos mudamos al suburbio, los vecinos nos invitaron a participar en las Posadas. Al caminar los miembros de la familia a los hogares de los vecinos por calles alumbradas con luces navideñas y luminarias, cantábamos canciones navideñas en ambos inglés y español. Mi esposo guiaba al grupo mientras tocaba su trompeta. En nuestra primera parada, tocamos la puerta, y cuando los vecinos la abrieron, cantamos las Posadas. Ya que estaban celebrando su propia reunión familiar, nos invitaron a pasar y compartir unas galletas y algo para tomar. Les deseamos una feliz Navidad y luego seguimos a la siguiente casa vecina. Nuestra casa fue la última parada, donde todo el grupo entró después de cantar, para disfrutar de mucha comida y alegría. Pero antes que nada, todos nos arrodillamos ante el nacimiento, con el niño Jesús en su pesebre, donde permanecía hasta el día de los Tres Reyes Magos.

Justo antes de la medianoche, generalmente toda la familia acude apresuradamente a la Misa de Gallo, llamada así por la legendaria historia de dos gallos, uno que se paró en el pesebre en la primera Navidad y anunció: "¡Cristo nació!" mientras el otro contestó: "¡en Belén!" En la Misa de Gallo recibimos la Eucaristía, miramos una representación del nacimiento de Cristo, y cantamos populares canciones navideñas, tales como *"Noche de paz"*.

Noche de paz

Noche de paz, noche de amor,
Todo duerme en derredor,
Entre los astros que esparcen su luz,
Bella, anunciando al niñito Jesús,
Brilla la estrella de paz, brilla la estrella de paz.

Noche de paz, noche de amor,
Todo duerme en derredor,
Sólo velan en la oscuridad
Los pastores que en el campo están;
Y la estrella de Belén, y la estrella de Belén.

Usted puede crear alegres recuerdos cuando adorna su casa para la Navidad, con sus niños. En mi casa, Steven se enorgullece de construir el nacimiento, adornado con musgo, luces navideñas, ángeles, pastores, animales, y estatuillas de la Virgen María y José, el cual se coloca en un lugar prominente de la casa. Al lado del nacimiento está un pueblito cubierto por nieve que se convierte en el proyecto familiar, y todo el mundo decide dónde poner las muchas casas, los edificios, y la gente que he coleccionado a través de los años. Algunos "pueblitos" en casas latinoamericanas ocupan toda una pared, del piso hasta el cielo raso, con animales, pastores, y gente del pueblo, un cuadro de la imagen que tienen de aquella noche especial. Trate de construir uno con sus niños. Le aseguro que esta experiencia les dejará recuerdos duraderos a todos los involucrados.

Bellos adornos como angelitos, bolas de nieve, velas, y arreglos florales se pueden utilizar para crear un espíritu navideño. Unas guirnaldas engalanadas con las piñas del pino, unos ángeles, y otros adornos pueden embellecer la repisa de la chimenea y las escaleras. Ponemos un majestuoso árbol de Navidad en mi sala y lo cubrimos de todos los angelitos posibles además de flores y pájaros. El segundo arbolito que tenemos lo ponemos en el cuarto de juego y se adorna con solamente adornos mexicanos, hechos de estambre y brillantes cuentas coloridas.

Puede tener otro memorable proyecto familiar al crear la escena del nacimiento en su patio delantero. El orgullo de mi esposo es un gran pesebre que todos los de la familia construyen cada año, adornado con luces navideñas, nochebuenas, y una enorme estrella que ilumina el cielo. También hay estatuillas plásticas de tamaño natural de María, José, y el niño Jesús, dentro del pesebre, con figuras cortadas de madera de reyes, un pastor, un camello, un burro, además de ángeles de hierro forjado iluminados. Esta escena exterior navideña siempre atrae atención y hace que los carros se paren para echar una segunda mirada. Usted también puede ayudarles a sus niños a construir algunos de estos personajes religiosos o aun un Santa Claus con sus renos. Ponga al niño que posee talento artístico a trazar las figuras en madera (contrachapado) y consiga que un adulto las corte. Luego, permita que sus niños pinten y adornen los personajes. Aun yo tomé parte en el proceso de adornar a los Tres Reyes Magos con joyería de fantasía y al camello con una montura de mentira, con todo y borlas. Este tipo de actividades son muy divertidas y entretenidas y aseguran hacer de sus Navidades unos momentos extremadamente memorables.

EL DÍA DE NAVIDAD

Nuestra familia celebra la Navidad dos veces: en Nochebuena con la familia extensa de mi esposo y en el día de Navidad con la mía. Ambos días pueden producir momentos excitantes y encantadores, llenos del sonido de risas alegres, el aroma de comidas deliciosas, y el resplandor de luces navideñas. Arreglamos una mesa bien puesta, llena de tamales, arroz, frijoles, chilitos, ensaladas de verduras, y un rico surtido de deliciosos postres, desde el pastel de nueces, hasta los bizcochitos y las empanadas.

Tamales

Una tradición que está volviendo de gran manera entre los hispanos durante la temporada navideña es la de hacer tamales. Es un evento familiar o un momento cuando las amigas y las familiares se reúnen para cumplir esta tarea laboriosa. Cada vez más hombres se están uniendo a la confección de los tamales caseros. Es una tarea ardua y un acontecimiento que toma todo un día para completar. Sin embargo, también puede ser un momento para ponerse al día con todo el más reciente chisme. Algunas personas tienen la tradición de hacer tamales en Nochebuena para tener su cena principal esa noche con tamales calientitos. Otras los cocinan días o semanas por adelantado y los congelan. Los tamales son muy sabrosos, pero también engordan mucho. Pero, bueno, como dice el dicho, *Una vez al año no hace daño, una vez al mes, tal vez.* Si quiere hacer unas comidas tradicionales para la temporada navideña, pruebe estas recetas para hacer empanadas y tamales. En esto también sus niños pueden ayudar a hacer las bolitas, estirarlas, o picar las empanadas. Ponga a sus niños a separar las hojas para los tamales, remojarlas en agua, y sacarlas cuando están listas. Los niños mayores pueden ayudar a embarrar la masa. Hacer tamales cuesta mucho trabajo, pero los tamales caseros son tan ricos, y la tradición de hacerlos tiene que seguir. Sería maravilloso si su hijo disfrutara de la experiencia de hacer tamales cuando menos una vez, para que pueda seguir esta tradición con sus propios niños.

Hay tantas variedades de tamales. Se pueden hacer los tradicionales, hechos de cabeza y patas de puerco, o bien de carne de puerco o de res, los cuales están ganando popularidad. También se pueden conseguir tamales de venado, frijoles, pasas con canela y azúcar, o para aquéllos que están más conscientes de su peso, reemplace la manteca de puerco con la vegetal, y la carne con verduras frescas, tales como calabacitas o elote. Por supuesto, siempre hay una pila de tamales que contienen chiles y otra de los que no los tienen.

Mi hermana Rosa Linda y su familia hacen entre veinte y veinticinco docenas de tamales cada año para la Navidad; guarda algunos en el congelador y los vuelve a calentar cuando llegan de visita los amigos o parientes. Sus tamales son más grandes y contienen más carne que lo normal. Ha aprendido ciertas reglas generales sobre el proceso de hacer tamales. Según dice, ella utiliza una libra de carne para hacer una docena de tamales. Para cada libra de masa, ella usa una cucharadita de sal y una de chile colorado en polvo y ½ cucharadita de paprika. Nunca permite que el agua toque los tamales cuando se están cociendo. Ya no hace todas las veinte docenas en un solo día como solía hacerlo antes, sino que los completa en dos días. Prepara toda la carne el primer día y hace una tanda el primer día, y la otra al día siguiente.

La mayoría de las familias hispanas que yo conozco no harán el esfuerzo de hacer tamales a menos que hagan suficientes para congelar. Por lo mismo, las siguientes recetas son para grandes cantidades. En la primera receta, se pueden dividir todos los ingredientes por la mitad para hacer entre 10 y 12 docenas, o por cinco para hacer cinco docenas. La segunda receta utiliza chiles secos y remojados que se licuan en la licuadora, en lugar del chile colorado en polvo, y los tamales se colocan parados en lugar de acostados.

Receta para hacer entre veinte y veinticinco docenas de tamales

- 10 libras de asado de puerco
- 10 libras de asado de res
- 5 cucharaditas de sal (o al gusto)
- 2 a 3 tazas de agua
- 1 taza de manteca de puerco para cada olla
- ½ taza de harina (2 cucharadas grandes para servir la comida) para cada olla
- 3 tazas de agua caliente para cada olla
- 3 cucharaditas de sal para cada olla
- 2 cucharaditas de pimienta para cada olla
- 2 onzas de chile colorado en polvo (Gebhardt) con especias, para cada olla
- 2 cucharadas soperas de paprika para cada olla
- 2 cucharadas soperas de cominos para cada olla
- 4 cabezas de ajo, en trozos pequeños, para cada olla
- ⅓ del caldo de res para cada olla

  chile colorado en polvo (opcional, al gusto)

La carne

Precaliente el horno a 350 grados. Corte el asado en trozos de una libra. Coloque los asados de puerco y de res juntos en una fuente de horno grande (suficientemente grande para un pavo de veinte libras). Añada sal y agua y hornee por tres horas. Voltee el asado y hornee por otra hora, hasta que esté muy tierno. Luego apague el horno y déjelo hervir lentamente por treinta minutos. Desmenuce y mezcle la carne de los dos asados. Aparte más o menos dos tercios del caldo de la carne para mezclar con la carne y un tercio para mezclar con la masa.

En dos ollas grandes de hierro grueso, de 5 litros de capacidad, ponga la manteca de puerco y caliéntela sobre fuego lento hasta que derrita. Añada harina a cada olla, removiéndola hasta que se dore. Añada agua a cada olla para hacer una salsa espesa, removiéndola y rascando el fondo con la espátula, hasta que comience a hervir. Añada la sal, pimienta, chile colorado en polvo Gebhardt, paprika, cominos, y ajo, y cocine a fuego lento por treinta minutos. Añada un tercio del caldo de carne a cada olla mientras está hirviendo. Si se pone demasiado espesa, añada un poco más de agua y hierva a fuego lento por diez minutos más. Añada sal si es necesario. Añada la carne a la salsa, poco a poco, removiéndola constantemente. No deje de remover con la espátula, o se pegará en el fondo. Añada agua si es necesario. Baje más el calor y deje hervir suavemente por entre veinte y treinta minutos. Apague el fuego y déjela enfriar, removiéndola cada quince minutos hasta que se enfríe lo suficiente para tocar la olla con las manos. Luego meta las ollas en el refrigerador toda la noche, con la tapadera ligeramente abierta. Saque una olla a la vez cuando la masa y las hojas están listas.

La masa

20	libras de masa preparada para tamales
4	libras de manteca de puerco
⅓	del caldo de res
10	cucharaditas de sal
10	cucharaditas de chile colorado en polvo (de un sobre)
5	cucharaditas de paprika

Derrita la manteca de puerco y deje enfriar. En un recipiente grande, mezcle la masa con la manteca a temperatura ambiental, poco a poco con la mano hasta que quede bien mezclada—aproximadamente de treinta minutos a una hora. Añada el resto del caldo de res, sal, chile colorado en polvo y paprika a la masa a la mitad del proceso. Cuando ya está bien mezclada la masa, dibuje una raya por la mitad de la masa para designar la porción que se usará para la mitad de la carne, como manera de orientarse.

Limpie las hojas y extienda la masa

Quite todas las barbas del maíz de las hojas. Justo antes de extender la masa, enjuague las hojas dos veces y remójelas por treinta minutos en agua limpia y tibia, aproximadamente seis a ocho docenas a la vez. Saque una hoja a la vez y colóquela en la mano con la punta hacia arriba. Extienda una cucharada sopera de masa en el lado liso de la hoja. Extienda del centro hacia afuera, mientras voltee la hoja, hasta cubrir uniformemente los dos tercios inferiores de la hoja. NO le ponga masa al tercio de la hoja donde está la punta. Ponga una cucharada sopera de carne preparada en el centro de la masa, y use los dedos para formar una tira de carne por el centro. Doble un tercio de la hoja para cubrir la carne. Doble el otro tercio. Con el dedo, aplane un poco el tamal y doble la punta de la hoja para cubrir las otras partes dobladas. Póngalo a un lado con la parte doblada hacia abajo. Haga tandas de cinco docenas antes de colocarlos en la olla.

Cocine los tamales

En una olla con capacidad de 5 galones, con una rejilla de alambre, cubra la rejilla con hojas, dejando una apertura de dos pulgadas en el centro y una apertura continua de una pulgada por las orillas de la olla para permitir que suba el vapor para cocinar los tamales. Coloque los tamales acostados, con la parte doblada hacia abajo y la parte abierta hacia el lado opuesto del centro. Deje la parte doblada hacia el centro. Deje una apertura de ¼ pulgada entre cada tamal, trabajando en un círculo, dejando el centro abierto. Se comienza la segunda capa al colocar un tamal encima de una de las aperturas de ¼ pulgada en la primera capa, de nuevo dejando una apertura de ¼ pulgada entre los tamales y colocándolos con la parte doblada hacia abajo. Siga este proceso hasta completar el círculo, dejando el centro abierto. Continúe hasta colocar las cinco docenas. Añada más o menos seis tazas de agua, suficiente para tener ¾ pulgada de agua en el fondo de la olla. Cubra y cocine por una hora y quince minutos a fuego medio. Para permitir que se escape lentamente el vapor, cubra dos tercios de la orilla con papel aluminio. Saque la docena y media que están encima y ya cocidos, añada otra taza de agua y deje que el resto se cueza por otros treinta minutos para asegurar que los tamales en el centro queden bien cocidos. Repita el mismo proceso para cada cinco docenas de tamales. Cuando abre el tamal, déjelo por un minuto y luego saque la hoja. Si el tamal cocido no se pega a la hoja y se resbala fácilmente, está bien cocido. Si el tamal tiene manchas blancas de masa, necesita cocerse un poco más. Buen provecho.

Otra manera de hacer los tamales
Para hacer 14 docenas

La carne
7   libras de carne de puerco para asar
5   dientes de ajo
2   cucharaditas de sal
    suficiente agua para cubrir la carne (guarde el caldo para usar en la masa)

Ponga la carne en una asadera grande de tres litros de capacidad y añada agua. Añada los dientes de ajo y sal y cocine por 2 horas a fuego medio, o hasta que esté bien cocida y tierna. Saque la carne y aparte cuatro tazas de caldo. Desmenuce la carne.

El chile

15 ó 16 de chile colorado
agua caliente
1 cucharadita de comino
4 dientes de ajo

Remoje los chiles en agua caliente por una hora. Deseche los tallos y las semillas. Llene la licuadora hasta la mitad con los chiles, añada una taza de agua y licue. Repita este proceso hasta licuar todos los chiles. Licue el comino y los dientes de ajo con la primera tanda de chiles. Ponga cada tanda en un tazón y revuelva bien. Añada la carne desmenuzada y mezcle. Deje que hierva y luego apague el fuego.

La masa

3 libras de manteca de puerco (a temperatura ambiental)
1½ cucharaditas de polvo de hornear
10 libras de masa de maíz, ya preparada
2 cucharadas soperas de sal
4 tazas del caldo de puerco tibio

Con una batidora eléctrica, en un recipiente grande, mezcle la manteca y el polvo de hornear por 30 minutos, hasta que esté esponjosa la manteca. Por tandas, añada la masa y el caldo tibio poco a poco, y mezcle con la mano hasta que esté lista. (Llene un vaso con agua fría y meta un trocito de masa al agua. Si sube la masa hasta arriba, está lista.) Añada la sal.

Remoje las hojas para 14 docenas de tamales

Remoje en agua caliente toda la noche. Enjuague las hojas, asegurando quitarles todas las barbas del maíz. También puede limpiar las hojas justo antes de hacer los tamales, pero asegúrese que se hayan enfriado antes de usar.

Extienda la masa

Coloque una hoja en la mano con la punta hacia afuera. Extienda una cucharada sopera de masa en la hoja. Extienda de lado a lado en forma rectangular, asegurando dejar una margen de ¼ de pulgada, a los lados y abajo, sin masa. NO ponga masa en la punta superior de la hoja. Coloque una cucharada sopera de la mezcla de carne con chile en el centro de la masa. Doble los lados de la hoja en tercios, para cubrir la masa, luego doble el punto superior hasta la mitad, hacia abajo.

Cocine los tamales

En una olla de 5 galones de capacidad, coloque suficientes hojas para cubrir el fondo. Coloque una rejilla de alambre encima de las hojas. Añada 4 tazas de agua. Pare los tamales encima de la rejilla, con la punta abierta hacia arriba. Comience en el centro y dé vueltas hasta terminar (no deje que se queden tumbados). Coloque hojas encima de los tamales y luego dos estopillas (telas) para contener el vapor. Cubra la olla y cocine a fuego alto por la primera ½ hora, y luego baje el fuego y cocine a fuego medio por 45 minutos. Apague el fuego y mantenga cubierta la olla por lo menos 30 minutos más. Si el tamal se resbala fácilmente de la hoja, está cocido. Rinde 14 docenas.

Empanadas de calabaza fresca

El relleno
una calabaza de tamaño mediano, de 7 a 10 libras, para hacer 1¾ tazas de calabaza cocida
2   tazas de azúcar moreno
1   cucharadita de canela
1   cucharadita de clavos molidos
1   pizca de sal

La masa
1   paquete de 4 onzas de semillas de anís, ó ¼ taza
2½ tazas de agua
7½ tazas de harina

2½ tazas de mantequilla o margarina
½   taza de azúcar
1   cucharada sopera de sal

Precaliente el horno a 375 grados. Lave la calabaza por fuera primero. Después de sacar las semillas, corte la calabaza en pedazos de 5"x 3". Coloque en una olla grande, con la cáscara hacia arriba, y cubra con agua. Deje hervir y luego cocine a fuego lento hasta que esté cocida. Quite del fuego y deje que se enfríe. Quite la cáscara al sacar la calabaza con una cuchara y colocarla en una olla. Haga puré la calabaza. Añada el azúcar moreno, la canela, los clavos y la sal. Cocine la mezcla hasta que se mire pastosa. Póngala a un lado.

Para la masa, hierva el anís en agua por varios minutos. Quite del fuego y aparte a un lado. Mezcle la harina, la mantequilla o margarina, el azúcar, y la sal. Añada poco a poco el té de anís a la mezcla de harina y amase hasta que tenga una consistencia firme. Forme bolitas de 2 pulgadas y estírelas a un grosor de ¼ pulgada. O bien, estire toda la masa hasta que tenga un grosor de ¼ pulgada y corte círculos de 3 pulgadas. Ponga una cucharada sopera de relleno en el círculo, pero un poco descentrado. Doble a la mitad, cubriendo el relleno, selle las orillas con un tenedor, y píquela tres veces con el mismo. Colóquelas en una bandeja de horno sin engrasar y hornéelas por 20 a 25 minutos o hasta que se doren. La receta rinde alrededor de 25 empanadas.

Empanadas fáciles de hacer

El relleno
1   taza de calabaza
⅔   taza de azúcar
1   cucharada sopera de semillas de anís
1   cucharada sopera de trozos de canela finamente molidos

La masa
⅔   taza de agua
2   cucharadas soperas de azúcar
½   cucharadita de sal
1   ó 2 pizcas de trozos de canela finamente molidos
1¼ tazas de manteca vegetal
1   gota de colorante vegetal amarillo

3½ tazas de harina
2 cucharaditas de polvo de hornear

Precaliente el horno a 375 grados. Mezcle los ingredientes para el relleno hasta que se disuelva el azúcar. No cocine la mezcla. En un tazón mezcle el agua, el azúcar, la sal, los trozos de canela molidos, la manteca vegetal, y el colorante vegetal. En otro tazón mezcle la harina y el polvo de hornear, y después añada a la mezcla. Mezcle para formar una masa. Si se siente pegajosa, añada más harina. Evite mezclar de más. Corte para formar bolas un poco más grandes que una bola de golf. Estire y coloque el relleno en el centro del círculo, doble y selle con un tenedor. Hornee por 20 a 25 minutos.

▼▲▼▲▼▲▼▲▼▲▼▲▼▲▼▲▼▲▼▲▼▲▼▲▼▲▼▲▼▲▼

Tenemos la tradición en nuestra familia de disfrazar a algún miembro de la familia como Papá Noel, o Santa Claus, para repartir los regalos navideños. Al ser traídos los niños enfrente del árbol de Navidad, mi hermana Susie y yo, las dos maestras de escuela, dirigimos a los niños para cantar canciones navideñas tales como "Feliz Navidad" y "Noche de paz". También cantamos *Jingle Bells,* "Frosty the Snowman", y *Santa Claus Is Coming to Town*". Al escuchar su pie de entrada, al final de esta canción, Papá Noel baja las escaleras con su barba blanca, la cual a veces revela su bigote negro, y su barriga rellena y desproporcionada. Se sienta en su silla mecedora especial al lado del árbol de Navidad, y se une a los niños emocionados para cantar una o dos canciones navideñas antes de distribuir los regalos. Los niños muy pequeños están cautivados por este personaje, mientras tratan de descifrar si es verdadero. Los niños mayores generalmente siguen la corriente. Cada año los adultos esperamos ilusionadamente el momento de ver a la novia o esposa de Santa Claus sentarse en su regazo para recibir su regalo, en adición a su beso, claro.

Luego viene el final, el momento cuando algunos niños "suben al escenario" para demostrar sus talentos musicales. Tenemos a Iris, quien cada año canta canciones de Selena. Otros años hemos sido entretenidos por Sal, Monica, y Marisa, quienes han tocado el piano; René, el violín; Tony y Miguel, la guitarra; y Steven, el acordeón. Si sus niños tienen algún talento musical especial, hágalos sentirse importantes al pedirles tocar sus instrumentos, cantar una canción, o representar un papel en alguna festividad navideña.

Requiere de tanta preparación y esfuerzo producir la aparentemente perfecta y memorable celebración navideña. Es importante que todos los miembros de la familia cooperen y cumplan su parte. Sin embargo, en muchos hogares, las mujeres de la familia todavía hacen más que les corresponde de la limpieza y preparación de comida, con poca ayuda de los hombres. Es importante que todos los miembros de la familia cumplan con su parte de crear momentos encantadores. Sin embargo, me doy cuenta de que si algunas mujeres no están determinadas ni dispuestas a mantener vivas ciertas tradiciones, éstas seguramente van a desaparecer. Es muy cierto cuando la gente dice que *la mujer hace el hogar*. Ella es el pegamento que mantiene unida la familia.

Los Pastores

Los Pastores es una obra popular religiosa que originó en el doceavo siglo en Europa, y los misioneros españoles la trajeron al Nuevo Mundo como una manera de cristianizar a la gente indígena. Ya que los españoles no hablaban el mismo idioma que los indios, trataban de enseñar muchas de sus creencias religiosas a través de drama popular y tradiciones. El drama del nacimiento de Jesús, basado en una versión en Lucas 2, todavía se mantiene vivo en la actualidad. Esta obra sobre pastores, en parte comedia, está realizada por hispanos en los patios de sus casas, las iglesias, y los patios comunitarios durante el mes de diciembre y la primera parte de enero. Estos personajes incluyen a un ermitaño, un anciano espiritual con una barba blanca quien lleva un rosario y una cruz, varios demonios, San Miguel el Arcángel, y algunos pastores. El tema gira alrededor de los demonios que vienen al mundo terrenal para atacar a los hombres mientras Jesús todavía es un bebé. Al final, prevalece el bien.

La obra comienza con un ángel de Dios que les dice a los pastores las *buenas noticias* del nacimiento de Cristo. Los pastores se alegran mucho y se ponen en marcha para ir a ver al niño Jesús en el pesebre. Uno de los pastores se encuentra con un ermitaño anciano y le dice que ha llegado el Mesías. El pastor invita al ermitaño anciano a su campamento para informar a los demás acerca del Mesías. Allí encuentran a los pastores riñendo y discutiendo, especialmente una pareja de casados. Los demonios se le aparecen a uno de los pastores que se había alejado del campamento. Asustado, vuelve corriendo al campamento para contarles a los otros sobre los demonios. El complot de los demonios en contra de los hombres comienza cuando tientan al ermitaño a secuestrar a una de las pastoras. Mientras los pastores están golpeando al ermitaño, el Arcángel San Miguel lucha contra los demonios y los manda de vuelta al infierno. La obra culmina con la representación del nacimiento de Cristo, una canción de cuna, y una despedida. Si no se encuentra esta celebración en su comunidad, vaya a la tienda de vídeos y rente el vídeo de Linda Ronstadt y Los Lobos, titulado *Los pastores*. Ha llegado a ser un clásico, y que ponen al aire cada año en PBS durante la temporada navideña. Una canción tradicional sobre los pastores es "Amigos pastores".

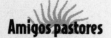

Amigos pastores

Amigos pastores, es tiempo de ver
a la Virgen Pura y al Niño también.
Venid, venid, venid a Belén.
Venid, venid, venid a Belén.

Amigos pastores, vamos a Belén,
ha nacido un Niño llamado Emmanuel.
Venid, venid, venid a Belén.
Venid, venid, venid a Belén.

Los Tres Reyes Magos

En algunas familias hispanas, especialmente entre los puertorriqueños, el día de los Tres Reyes Magos, el cual cae en el 6 de enero, doce días después del nacimiento de Cristo, se celebra tan fielmente como la Navidad. Y no es de sorprenderse. Este día conmemora el día cuando los Tres Reyes Magos siguieron la brillante estrella del norte hasta llegar a un pesebre en Belén para traerle regalos al niñito Jesús, el Mesías. Este día también es llamado el día de la Epifanía. Para los hispanos, esta historia se ha transformada en una tradición que se convierte en un día de más regalos y lecciones para los niños después de la Navidad. Los miembros de la familia esperan para hacer el intercambio de regalos, unos a otros, y los niños reciben hasta tres regalos especiales de los Reyes "visitantes", en muchos sentidos, igual a como los niños americanos reciben de Santa Claus.

El 5 de enero, mande a sus niños a poner paja para los camellos, en botas o zapatos que dejan afuera de su puerta o debajo de su cama.

Dígales que pongan un vaso de agua y frutas para los Reyes. Durante la noche, reemplácelos con golosinas que a ellos les gustan. Cuando los niños se despiertan, encontrarán que la paja, el agua, y las frutas se han desaparecido, y en las botas o zapatos encontrarán regalos y golosinas.

Los padres deben intentar hacer de esto un día alegre para sus niños, al mismo tiempo de enseñarles su verdadero significado religioso. En México, éste es el día en que la madrina, la que meció al niño Jesús en Nochebuena, tiene el honor de "levantar" al niño del pesebre, y lo viste como al *Niño de las Palomas* y el *Niño de Atocha* para ser bautizado en una iglesia. Algunos visten con esplendidez al niño con un extravagante faldón bautismal, un largo y hermoso vestido blanco, hecho de encaje. En el tercer año de la madrina, el bebé es coronado con una corona de rey y una capa. El Santo Niño, recién bautizado, se trae de vuelta de la iglesia y se coloca en una silla especial o en un altar donde permanece hasta el 2 de febrero, cuando es guardado y oficialmente termina la temporada navideña. Personas de México que han emigrado a los Estados Unidos se han traído esta tradición y la han enseñado a otros. "Las mañanitas" se cantan al levantar al Niño. En lugar de llevar al Niño a la iglesia, quizá pueda invitar al padre a su hogar para dirigir a un grupo de personas en la recitación del rosario y para oficiar durante la ceremonia de levantar al Niño. Quizá solamente quiera construir o comprar una silla especial y otorgarle el privilegio a uno de sus niños, de colocar al Niño en su sitio de honor.

Entre algunos México-americanos, el día de los Tres Reyes se celebra con la familia o con los vecinos, y con champurrado, un atole hecho de harina de maíz, canela, azúcar, chocolate y leche, o agua de horchata, la cual se hace con agua de arroz, leche, canela, y vainilla. A veces, entre los puertorriqueños, el acontecimiento incluye una gran comida con un festín de pasteles, arroz con grandules, lechón asado, y tostones (plátanos machos fritos). Pruebe estas recetas con sus niños en un día lluvioso y frío.

Champurrado

2   tazas de Masa Harina de Maíz de Quaker
4   tazas de leche
4   cuadros de chocolate mexicano, de una onza cada uno
1   cucharadita de azúcar
1   palito de canela

En un tazón grande mezcle la masa harina con la leche, utilizando las manos para desbaratar los grumos y disolver completamente. Añada el azúcar y vierta la mezcla a una olla de 5 litros de capacidad. Cocine a fuego bajo por 15 minutos. Cuando comienza a hervir, añada los cuadros de chocolate, revolviendo constantemente para que no se pegue en el fondo. Añada leche al gusto. Si le gusta espeso, añada poca leche, o quizá nada. La receta rinde seis tazas.

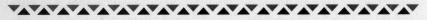

Se les puede cantar la siguiente canción "Chocolate" a sus niños mientras está preparando el champurrado.

Chocolate

¡Uno, dos, tres–cho!
¡Uno, dos, tres–co!
¡Uno, do tres–la! ¡Uno, dos, tres–te!
(Frótese las manos como si estuviera usando un molinillo.)
¡Cho–co–late, cho–co–late!
¡Bate, bate el cho–co–late!

Champurrado
Variación

  2 tazas de harina de maíz
8½ tazas de agua
  1 trozo de canela
  1 taza de leche
  1 taza de azúcar

Ponga la harina de maíz en una cacerola grande. Añada 1½ tazas de agua, amasando hasta conseguir una consistencia firme. En una olla grande, ponga a hervir 5 tazas de agua y el trozo de canela. Vierta las 2 tazas restantes de agua fría en un pequeño tazón. Separe la masa en pequeños pedazos y échelos al agua fría para disolverlos. Vierta lentamente la mezcla de masa disuelta, a través del colador, adentro del agua hirviendo con canela, revolviendo constantemente hasta que se espese ligeramente—alrededor de 30 minutos. Quite del fuego y añada la leche y el azúcar; revuelva. Vuelva al fuego y deje hervir a fuego lento antes de servirlo. (Para hacer el champurrado de chocolate, sustituya 1 taza de azúcar moreno por la de azúcar blanco, y añada tres cuadros de 1 onza de chocolate sin azúcar.) Rinde 12 tazas.

Algunas personas sirven un pan de Tres Reyes, el cual es llamado Rosca de Reyes por algunos hispanos y Marzán por otros. Este pastel de rosca está adornado con joyas confeccionadas de fruta seca y cerezas frescas en la forma de una corona y con un pequeñito niño Jesús hecho de porcelana, horneado dentro del pastel. Permita que sus niños ayuden a adornar el pastel o poner al muñequito adentro del pastel al hacer una corte en el costado y empujarlo para adentro. Luego cubra la corte con el glaseado.

Pan de Rosca de Reyes

2	sobres de levadura
½	taza de agua tibia
2	barras de mantequilla sin sal
½	taza de azúcar
4	huevos ó 6 yemas de huevo
½	cucharadita de sal
5	tazas de harina
1	taza de fruta confitada
½	taza de nueces picadas
½	taza de pasas
2	pequeños muñequitos que no se derretirán
1	huevo
1	cucharada sopera de agua

Glaseado

4	cucharadas soperas de mantequilla sin sal
½	taza de azúcar
	o
½	taza de jugo de naranja
2	tazas de azúcar glas

En un tazón grande, disuelva la levadura en agua. Derrita la mantequilla y deje enfriarse. Mezcle la mantequilla, la sal, el azúcar, los huevos o yemas de huevo, ligeramente batidos, y la mezcla de levadura, y bata todo bien. Añada 3 tazas de harina y bata otra vez. Poco a poco, añada el resto de la harina hasta que tenga una consistencia firme, y no pegajosa. Amase en una tabla enharinada, añadiendo un poco más de harina hasta que tenga elasticidad. Cubra y deje que la masa se levante hasta el doble de su tamaño, alrededor de 1½ horas. Desinfle la masa en una superficie enharinada y divida en dos porciones para hacer dos panes. Separe las frutas confitadas, las pasas, y las nueces en dos mitades y distribúyalas a cada masa. (Aparte un poco de cada uno para decorar los panes al final.) Estire la masa y una las puntas de cada una, para formar dos ruedas gruesas. Empuje un muñequito adentro de cada pan.* Ponga cada rosca en una bandeja de horno engrasada con mantequilla. Cubra los panes y déjelos levantarse por una hora. Justo antes de hornearlos, pinte la masa con huevo batido que hará al mezclar 1 huevo ligeramente batido con 1 cucharada sopera de agua. Coloque las roscas en el horno previamente calentado a 375 grados, por 30 minutos o hasta que se dore. Prepare un glaseado al mezclar la mantequilla con el azúcar, o bien, al mezclar el jugo de naranja con el azúcar glas. Vierta el glaseado en el pan mientras esté caliente y adorne con las nueces, las pasas, y la fruta confitada que usted apartó.

*Se puede meter el muñeco adentro del pan después de hornearlo al cortarle una raya y luego adornar encima para taparla.

Un miembro de cada familia corta el pan en porciones iguales. Si no se encuentra al niño Jesús, entonces el miembro mayor de la familia sigue cortando hasta que se encuentre. La persona que encuentra al bebé en el pastel es la madrina o el padrino y se dice que tendrá buena suerte por el resto del año. Esa persona viste al pequeño bebé de porcelana que se encontró dentro de la rosca, en una vestidura blanca hecha de tela o papel de seda. La persona que encuentra al niño Jesús es responsable de llevar a cabo otra celebración en su hogar cuarenta días más tarde, el 2 de febrero, fecha también conocida como la Candelaria. Esta tradición es semejante a la cuarentena, una tradición observada por mujeres hispanas que se quedan en cama por cuarenta días después del nacimiento de un niño. Esta tradición quizá haya originado de la Fiesta de Presentación que se celebra el 2 de febrero, y que tiene como significado los cuarenta días que María tuvo que esperar hasta poder presentar a Jesús al Señor del Templo. De acuerdo a la ley de Moisés, a la mujer judía que diera a luz a un hijo varón, no se le permitía tocar nada sagrado ni entrar al templo hasta cuarenta días después del nacimiento, ya que para esa fecha se ha purificada del flujo de sangre (Lev. 12, 2–8).

Entre los puertorriqueños, el día de los Reyes Magos también se celebra con parrandas, cuando un grupo de personas va a los hogares de otros cantando aguinaldos. Los aguinaldos son unas canciones que frecuentemente son improvisadas espontáneamente al tomar coquito (ponche de huevo, rompope), u otras bebidas de días festivos. Mi amiga puertorriqueña, Isaura Santiago Santiago, compartió conmigo dos de estos versos improvisados.

Si me dan pasteles, dénmelos calientes
Pues pasteles fríos empachan a la gente.

De las montañas venimos a invitarles
A comer ese lechoncito en su barra
Y Don Pitorro* a beber.

*ron casero

La segunda se canta con la misma melodía que la tradicional canción navideña americana *"We Three Kings"*.

Los Reyes de Oriente

Reyes de Oriente son,
Van en busca de Jesús,
Por la tierra van guiados
Por una estrella.

O bella es la santa luz,
la maravillosa luz
Que los guía al pesebre
Del divino Rey Jesús

Día de los Muertos

El día de los Muertos es otra tradición que es celebrada por los latinos a través de los Estados Unidos y Latinoamérica. Con sus raíces en épocas antiguas en Mesoamérica, la tradición evolucionó simultáneamente con *All Saints Day* y *All Souls Day*, ambos de los cuales son celebrados en muchos países. Igual que los aztecas, los españoles creían que se debe mostrar respeto por los muertos. Ellos creían en el continuo entre la vida y la muerte y que, una vez al año, los espíritus de los muertos se unen a los vivos. En Puerto Rico, la tradición española se combinó con las tradiciones de los indios taínos del Caribe, y el resultado fue el día de los muertos. Los indios taínos creían que cuando los espíritus familiares se unían a los vivos, ellos volvían a visitar aquellas cosas de las cuales disfrutaron cuando estuvieron vivos.

El día de los Muertos se celebra dos veces. Primero, en el 1 de noviembre los seres queridos van al cementerio para recordar a los niños pequeños que fallecieron, y el día se llama día de los Angelitos. El siguiente día, el 2 de noviembre, es reservado para seres queridos que eran adultos cuando fallecieron. El día festivo proporciona una extensión más cultural y menos comercializada de las festividades del día de Todos los Santos (*Halloween*). La tradición del día de los Muertos ayuda a los hispanos a enfrentarse a la muerte y aceptarla como una parte natural de la vida. Enseña que la muerte no es una tragedia ni algo a que temer, sino una parte de nuestro viaje a la próxima etapa de vida. Es el punto en que el mundo de los vivos y el mundo de los muertos se cruzan en un festival de cosas dignas de verse y sonidos. El rito del día de los Muertos nos une con los espíritus de nuestros antepasados y con los espíritus de aquéllos que amamos. Se dice que el valor de la vida de una persona se puede determinar por su muerte, y que la ocasión que marca su fallecimiento mantiene viva a esa persona. Los niños que participan en este rito observan la importancia de la vida de esa persona y aprenden cómo una vida puede tocar a muchas otras. Les enseña a ser compasivos y a honrar a los vivos, tal como uno debe honrar a los muertos. Los niños también aprenden que la gente posee valor. Los hace reflejarse sobre cómo les gustaría ser recordados después de fallecer, y lucharán por vivir su vida de acuerdo a eso.

En el día de los Muertos, un colorido altar llamado *ofrenda*, se construye en cierta sección de la casa donde las fotos de todos los familiares y personas estimadas que han fallecido están colocadas, junto a votivos y un incensario. Un arco encima del altar hecho de carrizo o plástico maleable está cubierto de caléndulas. La caléndula (o *cempasúchil*) es la flor de la muerte. Se cree que con su aroma fuerte y su brillante color anaranjado, la flor ayudará a los espíritus a encontrar su camino a casa. Al lado de las fotos, se colocan objetos en el altar que ilustran la vida de una persona, tal como una guitarra, un juguete, o alguna prenda de vestir. El año en que falleció Selena, la cantante de música tejana, se construyeron altares a través de México y los Estado Unidos en recuerdo a ella. En Texas, una familia adornó un altar con unos aretes grandes, un bote de Coca-Cola y una hamburguesa de What-A-Burger, todos los cuales a ella le encantaban. Quizá usted quiera construirle un altar a alguien especial a quien admiraba o a algún pariente a quien amaba verdaderamente y que ya no se encuentra entre los vivos, tal como un abuelito o una abuelita que falleció. Ésta es una forma especial de hacer una conexión entre sus niños y sus antepasados.

En el altar, uno también puede encontrar coloridas calaveras, con los nombres de los muertos escritos en la frente, al lado de ataúdes de chocolate. Junto al altar, las familias colocan coloridas calaveras, esqueletos, y brillantes flores hechas de papel de seda. Añaden máscaras de papel majado y papel picado de bellos diseños geométricos. Una ofrenda no estaría completa sin un pan de muerto, un pan grande y redondo, el cual a veces tiene forma de persona. A lo siguiente está una receta para hacer este delicioso pan que le hace a uno agua la boca. Los padres y los niños se pueden entretener y divertir adornando el pan con azúcar de colores espolvoreado o con calaveras hechas de glaseado.

Pan de muerto

½ taza de mantequilla
½ taza de leche
½ taza de agua
5 a 5½ tazas de harina
2 sobres de levadura seca (½ onza cada uno)
1 cucharadita de sal
1 cucharada sopera de semillas enteras de anís
½ taza de azúcar
4 huevos

Mezcla de huevo
1 huevo
1 cucharada sopera de agua

Glaseado
4 cucharadas soperas de mantequilla sin sal
½ taza de azúcar

En una cacerola, caliente la mantequilla, la leche, y el agua hasta que estén calientes. En un tazón muy grande, mezcle 4 tazas de la harina, la levadura, la sal, las semillas de anís, y el azúcar. Añada el líquido caliente, batiendo hasta mezclarse bien. Añada los huevos y otra taza de harina, batiendo bien. Continúe añadiendo más harina hasta que la masa esté suave y no pegajosa. Amase en una tabla ligeramente enharinada por diez minutos hasta que esté suave y elástica. Coloque la masa en un tazón ligeramente engrasado, cubra la masa, y deje reposar hasta que crezca al doble de tomaño.

Corte la masa en dos porciones que se parezcan a personas, calaveras, o simplemente redondas. Separe un pedazo de masa, aplánela y dele vuelta con las manos hasta que tenga forma de una cuerda y úsela para formar una calavera en el centro del pan redondo. Cubra el pan y deje que se levante, por una hora.

Bata ligeramente un huevo con 1 cucharada sopera de agua. Pinte la masa con esta mezcla justo antes de hornearlo. Engrase ligeramente con mantequilla unas bandejas de horno y hornee los panes en un horno previamente calentado a 350 grados, por 30 a 40 minutos, o hasta que se doren. También puede dejar que sus niños adornen los panes después de que se enfríen, con el glaseado que se hace al mezclar 4 cucharadas soperas de mantequilla derretida con ½ taza de azúcar.

La gente celebra el día de los Muertos de diferentes maneras a través de los Estados Unidos. La visita al panteón es quizá el rito más elaborado. En comunidades hispanas a través de América, estos ritos se pueden convertir en eventos organizados de la comunidad que dan participación a la iglesia, o bien pueden ser ocasiones privadas para la familia solamente. Lleve a sus niños al panteón el 1 de noviembre, a rezar por los angelitos que fallecieron. Limpie sus tumbas y lápidas y coloque flores frescas y velas o votivos. Tal como en la época de los aztecas, las tumbas se pueden adornar con flores blancas para los niños y caléndulas amarillas o anaranjadas para los adultos. A veces se forman cruces en las tumbas, utilizando los pétalos de las caléndulas. En el 2 de noviembre, lleve a su familia al panteón a rezar, cantar, y comer los platillos y alimentos favoritos de los adultos que han fallecido, y platicar acerca de lo especiales que fueron sus vidas. En México y América Central, se encuentran muchísimas familias haciendo vigilias en el panteón, para los muertos, que duran toda la noche. El día de los Muertos es una ocasión para reunir a amigos y familiares, jóvenes y ancianos, para inculcar un sentido de cultura, espiritualidad, y continuidad.

En algunas comunidades, especialmente aquéllas al lado de la frontera con México, son comunes los acontecimientos elaborados con grandes grupos de personas en el día de los Muertos. La gente se encuentra enfrente del panteón con máscaras de papel maché, instrumentos musicales tales como cascabeles, tambores, y guitarras, además de incensarios y grandes coronas cubiertas de caléndulas, representando a los parientes que han fallecido. Los que participan en la procesión se visten como la muerte, lucen máscaras coloridas, y sostienen un arco de flores del altar. A veces cargan un ataúd con un esqueleto de mentiras que se levanta como resorte y saluda con la mano, como burlándose de la muerte. Con las caras volteadas hacia el norte, rezan por los ancianos; hacia el oeste, honran a las mujeres; hacia el sur, rezan por los angelitos, los niños pequeños y bebés; y hacia el este, rezan por los hombres, especialmente los hombres, padres, hijos, y aun abuelos que han muerto en alguna guerra. Se pueden encontrar a mariachis en los panteones, dándoles serenata a los espíritus de los que han fallecido. Una persona hace sonar una concha en honor a los espíritus. Luego la gente esparce pétalos de caléndulas por el camino, desde el panteón hasta el altar de su casa. Una vez que vuelvan a su casa, cuelgan la corona de caléndulas en la pared y participan en rezos y luego en un gran festín, en recuerdo a los que han fallecido. También se llevan a cabo misas para los que han fallecido, y, tal como en épocas antiguas, los Matachines y los Concheros bailan danzas rituales, luciendo brillantes y coloridos disfraces con tocados de plumas y cascabeles en los tobillos. Quizá pueda convencer a su iglesia a organizar un evento así para su comunidad.

Día de Pascua

La temporada de Pascua, en algunas partes de Latinoamérica, comienza con una semana de carnavales, desfiles, música, disfraces, fuegos artificiales, y una gran cantidad de comida, antes del período de cuarenta días que compone la Cuaresma. Comienza con cenizas en miércoles de cenizas. Durante este período de cuarenta días, las personas mayores de doce años de edad hacen penitencia al renunciar a algo que les gusta tal como los dulces, la carne, los refrescos, la televisión, o los vídeos. Algunas personas tal vez hagan un ayuno parcial, excluyendo los platillos tradicionales de nopalitos y albóndigas. Muchas familias participan en las tradicionales misas de Viernes Santo y Domingo de Pascua para conmemorar la muerte y resurrección de Cristo. Éste también es el momento cuando los niños, vestidos de blanco, hacen su Primera Comunión, y los niños y adultos se engalanan con sus mejores trajes.

Yo recuerdo que mi madre se pasaba los fines de semana cosiendo nuestros bellos vestidos para Pascua cuando éramos niñas. Con nuestras enaguas, sombreros, y guantes, nos sentíamos bastante especiales ese día. Si usted va a la iglesia en Domingo de Pascua, conviértalo en una gran ocasión para sus niños al endomingarlos con su mejor ropa. Ellos lo recordarán y usted también con todas esas fotografías que atesorará para siempre.

Para muchos hispanos en Texas, las festividades comienzan al volver de la iglesia, con un día de campo completo con parrillada, ensalada de papas, y capirotada. Luego organizamos la tradicional búsqueda de huevos de Pascua para los niños y una batalla de cascarones entre los adultos y niños mayores. Por semanas antes del Domingo de Pascua, guardamos las cáscaras enteras de los huevos para hacer los cascarones. Si está cocinando u horneando con huevos, corte un pequeño agujero en la punta y saque el contenido a través de esa abertura, en lugar de quebrar el huevo en dos. Enjuague las cáscaras y déjelas secar. Se pintan las cáscaras de diferentes colores pasteles, tal como se hace con los huevos de Pascua. Luego las cáscaras se llenan con confeti y se sellan con un pedazo de papel de seda de color, el cual se pone con pegamento para tapar el agujero y evitar que se tire el confeti. Algunos cascarones se convierten en obras de arte con papel de china, listones, plumas, y espumillón. Algunos se destacan con unos muy elaborados diseños artísticos geométricos de muchos colores; otros asemejan cabezas humanas, personas, o animales y se obsequian como regalos o se exponen como arte popular hispano.

Pero, el verdadero propósito de hacer y quebrar los cascarones es que es una encantadora y divertida tradición. Nada se puede comparar con la risa y la sorpresa de la "víctima" de un ataque de cascarón. En nuestra familia, los adultos y los niños se persiguen alrededor del patio tratando de suavemente romper el cascarón lleno de confeti en las cabezas de los demás. Hay tanta risa y alegría para los jóvenes y para los mayores también. Nosotros celebramos esta feliz ocasión de la Resurrección del Señor con una reunión de la familia extensa que siempre incluye risas, pláticas, comida, y juegos.

No sería Pascua sin capirotada. Mientras que la capirotada tradicional contiene principalmente el pan, queso, pasas, manzanas, y cacahuates, a mi tía Lupe le encanta añadir más ingredientes para hacerla más dulce. Algunas personas le echan tres tipos de frutos secos: cacahuates, almendras, y nueces. Puede hacer la capirotada tan dulce como desee al añadir cualquier ingrediente que su niño le pueda ayudar a picar o simplemente echar para dentro. Ambos pueden arreglar y componer cada capa o pueden turnarse. Sigue la receta para capirotada que ha estado usando la familia Rodríguez por muchas generaciones.

Capirotada

1   piloncillo, ó 1½ tazas de azúcar moreno
2   tazas de agua hirviendo
¼   cucharadita de canela en polvo ó 1 trozo de canela
½   taza de pasas
6   rebanadas de pan tostado (se pueden usar 4 tazas de pan francés, cortado en cuadritos)
1   taza de queso cheddar rallado
½   taza de piña bien picada
½   taza de manzanas, peladas y cortadas en rebanadas delgadas
½   taza de nueces, finamente picadas
½   taza de plátanos en rebanadas
½   taza de coco rallado

Disuelva el piloncillo en una cacerola pequeña, con el agua, la canela y las pasas. Aparte a un lado. En una fuente rectangular para el horno, coloque una capa de pan. Esparza el queso en el pan, luego esparza la piña, las manzanas, las pasas hervidas de la cacerola, las nueces, las rebanadas de plátano, y el coco. Vierta la mitad del líquido de piloncillo encima de los ingredientes y luego repita el proceso. Hornee, sin tapar, en un horno previamente calentado a 350 grados por 20 minutos o hasta que el pan se haya dorado ligeramente pero no está seco. Se puede comer caliente o fría.

La noche de Fin de Año

El Año Nuevo es otro día que reúne a la familia y los amigos, esta vez para despedirse del año viejo y dar la bienvenida al nuevo con diversión, risa, y alegría. Algunas personas tienen sus tradiciones de aventar un balde de agua, asegurarse de que su casa esté limpia, o asistir a fiestas de Año Nuevo. Pero para nosotros es otro día para ir a misa y celebrar después con música, fuegos artificiales, comida, y juegos, con la familia extensa. Al volver a casa de un día muy alegre y agotador, mi familia se arrodilla enfrente del árbol de Navidad. Tomados de las manos, le rezamos a Dios y le damos gracias por Sus bendiciones durante el año anterior y le pedimos que nos proteja y nos oriente durante el año venidero.

En lugar de tratar de describir el día, he incluido un pasaje de un ensayo corto que mi hijo mayor, Sal, escribió como tarea para una clase de inglés, recordando cómo su familia pasó la noche de Fin de Año cuando él tenía doce años. Como un niño de doce anos, él recuerda la excitación al reunirse familiares y amigos y sentir lo que el Señor representa: amor, paz, y alegría. Su maestra escribió en el ensayo de mi hijo: "Sal, ésta es una historia tan alentadora. Le mueve al lector a darse cuenta lo que una familia realmente significa y que tú te das cuenta de lo especial que fue crecer en la forma que creciste".

Siendo un niño de doce años de edad, no había nada que esperaba con más ganas que la noche de Fin de Año. Yo disfrutaba de la comida, la familia, la diversión, y los fuegos artificiales, pero más importante, aunque no lo sabía en ese momento, lo que verdaderamente era más significante y querido para mí, era la tradición. Todos los acontecimientos que transcurrieron ese día fueron pasados a nosotros por generaciones anteriores. Lo que yo sentía al ser un niño, y que solamente podría describir como un pequeño nudo en la garganta y un cosquilleo en el corazón, en realidad era orgullo. Estaba orgullo de mi familia, y de mi cultura.

La mañana de la noche de Fin de Año es una de caos y desorden para mi familia. "Salvador Julián Rodríguez, levántate de la cama y meta estas cosas al carro", grita mi madre al estirarme yo en mi cama. "...Steven y Vanessa, ¡apaguen la televisión y ayuden!" Mi padre siempre reunía su cámara y los rollos de fotos. Él adoraba tomar fotos, y no era poco usual que él se llevara seis o aun siete rollos de fotos para ir a alguna reunión familiar.

Ya para alrededor de las diez u once, íbamos en camino a casa de mi abuela. Su casa estaba ubicada en lo profundo del lado oeste de San Antonio. Una cosa en que me fijé sobre ese lado de la ciudad era que había tantos perros. Algunos se sentaban a mitad de la calle y no se movían, así que tuvimos que darles vuelta. Otros atacaban el carro.

Exclamaron todos al mismo tiempo: "¡Eh, miren quiénes están aquí!" Siempre éramos los últimos para llegar a cualquier reunión familiar. Eso quería decir que yo tenía que ir y saludar a todos en la casa, todos las tías, los tíos, y los primos. Debe haber habido más de cincuenta personas metidas en esa pequeña casa de tres recámaras, pero de alguna manera, todos parecían estar muy cómodos.

Después de cumplir con todas las formalidades, todos los niños varones y hombres salieron para afuera a jugar un partido de fútbol americano. Ya que teníamos suficientes jugadores para completar dos equipos, y el patio era tan pequeño, nos pusimos a jugar en la calle. La anotación se hacía de un buzón de correo a otro y cada jugador tenía su propia sección de aplausos y animadoras cuando anotaban un "touchdown", ya sean sus esposas o novias, o sus madres y hermanas. Alguien siempre se lastimaba de alguna manera, y eso generalmente significaba el fin del juego.

Más de veinte hombres cansados y agotados se fueron derechos a la cocina. Había todo tipo de comida mexicana imaginable. Había pan dulce, polvorones, bizcochitos, enchiladas, tamales, arroz, frijoles, caldo o menudo, chalupas, y mucho más. Pero lo que le enorgullecía más a mi abuela eran sus buñuelos. Ella poseía una receta de familia que se había pasado de generación en generación. Había hileras e hileras de buñuelos apilados hacia arriba en grupos de alrededor de veinte. Así que después de darnos un atracón todos, nos salimos para afuera. Se aparecieron las guitarras, las maracas, las claves, y las trompetas, y siguió la música mexicana. Todos mis tíos tocaban los instrumentos y cantaban mientras los niños y las esposas solamente nos sentábamos y escuchábamos. Sonaba de maravilla. La música siguió hasta que oscureció.

Entonces era el momento para los fuegos artificiales. Antes de que prohibieran los fuegos artificiales, todos nos subíamos en un par de carros e íbamos a las orillas de la ciudad para comprar todo tipo de fuegos artificiales imaginables, desde gatos negros a luces de Bengala, a los "especiales de medianoche". Si ha estado usted alguna vez en el lado oeste de San Antonio en Año Nuevo, pensaría que estábamos en medio de una zona de batalla. Parecía que cada casa trataba de superar a sus vecinos. ¡Bum! Yo podía sentir que el corazón dejaba de latir por un par de segundos cuando mi tío Ramiro, un veterano de la guerra de Viet Nam, hacía explotar sus pequeñas bombas caseras. A exactamente las doce de la medianoche, mi papá volvió a sacar su trompeta y tocó *Auld Lang Syne* lo más fuerte y claramente que pudo, y todos cantaron, besándose y abrazándose. Yo paré por un breve momento de prender los fuegos artificiales y simplemente miré a todos a mi alrededor. Yo escuchaba la música y los fuegos artificiales, la gente cantando, y yo sentí, sólo por un instante, que todo en el mundo era perfecto.

Los buñuelos y el menudo son indispensables en muchos hogares hispanos en la noche de Fin de Año. Sigue la receta favorita de mi suegra para los deliciosos buñuelos que todos añoramos cada noche de Fin de

Año. El secreto radica en estirarlos muy delgaditos y en tener el aceite bien caliente. Haga que participen sus niños al ponerles a espolvorear la mezcla de azúcar con canela. El dicho de *una vez al año no hace daño, una vez al mes, tal vez*, se aplica tanto al menudo como a los tamales. Ambos platillos engordan mucho, pero son tan sabrosos, y una parte íntegra de nuestras tradiciones culturales. El aroma de una olla de menudo, con todas sus especias, se puede oler escapándose de muchos hogares al pasar por los barrios en la noche de Fin de Año.

Buñuelos

3	tazas de harina
1	cucharadita de sal
¼	taza de mantequilla
¼	taza de azúcar
1	cucharada sopera de canela molida
2	huevos
3	trozos de canela
1	taza de agua
4	a 5 tazas de aceite vegetal para freír, o llene el sartén hasta una pulgada de profundidad
½	taza de azúcar mezclado con 2 cucharaditas de canela para espolvorear

En un tazón grande, cierna la harina con la sal. Añada la mantequilla, mezclando con las manos hasta que se disuelva y la mezcla sea parecida a unas migas gruesas. Con las manos, mezcle el azúcar y la canela molida a la mezcla de harina. En un tazón pequeño, bata los huevos ligeramente y revuelva con la mezcla de harina. Hierva los trozos de canela en una taza de agua por diez minutos. Añada de 5 a 6 cucharadas soperas de este agua de canela a la mezcla de harina y amase hasta formar una masa firme. Vierta la masa en una tabla ligeramente enharinada y amase hasta que esté firme y no pegajosa, añadiendo un poco más de harina o agua de canela si es necesario. Cubra la masa con una toalla de cocina húmeda y aparte a un lado por entre 20 y 30 minutos. Ponga la masa en una tabla ligeramente enharinada y forme doce bolas de dos pulgadas de diámetro cada una. Comenzando por el centro, aplane cada bola al hacer presión por las orillas, dándole vuelta con las palmas de las manos para formar una bola plana de tres pulgadas. Forme todas las bolas primero.

(Para evitar la formación de burbujas, algunas personas dejan reposar de nuevo las bolas, por veinte minutos.) Luego, con un palote de amasar, estire cada bola aplanada hasta que esté muy delgadita, elástica, y casi transparente. (También puede seguir estirando la bola aplanada utilizando las palmas de las manos como descrito antes.) Probablemente se desgarre un poco la masa durante el proceso de estirarla al punto delgado y transparente necesario. Los buñuelos necesitan freírse en bastante aceite muy caliente—de más o menos 360 a 375 grados. Pruebe el aceite para asegurar que esté suficientemente caliente al echarle un pequeño trozo de masa. Si se infla la masa, está listo. Si se queda plana, no está listo y se necesita subir el calor. Levante la masa estirada con mucho cuidado de la tabla, evitando desgarrarla más, y déjela resbalar lentamente al aceite. Deje freírse entre 10 y 15 segundos por cada lado o hasta que se dore. Sáquela del aceite con unas tenacillas o un tenedor y deje escurrir por unos cuantos segundos encima de varias servilletas y luego espolvoréelas con la mezcla de azúcar y canela. Se puede crear una "cadena de montaje" con amigos y familiares para completar la tanda de buñuelos. Mi cuñada, Dolores Garza, me dio esta receta. Ella recuerda cómo su abuela solía estirar los buñuelos sobre la rodilla para lograr hacerlos sumamente transparentes.

Menudo

2   libras de pancita (mondongo), cortada en trozos pequeños
2   libras de codillo, paletilla, o pernil de puerco, cortado en trozos
     de 2 pulgadas (opcional)
2   ó 3 patas de puerco (opcional)
     agua
1   ó 2 cucharaditas de sal (al gusto)
1   cebolla blanca o amarilla picada
3   dientes de ajo picados
2   cucharadas soperas de chile colorado en polvo
2   cucharadas soperas de orégano
2   cucharadas soperas de paprika
1   cucharadita de pimienta
1½ tazas (o una lata de 28 ó 30 onzas) de maíz blanco
     descascarillado
     rodajas de limón

> cebolla o cebolletas picadas
> tortillas de maíz calientitas

Coloque los trozos de pancita y pernil y las patas de puerco, todo bien lavado, en una olla grande de agua, más o menos cuatro pulgadas por encima de los ingredientes. Deje que hierva. Añada sal. Baje la llama. Cocine por 1½ horas. Añada la cebolla, el ajo, el chile, el orégano, la paprika, y la pimienta. Cocine por 1 hora, o hasta que la carne esté tierna. Añada el maíz descascarillado, escurrido, 30 minutos antes de estar listo y más agua y sal si es necesario para mantener suficiente caldo. El menudo se sirve caliente, con limón, cebolla, y tortillas de maíz.

CELEBRACIONES RELIGIOSAS CENTRADAS EN NUESTROS NIÑOS

El bautismo

Un bautismo es otra ocasión para celebrar un importante acontecimiento religioso en la vida de un niño. Los compadres, los cuales son parientes o buenos amigos de los padres, son escogidos por los padres para bautizar al niño ante la familia y la comunidad. Generalmente son escogidos los compadres porque los padres los quieren bien y porque son buenos modelos espirituales para el niño. Ellos se convierten en los padrinos de los niños, quienes, por tradición, compran el faldón o traje bautismal además de la vela que se debe volver a prender cada año para renovar el sacramento del bautismo. Ellos se paran al lado de los padres durante la ceremonia en la iglesia. Después del bautismo, hay una comida en la casa para los padrinos, los parientes, y los amigos especiales.

En Puerto Rico, los bautismos son celebrados con capias, o recuerdos, que se prenden en la ropa de los invitados. Podrían hacerse de una moneda pegada a un listón que tiene el nombre del niño. En México, un padrino avienta monedas a los niños vecinos afuera de la iglesia. Ambas tradiciones simbolizan la esperanza de una seguridad económica para el niño.

Los padrinos forman una parte importante del sistema social de apoyo de los padres y del niño. Ellos aceptan el gran honor de ser los padrinos espirituales del niño, para ayudar a fortalecer el crecimiento espiritual del niño. Pero también sirven un propósito mayor, el de ayudar al niño a sentirse amado y especial. En los primeros años de la vida de un niño, los padrinos le colmarán a su ahijado de regalos en su cumpleaños y una canasta especial para Pascua. En algunos casos, cuando los compadres no tienen hijos propios, el ahijado recibe todo, desde ropa hasta vacaciones. A veces los padrinos aun ayudan a pagar los gastos de una quinceañera, o una educación universitaria, o una boda. Durante épocas difíciles, los padrinos pueden intervenir y actuar de mediadores cuando los padres tienen problemas con la crianza de su niño. Ellos comprenden que en el caso de que ambos padres fallecieran y si nadie de la familia extensa pudiera asumir la responsabilidad de criar al niño, los padrinos podrán cumplir con esa responsabilidad hasta que el niño tenga edad suficiente para cuidarse solo.

¿Ustedes tienen padrinos para sus niños? Ser un padrino requiere una comunicación de ambos participantes, lo cual significa tener un contacto estrecho con sus compadres para que ellos puedan llegar a conocer, amar, y apoyar el desarrollo espiritual y moral de su niño. Los beneficios de mantener esta tradición cultural son importantes tanto para usted como para sus niños. Si usted es padrino o madrina de alguien, tome su papel en serio. Mantenga un contacto estrecho con su ahijado, y conviértase en su mejor amigo(a) y mentor(a).

La Primera Comunión

La Primera Comunión, la primera vez que un niño recibe la Eucaristía, es celebrada durante la Cuaresma, generalmente cuando los niños están en segundo año de primaria. En algunas partes de México, la Primera Comunión se celebra el 8 de diciembre, el día de la Inmaculada Concepción. Los niños y las niñas por tradición lucen trajes y vestidos blancos, aunque esta tradición está cambiando en algunas iglesias. Mis niños varones llevaron trajes blancos y mi hija lució un hermoso vestido blanco de satén bordado, con una larga vela blanca y guantes blancos. Ella parecía una pequeña Madona. Muchos hogares hispanos muestran fotos de sus niños, arrodillados en un banco, sosteniendo el rosario y los libros de rosario que le fueron obsequiados por sus padrinos. Los padrinos prometen orientarlos y apoyar su desarrollo religiosa. Igual a los padrinos de bautismo, ellos recuerdan a sus ahijados durante días festivos y en sus cumpleaños.

La quinceañera

La quinceañera es un acontecimiento muy especial para una niña hispana de quince años. Es el día en que ella se convierte en mujer y se efectúa su "rito de paso" de niña a adulta. Por medio de una misa especial y una celebración, una niña establece públicamente su relación con sus padres, su comunidad, y su Creador. Aparte de la pompa y solemnidad, el aspecto más importante de la quinceañera es la ceremonia religiosa, durante la cual los padres expresan su cariño hacia su hija y ella, a su vez, reflexiona sobre su relación con sus padres, con Dios, y con la Virgen María. Uno de los momentos más encantadores de la ceremonia ocurre cuando la debutante presenta quince rosas frescas a la estatua de la Virgen de Guadalupe mientras se cante la Ave María. La jovencita es presentada por sus padrinos para recibir la bendición, un collar con una cruz, unos aretes de perlas, un anillo, una Biblia, una corona de perlas, un álbum para fotos, y su "última" muñeca, la cual generalmente es de porcelana y lleva un vestido idéntico a aquélla que luce la quinceañera.

La invitación a una quinceañera frecuentemente incluye una foto de la debutante de niña y también de jovencita de quince años. Es aun otra ocasión para reunir a la familia extensa y a los amigos para celebrar, bailar, y capturar uno de los días más importantes en la vida de una niña con unas fotos memorables. Algunas quinceañeras son acontecimientos elaborados con esculturas de hielo, globos, pasteles de cumpleaños de muchos pisos, limosinas de las más grandes, enormes retratos de la quinceañera, vídeos o una proyección de diapositivas de la quinceañera, carruseles, y elegantes capias, o regalos de recuerdo para los invitados. Y no se nos vaya a olvidar mencionar la música, la comida, el salón, y la iglesia. Este acontecimiento puede ser tan costoso como una boda y es pagado por los padres y a veces algunos patrocinadores, quienes generalmente son padrinos y miembros de la familia.

La debutante tiene un cortejo de honor, el cual puede consistir de su propio acompañante, el chambelán de honor, y catorce amigas o parientes mujeres, todas luciendo vestidos iguales. Están acompañadas por jóvenes varones luciendo trajes de esmoquin. A las jovencitas les llaman damas y a los jovencitos les llaman chambelanes, lo cual significa "señores" (a veces también son llamados acompañantes, o galanes). A veces hay un cortejo de honor que consiste en niñas pequeñas que van arrojando pétalos de rosas al caminar ella hacia el altar de la iglesia. El cortejo de la quinceañera a veces se va de la iglesia en unas limosinas o en un autobús especial. Éste es un día en que la jovencita recibe trato de realeza y se le hace sentir muy importante. Se convierte en "princesa" por una noche al pasar con su cortejo debajo del arco adornado, luego bajo otro arco hecho de listones que están conectados a rosas, sostenidas por el cortejo. Ella se pasa al centro de la pista de baile en un despliegue de gracia, hace una reverencia, inclinándose hasta el piso, y luego una nueva diadema de joyas de fantasía se le coloca en la cabeza. En algunas celebraciones, en ese momento se acompaña a la debutante a una silla de respaldo alto y elaborados adornos, donde el padre se arrodilla enfrente de su hija y le cambia los zapatos bajitos a su "primer par" de zapatos de tacón alto, los cuales son llevados en un cojín de satén por la madre. La debutante luego se para y baila la primera pieza de la noche, un vals, con su padre. El padre baila el vals con ella primero, y luego la entrega a sus hermanos y después a su príncipe azul, el chambelán de honor. Continúan el vals junto con el resto del cortejo. Al final del vals, el cortejo cambia a un ritmo latino, como salsa o merengue.

Más entrada la noche, antes de cortar el pastel, se atenúan las luces y las catorce jovencitas sostienen una vela adornada encendida para que la quinceañera formule catorce deseos. El padre, abuelo, padrino, o hermano mayor hace un brindis. En este momento entran los mariachis o un trío, cantando "Las mañanitas". Casi nunca hay ningún ojo sin lágrimas en todo el salón cuando la debutante baila a la música de la tradicional canción, "La muñequita", con su padre. Al escuchar las palabras los espectadores admiran el afecto entre padre e hija y reflexionan sobre la rapidez con que se han pasado los años, al pasar su muñeca de la cuna a la escuela y convertirse en toda una señorita.

La muñequita

Llegaste tú, mi bien, llenando de ilusión,
mi corazón, también el de mamita.
Con gusto celebré y a todos les conté
Dijeron qué bonita.

Los días pasaron ya, creciste un poco más
Y ahora estás dormida en tu cunita.
Por nombre al bautizar, les dije llevará
por nombre muñequita.

Los años han pasado, ya recuerdo estos momentos
que fueron en mi vida de una gran ilusión.

Muy pronto partirás a la escuela a estudiar,
Y cumplirás del destino nacida
Y todos al pasar con gusto te dirán,
qué linda, qué bonita.

Y cuando vayas ya a la universidad,
Preguntarán, ¿Quién es la señorita?
Y tú contestarás por gusto de papá,
me llamo muñequita.

Las quinceañeras no tienen que ser lujosas para ser significativas. Yo no tuve una quinceañera porque no teníamos los recursos, ya que éramos ocho niños en la familia. Sin embargo, mis dos hermanas mayores fueron afortunadas y tuvieron una modesta quinceañera con madrinas, una diadema, y muchos amigos, familia, música, y comida.

Espero con ansias el día en que mi hija cumple los quince años y tendrá la oportunidad de celebrarlo de manera especial. Algunos padres comienzan las preparaciones para la quinceañera por lo menos dos años por adelantado. Planear una quinceañera puede ser una manera maravillosa en que los padres y su hija exploren su experiencia de ambas culturas al añadir elementos de ambas, por ejemplo, al escoger una mezcla de música tradicional latina y música moderna, o bien, una combinación de platillos hispanos y americanos. Es el momento apropiado para aprender modales, y aprender sobre su cultura, incluyendo el baile latino.

No se sorprenda si su hija le dice que no quiere tener una quinceañera si es que tiene amigas que no celebran sus quince años de esta manera. Algunas de mis sobrinas no tuvieron quinceañeras. En lugar de eso, prefirieron recibir el dinero que sus padres hubieran gastado en la celebración, para comprar un carro. Muchos hispanos optan por hacer una fiesta de los dieciséis años (Sweet Sixteen). Una de mis amigas me contó que no quería una quinceañera porque sus amigas no iban a tener una y ella pensaba que toda esa "cosa cultural" hispana no era muy buena onda. Sin embargo, cuando ella creció y fue a la universidad, cobró consciencia de su etnicidad y sus raíces culturales. Se enojaba tanto cuando iba a casa de sus tías y miraba los lindos retratos de sus primas, con sus vestidos de quinceañera, orgullosamente expuestos. Ahora mi amiga desea haber tenido una quinceañera y quiere asegurarse de que sus hijas tengan un glorioso cumpleaños al cumplir los quince años—a la manera latina.

La más importante sugerencia para ayudar a animar a su hija a tener una quinceañera es que debe comenzar desde pequeña. Cuando su hija es joven, llévela a quinceañeras, póngala a servir en otras celebraciones de quince años, ya sea como miembro del cortejo cuando es pequeña o como dama cuando es más grande. Llévele libros sobre el tema, como el de Mary D. Lankford titulado *Quinceañera: A Latina's Journey to Womanhood*, y el de Sister Angela Erevia, *Quince años celebrando una tradición*, y el de Michele Salcedo, *Quinceañera*. Además, asegure que su hija se asocie con amigas cuyos padres tienen la intención de hacerles una celebración de quince años. Si su hija mayor tuvo una, tiene mejor probabilidades con las menores. Los hermanos también pueden ayudar. Steven se ha parado en numerosas quinceañeras como chambelán y cada vez le ha dicho a Vanessa que espera ansiosamente el día especial cuando ella será la "reina de la fiesta".

OTRAS CELEBRACIONES

El día de la Madre

Como en todas las culturas, las madres del mundo hispano son honradas, amadas, y conferidas el mayor respeto. En el día de la Madre, la familia completa se reúne para mostrar gratitud por los muchos sacrificios y el amor tan abundante que una madre muestra a través de todo el año.

El día comienza para muchas afortunadas madres hispanas, a las altas horas de la madrugada, con una serenata. En San Antonio y en muchas comunidades latinas, un grupo de mariachis les da serenata a las madres, afuera de sus ventanas o en su porche. Mi esposo, que es un músico con un traje de mariachi, antes solía unirse a otros músicos para cantar "Las mañanitas" a las madrecitas queridas. Esta tradición se originó en España, donde los hombres les daban serenata a las mujeres afuera de sus ventanas. A pesar de que mi esposo tenía que ahuyentar a los perros del barrio para llegar al porche o a la ventana, él siguió haciéndolo por muchos años porque estaba tan conmovido al ser testigo de las lágrimas de gusto en las caritas de las viejitas, cuando él comenzaba a rasguear la guitarra.

Generalmente, los niños mayores, quienes pagaban a los mariachis, se congregarían a cierta hora en la casa de la madre para darle besitos y abrazos y para decirle cuánto la quieren y la aprecian. A veces las madres salían al porche cuando los mariachis llegaban o los invitaban para dentro a tomarse un cafecito. Otras veces, dependiendo de la hora, las madres simplemente prendían y apagaban las luces, o aparecían brevemente en la ventana como muestra de agradecimiento por tales canciones como "Madre querida", "Canto a la madre", y "Las mañanitas" que tocan tan calurosamente el corazón y el alma de cualquier mujer. Cuando mi esposo y los mariachis vinieron a mi casa a traerme serenata, mis niños corrían a mi lado a besarme y abrazarme, igual que mi esposo hacía. No hay ninguna posibilidad de que una madre latina no se emocionara a escuchar estas clásicas canciones para el día de la Madre:

O madre querida

O madre querida, O madre adorada
Que Dios te bendiga, aquí en tu morada.
Que Dios te conserve mil años de vida
Feliz y dichosa, O madre querida.

Si estás dormidita, escucha este canto
Que todos tus hijos convierten en llanto
Tú que por tus hijos vives implorando
En ti, Madrecita, vivimos pensando.

Recibe el cariño de todos tus hijos
Que nunca en la vida podrán olvidarte
Hoy día de las Madres venimos a darte
Perfumadas flores para consolarte.

O madre querida, O madre adorada
Que Dios te bendiga aquí en tu morada
Tu nombre es (María)*, y no hallan que darte
Se sienten dichosos al felicitarte.

*use su nombre

Canto a la madre

Madre querida en este día,
Las Mañanitas quiero cantar.
Recibe madre mil bendiciones,
Que Dios del cielo te mandará.

En este día todos tus hijos,
aquí reunidos estamos ya.
Trajimos flores de primavera
Y todas ellas te adornarán.

Madre querida, despierta madre
Si estás dormida, despierta ya.
Que desde el cielo una corona
Hecha de estrellas te adornará.

Todos los campos ya florecieron
Y sus aromas te brindarán.
Mientras que un coro de pajarillos
Alegremente te cantarán.

Madre querida, despierta madre
Si estás dormida, despierta ya.
Que desde el cielo una corona
Hecha de estrellas te adornará.

Las mañanitas

Éstas son las mañanitas que cantaba el Rey David
Hoy que es día de la madre*
Te las cantamos así

Despierta, mi bien, despierta, mira que ya amaneció.
Ya los pajarillos cantan, la luna ya se metió.

Qué linda está la mañana en que vengo a saludarte.
Venimos todos con gusto, y placer a felicitarte.
El día en que tú naciste, nacieron todas las flores
Y en la pila de bautismo, cantaron los ruiseñores
Ya viene amaneciendo, ya la luz del día nos dio.
Levántate de mañana, mira que ya amaneció.

*para cumpleaños cante "de tu cumpleaños" o "de tu santo"

LOS CUMPLEAÑOS Y LAS PIÑATAS

Los cumpleaños hispanos frecuentemente son celebraciones de generaciones múltiples, con las casas repletas de comida, regalos, canciones, y familia. Los primos, juntos con los abuelitos, se unen a los amigos alrededor del pastel para cantar "Las mañanitas", seguidas por "Happy

Birthday" al niño del cumpleaños. Uno de los momentos culminantes del día es cuando los niños rompen la piñata, una figura de papel maché, rellenada de dulces. Los dos tipos más conocidos de piñatas provienen de México y de Cuba, y pueden hacerse en casa o comprarse en una tienda de especialidades.

La piñata cubana es diferente a la mexicana en tamaño, estructura, y en el método usado para sacar los dulces de adentro. La piñata cubana generalmente es más o menos del tamaño de una canasta cuadrada de tres pies de ancho, con una plataforma que se adorna con alguna escena que ilustra algún personaje o héroe de los niños, tal como *Winnie the Pooh* o *Barney*. La diferencia principal entre las dos piñatas es que la cubana no se rompe. En el fondo de la bella obra de arte está un recipiente rectangular que se llena de dulces. Coloridos listones se cuelgan del fondo y cada niño jala un listón que abre el recipiente para que se caigan los dulces. La parte principal de la piñata se mantiene intacta para poder volver a usarse.

La piñata mexicana fue traída al nuevo mundo por los misioneros españoles para ayudar a convertir a los indios al cristianismo. Las primeras piñatas de adobe se construyeron en formas de demonios o en una figura de siete conos, los cuales representaban los siete pecados cardenales que los niños rechazarían simbólicamente con cada vez que le pegaban a la piñata. Al romper la piñata los niños, les llovían frutas y nueces, los cuales significaban la gracia que trae el haber rechazado a Satanás. Al pasar el tiempo, las piñatas se transformaron de un símbolo religioso a uno utilizado para entretenimiento y diversión durante las Posadas y las fiestas de cumpleaños. La tradicional estrella evolucionó para convertirse en formas de animales y luego en personajes populares como *Mickey Mouse* (el Ratón Miguelito). Construir una piñata mexicana puede ser una manera maravillosa para atraer la participación de sus niños en la preparación para la fiesta además de una forma de conectarlos a su cultura. Si vive usted en una comunidad hispana, puede comprar piñatas ya hechas llenas de dulces y juguetes.

Ambas piñatas cubanas y mexicanas son una gran fuente de diversión para los niños. Proporcionan impresiones duraderas, maravillosos recuerdos, y muchas ricas golosinas. Sin embargo, en el caso de la piñata mexicana, la diversión dura más y los niños participan de una manera más activa. La construcción de una piñata mexicana puede ser tan divertida como romperla. Compre un palo que le haga juego o adorne un viejo palo de escoba con los mismos colores de la piñata. Simplemente corte un agujero en la parte de arriba de la piñata y llénela con dulces. También puede añadir monedas y confeti. Utilice una cuerda larga para

Instrucciones para hacer una piñata

Haga una pasta pegajosa en una vasija grande al mezclar dos partes de agua por cada parte de harina. Haga tiras de varios periódicos. Meta cada tira de papel periódico en la vasija de pegamento (pasta) y saque el exceso de pasta al deslizar la tira entre dos dedos. Cubra un globo inflado, entre más grande mejor, con las tiras, poniendo cuatro o cinco capas. Cuando se seca la pasta, desinfle el globo y haga un agujero en la parte superior de la forma. Utilice un cordel (mecate) para formar un lazo encima de la forma, sujetándolo con un pedazo de cinta adhesiva protectora. Cubra la cinta con el resto de las tiras de periódico y pasta.

La base de la piñata se puede transformar y convertir en una estrella o un personaje especial, con el uso creativo de papel periódico. Pegue dos orejas y una cola hechas con varias capas de periódico en la base del globo para hacer la piñata de Mickey Mouse, o puede hacer de tres a cinco conos de periódico o cartulina y pegarlos en la base para formar las puntas de una estrella. (Puede formar cualquier animal al enrollar varios pedazos de papel para hacer patas, cola, o trompa). Adorne la piñata con tiras de colorido papel crepé o papel de seda. Use papel negro, blanco, y rojo para hacer una de Mickey Mouse y cualquier color brillante para hacer una estrella.

Para hacer cualquier piñata, corte papel de seda doblada en tiras de dos pulgadas, y luego haga un corte a ½ pulgada de la orilla en la parte doblada, para hacer un fleco, dejando la parte superior sin cortar. Desdoble el papel de seda y voltéelo al revés para formar flecos de lazos doblados que se pegarán, una tira a la vez, hasta cubrir completamente la piñata. Si utiliza el papel crepé, corte la parte doblada en dos y extienda la tira de fleco de papel crepé. Utilice la hoja de unas tijeras para rizar el fleco. Pegue la parte sin cortar de la tira a la piñata con pegamento, una tira a la vez, para cubrirla toda, con los rizos volteados hacia arriba o hacia abajo, como guste. Para hacer la piñata de estrella, pegue seis tiras largas y delgadas de papel de seda, pasándolas para dentro y sacándolas del punto de cada cono.

colgar la piñata de una rama de árbol y amarre una segunda cuerda a la piñata para jalarla cuando los niños tratan de romperla, mientras los otros gritan o cantan: "Dale, dale, dale". Quizá quiera, o quizá no, vendarles los ojos a los niños mayores que van a tirar un golpe a la piñata, pero esté consciente de que va a tener a un montón de niños gritando, apilados unos encima de otros, una vez que la piñata se rompa y los dulces caigan. Para hacer aun más divertido el acontecimiento, quizá quiera enseñarles a sus niños y a sus invitados la popular canción que generalmente acompaña el turno de cada niño:

Dale, dale, dale
no pierdas el tino
mide la distancia
que hay en tu camino.

Que si le das
de un palo te tiro.
Que si no le das
de un palo te tiro.
Dale, dale, dale.

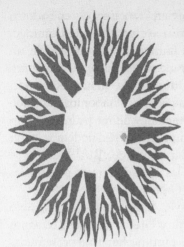

Capítulo III

Modelos de conducta hispanos

Nuestras estrellas brillantes

Tal vez haya escuchado acerca de los genios de la física, la medicina, o la química, que descubrieron o inventaron algo que avanzó nuestra comprensión de la medicina, la ciencia, o de nuestro mundo físico. Muchos se maravillan ante aquellos individuos cuyos talentos pueden crear bellas obras literarias o aquéllos que demuestran unas habilidades diplomáticas astutas, o valentía excepcional para lograr la paz mundial. También hay aquéllos que están bendecidos con los conocimientos y las habilidades para poder explorar otros planetas o crear bella música. Tal como el mundo europeo produjo un Beethoven, un Michelangelo, un Einstein, y un Pasteur, el mundo hispano también ha cultivado a individuos excepcionalmente brillantes.

Considere la amplia gama de especialidades donde han sobresalido los hispanos. El mundo de la música y el entretenimiento ha tenido estrellas tales como Edward James Olmos, José Ferrer, Jennifer López, Anthony Quinn, Raul Julia, Jimmy Smits, Julio Iglesias, Martin Sheen, Vicki Carr, Gloria Estefan, Andy García, Rosie Pérez, Celia Cruz, Cristina Saralegui, y John Secada, entre muchos otros. Luis Valdés, el dramaturgo hispano, produjo *Zoot Suit* y *La Bamba*. El niño de usted podría ser como Rafael Méndez, el primer trompetista a ejecutar un solo en Carnegie Hall; o como Pablo Casals, el famoso violincelista; o Evelyn

Cisneros, la primera bailarina del Ballet de San Francisco, quien bailó en la Casa Blanca. Podría poseer talento operístico como Plácido Domingo, Daniel Catán, Ramón Vargas, o Suzanna Guzmán. Linda Ronstadt, un artista hispana que ha alcanzado al estatus de ganadora de discos de oro y platino y que fue invitada a cantar durante la inauguración del Presidente Carter, le otorga el mérito a su padre por haber influenciado su carrera musical. Su disco titulado "Canciones de mi padre", fue un tributo a su padre y también a su cultura. Los latinos nos podemos jactar de tener una buena cuota de estrellas, sin embargo, Rita Moreno se destaca por haberse ganado cada uno do los cuatro premios principales de la industria: los *Oscar, Emmy, Tony, y Grammy.*

Tenemos muchos artistas hispanos del ayer, como Diego Rivera, Pablo Picasso, Frida Kahlo, Salvador Dali, Goya, y Greco. También tenemos los más actuales como Jesse Treviño, cuyas pinturas han sido presentadas al príncipe Carlos y a Hillary Rodham Clinton, y el artista Manuel Acosta de César Chávez, cuyo retrato adornó la portada de la revista *Time.* Modistas hispanos como Carolina Herrera, Paloma Picasso, Oscar de la Renta, y Adolfo han dejado su huella en la vida y en sus diseños singulares y exquisitos. Todos estos hombres y mujeres se cuentan entre los muchos hispanos que han cultivado sus habilidades y talentos divinos y llegaron a ser modelos brillantes para nuestros niños hispanos.

Las escritoras y ganadoras del premio *McArthur,* Sandra Cisneros y Ruth Behar, se destacan en el mundo literario, juntas con otros escritores hispanos tales como Julia Alvarez, Rudolfo Anaya, y el ganador al *Hispanic Heritage Award,* Luís Rodríguez. Los atletas como los jugadores de golf, Lee Trevino, Chi Chi Rodíguez, y Nancy López; y los jinetes, Ángel Cordero y Jorge Velásquez probaron que los latinos podían ser campeones en los deportes que eran dominados por anglosajones y negros. Otros excepcionales personajes deportistas hispanos incluyen al entrenador de fútbol profesional, Tom Flores; el futbolista (de fútbol americano) profesional que cuenta entre los talentosos de los anales del atletismo, Anthony Muñóz; y los boxeadores, Oscar de La Hoya, y Julio Caesar Chávez. La leyenda de béisbol, Roberto Clemente, demostró que con mucho esfuerzo y determinación, los latinos pueden ser héroes además de tener un puesto en los anales del atletismo, en el *Hall of Fame.* Aun en nuestra época, hemos sido testigos de la temporada histórica de bésbol de 1998 cuando Sammy Sosa, de la República Dominicana, jugador de los Chicago Cubs, hizo sesenta y seis cuadrangulares y sobrepasó el récord de Roger Maris de 1961, al lograr cinco cuadrangulares más que él. Éste fue un increíble año para los latinos y para el bésbol. Sammy Sosa y Mark McGwire compitieron por sobrepasar el récord de Maris, y ambos Sammy Sosa y Juan

González, de Puerto Rico, ganaron el título del "jugador más valioso" de la Liga Nacional y la Liga Americana, respectivamente.

Aqéllos que han luchado para darnos una voz más fuerte a los latinos en la arena política y más allá, incluyen a Joseph Marion Hernández, quien fue el primer congresista hispano de los Estados Unidos en 1822, y Octavio A. Larrazolo, quien fue el primer senador hispano de los Estados Unidos en 1928. Aquellos líderes abrieron el camino para otros como Henry B. González y Edward R. Roybal. Los primeros hispanos que ocuparon puestos en el gabinete incluyen a Lauro Cavazos, Henry G. Cisneros, y Federico F. Peña. Antonia C. Novello fue la primera hispana para encabezar la Dirección General de Salud Pública en Estados Unidos en 1990. Franklin Chang-Díaz, nacido en Costa Rica, habló en español desde el espacio en 1986 y fue el primer astronauta hispano en los Estados Unidos. Lo siguieron Sydney Gutiérrez y Ellen Ochoa, quien fue la primera astronauta latina en 1993. Treinta y ocho hispanoamericanos, incluyendo a Cleto Rodríguez y Roy Benavídez de Texas, y Eurípedes Rubio y Héctor Santiago-Colón de Puerto Rico recibieron la Medalla de Honor del Congreso. Las personas que lucharon por la libertad y democracia de los Estado Unidos en numerosas guerras, también incluyen a personas nacidas en Chile, México, y España.

Tenemos muchísimos campeones que han asumido papeles de liderazgo para mejorar la calidad de vida de los hispanos. El líder de derechos civiles, César Chávez; el fundador del American G.I. Forum, el doctor Hector Pérez García; el poeta, José Marti; y el periodista, Rubén Salazar, fueron activistas que lograron producir una consciencia social. Reies López Tijerina, Rodolfo "Corky" González, y José Ángel Gutiérrez fueron los líderes del movimiento chicano y provocaron un orgullo étnico en los años sesenta. La doctora Blandina Cárdenas, Antonia Hernández, y Raul Yzaguirre han luchado incansablemente por resolver problemas educativos, sociales, y de derechos civiles para los hispanos. Willie Velásques, a través de la organización que él fundó, *Southwest Voter and Education Project*, fue responsable por el aumento en la cantidad de votantes hispanos, lo cual hizo un impacto en el número de políticos hispanos.

Eugenio María de Hostos y George I. Sánchez se encuentran entre nuestros grandes educadores. El doctor José A. Cárdenas y la doctora Gloria Zamora son de los primeros campeones de la educación bilingüe para hispanos. Estamos sumamente orgullos de Mario Obledo, quien en 1998 recibió la Medalla de Libertad del presidente Bill Clinton por ayudar a establecer MALDEF y las Organizaciones Nacionales Hispanas, y el doctor Manuel Berriozabal implementó un programa modelo para niños de minorías de nivel secundario en los campos de matemáticas y ciencia, el cual lo hizo acreedor al *Presidential Freedom Award in Science*. Ernesto Cortez ha recibido reconocimiento a través de los premios MacArthur y Heinz, por sus habilidades de organización en la comunidad y su liderazgo al fundar la organización conocida como *COPS*.

Latinos a través del mundo entero han recibido reconocimiento con los premios Nobel y Pulitzer, o las Medalla de Honor del Congreso. Para comenzar, en 1906 Santiago Ramón y Cajal de España ganó el premio Nobel de la Medicina por su trabajo sobre la estructura del sistema nervioso. Conocido como el "padre de la neurociencia", sus investigaciones han proveído los cimientos para la actual neuroanatomía, y han inspirado el interés actual por el funcionamiento del cerebro. En 1959, el doctor Severo Ochoa de España ganó el premio Nobel de la Medicina y Fisiología por su descubrimiento de ARN (ácido ribonucleico), uno de los componentes básicos de la vida. En 1968, Luis Alvarez de los Estados Unidos, un físico, recibió el premio Nobel por su creación de la cámara de burbujas de hidrógeno. Al argentino, César Milstein y al venezolano, Baruj Benacerraf también les otorgaron éste, el más alto de los honores, por su trabajo en el campo de inmunología. Otro argentino, Luis Federico Leloir, recibió el premio Nobel de la Química. En 1995, Mario J. Molina de los Estados Unidos, quien reconoció los peligros que las sustancias químicas hechas por el hombre, implican con respecto a la capa de ozono de la tierra, también fue ganador del premio Nobel de la Química. Algunos hispanos que han ganado un premio Nobel de Literatura, incluyen a Octavio Paz, de México; Gabriel García Márquez, de Colombia; y Miguel Ángel Asturias, de Guatemala. Ganadores múltiples de este distinguido honor literario, de un solo país, incluyen a Pablo Neruda y Gabriela Mistral, de Chile; y Juan Ramón Jiménez, Camilo José Cela, y Vicente Aleixandre, de España. Han habido por lo menos cinco ganadores hispanos del premio Nobel de la Paz. Entre ellos figuran el autor guatemalteco, Rigoberta Menchú; Óscar Arias, de Costa Rica; y Alfonso García Robles, de México. Ganadores múltiples de Argentina incluyen a Adolf Pérez Esquivel y Carlos Saavedra Lamas. Oscar Hijuelos, un cubano, ganó el premio Pulitzer por su novela *The Mambo Kings Play Songs of Love (Los reyes mambos tocan canciones de amor)*.

Cada niño, en algún momento de su vida, desarrolla metas o sueños acerca de lo que quisiera lograr en su vida. A una mente inocente y joven, nada parece imposible de lograr. Desde héroes deportistas hasta estrellas favoritas de la televisión y del cine, los modelos de conducta surgen para fascinar al niño influenciable. Todo niño hispano debe aprender acerca de los logros y las contribuciones excepcionales de otros hispanos, como aquéllos previamente mencionados. El niño entonces puede identificarse con ese modelo y su sueño no le parecerá tan imposible de lograr.

De joven, mi esposo estaba interesado en matemáticas y ciencia, y fue apoyado y alentado por sus padres a meterse en ese campo. Sin embargo, al ser el primer miembro de su familia de conseguir una licenciatura, no había nadie con quien podía platicar acerca de dedicarse a una carrera en ingeniería. Hoy en día, se han formado muchas organizaciones por hispanos profesionales de varios campos, tales como la ingeniería, la medicina, y la ley, para llenar este vacío, inspirar a jóvenes hispanos que desean dedicarse a esas carreras, y servir de mentores. Algunas de dichas organizaciones son: *National Hispanic Medical Association, Society of Hispanic Engineers—SHPE, Society of Mexican American Scientists and Engineers—MAES, Hispanic Nurses Association, National Society of Hispanic MBAs, Hispanic Dental Association, Hispanic Lawyers Association, National Association of Hispanic Publications, National Association of Hispanic Journalists, U.S. Hispanic Chamber of Commerce, National Hispanic Business Association, National Coalition of Hispanic Health and Human Services Organizations, Hispanic American Association—HAA—of Dancers, Hispanic Communications Association—HCA.*

Claramente, los hispanos han demostrado excelencia en una amplia gama de áreas. Yo los menciono aquí, además de una lista de organizaciones profesionales, para ilustrar las posibilidades que les esperan a sus niños. Leer sobre cualquier de estas personas, en la biblioteca o en el Internet, o ponerse en contacto con estas organizaciones puede revelar una riqueza de información e inspiración. También le proporcionará una comprensión acerca de cómo muchos hombres hispanos y muchas mujeres hispanas han logrado aplicar sus talentos, muchas veces en contra de las probabilidades, para alcanzar el éxito y hacer que el mundo sea un lugar mejor, sin haber olvidado quienes son.

Segunda parte

Las necesidades básicas

del desarrollo de los niños

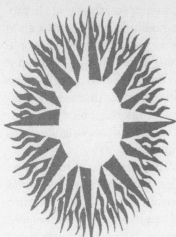

Capítulo IV

Nuestros niños son únicos y especiales

Como los dedos de la mano

Mi suegra, quien crió a ocho niños, solía levantar la mano y decir: "Mira mis dedos. ¿Ven como todos son diferentes? Mis dedos son como cada uno de mis hijos". Desde un conjunto complejo de ADN y huellas digitales, hasta una personalidad y una estructura de cuerpo singulares, cada niño nace con habilidades, intereses, talentos, y un carácter que lo distingue de todos los demás en el planeta. El propósito de esta sección es ayudarle a usted, como padre, a reconocer que aquellas diferencias existen y que usted las debe comprender, aceptar, y cultivar, y no lamentarlas ni temerlas.

Cuando mi suegra me pasó esas palabras, ella ya se había dado cuenta que sus niños exhibían ciertas características únicas que, con un poco de orientación y apoyo, llevaría a cada uno en cierta dirección. "Voy a tener un doctor, un abogado, un ingeniero, y un maestro", ella les declaró a sus vecinos. De hecho, uno de sus hijos llegó a ser médico, otro llegó a ser maestro, y dos llegaron a ser ingenieros. Lo único que no produjo fue el abogado, pero fue bendecida con un consejero universitario en su lugar. ¿Cómo ocurrieron estos logros? ¿Fueron las altas aspiraciones y expectativas que ella les inculcó a sus niños, o fue que ella verdaderamente se dio cuenta de que cada uno tenía un don especial y ella fue capaz de extraerlo y cultivarlo? Cuando yo le hice esta pregunta a mi suegra, ella respondió que fueron ambas cosas, sus expectativas y su aliento. Como educadora, primero pensé que tal logro era lo que nosotros en el campo educativo llamamos una "profecía que acarrea su propio cumplimiento", que los niños eventualmente reaccionan a, o llegan a ser, lo que se espera de ellos. Yo comencé a comprender lo que ella quiso decir al tomar consciencia de, y apoyar, los talentos, intereses, y temperamentos singulares de mis propios hijos. Yo, también, hice tales profecías acerca de mis niños, basadas en sus características singulares, las cuales se hicieron evidentes desde muy temprano.

Mucho antes de convertirse mi esposo en ingeniero, él tenía sumo interés en los misterios de la electricidad y en desarmar cosas y volverlas a armar. De niño, él construía radios y renovaba la instalación eléctrica de muchos aparatos eléctricos. Tal como mi suegra predijo que mi esposo llegaría a ser ingeniero, mi abuelo predijo que yo sería una maestra cuando él me observaba acomodando a todas mis muñecas en un salón de clase de mentiritas. Él decía: "Ahí viene la maestra". El reconocimiento y el aliento de estas dos personas jugaron un papel influyente en nuestras vocaciones futuras. ¿Puede usted recordar qué le interesaba cuando era niño? ¿Cómo le alentaron o apoyaron sus padres para que llegara a ser la persona que es hoy en día? ¿Puede identificar la singularidad en sus propios niños y en los intereses que están mostrando? Su forma de responder tendrá una influencia decisiva. Como padres, necesitamos apreciar y respetar la singularidad del temperamento, los intereses y las habilidades innatas de nuestros niños, por medio de paciencia, apoyo, y aliento.

DE PERSONALIDAD SINGULAR

La personalidad de un niño se hará notar temprano. Mi madre solía decirme que yo era "bien risueña y bien lista". Yo era una verdadera extrovertida, siempre sonriendo, amistosa, y platicadora, aun con los extraños. Mi carácter fuerte y mis características de liderazgo se manifestaron muy temprano en mi vida. Con frecuencia se me ha dicho que soy muy aferrada a mis ideas, muy creativa, y tenaz, además de que me atrevo a tomar riesgos, analizo todo y me gusta organizar. Estas características fueron cultivadas a través de los años por medio de una serie de actividades y puestos de liderazgo, desde patrullera de seguridad y columnista del periódico escolar hasta la directiva de algún club, animadora, y *Sweetheart Queen* en la escuela preparatoria. En la universidad, me eligieron Miss Fiesta, reina del desfile nocturno de San Antonio, lo cual me permitió representar a mi ciudad en varios desfiles fuera de la ciudad, incluyendo el desfile para el Torneo de las Rosas en California. Originaria del barrio, nunca había asistido a escuelas de cotillón, sin embargo aprendí al observar a otros. En aquellos días, mi lema era *Cuando en Roma, haz como los romanos*. El carácter con el que nace cada persona se sigue formando por medio de innumerables experiencias.

Todas las personas poseen distintas disposiciones y personalidades. Las personalidades individuales de mis niños se hicieron evidentes desde el momento de emerger de la matriz. Durante el nacimiento de mi primer hijo, tuve la oportunidad de observar a Salvador Julián Rodríguez entrar al mundo, mirando silenciosamente a su alrededor con enormes ojos obscuros, observando curiosamente cada detalle de su medio ambiente. Sus ojos inmediatamente se detuvieron al encontrarse con los míos, tal como si estuviera programado para reconocer una cara humana. En ese momento, con profunda emoción, comenzó a llorar suavemente. Desde su nacimiento, Sal siempre ha sido sensible y de voz suave. Desde el momento en que su niño entre al mundo, observe sus primeros gestos y movimientos, acarícielo e inmediatamente sosténgalo cerca de su cuerpo. Aprenderá mucho de su personalidad, y al sostenerlo y acariciarlo, comenzará a desarrollar los vínculos afectivos entre el padre o la madre y el hijo, los cuales son esenciales para la formación de futuras relaciones sociales.

Cuando era niño, Sal generalmente trataba de evitar los problemas, las confrontaciones, y la falta de harmonía al mantener sus emociones escondidas adentro, nunca mostrándose mal educado ni descortés ni aparentemente irrespetuoso. Al crecer, reaccionaba al conflicto por medios pasivo-agresivos, nunca expresando sus sentimientos verdaderos. Por ejemplo, un día cuando él tenía alrededor de siete años, yo le estaba reprendiendo por no querer practicar sus lecciones de piano. Al hablar, me escuchó silenciosamente, pero luego lentamente metió los pulgares en los oídos y me hizo caso omiso.

Para una madre denominada como "tipo A" personalidad extrovertida, como yo, que es tan activa, agresiva, y tiene más deseo de control que otras personas, es sumamente difícil criar a un niño que va tan en contra de esa corriente. ¿Usted es extrovertido? ¿Lo es su niño? Si usted y su niño poseen personalidades opuestas puede ser un enorme desafío. Si sus respuestas a estas preguntas son afirmativas, se ha dado cuenta que tiene que ser muy paciente, comprensivo, y flexible. Por ser una persona extrovertida, al crecer yo requería mucha disciplina firme de parte de mi madre y mi abuelo. Puede que encuentre que disciplinar a un niño como

Sal sea parecido a caminar sobre cáscaras de huevo, nunca sabiendo cuándo quizá haya pasado a la zona de incomodidad del niño, y siempre sienta el temor de que si dice o hace algo equivocado pueda afectar negativamente su relación para siempre. Con este tipo de personalidad, quizá tenga que ser firme pero calmado. Háblele a su niño con una voz baja y racional, al darle explicaciones y razonar con él. Los niños aprenden mejor cuando uno les explica lógicamente el porqué de las cosas. Evite usar una voz de tono agudo, dar mensajes negativos con gestos o movimientos de su cuerpo, y utilizar amenazas. Éstas no funcionan. Todos los niños necesitan tener límites claramente definidos con consecuencias firmes. Llegará un momento, al crecer más su niño, cuando tiene que soltarlo, tal como lo hice yo, y dejarlo aprender a través de sus errores.

Un año, a pesar de que calificó dentro del percentil 99 en un examen estandarizado de la escuela, Sal estaba a punto de repetir el año porque se negaba a entregar sus tareas. Yo atribuía su falta de motivación a un conflicto de personalidad entre mi hijo y su maestra firme, quien no era muy flexible. *El agua y el aceite no se mezclan*, y así eran ella y Sal. Ella compartía conmigo una personalidad muy fuerte, pero no aprendió por el camino a relajarse y ser más sensible a las necesidades de Sal. Era estricta y exigía que los niños asumieran responsabilidad por sus acciones. En pocas palabras me dijo que "lo estaba mimando".

En términos generales, las madres hispanas tienden a hacer demasiado por sus niños, especialmente los varones. Tal como declaré antes, nuestros niños son el centro de nuestra existencia. Estamos constantemente motivados por la idea de que tenemos que hacer algo para nuestros niños. Esto es cierto, especialmente en el caso de nuestros niños varones, aunque sabemos que hacer demasiado no es bueno para ellos. Esto puede provocar un choque cultural con maestros que a veces exigen independencia y responsabilidad a una edad mucho más joven de lo que estamos acostumbradas algunas madres hispanas. Tal como dice el dicho, *si nos chocamos, nos rompemos*. Yo sentí que era mi deber de madre tratar de trabajar con la maestra para prevenir un desastre total.

Yo recuerdo que cuando nos reunimos para una conferencia, su maestra me dijo: "Si usted no hace algo con respecto a su actitud y conducta ahora que tiene doce años, Sal va a depender de usted por el resto de su vida". ¡Ni lo mande Dios! Ésa era toda la motivación que yo necesitaba para trabajar con ella para ayudarle a Sal a comprender que él tenía que ser responsable y enfrentarse a los hechos concretos, y tal vez crueles: que no todos van a tener presente ni satisfacer su singular personalidad sensible. A Sal se le dieron dos opciones: o seguiríamos tras de él para que entregara sus tareas, o no le molestaríamos para entregarlas y el aceptaría las consecuencias. Él escogió la segunda opción. Juntos, mi esposo y yo firmamos un contrato con su maestra acordando que ya no le íbamos a fastidiar y que se le iba a ser responsable de sus acciones. Su maestra se mantuvo fuerte y exigente, y Sal puso a prueba los límites.

Es difícil para cualquier padre mirar a su niño ir por el camino equivocado, especialmente después de haber tratado de hacer todo lo posible para modificar su conducta. A pesar de haberse calificado más allá del nivel preparatorio en los exámenes estandarizados ese año, Sal volvió a cursar el séptimo año. Como dice el dicho, *el error sólo es fracaso cuando no se convierte en experiencia.* Él aprendió una lección valiosa a base de cometer un error. Pero ya nunca más tuve que recordarle de ser responsable y entregar su tarea. Aprendió que sus acciones le perjudicaron más a él que a su maestra (o padres), al mirar a sus amigos pasar al siguiente año sin él.

Sin embargo, era importante que mi esposo y yo le apoyáramos durante esta experiencia desagradable de aprendizaje. Hubiera sido tan fácil haberle forzado a completar sus tareas, pero no hubiera aprendido su lección. Nosotros demostramos nuestro amor incondicional, el cual no estaba basado ni en sus calificaciones ni sus logros, ni tampoco en lo que otros opinaban acerca de mí como educadora o como "experta" en la crianza de los niños. Era más importante que él aprendiera que necesitaba ser responsable de *sus* propias acciones y que el aprendizaje a través de cometer errores es una parte normal del crecimiento.

Quizá observe muchas características en sus niños que se parezcan a usted o a su pareja. Yo veo muchas de las características de mi esposo cuando pienso en como mi hijo adora pasar horas de soledad, pescando, acampando, o simplemente meditando. Además, son similares en su manera de reaccionar a cosas tales como compromisos, horarios, y quehaceres. Sal personifica el viejo refrán *de tal palo, tal astilla.* Cada uno, padre e hijo, tiene su propio reloj y hará ciertas cosas de acuerdo a cuando él quiere hacerlo. Esto puede causar trastornos o disgustos cuando no se hacen los quehaceres de la casa, o cuando Sal se escabullía de practicar el piano. A veces mi esposo y yo teníamos diferentes expectativas con relación a los quehaceres de la casa y la disciplina. No siempre estábamos de acuerdo en los límites que les imponíamos a los niños. Sin embargo, es tan importante que usted y su esposo transijan y se pongan de acuerdo en cuando menos los asuntos principales, tal como nosotros lo hicimos.

La maestra de piano de Sal se disgustaba con él porque sabía que tenía un buen oído para la música y talento para tocar el piano, pero no con-seguía hacerlo practicar. Y sin embargo, durante los recitales, ¡era fantástico! Lucía como un pianista maestro, tal como mi esposo lo predijo. Mi esposo sentía que si Sal verdaderamente sentía amor por la música, nosotros no tendríamos que forzarlo a practicar.

Ponga a sus niños en contacto con tantas actividades como sea posible, para que puedan surgir aquéllas que realmente les interesen. Puede tratar de modificar la conducta hasta cierto punto, por ejemplo al dar premios y privilegios a cambio de conducta deseable, pero debe darse cuenta de los límites de ese método. Yo sentí que seis años de lecciones de piano era suficiente tiempo para establecer unos buenos cimientos. Le dije a mi hijo, "Sal, cuando ya no quieres seguir con tus lecciones de piano, dime". Inmediatamente él respondió, "¡YA NO QUIERO MÁS LECCIONES DE PIANO!" Comprendí el mensaje perfectamente y paramos las lecciones. Sin embargo, poco tiempo después de su fuerte declaración, Sal volvió de cuando en cuando a tocar el piano por placer. Él podía hacerlo debido a sus sólidos cimientos, construidos a través de años de práctica, y yo sabía que si él decidía que quería seguir sus lecciones, él me diría.

El solo hecho de que los niños muestren tener talento en cierta área, no significa necesariamente que tengan un gran interés en eso. Uno nunca sabe cuál interés surgirá. Si uno los presiona a participar en cierta actividad, aun si les gusta, un pasatiempo se puede convertir en un trabajo, y bien pueden llegar a odiarlo. Lo único que puede hacer es proporcionar las oportunidades y esperar para ver cuál pega en el blanco, y estar preparado a dejarlo a un lado cuando ellos mandan el mensaje de que ya fue suficiente. Sal probó la gimnasia, los deportes, las artes, y las artesanías, y varios instrumentos musicales.

Por contraste, cuando se trataba de computadoras, equipos eléctricos, y deportes acuáticos, ¡Sal irradiaba alegría! Ésta fue la misma sensación que tuvo mi esposo la primera vez que sostuvo su adorada trompeta. No la soltaba. Mi suegra nunca tuvo que decirle que practicara. De hecho, él tenía que practicar afuera de la casa porque ella no soportaba el ruido. Esto me recuerda a un hijo de una graduada de AVANCE que un día escuchó a un hombre practicando el piano en el barrio. El niño corrió a casa, les dijo a sus padres que él quería aprender a tocar el piano, y ellos juntaron a duras penas el dinero para comprarle uno. Él practicaba cada minuto que podía y esperaba con ansias las lecciones que le daba el mismo hombre que se lo había introducido.

De manera similar, la primera vez que Sal puso las manos en una computadora, ya no la quiso dejar. Ya para los cuatro años de edad, sabía usar la computadora mejor que yo. Yo me sentí tan frustrada cuando su interés y su habilidad no encontraron su equivalencia en un programa de estudios apropiado en la secundaria. Su escuela no podía saciar su sed de aprendizaje. Sin embargo, como la escuela insistía que todos los niños pasaran por un programa requerido de estudios, Sal se aburría muchísimo. Yo intenté ponerlo en una clase avanzada de computadoras, pero el maestro respondió con: "No, hasta que cumpla los requisitos de esta clase de introducción". Mientras tanto, Sal rehusaba comunicar sus sentimientos. Su maestro y el director de la escuela se negaron a escuchar cuando yo les expliqué que él ya estaba aprendiendo programación mientras el resto de la clase estaba aprendiendo las habilidades básicas de las computadoras. Más adelante, Sal se metió en problemas con su maestro porque obtuvo acceso a su computadora e intentó ver cómo funcionaba un nuevo programa sin su permiso. Él sabía las reglas y las consecuencias pero estaba tan empeñado en dominar el nuevo programa que estaba dispuesto a sufrir las consecuencias. Por fin en la preparatoria, su maestro de noveno año reconoció sus talentos y habilidades y no solamente lo puso en clases para estudiantes sobresalientes, sino también le pidió que le ayudara a enseñar una clase de computadoras. ¡Él sobresalió!

Esta experiencia me hizo darme cuenta que los padres necesitan trabajar estrechamente con la escuela e insistir que sus niños reciban apoyo y desafíos académicos. Los padres y los maestros deben trabajar en conjunto para ayudar a los niños a progresar en su desarrollo y alcanzar su potencial. Como educadora, yo aprendí que las escuelas necesitan descubrir el nivel de desarrollo de cada niño y comenzar a trabajar desde ese punto. Los maestros tienen que evaluar dónde se encuentra cada niño en el continuo educativo. Deben comunicarse con los padres y apoyarles, ya que los padres conocen mejor a sus niños. Los padres también deben cumplir su parte de apoyar a los maestros al reforzar y aumentar el programa de estudios en el hogar. De esta manera, los padres y los maestros se convierten en socios educativos. Juntos cultivan el interés y los talentos de los niños. Si no se realiza esta asociación, los padres deben aprovechar las avenidas disponibles al quejarse con el director o con un miembro de la mesa directiva local. Cuando todo lo demás falla, en última instancia depende de ustedes asegurarse de que sus niños no queden atrás en su desarrollo. Quizá considere complementar el programa de estudios de la escuela al matricular a sus niños en algún programa privado de enriquecimiento de fines de semana, o al hacer que su hogar sea lo más estimulante y enriquecedor posible.

Desde que era niño, Sal ha sido muy curioso y analítico como su padre, siempre tratando de desarmar cosas y luego volverlas a armar. No sé con cuántos aparatos eléctricos experimentó para averiguar cómo funcionaban. Fue entonces cuando yo me di cuenta de lo que se refería mi suegra cuando describía "los dedos de la mano". Yo sabía que yo también tendría a un ingeniero en la familia. Esta idea se reforzaba constantemente a través de los años. Tan temprano como el tercer año de primaria cuando Sal asistía a una escuela para niños superdotados, el director de la escuela también predijo que él llegaría a ser ingeniero. Dijo: "Él es un soñador y siempre está analizando las cosas. A los niños como Sal no les gusta un ambiente estructurado ni que nadie los esté presionando. Ellos necesitan tiempo y espacio".

Si usted se da cuenta que sus niños tienen un interés en llegar a ser ingenieros, doctores, astronautas, o científicos, apóyelos en casa al proveerles objetos seguros como *Tinker Toys*, cuadritos de madera, y aeromodelos. Aliente a su niño a jugar con arena y agua y todo tipo de recipientes. Bajo su supervisión, permítale a su niño construir cosas y desarmarlas, utilizando viejos aparatos eléctricos, madera, martillos, y clavos. Sal construyó varios fuertes con su hermano y su hermana y ayudó a su padre a construir una cama en la forma de un carro. Una vez, en el día de Todos los Santos (Halloween), ayudó a su padre a hacer su propio disfraz de robot que se prendía.

Las computadoras, ahora más que nunca, forman una parte principal de nuestras vidas. Es crítico que usted asegure que sus niños tengan contacto con computadoras, porque estamos en la edad de la información, donde todo el mundo tendrá que operar una computadora en su trabajo, sin importar el tipo de trabajo que tenga. Pero también es importante asegurarse de rodearles de todo tipo de libros que abrirán sus mentes a las maravillas y las cosas fascinantes que existen en el mundo a su alrededor.

Sal nunca se desvió de su pasión por matemáticas, ciencia, y computadoras, a pesar de los contratiempos. Fue nominado por su congresista y senador para la Academia Naval (*Naval Academy*), la Academia de la Fuerza Aérea de los Estados Unidos (*U.S. Air Force Academy*), la Academia Militar de los Estados Unidos (*U.S. Military Academy*), y la Marina Mercante (*Merchant Marines*). Él escogió la Academia Naval y había tomado y pasado todos los exámenes, excepto el físico. Antes de ir por su examen físico, rompió la pierna jugando fútbol americano en la preparatoria. Huelga decir que Sal tuvo que cambiar sus planes y decidió asistir a Texas A&M para estudiar ingeniería e informática. Sal quería ser un *Aggie* a pesar de que ambos su padre y yo nos graduamos de la escuela rival, la Universidad de Texas en Austin. De nuevo, Sal quería ser diferente y único.

¿Qué tal si su niño es el extrovertido energético y expresivo con quien es menos difícil lograr comunicarse? De hecho, ¿qué tal si es muy travieso y da mucho trabajo? Mi segundo niño, Steven René Rodríguez, era la antítesis de Sal y de su padre. Era un poco más atrevido, mucho más agresivo, activo, y fuera de control. ¡Bien bárbaro! ¿Cómo puede una madre lidiar con un niño tan difícil de controlar?

Aun antes de nacer, Steven se las arreglaba para salirse con la suya. Mientras todavía estaba dentro de la matriz, me despertaba a medianoche, dándome unas pataditas tan fuertes que verdaderamente me hacía voltear hacia el lado izquierdo. Al nacer, ¡Steven salió con un estallido! ¡Me dio un buen susto! Yo estaba terriblemente asustada porque nació con un tono morado, y yo pensé que tenía dificultades para respirar. Pero tenía ese tono de piel porque estaba a punto de dejar salir un fuerte grito, para informarles a todos que él estaba muy enojado porque fue despertado de un sueño cálido y cómodo. De bebé, Steven se despertaba de pequeñas siestas, daba la vuelta repentinamente, se asía de la almohadilla de la cuna, y encontraba gran placer en aventarla de un lado a otro, para arriba y para abajo, hasta casi dejarla hecha trizas.

Por muchos años, ese niño lleno de energía no cambió. Cuando era pequeño, era un bulto de energía pura, curioso, aventurero, y me volvía loca. Yo pensaba que ni él ni yo sobreviviríamos más allá de su sexto cumpleaños. Steven siempre ha sido expresivo y determinado, y pone en duda lo que dicen todos y pelea por sus derechos y los de otros. Él tiene que tener la palabra final. Él siempre tiene su opinión y puede construir un caso sólido para cualquier asunto en el cual él cree. ¡Al estar creciendo, yo siempre sabía más de lo que quería saber y siempre sabía lo que *él* estaba pensando!

Los niños así no están siempre tratando de volver locos a sus padres. Steven podía oscilar entre una emoción extrema y otra. Por un lado podía ser el niño más dulce, más gracioso, y más sensible, y luego ser completamente lo opuesto. Si quería atención, tan sólo tenía que decir amorosamente: "Mamá, ráscame la espalda", y él recibía ese cálido tacto humano que él deseaba. Si se le daba un micrófono a Steven, él actuaba, cantaba, y recitaba sin que se lo pidieran siquiera. Siempre era el centro de atención, ya sea de payaso, de artista, o de líder autoproclamado. Nunca hay un momento de aburrimiento cuando los Stevens del mundo están cerca. Aun nos dejan admirados con sus talentos. El lado derecho del cerebro, el cual controla la creatividad y expresión, siempre estaba trabajando al dedicarse a sus talentos para el dibujo, la exploración, y la experimentación.

Como padres, debemos apoyar y amar a todos nuestros niños, pero especialmente a estos *caranchitos*, estos diablitos, hasta transformarlos en angelitos. Lo único que necesitan es nuestra aprobación, orientación, amor incondicional, y mucha paciencia. Su niño tenaz necesita saber que siempre podrá depender de usted. Con una guía apropiada, probablemente se llegue a ser un muy exitoso empresario o abogado, o un gran líder de la comunidad—aun el presidente de los Estados Unidos, especialmente si usted les dice que es posible. No debe matar el espíritu impulsor que los provoca a ser tan determinados. Solamente tenemos que canalizarlo hacia el camino apropiado y estar siempre vigilantes y atentos, para saber dónde están y qué están haciendo.

Yo pasé muchos momentos inolvidables y alarmantes con Steven. ¿Ha perdido usted a su niño por unos cuantos minutos en el centro comercial? ¡Esos minutos parecen una eternidad! Poco antes de cumplir los dos años de edad, Steven se fue a explorar el barrio, ¡y no lo pudimos encontrar por tres horas! ¿Se imagina por lo que pasé? Una madre joven en ese entonces, yo me acuerdo que las rodillas temblorosas se me volvieron tan débiles por la desesperación y el temor, que me caí al suelo llorando. Pensé que nunca más lo iba a ver. Teníamos a policías, bomberos, y todos nuestros parientes buscándolo. Por fin, mi cuñada Lupe lo encontró a seis casas de donde vivíamos, jugando dentro del garaje de una casa vacía. Yo he pasado por mil muertes con este niño. Cuando él tenía tres años, fuimos a acampar en Colorado. Un momento estaba a mi lado, y al siguiente, estaba persiguiendo a una ardilla listada, hasta lo profundo del bosque. Parecía ser que Steven necesitaba estar sujetado a una correa durante los primeros seis años de su vida.

Estos niños representan un desafío para cualquier padre. Tal como antes mencioné, yo soy extrovertida y también lo es Steven, sin embargo, ha sido abrumador para mí en muchas ocasiones. Yo me imagino como habría sido para padres que tienen la personalidad opuesta. No se desesperen. ¡El truco es mantenerlos *ocupados*! Mi esposo y yo sabíamos que teníamos que soltar algo de esa energía desbordante. Inscribimos a Steven en clases de natación cuando tenía nueve meses de edad y lecciones de karate a los tres años de edad. Siempre ha sido competitivo y alguien que desarrolla al máximo su potencial, luchando por alcanzar la perfección. Su niño o niña quizá le sorprenda con su espíritu competitivo. Cuando tenía tres años, nosotros fuimos a una feria en el YMCA donde acababa de ganar varios galones en una competencia de natación. Nos íbamos del terreno cuando detuvo a toda la familia para mirar una competencia de *breakdance*. Inmediatamente quiso competir Steven. Mi esposo estaba renuente a permitirle competir porque los otros competidores, quienes eran mucho mayores, lucían trajes especiales y habían practicado sus rutinas por semanas, pero yo lo convencí que le permitiera hacer el intento. Steven estudió los movimientos de los niños al practicar sus rutinas y en el tiempo tan corto que pasó observando, aprendió como hacer el *moon walk* y girar sobre su cabeza. Se metió al concurso y volvió a casa con el trofeo de primer lugar.

De nuevo, es importante que usted sepa dónde están sus niños activos en todo momento del día y de la noche. La niñera también tiene que ser muy atenta, ya que este tipo de niños siempre están dentro de un mundo de fantasía, fantaseando y actuando los papeles de sus héroes y personajes favoritos. Como el día que quiso ser un *ninja*. Mi esposo y yo estábamos en Puerto Rico en viaje de negocios que sirvió también de escapada para celebrar nuestro aniversario. Contratamos a una niñera que se quedara en casa y cuidara a los niños. Una noche, Steven, de alrededor de ocho años de edad, salió a escondidas, furtivamente, al patio de atrás vestido con su traje de karate, con la cara y las manos pintadas de negro. Se escondió debajo de uno de los muchos carros que estaban estacionados en *nuestra* propiedad con el motivo de un concierto de los *Beastie Boys* que estaban dando a un lado de nuestra casa. Él quería ver de qué se trataba todo el "borlote". Recibimos una llamada de la niñera esa noche y nos dijo que un policía acababa de traer a Steven, con esposas puestas, a la puerta de entrada. El policía bien pudo haberle disparado a Steven, al andarse arrastrando por la oscuridad. ¡Volvimos inmediatamente a casa! Si usted tiene a un niño semejante al mío, necesita poner a prueba de niños su casa. La razón no es para hacer prisionero a su niño, sino disuadirlo de dejar que su curiosidad tome control.

Las monjas de la escuela primaria católica de Steven nos dijeron que rezarían mucho por él después de que él dejó de asistir a la escuela. Años más tarde, ellas me preguntarían: "¿Cómo está Steven?" A esta pregunta siempre la seguía una mirada de "pobrecitos", como si sintieran lástima por mi esposo y por mí. Yo les respondía: "Ya verán. Algún día Steven será un gran líder. Yo tengo fe en mi hijo especial".

Los rezos han de haber funcionado, porque al entrar Steven a la secundaria, verdaderamente maduró y se volvió más calmado y con más dominio de sí mismo. Su participación en el fútbol americano le ayudó, y eso o cualquier otra actividad física y deportista quizá les ayude a sus niños que tienen mucha energía. El fútbol proveía todo lo que Steven necesitaba: excitación, aventura, competencia, prestigio, y un sentido de pertenecer. ¡Y los entrenadores verdaderamente lo hicieron trabajar! Para poder jugar fútbol él tenía que mantener sus calificaciones y no podía meterse en problemas. El fútbol le enseñó el significado de la cooperación y el espíritu deportivo. Le levantó su confianza, su valor, su fortaleza, y su imagen propia.

Muchos hispanos tienen una estatura menor del promedio, son bien chaparritos—Steven forma parte de este grupo. ¿Qué puede hacer uno si le hacen burla a su niño a causa de su estatura? Nosotros le dimos a Steven un poco de munición para defenderse—los dichos y los cuentos. Aunque Steven era más pequeño en tamaño que muchos de sus compañeros de equipo, Steven le respondía a cualquier que trataba de menospreciarlo por su estatura, con el dicho: *como un chile piquín, soy chiquito pero picoso*. También había escuchado el cuento popular mexicano de la carrera entre el caballo arrogante y la pequeña abeja, en el cual la abeja ganó la carrera al encaramarse en la punta de la nariz del caballo. Steven solía decir: "Lo que cuenta no es tu estatura, sino tu astucia, tu agilidad, y tu dedicación y compromiso a algo". Como resultado de este tipo de actividad, creo que Steven algún día va a llegar a ser un político o un líder de la comunidad o un abogado.

Su propia versión de una ley común de física para la fuerza es: la fuerza = la masa x aceleración + ganas. Más adelante, al ser uno de los jugadores que comenzaba el juego, en el equipo defensivo *varsity* de preparatoria de categoría de 5A, su cuerpo de 5 pies con 6 pulgadas, y 150 libras de peso, junto con su fuerte empuje y determinación, hicieron posible que él tacleara a enormes jugadores que constaban de seis pies de estatura y doscientas libras de peso. El hacer pesas todos los días le ayudaba. Él estaba determinado a ser como el personaje de la película *Rudy*, una historia sobre un pequeñito jugador de fútbol que finalmente logra jugar fútbol universitario en Notre Dame, a través de la perseverancia y el arduo trabajo. Steven siempre estaba jugando en contra de las probabilidades. A las personas que le dijeron que nunca podría ser un jugador de fútbol en el equipo *varsity* a causa de su estatura, les probó que *él que quiere, puede* y también probó que *más hace él que quiere, que él que puede*.

Las buenas calificaciones serán fáciles de lograr para algunos de sus niños; para otros, como Steven, les costará mucho esfuerzo lograrlas. No compare a sus niños. Todos son diferentes y tienen diferentes necesidades, deseos, y aspiraciones. Un niño quizá necesite más ayuda con sus tareas y con estudiar para los exámenes. Nos pasamos muchas horas con Steven repasando listas de palabras para ortografía, o preguntas de historia. Muchas veces los maestros trataron de desanimarlo de tomar las clases para estudiantes sobresalientes (*honors classes*), pensando que él no podía hacerla en esas clases. Como padres, ustedes tienen que estar allí para apoyar a sus niños y asegurarse que reciban las oportunidades que necesitan para conseguir una buena educación. Aunque era inteligente y lograba sacar calificaciones de "A" y "B", generalmente una "C" le impedía muchas veces alcanzar a figurar en el cuadro de honor.

Pero les mostró a los maestros que sí podía hacerla en la clase de matemáticas para estudiantes sobresalientes. A Steven le encantaban la lógica y la utilización de la analítica para resolver problemas, ambas de las cuales usaba astutamente y con habilidad, para alcanzar sus metas.

Los niños de espíritu muy fuerte y llenos de energía, requieren de firmeza, reglas consistentes y vigilancia de parte de los padres, hasta que puedan lograr mayor dominio de sí mismos. Con Steven, no pude soltarle ni un poquito las riendas, por muchos años. Aunque mi esposo y yo estuvimos de acuerdo en no utilizar el castigo corporal como forma de disciplina, tengo que admitir que en algunas ocasiones Steven hizo cosas que estaban fuera de los límites, cosas que podían haber lastimado a otros o a él mismo. Criando a Steven, frecuentemente recuerdo las famosas palabras de mi madre: "Vas a pagar todas las que debes con este muchacho". Yo no podía quejarme demasiado porque mi madre toleró mi conducta expresiva y curiosa. Era fuerte y estricta, pero nunca mató ese espíritu que me impulsaba y que eventualmente me ayudó a llegar a ser una líder de la comunidad más tarde en mi vida. Yo, como mi madre, he tratado de usar todos mis recursos y toda mi fortaleza para mantener a mis niños seguros y en el camino apropiado, pero al mismo tiempo, preservar sus personalidades singulares.

Si usted tiene un niño como Steven, probablemente le reconforte saber que no se encuentra solo en aquellos episodios por los cuales tiene que pasar. Aunque nos salgan canas con las cosas increíbles que hacen, también nos pueden proporcionar muchos recuerdos alegres. Disfrute de su espíritu radiante, eventualmente crecerá y más tarde usted se reirá de las cosas que le hicieron llorar.

Cada uno de sus niños es tan diferente. Le he dado una descripción de dos personalidades distintas. Ahora le ofrezco la tercera, la niña obstinada, tenaz. El parto de mi niña, Gloria Vanessa Rodríguez, me sirvió como seña de lo que estaba por venir, y del tipo de personalidad que poseería. Aun antes de su nacimiento, ella era diferente a los niños varones. Cuando llegaba al hospital, los niños varones nacieron en menos de una hora. Con Sal pasaron cuarenta y cinco minutos y con Steven, treinta minutos. Cuando se me rompió la bolsa de aguas, yo sabía que iba a tener a Vanessa dentro del elevador. Les advertí a todos que tendría a mi bebé en menos de treinta minutos. Después de todo ese borlote, duré doce largas horas para dar a luz a Vanessa. Tres diferentes mujeres entraron y salieron de la sala de partos para tener a sus bebés, y yo, nada. ¡Qué vergüenza! Después de que el doctor tuvo que inducir el parto, comenzamos a pensar que tal vez era una señal de lo que se nos esperaba: el carácter de Vanessa sería siempre imprevisible y terco.

Con sólo la cabeza afuera, el doctor concluyó prematuramente que era un niño porque sus facciones se parecían a las de Steven. Engañó al doctor. Resultó ser la niña más hermosa, tan rosada como las rosas que mi esposo me obsequió. A lo largo de su vida, Vanessa ha seguido siendo imprevisible. Tiene una personalidad expansiva que incluye muchos intereses y habilidades. Es inteligente, tenaz, amistosa, y empática. Es tímida, pero muy agresiva y competitiva. Estas características le han ayudado a sobresalir en variados deportes, particularmente en básquetbol, el cual ha jugado con fervor desde edad preescolar. Mi esposo fue su entrenador y la matriculaba en cada liga de básquetbol que podía para ayudar a desarrollar su interés.

Mientras que el interés de Vanessa por matemáticas, ciencia, y deportes igualaba al de sus hermanos, ella en contraste aparentaba poseer una personalidad más cariñosa y comprensiva. Muchas veces Vanessa me ganaba en ir al botiquín a traer jarabe para la tos o una curita (*Band-Aid*) cuando los niños se enfermaban o se lastimaban. También les dedicaba bastante atención a los animales enfermos. Quizá eran sus instintos maternales naturales que la hicieron ser así, porque estas características eran menos frecuentes en la conducta de los niños.

¿Usted tiene a una niña que es la menor y se ha criado con solamente hermanos varones? Si la tiene, probablemente se habrá dado cuenta que esto la ha hecho ser fuerte y firme, simplemente para poderse defender. Sin embargo, ¿vio también el cariñoso lado femenino en ella, aun si resultó ser menos femenina que el de muchas niñas? ¿Se ha preguntado alguna vez si las niñas son diferentes a los niños por naturaleza?

La forma de jugar de Vanessa siempre fue diferente a la de los niños. Sus juegos de imaginación siempre fueron mas realistas. Ella acomodaba a sus muñecas y se convertía en maestra o doctora, tal como yo hacía cuando era niña. Ya sea enseñando u "operando" a sus hermanos, niños vecinos, o primos pequeños, Vanessa siempre mostró una preferencia por ayudar a otros. Más adelante, al ser niñera, ella mostraba su amor por los niños con su paciencia y su capacidad de llegarle al más terco de los niños.

Yo oigo a los padres del barrio decir que sus niños varones son "puros hombres", y si bien no me gusta generalmente catalogar las cosas así, en realidad yo veía una diferencia definitiva entre las formas de jugar de mis niños. Los juegos de mis niños varones nunca mostraron la conducta cariñosa que miraba en los de Vanessa. Mientras que ella cuidadosamente jugaba con sus muñecas o las cuidaba, Steven les quitaba la ropa, el cabello, y los brazos o los usaba como si fueran pelotas de fútbol. Me encontré con que a pesar de que les compré muñecos de ambos sexos para todos mis niños para quitar el énfasis que hay en los estereotipos y los papeles que juegan, a veces las diferencias se manifestaban por su propia cuenta.

El libro *In a Different Voice*, de Carol Gilligan, confirma estas diferencias. Ella cita investigaciones que han concluido que se encontraron diferencias entre los sexos en los juegos de los niños durante el recreo y en las clases de educación física. Se estableció que los niños varones juegan afuera con más frecuencia que las niñas. Juegan más frecuentemente en grupos grandes y de edades variadas, juegan juegos competitivos con más frecuencia, y sus juegos duran más tiempo que los de las niñas. Los juegos duran más tiempo no solamente porque sus juegos son más complejos y requieren más habilidades para organizar, sino también porque cuando ocurre algún conflicto, los niños resuelven más efectivamente sus problemas que las niñas. Cuando las niñas tenían un conflicto, mejor dejaron de jugar porque les importaba más mantener una relación que ganar. Los juegos de las niñas se constituían de grupos más pequeños, más íntimos, cooperando y turnándose, y por la mayor parte, se llevaban a cabo en lugares privados. Gilligan afirma que para niñas pequeñas, la intimidad y la identidad van juntas, ya que las niñas llegan a conocerse a sí mismas por medio de sus relaciones con otros. Los niños adquieren su sentido de identidad por medio de su posición particular en el mundo, sus habilidades, sus creencias, y sus características físicas. En su libro titulado *Your Child's Growing Mind*, teórica de aprendizaje Jane M. Healy cita investigaciones que concluyeron que la mayoría de las niñas hablan, leen, y escriben a una edad más temprana que los niños varones y también sacan mejores calificaciones en exámenes que miden habilidades verbales, incluyendo la lectura, la escritura, la gramática, y la ortografía. Generalmente tienen mayores habilidades motrices refinadas (utilización de las manos para tareas delicadas, intrincadas), y para cálculos matemáticos. Se piensa que las niñas son más sensibles a expresiones faciales y a señales o pistas en su medio ambiente, lo cual, según creen algunos investigadores científicos, las hace ser más intuitivas. Se sabe que las niñas son diferentes a los niños en que buscan la opinión de otros antes de actuar. ¿Ha encontrado que esto sea cierto con respecto a sus niñas? La mayoría de los niños, de acuerdo a Healy, son más diestros en las habilidades espaciales, el razonamiento matemático, el pensamiento abstracto, y las habilidades motrices mayores. Algunas investigaciones científicas afirman que los niños son mejores que las niñas para resolver los laberintos, y que al llegar al décimo año escolar, generalmente superan a las niñas en matemáticas.

Tal vez estas diferencias, hasta cierto punto, tengan que ver con cómo los adultos tratan a sus niños. Los hispanos somos iguales a otros grupos étnicos en que muchas veces tenemos diferentes expectativas de las niñas que de los niños. Cuando hacemos esto, estamos transmitiendo mensajes no verbales a las niñas que a la larga pueden afectar su imagen propia y su conducta. ¿Usted trata a sus niños varones de una manera y a sus niñas de otra? En el caso de Vanessa, mi esposo y yo nos hemos esforzado mucho por exigir y esperar tanto de ella como de los niños, razón por la cual creo que se ha mantenido agresiva y competitiva. Su naturaleza firme no nos permitía tratarla de otra manera, ya que ella inmediatamente decía: "¿Y los niños qué?" O, tal vez: "Espera un momento, ¿hay algo de sexismo aquí?"

Si usted tiene una niña, hágale saber que ella merece igual oportunidad en un mundo competitivo. Proporciónele bastantes experiencias y oportunidades para observar a muchos tipos de modelos de conducta. Al mismo tiempo, ayude a sus niños varones a volverse más cariñosos y sensibles, al pedirles que sean más serviciales, más empáticos, y más comprensivos. Ellos necesitan comprender cómo afectan a otros, y tener la mente más abierta a los puntos de vista de otros. Cuando la maestra de Sal me dijo que lo estaba mimando, me hice más consciente de mis acciones y me esforcé mucho por no dejar que él me manipulara para conseguir que yo hiciera cosas por él. Yo me sentía ir contra la corriente de una cultura donde las madres tienden a hacer más por los hombrecitos. Pero, mi esposo y yo tuvimos que hacer un gran esfuerzo para tratar de manera justa e igual a todos nuestros niños.

La personalidad bondadosa y cariñosa de Vanessa le ha ganado muchas amistades, pero también le ha metido en problemas. Por ejemplo, cuando estaba en el kinder, su maestra me dijo: "Vanessa es muy metiche. Ella se hace responsable de ver quién necesita ayuda. Se pasa demasiado tiempo fuera de su asiento, platica con sus compañeros demasiado, y no me escucha a mí como debe. Yo sé que tiene buenas intenciones, y que los niños la quieren mucho, pero como maestra, ¡yo quiero que se quede sentada y que no se meta en lo que no le importa!" El ser metiche y sociable fue el tema de muchas conferencias entre los maestros y nosotros hasta la secundaria. Le acarrearía ambos elogios y castigos. En cuanto a los niños, la miraban como una líder, y la buscaban como un recurso y como una compañera. En casa, ella asumía el papel de mandona al decirles a todos lo que debían hacer. Sus habilidades de liderazgo surgieron desde el kinder, cuando su clase la eligió "líder de su clase". Como padres, debemos reforzar y apoyar estas características de liderazgo, además de enseñarles más habilidades sociales positivas. Debemos enseñarles cómo su conducta afecta a otros, incluyendo a la maestra.

Aunque las investigaciones demuestran que los niños son mejores que las niñas en matemáticas, Vanessa tenía fuertes habilidades analíticas y matemáticas, pero también tenía un sentido natural de creatividad, el cual expresaba por medio de caricaturas y figuras a escala. Siempre era aplicada y sacaba buenas calificaciones y figuraba en el cuadro de honor cada año antes de entrar a la secundaria. Nunca tenía que recordarle de hacer su tarea, y siempre la completaba a tiempo, además de pulcra y ordenadamente, bueno, hasta la edad de doce años.

Si no ha notado la diferencia entre los niños varones y las niñas cuando eran pequeños, seguramente la notará al acercarse a los doce años de edad. Algo le pasó a Vanessa cuando cumplió los doce años. Quizá eran las hormonas o el cambio de una pequeña escuela católica a una escuela pública más grande que hizo surgir una personalidad más fuerte, y algo rebelde—una personalidad *carancha*. Se había convertido en una total extraña. Vanessa siempre había sido casi perfecta: dulce, bondadosa, y respetuosa, siempre haciendo lo debido y nunca metiéndose en problemas reales (excepto cuando estaba Steven detrás de ello). Ella era la "princesa" de Papi y Mami. Pero cuando cumplió los doce anos, se convirtió en una persona que no reconocíamos. Tal como su alumbramiento fue imprevisible, tampoco esperaba un cambio tan abrupto de personalidad. No vi ese cambio tan abruptamente con mis niños varones. Les estoy previniendo a todos los padres: *cuidado con esas listas y calladitas, pueden saltar y picarte*. Si usted siente que tiene a la niña perfecta, una perfecta princesita, prepárese. Algunos niños parecen comenzar los tumultuosos años de adolescente con pocas erupciones tempranas.

Vanessa, igual a muchos preadolescentes, deseaba agradar y parecerse a otros. Por lo tanto, si sus mejores amigos no estaban sacando buenas calificaciones, ella no quería ser catalogada como "la inteligente" o "la gansa". Estaba muy acomplejada acerca de su apariencia, especialmente cuando tenía frenos en los dientes, y no quería ser diferente a los demás. Al cambiarse su apariencia para "encajar", así también cambió su actitud, su dignidad, y su forma de relacionarse con otros. Se ponía las camisas grandes de su hermano y luego se volvió discutidora, rebelde, grosera, insensible, e irrespetuosa—una adolescente típica, sin embargo, unos cuantos años antes de su tiempo.

De nuevo, el ser padre tiene sus momentos buenos y no tan buenos, sus cimas y sus valles. No es fácil ser padre, o madre, de un preadolescente. Siendo una madre hispana, es tan difícil enfrentar y lidiar con el egoísmo y las faltas de respeto que surgirán.

Una fría mañana de invierno, por ejemplo, me desperté temprano para hacerle un poco de cereal calientito a Vanessa antes de salir ella para la escuela. Bajó por los escalones con pantalones cortos y dijo: "No quiero desayunar". Horrorizada al verla con ropa de verano, mandé a Vanessa a volver a su cuarto para ponerse algo más abrigado. Ella respondió con palabras que nunca antes había usado. "Ay, madre, vete a dormir", dijo al salir de la casa, dejándome completamente anonadada. "¿Qué pasó?" me pregunté. ¿Por qué fue tan irrespetuosa? ¿Debo correr tras de ella o dejarla morir de frío? Antes de poder tomar una decisión, ella ya estaba a bordo del camión de la escuela.

Para madres tradicionales hispanas que valoran el respeto, lidiar con este tipo de conducta puede requerir un esfuerzo tremendo. Por un lado, quería que me mostrara respeto, pero por el otro, yo sabía que le había enseñado a poner en duda las cosas y a ser firme. Cuando ella tenía una opinión se volvía inflexible. Vanessa sentía tanta presión por comportarse como los demás adolescentes. Está claro que los valores que se le habían enseñado estaban siendo puestas a prueba durante este período crítico. ¿Qué hace uno durante estos episodios?

Esta experiencia me enseñó que algunas personalidades son más vulnerables a la presión a la que se ven sometidos los adolescentes, que otras. Como padres, necesitamos ser muy pacientes, atentos a lo que hacen y dicen, y apoyarlos. También necesitamos estar conscientes de las personas con quienes se asocian nuestros niños, porque cada uno puede ejercer una tremenda influencia sobre ellos. Tal como dice el dicho, *dime con quién te juntas y te diré quién eres*. Nuestros niños pueden aprender fácilmente cosas que escuchan y miran, de aquéllos con quienes se asocian. Si su niño o niña aparece muy distante o si asocia con un grupo de gente mala, no trate de resolverlo solo. Trabaje en conjunto con el personal de la escuela. Quizá puedan aconsejar a su niño, permitirle a usted observar una de sus clases si es que están preocupados por los niños con quienes está asociando, o quizá usted pueda servir como chaperón(a) durante actividades escolares. Esfuércese por conocer a los padres de los niños que son compañeros de clase de su niño, y lo más importante a esta edad, mantenga a su niño ocupado en actividades de la escuela, la iglesia, y la comunidad, donde puede conocer a una variedad de amigos.

Yo tuve que trabajar en conjunto con la escuela para hacer algo sobre el cambio en la conducta de Vanessa. Sus maestros presentían que ella estaba comenzando a sentirse abrumada al tratar de pertenecer a un grupo de niñas que tenían valores diferentes a los suyos. Todos los niños tienen que enfrentarse a esta presión de otros que quieren que sean como ellos, y como padres, tenemos que ayudarles a lidiar con esto y resolverlo. Esta presión hizo que el exterior de Vanessa cambiara, pero adentro, todavía añoraba ser ella misma. Los cimientos que se construyeron cuando era pequeña estaban en conflicto con su necesidad de pertenecer y de agradar.

Eventualmente, Vanessa volvió por voluntad propia a la pequeña escuela católica donde había asistido desde kinder hasta tercer año de primaria. Las clases eran más pequeñas y yo conocía a los niños y a las familias con quienes se estaba asociando. Volvió a un ambiente que reforzaba los valores con los cuales ella había crecido. Miré una transformación en su apariencia cuando ella comenzó a asociarse con amigos que tenían valores similares, y cuando volvió a usar uniformes. Se enorgullecía de su apariencia y su conducta volvió a ser la de aquella persona compasiva y servicial que siempre había sido, bueno, por la mayor parte. ¡Gracias a Dios!

En este capítulo, he compartido con ustedes tres personalidades separadas en un intento de demostrar las diferencias tan marcadas que pueden haber entre los niños, aun los de una misma familia. He ofrecido algunas estrategias que pueden utilizar los padres para sacar lo mejor de esas personalidades. Como padres, no debemos mostrar favoritismo hacia cierto niño, ni compararlos entre sí, porque *cada quien es como Dios lo hizo*. Cada uno de sus niños es único y especial, como los dedos de la mano.

ÚNICOS EN SUS CARACTERÍSTICAS FÍSICAS

Los niños también son diferentes y únicos en las características físicas que son pasadas de generación en generación. Los hispanos vienen de todas formas, tonos, y tamaños. Sangre india, europea, africana, y de Asia han añadido muchas dimensiones a como nos miramos. Aun dentro de una misma familia, las diferencias físicas entre los niños pueden ser profundas.

Por ejemplo, en las familias de mis padres se pueden encontrar a personas de cabello lacio, ondulado, y muy chino, estilo afro. Puede encontrar a personas que tienen la piel muy blanca además de aquéllas de tez aceitunada o morena. Encontrará ojitos chinitos y negros, y también ojos grandes y redondos azules, cafés, o verdes. En el lado de mi esposo, hay siete niños con ojos verdes y uno con ojos cafés obscuros. Todos nuestros niños tienen que ser aceptados y respetados tal y como los creó Dios. Yo he escuchado a hispanos decir de los niños de otros: "Ay, pobrecito, salió morenito", como si la piel morena fuera una desgracia o una maldición. Un día mi hija me dijo que otros niños le estaban llamando nombres en la escuela por la forma chinita de los ojos. El amor propio de un niño se forma y se refuerza con la comunicación verbal y no verbal de los padres. El niño a quien se le dice "morenito", "chinito", o "negrito", todos los cuales se utilizan frecuentemente como sobrenombres de cariño, debe saber, por sus palabras y acciones, que es amado y admirado tanto como sus hermanos. Necesitamos recordarles a nuestros niños que son bellos, diferentes, y especiales, y que los amamos a todos por igual.

ÚNICOS EN SU INTELIGENCIA

Cada uno de sus niños, tal como los míos, posee puntos fuertes y habilidades que lo distinguen, cada uno nace con ciertas tendencias o preferencias, y cada uno posee un gran potencial que está a la espera de ser descubierto y cultivado. Tal como dice el dicho *el que nace para tamal, del cielo le caen hojas*, cada persona está dotada de ciertos rasgos de personalidad y habilidades innatas singulares. Howard Gardner, un neuropsicólogo, se refiere a estas habilidades como inteligencias múltiples. De acuerdo a Gardner, todos somos capaces de demostrar conocimientos de nueve maneras. Él explica que toda persona posee todas estas inteligencias hasta cierto grado, sin embargo unas simplemente son más fuertes que otras.

Ellas son:

1. lingüística, o una habilidad para el lenguaje (especialmente escritores, poetas)
2. lógica y matemática, la capacidad de resolver problemas, por ejemplo, por medio del razonamiento y la deducción, y distinguir o encontrar las pautas (científicos, ingenieros)
3. espacial, la capacidad de visualizar el dibujo físico de un objeto o del ambiente y navegar o diseñar (arquitectos, jugadores de ajedrez, artistas)
4. musical, la capacidad de orquestar y producir ritmos y canciones (compositores, cantantes)
5. cinética del cuerpo, utilizando el cuerpo de uno para expresarse, crear o encontrar una solución a un problema (atletas, bailarines)
6. interpersonal, el poseer una comprensión de otros seres humanos, sus pensamientos y sus emociones (maestros, políticos)
7. intrapersonal, el conocer el ser interno de uno mismo, los sentimientos de uno mismo y cómo éstas afectan la conducta, saber

resolver problemas o sobrevivir a situaciones difíciles (estrategas, analistas militares)

8. naturalista, alguien que ama y aprecia la naturaleza (ecologistas)
9. espiritual, una conexión a aspectos de la vida que son "del otro mundo" (religión, filosofía, y hipnotismo)

Un niño puede ser dotado de ambas inteligencias lingüísticas y lógica matemática. Puede que sea un genio para la computadora o un escritor talentoso. Un niño con una habilidad viva de resolver problemas a través de asociaciones y relaciones es un niño con buenas habilidades intrapersonales. ¿Qué tal sus propios niños, cuáles son sus puntos fuertes intelectuales? ¿Qué es lo que verdaderamente les gusta hacer? Su hijo o hija quizá sobresalga en el área de inteligencia cinética del cuerpo al ser una bailarina o un atleta. Quizá sea una combinación de varias de éstas. Gardner pone énfasis en el hecho de que inteligencias múltiples no se cancelan. El tener habilidad para las matemáticas y también para el dibujo no necesariamente significa que uno no tenga habilidad para jugar básquetbol, tal como nos dimos cuenta con Vanessa. Un niño que se asocia bien con la gente y posee un talento especial para negociar y lograr lo que quiere, posee fuertes habilidades interpersonales.

La frase *cada cabeza es un mundo* nos recuerda que las experiencias, los pensamientos, y las habilidades de cada persona son diferentes y singulares. Si los padres comprenden que los niños poseen una variedad de habilidades innatas tal vez les ayude a apoyar y cultivar la individualidad de sus niños. Ha requerido mucha observación crítica y escuchar atentamente para reconocer los dones que posee cada uno de mis niños. Se necesitará el esfuerzo de los padres, maestros, entrenadores, parientes, y amigos para descubrir y cultivar sus dones divinos. Desdichadamente, demasiadas escuelas en los Estados Unidos están diseñadas para los niños que tienen fuertes habilidades para el lenguaje y la lógica, aquellas habilidades que se dicen emerger del lado izquierdo del cerebro. Necesitamos apoyar y valorar al artista creativo, a aquéllos que tienen una inclinación musical y a aquéllos que piensan de una manera poco convencional, que no siguen la corriente.

Muchas escuelas de hoy están tratando de cambiar y, ojalá, hacer un mejor trabajo con relación a reconocer y cultivar los talentos en ciernes, con miras a nuestra cultura. Como padres debemos trabajar con los maestros de nuestros niños para ayudarles a reconocer su singularidad y trabajar con ellos para sacar sus patrones de conducta e intereses innatos. Cultive sus puntos fuertes en casa para que los maestros los puedan reforzar en clase.

Cada año se escoge a una cierta cantidad de niños para participar en los programas para los niños superdotados en las escuelas a través del país. Como miembro de la Comisión Presidencial para la Excelencia Educativa para los Hispanoamericanos, yo puedo confirmar que los niños hispanos no tienen la representación que les corresponde en estos programas. Como padre, es su responsabilidad inquirir e informarse sobre estos programas y asegurar que sus niños no son excluidos, que participen en ellos. Las escuelas *"magnet"* son diseñadas para tratar de satisfacer los diferentes intereses y talentos de los niños. Inscriba a sus niños en clases que les ayudarán a desarrollar sus talentos. Mi hermano tenía diez años cuando mi madre se dio cuenta de que tenía una afinidad y un talento para el arte. Lo inscribió en clases de arte por correspondencia. Ya para cuando cumplió los once años, sus pinturas religiosas y culturales estaban expuestas a través de su escuela.

Si a sus niños les gusta desarmar cosas, permítalos experimentar y explorar con radios y tocadiscos viejos, y al mismo tiempo asegúrese de que no se electrocuten al desenchufar los aparatos mientras estén experimentando. Si sus niños tienen preferencias musicales, consígales instrumentos, aliéntelos a cantar, o llévelos a clases de baile. Cómpreles un piano o un trompeta. Haga ese esfuerzo especial de ayudar a sus niños a lograr sus destinos. Usted juega un papel importante en lo que sus niños lleguen a ser, por medio del tipo de medio ambiente que usted provee y los estímulos que éste ofrezca.

ÚNICOS EN SUS ESTILOS DE APRENDIZAJE

Otra forma de pensar acerca de la singularidad de los niños es determinada por cuál lado del cerebro es más dominante, el derecho o el izquierdo. Algunos niños procesan la información con el lado izquierdo del cerebro, mientras que otros la procesan con el derecho. A los niños cuyos cerebros son dominados por el lado izquierdo, les gusta desbaratar, desentrañar, analizar cada parte de las cosas con su mente, mientras que a los niños cuyos cerebros son dominados por el lado izquierdo les gusta mirar el "cuadro completo". El del lado izquierdo es alguien que aprecia los detalles y es bueno para escribir y escuchar. Yo pienso en cómo Sal sobresale al escribir y al utilizar una amplia gama de habilidades motrices refinadas, al cambiar rápidamente entre usar la computadora a trabajar en juegos de vídeo complicados, al demostrar su agilidad para el piano. Su estilo de aprendizaje es más como el que utiliza el lado izquierdo del cerebro. Esto no quiere decir que alguien que tiene el lado izquierdo dominante no podrá sobresalir en otras cosas, tal como lo demostró el talento de Sal para jugar fútbol americano, fútbol, y béisbol. Una persona que es dominada por el lado izquierdo del cerebro puede poseer una mente muy analítica y lógica, pero sólo hará una cosa a la vez y tiene que seguir una orden secuencial. ¿Usted tiene a alguien así en su casa? Observe cómo resuelven los problemas sus niños. Por ejemplo, cuando Sal se encontraba frente a algo nuevo, como la vez que comenzó su acuario para peces, él tenía que analizar todo acerca del proceso. Primero comenzó con un acuario para peces de agua dulce, y luego, metódicamente, siguió con el acuario para peces de agua salada.

Mientras que aquéllos dominados por el lado izquierdo del cerebro tienen más habilidad para lo concreto y las fórmulas matemáticas, los que son dominados por el lado derecho tienen habilidad para los problemas matemáticos, la geometría, los mapas, y los cuadros y gráficos de estadísticas. Aquéllos gobernados por el lado derecho son más intuitivos y creativos. Ellos son los llamados visionarios y aprenden por medio de hacer y crear. Similar a Steven, quizá sobresalgan en arte o drama con su poderoso estallido de creatividad. Son afectados por imágenes sensoriales, especialmente si éstas se relacionan con la interacción entre personas. Cuando Sal leía, estaba fascinado por las palabras, mientras que Steven, el que está dominado por el lado derecho del cerebro, estaba más interesado en las relaciones y el significado detrás de la historia. A Sal le gustaba la rutina, y a Steven le encantaba la novedad y la excitación. Los que son dominados por el lado derecho del cerebro van en contra de la corriente, hacen todo a su particular y singular manera.

Yo sé que Sal puede ser clasificado como dominado por el lado izquierdo del cerebro, y Steven por el lado derecho, pero catalogar a Vanessa no fue tan sencillo. Sus habilidades naturales la hicieron fuerte por ambos lados. Tiene buenas habilidades para las matemáticas, las relaciones personales, y la creatividad. Es muy parecida a su padre, que es ingeniero, músico, y poeta.

¿Cómo clasificaría usted a sí mismo(a) o a sus niños? Como padres, debemos ser pacientes y comprensivos y apoyar los estilos singulares de aprendizaje de nuestros niños y sus puntos fuertes. Al mismo tiempo, tenemos que proveer una variedad de experiencias para estimular y equilibrar ambos lados del cerebro. Vamos a explorar este punto detalladamente en el próximo capítulo. Aunque los niños nacen con ciertas tendencias y patrones de conducta, en última instancia su medio ambiente más cercano será el factor determinante para alcanzar su potencial, formar su personalidad, y desarrollar sus habilidades, talentos, e intereses.

LA NATURALEZA FRENTE A LA CULTIVACIÓN

¿Nacen algunas personas con más potencial o capacidad intelectual que otras, o es el medio ambiente el factor decisivo? Hace algunos años, tuve la fortuna de conocer al astronauta Franklin Chang-Díaz en el Centro Espacial de NASA, donde pronunció un discurso ante un grupo de científicos y matemáticos. Yo fui invitada para hablar en esa conferencia sobre maneras de aumentar la cantidad de niños hispanos que entran a los campos de ingeniería y ciencia. Mi tema era la importancia de los estímulos durante la primera infancia y el papel de los padres como los primeros maestros. Durante el periodo reservado para preguntas y respuestas, yo le pregunté al doctor Chang-Diaz: "¿Por qué quiso usted ser astronauta? ¿Quién lo motivó a seguir ese sueño?" Después de meditar un momento sobre las preguntas, él luego respondió enfáticamente que su madre merecía el crédito por el camino que él escogió para su vida. Yo sentía ganas de pararme en la silla y gritar: "¡Sí! ¡Dame cinco!" Contó al grupo que cuando era niño, siempre sentía curiosidad acerca de la luna y las estrellas, y su madre iba a la biblioteca para sacarle todos los libros que encontraba sobre ese tema. Ella llevó a la casa unas enormes cajas vacías que habían contenido muebles, las juntó y lo alentó a que se imaginara que fuera una nave espacial. Esto le hizo posible soñar que algún día él podría llegar a ser un astronauta. Su sueño se convirtió en realidad gracias a sus genes y a la gente a su alrededor que lo alentó.

Selena, la adorada cantante de la música tejana, es otro ejemplo de lo que puede occurrirles a los niños con el tipo apropiado de apoyo de parte los padres. Sus padres reconocieron su talento para cantar cuando ella era sólo una niña pequeña y lo cultivaron por medio de aliento y apoyo, aunque ella inicialmente se resistió. Ellos le enseñaron a cantar en español y le recalcaron la importancia de su experiencia en ambas culturas. Impulsados por un ambiente amoroso y de apoyo, los talentos de Selena florecieron y ella llegó a ser una artista fabulosa.

Por generaciones ha existido un gran debate entre los llamados teóricos, entre la "naturaleza" y la "cultivación", que cuestiona si es la herencia o el medio ambiente que determina el potencial intelectual y la personalidad de uno. En mi opinión, una persona nace genéticamente con cierta determinada potencial, capacidad intelectual, y temperamento, pero este hecho no garantiza que el potencial, la capacidad, o las características de personalidad de uno serán completamente desarrolladas si el medio ambiente no es favorable.

El niño será afectado de manera positiva o negativa, por su medio ambiente, antes y después de nacer. Por ejemplo, la conducta de una mujer embarazada que no come bien, que toma alcohol o drogas no recetadas por su médico, o se expone a infecciones virales antes de dar a luz, puede ser la causante de algunas formas de epilepsia, retraso mental, autismo, y esquizofrenia en el recién nacido. Con demasiada frecuencia, el desarrollo de los niños sufre por problemas de visión y audición que pudieron haberse prevenidos, por accidentes, o por problemas que se pueden tratar como la dislexia. Es importante que los niños reciban sus exámenes físicos anuales y sus inmunizaciones. Si no, su mala salud puede invalidar sus habilidades innatas. A veces el desarrollo y el aprendizaje de los niños son atrofiados porque necesitan anteojos, porque tienen hambre, o porque crecen en un ambiente de violencia y temor.

Algunas personas todavía creen que es inútil tratar de cambiar la naturaleza de una persona. Ellos usan el dicho, *lavar puercos con jabón es perder el tiempo y jabón*. Muchas otras personas no están de acuerdo. La genética y el medio ambiente trabajan en conjunto para afectar el temperamento y la personalidad de una persona. Uno influye al otro. Por ejemplo, los padres pueden modificar la conducta fuera de control y potencialmente peligrosa de sus niños al restringir un poco su medio ambiente hasta que aprendan a moderar su propia conducta, tal como tuvimos que hacer mi esposo y yo con Steven. A la vez los padres pueden canalizar la energía desbordada y la personalidad determinada de sus niños hacia algo positivo que les ayudará a llegar a ser grandes líderes más tarde en su vida. Similarmente, tienen la capacidad de sacar a relucir lo mejor de sus niños. Sal creció y dejó atrás su personalidad tímida al alentarlo nosotros a participar en deportes y otras actividades en las que tenía que tratar con otras personas. Sus compañeros le eligieron presidente de su clase en la preparatoria y vicepresidente del consejo estudiantil. Todo esto le dio confianza en sí mismo. Muchos grandes líderes y exitosos presidentes de compañías y organizaciones que eran tímidos por naturaleza han aceptado el desafío y tenido éxito en puestos que generalmente se reservaban para los extrovertidos.

Los padres pueden alterar el destino de sus niños al cambiar su medio ambiente. Si los padres reconocen que sus niños van por mal camino, tal como vimos en el caso de Vanessa, pueden alterar el medio ambiente de sus niños, al remover las influencias negativas y, al fin de cuentas, cambiar su conducta y su futuro. Muchos niños que no son supervisados, ni enseñados valores morales ni límites, se convierten en delincuentes. En adición, los niños que son víctimas del abuso y no reciben muestras de amor, tienen dificultad para ser bondadosos y compasivos.

Usted, como padre, puede provocar un revés o una aceleración en el progreso del lenguaje o el desarrollo cognoscitivo o motor al modificar el medio ambiente. Las investigaciones han concluido que los niños que son privados del afecto y los estímulos intelectuales durante este período crítico pueden quedar seriamente afectados intelectual, social, y emocionalmente. Los niños que tienen menos potencial intelectual pero que son motivados y se esfuerzan mucho pueden lograr más que los niños con más potencial intelectual que no son tan motivados a sobresalir ni a tener éxito. Por lo tanto, la "cultivación" (o el medio ambiente) juega un papel tan importante como la "naturaleza" (o la herencia) en el desarrollo y los logros de uno. De todos modos, no hay duda que después de su nacimiento, los niños necesitan tener un medio ambiente que continuamente los enriquece, cultiva, y estimula para que puedan alcanzar sus potenciales.

EDADES Y ETAPAS: SU NIÑO ES NORMAL Y SU CONDUCTA ES PREVISIBLE

Aunque cada niño es diferente y único, todos ellos, sin tomar en cuenta su raza, clase social o económica, o sexo, pasarán por pautas normales y previsibles de crecimiento y desarrollo. Esto es lo que comúnmente se llaman "edades y etapas", las etapas en el desarrollo de los niños. Incluyen las conductas y las características típicas que han sido observadas en la mayoría de los niños a cada edad, sin embargo, no todos los niños encajan exactamente. Cada etapa está basada en promedios. Esto significa que aproximadamente el 50 por ciento de los niños están en la misma etapa a cierta edad, un 25 por ciento están más adelante, y un 25 por ciento todavía no han alcanzado dicha etapa.

Los expertos en el desarrollo de los niños hace mucho explicaron esta pauta de crecimiento, la cual es caracterizada por períodos de buena conducta seguidos por períodos de mala conducta, llamados *equilibrio* y *desequilibrio*, respectivamente. Cuando los niños están luchando por alcanzar una nueva habilidad de su desarrollo tal como caminar, pero no la han dominado por completo todavía, entran a un estado de desequilibrio y se vuelven ansiosos, temerosos, sensibles, e irritables. Quizá hagan berrinches o sufran de problemas para dormir o comer. Al aprender nuevas habilidades, tal vez experimente un retroceso a un estado de dependencia, donde una vez más se aferra de la falda o la pierna de su madre.

Entran a un estado de desequilibrio cuando no han dominado por completo una habilidad que es necesaria para el aprendizaje de una más avanzada. Por ejemplo, un niño que ha entrado a la etapa de juegos imaginarios pero quien todavía no ha desarrollado suficientemente su lenguaje, se sentirá sumamente frustrado. Un niño que quiere correr pero no ha dominado la habilidad de caminar se irritará. Cuando los niños intentan aprender muchas habilidades al mismo tiempo, tales como caminar, hablar, apilar, andar en triciclo, es comprensible que quizá se sientan abrumados y se comporten de manera terrible. Se volverán temerosos, se aferrarán a uno, y se volverán dependientes al utilizar toda su energía para tratar de comprender y lidiar con lo que está ocurriendo. Es importante que los padres comprendan y expresen su consuelo y apoyo a sus niños. Ellos necesitan ayudarles a resolver sus problemas y a dominar sus habilidades. Manténgase cerca de sus niños y pase tiempo adicional con ellos durante este período, para transmitirles un mayor sentido de seguridad.

Cuando por fin dominan la habilidad, se sienten mejor y una vez más entrarán al estado de equilibrio. Son los angelitos que se convierten en el centro de atención al demostrar sus talentos recién adquiridos. Cuando están en desequilibrio, ¡*mucho cuidado*! Tengan cuidado, porque estarán empeñados en dominar la habilidad, ¡sin tomar en cuenta a quién le estorban!

El período de los dos años hasta los dos años y medio es el punto crítico, el momento de mayor desequilibrio, el cual llamamos los terribles dos años (*terrible twos*). Verdaderamente existe una oscilación entre la conducta buena y la mala. Pero puede estar seguro de que a la etapa negativa le seguirá una etapa más agradable. Justo cuando los padres están disfrutando a sus niños, comienza otra etapa de desequilibrio y los padres tienen que prepararse una vez más para lo que vendrá.

Mientras todos los niños pasan por las mismas etapas secuenciales de desarrollo, los perciben y los encaran de diferente manera, dependiendo de la cultura. Uno de los peores insultos que una persona hispana puede lanzarle a otra es llamar a su niño revoltoso un *hijo malcriado*. Frecuentemente se llega a esta conclusión sin tener una comprensión clara del proceso normal de desarrollo por el cual pasan todos los niños. Sin tener estos conocimientos, los padres quizá pasen por momentos de mucha pena e ira cuando su niño se vuelve más agresivo y terco. Pero después de aprender el porqué y el cómo del desarrollo, serán más pacientes y comprensivos cuando sus niños entran al estado de desequilibrio. Ellos sabrán que esta conducta indeseable es temporal y que la buena conducta está esperando a la vuelta de la esquina.

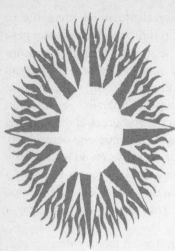

Capítulo V

Ayudar a sus niños a desarrollarse intelectualmente

Cada cabeza

es un mundo

EL IMPULSO NATURAL DE APRENDER: ¿QUÉ? ¿POR QUÉ? ¿CÓMO?

Nuestros niños, como todos los niños, nacen con un impulso y una necesidad de aprender y crecer intelectualmente. Poseen un deseo natural de explorar, experimentar, y dominar el cuerpo y el medio ambiente. Los niños necesitan sentir que son competentes y que pueden lograr sus metas. Desde el momento en que nacen, aprenden activamente, absorben información, y tratan de descifrar el mundo al utilizar sus sentidos de la vista, el oído, el tacto, el olor, y el gusto. Al encontrarse los niños con nueva información en su medio ambiente, su curiosidad natural les provoca a hacer preguntas tales como: "¿Qué es? ¿Cómo funciona? ¿Qué hace?" Esta curiosidad los impulsa a hacer preguntas, investigar, y buscar, hasta descubrir, comprender, o encontrar una solución. Todo les provoca a los niños pequeños una sensación de asombro y maravilla. Es una aventura.

La incontrolable urgencia y presión para aprender, con la cual nacen todos los niños, es lo que fomenta la inteligencia. ¿Qué es la inteligencia? Es lo que ocurre en la mente: la adquisición de conocimientos y lenguaje, y el desarrollo de las habilidades motrices refinadas y mayores. Es la capacidad de pensar, percibir, y recordar. Incluye la capacidad de entender, resolver problemas, razonar, planear, evaluar y juzgar, inventar, y crear. Una persona inteligente es alguien listo. Tiene *buena cabeza*. Sin embargo, la mente de cada niño es como un mundo propio y único. Tal como el dicho nos recuerda, *cada cabeza es un mundo*. La mente de cada niño puede imaginarse como un rico almacén de focos, los cuales se relacionan con sus experiencias singulares de aprendizaje.

Los niños que continuamente construyen sobre esas experiencias tienen una ventaja porque producen conocimiento, y *el conocimiento es poder*. Los padres o pueden ayudar a sus niños a utilizar y aprovechar el poder, o pueden extinguirlo. Si los padres no comprenden que los niños poseen un impulso natural de ir en busca del conocimiento, las acciones de los niños pueden ser interpretadas como travesuras y los niños mismos pueden ser catalogados como groseros, rebeldes, o malcriados. Por consiguiente, esta curiosidad natural puede causarles a los padres una gran frustración e ira y ganas de gritar. No es fácil seguir el ritmo de energía sin límite de sus niños, y su necesidad de aprender. Pero entre más comprenda lo que hay detrás de sus acciones, más paciencia y comprensión podrá ejercer.

¿Cómo manifestaron sus niños su natural curiosidad y necesidad de aprender? Mis propios niños mostraron su curiosidad natural de muchas maneras. Las más memorables eran las lecciones que aprendieron al estar sentados en sus sillas altas cuando eran pequeños. Les encantaba aventar la cuchara al piso una y otra vez. Un padre frustrado quizá responda con un "¡Ay, Dios mío! ¿Qué hace este niño?" cada vez que se tiene que agachar para recoger la cuchara y luego lavarla. Sin embargo, cuando se ponga a pensar en lo mucho que puede ser aprendido por el niño con esta simple acción, por ejemplo el sonido singular que hace al pegar contra el piso, o las leyes de la gravedad, tal vez ya no le moleste el esfuerzo adicional. Cuando mis niños se quedaban absortos en esta actividad, yo hacía que la lección fuera más efectiva al decir: "¡O! ¿Dónde está?" cada vez que la cuchara caía al piso. Yo me imaginaba que ellos se preguntaban adónde se había ido la cuchara y por qué se caía para abajo en lugar de para arriba.

Otro ejemplo de la curiosidad insaciable de los niños tiene que ver con la leche que inevitablemente termina en el piso cada vez que el niño come. Después de aventar la taza de leche al piso, mis niños exigían que la volviera a llenar. En cuanto la volvía a llenar, inmediatamente dejaban caer la taza de nuevo. Aunque tales escenas pueden exasperar y sacar de quicio a cualquier padre, necesitamos recordarnos que nuestros niños están experimentando con el concepto de causa y efecto. Se están preguntando: "¿Qué va a pasar? ¿Produciré el mismo efecto si lo vuelvo a empujar?" A veces sus niños prueban esta hipótesis de causa y efecto con sus hermanos cuando les pellizcan, muerden, o pegan, y luego simplemente les provocan gracia las respuestas y reacciones que causaron. Cuando usted corrige este tipo de conducta, sus niños están aprendiendo los límites y parámetros que tiene su curiosidad natural.

Los niños tienen una tremenda necesidad de repetir las cosas. Yo recuerdo a un niño en el barrio de AVANCE que se entretenía al meter una piedra por las aberturas de la alambrada. Empujaba la piedra por una abertura, caminaba al otro lado de la alambrada y empujaba la misma piedra de nuevo por una abertura, y repetía esta acción una y otra vez. Él estaba aprendiendo el concepto de "por" mientras desarrollaba sus habilidades de coordinación entre los ojos y las manos. A veces se puede probar la paciencia de los padres cuando sus niños andan por el mundo adquiriendo habilidades esenciales, si es que los padres no comprenden la importancia de la necesidad de aprender de sus niños.

¿Se ha preguntado alguna vez si sus niños realmente están decididos a romper o destruir todo en la casa, al ir de los botones de la televisión, al manivela de la taza de baño, a los botones del radio, al apagador de luz, y a todos los demás objetos movibles de la casa? De nuevo, debe tener paciencia y recordar que sus niños adquieren información al tener interacción con el mundo a su alrededor. Necesitan tener una sensación de control sobre su medio ambiente y sobre el cuerpo. Es algo fenomenal cuando un niño puede decir: "Yo hice que 'esto' pasara". Apoyar este proceso de descubrimiento y experimentación puede proveerles a sus niños la posibilidad de inventar, crear, o hacer algo excepcional que algún día pudiera cambiar el mundo. Los cimientos para el aprendizaje deben ser construidos por padres que demuestran paciencia y pueden proporcionar la información esencial que los niños requieren para comprender su mundo y crear su propio mundo de pensamientos y experiencias. Como el primer maestro de su niño, usted necesita proveer nombres para los objetos y para sus acciones, reforzarle, corregirle, y construir sobre lo que ya saben.

La curiosidad puede requerir un esfuerzo tremendo. Cada día los niños se despiertan con una enorme cantidad de energía, entusiasmo, y asombro, pensando en las aventuras que aún les faltan. Si usted ha observado a niños pequeños al jugar, sabrá que les encanta meter y sacar cosas de los cajones. También les encanta encaramarse y meterse en cosas. A Vanessa le encantaba sacar la ropa de los cajones y también subir por los anaqueles en la biblioteca. ¡Caramba! Varias veces estuvo decidida a subirse hasta lo más alto. ¡Qué sustos pasé! Tuve que colocar una barrera enfrente de los anaqueles o ayudarle a alcanzar su meta por medio de guía y apoyo. ¿Qué aventuras han tenido sus niños con los rollos de papel higiénico? Ambos Vanessa y Steven, a más o menos la misma edad, descubrieron que podían arrastrar el papel alrededor de la casa hasta que se desaparecía del rollo. Vanessa lo usaba para cubrirse como momia. Steven metió todo el rollo en el excusado y ya iba a tirar de la cadena cuando yo lo detuve. Sus niños quizá hagan las cosas más graciosas, creativas, e interesantes, no solamente con cosas como el papel higiénico, sino también con la pasta dental, y con el agua del excusado, entre otras. Los cuartos de baño son una gran fuente de asombro y descubrimiento, pero también pueden ser trampas peligrosas cuando objetos como navajas de afeitar, productos de limpieza, y medicinas están al alcance de sus niños inquisitivos. Es importante que ponga a prueba de niño su casa para prevenir que sus niños se hagan daño.

El aprendizaje de los niños puede ser desordenado. Si usted es una persona muy ordenada que espera tener todo en su lugar, puede angustiarse cuando su niño pequeño descubre la alacena o los gabinetes de la cocina. Meterá las ollas unas dentro de otras, y las golpeará unas contra otras, o contra el piso. Apilará las latas una encima de otra, y las pondrá en fila, o las rodará por todo el piso. Aun puede encontrarlo todo cubierto de harina, o encontrar un caminito de sal que hizo por el piso de la cocina. Mientras sí le puede causar un disgusto tener que limpiar el desorden, es importante darse cuenta que los niños están practicando y aprendiendo la coordinación entre los ojos y las manos, algunos principios matemáticos, causa y efecto, sonidos y texturas. Qué episodio pasamos cuando Sal, quien tenía menos de un año de edad, quedó fascinado con el color rojo, el cual descubrió en un tazón de salsa para espagueti. Embarró la salsa por toda su camisa, los brazos, las piernas, la cara, y como remate, se volteó el tazón con el resto del espagueti encima de la cabeza. ¡Qué espectáculo!

¿Han tenido sus niños alguna experiencia con lodo, tal como hacer y tratar de comer tortillas o taquitos "de mentirillas"? ¿Qué tal construir castillos o animales o monitos de lodo? Un día caluroso de verano, cuando Steven estaba jugando afuera con la manguera de agua, se estaba deleitando con la sensación del lodo al apretarlo y hacerlo salir por entre los dedos de la mano. Agarró la manguera de agua e hizo un gran charco de lodo justo enfrente de la resbaladilla donde estaba jugando. Luego se quitó toda la ropa y, totalmente desnudo, se bajó por la resbaladilla para caer dentro del charco que había creado. Al salir de la casa, riéndome a carcajadas con la cámara en la mano, este monstruo cubierto por lodo vino hacia mí como si me iba a comer. Siempre debe mantener una cámara lista y a la mano, para aprovechar los momentos inolvidables como estos. Hasta la fecha, miramos esas fotos invalorables y nos reímos,

¡rememorando las muchas cosas increíbles que ellos hicieron! Usted puede anticipar pasar por muchos de sus propios episodios maravillosos, durante los cuales sus niños harán cosas locas y difíciles de creer al explorar y descubrir su mundo.

Los niños no tienen ningún horario ni compromiso cuando se trata de descubrir, experimentar, y aprender. El día que necesita llegar a algún lado de prisa, será el día cuando sus niños querrán observar al más pequeño escarabajo, o seguir a algún chapulín por las largas briznas de hierba. Nuestros días de campo generalmente se interrumpían cuando teníamos que ir frenéticamente en busca de Steven, quien estaba con nosotros un momento y luego al siguiente desaparecía, al ir a perseguir a las ardillas. Necesitaba hacer acopio de toda mi paciencia y fortaleza simplemente para seguir el ritmo de la inmensa curiosidad de Steven. Pensamos que no vamos a sobrevivir, pero de alguna manera sí lo hacemos, especialmente si comprendemos su pasión por el aprendizaje.

La curiosidad de los niños necesita ser apoyada, no reprimida. Si los padres les gritan a sus niños, constantemente les dicen "no", o les pegan la mano cada vez que son curiosos, su impulso natural para aprender disminuirá. Una vez que se dé cuenta de que los niños serán curiosos por naturaleza y conseguirán meterse en todo, aprenderá a ser más vigilante y pondrá su casa completamente a prueba de niño, por dentro y por fuera. Usted debe crear un ambiente seguro, que enriquece y estimula, y que podría satisfacer la mente más determinada y curiosa.

Los niños también poseen un fuerte impulso para dominar y controlar el cuerpo, por medio del desarrollo de las llamadas habilidades motrices mayores, el uso de los músculos grandes. Utilizan estos músculos grandes para caminar, correr, brincar, tirar, andar en sus triciclos, y treparse a los arboles. Sus habilidades motrices refinadas, o el uso de los músculos más pequeños de las manos, se utilizan para cosas tales como escribir, cortar, pegar, y jugar con plastilina. Para algunos niños que tienen talento especial atlético, las habilidades motrices mayores se coordinarán con sus habilidades visuales para ayudarles a algún día ganar una competencia de atletismo en pista, o romper un récord mundial Olímpico. Aquéllos que poseen fuertes habilidades cinéticas combinarán sus habilidades motrices refinadas con sus habilidades visuales o auditivas, para llegar a ser cirujanos o violinistas.

Al desarrollar sus niños sus habilidades de lenguaje, anticipe ser bombardeado con millones de preguntas: "¿Qué es esto?" Al crecer un poco, entrarán a la etapa cuando el "por qué" y el "cómo" son abundantes. ¿Cómo funciona? ¿Cómo hiciste eso? ¿Por qué está triste mi abuelita? ¿Por qué es azul el cielo? ¿Por qué no se cae la luna? ¿Por qué se derrite el hielo? ¿Qué hace brillar tanto el foco? Sus niños necesitan que usted intente contestar todas sus preguntas interminables. Si usted no sabe la respuesta a una de sus preguntas, está bien. Si su niño es bastante mayor, sugiera que juntos busquen la respuesta por medio del uso de enciclopedias, diccionarios, libros de recursos, o la Internet. Explore las respuestas en la biblioteca, el museo, o el planetario. Consiga un profesor particular. Estimule los pensamientos de sus niños y satisfaga su búsqueda de conocimientos. Ayudar a sus niños a alcanzar su máximo potencial requerirá una gran cantidad de paciencia, energía, comprensión, y el compromiso de su parte de ayudarlos a aprender y a crecer.

Son grandes las expectativas de aprendizaje que se tienen de sus niños antes de entrar a la escuela. Como su primer maestro, usted necesita saber qué es lo que necesita hacer para prepararlos para entrar a la escuela. Por ejemplo, se espera que los niños sepan sus nombres completos, además de los nombres de los colores básicos y las formas tales como el triángulo, el cuadrado, el círculo, y el rectángulo. Deben estar familiarizados con armar rompecabezas. Deben haber tenido suficientes experiencias dibujando y garabateando con crayolas grandes, gises, o lápices. Deben poder dibujar un hombre o una mujer con muchos detalles, incluyendo las partes de la cara, el cabello, el cuello, los dedos de las manos y la ropa, y algunos niños muy listos aun dibujarán un anillo, un sombrero, o espuelas en las botas. Deben poder contar cuando menos diez objetos, amarrarse las agujetas de los zapatos, abrocharse los botones, cerrar los broches de presión, colorear, cortar, pegar, sentarse silenciosamente por períodos cortos de tiempo, escuchar, y seguir instrucciones. Quizá lo más importante—tienen que poder expresar sus necesidades en inglés o en español. Para la edad de tres años, un niño generalmente tiene un vocabulario de 1,000 palabras. Para los cuatro años, este almacén de palabras aumenta a 1,500 palabras y para los cinco, la mayoría de los niños han aprendido alrededor de 2,000 palabras. No puedo enfatizar demasiado la importancia de hablarles a sus niños. Entre más les habla, más palabras aprenderán.

Como maestra de primer año de primaria, yo estaba muy preocupada porque había niños entrando a mi escuela a los seis años de edad, con muy pocos conocimientos, experiencias, y habilidades. Por medio de un cuestionario que les di a los padres de mis estudiantes, yo me enteré que los padres no sabían qué se esperaba que ellos hicieran durante los primeros años de vida de sus niños, ni tampoco se percibían como maestros de sus niños. Por ejemplo, muchos padres creían que el aprendizaje comenzaba entre "los cinco y siete años de edad".

Este descubrimiento me llevó a pensar que tal vez no hablaron lo suficiente con sus niños ni les permitieron jugar libremente durante los años más críticos. Quizá no apoyaron el impulso natural de sus niños de aprender, ni contestaron sus muchas preguntas. Como muchos de los niños en mi clase de primer año no podían sostener un lápiz ni dibujar un círculo, yo sabía que sus padres o las personas que los cuidaron no les habían proporcionado herramientas tan sencillas como unas crayolas. Al pedirles que dibujaran un hombre, algunos niños dibujaron dos líneas en un círculo que no estaba completamente cerrado.

Algunas escuelas catalogan a los niños con nombres, de acuerdo a sus dibujos o el nivel de conocimientos que tengan al entrar a la escuela. Los niños que me fueron asignados habían sido catalogados como "lentos para aprender", "retrasados mentales", y "vegetales" por los maestros. Estos niños eran inteligentes y sanos, pero a algunos les faltó adquirir los conocimientos, las habilidades, y las experiencias esenciales antes de entrar a la escuela. Ellos requerían más tiempo y asistencia de lo que la escuela podía o estaba dispuesta a proveer. Porque estaban tan atrasados cuando entraron a la escuela, habían sido dejados a un lado y hecho caso omiso por la primera mitad del año. Bajo estas condiciones, estaban destinados a fracasar. Cuando fui asignada como maestra bilingüe de estos niños, ya muy avanzado el año escolar, me dijeron simplemente que hiciera "lo que podía" para ayudarles. Más tarde recibí otro grupo de niños maltratados de manera similar. ¡Basta!—me dije a mí misma.

Yo sentí tan frustrada que no podía seguir como maestra a sabiendas que había tantos niños entrando a la escuela tan mal preparados y que los padres no sabían lo que se esperaba de ellos antes de que sus niños entraran a la escuela. Yo sabía también que el abismo entre aquéllos que entraban a la escuela preparados y aquéllos que no, sólo se iba a hacer cada vez mayor. Yo quería hacer algo para resolver este problema. Yo decidí dejar mi carrera de maestra para ayudar a los padres a comprender la importancia de los primeros cuatro años de vida y orientarlos para llegar a ser los mejores padres y maestros que podían ser. Yo quería que los padres les proporcionaran a sus niños un medio ambiente que estimulaba y enriquecía, para que cuando sus pequeños entraran a la escuela, ellos se encontrarían entre los "listos", aquéllos que tendrían éxito. Y con esa motivación, AVANCE llegó a ser.

En las clases de crianza de AVANCE, las madres hacen títeres hechos de calcetines o caballitos hechos de viejos palos de escoba, calcetines, y estambre. Hacen coloridos recipientes de diferentes tamaños que se colocan unos dentro de otros, cubiertos por papel de contacto en colores vívidos. También hacen libros, muñecos, figuras recortadas de esponja, y otros juguetes que estimulan la mente. Durante el programa de nueve meses tienen muchas experiencias. Llevamos a las madres y a los niños a la biblioteca a sacar libros, al supermercado para enseñarles lo que pueden aprender los niños en un simple pasillo allí, o a lugares como el aeropuerto donde pueden aprender cómo funcionan los sistemas. Igual a los niños a quienes les faltaban experiencias, yo descubrí que también a muchas madres les faltaban. Algunas de las madres que participaban en el programa nunca habían tenido las experiencias básicas de colorear, cortar, y pegar. Un día, durante una excursión de AVANCE a un gran almacén para mirar los adornos navideños, me quedé desconcertada cuando una madre vacilaba para subirse a una escalera mecánica porque nunca antes se había subido a una. Las madres se preguntaban: "¿Qué es esto?" Muchas madres pudieron ganar lo que ellas mismas habían perdido al hacerles a sus niños juguetes no costosos, pero que los estimulaban, y también pudieron captar algo que les había faltado al participar con sus niños en las excursiones.

Desde 1973, AVANCE ha ayudado a muchos miles de padres con niños pequeños a construir esos cimientos sólidos y firmes para el aprendizaje. La gente no nace con estos conocimientos. Como ya he repetido muchas veces, una crianza efectiva es una habilidad que debe ser aprendida, sin tomar en cuenta las condiciones socioeconómicas de los padres. Ya sea en los suburbios o en el barrio, uno encontrará a padres que proveen experiencias que estimulan a sus niños, y aquéllos que no las proveen.

Como trabajadora doméstica, mi suegra solía observar lo que una madre anglosajona de la clase media hacía con sus niños diariamente y aplicaba estos conocimientos con sus propios niños. Les compraba a sus niños rompecabezas, damas, ajedrez, y juegos de mesa. Los llevaba a lugares como museos, playas, y parques. Les hablaba y leía constantemente. Mi suegra pertenecía a un club de revistas de historietas que les proporcionaba una amplia gama de libros de historietas de aventuras y ficción científica, las cuales ayudaron a sus niños a aprender a leer. También tenía una colección de enciclopedias y jugaba un papel muy activo en los eventos escolares. Siempre tenía madera a la mano para que sus niños construyeran cosas, como fuertes, o jaulas para los animales que ella les permitía tener. Mi madre también sabía la importancia de un medio ambiente que estimula, por su propia madre y por las enfermeras que hacían las visitas a casa después del nacimiento de cada uno de sus niños. Ellas le proveín información sobre el crecimiento y desarrollo de los niños. Teníamos trompos, baleros, y lotería mexicana, además de muñecas, libros, rompecabezas, crayolas, marcadores, libros para colorear, muñecas de papel, y juegos de mesa. Mi madre nos daba retazos de tela, agujas, e hilo para coserles ropa a nuestras muñecas. Todavía recuerdo los aros (hula-hoops), y cómo jugábamos a las tabas y las canicas de todo tamaño, color, y diseño, para entretenernos. El terreno baldío al lado de nuestra casa se convertía en una selva para nosotros y las calles se convertían en campos de béisbol.

Cuando estaba creciendo en el barrio, una niña de trece años asumía muchas responsabilidades. A esa edad, se esperaba que mi hermana Julia nos llevara de excursión. Éramos semejantes a la mamá pata con sus patitos a la zaga, caminando en pares por los parques y los museos. En los Jardines Japoneses en San Antonio, mis hermanos y yo pasábamos tardes enteras andando por los caminitos, y juntos a los estanques llenos de hermosos peces anaranjados que nadaban entre los lirios con sus grandes hojas verdes. Explorábamos al pie de una majestuosa cascada, y subíamos por un camino serpenteante para llegar a lo que a una niña pequeña le parecía la cima del mundo. También anticipábamos el momento de rodar por la pequeña loma cubierta por hierba, llenos de júbilo por tanta risa y excitación.

Mi niñez estuvo repleta de experiencias agradables y educativas. Estábamos bendecidos al tener a tíos que nos llevaban a la granja familiar cuando éramos jóvenes. Esas experiencias influenciales de cuando ordeñábamos una vaca o una cabra, juntábamos los huevos, o simplemente nos quedábamos mirando el cielo lleno de estrellas por la noche, con el sonido de grillos en el fondo, están firmemente grabadas en mi memoria y mi alma. Aun cuando no salíamos de la casa, siempre había bastante que hacer. Todos los niños en el barrio se juntaban para jugar varios juegos como "La les", "Los colores", y "La orna". Jugábamos a "La víbora de la mar", la versión hispana de *"London Bridge"*, y también a "Las escondidas" y "Naranja dulce". Jugábamos los más complicados juegos con la cuerda. Ya para cuando entramos a la escuela, mis hermanas y yo teníamos muchas experiencias y conceptos, muchos focos que se nos prendían cada vez que teníamos una nueva experiencia que más adelante nos ayudaría a lograr el éxito en la escuela y en la vida.

¿Usted recuerda haber jugado estos juegos? Muchos de mis amigos sí recuerdan, sin embargo, por alguna razón no se los enseñaron a sus niños. No es demasiado tarde para sus niños. Enséñeles estos juegos si usted los sabe. Si no los sabe, vaya a una tienda de útiles escolares para maestros bilingües. Tienen discos y cassettes para ayudarle a aprender. Usted también puede crear este tipo de experiencias que iluminan, y puede construir unos firmes cimientos de aprendizaje para sus niños. Al hacerlo, puede ayudarles a desarrollar su capacidad intelectual, además de ponerlos en contacto con su rica cultura hispana. Como el maestro principal de sus niños, usted juega un papel vital al proporcionar un medio ambiente rico, donde sus niños pueden aprender y crecer. Usted es el principal responsable de construir esos cimientos sólidos que fomentarán el éxito en la escuela y en la vida. Los siguientes son unos temas importantes acerca del aprendizaje, los cuales le ayudarán a realizar el desarrollo intelectual de sus niños.

Cuándo se inicia el aprendizaje: La inteligencia comienza dentro de la matriz

El aprendizaje de los niños se inicia dentro de la matriz donde ya son capaces de percibir, escuchar, y aprender. ¿Usted se comunica con su niño cuando está adentro de la matriz? Yo recuerdo que mi hija solía moverse al ritmo de la música clásica suave durante el último trimestre de mi embarazo, como si pudiera apreciar más una cierta pieza musical que otra. Al hablar a cada uno de nuestros niños mientras ellos se encontraban todavía dentro de la matriz, ellos parecían responder a mi voz. Los investigadores han concluido que los bebés, dos o tres días después de nacer, responderán más a una canción o voz conocida, que escucharon cuando estaban dentro de la matriz, que una que no han escuchado. También pueden distinguir entre diferentes aromas aun a los dieciséis días después de nacer. Durante el embarazo, puede comenzar a estimular el medio ambiente de su niño con música suave y aromas fragantes. No tenga vergüenza, no sea tímido con relación a hablarle y cantarle a su bebé. ¡Anímese! Usted y su pareja deben tener sus propias pláticas con su niño y acariciar suavemente su pancita. Ambos pueden comenzar a establecer una cálida relación con su bebé aun antes de poderlo ver y tocar.

LOS CIMIENTOS PARA EL APRENDIZAJE: EL PERÍODO CRÍTICO

Los primeros cuatro años de vida se consideran los años más críticos para el aprendizaje. Si un niño aprende muchas cosas durante sus primeros cuatro años de vida, él tendrá unos cimientos sólidos sobre los cuales podrá construir en el futuro. Todo nuevo conocimiento tiene que asociarse con conocimientos previos. *De un éxito, nacen otros éxitos.* El aprendizaje es un proceso donde se agrega una cosa a otra. Si los cimientos son demasiados estrechos o débiles, entonces su capacidad futura para el aprendizaje será sofocada por aquellas experiencias limitadas que adquirió temprano en su vida.

De acuerdo al teórico Benjamin Bloom, la mitad de todos los conocimientos que un niño adquiere desde el nacimiento hasta los diecisiete años de edad, será aprendida ya para los cuatro años de edad. Durante los tres primeros años de vida, hay un desarrollo rápido de lenguaje y aprendizaje. Los valores, los principios, y el autoestima se comienzan a formar ya para los tres años de edad. Aun el desarrollo de ciertas funciones, tal como la visión, puede ser obstaculizada, dependiendo de lo que ocurre durante los primeros meses de vida. Por ejemplo, un niño que nace con cataratas en ambos ojos será permanentemente afectado si las cataratas son operadas después de los seis meses de edad. Las conexiones visuales en el cerebro son tentativas y necesitan estímulos del medio ambiente para mantenerse activas. Si no reciben los estímulos apropiados durante este período crítico del desarrollo, estos sistemas dejarán de funcionar o bien, no funcionarán tan bien como deben. *Lo que se aprende en la cuna, siempre dura.* Todas sus futuras relaciones sociales se relacionan con los vínculos afectivos que se forman entre el niño y sus padres durante los primeros meses de vida.

¡EL FENOMENAL CEREBRO HUMANO!

¡Sabía usted que el proveer un medio ambiente estimulante también podría afectar el tamaño, el peso, la composición química, y las estructuras neurológicas del cerebro de su niño? Un bebé nace con alrededor de cien billones de neuronas en el cerebro, la cantidad total que tendrá por el resto de su vida. Inmediatamente después de nacer, con los estímulos apropiados, el cerebro desarrolla trillones de sinapsis entre las neuronas para organizarlas para componer las diferentes facetas de la inteligencia. Algunas de estas sinapsis se unen en grupos para formar funciones tan básicas como las del oído, la vista, el caminar, y el habla. Para poder sobrevivir, estas sinapsis necesitan ser estimuladas por cosas que ve, olores, sonidos, sabores, y el tacto. Si no hay experiencias para fortalecer estas redes, las sinapsis comienzan a morir. Por contraste, entre más experiencia tenga uno, más fuertes se vuelven las sinapsis. Lo opuesto también es cierto. Las experiencias negativas, o la ausencia de experiencias estimulantes, pueden provocar efectos dañinos y duraderos.

Mientras algunos de estos efectos negativos pueden quizá cambiar, tal vez requieran de una terapia costosa y una intervención extensiva de parte de los directores de la escuela, y los funcionarios de la salud y de la salud mental, para intentar remediar los problemas.

La publicación del innovador reporte de 1994 de la Corporación Carnegie llamado *"Starting Points Report"* puso énfasis en la importancia del desarrollo del cerebro durante los tres primeros años de vida. Como miembro del equipo operativo que produjo ese reporte, yo estaba asombrada ante la reacción del público a la información que muchos de los que formamos parte de los campos educativos y del desarrollo de los niños hemos sabido por décadas. Cuando yo asistí a la universidad de Our Lady of the Lake, en los años sesenta y setenta, aprendimos acerca de investigaciones exhaustivas sobre el cerebro, que se habían conducido utilizando a animales. Por ejemplo, en uno de los experimentos, hubo un grupo de ratas que fue permitido a jugar con una variedad de juguetes y alentado a resolver los laberintos, y las ratas de otro grupo no fueron permitidas a tener nada con que jugar en su medio ambiente. Después de cierto tiempo, los investigadores mataron a las ratas, examinaron los cerebros de aquellas ratas de un grupo, y los compararon con los del otro grupo. La investigación demostró que los cerebros de aquéllas que fueron permitidas a jugar y explorar eran más grandes y pesados y produjeron un 25 por ciento más de sinapsis entre las células del cerebro (las neuronas). Las investigaciones han demostrado que las ratas que fueron permitidas a jugar y ser más activas tenían un tejido cortical más grande y más pesado que aquéllas que recibieron pocos estímulos. Las ratas que fueron permitidas a tener objetos estimulantes y actividades tenían 15 por ciento más neuronas que las ratas que se dejaron dentro de jaulas desprovistas de todo estímulo. El peso del cerebro puede doblarse durante el primer año de vida al proporcionarle al niño muchas experiencias.

Con nueva tecnología llamada escanograma de topografía de la emisión de positrones (PET scans) que permite el examen detallado de la actividad del cerebro, ahora podemos ver los mismos resultados y efectos del estímulo en el cerebro de los niños. Las investigaciones están demostrando que la mayor parte del desarrollo del cerebro ocurre fuera de la matriz y que tiene una relación directa con las experiencias que un niño adquiere de su medio ambiente externo. Entre más estímulos reciba el niño, más sinapsis se formarán, y más pesado será el cerebro. Harry Chugani y sus colegas del Hospital para Niños en Michigan, usando *PET scans*, pudieron demostrar resultados sorprendentes relacionados a la actividad del cerebro en la corteza cerebral, la parte del cerebro de donde salen las funciones cognoscitivas complejas, por ejemplo el lenguaje y la orientación espacial. Desde el nacimiento hasta un año de edad, esta área del cerebro apenas muestra actividad, pero justo después del año, se estalla con actividad. Al completar los tres años de edad, el cerebro muestra dos veces y medio más actividad que el cerebro de un adulto. La mayoría de las sinapsis se producen durante los tres primeros años de vida y se mantienen muy densas hasta alrededor de los diez años de edad. En este momento, la densidad comienza a disminuirse lentamente a alrededor de quinientas trillones durante la última etapa de la adolescencia, y se mantiene sin cambio después de eso.

Aunque el peso de tal órgano tal vez no parezca significar mucho por su propia cuenta, la diferencia se puede notar claramente durante observaciones cotidianas a los niños. Yo vi la transformación en algunos casos de niños que "no se desarrollaban", después de que los padres de unos niños flaquitos y letárgicos, quienes habían sido referidos a AVANCE, comenzaron a aplicar con sus niños lo que aprendían. Aprendieron la importancia de hablar, abrazar, y acariciar a sus niños, en adición a proveer un medio ambiente sano y con buena nutrición. Después de recibir los estímulos y cuidados apropiados, sus niños comenzaron a subir de peso, desarrollarse, y aun comenzaron a sonreír. Una investigación llevada a cabo con unos huérfanos de Rumania, quienes prácticamente no fueron tomados en cuenta por las personas que los cuidaban, demostró que muchos fallecieron como resultado de esta privación. Se satisfacían sus necesidades físicas, tales como el alimento y el agua, pero porque no se les hablaba, ni tocaba, ni recibieron ningún estímulo mayor, su desarrollo deterioró.

En el programa de estudios de AVANCE, enseñamos una lección sobre el cerebro que incluye un diagrama que ilustra todas las partes del cerebro y sus principales funciones. Yo solía bromear con las madres de AVANCE y decirles que entre más estimulaban el de sus niños a través de un medio ambiente enriquecedor, más largas aquellas ramas en el cerebro (las dendritas) crecerían, hasta que les salieran por los oídos. Las madres comprendían el mensaje. Yo no tenía que darles un examen sobre los términos científicos (las neuronas, las dendritas, los neuroejes, y las sinapsis) ni los procesos eléctricos y químicos exactos a través de los cuales ocurre el aprendizaje en el cerebro. Ellas simplemente aprendieron que con más estímulos la estructura, el peso, el tamaño, y la composición química del cerebro cambiaban. Ellas se daban cuenta que al fin de cuentas, la calidad de los pensamientos, la conducta, y la capacidad de una persona también serían afectados por el medio ambiente que los padres proveyeran, especialmente durante los años críticos de la formación.

En una investigación científica sobre las familias de AVANCE, fundada por la Corporación de Carnegie de Nueva York, se encontraron diferencias significativas entre el medio ambiente de los niños que asisten a AVANCE y aquéllos que no asisten. Las madres que son participantes de AVANCE proporcionan un medio ambiente en su hogar que es más organizado y responsivo, que cultiva más y contiene más estímulos. El medio ambiente es estructurado de una manera que permite que los niños aprendan, exploren, y experimenten. Tienen más juguetes apropiados a su nivel de desarrollo, muchos hechos por las mismas madres. Ellas tienen interacción con sus niños utilizando un lenguaje que fomenta el aprendizaje, y los elogian más. Alientan y apoyan el aprendizaje de sus niños y participan activamente al leerles y hablarles además de enseñarles y jugar con ellos. Las madres cambian sus actitudes con respecto a castigo físico. Comienzan a percibirse como maestras al aprender más acerca del crecimiento y desarrollo de los niños y acerca de cómo aprovechar los recursos de su comunidad.

CONCEPTOS: FOCOS E IDEAS EN LA MENTE

Toda inteligencia está construida sobre conceptos, ideas, o imágenes en la mente que organizan y unen todo lo que un niño aprende de su medio ambiente. Cierre los ojos. Imagine el concepto de un gato. ¿Qué tipo de imagen tiene en su mente cuando piensa en un "gato"? Yo quizá haya imaginado algo un poco diferente a lo que usted imaginó, pero ambos tenemos una idea general de lo que es un gato. Un concepto es similar a una canasta, dentro de la cual se ponen juntas las cosas con propiedades semejantes. Por ejemplo, el concepto de "gato" puede definirse como la canasta que contiene las características que describen los gatos, desde los sonidos que emiten hasta sus pelos, su cola larga, y sus bigotes. Al ver a una variedad de gatos, un niño aprende que hay gatos de diferentes colores, formas, y tamaños. Estas experiencias agudizan su concepto del gato.

Si un niño mira a un animal pequeño y peludo que se parece a un gato, pero no tiene los largos bigotes y no dice "miau" sino que ladra, se confunde. Hay una discrepancia entre lo que él sabía acerca de los gatos y lo que él ve en este nuevo animalito. Por consiguiente, esta experiencia lo motiva a aprender un nuevo concepto llamado "perro". Después de esta experiencia, su niño ve a otro animal que se parece al primer

perro, pero es mucho más grande y tiene diferente tipo de orejas. Este
animal también dice "guau" y tiene cuatro patas, una cola, y pelos
suaves. Porque ha aprendido algunas características de los perros, él se da
cuenta que tiene algunas de las mismas propiedades. Con muchas más
experiencias, él puede ampliar y refinar su concepto de perro. Él añadirá
más información a su "canasta", o concepto de perro, o se dará cuenta de
que tiene que crear un nuevo concepto porque la información nueva no
encaja con la vieja. Al crecer su niño, las categorías se vuelven más
amplias y su pensamiento se vuelve más preciso, lógico, y abstracto. El
niño organiza su mundo y sus experiencias a través de conceptos, lo cual
le posibilitará a adquirir habilidades intelectuales más elevadas, tales
como planear, analizar, crear, y resolver.

En un mundo bilingüe y de dos culturas, un niño pasará por los mismos procesos en ambos idiomas. Inicialmente, mientras está intentando
aprender el concepto, quizá lo nombre mal al combinar una parte de la
palabra en un idioma con otra parte del otro idioma. Por ejemplo, cuando yo primero aprendí el concepto de "broom", yo decía "escroom", com-
binando la primera parte de la palabra en español, "escoba", con la parte
final de la palabra en inglés, "broom". Con suficientes experiencias de
escuchar y repetir estas palabras, el niño bilingüe eventualmente dejará
de usar palabras como "chequear", "chusiar", "mistiar", "dostear", y "par-
quiar", a menos, claro, que es esto lo que escucha a su alrededor y se convierte para él en la manera apropiada de hablar, en lugar de revisar, elegir o escoger, extrañar o echar de menos, sacudir, y estacionar. Los niños
tienen la capacidad de aprender muchos conceptos y de aprender diferentes nombres para cada concepto en más de un idioma. Ellos desarrollarán la habilidad de cambiar de un idioma al otro, dependiendo de la
señal apropiada que el cerebro recibe en una situación en particular. Tal
como discutiré más a fondo más adelante en este capítulo, los niños
pueden aprender muchos idiomas, especialmente si tienen contacto frecuentemente con ellos cuando son pequeños.

EL AMBIENTE PARA APRENDER

Tal como he dicho antes, todo lo que aprende un niño está basado en
conocimientos que ya ha recogido de experiencias previas. Permítame
reiterar que todos los conocimientos deben ser conectados y relacionados, o se olvidarán. Al aprender nuestros niños, ellos avanzan de lo sencillo a lo complejo, de lo concreto a lo abstracto, y de lo general a lo

específico. Por ejemplo, ellos aprenderán a meter algo por un agujero antes de poder coser. Aprenderán el concepto de pelota antes de aprender el concepto de fútbol. Aprenderán el concepto de perro antes de aprender qué es un caniche. Aprenderán el concepto de hermano o hermana antes de aprender el significado de amor. Un niño aprenderá mejor cuando hay una *ligera* diferencia entre la información nueva y la que ya sabe. El concepto nuevo no debe ser demasiado nuevo ni demasiado familiar. Recuerde el ejemplo de un gato y la manera en que un niño recordará sus características cuando se encuentra ante otro tipo de animal por primera vez. Si una actividad es demasiado familiar, o ya la ha dominado, se aburrirá. Si es totalmente diferente a cualquier cosa que conoce, fácilmente puede pasar de largo o hacerle caso omiso. Si es demasiado y con demasiada rapidez, ni siquiera hará el intento de entenderlo. Es un reto para los padres proveer el tipo apropiado de medio ambiente para sus niños para fomentar el máximo aprendizaje. La clave es observar y fijarse si su niño responde y muestra interés en lo que está tratando de enseñarle.

El aprendizaje también se ve muy afectado por cómo se sienten sus niños. Tal como declaré anteriormente, sus niños no podrán aprender si tienen hambre, o están asustados, nerviosos, con tensión, o enojados. Si los niños se sienten amenazados, o llenos de emoción, la parte inferior del cerebro, el cerebelo, manda un mensaje de "huir o pelear" al sistema nervioso. Ellos opondrán resistencia a o desearán huir de una situación emocional, lo cual prevendrá el aprendizaje. Muchos niños comienzan a tener problemas de aprendizaje cuando sus padres están en medio de un divorcio, cuando ellos o alguien más en la familia es víctima del abuso, o cuando son testigos de violencia en su barrio. Los niños que reciben un exceso de estímulos y son forzados a pasar de una lección a otra sin ningún control sobre lo que está ocurriendo, a veces están tan exhaustos que no pueden pensar ni procesar información. Ellos tienen que tener control sobre su medio ambiente. Nosotros, como padres, necesitamos estar atentos a sus señales e indicios para mantener viva esa natural sed de aprender.

El mejor medio ambiente para el aprendizaje se establece cuando los niños se sienten felices, seguros, y bien descansados. Pueden aprender mejor si tienen un medio ambiente bastante limpio, organizado, y seguro. El aprendizaje también ocurre si la experiencia de aprendizaje está acompañada de sentimientos positivos. Se puede fomentar un amor a la lectura al compartir el libro de cuentos con su niño mientras se acurruca junto a usted y usted lo acaricia y lo abraza cariñosamente. El niño asociará esta experiencia agradable con la lectura. Al mismo tiempo, también está estableciendo una sólida relación con sus padres que perdurará toda la vida.

En un mundo bilingüe, de dos culturas, donde abundan las imágenes cálidas y coloridas y el contacto humano estrecho, no existen límites a lo que los niños hispanos pueden aprender y a las habilidades que pueden adquirir con los estímulos apropiados. Ellos tienen la capacidad de desarrollar sus talentos e intereses innatos, y de descubrir y eventualmente crear cosas inimaginables. Con los estímulos apropiados, ellos tendrán la capacidad de pensar, resolver problemas, distinguir entre el bien y el mal, y crear el tipo del mundo en el cual a ellos les gustaría vivir. Es crítico que usted desarrolle y mantenga una sólida relación con sus niños si quiere que lleguen a ser adultos responsables, con buenos principios, y con confianza en sí mismos. Al crecer los niños, su aprendizaje depende en gran parte en cómo se sienten acerca de sí mismos y de otros.

El aprendizaje también ocurre a través de los modelos de conducta. Si los niños ven a una persona que ellos admiran y esa persona está fumando, tomando, o usando drogas, ellos querrán hacer lo mismo. Por el otro lado, si los padres, los parientes, o las celebridades que ellos admiran, demuestran buenos modales y valores positivos, los niños los emularán al crecer. Si sus niños ven a usted leer, quizá quieran leer también. Tal como dice el dicho, *él que bien vive, bien cría.* Como padres, tenemos que enseñar y vivir lo que deseamos para nuestros niños. Todo lo que rodea a su niño, incluyendo programas de televisión, música, y amigos nuevos, puede afectar positiva o negativamente su desarrollo.

REFUERZOS Y CASTIGOS: ¡PÓRTATE BIEN! DULCES, SONRISAS Y CASTIGOS

Mientras un niño posee un impulso natural de aprender, a veces su necesidad de descubrir o de retraerse puede ser dirigido o influenciado por refuerzos. Los refuerzos funcionan para entrenar a animales para hacer todo tipo de trucos. También pueden funcionar con los niños. Una sonrisa, una palmadita, o un guiño, todos son refuerzos que fortalecerán la conducta. Los refuerzos son aquellas cosas que le gustan al niño o que él desea, y pueden ser utilizados para lograr que su niño haga lo que usted quiere. Incluyen: darle un gusto especial ocasional, mirar la televisión, o una excursión al zoológico o al cine. "Cuando terminas de guardar tus juguetes, iremos a comprar pan dulce o un helado" es un ejemplo de cómo se utilizan los refuerzos. Otra manera es premiar a su niño que sacó buenas calificaciones con una excursión al parque. Lamentable-mente, la modificación de la conducta, el nombre de este método, no siempre funciona a menos que utilice el refuerzo apropiado. Los refuerzos no tienen que ser costosos ni tienen que ser cosas de las cuales usted no aprueba. Una advertencia de precaución: a veces los refuerzos pueden provocar los resultados contrarios y matar el impulso natural de aprender. Los niños pueden perder el deseo de hacer algo bueno por la simple satisfacción que se deriva de aprender o dominar una habilidad. Es más importante que sus niños se sientan bien cuando hacen algo positivo en lugar de simplemente tratar de agradar a Mamá. Mientras sí debe elogiar y premiar la buena conducta, en última instancia, los niños tienen que desarrollar una consciencia y un sentimiento positivo acerca de hacer lo correcto, aun cuando usted no está presente para darles premios o elogios.

Aun así, los refuerzos positivos son mejores que los castigos. El castigo (que causa un dolor físico) puede apagar, o extinguir, el impulso natural del niño de aprender y puede provocar resentimientos. Un ejemplo que ya mencioné es pegarle la mano al niño cada vez que quiere tocar algo. En experimentos de laboratorio con animales, los investigadores encontraron que las ratas que fueron dadas descargas eléctricas cada vez que se portaban de cierta manera eventualmente eliminaron esa conducta particular. Sin embargo, si las descargas continuaban sin importar lo que hacían, las ratas se daban por vencidas. Como aprenderán en el capítulo sobre las necesidades emocionales de los niños, la atención negativa es preferible a ninguna atención. A nadie le gusta que le hagan caso omiso. Si un niño quiere aprender algo y sus preguntas no son contestadas, se dará por vencido. Si le hacen caso omiso, quizá prefiera un castigo a su silencio. La falta de responsividad y atención de los padres puede impulsar a sus niños a romper la tarea de su hermana o quebrar una ventana. Mi madre sabía exactamente cómo maniobrar mi carácter obstinada con métodos positivos. Ella sabía que unas nalgadas no producían los resultados que ella deseaba, así que me hacía caso omiso por suficiente tiempo como para llamarme la atención para que yo hiciera lo que ella quería. Luego, inmediatamente (y consistentemente) me premiaba. Hacía un pastel o me daba un abrazo o una sonrisa. Estos eran los premios que yo quería y disfrutaba.

Yo no estoy diciendo que la curiosidad y las acciones de los niños no pueden tener límites. Usted debe imponer límites para el desarrollo sano y seguro del niño. Puede alterar su curiosidad que está fuera de los límites y potencialmente peligrosa al restringir su ambiente un poco hasta que aprenda a moderar su propia conducta. Se cubrirá más sobre este tema en la sección sobre disciplina.

Niños activos: El aprendizaje por medio de los sentidos y las actividades motrices—del nacimiento a los veinticuatro meses de edad

Los niños nacen con la capacidad de ver, oír, probar, tocar, y oler, todo lo cual le posibilita a juntar información del mundo a su alrededor. Desde el momento de nacer, pueden enfocar objetos que están a una distancia de hasta trece pulgadas. Disfrutan al mirar fijamente, especialmente a caras humanas además de objetos de colores brillantes que contrastan. Cuando nacen, los bebés usan actos reflejos, tales como chupar, agarrar, y alcanzar. Ellos se quieren llevar todo a la boca, desde su propio pulgar hasta el mentón de usted. Cuando aún son bebés pequeñitos por naturaleza quieren andar. Si coloca los pies de su bebé en una superficie dura, las piernas automáticamente se mueven, como para caminar o correr, pero el resto de su cuerpo no puede. Estos actos reflejos son todos programados al momento de nacer, juntos con el impulso innato de explorar y aprender. Utilizando estos reflejos rudimentarios, ellos comienzan a descubrir el mundo a su alrededor. Al crecer los niños, ellos practican estos reflejos hasta que aprendan a controlarlos, luego aprenden a adaptarlos y coordinarlos. Sus acciones se vuelven más deliberadas y más resueltas y sus conocimientos se vuelven más refinados y organizados.

Los niños pequeños siempre tienen interacción con su medio ambiente al utilizar sus sentidos, agarrar, empujar, agitar, aventar, y otras cosas por el estilo. Los bebés se meten casi todo a la boca para ver a qué sabe. Agitan sus pequeños brazos para pegar los móviles, y tratan de agarrar los objetos. Al aprender a controlar el cuerpo, comienzan a tener una interacción intencional con el medio ambiente. Se sienten atraídos por cosas novedosas, y utilizarán todas las herramientas innatas que tienen a su disposición para aprender activamente acerca de ellas, utilizando sus cinco sentidos.

Los niños son muy activos para aprender. Los niños tienen que tener una interacción con el medio ambiente para aprender de él. Por ejemplo, un día en una clase de crianza de AVANCE, una madre cargaba a su bebé de seis meses de edad. Yo le di al bebé una bella rosa roja, sin espinas, para ilustrarles a las madres cómo aprenden los niños por medio de los sentidos. Tal como yo había predicho, en cuanto el niño miró la rosa, la agarró. Tocó sus suaves pétalos, la olió, y luego la agitó para ver si producía algún sonido. Inevitablemente, se metió algunos pétalos a la boca. Luego siguió sintiendo la textura al hacer trizas los pétalos.

Observe a su niño mientras juegue. Anote y mantenga un registro de lo que hace. En otra ocasión yo observé a mi hijo reaccionar a un nuevo columpio de llanta que mi esposo y yo le acabábamos de colgar en el patio de atrás de la casa, de esa misma manera inquisitiva. Cuando Sal, quien tenía alrededor de seis años de edad, recién miró el columpio, corrió hacia él, lo olió, y lo tocó. Trató de levantar la llanta para ver qué tan pesada era. Se la colocó de una manera, dio la vuelta y se la colocó de otra manera. Se le paró encima, metió la cabeza adentro del agujero, lo empujó y permitió que le pegara suavemente. Después de aprender todo lo que podía a través de tener una interacción activa con la llanta, Sal disfrutó del puro placer de columpiarse. Dejaba que la cabeza se le fuera para atrás lo más que podía al empujarse con las piernas cada vez más alto. Ya cuando se cansó de eso, intentó varias veces brincar del columpio en movimiento y caer parado. Estaba tan orgulloso de que había dominado todos los aspectos que él podía imaginar del columpio. Lo fascinante era que todas estas actividades ocurrieron en menos de una hora.

Los niños tienen la necesidad de explorar y experimentar con una variedad de cosas. Necesitan sentir los cuerpos en el espacio. Un maravilloso proyecto familiar sería construir una estructura de columpios y otros equipos de juego en su patio de atrás. Puede sacar libros de la biblioteca que le puedan servir de recurso si parece demasiado difícil de construir. Yo asistí a una clase sobre la construcción de equipos de juego para niños enseñado por el doctor Joe Frost de la Universidad de Austin, y mi esposo y yo construimos uno detrás de la casa. La estructura que les construimos a nuestros niños consistía de una resbaladilla, una barra de descenso de bombero, un puente que se bamboleaba (a propósito), un cuarto encerrado con ventanas cortadas de diferentes formas, y un cajón de arena. Nuestros niños se pasaban horas enteras corriendo, subiéndose, columpiándose, resbalándose, riéndose, ¡y *aprendiendo*! Los niños aprenden cuando juegan. Tenían varios fuertes en nuestro patio tan grande además de un sendero donde se paseaban en su carrito. Tenían un pony y todo tipo de animales. Cortar el césped era toda una aventura cuando le sujetamos un pequeño remolque a la cortadora de montar, y lo llenamos con la hierba recién cortada. A los amigos, primos, y primas les gustaba venir a las fiestas de cumpleaños de mis niños porque había tantas cosas emocionantes que podían disfrutar.

Un niño a quien no le permiten explorar y experimentar, sino que le mandan a estar quieto o silencioso, está siendo privado del aprendizaje. Aunque los columpios para bebés son reconfortantes emocionalmente y ayudan a establecer el equilibrio en los bebés, pueden volverse, igual que los corralitos, muy restrictivos. La televisión puede prevenir que sus niños aprendan activamente. Los niños necesitan experiencias reales de la vida que les permiten absorber información a través de los sentidos y conectarla a todas las partes posibles del cerebro. Al crecer los niños, los padres necesitan controlar cuánto tiempo se pasan mirando la televisión, y jugando videojuegos y con la computadora, al mismo tiempo de alentarlos a jugar libremente. Yo recuerdo con cuánta frecuencia mi madre solía decir: "Váyanse afuera a jugar". Quizá lo haya dicho motivada por la frustración cuando le poníamos de nervios, pero también sabía la importancia del juego y el ejercicio para el desarrollo del cuerpo y la mente.

Del nacimiento a los veinticuatro meses de edad es un período cuando los niños aprenden a través de los sentidos y por medio del contacto físico con objetos concretos. Los estímulos que reciben necesitan ser los apropiados. Los colores brillantes, formas y contornos, y diferentes diseños geométricos, todos los cuales se encuentran en el arte popular hispano, proveen a los niños el apropiado telón de fondo. Los bebés se pueden quedar fascinados, como hipnotizados, mirando fijamente unos lunares o diseños geométricos negros contra un fondo blanco. Ellos responden a voces de timbre alto y sonidos suaves. Decore el cuarto de su niño con colores brillantes que contrastan. Las madres que asisten a clases de AVANCE hacen bellos diseños para la pared, al calcar dibujos de libros para colorear de flores, animales, u otros objetos, en cartulina. Después los colorean y ponen un laminado con papel de contacto transparente. También hacen unos coloridos móviles llamados "ojos de Dios", hechos de estambre, palitos, y tapaderas de frascos. Puede alternar diferentes tonos de estambre para crear un arcoiris de colores. A lo siguiente están las instrucciones para hacer un hermoso y colorido móvil "ojo de Dios". Su niño disfrutará al mirar el diseño de muchos colores—el mismo diseño que sus antepasados utilizaron hace muchas generaciones.

Móvil de ojo de Dios

Necesitará dos palitos de madera de 24 pulgadas de largo y cuando menos dos diferentes colores de estambre. Forme una cruz con los dos palos. Seleccione un color de estambre. Amarre un cabo de estambre a alguno de los palos cerca del centro donde se juntan los palos. Dé vuelta alrededor de ambos palos para formar una X, cruzándolos por el centro varias veces, hasta quedar bien sujetos los palos. Sostenga los palos cruzados con una mano y utilice la mano libre para comenzar a tejer el diseño del ojo de Dios. Meta el estambre por debajo y alrededor de cada palo dos veces, formando una X, y repita el proceso aproximadamente veinticinco veces (haga veinticinco X). Comience un nuevo color al amarrar un nuevo pedazo de estambre al primero (corte cualquier sobrante) y repita este proceso de "tejer" cuando menos veinticinco veces más, o hasta que consiga un diseño que le guste (o se le acabe el estambre). Puede crear su diseño al determinar cuántas veces cambiar los colores. Pare de tejer cuando llega a la última pulgada de cada palo. Amarre el estambre al hacer un nudo fuerte en la punta de cualquier de los palos, y cortar el sobrante.

Puede hacerle una borla en la punta de cada palo al enredar el estambre alrededor de su mano veinte veces permitiendo que el cabo más largo se amarre del palo. Saque la lazada y amárrela en el centro con un pedazo de estambre de tres pulgadas de largo. Corte las lazadas y recorte cualquier sobrante. Amarre una borla a la punta de cada palo. Puede utilizar palos de cualquier longitud, y un solo color hasta todos los colores de estambre que usted desea.

Unas bellas y brillantes mariposas y unas coloridas flores también proporcionan una variedad de imágenes a cualquier hogar. Es importante cambiar periódicamente la vista que tiene el niño. El arte popular hispano, desde tapices hasta el papel picado (papel de seda cortado para formar bellos diseños), pueden verdaderamente fascinar a una mente joven y son perfectos y estimulantes como adornos. Además de poner cosas bellas e interesantes que el bebé puede mirar, también puede ponerle música suave y reconfortante. Como padres, necesitamos saber cuánto estímulo es apropiado y cuánto es demasiado, o quizá tengamos como resultado un niño necio y enojadísimo. Si se estimula demasiado a los niños, se duermen, se retraen, o hacen berrinche.

DEBE SER RESPONSIVO A LAS NECESIDADES DE SU NIÑO: ¿QUÉ QUIERES, MI HIJO?

Durante este período, los niños creen que si no ven un objeto, no existe: *fuera de vista, fuera de mente.* Ellos suponen que todo está conectado a ellos. A alrededor de los ocho meses de edad, los niños adquieren el conocimiento de la "permanencia de un objeto", o sea la creencia que los objetos o las cosas siguen existiendo aun si ellos no los ven. Para la edad de dos años, los niños dominan este concepto y pueden anticipar la relación entre acciones y futuras consecuencias. Un niño puede anticipar que su mamá volverá cuando sale del cuarto o que un objeto seguirá existiendo aun cuando no está a plena vista. Éste es un logro importante en el aprendizaje, porque señala el momento cuando surgen la memoria, el pensamiento psicológico, y el lenguaje. Durante este período, su niño comienza a pensar que sus acciones provocan ciertos efectos, sin tener que "actuarlas". Si hago esto, piensa el niño, entonces esto ocurrirá. Comienza a pensar que es un ser separado y que las personas y las cosas existen aparte de él. Es un período durante el cual muchos focos se prenden en el cerebro del niño, con muchos tipos de conocimientos nuevos.

Es importante que usted sea responsivo a los sentimientos de sus niños y a sus necesidades físicas, emocionales, sociales, y de aprendizaje. Si su niña llora por hambre, dele de comer. Si su niño llora porque presiente que usted se va, asegúrelo que va a volver. Asegúrese de que su medio ambiente sea tan familiar posible al escoger a una niñera con quien él se siente cómodo. Si quiere un juguete, déselo. Si está aburrido, hable o juegue con él. Si usted no hace estas cosas, su niño aprenderá que no importa lo que él haga, se dará por vencido. Se dará por vencido porque no puede provocar un efecto o cambio deseado en su medio ambiente. Inevitablemente dejará de intentar si las personas le hacen caso omiso. (En los casos de niños que han sido víctimas de negligencia severa, los niños se vuelven letárgicos, se niegan a comer, y algunos aun llegan a fallecer.) Desatender la necesidad de sus niños de aprender y tener un medio ambiente estimulante puede afectar su futuro potencial para el aprendizaje y sus futuras relaciones sociales con otras personas. A través de su responsividad y su atención, usted está apoyando su bienestar, enseñándoles a tener confianza en usted y en otros, y de tener un sentido de seguridad.

Las primeras formas de comunicación a través de las cuales se construyen estos cimientos ocurren cuando el niño se le queda mirando a los ojos y usted trata de adivinar qué necesita: "¿Tienes hambre, mi hija?" "Te ves tan triste, ¿qué quieres, mi amor?" "¿Quieres tu biberón?" "¿Quieres que te levante?" Cuando usted responde a las necesidades de su niño, está comunicando con él. Usted está recibiendo el mensaje que él está tratando de transmitir. Si usted responde a sus necesidades, entonces él adquirirá la confianza necesaria para ayudarle a aprender activamente. Tenga contacto con su niño y lea sus expresiones faciales. Si su bebé saca la lengua o hace burbujas, imítelo. Encontrará que el bebé a su vez imitará a usted. No solamente está aprendiendo el niño, sino que está mandándole mensajes. Hay un dicho que dice que *la mejor palabra es la que no se dice.* Esta pequeña perla de sabiduría se aplica a estos primeros meses cuando se comienzan las formas básicas de comunicación. Cuando su niño hace un sonido y usted trata de repetirlo, usted está comunicando. Los primeros "arrullos" se convertirán en palabras, frases, y más tarde en cuentos. Sus niños llegarán a darse cuenta que la comunicación es una acción recíproca y sincronizada entre dos o más personas, que abarca todo, desde las expresiones faciales y las palabras, hasta los gestos y movimientos del cuerpo.

JUGANDO Y APRENDIENDO

Los niños pequeños poseen una necesidad innata de jugar. Para ellos, el juego no solamente es divertido, sino que es serio. Los niños aprenden con todas estas alegres actividades de juego. Desde el momento cuando se dan cuenta que tienen manos y pies, pasarán muchas de sus horas despiertas jugando con ellos y aprendiendo qué pueden hacer con ellos. No pasará mucho tiempo antes de que se meten las manos y los pies dentro de la boca. Pronto se dan cuenta que sus bocas y otros órganos vocales producen sonidos y se pasan mucho tiempo entreteniéndose a sí mismos, y a otros también, con estos nuevos descubrimientos. Cuando su niño gorjea, arrulla, y balbucea, no está sólo jugando, está creando sus sonidos, tonos, y timbres básicos, los cuales con el tiempo conducirán a la construcción de palabras y frases.

Durante los primeros meses de la vida, una madre y un padre son los compañeros de juego favoritos de sus niños. Muchos expertos del desarrollo de los niños describen este período como un "dar y recibir" entre padres y niños. Cuando su niño arrulla o le sonríe y usted le arrulla y le sonríe de vuelta, no sólo se está divirtiendo, sino que también está aprendiendo a confiar en usted y a desarrollar una importante relación que le ayudará a relacionarse con otras personas más adelante. Otra interacción de juego ocurre cuando su pequeño bebé imita los diferentes sonidos, gestos, y expresiones que usted hace. Por ejemplo, yo a veces hacía un sonido como "ba, ba" a mi niño y él imitaba el sonido. Luego le cambiaba el sonido a "da, da", y él repetía ese sonido también. Yo le decía: "Ojitos, mi hijito" (y entrecerraba los ojos), y él, a su vez, me entrecerraba los suyos. Si yo le decía: "Dame un besito", él me complacía al tirarme unos besitos. Si yo le pedía que me dijera "adiós", me hacía adiós con la mano. Si le sacaba la lengua o le hacía burbujas, él hacía lo mismo.

Otra cosa que les encantaba a mis niños era cuando les picaba la pancita al recitar rimas como *Pin marín de Don Pifuel, cúcara mácara, títere fue él.* Con la última estrofa, les soplaba o les hacía cosquillas en la pancita. A veces les decía: "Te voy a hacer cosquillitas", y se reían aun antes de tocarles siquiera. Aun el niño muy pequeño sabe cómo advertirnos que ya ha sido suficiente. Es capaz de regular la cantidad apropiada de estímulos que puede soportar al voltearse y mirar otra cosa. Después de un pequeño descanso, quizá quiera reanudar el juego. Nosotros, como padres, debemos responder a esas señales.

Las investigaciones científicas han relacionado altas calificaciones en los exámenes de inteligencia y logros académicos excepcionales en la lectura y las matemáticas con la presencia de materiales de juego interesantes y que constituyen un desafío intelectual, que los niños utilizan en su hogar después del primer año de vida. Los juguetes tales como las sonajas, los móviles, y los suaves animales de peluche los motivarán a manipular su medio ambiente físico. Materiales de juego tales como la arena, el agua, los rompecabezas, y los cuadritos de madera ayudan a los niños a aprender conceptos tales como las formas y los números, y habilidades como la coordinación entre los ojos y las manos. Los juegos con pelotas, triciclos, y cuerdas ayudan a los niños a desarrollar sus habilidades motrices. Los muñecos, los muebles en miniatura, y la ropita crean un mundo imaginario para su exploración.

Cuando su niño tenga la edad suficiente, dele juguetes y objetos de diferentes colores, tamaños, y texturas que pueda manipular. Cuando comience a gatear, su niño necesitará suficiente espacio para explorar y experimentar. Sin embargo, al crecer y volverse más fuerte y más activo, usted debe poner a prueba de niño la casa y estar más atento a dónde está el niño y qué está haciendo, ya que deambulará por todas partes en busca de cosas interesantes que todavía no ha descubierto. Objetos ordinarios en la casa servirán para satisfacer su interés al prender y apagar cosas, moverlas para adentro y para afuera, o pasarlas "a través" de otros objetos.

La música frecuentemente es un medio poderoso para el juego. Aun en la cuna, los niños responden a sonidos rítmicos. En las tiendas se venden discos y discos compactos con el sonido del latido de corazón de la madre, los cuales algunos padres, especialmente aquéllos de bebés que nacieron prematuramente, tocan para recordarles a sus bebés la cálida y tierna comodidad de la matriz. Proporcióneles a sus niños tambores de mentiritas y xilófonos en miniatura para que puedan comenzar a desarrollar un oído musical. Trate de combinar la música con el momento del baño y tendrá a un bebé muy contento, aunque la mayor parte del agua terminará en el piso. Cuando era un bebé, mi hermano Eddie le hacía a mi madre tocar su canción favorita, "*Soldier, Soldier, Would You Marry Me*", constantemente y cada vez se dejaba llevar y se ponía a bailar con la música. Igualmente, cuando yo era una jovencita, yo me convertía en el centro de atención al moverme los hombros para adelante y para atrás cada vez que se tocaba la canción "Mambo, qué rico el mambo". A los niños les encanta moverse al son de la música. En el mundo hispano, se puede observar a niños pequeños a mitad de la pista de baile en bodas, moviéndose al compás de la música. Muchos padres inscriben a sus niños en clases de baile folclórico a una edad muy pequeña para ver si tienen interés por el baile. Así como la música puede utilizarse para infundirle al niño creatividad, una música suave también puede tener un efecto calmante después de un día repleto de exploración.

Ya sea escuchando la canción de cuna en inglés "*Hush Little Baby*" o "Señora Santa Ana" o "A la rurru niño", a los niños les encanta ser arrullados en la mecedora con canciones de cuna. Tal como mi abuela le cantó "Señora Santa Ana" a mi madre, quien a su vez la cantó a nosotros, mis hijos probablemente compartirán esta melodía con sus propios niños. Hasta la fecha, esa canción nos provoca emociones positivas a mis niños y a mí. (Véase el siguiente capítulo para encontrar más canciones de cuna.) Si usted no sabe la canción "Señora Santa Ana", pregúntele a una persona mayor de México si sabe la melodía de esta muy popular canción de cuna. Cántesela a su bebé y estará comenzando una tradición que seguirá a través de las generaciones. "A la rurru niño" tiene la misma melodía que "Señora Santa Ana".

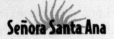

Señora Santa Ana

Señora Santa Ana, ¿Por qué llora el niño?
Por una manzana que se le ha perdido.

Iremos al huerto, cortaremos dos,
una para el niño y otra para Dios.

Manzanita de oro, si yo te encontrara
se la diera al niño para que callara.

Santa Margarita, carita de luna,
méceme este niño que tengo en la cuna.

Duérmese mi niño, duérmese mi sol,
duérmase, pedazo de mi corazón.

María lavaba, San José tendía,
eran los pañales que el niño tenía.

A la rurru niño

A la rurru niño, a la rurru ya,
duérmase mi niño y duérmase ya.

Este niño lindo, que nació de día,
Quiere que lo lleven a pasear de día.

Este niño lindo que nació de noche,
Quiere que lo lleven a pasear en coche.

A los niños muy pequeños también les encanta hacer "tortillitas" y otros juegos de manos. Por medio de estos juegos ellos adquieren habilidades de lenguaje, desarrollan sus habilidades musicales, y forjan una relación estrecha con usted. Los siguientes son algunos juegos de manos tradicionales favoritos en inglés y español que han deleitado a los niños por muchas generaciones. Siéntese en el piso con su niño y juegue estos juegos de mano tradicionales. Si no sabe la melodía, invente una. Intente actuar las palabras, tal como moverse los dedos lentamente cuando dice "dedos", y luego moverlos muy rápidamente cuando dice "que gire, que gire, como un girasol".

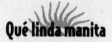

Qué linda manita

Qué linda manita que tiene el bebé.
Qué linda, qué mona, qué bonita es.
Pequeños deditos, rayitos de sol.
Que gire, que gire, como un girasol.

Las hojitas

Repita pero con la palabra "bailar" al final. El niño agita las manos en el aire y baja las manos cuando la mamá dice "caen", luego las vuelve a levantar.

Las hojitas, las hojitas
De los árboles se caen
Viene el viento, y las levanta
Y se ponen a cantar.

Pon pon pon

Péguele suavemente al niño con el dedo en la palma de la mano mientras recite esta rima.

Pon pon pon la manita en el bordón.
Dame un veinte para el jabón
Para lavar el pantalón de tu tío Simón.

Pat-a-cake

Pat-a-cake, pat-a-cake, baker's man.
Bake me a cake as fast as you can.
Pat it, roll it, and mark it with a B,
and put it in the oven for baby and me.

Papitas

Papitas, papitas
Para Mamá.
Las quemaditas,
Para Papá.

Papas

Otra versión, ésta favorece al papá en lugar de la mamá:

Papas y papas para Papá,
papas y papas para Mamá;
las calientitas para Papá,
las quemaditas para Mamá.

La pequeña araña

La pequeña araña, subió, subió y subió.
Cayó la lluvia, y se la llevó.
Salió el sol, y todo lo secó.
Y la pequeñita araña subió, subió, subió.

Sigue la versión en inglés de "La pequeña araña":

Itsy, bitsy spider

Itsy, bitsy spider went up the waterspout.
Down came the rain and washed the spider out.
Out came the sun and dried up all the rain.
And the itsy, bitsy spider went up the spout again.

Mis niños adoraban el siguiente juego de mano llamado "La viejita", el cual es similar a *"This Little Piggy Went to Market"*. Para jugarlo, comienza por hacerle cosquillas a la palma de la mano de su niño. Cuando recita la frase de la "leñita", uno hace como si cortara cada dedo de la mano de la misma manera que cortaría la leña con un serrucho. Luego, cuando llega a la parte de "llover", haga cosquillas en la palma de la mano otra vez. Mueva los dedos lentamente para arriba del brazo del niño como si fuera la "viejita corriendo para meterse en su casita", y luego le hace cosquillas al niño debajo del brazo, en la axila. Mis niños me pedían repetir este juego una y otra vez. Ellos adoraban la anticipación de lo que sabían que iba a ocurrir al final de la rima.

La viejita

Había una viejita
que cortaba su leñita,
y comenzó a llover,
y no hallaba donde correr,
y se metió en su casita.

This Little Piggy Went to Market

This little piggy went to market.
This little piggy stayed home.
This little piggy had roast beef.
This little piggy had none.
This little piggy cried wee wee wee all the way home.

Sus niños comienzan a aprender a una edad muy pequeña que sus acciones causan ciertos efectos. Son capaces de decir: "Si yo hago esto, entonces esto ocurrirá". Las cajas de sorpresas (*Jack-in-the-boxes*) y los teléfonos son muy populares durante esta etapa. A través de estos juguetes, los niños provocan una respuesta a una acción, ya sea algo que salta de una caja o una voz en el teléfono. Les provoca una agradable sensación ver la reacción. Están aprendiendo que pueden tener algún control sobre diferentes aspectos del mundo. Como ya han aprendido, los niños menores de ocho meses de edad generalmente no se disgustarán tanto cuando usted sale del cuarto. Sin embargo, después de esa edad, ellos saben que usted y los objetos existen aun si no son visibles. Éste es un momento maravilloso para jugar "a las escondiditas". Con una cobijita, puede entretener a su niño diciendo: "Te veo". Durante este juego, mis niños se tapaban la carita con las manos, como escondiéndose, y yo les seguía la corriente al decirles: "¿Dónde está mi hijito(a)?" hasta que bajaban las manos. Cuando yo les decía: "Allí está mi hijito(a)", siempre se soltaban riendo.

EL MUNDO DE LA FANTASÍA: EL JUEGO DRAMÁTICO E IMAGINARIO– DE LOS DOS A LOS CINCO AÑOS DE EDAD

Durante este período, los juegos del niño consisten en un mundo imaginario. Los niños actúan relaciones al jugar juegos como las comadritas, la casita, o la escuela. Se pueden imaginar como médicos o como policías. Permítales a sus niños suficiente tiempo para sus juegos imaginarios. Proporcione los accesorios necesarios como, por ejemplo, sombreros, ropa, cuadritos de madera, muñecos, camionetas, juegos de té, herramientas en miniatura, y aparatos eléctricos caseros de mentiritas. Después de que su niño le haya observado durante dos años, usted verá todo lo que usted mismo hace y dice representado en su juego. ¡Cuidado! *Lo que no puedes ver en tu huerto, ha de crecer*. Le imitan al ir a la oficina o al discutir con su pareja o una vendedora. Por esto uno tiene que tener cuidado con todo lo que hace y dice. En sus juegos, los niños interpretarán las cosas que agitan sus emociones, como ir por sus vacunas, ir a la guardería, o los pleitos entre Mami y Papi.

Había una sección en el cuarto de mis niños que estaba designado como su "rincón imaginario". Tenía un buen surtido de sombreros, ropa, artículos caseros, y disfraces de Halloween. Al observar a los niños en juego, casi puede "ver" al cerebro funcionando. Los niños piensan en voz alta al tratar de resolver problemas o al construir edificios de bloquecitos. Continuarán jugando con algo hasta aprender todas sus propiedades y cómo funciona. Entonces seguirán con la siguiente cosa que les fascina o que simplemente les proporciona placer.

Mientras el niño juega y aprende conceptos, los padres deben aprovechar la oportunidad de meterse al proceso y ponerles nombres a los objetos y las acciones. ¿Recuerda al niño de AVANCE que estaba metiendo piedras por las aberturas de la cerca? Esta actividad le ofrecía una excelente oportunidad a su madre para decir: "Ah, yo veo que estás metiendo una piedra *por* el agujero". Los padres necesitan estar cerca de sus niños cuando ellos están creando y explorando. No interrumpa el juego, facilítelo. Reálcelo con un ambiente seguro y enriquecedor. Intervenga en el momento apropiado y responda, como cuando su niño necesita ayuda para nombrar los conceptos y acciones con las palabras correspondientes apropiadas. Por ejemplo, cuando está jugando con bloquecitos y carritos, dígale: "Ese *carro* va *alrededor* del edificio. ¿Adónde va el carro *azul?*" Ponga énfasis en las palabras "carro", "alrededor", y "azul".

Los niños requieren una variedad de actividades y materiales para explorar y experimentar cuando juegan. Por ejemplo, cuando están afuera, provee agua, arena, botes, palas, coladores, embudos, y recipientes de diferentes tamaños y observe lo que pasa. Por medio del descubrimiento, los niños aprenderán habilidades matemáticas tales como el volumen y el peso. Aprenderán el significado de "más que", "menos que", "igual a", y "la mitad de". Este tipo de juego construye los cimientos para que sus niños luego sobresalgan en matemáticas y ciencia.

Deles bloquecitos para que puedan construir edificios, puentes, casas, y torres. No solamente aprenderán algunos aspectos de matemáticas, física, y arquitectura, sino que también se divertirán creando objetos. Los niños también necesitan estar afuera para correr, pasear, subirse en cosas, columpiarse, rodar, saltar, deslizarse, y caminar. Construya o compre unas barras de equilibrio y/o una estructura de juego en el patio de su casa, tal como discutimos anteriormente. Cómpreles juguetes con ruedas, cuerdas, y gises. Llévelos de excursión, a caminar, y a comer al campo. Ellos necesitan oportunidades para explorar el mundo y dominar el cuerpo.

Acercándose al final de esta etapa, los niños pueden separar cosas en categorías—animales, frutas—y por formas, colores, y tamaños. Pueden armar rompecabezas y crear cosas con plastilina. Déles a sus niños bastantes crayolas y lápices y mucho papel y aliéntelos a dibujar, garabatear, conectar los puntos, y calcar las líneas. Ponga grandes hojas de papel alrededor del cuarto para que puedan garabatear en el papel y no en las paredes. Deles artículos de arte, pero cuidado. Permítame advertirle que debe colocar papel periódico por todo el piso para cuando el niño tenga su arrebato de energía y expresión artística y también que debe asegurar que el futuro Diego Rivera se ponga ropa vieja al crear sus obras maestras. Al crecer, siga alentando a sus niños a expresar su creatividad al darles papel para dibujar. Vanessa está fascinada con los monos de historietas y caricaturas. Comenzó a trazarlos del periódico. Como yo sabía que a ella le interesaba el dibujo, yo le compré un caballete, pintura, gises de colores, y mucho papel de dibujo, para que los tuviera a la mano cuando-quiera que ella quería dibujar. Al exponer yo sus obras maestras, la motivaba a seguir dibujando. Sus amigos descubrieron su talento artístico y pronto comenzó a crear dibujos para ellos. Asegúrese de tener bastantes materiales que pueden usarse para crear piezas de arte, tales como tijeras, marcadores, pegamento, papel de colores y papel de seda, plumas, piedritas de fantasía, botones, calcomanías, serpentinas, etc. Organice un proyecto de arte para toda la familia, para hacer sombreros, dibujos, o barquitos. ¡Esto puede ser muy divertido!

Si su niño se interesa por la música, ésta es la etapa durante la cual tratará de imitar ciertas melodías y aprender canciones repetitivas. En adición, éste es el momento perfecto para enseñarles a sus niños rimas, canciones, y juegos que les ayudarán a aprender los números, los días de la semana, y las partes del cuerpo. Siguen unos cuantos juegos, rimas, y canciones tradicionales que yo les cantaba a los niños en la escuela y a los míos propios en casa. Quizá los quiera usar con sus niños. Puede encontrar grabaciones de estas canciones hechas por algunos de los artistas nombrados en la Lista de Recursos al fin de este libro. Tal vez encuentre éstas u otras canciones que les encantarán a sus niños. Mis niños todavía recuerdan los discos del Grillito CriCri que yo solía tocar para ellos, especialmente "El ratón vaquero". Su niño que vive en un mundo bilingüe puede aprender los números en ambos inglés y español a través de estas canciones y rimas.

Acitrón de un fandango

Acitrón de un fandango
Sango, Sango, Sango
Savaré
Savaré que va pasando
Con su triqui triqui trán.

Matarilli-rili-rón

Este juego se trata de un niño que está tratando de casarse con la hija de una mujer llamada Ambo Gato. La madre (M) le hace al niño (N) una serie de preguntas, incluyendo qué será su profesión. Él nombra varias profesiones hasta encontrar una que ella acepta (cancionero). Ella acepta el matrimonio y todos los niños dicen juntos la última estrofa. En este momento, la hija se pasa al otro lado, con el niño. Cada estrofa de la canción se repite dos veces. Todos los niños que están en el mismo lado de la madre van al lado del niño, al mismo tiempo que hacen la pregunta; vuelven, de espaldas, a su posición original, repitiendo la pregunta. Luego, los niños que están en el mismo lado del niño van al lado de la madre, al mismo tiempo que contestan la pregunta; vuelven, de espaldas, a su posición original, repitiendo la respuesta. Cambian las profesiones y eventualmente termina el juego cuando la madre se queda sola.

N: Ambo Gato, Matarili rili rón
M: ¿Qué quería usted? Matarili rili rón
N: Yo quiero un paje, Matarili rili rón
M: ¿Qué oficio le pondremos? Matarili rili rón
N: Le pondremos carpintero. Matarili rili rón
M: Ese oficio no me agrada. Matarili rili rón
N: Le pondremos cancionero. Matarili rili rón
M: Ese oficio sí me agrada. Matarili rili rón
Todos: Celebramos todos juntos, Matarili rili rón

Un elefante

Para jugar este juego, utilice varios dibujos de elefantes cortados de papel y con un número distinto en cada uno. Utilice el elefante correspondiente al número que está cantando. La canción también se canta al reemplazar "balanceaba" con "columpiaba".

Un elefante se balanceaba (columpiaba)
sobre la tela de una araña.
Como veía que resistía,
fue a llamar a otro elefante.

(Repita utilizando otros números)

Dos elefantes se balanceaban (columpiaban)
sobre la tela de una araña.
Como veían que resistía,
fueron a llamar a otro elefante.

Tres elefantes…etc.
Cuatro elefantes…etc.

El barquito

Cuente con los dedos al decir los números.

Había una vez un barco, un barco chiquitito.
Había una vez un barco, un barco chiquitito.
Había una vez un barco, un barco chiquitito
Tan chiquitito, tan chiquitito que no podía navegar.

Pasaron una, dos, tres, cuatro, cinco, seis, siete semanas.
Pasaron una, dos, tres, cuatro, cinco, seis, siete semanas.
Pasaron una, dos, tres, cuatro, cinco, seis, siete semanas.
Y el barquito, el barquito, no podía navegar.

Zapatito

Zapatito blanco, zapatito azúl
Dime, ¿cuántos años tienes tú?
Seis. Uno, dos, tres, cuatro, cinco, seis.

One Two, Buckle My Shoe

One, two, buckle my shoe
Three, four, shut the door
Five, six, pick up sticks
Seven, eight, lay them straight
Nine, ten, a big fat hen.

¿A qué hora?

A la una, miro la luna.
A las dos, miro el reloj
A las tres, no me ves
A las cuatro, miro el sapo
A las cinco, pego un brinco
A las seis, tarde es
A las siete, sale un cohete
A las ocho, como un bizcocho
A las nueve, voy a la nieve
A las diez, comienzo otra vez.

Los días de la semana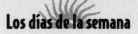

Lunes y martes, miércoles y jueves, viernes y sábado—
domingo es la semana.

EL CUIDADO DE LOS NIÑOS: ¿QUIÉN CUIDARÁ A MI NIÑO?

Usted tiene que volver al trabajo, ¿pero quién cuidará a su bebé? Quizá tenga que llevar a su niño a una guardería. La guardería juega un papel muy importante en el crecimiento y desarrollo cognoscitivo de su niño pequeño. Las guarderías pueden ser lugares donde los niños se pasan mucho tiempo aprendiendo y jugando. En la actualidad, muchos padres tienen dificultad para encontrar una guardería de calidad que es buena para sus niños. Los latinos no son la excepción. Se da por hecho entre muchos hispanos que no hay mejor niñera que la abuelita o algún miembro de la familia extensa para cuidar a los niños, especialmente cuando son muy pequeños. Mucha gente, sin embargo, no tiene la buena fortuna de tener a esas personas cerca. Aun si usted no trabaja, quizá quiera proporcionarle a su niño la oportunidad de jugar con otros niños, especialmente después de los tres años de edad. Es su responsabilidad encontrar el tipo de cuidado para su niño que satisface sus necesidades y su presupuesto. Querrá que sea un lugar donde usted puede sentirse cómodo al dejar a su niño precioso al cuidado de alguien en quien puede confiar y quien proveerá un medio ambiente seguro y propicio al aprendizaje.

Una vez que se decida por un arreglo que satisface sus requisitos, prepare a su niño para estar alejado de usted por unas horas y facilita suavemente la transición a su nuevo ambiente. Háblele acerca del nuevo lugar que él visitará todos los días. Léale libros y cuentos sobre niños que están pasando por experiencias similares. Visite el lugar por unas cuantas horas cada día. Propicie que la educadora lo conozca. Asegúrese de que su primer día no es uno de tensión ni para él ni para usted. Si es posible, quédese en la guardería con él por parte del día, por dos o tres días. Estas actividades deben ayudarle a hacer la transición.

Quizá lo considere importante que el centro proyecte algo de su cultura a través de comidas, canciones, juegos, y lenguaje. Si no están dispuestos o equipados para hacerlo, quizá el centro le permita a usted llevar algunos artículos que reflejan su cultura, tales como cassettes de canciones en español y arte popular hispano. Enséñele a la maestra o a los estudiantes cómo hacer una piñata, un móvil de "Ojo de Dios", cascarones, o un altar para el día de los Muertos. Describa el significado cultural de la celebración. Prepare y contribuya un platillo tradicional como arroz con habichuelas o buñuelos para algún acontecimiento en el centro. Comparta algunas de sus creencias y tradiciones culturales con la clase. Podría iluminar un poco a los compañeros de clase de su niño acerca de los muchos aspectos bellos de nuestro patrimonio cultural por medio de otras maneras que no sean simplemente llevar objetos y hablar acerca de ellos.

Aun aquéllos que han logrado mantener su primera selección para el cuidado de su niño, o sea la familia, se enfrentan a sacrificios y compromisos. Mi hermana Rosa Linda dejó su trabajo para cuidar a sus nietos en su hogar. Ella creía firmemente que nadie podría darles a sus nietos el amor y el cuidado que ella les daría, y además le encanta hacerlo. Ella lo considera una inversión de su tiempo a cambio de establecer una relación con sus nietos. Mi suegra y mi madre cuidaron a mis niños, un hecho que me hizo más fácil la vida.

Tales arreglos pueden, claro, tener ciertas desventajas cuando "la doña" tiene diferentes conceptos con respecto a la crianza de los niños. *Cuando los abuelos entran por la puerta, la disciplina sale por la ventana.* Sin embargo, yo sentí que los vínculos afectivos que formaron mis niños con sus abuelas bien valía la pena de algunas concesiones que yo tuve que hacer, como dejar que los niños se salieran con lo suyo de vez en cuando, o aceptar los dulces que les daban, o las ocasionales "piedras", o comentarios que mi suegra me aventara acerca de como *ella* se quedó en casa cuidando a *sus* niños. Ya sea pariente o no, es importante que usted se sienta cómodo con la persona que cuida a su niño y el arreglo que han hecho. Hasta la fecha, mis niños recuerdan las maravillosas aventuras que pasaron con su abuelita Dolores, quien los llevaba a días de campo y de excursión a los parques de diversión. Mi hija, Vanessa, se sintió muy agradecida con su abuelita Lucy, quien la recogió un día de la escuela porque se sentía mal, y le dio a comer caldito y le hizo té para beber. La comadre casi se convierte en miembro de la familia cuando se trata de cuidar a los niños. Vanessa llegó a conocer muy bien a su madrina Carmen por las mañanas cuando la llevaba a la escuela. Nuestra familia llegó a conocer muy bien a su hijo, Adam, al llevarlo de la escuela a su casa.

Cualquier que haya sido el arreglo que yo tenía para el cuidado de mis niños, había ocasiones cuando, a causa de días festivos de la escuela, o las vacaciones de una niñera, tenía que llamar a otra persona. Una buena estrategia es mantener una lista de varias personas de quienes puede depender, comenzando con la familia extensa, las comadres, las vecinas, y cualquier otra persona que quizá esté dispuesta a sacarle de un apuro.

EL DESARROLLO DE LENGUAJE: APRENDIENDO A HABLAR

La manera en que los niños desarrollan el lenguaje es uno de los aspectos más fascinantes de su crecimiento. Cuando oye a su niño arrullar a alrededor de los tres meses de edad, él hace los mismos sonidos que están incluidos en todos los idiomas del mundo, ya sea alemán, español, inglés, o japonés. Todos los niños tienen la capacidad de aprender todos estos sonidos. De acuerdo al psicólogo James Deese, a los seis meses de edad, un niño gradualmente comienza a distinguir y favorecer algunos sonidos más que otros. Al paso del tiempo, dejará a un lado aquellos sonidos que no escucha en su medio ambiente y practicará sólo aquéllos que sí escucha. Si el niño que habla español escucha la palabra "perro", continuará practicando hacer vibrar las erres. Si se cría en un ambiente bilingüe, también escuchará y continuará diciendo los sonidos que se utilizan para hablar inglés, como "th", "sh", "ch", y los doce sonidos de los vocales, algunos de los cuales no se encuentran en el idioma español. Sin embargo, los sonidos como la "ch", como se pronuncia en las palabras alemanas como "Bach", se quedarán por el lado si el niño no sigue escuchándolos. Poner a los niños en contacto con una amplia gama de sonidos a una edad muy pequeña tal vez facilite su habilidad de llegar a ser multilingüe. El niño que habla inglés aprenderá cuarenta y cinco sonidos básicos que se pueden hacer usando las veintiséis letras del abecedario inglés, y el niño que habla español aprenderá los veintidós a veinticuatro sonidos del abecedario español.

El niño practicará sus sonidos al arrullar, reírse, y gorjear. A los seis meses de edad, el niño balbucea al unir los sonidos de las consonantes y las vocales para formar sonidos como "ma", "ta", y "pa". Practica la producción de una variedad de sonidos, y trata de explorar cómo funcionan las diferentes partes de la boca para producir estos sonidos. Repita los balbuceos que su niño produce. Sonríale y abrácele cuando repite los sonidos que usted hace.

Es importante que usted le hable a su niño y platique con él. Utilice el lenguaje afectuoso que usan los padres cuando les hablan a los bebés. Las madres hispanas conocen estas palabras afectuosas por el nombre de "cariños", y en inglés se llama "parentese" o "motherese". Es más fácil para el bebé encontrar, entender, y reconocer las palabras de este tipo de lenguaje. Las madres por naturaleza tratan de hacer una conexión con sus bebés al mirarlos a los ojos, hablar más lentamente, y utilizar un timbre alto de voz. Hacen una pausa entre una frase y otra para ponerles énfasis a palabras importantes. Las frases en este lenguaje de cariños son cortas y sencillas. Hay mucha repetición y muchas preguntas insertadas en las palabras. Al mirarle a su hijo a los ojos, sonríale y suba suavemente el timbre y con una voz cantarina diga cosas como: "¡Ay, qué liiinda, mi hijita! ¡Qué chuuula! ¿Dormiste bastante? Dale un besiiito a Mamá. Mamá quiere muuuucho a su angeliiito. Dame una sonrisa. Ay, qué preciooooosa, mi luna de miel". Ya sea en español o en inglés, esta forma de hablar suena muy parecido: *"Hiiiii. How's my precious doooing? Did you have a good naaap? Yeaaaa! You diiiid have a good nap. You are sooooo preeeetty. Give Mama a biiiig smile"*. Después de platicar con su bebé de esta manera, estará tan entusiasmado que se volverá muy atento y receptivo a cualquier cosa que le quiera enseñar. Mantenga en mente que este lenguaje de cariño, el cual puede continuar hasta los tres años de edad, es muy diferente a "baby talk", cuando uno habla como bebé y distorsiona la pronunciación de las palabras. Es importante que pronuncie las palabras con precisión. Aun si su bebé dice "bibi" o "baba", usted debe repetir las palabras en su forma correcta al decir "biberón" o "bottle".

LENGUAJE RECEPTIVO Y EXPRESIVO: ENTENDER Y HABLAR

Todos los niños pasan por dos tipos de lenguaje: primero el receptivo y luego el expresivo. Ambos son componentes básicos de la comunicación. Durante el primer año de vida, nuestros niños pueden entender lo que les decimos, pero generalmente no pueden expresarse. A esto se le llama lenguaje receptivo. Por ejemplo, cuando usted le pide a un niño de diez meses de edad que le dé la pelota y él se la da, él está demostrando que entiende. El lenguaje expresivo, en cambio, significa que él puede verbalizar lo que él quiere. El lenguaje expresivo se aprende por etapas. La primera etapa comienza con los arrullos y balbuceos, sonidos de una sílaba consistente en consonante y vocal, como "ma", "ta", "pa". Es importante hablarle y leerle a su niño aun antes de que él pueda decir su primera palabra. La primera palabra expresiva del niño aparece a aproximadamente un año de edad y aumenta rápidamente si usted continúa hablándole y proporcionándole nombres para los objetos y las acciones. A alrededor de los dieciocho meses de edad, el niño unirá dos palabras— un sujeto y un verbo—para formar pequeñas frases. A esto se le llama habla telegráfica. Deja fuera los artículos, las preposiciones, las partes finales de los verbos, o los verbos auxiliares. Por ejemplo quizá diga, "perro come", "yo come", "arriba yo", "arriba pelota", "más jugo", "perro grande", "bebé grande", o "carro grande". Al cumplir los dos años de edad, su vocabulario aumenta de alrededor de 200 palabras a 300 palabras. A los tres años, ya sabe alrededor de 1,000 palabras. A los cuatro,

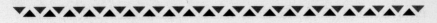

Logros importantes en el desarrollo del lenguaje

2 meses	se comienzan los balbuceos
3 meses	se comienzan los arrullos, sonidos (no palabras) de dos sílabas
4 meses	el bebé hace sonidos compuestos por 4 o 5 sílabas
6 a 9 meses	patrones de entonación
9 meses	sílabas de vocalización—puede hacer "tortillitas", "adiós"
9 meses a 1 año	el niño demuestra una variedad de timbres
12 meses	sigue mandatos sencillos, dice una palabra
14 meses	el niño puede decir 3 palabras
16 a 18 meses	el niño puede decir de 5 a 25 palabras; reconoce dibujos; responde a mandatos
18 a 24 meses	el niño posee un vocabulario de 200 a 300 palabras
24 meses	se comienzan las frases de dos palabras ("carro va"); el niño le jala hacia algo para mostrárselo; usa algunas palabras espaciales y "yo" y las conjugaciones con "iendo" y "ando"
24 a 30 meses	el niño tiene un vocabulario de 400 palabras, "mi", "mío", "tu"
30 a 33 meses	hace preguntas de "qué", "dónde", "por qué", "quién", y "cómo"; usa las palabras "él", "ella", "nosotros", "tuyo", "tuyos"
3 años	frases de 3 a 4 palabras; un vocabulario de 1000 palabras; juego dramático; tiene dificultad con la *s*, *z*, *r*, y *l*; pregunta "cuándo"; usa las palabras "suyo", "él", "nuestro", "debajo"
4 años	tiene un vocabulario de 1,500 palabras; usa las palabras "detrás", "enfrente", "arriba", "abajo", "al fondo"; repite los cuentos
5 años	tiene un vocabulario de 2,000 palabras y comienza a usar pensamiento lógico

ha aprendido 1,500, y a los cinco, ha alcanzado la cifra de 2,000 palabras. Usted propicia el aumento de la lista al seguir el interés de su niño y ponerles nombres a las cosas que le interesan. Si él le apunta a un objeto, dígale la palabra. Cualquier cosa que le interesa (pelota, perrito), descríbala. Los niños se hablarán solos al andar por allí experimentando y practicando con palabras nuevas. Proporcióneles nuevas palabras a través de rimas, cantos, y juegos.

Una explosión de desarrollo de lenguaje: ¡Mío! Yo hacerlo—De los dos a los siete años de edad

¿Ha estado usted asombrado de cómo el lenguaje de su niño aumenta con la fuerza y rapidez de una explosión al acercarse a su segundo cumpleaños? Su niño ha tenido mucho tiempo para jugar, explorar, experimentar, tocar, oír, y observar. Ha creado muchas imágenes, numerosos conceptos, y comprende el significado de muchas palabras. Ahora está listo para aumentar rápidamente su lenguaje verbal. Ahora puede nombrar los conceptos que representan imágenes y palabras. Puede visualizar imágenes, memorizar, y reconocer palabras. Usted quería que su niño hablara, pero ahora se pregunta cómo hacerle tomar un respiro.

Cuando su niño de dos años le dice "yo lo hace", aun si usted no cree que él puede hacerlo, permítale intentar. Quizá le sorprenda. Cuando los niños cumplan dos años de edad, entran a la etapa de "mío" y "yo". A veces dicen su nombre en lugar de decir "mi". Ellos les avisarán a todos que todo es "mío". Ellos creen que pueden hacer todo y que todo les pertenece. En un vídeo familiar que le tomamos a mi hijo Steven, donde recitaba unas rimas infantiles, se podía escuchar a Vanessa, de dos años de edad, al repetir una y otra vez: "¡Yo también! Yo lo hace. Yo puede hacerlo". Después de que Steven recitó "Jack and Jill", ella quería hacerlo también, así que inmediatamente siguió con: "Jack and Jill went up the hill to get aaaaawa. Fell down. Broke crown. Jill…ah…ah…er!" Luego Vanessa rodó por el piso para mostrarme lo que pasó en seguida. Ella poseía un fuerte concepto mental de cómo ocurría la historia y su secuencia, pero tenía algunos de los nombres para los conceptos en inglés y otros en español, y luego no tenía las palabras para algunos otros conceptos, los cuales me mostró a través de sus acciones.

A esta edad, los niños siguen con su habla telegráfica, componiendo frases de dos o tres palabras. Tienen dificultad para pronunciar los sonidos producidos por las letras *s, z, r,* y *l.* Escuchará frases como "dame etho", "vatho de agua", "I wuv you", "I wun fast".

Después del habla telegráfica, su niño añadirá artículos (el, la, los, las, un, una, unos, unas), preposiciones (en), pronombres (él, ella), además de las formas plurales y posesivas de ciertas palabras. También comenzará a utilizar correctamente los verbos irregulares y las contracciones. A alrededor de los cinco años de edad, su niño comenzará a usar el tiempo futuro. Sus frases incluyen una declaración afirmativa seguido por una pregunta, pidiendo reafirmación. Por ejemplo: "Papi está en la casa, ¿verdad que sí?" "Está lloviendo, ¿verdad?" Los niños han aprendido ya que el pronombre tiene que estar de acuerdo con su objeto en persona, número, y género. De aquí en adelante, las frases de los niños se vuelven más largas y más complejas al combinar dos pensamientos y luego dos ideas independientes en una sola frase, por ejemplo: "Yo quiero una manzana", y "Yo quiero mirar la televisión".

Al cumplir los cinco años de edad, los niños casi habrán dominado la estructura lingüística necesaria para toda la vida. Los niños aprenden el lenguaje por métodos naturales a través de escuchar, y por medio de ensayo y error, y la experimentación y la práctica. Cometerán errores al tratar de aplicar las reglas que aprenden, tal como cuando dicen "pieses" y "yo sabo". No les haga burla cuando dicen estas cosas. Simplemente corríjalos, utilizando la palabra correcta. Los niños aprenden las reglas complejas y la estructura del lenguaje a través de escuchar lo que se dice a su alrededor. Entre más habla con su niño, mayor será su habilidad de lenguaje y pensamiento. Si usted le señala las cosas, él recordará mejor. El lenguaje les ayuda a los niños a entender, pensar, y resolver problemas al desarrollarse intelectualmente.

Tenga en mente, al observar a su niño pasar por este proceso, que aunque no parezca estar aprendiendo, está adquiriendo "lenguaje receptivo", el lenguaje que sabe y entiende pero todavía no puede verbalizar. Cuando usted dice "tráeme el biberón" y él lo trae, usted sabe que él entiende lo que significan "trae" y "biberón". Él sabe que quiere que lo traiga a usted, no a otra persona. Los niños necesitan escuchar muchas veces las palabras para comprender su significado.

Si el niño apunta hacia algo, recalque la palabra para el objeto al decirla y pedirle a él que la repita. Aunque se niegue a hacer eso, asegure que escuchó el nombre. Su lenguaje verbal crecerá con muchísima rapidez a los dos o tres años de edad si le empieza a hablar desde un principio. Las investigaciones han demostrado que los niños a quienes se les habla con frecuencia, desarrollan un vocabulario más amplio y eventualmente sacarán mejores calificaciones en las pruebas de inteligencia más adelante en su vida. Así que, póngale nombres a todo—¡Nombre, nombre, nombre! ¡Hable, hable, hable! ¡Lea, lea, lea! La única manera en que su niño aprenderá a hablar es si está rodeado de palabras.

Después de poner un nombre a algo, haga una pequeña pausa y permita que su niño responda. Refuerce cualquier sonido que salga de su boca, y repita la palabra en una frase completa: "Sí, mi hijo, ésa es una pelota, una pelota roja y grande". Use la misma palabra en diferentes frases. Ponga letreros en objetos conocidos para que el niño comience a asociar la palabra hablada con la palabra escrita. Piense en voz alta acerca de lo que está haciendo, para que el niño pueda aprender palabras nuevas: "Ay, tengo que tener cuidado porque me puedo cortar".

Al cumplir con su rutina diaria, deje que su niño lo acompañe. Nombre y describa los objetos que está usando y explica lo que está haciendo: "Los vasos van aquí y los platos acá". Al darle de comer, diga cosas como "Come tus chícharos. Los chícharos son verdes". Ponga énfasis en las palabras "chícharos" y "verdes", y aliéntelo a repetir las palabras. Cuando está doblando la ropa, hable en voz alta acerca de lo que está haciendo: "Las toallas van aquí. Las faldas van acá". Hágale preguntas: "¿Qué es esto? Es una toalla. Di *toalla*". (Permita que responda.) "¿De qué color es esta toalla? Azul". Permítale al niño repetir la palabra. "Azul". Si el niño dice "azul", repita la palabra en una frase completa: "Sí, la toalla es azul, es una toalla azul. Encuentra otra cosa en el cuarto que es azul. Eres tan inteligente por traer la pelota azul. ¿De qué color es?" Espere la respuesta. Abrácelo y dígale: "Sí, tú sí sabes. Es azul. Es una pelota grande y azul. ¿Qué es esto? Es la *camisa* de Papá". Puede repetir el proceso. El niño aprenderá muchas palabras para aumentar su vocabulario, además de estructura y reglas gramaticales. La fórmula es sencilla. Nombre algo, y luego pídale a su niño que repita la palabra. Haga una pausa y espere una respuesta. Prémielo con una sonrisa o un abrazo. Repita y elabore. El proceso es igual en inglés que en español.

SI HABLA DOS IDIOMAS: LOS BENEFICIOS DE SER BILINGÜE

En la actualidad, muchos padres hispanos luchan al tratar de decidir si enseñarles a sus niños a ser bilingües, o no. Se preguntan: "¿Tendrán dificultades para aprender dos idiomas?" "¿Enfrentarán discriminación en la escuela y en la sociedad si hablan español?" "¿Por qué debe ser bilingüe mi niño?" Sin duda, las preguntas como éstas son muy importantes, pero a veces pueden abrumar a los padres que están expuestos a información equivocada que eclipsa a los muchos beneficios de ser bilingüe. No puedo recalcarles lo suficiente a mis niños y a todo el mundo, la importancia de saber dos o más idiomas. El ser bilingüe es uno de los atributos más valiosos que una persona puede tener.

Saber es poder, y eso se refiere a saber dos idiomas, porque *él que habla dos idiomas vale por dos.* Hoy en día, la mitad de la población del mundo es cuando menos bilingüe. Muchas personas hablan varios idiomas. Debe recordarle a su niño, al crecerse, que las personas que son multilingües podrán comunicarse con más personas. Los niños que hablan dos o más idiomas podrán comunicarse mejor con sus parientes que no hablan inglés, y podrán apreciar y valorar mejor su cultura y a sí mismos. Tendrán un amor propio más fuerte al poder responder a las personas que quizá esperen que ellos hablen el idioma por su apellido hispano o sus características físicas. Podrán tener más amigos. El idioma forma parte de la cultura, identidad, y sentido de pertenecer, de una persona. En adición, pueden crear un almacén mental mayor de literatura, música, y recuerdos. Cuando nuestros niños pequeños crezcan y los hispanos lleguen a ser el grupo étnico más grande de los Estados Unidos ellos tendrán que saber hablar español si van a ser líderes porque necesitarán relacionarse con y comprender a una mayor cantidad de personas. El conocimiento es poder, y la persona que entiende y es capaz de comunicarse con más personas, tendrá el poder.

En el mercado global de hoy en día, aquéllos que hablan dos idiomas se consideran recursos valiosos. Por el hecho de que la población hispana está aumentando tan rápidamente, muchas empresas de servicios en los campos de la salud, el servicio social, el espectáculo, la mercadotecnia, y comercio requerirán que sus empleados sean bilingües. Aun hoy, yo me encuentro sirviendo de traductora e intérprete a otras personas cuando-quiera que estoy en los aeropuertos, hospitales, tiendas de departamentos, hoteles, y restaurantes. Se busca ávidamente a las personas bilingües por su doble conocimiento. Hasta en las escuelas hay una escasez tan grande de maestros bilingües que faltan doscientos cincuenta mil maestros bilingües en el ámbito nacional. En California, los representantes de los distritos escolares tienen la necesidad de ir hasta los países de habla española para combatir la escasez de maestros.

Si los empresarios quieren servir efectivamente a sus clientes y competir en el mundo actual, necesitarán tener más empleados bilingües. A los maestros bilingües, las operadoras telefónicas bilingües, y vendedores telefónicos bilingües (telemarketers) se les paga más debido a sus habilidades bilingües. Los niños que saben dos idiomas podrán llegar a ocupar puestos de supervisor debido a su capacidad para comunicarse, resolver problemas, y hacer ventas en dos idiomas. Junto con el idioma, una comprensión de los matices culturales entre los hispanos que hablan español también puede ser una gran ventaja. Por ejemplo, en Latinoamérica, hacer su argumento de vendedor a una persona que habla español puede requerir más que ser hábil para hablar. Puede requerir una comprensión de costumbres, tradiciones, creencias, y preferencias, todas las cuales pueden variar considerablemente entre diferentes grupos étnicos.

A pesar de que algunos de nosotros sí valoremos el bilingüismo, muchos padres hispanos, yo incluida, somos culpables de no ser persistentes y consistentes al hablarles a nuestros niños en español. Les hemos privado a nuestros niños de gozar del pleno patrimonio rico que ellos merecen, al no ser tenaces con relación a mantener al idioma español como un aspecto siempre presente en nuestros hogares. No ha sido fácil para los hispanos que viven en una sociedad donde existe la discriminación, el rechazo, y una insistencia de hablar inglés solamente. Esto ha tenido un impacto negativo en el deseo que sienten nuestros niños de aprender y en la buena voluntad de los padres de enseñar su lengua materna. Algunas suposiciones acerca del bilingüismo han impedido a los padres ofrecerles a sus niños su patrimonio, y el regalo de poder vivir en dos mundos.

Mitos acerca del bilingüismo

La sociedad está repleta de ideas exageradas y negativas acerca del bilingüismo. Algunas de estas creencias son las siguientes:

- El bilingüismo es perjudicial a los niños ya que no aprenden bien ninguno de los dos idiomas
- El ser bilingüe puede traer como resultado un prolongado y permanente atraso en el desarrollo de lenguaje
- El bilingüismo confunde a los niños
- El mezclar dos idiomas es malo y significa que los niños no han aprendido a comunicarse
- Si uno quiere enseñar a sus niños a ser bilingües, es mejor hacerlo cuando están más grandes
- Los niños tienen la capacidad de aprender bien sólo un idioma
- Si les enseña a sus niños el idioma español primero, aprenderán inglés con un acento
- No tiene sentido hablarles a sus niños en español si ellos no tienen interés en aprender el idioma

- La única manera en que los niños hispanos pueden tener éxito en los Estados Unidos es si hablan sólo inglés
- Los niños deben hablar solamente inglés o no serán aceptados en esta sociedad

Éstos son mitos que han sido retados por los expertos y la experiencia una y otra vez. El ser bilingüe no es perjudicial para los niños. No los confunde. El ser bilingüe no provoca atrasos permanentes en el aprendizaje ni en el desarrollo de lenguaje. Al llegar a la edad de ocho años, al niño se le considera adulto con relación al lenguaje. Esto significa que los niños menores de ocho años son más capaces de aprender muchos idiomas con el acento apropiado. Los niños de esta joven edad son como esponjas, capaces de aprender muchos idiomas. Si nosotros no hacemos un esfuerzo coordinado para ayudar a nuestros niños a llegar a ser bilingües, el tiempo pasará tan rápidamente que nuestros niños perderán una gran oportunidad de aprender el idioma. Aunque no los puede uno presionar para aprender español, tiene que encontrar la forma de hacerlo parte de sus conversaciones diarias.

Su niño necesita experiencias ricas, variadas, y continuas de lenguaje. Es un desafío para los padres tratar de ayudar a sus niños a aprender un idioma que no escuchan con tanta frecuencia. Es nuestro deber ponerles en contacto con el idioma español, aun si aparentan no tener interés. No debe alarmarse si oye a su niño mezclando los idiomas al principio. Eventualmente él distinguirá entre los dos. Un niño bilingüe quizá experimente un retroceso o progrese más lentamente en su desarrollo linguístico mientras está aprendiendo otro idioma, pero esto es temporal. Eventualmente alcanzará el nivel donde debe estar y se desempeñará igual de bien en ambos idiomas. Si se le proporcionan experiencias ricas, constantes, y variadas en ambos idiomas, hablará ambos con fluidez. Muchos padres no hispanos y no pertenecientes a alguna minoría, se están dando cuenta de la importancia de saber dos idiomas y están haciendo todo lo posible por ayudarles a sus niños a ser bilingües. Desdichadamente, ya para la tercera generación muchos hispanos en los Estados Unidos pierden su más valioso atributo cultural. En la actualidad, un tercio de los hispanos sabe solamente español, un tercio sabe solamente inglés, y un tercio sabe ambos idiomas. Nosotros, por ser padres que hablan español, con fluidez o no, tenemos una facilidad natural para enseñarles a nuestros niños a ser bilingües. Lo único que necesitamos es tener la voluntad, o las ganas, de darles esta valiosa herramienta.

Consejos prácticos para ayudarles a sus niños a llegar a ser bilingües

Hay muchas razones por las cuales es importante que su niño sea bilingüe. ¿Cómo se hace, o qué debe hacer uno, cuando hay tanta presión exterior de negarles a nuestros niños la gran oportunidad de aprender dos idiomas? Primero, haga caso omiso a la gente que intenta disuadirle de ayudarle a su niño a ser bilingüe. Dígale que usted sabe lo contrario cuando trata de contarle algún mito sobre ser bilingüe. Manténgase enfocado y determinado.

¿Qué ocurre si su niño siente la presión de no aprender y dice que no tiene interés? Poner a su niño en contacto con el idioma significa hacerlo aun cuando él parezca resistirse a su esfuerzos. Recuerde que el lenguaje receptivo ocurre antes del expresivo. Mientras les hable desde el principio, cuando son pequeñitos, está construyendo los cimientos para el momento cuando están más grandes y se dan cuenta de la importancia de ser bilingües. Aun si se quejan y dicen que no quieren oír el idioma, siga hablándoles en español. Le darán las gracias más adelante. Igual que con todo lo demás, el aprender español es algo que tiene que llegar a querer y sentir la necesidad de hacer. Si acaso puede, vaya con sus niños de vacaciones a México, Puerto Rico, Centro o Sudamérica, o España para darles la oportunidad de practicar el idioma. Permita que sus niños se queden por períodos largos con parientes que hablan español para que practiquen en un medio ambiente donde están forzados a usar el idioma para poder comunicarse. Cuando yo iba a la universidad, fui a México por varias semanas y recuerdo que me tomó un par de días para soltarme la lengua y hablar como nativa. Con qué rapidez avancé de los primeros días cuando me llamaban "pocha", una hispanoamericana que había olvidado sus raíces.

La única manera en que los niños podrán aprender ambos idiomas es si ambos son hablados naturalmente y producen igual placer, respuesta, y premios. Medite sobre el proceso natural, descrito anteriormente, a través del cual un niño aprende a hablar cualquier idioma. Los mismos principios se aplican al aprender dos o más idiomas. Los niños necesitan escuchar muchas veces las palabras asociadas con objetos, personas, o acciones. En el curso normal de interacción, los padres deben decir las palabras que quieren que sus niños aprendan y alentar al niño a repetirlas. Cuando el niño finalmente intenta hablar las palabras, los padres deben repetir la palabra, elaborar, y premiar al niño por su esfuerzo. Enseñando se aprende. Si usted puede hacer esto en ambos idiomas, estará ayudando a sus niños a aprender ambos idiomas.

El niño posee una necesidad natural de comunicarse, de entender, y de ser entendido. Si la madre habla solamente un idioma, y el niño quiere interactuar con ella, el niño tendrá un fuerte deseo de aprender ese idioma para poder comunicarse con ella. Usted debe comenzar por enseñarles a sus niños el idioma que domina mejor. Si es español, háblele en español. Si es inglés, háblele en inglés, y luego comience a hablarle español al aprenderlo usted, y pídales a aquellos parientes que hablan con más soltura que le ayuden a enseñárselo. Algunos de mis colegas y amigos hispanos han enseñado a sus niños a ser bilingües al dividir la tarea con sus parejas. Uno de los padres le habla al niño totalmente en español, y el otro totalmente en inglés. Otros padres les enseñan a sus niños primero un idioma y luego, varios años más tarde, introducen el otro. Como saben que sus niños aprenderán el idioma inglés a través de la televisión, los amigos, o en la escuela, les enseñan primero el español y luego el inglés. Ambos son métodos aceptables. A veces ambos padres hablan solamente español y le enseñarán al primogénito español primero. Después de que él aprenda inglés en la escuela, probablemente les hable a sus hermanitos en inglés y a sus padres en español. De esta manera, el niño mayor se convierte en un modelo y una especie de puente que ayuda a pasar el idioma dentro de una familia.

El aprender un nuevo nombre para una palabra no es tan difícil como aprender su concepto, o significado. Una vez que se aprenda el concepto, una persona puede aprender diferentes nombres para el mismo concepto. Por ejemplo, "manzana" es simplemente otro nombre para "apple", de la misma manera que utilizamos muchos nombres para referirnos a nuestras hijas. Yo le llamo a mi hija "mi hijita", "mi corazón", o "mi princesa". Un carro puede ser llamado "carro" o "coche", dependiendo de quién está hablando. Pueden haber muchos nombres para el mismo concepto. Cuando yo era maestra, yo descubrí que los niños que venían de México con muchos conceptos en español, hicieron la transición al idioma inglés con más facilidad que el grupo de niños que hablaban español, pero que nacieron en los Estados Unidos, quienes tenían menos conceptos en cada idioma porque no se les habló suficiente en ninguno de los dos idiomas. Mientras que el grupo de México estaba aprendiendo un nuevo nombre, el grupo nacido en los Estados Unidos todavía estaba aprendiendo conceptos, lo cual requiere de mucho más tiempo. Por medio de estas experiencias, yo me di cuenta de lo importante que es comunicarse con su niño primero en el idioma con que se siente más cómodo y tiene más dominio. Una vez que el niño tenga unos cimientos sólidos en un idioma, puede aprender más adelante un nuevo nombre para el mismo concepto. Si usted hace esto antes de que su niño cumpla los cinco años de edad, o a más tardar, los ocho años, su niño puede llegar a ser bilingüe más fácilmente y con menos esfuerzo.

Sin embargo, en muchos hogares hispanos en los Estados Unidos en la actualidad, los niños han aprendido conceptos en ambos idiomas, pero son verbales en inglés porque ése ha sido el idioma dominante en el hogar. Aun si su niño habla solamente inglés, continúa hablándole en español. Ayúdele a adquirir el lenguaje receptivo, para que cuando menos pueda entender el español. Enseñarles a sus niños rimas infantiles, adivinanzas, canciones, juegos, y cuentos populares en español les ayudarán a apreciar y a aprender el idioma español. A continuación están algunos que usted puede enseñarles a sus niños. Las instrucciones quizá le ayuden a recordar los juegos divertidos en los cuales participó en su país cuando era joven. Compártalos con sus niños. Si no los sabe, pregúntele a algún hispano de primera generación o a sus padres si los saben.

Juegos

Los pollitos

Uno de los niños hace el papel de la mamá gallina y los demás son los pollitos que caminan alrededor de la gallina en un círculo moviéndose los codos para arriba y para abajo. Los niños se paran mientras la madre los alimente. Luego los niños se sientan y cierran los ojos y la mamá gallina va y abraza a todos.

Los pollitos dicen, "pío, pío, pío",
cuando tienen hambre, cuando tienen frío.

La gallina busca el maíz y el trigo
les da de comer y les busca abrigo
(o les da la comida y les presta abrigo)

Bajo sus dos alas acurrucaditos
hasta el otro día duermen los pollitos.

Arroz con leche

Una niña en el centro. Los niños varones en un círculo alrededor de ella. La niña selecciona a un niño y cambia de lugar con él, luego el juego comienza de nuevo, con la niña seleccionando a otro niño, etc. En lugar de "sociedad", algunos dicen "capital".

Arroz con leche.
Me quiero casar
Con una señorita de la sociedad (capital)
Que sepa coser, que sepa bordar
Que ponga la aguja en la campañar.
Tilín, Tilán, sopitas de pan.
Allá viene Juan comiéndose el pan.
Yo soy la Señorita, la hija del Rey.
Me quiero casar y no encuentro con quién:
Contigo sí, contigo no, contigo mi vida, me casaré yo.

Los colores

Los niños se sientan formando un círculo. Cada niño escoge un color. Luego el niño "A" se mete dentro del círculo y les dice a los demás: "Quiero un listón". Ellos le preguntan: "¿De qué color?" El niño "A" trata de adivinar el color. Cuando ha adivinado el color que alguien escogió, ese niño, niño "B", se levanta y niño "A" le pregunta: "¿Cuanto cuesta?" El niño "B" contesta, "Cinco", y saca la mano para recibir cinco palmadas. Después de pagar la suma debida, el niño "B" corre y el niño "A" lo persigue. Si al niño "B" lo alcanza, éste vuelve al círculo y no recibe un color. Si no lo alcanza, vuelve a su lugar en el círculo y recibe un nuevo color. El proceso se repite.

La muñeca

VERSIÓN MEXICANA

Tengo una muñeca vestida de azul,
Zapatitos blancos, delantal de tul.
La saqué a paseo y se me constipó,
la tengo en la cama con mucho dolor.
Esta mañanita me dijo el doctor
que le diera jarabe con un tenedor.
Dos y dos son cuatro
Cuatro y dos son seis
Seis y dos son ocho

y ocho diez y seis.
Brinca las tablitas, yo ya las brinqué,
brincalas de nuevo, yo ya me cansé.

La muñeca

VERSIÓN ESPAÑOLA

Tengo una muñeca vestida de azul,
Con su camisita y su canesú.
La saqué a paseo, se me constipó,
la metí en la cama con mucho dolor.
Una mañanita le llamé al doctor,
que le dé jarabe con un tenedor.
Dos y dos son cuatro,
Cuatro y dos son seis,
Seis y dos son ocho
y ocho, diez y seis,
y ocho, veinticuatro
y ocho, trienta y dos,
Ánima bendita, me arrodillo yo.

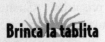

Brinca la tablita

En este juego, un círculo de niñas rodea a una niña meciendo a un bebé, luego ella representa las acciones que las otras le digan: lavar, planchar. Durante la mayor parte de la canción las niñas en el círculo están de rodillas. Cuando se llega a la parte de "brinca la tablita", se levantan de un salto, brincan para adelante y luego para atrás. Otra niña se mete al centro del círculo, y el proceso se repite hasta que todas alcancen su turno.

Brinca la tablita, yo ya la brinqué.
Bríncala de vuelta, yo ya me cansé.

Lava la ropita, yo ya la lavé.
Lávala de vuelta, yo ya me mojé.

Dos y dos son cuatro y cuatro y dos son seis
Seis y dos son ocho y ocho diez y seis.

Plancha la ropita, yo ya la planché
Plánchala de vuelta, yo ya me quemé.

Dos y dos son cuatro y cuatro y dos son seis
Seis y dos son ocho y ocho diez y seis.

Osito, osito

Esta canción se canta cuando los niños brincan la cuerda. Cada niño tiene una piedra. Dejan caer la piedra cuando dicen "tira", la levantan cuando dicen "levanta", se dan la vuelta cuando dicen "date", y se salen cuando dicen "salte".

Osito, osito, tira la piedrita.
Osito, osito, levanta la piedrita.
Osito, osito, date una vuelta
Y salte para afuera.

Juan Pirulero

Varios niños echan suertes para ver quién va a ser Juan Pirulero, él que simula tocar un clarinete al comenzar el juego. Juan Pirulero le asigna a cada niño un instrumento para "tocar" por ejemplo, una guitarra, los tambores, el órgano, la marimba, el bajo, el bandolón, o el acordeón, o bien, le asigna una tarea, como lavar los platos, escribir a máquina, manejar un carro, planchar, pintar, etc. Juan Pirulero canta la canción dos veces, simulando tocar el clarinete. Luego para de tocar y dice, "Y ahora le toca al órgano", etc. Juan Pirulero imita las acciones del niño, quien a su vez, lo imita a él, tocando el clarinete. Entonces, Juan Pirulero comienza a cantar la canción de nuevo; el primer niño vuelve a su acción original si Juan Pirulero escoge a otro niño u otra acción, de lo contrario, él continúa con la misma acción. De nuevo canta dos veces la canción, para de cantar e imita las acciones de otro niño. Cuando menciona los tambores, todos cantan "la, la, la", etc. a la tonada de Juan Pirulero. Se el niño no puede mantener el ritmo de los cambios, tiene que pagar el precio que Juan Pirulero le pide, por ejemplo, simular ser un gorila o un gato, etc. Este juego puede causar mucha confusión, pero es muy divertido.

Las adivinanzas

Los adivinanzas son maneras ingeniosas de utilizar palabras descriptivas para adivinar ciertos objetos.

Blanca es de pequeña,
La adornan con verdes lazos,
Lloro con ella de ver
Que la hacen mil pedazos.
(la cebolla)

Adivina, adivinanza,
qué se pela por la panza.
(la naranja)

Negro por fuera,
verde por dentro
y con hueso de aguacate adentro.
(aguacate)

Colorín, colorado,
chiquito, pero bravo.
(el chile)

Adivina, adivinanza,
qué tiene el rey en la panza.
(el ombligo)

Allá en el llano
está uno sin sombrero.
Tiene barbas, tiene dientes,
Y no es un caballero.
(el helote)

Doce señoritas en un corredor;
todas tienen medias, pero zapatitos
no.
(las horas)

Oro no es.
Plata no es.
Abre las cortinas
y verás lo que es
(el plátano)

Una vieja flaca
y la escurre la manteca
(una vela)

¿Qué le dijo la luna al sol?
(Tan grande y no te dejan que
salgas de noche.)

Una vieja, flaca y seca,
que arrastra las tripas.
(aguja e hilo)

Una versión más sencilla de este juego es que Juan Pirulero le dice a un niño a la vez cuál instrumento tocar o qué acción imitar, y al final todos los niños tocan juntos sus instrumentos y realizan sus acciones.

Éste es el juego de Juan Pirulero.
Que cada quien atienda a su juego.
Éste es el juego de Juan Pirulero.
Que cada quien atienda a su juego.
Y ahora le toca a tocar la guitarra—

(Repita y cambie los instrumentos—y ahora al órgano, a los tambores, a la marimba, al bajo, al bandolín, al acordeón, etc.)

Cuando Juan Pirulero señala el turno de los tambores, todos los niños cantan con él.

Lalalalalalala, lalalalalalala. Lalalalalalala, lalalalalalala.

Cancion tradicional

Allá en el rancho grande

Allá en el rancho grande, allá donde vivía
Había una rancherita que alegre me decía, que alegre me decía.

Te voy a hacer tus calzones, como los que usa el ranchero.
Te los comienzo de lana y te los acabo de cuero.

Cuentos

Hay muchos cuentos especiales que se han pasado de generación en generación, pero uno de los favoritos sobre fantasmas es "La Llorona", del cual existen muchas versiones y se ha estado contando desde la época de los aztecas.

La Llorona

La Llorona es el cuento de una madre que cae en un profundo estado de depresión después de que su marido abandona a ella y a sus dos niños pequeños. El marido vive al otro lado del río. La mujer está tan abrumada por la pena que ahoga a sus dos pequeños niños en el río que la separa de su marido. Cuando se le vuelve el juicio y se da cuenta de lo que hizo, se enloquece. "¿Dónde están mis hijos?" ella llora. Cuando se les cuenta a los niños, la leyenda les advierte que necesitan estar fuera de la calle y en sus camas temprano, o la Llorona los va a agarrar. La leyenda dice que un día un niño que no creía en la Llorona fue al río donde se dice que ella camina sin rumbo fijo. Él vio al fantasma y escuchó los gemidos de la madre que todavía buscaba a sus niños. La Llorona agarró al niño, pensando que era uno de sus hijos, pero sonaron las campanas de la iglesia y ella lo soltó. El niño corrió aterrorizado a su casa y le contó a su madre lo que había visto y escuchado. Al principio la madre no le creyó, hasta que miró las huellas ensangrentadas de la Llorona en la camisa del niño.

La Chupacabra

La Chupacabra se está convirtiendo en un cuento de terror tal como el de la Llorona. La Chupacabra es una criatura parecida a un pequeño lagarto gris o verde con ojos grandes de monstruo y una espalda con púas, y que camina sobre dos patas. Derivó su nombre por su costumbre de chuparse casi toda la sangre de algunos chivos en Puerto Rico, dejando dos heridas de punción en el cuello de las víctimas. La Chupacabra primero fue divisada en Puerto Rico en 1994, y se dice que ha emigrado a los Estados Unidos y a América del Sur. La leyenda dice que ahora está chupando la sangre y los órganos vitales de animales como perros y borregos, dejando los dos agujeros de punción. Se les ha aparecido a varias personas, a veces caminando, y a veces volando o saltando como un canguro, y tiene una estatura que varía entre los tres y seis pies. Algunos suponen que es un extraterrestre.

Mis experiencias al ser bilingüe: Las luchas para mantener el idioma español

Piense en el pasado por un momento y medite sobre cómo se ha manifestado el idioma español en su vida a través de los años. Al rememorar yo, tengo que pensar en lo diferente que era mi mundo en mi hogar comparado al mundo de la escuela donde yo asistía. Igual a muchos hispanos de mi edad, el sistema escolar hizo todo lo posible por hacerme rechazar mi idioma dominante. Sin embargo, a pesar de la agonía y el dolor, logré mantener mi idioma español.

Durante los primeros seis años de mi vida, yo hablé principalmente español pero podía entender un poco el inglés. Aunque en ocasiones combinaba ambos idiomas, yo podía comunicarme con todos a mi alrededor porque todos hablaban de la misma manera. Yo sabía, sin embargo, que si yo les hablaba a mi madre o a mi abuelo tendría que hacerlo exclusivamente en español, porque ése era el único idioma que ellos sabían. Después de entrar a la escuela, sufrí un choque cultural cuando los maestros no permitían que los niños de esa primaria se comunicaran usando el idioma que sabían mejor. En esa época, las escuelas creían en el método de inmersión para aprender inglés y se eliminaba completamente el uso del idioma español. Los golpes que recibí en la mano y la humillación que sufrí al tener que estar con la nariz metida en un círculo cada vez que un maestro me escuchaba hablar español, me provocaron una gran dificultad para aprender. Cuando me hablaban completamente en inglés, no entendía lo que trataban de enseñarme. Nos estaban forzando a aprender un idioma y una materia por medios no naturales y punitivos. Esas experiencias traumáticas que sufrí de niña, me afectaron por mucho tiempo. Yo me sentía muy incómoda al hablar español en público, por temor de que era algo indebido. Mientras que muchos sí logramos aprender el inglés y al mismo tiempo mantener el español, ¡fue a costa de mucho sufrimiento emocional! Me retuvieron en mis estudios básicos de lectura el primer año escolar, ya sea por mi falta de aprender el inglés durante ese año o por mi inmadurez emocional, ya que literalmente me salí del salón de clase, por la ventana, para ir en busca de mi hermana mayor. La escuela era un lugar aterrador para una niña que se sentía rechazada por el idioma que hablaba.

Muchos hispanos trataron de evitarles ese trauma a sus niños al impedir totalmente que hablaran español aunque el inglés no era su idioma dominante. Otros sentían que al saber sólo inglés, sus niños tendrían la mayor posibilidad de lograr éxito en la escuela y en los Estados Unidos. Ellos no se daban cuenta que sus niños podían absorber ambos idiomas si les daban la oportunidad, especialmente cuando eran pequeños. Algunos padres hispanos mandaban a sus niños a la escuela hablando solamente español, y les pedían a los directores de la escuela que les hablaran sólo en inglés, sin darse cuenta que si se les enseña a los niños primero en su lengua materna, es más fácil para ellos aprender el inglés, sin las cicatrices emocionales.

Igual a muchos hispanos de mi generación, podía haber evitado ir a clases de español en la universidad porque pasé los exámenes necesarios, sin embargo me negué a aceptar los créditos. Yo sentí que me beneficiaría conseguir la instrucción formal en mi lengua materna que nunca había recibido. También sentía la necesidad de ampliar mis conocimientos del idioma, ya que pareció detenerse mi progreso en cuanto entré a la escuela. A través de los años, he hecho un esfuerzo especial por aumentar mi vocabulario y he tenido la oportunidad de practicar mi español con las familias de AVANCE y con los medios de comunicación hispanos. Mientras mantenga una conversación formal en mi área de especialidad o sobre un tema conocido, me siento con más confianza.

A través de mi vida, he mezclado los idiomas con facilidad. Cuando estoy hablando con un amigo o pariente que sabe ambos idiomas, me encuentro usando una mezcla de palabras. Cuando estoy disgustada, cansada, preocupada, o nerviosa, me siento con ganas de hablar español. Cuando mi esposo y yo no queríamos que nuestros niños pequeños entendieran lo que decíamos, hablábamos en español. Claro que esto no funcionó muy bien una vez que los niños comenzaron a comprender más el idioma.

¿Se cuenta de que el idioma que utiliza en ese momento particular frecuentemente se relaciona con el contexto de la conversación? Puede variar dependiendo de la persona con quien está hablando uno, su edad, si es hombre o mujer, su trabajo/profesión, su nivel social y económico, su país de origen, su origen étnico, y el tema que se está discutiendo. Cuandoquiera que mi madre o mi abuelo me hacía una pregunta, yo respondía con un español más formal y más respetuoso como "Mándeme" y "usted", comparado con el "¿qué?" y "tu" que usaba con mis amigos. Quizá hable inglés en una junta profesional, español para una entrevista con una estación local de televisión o a mi madre en la casa, y una mezcla de ambos idiomas a mi familia y amigos hispanos. Si veo a un bebé lindo, me dan ganas de decir algo en español como, "¡Ay, qué chulo!" Si estoy enojada con Steven, ¡le cambio su nombre a "Esteban"! Y, por supuesto, hay esas palabras emocionales, especialmente cuando uno está enojado, frustrado, y exasperado, que son más apropiadas en nuestra lengua. Éstas incluyen palabras y frases tales como "¡Se sale!" (para describir a alguien que hizo algo malo, injusto, o simplemente tonto) y "tonto" o "bobo" (para describir a alguien a quien le falta el sentido común). Aun si estoy en compañía de personas que hablan inglés, si yo me entero de algo que me perturba, las primeras palabras que me salen de la boca son, "¡Ay, Mamá!" o "¡Ay, Dios mío!" en español en lugar del inglés, "Oh, my God!" Estas palabras están tan cargadas de emoción que suelen ser las últimas de dejar de usarse, si uno no mantiene el español como su idioma principal.

Mi madre, quien hablaba solamente español, se sentía tan impotente al tratar de enseñarnos inglés. Tenía tantos anhelos de éxito para nosotros y de que no sufriéramos humillaciones. Tenía grandes deseos de hablar inglés y exigía que le habláramos en inglés mientras lo aprendiéramos nosotros. Claro, ya que no dominamos el idioma inglés inmediatamente, lo aprendió medio mocho. Cuando mi madre hablaba con un maestro hispano, se forzaba a hablar en inglés, aun cuando el maestro era bilingüe, y aun después de que se cambiaran las reglas de la escuela. Ella también ha de haber sido tan afectada como sus hijos. Estaba determinada a aprender inglés. Cuando unos miembros de la iglesia de los Testigos de Jehová venían a la casa para dejarle unos folletos, ella insistía que quería la versión en inglés, cuando bien podía haber leído los folletos en español. Ella consiguió un dominio de la lengua al leer y luego al evangelizar a otros en inglés con sus "hermanas" o amigas de la iglesia que hablaban inglés. Con toda su determinación y esfuerzo, le tomó muchos años aprender el idioma. Sin embargo, cuando les habla a sus hijos, especialmente sobre temas emocionales, vuelve a hablar su lengua materna, ocasionalmente mezclando los idiomas porque ella sabe que nosotros así le entendemos.

Al llegar a edad escolar mis niños, ellos no querían hablar español en la escuela porque sus amigos no hablaban la lengua. Nosotros nos dimos cuenta que estábamos perjudicándoles si no hacíamos el esfuerzo de hablarles en español, pero por mucho tiempo, cuando lo hacíamos, lo rechazaban. A pesar de esto, éramos persistentes al asegurar que nuestros niños adquirieran el acento, el vocabulario, y las habilidades de comprensión. Seguimos hablando español ocasionalmente en casa, aun si nuestros niños nos respondieran en inglés, porque sabíamos que eventualmente cuando crecían y querían averiguar más sobre sus raíces, tendrían los cimientos sobre los cuales podrían construir. Ya les había enseñando rimas infantiles en español, y juegos y canciones también. Teníamos muchos discos y libros en español para su uso, y al crecer, escuchaban la música tejana. Yo les leía en español y luego se lo traducía al inglés. Jugamos la lotería mexicana. Tenía letreros en inglés y español por toda la casa. Yo miraba telenovelas en español, planeaba viajes a México, y llevaba a mis niños a obras de teatro bilingües en un esfuerzo de que fueran bilingües. Teníamos varios cassettes de "How to Learn Spanish", y al crecer, discos compactos interactivos en español que han sido muy efectivos para proporcionarles información y respuestas inmediatas. Estas estrategias, combinadas con instrucción formal en la escuela, les han ayudado a aprender a hablar el idioma español, a cierto nivel. Hasta la fecha, mis niños siguen tomando cursos formales de español.

Tres cosas tuvieron un impacto significativo en el deseo de mis niños de abrazar la lengua española (y otros aspectos de nuestra cultura). La primera fue un viaje a Europa, donde mis niños conocieron a niños y niñas muy jóvenes que hablaban de dos a siete idiomas con soltura. Se dieron cuenta que el saber dos o más idiomas es un atributo valioso. Comenzaron a reexaminar la oportunidad que tenían en casa de aprender un segundo idioma. Comenzaron a preguntarnos a mi esposo y a mí qué significaban ciertas palabras y yo me fijaba que hacían un esfuerzo mayor por practicar el idioma con nosotros y con sus amigos. Otro gran factor que los motivaba fue el apogeo de la música tejana y de artistas tejanas como Selena. Nuestros niños sabían todas sus canciones en español. Cuando vieron que a sus amigos anglosajones que no hablaban español también les gustaba su música y estaban cantando sus canciones, se sintieron aun más motivados a aprender español. Ellos se sentían orgullosos porque tenían un acento perfecto y parecía que habían hablado español todas sus vidas. Pero a veces me preguntaba si realmente sabían lo que cantaban. Steven, el más competente de mis niños para hablar español, tuvo una niñera hispanohablante cuando era muy pequeño. También lo llevé, a los tres y cuatro años de edad, a un programa recreativo en el barrio para niños de edades mixtas. Aprendió rápidamente la lengua y también las matices sociales. Llegaba a la casa, moviendo la cabeza hacia adelante y los brazos de un lado para otro, diciendo: "¿Qué pasó, bato?" Del barrio, el interés de Steven extendió, al aprender a escucharlo en todas partes: en su escuela y en la casa de su abuelita, en la televisión y radio, en los restaurantes, y en el barrio.

Mis niños mezclaban los idiomas tal como lo hizo Vanessa cuando sustituyó "agua" por "water" cuando recitó "Jack and Jill". La palabra que le ayudó a aprender el concepto para agua fue la primera palabra que le salió de la boca. Su niñera y yo solíamos preguntarle: "¿Quieres agua?" Ella respondía con la palabra "agua" cuando quería agua. Luego yo repetía: "Do you want water?" Con el tiempo, ella aprendió a distinguir entre los dos idiomas.

Yo ahora creo que las escuelas y la sociedad pudieron haber realizado un esfuerzo común con familias como la mía, y pudieron habernos alentado a ser competentes en ambos idiomas. En cambio, existió por muchos años, tal como existe todavía, la actitud de que las personas que viven en este país deben hablar solamente inglés. Los hispanos deben mantenerse firmemente erguidos y defender sus derechos de hablar dos idiomas. Aun si el español es el único idioma que se habla en el hogar, las investigaciones científicas han demostrado que los niños adoptarán el idioma dominante, en este caso el inglés, porque es lo que escuchan en todas partes, desde la televisión hasta el patio de la escuela. Contrario a la opinión de algunas personas, los hispanos en este país tienen deseos de aprender el inglés, para poder conseguir trabajos y comunicarse con otros. Es crítico aprender el inglés, simplemente para poder leer recetas médicas, señales de tráfico, e instrucciones. Las madres participantes de AVANCE que asisten a clases de inglés, lo hacen por todas estas razones, y también para ayudarles a sus niños con su tarea. Cuando hay una necesidad para comunicarse y ser entendido, las personas son motivadas a aprender el inglés. Pero eso no significa que no deben valorar y mantener el idioma español.

El "Movimiento Chicano" de los años sesenta y primeros años de los setenta, tal como otros movimientos de la época de derechos civiles, provocó un orgullo por su cultura y por saber el idioma español. Sin embargo, hoy en día, las políticas del gobierno como el movimiento de "English Only" y el estigma asociado con ser inmigrantes han forzado a algunos hispanos a rechazar su lengua materna, motivados por el temor de ser humillados. Algunos padres, a causa de sus propias experiencias negativas asociadas con sus conocimientos de la lengua española, no quieren que sus niños aprendan español. A muchos se les hizo creer que el hablar español es malo, y no quieren que sus niños sufran. Tienen que darse cuenta que en la actualidad, con la educación bilingüe, los niños pueden mantener su idioma y su cultura mientras hagan la transición al idioma inglés. Ya no serán como nosotros, tratando de aprender el idioma inglés al mismo tiempo de aprender las habilidades básicas y el contenido en una lengua extranjera. Los padres deben alentar a sus niños a participar en programas bilingües que valoran igualmente a ambos idiomas. Deben apoyar la educación bilingüe y considerarla esencial para nuestra gente.

Aun así, por efectivo que sea un programa bilingüe, es importante recordar que las escuelas solamente construyen sobre los cimientos que los padres construyeron en el hogar. Los niños tienen que entrar a la escuela con una riqueza de experiencias en ambos idiomas. Además, si quiere alentar el bilingüismo, debe esforzarse por hablarles a sus niños en ambos idiomas. Cada experiencia refuerza a la otra.

EL LENGUAJE DEL CUERPO: LA CEJA, LOS BRAZOS, Y EL PIE

En cualquier cultura, el lenguaje del cuerpo se considera otra forma de comunicación. Hablamos por medio de palabras y gestos. Los padres aprenden las necesidades y los sentimientos de sus niños al interpretar sus movimientos y gestos, y viceversa. Por ejemplo, cuando se le sube la ceja o aprieta los labios, un niño sabe que usted está enojado. Cuando da golpecitos en el piso con el pie y se cruza los brazos, quizá esté diciendo que quiere que su niño se apure. Los niños saben cuando alguien está enojado, disgustado, tenso, o contento, basado en el lenguaje de su cuerpo.

Hay algunas diferencias culturales sutiles entre el lenguaje de cuerpo de algunas personas que hablan inglés y otras que hablan español. Por ejemplo, muchas personas que hablan inglés inmediatamente establecen un contacto con los ojos cuando comienzan a hablar con alguien. Si alguien no las mira directamente a los ojos, quizá piensen que está mandando un mensaje de que está tratando de evitar algo o de que no está siendo franco, directo. Pero a algunos hispanos tradicionales se les ha enseñado que mirar a alguien directamente a los ojos es una falta de respeto o mala educación. Por ejemplo, si están hablando con sus abuelos, quizá no quieran mostrar una falta de respeto al mirarles directamente a los ojos.

En adición, a los hispanos les encanta el tacto humano. Adoramos los abrazos, y abundantes besos. El psicólogo S. M. Jourard observó la conducta de parejas sentadas en cafés alrededor del mundo. Él descubrió que en una sola hora los puertorriqueños se tocaron 180 veces, mientras que las personas en París se tocaron 110 veces, las personas anglosajonas de clase media de Florida sólo se tocaron dos veces en una hora, y los londinenses a quienes estudió, no se tocaron siquiera. La investigación ilustra las diferencias culturales que pueden afectar la comunicación.

Muchos hispanos están acostumbrados a mantener menos distancia entre unos y otros cuando están conversando. Yo me he dado cuenta que a veces, cuando estoy conversando con alguien, yo me muevo un paso para adelante y la otra persona da dos pasos para atrás. Porque estamos tratando de enseñarles a nuestros niños a vivir en una sociedad de dos culturas, al crecer ellos, debemos enseñarles las diferencias y las semejanzas en el lenguaje de cuerpo de ambas culturas. Aunque no queremos que pierdan sus valores culturales en ciertas circunstancias, sí queremos que aprendan a ser flexibles y a estar preparados para adaptarse a nuevas situaciones. Uno puede vivir en ambos mundos, dependiendo de las circunstancias, y los deseos, preferencias y expectativas de uno.

LA LECTURA: AYÚDELE A SU NIÑO A LEER

La lectura debe ser un proceso continuo desde los primeros días de vida. Mis niños tenían muchos libros, algunos hechos en casa, otros comprados, y otros prestados de la biblioteca. Cuando eran muy pequeños, tenían libros del abecedario, libros de rimas infantiles, y libros que contenían dibujos que saltaban para arriba al voltear la página o abrir el libro. A los niños les encantan todo tipo de libros, grandes y pequeños, de tela, cartulina gruesa, o plástico. La lectura es para ellos una aventura—una aventura para los ojos, los oídos, las manos, y si se hace con amor, para el corazón.

Aparte y fije cuando menos quince minutos cada día para leerle a su niño pequeño. Siéntese junto a él cuando está leyendo para que esté bastante cerca para estudiar cada página. Hable acerca de los objetos y las actividades en el libro al apuntar hacia ellos su niño. Al leer, abrácele, acaríciele el brazo o el cabello, y mírelo a los ojos al examinar sus reacciones al cuento. Diga cosas como: "Ah, ¿qué crees que va a pasar ahora?" "¿Cómo se sintió el osito cuando se quebró la silla?" Después de terminar de leerles un cuento a mis niños, yo lo terminaba con "colorín colorado, este cuento se ha acabado", y les daba un abrazo. Esta experiencia cálida y placentera se asociará con un amor a la lectura.

Enséñele a su niño a comenzar desde el principio del libro hasta el final. Asegúrese de que su niño voltee las hojas de la derecha hacia la izquierda, y que cuando usted lee, él se dé cuenta de que lo hace de arriba hacia abajo y de la izquierda hacia la derecha. Después de observarle a usted, él querrá hacerlo por su cuenta. Permita que él voltee las páginas y apunte hacia lo que le interese. Describa cualquier cosa a la cual él le apunta con el dedo (gato, pelota, escarabajo). Dele tiempo para repetir lo que usted dijo. Compare lo que hay en el libro a objetos concretos en su medio ambiente. Nombre las letras e ilústrelas con letras de madera o magnéticas. Hágale preguntas acerca de las diferentes actividades en el libro, el tema, y cómo se desarrolla la historia. Pídale que le cuente la historia o le recite la rima. Cuandoquiera que usted le lee a su niño, le está diciendo que la lectura es importante y placentera. Trate de mantener periódicos, revistas, enciclopedias, y libros de consulta en su casa para poder contestar sus muchas preguntas. Diviértase con su niño mientras él aprenda a comunicarse y a leer. Entre más palabras y conceptos aprenda, mejor podrá pensar y lograr competencia intelectual.

Lleve a su niño periódicamente a la biblioteca. Ahora hay una mayor selección de maravillosos libros bilingües disponibles en casi todas las bibliotecas públicas de este país. Una sección grande en uno de los pisos de la Biblioteca Pública de San Antonio está dedicada a la colección latina, consistente en cientos de libros escritos por latinos y sobre latinos. Si su biblioteca tiene, pida que la bibliotecaria establezca una. Nuestra colección llegó a existir gracias a un grupo de mujeres dinámicas latinas que pidieron—no, exigieron—tener una en nuestra ciudad que consiste de un 60 por ciento de hispanos. Saque libros en ambos idiomas para sus niños.

Al crecer su niño, siga leyéndole y aliéntele a decirle cada vez más sobre cada cuento. Cubra las ilustraciones y pídale que cree su propia imagen para describir una historia. Enséñele un dibujo en el cuento y pídale que adivine lo que digan las palabras sobre el dibujo. Al leer una sección de la historia, pídale que le cuente sobre los personajes, el tema, y el escenario del cuento. Lea una sección de la historia y hágale preguntas para ver si entendió lo que le leyó. "¿Dónde estaba el niño al comienzo de la historia? ¿Dónde está ahora?" Si lee un libro como uno de los de la serie "Curious George", puede preguntarle: "¿De qué se trata este libro? ¿Es de un gato? No, éste es un cuento de un mono. ¿Qué tipo de mono era George? Era un mono muy curioso. Él quería saber todo". Si lee un libro bilingüe como *The Bossy Gallito, el Gallo de Bodas: A Traditional Cuban Folktale* por Lucía M. González, podría decirle: "Este libro es del gallito mandón. ¿Qué tipo de gallo era? Sí, era un gallito muy mandón. Le gustaba mandar a todos". Después de leer el libro favorito de su niño muchas veces, él podrá decirle lo que va a ocurrir en seguida o una parte de una frase o una sección de la historia. Quizá pueda decirle toda la secuencia de la historia sin siquiera mirar las palabras. Cuando el niño se hace como que está leyendo, esto solamente lo motiva más a hacerlo de verdad.

La lectura se trata de conectar un grupo de letras con sonidos correspondientes a un significado particular. Un niño no podrá comprender algo que lee si no ha tenido suficientes experiencias de interacción con otros y con el mundo a su alrededor para llenar su imaginación. Aquellas experiencias que le permitieron adquirir conceptos de lenguaje y formas ahora le serán muy útiles para ayudarle a entender lo que está leyendo. Todas esas experiencias observando pequeños detalles y distinguiendo entre objetos similares ahora le ayudarán a distinguir entre la "b" y la "d", y la "p" y la "q".

A alrededor de los dos y tres años de edad, la mayoría de los niños comienzan a reconocer letras. Nombre las letras en el libro y use letras de plástico, madera, o magnéticas para ilustrarlas. Escriba la letra en una hoja de papel. Escriba las palabras que él diga para que pueda aprender la asociación entre las palabras escritas y los pensamientos. Hay muchos libros para niños sobre el abecedario en ambos idiomas, que puede usar para enseñarles a sus niños las letras mayúsculas y minúsculas. Al llegar a la edad de cuatro o cinco años, la mayoría de los niños han aprendido las letras y están listos para conectar las palabras con objetos o actividades. Cuando mis niños eran pequeños, yo usaba tarjetas (de ayuda pedagógica) con los nombres de muchos objetos alrededor de la casa. Yo usé letras mayúsculas y minúsculas para que se dieran cuenta que había dos tipos de letras. Mis niños tenían un juguete con agujeros tallados en la forma de letras, que usaban para meter las letras correspondientes. Tenían letras hechas de plástico, madera, fieltro, y algunas que eran magnéticas que utilizaban para formar palabras en un tablero o en la puerta del refrigerador.

Algunas de las rimas que mis niños sabían en inglés y español les enseñaron los nombres de las letras y los sonidos que producen los animales. Una de estas rimas en inglés era la clásica "Old MacDonald", la cual les enseña a los niños los sonidos que los animales hacen. A lo siguiente, están algunos versos en español que enseñan a los niños acerca de palabras, sonidos, y las criaturas del mundo.

Los pollitos

Los pollitos dicen, "pío, pío, pío",
cuando tienen hambre, cuando tienen frío.
La gallina busca el maíz y el trigo,
les da de comer y les busca abrigo.

El sapito glo glo glo

Nadie sabe dónde vive.
Nadie sabe dónde vive.
Pero todos lo escuchamos
Al sapito: Glo…glo…glo…

Los tres cochinitos

Los tres cochinitos están en la cama.
Muchos besitos les dio su mamá.
Y calientitos todos en pijama.
Dentro de un rato los tres roncaron: oink, oink, oink.

Yo les recordaba a mis niños que igual que los pollitos, sapitos, y cochinitos en las rimas en español producen ciertos sonidos, así también las letras. Cuando mostraban un interés en jugar a la escuelita o simplemente jugar con las letras, yo elevaba la lección al siguiente nivel al enseñarles los nombres y los sonidos de las letras. Les enseñé a mis niños primero los sonidos de las letras en español porque los sonidos en español no varían como en el inglés. Una vez que aprendieron el proceso de unir los sonidos fonéticamente en español, pudieron transferir el mismo proceso al inglés.

Las rimas y los cantos que mis niños aprendieron y las veces que yo les alenté a escuchar música suave o el canto de los grillos, o la madera que crujía durante una noche en el campamento, les ayudaron a adquirir buenas habilidades para escuchar. Al enseñar a mis niños a leer en inglés y español, yo usaba las mismas técnicas que había utilizado con mis estudiantes de primer año de primaria. Comencé con las vocales en español, diciendo: "La 'a' en español suena como 'ahh'", y les enseñé un dibujo de una mujer que estaba gritando porque miró una araña. "¡Ahh, araña!" Continué con la letra "e". "La 'e' en español suena como 'ehh'", y levanté un dibujo de un hombre que no podía oír, mientras me ahuecaba la mano junto al oído diciendo: "¿Ehh?" La letra "i" vino con el dibujo de una ardilla que hacía el sonido "iiiii", que yo demostré al juntar las manos y hacer como si fuera una ardilla. La letra "o" significaba el sonido que hace el vaquero cuando trata de parar el caballo, "Ooooo, caballo", y la letra "u" era el sonido que hace un tren. "Chucu-chu, chucu-chu", les dije al jalar un cordón imaginario de un tren también imaginario. Terminé la lección con un canto que yo aprendí de niña:

> AEIOU, el burro sabe más que tú,
> a lo cual todos respondimos:
> "¡No, no sabe más que nosotros!"

Una vez que los niños aprendan los sonidos de las vocales, continuamos la lección con las consonantes. Conecté cada una de las vocales con las letras "m", "n", "c", "t", "d", "s", y "p" primero para formar palabras sencillas que ellos sabían como *mamá, papá, cama, toma, dedo, sopa*. Era fácil para ellos entender el proceso de leer cuando aprendieron cómo formar palabras fonéticamente en español. Luego les introduje a los sonidos de las vocales en inglés. Comparé los sonidos en inglés a los de español. Les pedí que me miraran la boca para aprender que se producían diferentes sonidos dependiendo de cómo abría yo la boca. Comencé con la "a" corta en inglés al hacer el sonido "Aaa", como en *aaapple*. Continué con el resto de los sonidos: "Eeeehh", como en *egg*; "Iiiihh" como en *Indian*; "Ohhhh", como en *orange*; y "Uhhh", como en *umbrella*. Luego combiné esos sonidos con los sonidos similares de las consonantes que ya sabían en español, poniendo énfasis en las vocales.

A, Aaa, Aaa. Apple.	M A D	Mad. I am so mad (make an angry face).
A, Aaa, Aaa. Apple.	C A T	Cat. The cat goes meow (make meow sound).
A, Aaa, Aaa. Apple.	S A T	Sat. I sat down (sit down).
A, Aaa, Aaa. Apple.	F A N	Fan. I fan myself (do it).
A, Aaa, Aaa. Apple.	F A T	Fat. I am very fat (exaggerate fatness).
E, Eeeehh, Eeeehh. Egg.	P E N	Pen. We write with a pen.
E, Eeeehh, Eeeehh. Egg.	P E T	Pet. A dog is a pet.
E, Eeeehh, Eeeehh. Egg.	G E T	Get. Get the ball.
E, Eeeehh, Eeeehh. Egg.	R E D	Red. This is red.
E, Eeeehh, Eeeehh. Egg.	N E T	Net. Something used to catch a fish.
I. Iiihh, Iiiihh. Indian.	K I S S	Kiss. Give me a kiss.
I. Iiiihh, Iiiihh. Indian.	S I T	Sit. I sit down.
I. Iiiihh, Iiiihh. Indian.	F I N	Fin. The fish has a fin.
I. Iiiihh, Iiiihh. Indian.	H I T	Hit. Do not hit anybody.
I. Iiiihh, Iiiihh. Indian.	M I T T	Mitt. You catch a ball with a mitt.
O, Ohhhh, Ohhhh. Orange.	M O P	Mop. I mop the floor.
O, Ohhhh, Ohhhh. Orange.	T O P	Top. The top spins.
O, Ohhhh, Ohhhh. Orange.	S O N	Son. You are my son.
O, Ohhhh, Ohhhh. Orange.	P O T	Pot. He cooks in a pot.
O, Ohhhh, Ohhhh. Orange.	C O T	Cot. I sleep on a small cot.
U, Uhhh, Uhhh. Umbrella.	S U N	Sun. The sun shines brightly.
U, Uhhh, Uhhh. Umbrella.	C U T	Cut. I cut my finger.
U, Uhhh, Uhhh. Umbrella.	N U T	Nut. Squirrels eat nuts.
U, Uhhh, Uhhh. Umbrella.	C U P	Cup. Baby drinks milk from a cup.
U, Uhhh, Uhhh. Umbrella.	P U P	Pup. A pup is a small dog.

Era fácil enseñar las palabras con vocales que tenían un sonido largo como "go", "so", y "no", hasta que llegué a palabras como "to", "put", y "do". Les dije a mis niños que podían aprender algunas palabras por vista. Las repetimos varias veces. Luego llegamos a palabras con un "e" mudo, como la palabra "came", y luego al doble "o", en "too". Les expliqué que las palabras "seat" y "pear" tienen la "ea" combinación, para mostrar algunas de las irregularidades en el inglés, y que simplemente tenían que memorizarlas. Luego continué enseñándoles todas las consonantes, incluyendo a las combinaciones como "bl", "st", y "gr". A estas alturas generalmente dejaba de enseñarles a leer, pero seguía ayudándoles cuando me pedían que les explicara cierta palabra. Al llegar a este punto, podían descifrar muchas palabras por sí solos, basándose en el contexto de la historia. Aunque mis niños sabían el proceso de leer y podían descifrar las palabras más sencillas, tuve que seguir recalcando la importancia de la comprensión de las palabras. Si un niño no tiene un buen vocabulario ni ha tenido suficientes experiencias para aprender acerca de su mundo, tal vez no pueda comprender lo que está leyendo. Yo solía crear dibujos divertidos para enseñarles a mis niños cómo leer frases cortas. Por ejemplo, había la frase, "fat man in a hat", o una similar en español podría ser, "el gato con tres patos" o "la vaca es muy flaca". Los libros de Dr. Seuss son ideales para este tipo de ejercicio de lectura. Las rimas infantiles y los libros sencillos en ambos idiomas, inglés y español, que los niños pueden memorizar, también les ayudarán a aprender a leer.

Si usted sigue algunas de estas técnicas de enseñanza, mandará a sus niños a la escuela con unos buenos cimientos para la lectura. Es importante que procuremos que la lectura sea divertida, no una tarea. El cerebro estará en su punto más preparado para la lectura alrededor de los seis años de edad, pero algunos niños comienzan tan temprano como la edad de cuatro años, o tan tarde como los siete años. Necesita observar las señales y estar atento a las pistas que le dan sus niños para avisarle que están listos, o pueden sentirse amenazados.

Mi hijo Sal comenzó a leer libros sencillos a los cuatro años de edad. Siempre tuvo un gran amor a los libros y unos anhelos de leer. Estaba rodeado constantemente de libros de la biblioteca o libros que le regalamos en su cumpleaños, o las enciclopedias. Tenía sus cuentos favoritos que yo le leía repetidamente. Algunos niños, como Vanessa, usan la lectura como un juego. Ella tomó el papel de "maestra" para sus muñecas, primos, y vecinos al leerles. Steven también disfrutaba de la lectura, pero solamente si yo le rascaba la espalda al leerle. Aunque cada uno de sus niños tal vez aborde la lectura con un enfoque diferente, todos pueden estar leyendo fonéticamente para cuando entran al kinder.

Los niños de mi cuñada, todos los cuales asistían a clases para niños superdotados, poseían habilidades avanzadas para leer antes de entrar a la escuela. Cuando sus niños tenían cuatro y cinco años de edad, ella estableció una rutina de ir a la biblioteca y sacar los libros que les interesaban. Les enseñó a escuchar muy cuidadosamente varias cosas: el título del libro, el autor, los personajes principales, y la trama de la historia. Luego les hacía preguntas. Sus niños aprendieron a ser muy atentos y podían fácilmente comprender lo que su madre les leía. Les preguntaba qué había ocurrido primero, segundo, y tercero. Al hacer todas estas cosas, ella les estaba enseñando que las palabras tienen significado, que los cuentos tienen una estructura particular, y que algún día ellos podrían escribir sus propios libros.

Al crecer más sus niños, juegue con ellos "Round Robin", un juego donde se turnan para leer las páginas de un libro. Sus niños realmente adquirirán un amor a la lectura si usted pasa tiempo de calidad con ellos, leyendo por turnos con ellos. Permítales sentir la alegría de descifrar palabras e imágenes por escrito. A veces, después de una excursión, pídales a sus niños que le digan lo que vieron ese día, y usando un marcador, crea una historia en una hoja de papel grande o en un caballete. Yo le daba un título a cada historia y escribía su nombre como autor de la obra. Les dejaba leer los cuentos y los elogiaba por sus esfuerzos. Nunca me disgusté si se equivocaban con las estructuras de sus frases. Yo sabía que los errores forman parte del proceso del aprendizaje. En otras ocasiones, pueden hacer tarjetas de cumpleaños o de Navidad, jugar "Scrabble", y escribir poemas, todo lo cual les ayudará a afinar sus habilidades de lectura y escritura.

A veces comparo el tipo de experiencias ricas y estimulantes que mi esposo y yo le proporcionamos a nuestros niños, con aquéllas de esos niños que no tuvieron a nadie para leerles, no se les permitió ni escribir ni garabatear, no les enseñaron ni canciones ni rimas, y rara vez los llevaron de excursión. Hay una diferencia notable entre los niños que han tenido estas experiencias antes de entrar a la escuela y los que no las tuvieron. Ellos saben más, hablan más, y están mejor preparados para lograr el éxito académico. Aunque no es imposible, sí es muy difícil para los niños alcanzar su nivel apropiado cuando no han tenido estas experiencias cuando eran pequeños. Aquellos niños cuyos padres construyeron los cimientos apropiados continuarán creciéndose y desarrollándose y construyendo sobre esos cimientos.

LA EXPANSIÓN DE SU MUNDO: DEL MUNDO CONCRETO AL MUNDO LÓGICO—DE LOS SEIS A LOS ONCE AÑOS DE EDAD

Un niño que se encuentra en esta etapa aprende a usar la lógica para resolver problemas, pero por lo general, está limitado a objetos y acontecimientos concretos en lugar de ideas abstractas. Reflexiona mucho. Ahora es capaz de aprender categorías más amplias de cosas como personas, alimentos, frutas, árboles, pájaros, y animales. Él puede ordenar o arreglar objetos y acontecimientos en una serie y encontrar las relaciones entre ellos. Es capaz de reconocer propiedades como la masa física a la edad de siete años. Al cumplir los nueve años, puede comprender los conceptos de volumen y peso, aun si el recipiente que está estudiando cambia de forma y tamaño. También a esa edad, un niño puede recordar y repetir cuatro o cinco números consecutivamente. Practica lo que ha aprendido y agudiza y aumenta el número de conceptos.

Durante estas edades, es bueno poner a sus niños en contacto con muchas actividades que pueden ampliar su vista y perspectiva del mundo. Ésta es la etapa durante la cual aprenden a desarrollar sus intereses y talentos innatos. Anímelos a participar en actividades que les gustan. Permítales comenzar una colección de estampillas, carros, estampas de béisbol, o monedas. Cómpreles telescopios y juegos de química. Los crucigramas, por ejemplo, quizá despierten su interés y les ayuden a aumentar su vocabulario.

Lleve a sus niños a los museos para niños y a vacaciones que les ayudarán a aprender acerca de diferentes gentes, culturas, y lugares. Si tiene la oportunidad de llevar a sus niños a un lugar como Washington, D.C., hágalo. Hay muchos museos educativos que son gratis, como el *National Museum of Natural History* (el Museo Nacional de Historia Natural), el *National Air and Space Museum* (el Museo Nacional del Aire y el Espacio), el *National Museum of American Art* (el Museo Nacional de Arte Americano), y el *Holocaust Museum* (el Museo del Holocausto). El *Smithsonian* publica un guía de recursos que describe las obras de latinos en sus colecciones además de programas diseñados por latinos. Explore la historia americana al visitar los monumentos a Jefferson y a Lincoln, la Casa Blanca, el Capitolio de los Estados Unidos y muchos otros importantes monumentos. Llévelos a aprender cómo se hace el dinero en la State Treasury (la Hacienda Pública del Estado). Llévelos a mirar una obra de teatro. Más cerca de la casa, puede llevar a sus niños a los museos locales, a los jardines botánicos, a la playa, a las montañas, al lago, o a los parques locales.

Ayude a sus niños con proyectos de investigación sobre sus raíces. Llévelos a la Basílica de la Virgen de Guadalupe, a la Pirámide del Sol en Teotihuacan en México o a ver las ruinas mayas en Chichén Itzá, Uxmal, y Palenque. ¿Y qué tal los fabulosos museos en la Ciudad de México donde sus niños pueden aprender tanto acerca de su cultura? Si pudiera llevarlos a Machu Picchu en Perú, ése es un fabuloso lugar para contemplar. Llévelos en una gira del sudoeste para visitar las reservaciones de los indios americanos. Éste es el momento en su vida cuando un viaje a las islas del Caribe para bucear con esnórquel sería no solamente placentero, sino educativo.

Permítales ser creativos. Aliente a sus niños a demostrar sus talentos al alentarlos a escribir sus propias obras y luego representar los papeles ellos mismos, con la ayuda de una cámara de vídeo. Mis niños crearon varias obras. Steven generalmente era el director. Algunas de sus producciones eran musicales en las cuales mis niños y algunos amigos suyos se vistieron como estrellas de rock. A veces las producciones eran dramas en los cuales los actores secuestraban a Vanessa. En otras ocasiones estaban montando un robo a un banco. Un día volví a casa del trabajo y los niños me agarraron la mano y me hicieron sentarme a mirar su más reciente producción. Estaba anonadada al ver en el vídeo a Sal, de quince años de edad y todavía sin carnet de manejar, manejando lentamente la camioneta familiar por el largo camino que llevaba a nuestra casa. La cámara se movió de una imagen de Sal en el asiento delantero hasta la parte de atrás de la camioneta para enfocar a Steven, de diez años de edad, colgándose de la orilla, con los pies arrastrando, al dramatizar su huida en la "camioneta de la fuga". Yo le grité a mi esposo: "¡SALVADOR, mira lo que hicieron tus niños!" Los niños me dijeron que no me preocupara. Ellos tenían el consentimiento de su prima Lisa, de veintiún años de edad, quien la estaba haciendo de niñera. De hecho, ella fue la que filmó el vídeo. A pesar de tales sustos, les alentamos a nuestros niños a ser creativos y a buscar los límites de su imaginación, pero con algunas precauciones necesarias.

Este es un momento apropiado para comprarle a su niña una muñeca Barbie, o mejor aun, una de las muñecas Josefina o Rosalba, las cuales vienen con sus respectivos libros en inglés y español. Para comprar estas muñecas latinas, remítase a la Lista de Recursos al final del libro (Niños Catalog para la muñeca Rosalba NS 4403, y el catálogo de la *Pleasant Company American Girls Collection* para la serie de libros y muñecas Josefina). Rosalba es una chica puertorriqueña que está explorando Nueva York con su abuela en el libro *Abuela* por Arthur Dorrios. En el libro *Isla*, del mismo autor, visita la isla de Puerto Rico con su abuela. Josefina Montoya es una niña México-americana de nueve años de edad que vive en la parte norte de Nuevo México en el año 1824, en los tiempos cuando se abrió el sendero de Santa Fe. Algunos de sus libros, escritos por Valérie Tripp, incluyen *Happy Birthday, Josefina: A Springtime Story; Josefina Saves the Day: A Summer Story;* y *Changes for Josefina* (Pleasant Co., $5.95). Su hija podría pasar horas innumerables jugando con los accesorios que también pueden encontrarse en el catálogo, por ejemplo los muebles, un piano, floreros, y utensilios para cocinar.

Durante este período, los niños aprenden a seguir las reglas. Los niños se han graduado de "hacer tortillitas", a jugar juegos de mesa y de barajas, y a jugar deportes organizados. A través de los deportes los niños que están pasando por esta etapa pueden aprender sobre las reglas, el juego limpio, y el trabajo en equipo. Con cuánta anticipación esperaba las excursiones donde salía toda la familia durante los fines de semana, para poder mirar a los niños jugando béisbol, fútbol, fútbol americano, o básquetbol. Nuestros niños esperaban que fuéramos, no solamente para ofrecer apoyo moral, sino para sacar fotos y filmar vídeos.

A los niños, ambos los niños varones y las niñas, hay que alentarles a participar en deportes competitivos organizados además de juegos cooperativos. Hay muchos juegos para los niños de esta edad que proveen lecciones acerca de cooperar, seguir las reglas, y tomar decisiones. Los siguientes juegos tradicionales hispanos son los mismos que aprendieron muchos padres hispanos cuando eran niños. Yo les enseñé algunos a mis niños y a los estudiantes en mi clase de primer año de primaria. Usted descubrirá al leerlos cuánto pueden contribuir a las experiencias de juego de sus niños.

Naranja dulce

Este juego generalmente lo juegan las niñas, pero los niños pueden unirse a ellas también. Los niños se paran formando un círculo y agarrándose de las manos; un niño, que hace de cuenta que es un soldado que va a la guerra, se para dentro del círculo. Los niños caminan alrededor del niño en el centro cantando *Naranja dulce*. Después de la estanza "Dame un abrazo que yo te pido", el soldado elige a una niña, la abraza, y la lleva al centro. El primer niño sale del círculo y se queda afuera. Los niños siguen dando vueltas y repitiendo la canción hasta que todos menos dos niños queden fuera del círculo.

> Naranja dulce, limón partido,
> Dame un abrazo que yo te pido.
> Si fueron falsos tus juramentos
> En poco tiempo, se olvidarán.
> ¡Tocan la marcha! Mi pecho llora,
> Adiós, señora, yo ya me voy.

La víbora de la mar
VERSIÓN MEXICANA

El siguiente juego tradicional es la versión en español de London Bridge. Hay dos personas, una es la sandía y la otra es el melón. Se agarran de las manos, parándose cara a cara, con los brazos levantados para formar una "cueva subterránea". La serpiente, que está compuesta por una fila de niños, agarrados de las manos, pasará por la cueva cantando la siguiente canción:

A la víbora, víbora de la mar, de la mar
por aquí pueden pasar,
los de adelante corren mucho,
y los de atrás se quedarán.
¡Tras, tras, tras, tras!

El niño a quien agarran debajo del arco, lo zarandean de un lado para otro, y le hacen escoger entre el melón y la sandía al cantar lo siguiente los otros niños:

Será melón, será sandía.
Será la vieja del otro día...día...día.

Luego continúa la canción y los niños siguen pasando por la cueva:

Una mejicana que fruta vendía
Ciruela, chabacano, melón o sandía,
Una mejicana que fruta vendía
Ciruela, chabacano, melón o sandía.

Día, día, día,
¡Será la vieja del otro día!

Verbena, verbena, jardín de matatena.
Verbena, verbena, jardín de matatena.
Campanita de oro, déjame pasar
con todos mis hijos, ¡menos el de atrás!
¡Tras, tras, tras, tras!

Otra vez, el niño a quien agarran debajo del arco, lo zarandean de un lado para otro, y le hacen escoger entre el melón y la sandía:

Será melón, será sandía.
Será la vieja del otro día...día...día.

Cuando yo era una niña, yo jugaba este juego, el cual incluía un juego de tira y afloja con una cuerda. El niño al que agarran es sacado del juego, llevado hacia un lado, y tiene que escoger a uno de los niños que están formando el arco y se convierte en "melón" o "sandía". La canción continúa hasta que se hayan agarrado a todos los niños y ellos se han formado en filas detrás de los dos niños que forman el arco. Luego hay un juego de tira y afloja con una cuerda, donde los niños se agarran de la cintura unos a otros. El lado que jala más fuerte y hace que el otro equipo cruce la línea gana, o si un equipo se cae, el otro gana. Algunas personas llaman a los ganadores "los angelitos" y a los perdedores "los diablos". En el pasado, este juego ha terminado con todos en el suelo, riéndose.

La víbora de la mar

VERSIÓN PUERTORRIQUEÑA

Dos niños guían:	La víbora, víbora del amor, De aquí podéis pasar,
Los demás niños:	Por aquí yo pasaré. Y una niña dejaré.
Los dos niños:	¿Y esa niña cuál será, la de adelante o la de atrás?
Los demás niños:	La de adelante corre mucho, la de atrás se quedará.
Dos niñas:	Pásame, sí, pásame, ya, por la puerta de Alcántara.

En otra versión de la "Víbora de la mar", la persona a la que se agarra ocupa el lugar del melón o la sandía (los jugadores que están formando el arco), para que él, o ella, pueda unirse a los demás niños y formar parte de la serpiente. Las reglas para este juego son similares a las de la primera versión, donde los dos niños que forman el arco son colores, frutas, o plata y oro. Luego termina con un juego de tira y afloja con una cuerda.

A la rueda de San Miguel

Un niño se para en el centro de un círculo de niños que están agarrados de las manos. El círculo se mueve en el sentido de las agujas del reloj al recitar los niños la rima. Cuando llegan a la parte de la rima que dice "que se voltee", el niño que está en el centro dice el nombre de uno de los niños en el círculo, y todos dicen juntos, "(el nombre del niño) de burro". El niño que fue escogido se voltea, volteado hacia afuera del círculo, manteniéndose agarrado de las manos con los otros niños. Se repite la canción, y el juego continúa hasta que todos los niños estén volteados. En otra versión del juego, la velocidad aumenta con cada repetición. El juego se vuelve a comenzar cuando todos se caen al suelo porque corrían tan velozmente.

A la rueda, rueda, de San Miguel, San Miguel
todos traen su caja de miel
A lo maduro, a lo maduro,
que se voltee
(Juan)* de burro.

*use su nombre

Doña Blanca

Los niños forman un círculo con Dona Blanca en el centro y el Jicotillo afuera del círculo. Después de cantar la canción dos veces los niños, el Jicotillo trata de romper el círculo para agarrar a Dona Blanca. Después de agarrarla, el Jicotillo se convierte en Dona Blanca y escoge un nuevo Jicotillo.

Doña Blanca está cubierta
con pilares de oro y plata.
Romperemos un pilar
Para ver a Doña Blanca.

¿Quién es ese Jicotillo
Que anda en pos de Doña Blanca?
¡Yo soy ése, yo soy ése
que anda en pos de Doña Blanca!

La raspa

Este baile folclórico mexicano se juega con parejas. En este baile, los niños se agarran de las manos. A veces el niño se sujeta las manos detrás de la espalda y la niña se agarra la falda en los dos extremos opuestos. Al recitar las palabras, cada niño se coloca el pie derecho enfrente, con el tacón en el piso, meneando el cuerpo hacia la derecha. Luego, con un salto, se cambian al pie izquierdo, con el tacón en el piso, meneando el cuerpo hacia la izquierda, y luego repite el paso con el pie derecho de nuevo. Ambos niños repiten estos pasos con el compás del tambor, da dun, da dun, da dun. Por ejemplo: La Raspa, la, bailó (pie derecho, pie izquierdo, pie derecho) un viejo, bi, gotón (pie izquierdo, pie derecho, pie izquierdo). Repiten la secuencia con las dos siguientes frases: y en medio, del, salón, —se le cae (cayó), el pan, talón. Cuando llegan a la parte que dice "¡Ay Mamá, pégale a María!" cada pareja va dando saltitos en un círculo, conectada a los brazos, los cuales están entrelazados por los codos, primero con el brazo derecho en una dirección con la primera "¡Ay Mamá, pégale a María!", luego con el izquierdo en la otra dirección con la segunda "¡Ay Mama pégale a María!", y luego se cambia de vuelta al derecho con la tercera línea y luego a la izquierda con "Porque trajo la leche fría". Los niños se agarran de las manos de nu y repiten los pasos desde el principio una vez más.

> La raspa la bailó
> Un viejo bigotón
> Y en medio del salón,
> Se le cae el pantalón.
>
> ¡Ay Mamá, pégale a María!
> ¡Ay Mamá, pégale a María!
> ¡Ay Mamá, pégale a María!
> Porque trajo la leche fría.

(Repita una vez desde el principio)

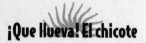

¡Que llueva! El chicote

Éste es un juego en el cual los jugadores caminan en una fila sujetándose de los hombros, mientras todos, menos el líder, miran al cielo. El líder trata de hacer que los demás se caigan, al jalarlos en diferentes direcciones. Cuando se cae la fila, la segunda persona en la fila se convierte en el líder y el líder anterior se va al final de la fila.

> ¡Que llueva! ¡Que llueva!
> la virgen de la cueva,

los pajaritos cantan,
las nubes se levantan.

¡Que sí! ¡Que no!
¡Que caiga el chaparrón!
Que sí, que no.
Le canta el labrador.

Pin Marín

Pin Marín es un verso que tradicionalmente se usa para elegir a una persona en un juego. La última persona a quien apunta uno al terminar el verso es el que uno quiere en su equipo o es el que "la para". La rima va así: Pin Marín de Don Pifuel, cúcara, mácara, títere fue él.

La campana

En este juego hay dos niños con los brazos entrelazados, con un tercer niño en medio de ellos, y cada uno se turna para mecer a esa persona como si fuera una campana que oscilaba.

San Serafín

En este juego, los niños forman un semicírculo y siguen las instrucciones y los movimientos del líder, de manera muy parecido al juego de "Simon Says".

San Serafín del Monte,
San Serafín Cordero,
Yo, como buen cristiano,
Me hincaré (sentaré, acostaré, pararé, brincaré).

LA PREPARACIÓN DE SU NIÑO PARA IR A LA ESCUELA: ¿ESTÁ LISTO?

La preparación de su niño para ir a la escuela abarca mucho más que simplemente comprar útiles escolares y zapatos nuevos. Si su niño tiene experiencias ricas y estimulantes en el hogar, si tiene oportunidades para jugar, hablar, escuchar, cantar, explorar, experimentar, leer, y escribir, tal como se ha mencionado a través de este capítulo, estará listo para lograr el éxito en el salón de clases. En algunas escuelas, a los niños se les da una serie de exámenes que sirven para catalogarlos en grupos. Con frecuencia, estos grupos son clasificados como el grupo "medio", el grupo "inferior", y el grupo "más acelerado". Los niños se desarrollan a diferentes ritmos, pero a ningún niño se le debe negar un programa educativo estimulante donde puede desarrollarse a su potencial máximo. Su papel como primer maestro incluye preparar a sus niños antes de entrar a la escuela. Éstas son algunas de las cosas que debe recordar:

- Desde el momento de nacer, háblele a su niño y enséñele cosas. Mantenga diálogos bilaterales con él.
- Asegúrese de que su niño tenga suficientes experiencias antes de entrar a la escuela, como por ejemplo, oportunidades para dibujar, cortar, jugar con plastilina, identificar las partes del cuerpo, leer, salir de excursión, y hacer otras actividades.
- Asegúrese de satisfacer sus necesidades físicas y alimenticias. Mande a su niño a la escuela con un buen descanso y un desayuno saludable.
- Hágale saber que es amado y ayúdele a sentirse seguro y con confianza.
- Asegúrese de que haya tenido experiencias previas de haber estado con otros grupos de niños, para que su primer día de escuela no sea del todo nuevo y aterrador.

EXPECTATIVAS ALTAS: LO ÚNICO QUE SE NECESITA ES TENER GANAS Y ESPERANZA

Una de las cosas más importantes que usted puede proporcionarles a sus niños es la capacidad de creer en sí mismos. Usted debe tener altas expectativas, aspiraciones, esperanzas, y sueños para sus niños. Hágales saber que usted cree que pueden tener éxito, que son listos, y que pueden llegar a ser, con determinación y mucho esfuerzo, cualquier cosa que desean, ya sea un médico, un astronauta o aun el presidente de los Estados Unidos. Tal como señala la película *Stand and Deliver*, lo único que hace falta es tener ganas, un deseo arraigado de lograr éxito en todo.

Por medio de la encuesta que completaron los padres de mis estudiantes, yo descubrí que muchas madres solamente tenían la expectativa de que sus niños llegaran al séptimo año escolar. No esperaban que sus niños lograran más de lo que ellas mismas habían logrado. Si los padres tienen bajas expectativas, pueden provocar algo que se conoce como "acarrear su propio cumplimiento". Esto quiere decir que si alguien cree que un niño solamente va a lograr llegar hasta cierto nivel, entonces él comienza a seguir ese camino porque empieza a creer que tiene razón. Lo contrario también puede ocurrir. Si las personas significativas en la vida de un niño creen que él puede lograr el éxito y se lo dicen con frecuencia, entonces él también lo creerá. Aunque mi madre sólo tenía una educación de nivel de tercer año de primaria, ella tenía esperanzas, sueños, y altas aspiraciones para todos sus niños. Mi madre hizo que tuviéramos fe en nosotros mismos, en nuestra capacidad, y en nuestro valor como seres humanos. Por lo mismo, nosotros creíamos firmemente que podíamos lograr cualquier cosa que quisiéramos. Desdichadamente, algunas investigaciones científicas han mostrado que algunos maestros tienen más bajas expectativas de los hispanoamericanos, afroamericanos, e indios americanos que de los anglosajones y asiáticos americanos, y esto se puede reflejar en cómo se relacionan con estos niños.

Aunque los padres pueden ayudar a los maestros a ganar consciencia de sus actitudes negativas y el efecto que estos tienen sobre sus estudiantes, primero tienen que asegurarse que sus niños vayan a la escuela con la creencia firme de poder alcanzar el éxito. Sus palabras y acciones tienen que ser persuasivas para que su niño pueda tener suficiente fortaleza para sobreponerse a las presiones que le pueden imponer aquéllos que quizá juzguen de antemano su potencial. Intente llegar a conocer bien a los maestros de su niño para que su presencia transmita el mensaje de que a usted sí le importa el tratamiento que recibe su niño y se preocupa por lo mismo.

Ayúdele a que sea organizado y preparado

Un lugar para todo, y todo en su lugar. La preparación para la escuela incluye ayudar a sus niños a organizar sus posesiones, tiempo, y ambiente de aprendizaje. Prepárelos. Asegúrese que sus niños tengan todos los materiales que necesitan para funcionar en la escuela. Éstos incluyen cuadernos, separadores, hojas de papel, plumas, lápices, diccionarios, cartulinas, una máquina de escribir o una computadora. Mientras una computadora puede significar una inversión fuerte, actualmente se ha convertido en una herramienta esencial para los niños. Es mucho más importante comprar una computadora para sus niños que una televisión. Asegúrese que sus niños se hagan responsables de completar todos sus proyectos, desde sus tareas diarias hasta sus proyectos científicos o de investigación. Asigne un lugar específico en la casa como el lugar donde sus niños pueden hacer sus tareas, o simplemente recostarse a leer un libro. Usted puede proveer un ambiente relajante al tocar música suave mientras están leyendo y aprendiendo. Además, ayuden a sus niños a organizar su tiempo para que puedan hacer sus tareas de la escuela, sus quehaceres de la casa, y sus actividades de después de clases y fines de semana.

Ayúdele con la tarea

Asegúrese de que sus niños establezcan una rutina donde terminan sus tareas antes de prender la televisión o comenzar a jugar. Puede ayudarles a repasar las palabras de vocabulario, las tablas de multiplicación, o las preguntas para un examen. Revise sus tareas y llévelos a la biblioteca para que aprendan a usar los materiales de recurso. Ayúdeles a sus niños a aprender a memorizar información mejor. Un método que utilicé para ayudarles a mis niños a aprender fórmulas, conceptos, o listas de nombres es a través de la ayuda nemotecnia. Simplemente memorice la primera letra de cada palabra y luego crea una nueva palabra con esas letras, lo cual les ayudará a recordar con más facilidad una serie de datos. En las familias hispanas, como en muchas otras culturas, los hermanos mayores juegan un papel importante en ayudar a los más pequeños a lograr el éxito en la escuela. No subestime el potencial que tiene el hermano o la hermana mayor para enseñar a su niño más pequeño cómo funciona el sistema y qué esperar de ciertos maestros. Ellos pueden modelar hábitos apropiados de estudio, y pueden ser excelentes tutores. Sin embargo, éstas son costumbres que se tienen que formar temprano. Mientras que usted o los hermanos de sus niños pueden proporcionar apoyo, asegúrese de no terminar haciendo la tarea por ellos. Los niños tienen que aprender que hay consecuencias si no entregan sus tareas a tiempo o si se niegan rotundamente a hacerlas. El sacar buenas calificaciones y tener éxito en la escuela principalmente se reduce a entregar las tareas correctamente y estudiar para los exámenes. Si tratan de reducir al mínimo lo que hacen o no esforzarse lo suficiente, lo notarán en sus calificaciones.

Controle y apague la televisión

Vigile los programas que miran sus niños además de la cantidad de tiempo que se pasan mirándola. Aliéntelos a mirar programas educativos como *Sesame Street*, *Barney*, *The Puzzle Place*, o el *Discovery Channel*. Se les debe limitar a los niños a mirar la televisión por no más de dos horas al día en los días de escuela. Si la televisión se queda prendida todo el día, puede prevenir que los niños hagan su tarea o adquieran buenas habilidades para escuchar, además de disminuir la probabilidad de que tengan experiencias más concretas y activas.

Antes de los siete años de edad, los niños no pueden distinguir entre la fantasía y la realidad y con frecuencia son afectados por lo que miran en la televisión, los vídeos, las películas, y los comerciales. Los niños a quienes se les permite mirar violencia en la televisión, aprenden a resolver sus problemas de una manera agresiva y se vuelven menos sensibles a los sentimientos ajenos. A esta edad, los niños pequeños que miran la violencia en la televisión pueden volverse temerosos del mundo a su alrededor. Los padres deben imponer límites y parámetros con relación a mirar la televisión. Siempre debe explicar por qué no aprueba los programas que sus niños miran. Debe alentar y participar en otras actividades con sus niños además de mirar la televisión, como tal vez jugar a las cartas o los juegos de mesa. Generalmente, como regla, la televisión debe mantenerse apagada en los días de escuela, como así también los juegos de vídeo y computadoras, y el teléfono, sin embargo, al crecer los niños, el reto aumenta para los padres.

La excelencia en la educación: Los programas de enriquecimiento y complemento

Como miembro del *College Board's Educational Excellence for All Students Task Force* (Fuerza de Trabajo para la Excelencia Educativa para Todos los Estudiantes de la Dirección de la Universidad), hemos discutido estrategias para ayudar a los hispanos, los negros, y los indios americanos a lograr excelencia educativa en la escuela, sacar mejores calificaciones en sus exámenes de SAT, y como meta final, sobresalir en la universidad. El mandar a sus niños a cursos de enriquecimiento y a academias especiales en los sábados puede realzar sus conocimientos en las matemáticas, en las ciencias, y en la resolución de problemas, entre otras cosas. Es importante que prepare a sus niños a tomar álgebra en la secundaria, porque eso les capacitará para hacer las clases preparatorias esenciales para la universidad, tales como el álgebra avanzado, la geometría, la química, y la física, más adelante en la preparatoria. Como padre, debe asegurarse que la escuela secundaria de sus niños ofrezca cursos de álgebra, y que ellos lo tomen. Con los ataques que se llevan a cabo contra la acción afirmativa, se está volviendo más difícil para nuestros niños entrar a la universidad de su elección—a menos que podamos abogar por ellos y ayudarles a construir unos sólidos cimientos al ir a clases adicionales de matemáticas, ciencias, inglés, computadoras, y aun clases que les enseñan cómo tener mejores resultados al tomar exámenes, cuando son jóvenes. Mi hijo una vez asistió a una clase durante el fin de semana para aprender cómo construir cohetes en miniatura. Otros niños asisten a academias de verano patrocinado por NASA, o participan en diversas actividades como explorar yacimientos arqueológicos o geológicos. Están aprendiendo mientras se divierten. Los programas de enriquecimiento pueden abarcar cualquier campo de interés, e incluyen la música, el arte, la danza, la gimnasia, y cualquier otro talento que poseen sus niños. Si nosotros les ayudamos a nuestros niños a desarrollar sus intereses y habilidades, tendrán éxito en la vida.

Las escuelas ofrecen programas especiales para los niños superdotados. Desdichadamente, los niños hispanos con demasiada frecuencia son excluidos de estos programas, y en cambio, un número desproporcionado se coloca en clases de educación especial. Como padre, usted puede insistir que sus niños reciban cada oportunidad posible de participar en estos programas enriquecedores. Sus niños merecen y tienen el derecho de estar incluidos. Además, entienda, si la escuela está tratando de negarle a su niño el derecho de participar en estos cursos, hay recursos a los cuales puede recurrir. Yo conocí a una joven hispana que tenía un CI (coeficiente intelectual) de 170 y sin embargo le negaron la entrada a una clase acelerada, aun después de que su padre pagó por su cuenta para que le hicieran un examen. Él llevó el asunto al superintendente de la escuela y, por último, a la mesa directiva local de la escuela para conseguir que le permitieran a su hija asistir al programa avanzado de la escuela. Más tarde se licenció con matrícula de honor de una de las universidades más prestigiosas de los Estados Unidos. Este ejemplo ilustra la razón por la cual los padres tienen que abogar por sus niños y exigir que sean tratados con justicia, y que tengan el mismo acceso al una educación de buena calidad.

Ponga en duda y formule preguntas a los maestros y a los administradores si sus niños son categorizados y catalogados, o si no son colocados en un programa apropiado a su potencial y a sus necesidades. Mientras los llamados "programas de recursos" o de "educación especial" son buenos para niños con necesidades especiales que tienen algún tipo de problema o discapacidad, a demasiados niños hispanos los colocan en estos programas inapropiadamente, y sin hacerles las pruebas adecuadas. Si su niño tiene un problema de aprendizaje, como la dislexia, la escuela debe proporcionar apoyo especial. Si no domina bien el inglés, es importante que sea colocado en un programa bilingüe que utiliza su idioma para hacer más fácilmente la transición al inglés y para facilitar su aprendizaje de otras materias como matemáticas y ciencia, en su lengua materna hasta que aprenda el inglés. Si lleva un atraso académico al entrar a la escuela, participe activamente en su aprendizaje. Enséñele usted mismo, consígale otros tutores, o inscríbalo en programas especiales que pueden ayudarle a alcanzar su nivel apropiado. Con demasiada frecuencia, nuestros niños son colocados en clases especiales, hechos a un lado, y olvidados. Con el tiempo, quizá abandonen sus estudios por completo. Hoy en día, casi la mitad de los jóvenes hispanos abandonan sus estudios. De aquéllos que se gradúan, sólo 10 por ciento de hispanos siguen y terminan sus estudios universitarios. Los padres juegan un papel vital en cambiar estas estadísticas alarmantes, desde antes de que el niño entre a la escuela, y a través de toda su educación formal.

Procure ser compañeros en la educación

Tal como mencioné antes, cada padre debe procurar conocer a los maestros de sus niños. Es sumamente importante que usted le haga saber a cada uno de ellos que a usted le importan y le preocupan los logros educativos de sus niños. Asista a la escuela en los días designados a los padres para ir a conocer y hacer preguntas (open house), y a conferencias con sus maestros, y ofrezca ser voluntario para actividades y acontecimientos especiales. Forje una relación de compañeros en el proceso educativo. Dígales a los maestros de sus niños que usted espera ser avisado inmediatamente si surge algún problema o preocupación para así poder tratar de ayudar a su niño a resolver cualquier problema académico o de conducta. El hacer esto le hará a un maestro pensar dos veces antes de perseguir a sus niños, darse por vencido con ellos, tratarlos injustamente, afectar su confianza propia, o dañar su amor propio. Yo solía decirles directa y francamente a los maestros de mis niños, desde un principio: "Mis niños son muy especiales para mí y yo haré todo lo que pueda para ayudarles a alcanzar éxito en la escuela. Dígame lo que yo puedo hacer para ayudarle a usted a ayudarles a ellos a alcanzar este éxito". Éstas son declaraciones que todos los padres deben sentirse cómodos para hacerles a aquéllos que comparten nuestra responsabilidad de educar a nuestros niños.

Cuando yo estaba trabajando para obtener mi doctorado, yo me sentí muy consternada al escuchar a una profesora de lenguaje de la universidad decirnos a sus estudiantes que las madres hispanas no les hablan a sus niños y que nosotros, como maestros, teníamos que respetar ese silencio como parte de la cultura. Como yo era la única hispana en la clase, yo le informé a la profesora que mi madre siempre me habló mucho, tal como lo hacen muchísimos padres hispanos que yo conozco. Yo le dije: "Aun si lo que dice fuera cierto, y no lo es, aun si fuera así, como educadores, ¿no cree usted que es importante enseñarles a los padres acerca de su importante papel como maestros, especialmente cuando se trata de la adquisición de lenguaje y de aprendizaje? ¿No cree que debemos ayudarles a los padres a ayudar a sus niños, especialmente durante el período crítico cuando el lenguaje y el aprendizaje se adquiere más fácilmente?" Ella respondió: "Yo estoy citando este libro". (El libro fue escrito por un anglosajón quien sabía poco de nuestra cultura. Fue en ese momento cuando yo me di cuenta de la importancia de que los hispanos escribiéramos y habláramos francamente sobre nuestra propia cultura y escribiéramos sobre nuestras necesidades especiales.)

Después, una estudiante en la clase, maestra por profesión, me dio las gracias por mis comentarios. Ella me contó que por las mismas razones que le fueron dadas por nuestra profesora que tenía mala información, ella había desperdiciado oportunidades para informarles a los padres hispanos lo que necesitaban hacer para ayudar a sus niños en la escuela. Ella dijo: "Me siento tan mal porque algunos padres hispanos se me habían acercado para preguntarme si había algo que ellos podían hacer para ayudar a sus niños. Yo dudé si decirles algo por lo que esta profesora nos enseñó. Yo sabía mejor, pero quise respetar su cultura. Me alegro que hayas hablado". Como proyecto para mi clase, el cual iba a ser el principal factor determinante para nuestras calificaciones, yo filmé unos vídeos de unas madres hispanas participantes de AVANCE que estaban jugando con sus niños y enseñándoles conceptos con los juguetes que ellas mismas habían hecho en su clase. Yo quise señalar y dejar en claro que en AVANCE enseñamos a los padres hispanos la importancia de hablarles a sus niños, especialmente cuando son muy pequeños, y también permitirles a los otros estudiantes ver por sí mismos que las madres hispanas de hecho sí les hablan a sus niños. Los estudiantes calificamos los proyectos de los demás, los cuales eran la base para la calificación del curso. A pesar de que recibí una "A" de los estudiantes, saqué una "B" en el curso. Ah, bueno, ¡planteé la cuestión y dejé bien clara la respuesta! Tuve que hacer esto sin tomar en cuenta las consecuencias.

De nuevo, no puedo recalcar demasiado la importancia de procurar conocer a los maestros de sus niños. Los hispanos, como muchos grupos, respetan las figuras de autoridad, especialmente a los maestros de nuestros niños. Sin embargo, necesitamos estar sensibles al hecho de que algunos maestros, francamente, no son calificados para ser maestros. Mientras que la mayoría de los maestros son dedicados y talentosos, algunos de ellos pueden lastimar a nuestros niños con su falta de preocupación o sensibilidad. Cuando yo era maestra de primer año de primaria, una de mis colegas forzó a tres niños hispanos a comer en el piso durante la hora de la comida, como castigo por estar pasando la comida de una charola a otra. Esa misma maestra aventó a una de mis antiguas estudiantes contra la pared, haciéndola caer dentro de un bote de basura, simplemente porque ella iba a mi salón a leerme después de clase. Yo me quejé con el director y luego les avisé a los padres de la niña lo que le ocurrió a su hija. Yo les dije que debían ir a la escuela a abogar por su hija. Lo que ocurrió ese día fue un comportamiento inapropiado. Yo me sorprendí cuando su padre trató de darme excusas para no ir. Me dijo: "Mi esposa y yo nunca hemos entrado a la escuela. No hablamos inglés. No tenemos ropa apropiada para ir a la escuela". Yo le expliqué al padre que no importaba cómo se expresara ni cómo se vestía, pero lo que sí era muy importante era que fuera para defender a su hija. Accedió ir. Me sentí tan orgullosa de él cuando al siguiente día fue y presentó una queja contra la maestra. Muchos años después, cuando estaba en la escuela preparatoria, su hija me llamó para decirme que nunca se le olvidaría el día cuando su padre y yo salimos en su ayuda. De nuevo, permítame volver a decir que aunque hay muchos maestros muy buenos, desdichadamente también los hay que no lo son, y que no deberían estar enseñando a nuestros niños.

Es importante que usted participe en la educación de sus niños y que se entere de lo que ocurre en la escuela. Cada día, al llegar de la escuela su niño, pídale que le cuente una cosa buena y una cosa mala que le ocurrió en la escuela. Un día cuando le hice esta pregunta a mi hijo, me quedé muda de asombro al escuchar su respuesta. Descubrí que el maestro de Sal lo había estado manteniendo afuera de la clase, en el pasillo, por dos semanas, sin mi conocimiento. El año escolar acababa de comenzar. Yo describo lo que hice para resolver este problema en la sección sobre "discriminación". Los programas de entrenamiento para maestros deben ayudar a los maestros a lograr consciencia acerca de sus parcialidades escondidas, porque sus prejuicios pueden surgir y afectar negativamente a nuestros niños.

LA PRESIÓN DE LOS COMPAÑEROS PARA NO TENER ÉXITO: DIME CON QUIÉN ANDAS Y TE DIRÉ QUIÉN ERES

Quizá haya crecido escuchando este dicho. Sus padres sabían que usted sería influenciado positiva o negativamente por las personas en cuya compañía se mantenía. Igual como los dichos *acompáñate con los buenos* y *serás uno de ellos*, y *él que anda entre la miel, algo se pega*, sus padres deseaban que escogiera la buena compañía para que algo bueno se le pegara. Pero cuando decían, *él que anda por malos caminos, levanta malos polvos*, le estaban diciendo que su actitud y sus acciones iban a ser influenciadas de manera adversa por aquéllos a su alrededor, los cuales ellos no aprobaban.

A través de los tiempos, los padres han deseado que sus hijos tengan amigos que poseen los valores que quieren para sus niños. Algo muy valioso para los americanos es el logro académico. Sin embargo, las investigaciones demuestran que algunos hispanos y afroamericanos rehusan sobresalir académicamente a causa de la presión de sus compañeros. Los jóvenes hispanos a veces tienen la creencia errónea de que solamente los niños anglosajones pueden sobresalir en la escuela y que si luchan para tener éxito, sus amigos hispanos quizá piensen que los están rechazando o haciendo a un lado para encajar bien en el "grupo anglosajón". Usted necesita asegurarles a sus niños y a los amigos de ellos que son tan inteligentes como cualquier otro niño y que tienen el potencial de sobresalir. Invite a los amigos de sus niños a venir a su casa con más frecuencia para que pueda alentarlos de manera sutil y ayudar a sus amigos también a tener éxito en la escuela.

Una manera de combatir los efectos de la presión negativa de los compañeros es pedirle a una persona exitosa que usted conoce y respeta que sea el mentor de su hijo. No necesita pasar más que unas cuantas horas al mes con su niño para tener una influencia sobre él. Si es buena la sintonía entre ellos, su niño tal vez aspire a ser como aquella persona y aprenderá más acerca de lo que hace falta para lograr el éxito. Maggie Comer, una madre que estaba criando a su niño sin pareja, solía lavarle las camisas a un médico a cambio de que él accediera a ser el mentor de su hijo, quien ahora es el reconocido psiquiatra de Yale, James Comer. El joven Comer se pasaba el tiempo en la oficina del doctor y simplemente platicaba con él acerca de la vida. ¡Y qué influencia tuvo! Usted también puede encontrar un mentor apropiado para sus niños para ayudarles a tener éxito en la vida.

Nuestros niños requieren modelos que valoran la educación, comenzando por usted. Si su niño lo mira leyendo y haciendo el esfuerzo de continuar su propia educación, le estará enseñando el valor del aprendizaje y los logros académicos. Llévelo consigo a la biblioteca de la universidad si usted asiste a la universidad. Mientras que sí se retarán los valores que usted trata de impartir en su casa, probablemente no serán cambiados por la presión negativa de compañeros si usted mantiene una relación positiva con sus niños, si ellos reciben cierta orientación de sus

mentores y si siguen escuchando las palabras de sabiduría que han o-
rientado a los hispanos a través de todos los tiempos.

Un conflicto en estilos de enseñanza y aprendizaje

En una frecuentemente citada investigación sobre niños hispanos, dos
investigadores reconocidos, Manuel Ramírez y Alfred Castañeda, concluyeron que los niños hispanos criados de acuerdo a los principios tradicionales, como, por ejemplo, el respeto a la autoridad, mostraron lo que
se han llamado estilos cognoscitivos "field-dependent". Las sociedades
hispanas tradicionales, dijeron, se adhieren a ciertas características:

1. Una creencia en el papel de fuerzas sobrenaturales en la creación
del universo. Lo que esto significa es que la religión, la fe, y las creencias
espirituales todavía son muy fuertes en la percepción que los hispanos
tienen de sí mismos y de otros.

2. Una identidad propia con relación a la familia, a la tribu, a la
religión, al grupo étnico o racial. Valoramos y somos leales a la familia,
a la comunidad, y a nuestro grupo étnico.

3. Una lealtad a las estructuras sociales jerárquicas en las cuales la
autoridad se designa por edad, derecho de nacimiento, o posición en la
familia o el grupo. Desde pequeño un niño le otorga respeto a todo aquél
que tiene autoridad, ya sea el abuelito, la madre, el padre, o el hermano
mayor. Aunque el padre sí es "quien manda", cuando la madre de él entra
al cuarto, a él se le asigna un papel menor. El honor y el respeto que ella
infunde quizá se transfieran a su esposo cuando *él* entra al cuarto.

Los estilos cognoscitivos que son "field-sensitive" o "field dependent",
[el aprender y pensar] como los explican Ramírez y Castañeda, son ca-
racterizados por una fuerte conexión a las relaciones entre las personas.
De acuerdo a esta teoría, el aprendizaje requiere mucha interacción y
participación en la comunicación. Los niños que son "field dependent"
prefieren premios sociales y tienen la tendencia de enfocarse en el aspecto global de las ideas y los problemas. Hablando en términos generales,
los hispanos tradicionales son personas muy sensibles. El lenguaje del
cuerpo y las señales que éste emite no son tan importantes como las palabras. Nos importa cómo se sienten las personas y cómo serán afectadas
por lo que decimos y hacemos.

Manuel Ramírez, quien también estudió la dinámica de los salones de
clases donde los estudiantes México-americanos eran enseñados por

maestros no hispanos, descubrió que la mayoría de los maestros mostraron más tendencias "field-independent" impersonales que sus estudiantes. Otras investigaciones demostraron que algunos maestros tienen una percepción más favorable de aquellos estudiantes que reflejaron su propio estilo cognoscitivo y les dieron mejores calificaciones que a los estudiantes cuyo estilo de aprendizaje era diferente.

En su investigación en 1980, Schultz, Florio, y Erickson encontraron diferentes estilos de enseñanza entre los maestros hispanos y los anglosajones. En el salón de clase de la maestra anglosajona, los niños fueron "alentados a trabajar independientemente, el logro individual era premiado por el adulto, una ligera distancia se mantenía en la relación entre maestra y niños, y se utilizaba la competencia entre los niños como motivación al éxito". Por el contrario, la maestra hispana "llamaba a los niños por sobrenombres, y con frecuencia los abrazaba y besaba y los sostenía en su regazo durante las lecciones". Esta clase alentaba que los logros de los niños fueran apreciados y era menos competitiva.

Los padres deben estar conscientes que los conflictos entre los estilos cognoscitivos y de enseñanza entre los estudiantes hispanos con valores tradicionales y los maestros no hispanos pueden entorpecer o ser un obstáculo para el éxito de su niño. Los salones de clase tradicionales, diseñados con sillas colocadas en filas rectas donde los niños son premiados por ser competitivos, individualistas, y agresivos, quizá sean contradictorios a lo que está acostumbrado un niño que se ha criado en un ambiente que refuerza la cooperación, el respeto, la lealtad al grupo, y la sensibilidad. Los niños hispanos en tales situaciones quizá se sientan rechazados y pueden eventualmente percibirse en términos negativos, lo cual lleva a una falta de autoestima. Es importante que los niños tengan maestros con quienes puedan entablar una buena relación e identificarse.

Eventualmente, debemos tratar de lograr que nuestros niños sean bilingües, tengan dos culturas, y dominen ambos estilos cognoscitivos. En los Estados Unidos, muchos hispanos han sentido que tienen que escoger entre una combinación de valores y la otra para que sus niños puedan lograr el éxito en la escuela y en la vida. Usted juega un papel importante en ayudar a sus niños a valorarse a sí mismos, a su cultura, a su familia, y a su origen étnico. Usted debe asegurarse que sus niños estén conscientes de las diferencias entre los idiomas, los valores, y los estilos cognoscitivos al ayudarles a entender que son únicos y especiales. Como latinos, somos diferentes porque podemos poseer dos culturas para satisfacer nuestras vidas, y dependiendo de la situación, podemos cambiar de una cultura a otra o combinarlas. Asimismo, nuestros niños deben crecer aprendiendo cómo actuar en ambas culturas. Nuestros niños no necesitan rechazar su idioma, sus valores, su cultura, ni su estilo cultural, para alcanzar el éxito en la escuela o para formar parte de la cultura dominante de los Estados Unidos. Al contrario, los valores hispanos capacitarán a nuestros niños a lograr el éxito en un ambiente multicultural donde las divisiones a veces son demasiado comunes y donde falta la cooperación. Nuestros valores hispanos y nuestra percepción del mundo deben ser reforzados en nuestros niños. Yo creo que este mundo sería un lugar mejor si más personas poseyeran los valores compartidos por los hispanos como el respeto, la cooperación, la sensibilidad, y la veneración a la familia y la comunidad.

Necesitamos enseñarles a nuestros niños a respetar la diversidad y las creencias de cada persona, aun cuando sean diferentes a las nuestras. También es importante que nuestros niños nos observen asociar con diferentes grupos étnicos y con hispanos tradicionales y no tradicionales. Debemos enseñarles a nuestros niños a ser flexibles y a adaptar a diferentes personas en diferentes situaciones. Necesitamos ayudarles a ser competentes socialmente y poder funcionar bien en muchos entornos sociales.

Igual como los padres pueden ayudar a sus niños a adaptarse a un ambiente tradicional de salón de clase, las escuelas también deben esforzarse más a tratar de tomar en cuenta las necesidades de los hispanos. Los programas de entrenamiento para maestros deben preparar a los educadores para responder a las necesidades de los hispanos, comunicarse con nuestros niños de una manera sensible e interpersonal, y participar en actividades de grupo. En el salón de clase, con demasiada frecuencia los conocimientos son presentados sin conectarlos a los antecedentes y a la cultura de los niños. En el aprendizaje, es crítico que toda nueva información sea conectada a experiencias o conocimientos previos. Las lecciones de la clase deben incluir actividades e imágenes culturales con las cuales el niño pueda identificarse. Ofrezca ayudar a enseñar la cultura hispana al cantar una canción o tocar un instrumento, enseñar un juego, cocinar, o hacer alguna artesanía. Las escuelas también deben darse cuenta de la importancia de la familia—los padres, los abuelos, la familia extensa, y la comunidad—y procurar que se sientan cómodos en las escuelas. Deben tener programas en los cuales los miembros de la familia pueden venir a observar la participación de los niños. Cuando era maestra, ayudé a hacer disfraces coloridos y económicos para los niños de mi clase cuando bailaron "La raspa" y otras canciones y danzas tradicionales durante las juntas para la asociación de padres y maestros—PTA. Les mandábamos invitaciones personales a los miembros de la familia para que pudieran mirar a sus niños bailar. Nunca antes asistieron tantos padres a una junta de la asociación de padres y maestros, además de los abuelitos, los tíos, y las tías de los niños.

A veces nuestros niños son castigados a causa de diferencias culturales. Acuérdese del episodio durante el cual mi colega forzó a tres niños hispanos a comer en el piso porque estaban compartiendo su comida. Esto podía haberse atribuido a un choque cultural entre el valor de compartir y el "cuidar al número uno". Por ser sólo una de ocho niños en mi familia, yo siempre compartí mi comida con mis hermanos. A los niños no se les debe humillar ni rechazar por sus valores y creencias.

El saber cómo comportarse y el tener respeto a la autoridad son atributos arraigados en nuestra cultura. Los padres quieren que sus niños sean bien educados, un atributo que tiene más relación con modales y saber comportarse. Una madre hispana le dice a su niño al salirse con rumbo a la escuela: "Pórtate bien". Para el niño esto quizá signifique que muestre respeto a la maestra y que no le mire directamente y que no haga preguntas, cosas que son exactamente contrarias a lo que la maestra espera de los niños.

Los padres hispanos deben entender que nuestros niños viven en dos mundos, los cuales no tienen que ser mutuamente exclusivos. Mientras que puedan haber diferencias entre los valores enseñados en el hogar y aquéllos enseñados en la escuela, unos no son mejores que los otros, ambos incorporan virtudes importantes. Aunque a los niños hispanos se les enseñe el valor del respeto a los mayores y a la autoridad, esto no quiere decir que no se les debe permitir expresar sus opiniones. Nuestro país está construido sobre la premisa de que todas las personas tienen el derecho de dudar o hacer preguntas, y de expresar sus creencias. Esto es cierto tanto para los padres como para los niños. Por esto necesitamos alentarles a nuestros niños a pensar, evaluar, analizar, preguntar, y expresar sus opiniones. Cuando nuestros niños dicen, "No es justo, yo quiero decir lo que pienso", permítales decirlo. Cuando uno de mis niños me decía esto, yo le respondía: "Si, puedes expresar tu opinión, pero es importante que lo hagas de una manera respetuosa. Yo estaré más dispuesta a escuchar lo que tienes que decir si lo haces de una manera cortés. Convénceme, dame una buena razón, y construye un buen caso de por qué debo cambiar mi forma de pensar y hacer lo que tú deseas". De más está decir que no tenía que empujar a Steven, el "abogado", para decir lo suyo. Él siempre tenía su postura y se mantenía firme a sus creencias. Tal como debe ser, en numerosas ocasiones nuestros niños han convencido a mi esposo y a mí a cambiar nuestro parecer tocante a ciertos temas.

A veces las personas que no están familiarizadas con nuestra cultura quizá interpreten mal nuestro silencio, bondad, y simpatía como señales de debilidad. Los padres necesitan preparar a sus niños para poder asociarse con personas que no son capaces de salir de su propio mundo cultural y aceptar diferentes estilos culturales. Yo una vez les platiqué a mis niños sobre un incidente cuando tuve que cambiar mi expresión facial y tono de voz para comunicarme más efectivamente con una persona que comenzó a volverse demasiada enérgica y grosera. Cuando lo hice, la persona se dio cuenta que el ser fuerte no siempre proviene de ser agresivo. Sin embargo, fui capaz de adaptarme a la situación y ajustar mi estilo de comunicación a uno más formal y más enérgico para que esa persona cambiara su conducta. Como hispanos, debemos enseñarles a nuestros niños a entrar y salir de ambos mundos dependiendo de la situación.

Tal como los padres, las escuelas tienen un papel para ejecutar para preparar a nuestros niños a vivir en un mundo armonioso, pacífico, y democrático, además de prepararlos para el mundo del trabajo. Por muchos años, las escuelas han preparado a los niños a entrar a la fuerza laboral al alentar una conducta individualista, competitiva, y agresiva. Sin embargo, en los negocios, el trabajo cooperativo en grupos, como en Japón, por ejemplo, puede ser igual de lucrativo. La sensibilidad a otros, habilidades positivas de interacción entre las personas, y la capacidad de trabajar en equipo son atributos esenciales de liderazgo. Nosotros queremos que nuestros niños se sientan orgullosos de los hermosos valores culturales que pueden llevar consigo a la escuela y aportar al mundo del trabajo.

LOS SÍMBOLOS Y LA LÓGICA: DE LAS OPINIONES A LOS VALORES— DE LOS ONCE AÑOS HASTA LA EDAD ADULTA

La última etapa del desarrollo cognoscitivo es cuando el conocimiento se adquiere y se estructura simbólica y lógicamente. Durante esta etapa, un niño tiene la capacidad de comprender conceptos abstractos tales como la hipótesis, las teorías, los cálculos, y las funciones matemáticas más complejas. Se ha vuelto más crítico acerca de diferentes situaciones y es capaz de considerar varios resultados antes de que estos ocurran. Al aislar diferentes aspectos del problema, él puede entonces escoger la mejor solución o el mejor camino a tomar. Al llegar a la adolescencia, los niños son capaces de analizar las posturas políticas y filosóficas además de las condiciones sociales a su alrededor.

Tienen una opinión acerca de todo. Esta etapa marca un período cuando los niños realmente comienzan a expresar sus puntos de vista y sus ideales. De repente escuchará a su niño diciéndole que la ropa que trae puesta no es la apropiada o que su carro está muy viejo y el color está mal. Les importa tanto lo que piensan los demás que quizá exijan que los deje a dos cuadras de la escuela para no arriesgarse a que alguien llegue a ver que su mamá los "dejó" o que llegaron en esa vieja carcacha. En mi casa, tratamos de encauzar esta firmeza y seguridad de nuestros niños al animarlos a examinar temas sociales. Les preguntamos sus formas de pensar o sus posturas acerca de la política de la inmigración, el movimiento de sólo inglés ("English Only"), la acción afirmativa, la educación bilingüe, la reforma de la asistencia social, y otros temas actuales que afectan a los hispanos. A esta edad, a los niños les gusta planear, evaluar, y resolver problemas. Éste es el momento perfecto para que ellos comiencen a participar en actividades para jóvenes y de la iglesia además de servicios para la comunidad. A través de estas actividades, ellos comenzarán a desarrollar habilidades de liderazgo al estar involucrados en la planeación, la organización, y la delegación de responsabilidades.

Durante este período, los niños comenzarán a desafiar sus valores y sus creencias. Yo recuerdo verme enfrentada con preguntas que comenzaban con: "¿qué tal si...?", o "¿qué harías si yo...?" Algunas de las cosas con que salieron mis hijos estaban en total desacuerdo con los valores que les enseñamos. Parecía que nos estaban poniendo a prueba a mi esposo y a mí para ver si realmente creíamos y practicábamos lo que predicamos.

Después de asegurarse de que sus hijos comprenden sus posturas con relación a ciertos temas, usted debe ayudar a sus niños a aclarar sus propios valores. Siga investigando para enterarse de sus pensamientos y sentimientos acerca de diferentes temas y circunstancias. ¿Qué harían ellos si se encontraran en cierta situación? ¿Qué son sus creencias con relación a ciertos temas? Los temas tales como el sexo, las drogas, el fumar, el alcoholismo, las armas de fuego, y la discriminación necesitan discutirse abiertamente. De acuerdo a recientes estudios sobre la conducta, un 31 por ciento de los jóvenes entre los diez y catorce años de edad están tomando bebidas alcohólicas y un 23 por ciento de los jóvenes en octavo año escolar han probado la marijuana. De acuerdo a *La Evaluación de la Salud de los Jóvenes Hispanos en Texas* (Texas Hispanic Youth Health Assessment) llevada a cabo por AVANCE y publicada en 1998, fuma un 15 por ciento de jóvenes hispanos que están cursando del noveno al doceavo año escolar. La edad promedia en que los niños comienzan a fumar es de 12.7 años. Con relación al sexo, un 45 por ciento de los hispanos menores de diez y siete años reportó tener relaciones sexuales, y sin embargo sólo un 45 por ciento de ellos utilizaron condones durante su más reciente experiencia sexual. En la misma encuesta, los resultados mostraron que hay más probabilidad de que los hispanos usen la cocaína crac y "freebase" al estar cursando del año noveno al doceavo, que ningún otro grupo étnico a esa edad, y un 9.4 por ciento de los hispanos en el octavo año escolar usó inhalantes un mes antes de la administración de la encuesta, lo cual muestra un nivel más alto que ningún otro grupo étnico.

Verdaderamente, la investigación subrayó la necesidad de que los padres vigilen y que la sociedad apoye a los padres al proveer mentores, más actividades positivas para ellos, y servicios educativos y de salud mental para sus hijos. Usted necesita informarles a sus hijos sus posturas sobre estos temas y por qué se siente así. Hábleles acerca de los efectos que tienen la televisión y el acceso incontrolado de la Internet sobre la conducta sexual. Explíqueles por qué tiene que vigilar los programas que miran en la televisión e instalar aparatos de control en la televisión y en la computadora. Monte una representación, un teatro improvisado con respecto a cómo se enfrentarían a ciertas situaciones, por ejemplo, lo que harían si alguien les ofreciera drogas, les animara a tener relaciones sexuales, o tratara de convencerles a unirse a una pandilla, para que ellos puedan practicar cómo responderían si se vieran enfrentadas a una variedad de situaciones difíciles. Las consecuencias de una decisión equivocada pueden ser devastadoras. Algunos juegos de mesa populares como "Life" y "Scruples" son buenos para ayudar a los niños a pensar acerca de tomar las decisiones apropiadas en la vida. Estos juegos realmente les han hecho meditar a mis hijos sobre sus valores y las consecuencias de sus acciones. Las investigaciones nos indican que el mejor indicador para predecir si un niño rechazará las drogas, el alcohol, el sexo, y las pandillas, es si tiene una sólida relación con su familia. Como padres necesitamos ser muy vigilantes durante estos años inquisitivos y con propensión a tomar riesgos. Establezca los límites y siga repitiendo lo que usted siente está bien o mal para que eventualmente esa voz interior de su niño se haga cargo y tome las decisiones apropiadas.

Éste es un período que constituye un desafío para los padres, pero debe ser divertido a la vez al observar a nuestros niños desarrollándose. Al acercarse a los doce años de edad, puede anticipar muchas preguntas acerca de lo que usted hizo a su edad. A veces sus respuestas pueden desatar una tumultuosa discusión. Puede ser difícil, especialmente para aquellos hispanos que realmente valoran el respeto. La construcción de unos sólidos cimientos morales y una sana relación entre padres e hijos le ayudarán a mantenerse firme en sus convicciones al mismo tiempo de aprender a ser flexibles y comprensivos. Escuchará cosas como: "nadie hace esto" o "todo el mundo hace aquello". Yo solía decirles como respuesta: "Sí, pero tú no eres cualquiera. Tú eres especial, y es por eso que yo te estoy diciendo que hagas esto (o que no hagas aquello), porque tú me importas". Después de decirles mis razones, terminaba con: "¡Punto final!" Muchas veces, ellos ya sabían la respuesta, pero querían probar la consistencia de mis respuestas.

Al madurar en su forma lógica y analítica de pensar, los niños comienzan a tratar de mejorar su autocontrol y desarrollar los valores y los principios que llevarán consigo por toda la vida. Yo me encuentro repitiendo las palabras de mi madre cuando le digo a Esteban: "¡No te descompongas!" A veces cuando está batallando con un problema le oigo decirse él solo, "No te descompongas, Esteban". El premio de ser padre es que cada uno de sus hijos llegue a ser una persona responsable, con autocontrol, moral, y compasiva. Con el tiempo harán aquello que han aprendido es lo correcto. Durante esta etapa, los niños se encuentran ante una encrucijada importante de su camino.

Todo lo que usted haga por cada uno de sus niños, al ser un padre responsable, para preparar y proveer el tipo apropiado de medio ambiente para el aprendizaje y para cultivarlo, durante sus primeros doce años de vida, le capacitará para tomar el camino que conduce hacia el éxito académico y el funcionamiento social apropiado. Usted es el primer maestro de sus niños, y ellos nunca tendrán un maestro más importante en su vida. El tiempo, la energía, y los recursos que usted les proporciona a sus hijos influirán en el tipo de estudiante, padre, trabajador, y ciudadano que llegarán a ser en el futuro. Su amor, compromiso, y esfuerzo serán ampliamente recompensados por muchas generaciones.

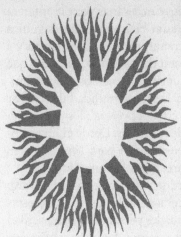

Capítulo VI

Las necesidades sociales y emocionales de los niños

El niño bien educado: Amor a manos llenas

El árbol que crece torcido nunca su tronco endereza. Con frecuencia recuerdo este dicho cuando considero el impacto de los primeros años de vida en el desarrollo social y emocional de un niño. La forma de interacción que tienen los padres con sus niños, cómo les enseñan, aman, orientan, y los límites que establecen para ellos, tendrán una gran influencia sobre su amor propio, carácter, y conducta, además de las habilidades personales que tendrán ellos más adelante en su vida. Al crecer el niño, se vuelve cada vez más difícil cambiar estos atributos.

La socialización es el proceso a través del cual un niño aprende a tener una interacción apropiada con otros seres humanos dentro de un grupo, bajo variadas circunstancias. La socialización comienza en el hogar y dentro de los confines de la familia, y continúa con las instituciones de la comunidad. El proceso comienza con el desarrollo de unos vínculos afectivos entre los padres y el niño, unos lazos a través de los cuales un niño aprende confianza y seguridad. Los padres tienen la responsabilidad principal de enseñarles a ser socialmente competentes. Los padres construyen los cimientos de la capacidad que tendrán los niños para portarse de una manera socialmente aceptable al enseñarles conductas aceptables y al ayudarles a sus niños a controlar la conducta alborotadora o demasiada impulsiva. El tener disciplina propia, posponer la gratificación, y regular las emociones son habilidades importantes, y necesarias para la interacción social y el funcionamiento social. El estar bien socializado significa saber cómo lidiar con los contratiempos, comunicarse efectivamente, y a la larga, mostrar preocupación por el bienestar de los demás. Mientras que las instituciones como la iglesia, las escuelas, los medios de comunicación, y la comunidad en general, tienen la responsabilidad de reforzar la buena moralidad, los valores, y la buena conducta social, los padres son los agentes principales de la socialización de sus niños. Desde el hogar, los padres proveen los cimientos esenciales necesarios para ayudarle a su niño a funcionar exitosamente desde la cuna hasta la comunidad.

Tal como mencioné antes, Howard Gardner, el psicólogo de Harvard, declara que los niños nacen con inteligencias múltiples. Una de estas inteligencias es el don natural de las habilidades personales, la capacidad de comprender a las personas, de discernir y responder a sus sentimientos y a sus necesidades. Este don se puede dividir en cuatro categorías: habilidades de liderazgo, habilidades de análisis social, habilidades de conexiones personales, y habilidades de resolución de conflictos.

1. Un buen líder es uno que puede influir sobre otras personas para que hagan lo que él quiere. Puede organizar a grupos de personas y motivarlos a realizar cosas.

2. Los niños que poseen buenas habilidades de análisis social pueden detectar y tener perspicacia con relación a los sentimientos, las motivaciones, y las preocupaciones de otras personas, un proceso que construye una buena relación de comunicación entre las personas.

3. Los niños que tienen la habilidad de cultivar las relaciones y mantener las amistades son aquéllos que pueden compenetrarse y establecer lazos de empatía con las personas con relación a sus sentimientos y preocupaciones. Son hábiles para "leer" las señales sociales como las expresiones faciales y el lenguaje del cuerpo.

4. Los niños que poseen buenas habilidades para negociar y mediar son aquéllos que pueden prevenir o resolver conflictos.

Sin embargo, las gentilezas sociales inherentes en los niños quizá no puedan florecer si su medio ambiente no cultiva su desarrollo.

La competencia social de un niño es directamente conectada a su desarrollo emocional y viceversa. Su conducta es un reflejo de cómo se siente, de su capacidad de comprender, controlar, y comunicar sus sentimientos además de interpretar e identificarse con los sentimientos ajenos. Aun si los niños no fueran dotados de gentilezas sociales naturales, pueden aprender estas habilidades personales sociales. De manera similar, aquéllos que por naturaleza son sociables no siempre demostrarán estas habilidades si son criados en un ambiente donde no se les cultiva emocionalmente.

El psiquiatra Stanley Greenspan describe seis etapas de desarrollo emocional en su libro *First Feelings: Milestones in the Emotional Development of Your Baby and Child*. Cada etapa coincide un poco con la otra y se construye *sobre* la otra para crear a un niño que podrá relacionarse mejor con diferentes personas y en variadas situaciones. Al conocer estas etapas, usted puede identificar en cuál está su niño y asistirlo en estos logros importantes. Yo presentaré dichas etapas con una perspectiva latina. Se requiere mucha paciencia, comprensión, energía, y amor de parte de los padres, para orientar apropiadamente a su niño desde su nacimiento hasta su madurez. Se vuelve más exigente si tienen a un niño que muestra atributos extremos: que sea muy activo y enérgico, o bien, muy tímido y silencioso. Una crianza efectiva en estos casos requerirá que los padres tengan mucha imaginación, ingenio, y creatividad para formar a sus niños para que lleguen a ser unos niños bien educados—niños que son respetuosos, considerados, compasivos, y autodisciplinados, además de agradables, fuertes, adaptables, y con confianza en sí mismos.

LAS ETAPAS DEL DESARROLLO EMOCIONAL DE GREENSPAN

PRIMERA ETAPA: CALMADO PARA APRENDER—AUTORREGULACIÓN E INTERÉS EN EL MUNDO—DESDE EL NACIMIENTO HASTA LOS TRES MESES DE EDAD

La primera etapa del desarrollo emocional de Greenspan concierne la capacidad del niño para regular sus sentimientos y para calmarse y relajarse inmediatamente después de su nacimiento. Después de haber estado en el ambiente perfecto dentro de la matriz, donde se satisfacían automáticamente todas sus necesidades, el bebé se encuentra abruptamente empujado a un mundo lleno de ruidos, olores, y muchas cosas para ver y probar. Es un lugar donde ahora depende de otros para la satisfacción de sus necesidades básicas. Al sentirse abrumado, la reacción inmediata del bebé es la de ponerse tenso y llorar. El papel de la madre es calmarlo y ayudarle a regular sus emociones intensas para que sienta deseos de observar y aprender lo que hay a su alrededor. Tiene que aprender a controlar lo que T. Berry Brazelton y Bernard G. Cramer llaman sus "sistemas de entrada (aportación) y salida (producción)" *[input and output systems]*. Deben aprender durante aquellos primeros momentos a no tomar en cuenta aquellos sonidos que distraen, y al mismo tiempo absorber otras sensaciones a su alrededor. Al hacer esto, aprenden a controlar los músculos, el latido del corazón, la respiración, y los reflejos. La madre juega un papel importante, antes y después del nacimiento, en ayudar a realizar esto. Las investigaciones demuestran que un bebé puede distinguir entre los sonidos dentro y fuera de la matriz y que puede identificar la voz de su madre siete días después de nacer. Su relación con su madre comenzó antes de que la viera. Por medio de sus caricias suaves y tiernas y sonidos reconfortantes, ella puede ayudar al recién nacido a hacer la transición de una matriz protectora y cálida a un mundo seguro, estable, y afectuoso.

El papel del padre también es muy importante durante este período. No sólo es importante que el padre le proporcione amor y apoyo a la madre para que ella pueda desempeñar su papel maternal, sino que él necesita fomentar unos vínculos afectivos con el bebé al sostenerlo, hablarle, y darle cariño. Un padre que le habla al bebé dentro de la matriz, y asiste a las clases de "Lamaze" (para facilitar el parto natural) con su esposa y la acompaña a sus visitas prenatales con el médico, demuestra que él quiere estar estrechamente relacionado con su bebé, aun antes de su nacimiento.

Todas sus futuras relaciones están arraigadas en las interacciones que comienzan con la primera persona que el bebé conoce al salir de la matriz. Los bebés necesitan ser tocados y necesitan ser hablados en un tono de voz suave y cariñosa. Las investigaciones mencionadas anteriormente, sobre los niños pequeños en los orfelinatos, subrayan lo que puede ocurrir cuando se satisfacen las necesidades físicas como el alimento, la ropa, y la vivienda, pero no satisfacen las necesidades emocionales a través del tacto físico y de hablarles. Estos niños no se desarrollaron bien, y algunos aun fallecieron debido a la falta del tacto físico, el calor humano.

Inmediatamente después de su nacimiento, una madre puede establecer unos lazos con su pequeño bebé al ponerlo afectuosamente contra sus pechos, mientras lo acaricia y lo mira a los ojos, sonriente y dándole la bienvenida a su nuevo y emocionante mundo. Permita que su bebé mire lo que está a su alrededor en la sala de partos. Háblele hasta que voltee la cabeza y le mire a los ojos. El bebé reconocerá la voz de su madre, se acurrucará entre sus brazos, se amoldará su cuerpo contra el suyo, e instantáneamente se aferrará al pecho, sintiéndose seguro en su nuevo ambiente.

Hace mucho años, el antropólogo David Landy observó que las madres en un pueblito puertorriqueño envolvían a sus bebés en una hamaca de tela llamada "coy", y los mantenían cerca de ellos en todo momento después de nacer. Esta práctica promovía una máxima vinculación afectiva entre el bebé y la madre. En la actualidad, ya sea en una sala de partos estéril o en un cuarto de alumbramiento más relajante, las madres todavía pueden aprovechar al máximo el período inmediatamente después del nacimiento de su bebé al establecer y estrechar los lazos entre ellas y sus bebés. En el pueblito puertorriqueño que estudió Landy, y ciertamente a través de Latinoamérica, las madres hispanas han tenido por costumbre cumplir con la cuarentena, un período de reclusión que dura cuarenta días después de dar a luz. Durante estos días cruciales, a una nueva madre se le exime de sus responsabilidades y quehaceres para que pueda descansar y establecer vínculos afectivos con su nuevo bebé, y a la vez darle tiempo a su cuerpo para aliviarse del parto. Hoy en día, las madres no mantienen la cuarentena como las mujeres hispanas lo hacían en el pasado. Sin embargo, esta tradición todavía recalca la importancia de permitir todo el tiempo posible durante las primeras semanas después del nacimiento, para tener una interacción con el bebé y ayudarle a aprender acerca de su cuerpo y el mundo a su alrededor.

Las primeras semanas de interacción con su niño son cruciales para ayudarle a regular sus emociones. Una vez calmado, se vuelve atento a las señales de sus padres y luego utiliza sus expresiones faciales, vocalizaciones, las manos, los pies, o el cuerpo, para provocar una respuesta de su madre o su padre. De acuerdo a Brazelton y Cramer, esta acción recíproca sincronizada y rítmica entre los padres y el niño produce la primera sonrisa social del niño al final del segundo mes. Es un proceso de dar y recibir, donde la madre o el padre recibe señales o pistas de su niño y luego responde con una serie de conductas que continúan el intercambio. Los ojos del bebé brillan al arrullar, sonreír, y deleitarse con lo que hace su madre o padre. El bebé luego espera que la madre o el padre responda con gestos similares que muestran su gusto. Al voltearse, el niño está avisándole: "Ya me cansé".

Durante esta primera etapa, sostenga a su bebé en una posición casi vertical, a una distancia de diez a doce pulgadas de su cara. Háblele afectuosamente, utilizando cariños. Proporciónele un medio ambiente estimulante y enriquecedor con colores fuertes que contrastan, sonidos suaves y tiernos, aromas dulces, y objetos que se mueven lentamente. La atención de un bebé durará sólo unos pocos minutos después de su nacimiento, y aumentará a alrededor de veinte o treinta minutos después de dos o tres semanas. Al utilizar los sonidos y las imágenes de su cultura, ya sea a través del vívido y colorido arte popular o con el ritmo suave de la música tradicional, usted puede ayudar a su niño a utilizar sus cinco sentidos. Él puede absorber, responder a, e interactuar con los diferentes aspectos de sus alrededores. Los niños necesitan el tipo apropiado de estímulos, que no sean demasiado ruidosos ni demasiado brillantes. Como ya mencioné antes, si un medio ambiente es demasiado estimulante, el bebé no lo tomará en cuenta o se pondrá disgustado y llorará. Las actividades que un bebé quizá disfrute cuando tiene un estado de animo silencioso, pero atento, son conductas donde imita, tales como hacer ojitos o burbujas. Él lo imitará cuando le saca la lengua o abre y cierra la boca. Si ambos padres participan activamente con su niño desde el comienzo de su vida, ambos tendrán la oportunidad de sentirse reafirmados y gratificados al saber que están influyendo exitosamente en el desarrollo de su niño.

La segunda etapa: Enamorarse—de los dos hasta los siete meses de edad

La segunda etapa de Greenspan se llama "enamorarse". Ésta es la etapa cuando el niño se pone radiante de gusto con sólo mirar a su madre o a otras personas que lo cuidan, como su padre o su niñera. Esta reacción refleja su amor además de su sensación de confianza y seguridad. Ya al cumplir los tres o cuatro meses de edad, el niño necesita haber establecido vínculos afectivos con los padres, y los padres con el bebé, de otra forma, la relación entre padres y niño y otras futuras relaciones están a riesgo. Cuando se le ilumina la cara de un niño cuando ve a su mami o papi, reafirma que existe un vínculo afectivo sano y armonioso entre el niño y esa madre o ese padre.

Todos los niños nacen con una gama de emociones. Aun de recién nacidos, pueden sentir alegría, entusiasmo, y satisfacción, además de tristeza, enojo, dolor, y desilusión. Los niños llorarán cuando tienen miedo, hambre, sueño, cólico, o indigestión. Desde el primer grito sano del bebé, al salir de la matriz, hasta las miradas alentadoras que le siguen a usted alrededor de la cuna, está mandando señales a aquéllos a su alrededor. Quizá esté avisándoles a sus padres que necesita alimentarse o que le cambien los pañales, que quiere que lo volteen, o que simplemente quiere ser arrullado en sus brazos. Por medio de las acciones sencillas de alimentar, cambiar, eructar, y mecerlo, los padres ayudan al bebé a sentirse competente en la expresión de sus necesidades. Establecen una relación amorosa con su bebé que provoca sonrisas radiantes y un refuerzo continuo de su papel como padres competentes y cariñosos. Al establecer los vínculos afectivos los padres con el bebé, ellos hacen un profundo e instintivo compromiso de continuar a cuidar a su niño y de preocuparse por su bienestar.

Es imposible que los padres consientan a un bebé de esta edad con demasiada atención. Los bebés necesitan que los padres les sonrían, los acurruquen, los besen, los acaricien, y les hablen con una voz suave y tierna. De todas las cosas en el medio ambiente que un niño mirará, escuchará, y olerá, el bebé se siente más atraído hacia la persona que le da más cariño, la que responde amorosamente a sus necesidades y deseos. A través de este proceso interactivo, durante el cual un padre y su niño se turnan para responderse y estimularse, surge el amor. Cuando uno colma a su bebé de cariño, con cálidos abrazos y aquellas dulces palabras de afecto que parecen fluir de la boca de las madres latinas, "¡Ay, qué linda, mi amorcito!", no puede sino enamorarse de uno. Cuando arrulla a su bebé con el dulce sonido de las tradicionales canciones de cuna, le está llegando al corazón y al alma. Las muy populares canciones de cuna que ya le mencioné en el capítulo V son "Señora Santa Ana" y "A la rurru niño". La siguiente canción de cuna, "A la rorro niño", la cual forma parte del cassette *Juegos infantiles* por Yolando del Campo y conjunto de Carlos Oropeza, con arreglos de Tío Nando e interpretada por Evangelina Elizondo. Esta canción es una adaptación de "Señora Santa Ana" y "A la rurru niño". Tish Hinojosa hizo lo mismo en su cassette llamado *Cada niño*. Usted también puede crear sus propias canciones de cuna al combinar algunas porciones de una canción con otras de su propia creación y creatividad.

A la rorro niño

Duérmete, mi niño, duérmete, mi amor.
Duérmete, pedazo de mi corazón.
Este niño lindo, que nació de noche,
Quiere que lo lleven a pasear en coche.

Señora Santa Ana, ¿Por qué llora el niño?
Por una manzana que se le ha perdido.
Yo le daré una. Yo le daré dos.
Una para el niño, y otra para vos.
Sh sh sh.

Duérmete, mi niño

Duérmete, mi niño, duérmete, mi sol,
duérmete, pedazo de mi corazón
Este niño lindo, se quiere dormir
Háganle la cama, en el toronjil
Y de cabecera, pónganle un jazmín
para que se duerma como un serafín.

Sleep my child, sleep, my sunshine,
Sleep, little piece of my heart
This beautiful child wants to sleep
Make his bed in the orange grove
And on his pillow, place a jasmine
So he can sleep like a cherub.

Muchas madres, yo incluida, han dormido a sus bebés con la canción tradicional de cuna en inglés *"Hush, Little Baby"*, aun cuando las palabras no son tan amorosas como las canciones anteriores en español.

Hush, Little Baby

Hush, little baby, don't say a word,
Papa's going to buy you a mockingbird.
And if that mockingbird won't sing,
Papa's going to buy you a diamond ring.
If that diamond ring turns to brass,
Papa's going to buy you a looking glass.
If that looking glass gets broke,
Papa's going to buy you a billy goat.
If that billy goat won't pull,
Papa's going to buy you a cart and bull.
If that cart and bull turns over,
Papa's going to buy you a dog named Rover.
If that dog named Rover won't bark,
Papa's going to buy you a horse and cart.
If that horse and cart fall down,
You'll still be the sweetest baby in town!

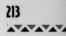

Amparo Ortiz, oriunda de Colombia, les cantaba estas siguientes canciones a sus niños al acostarlos:

Niñito Jesús, sal del copón
Da un brinquito y ven a mi corazón.
Ángel de la guardia, mi dulce compañía,
No me desampares, ni de noche ni de día
Hasta que me ponga en paz y alegría
Con todos los Santos, Jesús, y María.

Baby Jesus, come out of the Chalice
Take a jump and come into my heart.
Guardian Angel, my sweet companion,
Don't leave me, neither by night nor day,
Until I am in peace and happiness
With all the Saints, Jesus, and Mary

Antón Tiruliruliru

Duérmete, niño chiquito
Que la noche viene ya,
Cierra pronto tus ojitos,
Que el viento te arrullará.

Jesús al pesebre
Vamos a adoradar (bis),
Antón Tirulirula (bis)
Antón Tiruliruliru.

Duérmete, niño chiquito.
Que la madre velará,
Cierra pronto tus ojitos,
Porque la entristecerás.

Cuando los hispanos describen el afecto que un padre siente por su hijo, algunos lo llaman "amor a manos llenas". Aunque los padres tengamos muchos términos singulares para describir nuestro amor, como cuando nos referimos a nuestros seres queridos como *mi vida, mi cielo, mi alma,* o *mi luna de miel,* también podemos mostrar nuestro amor a través de otras incontables maneras. La vida cotidiana presenta a los padres con oportunidades para satisfacer las necesidades emocionales de su bebé, comenzando desde la cuna y continuando a través de la adolescencia. El doctor Urie Bronfenbrenner, de la Universidad de Cornell, una vez dijo que cada niño necesita tener a cuando menos una persona que está absolutamente loca por él. Un bebé siente la expresión de cariño por las cosas especiales que se le dicen o que hacen por él, como proveer un alivio a sus encías irritadas, o acariciar su cabello suave después de un baño, o sostenerlo en su regazo mientras le lea un cuento. Como padres, no podemos suponer que nuestros niños saben que los queremos. Necesitamos decirlo constantemente y continuar mostrando nuestro amor por medio de palabras y acciones. Las cosas afectuosas que hacemos por nuestros niños continuarán cuando les celebramos sus cumpleaños o cuando celebramos nuestras tradiciones, tales como la Navidad, el Día de los Reyes Magos, y Pascuas. Estos acontecimientos siempre los llevarán consigo. Al pasar los años, su amor por sus niños se demostrará con las noches que se queda tarde haciendo disfraces para *Halloween* o cuidándolos cuando están enfermos. Cuando una madre y un padre, con su tierno amor, curan la delicada piel irritada, un fuerte resfriado, o un molesto aire en el estómago, convierten a unos niños disgustados y de mal genio en unos niños agradecidos, que muestran su agradecimiento por medio de unas sonrisas de oreja a oreja.

A mi esposo y a mí nos encantaba mirar a nuestros niños jugar deportes o participar en una obra de teatro en su escuela o en sus recital. Pasar esos momentos especiales con sus niños es la mejor manera de demostrarles su amor. Escúchelos. Hágales preguntas. Mírelos a los ojitos lindos mientras hablan con usted.

Un niño no podrá dar algo que no tiene. Si no ha recibido amor, no podrá dárselo a otros. Es muy difícil tratar a alguien con afecto o ser bondadoso y considerado si nadie ha sido así con uno. Pero, si un niño es amado y recibe cuidados y cariños, será fácil para él más tarde en su vida, darles amor a usted y a otros a su vez. El amor es recíproco y contagioso. Usted puede sentir el cariño del niño no solamente con las risitas alegres que surgen al jugar a las escondidas o al caballito, sino también con un abrazo bien fuerte. Usted verá el agradecimiento de su niño o niña cuando le trae un ramito de flores silvestres y se las da con un besito cariñoso. Su intenso sentimiento emocional también se puede percibir cuando le acaricia suavemente la cara a usted. Lo verá también cuando se voltea a mirarlo con una sonrisa gozosa justo antes de pegar el jonrón o cuando sus ojos chispeantes se encuentran con los suyos justo después de un recital de piano. Se ha dicho que los ojos son las ventanas al alma. Los niños que se sienten amados irradian confianza, felicidad, y una alegría de vivir. Ellos sienten una sensación de seguridad, confianza, y compasión que les posibilitará dar cariño a otros.

Uno de los más bellos símbolos de los duraderos vínculos afectivos que existen en las familias hispanas es el cuidado y la atención que los niños les dedican a sus padres cuando son ancianos y delicados. A causa del cariño tan fuerte que los padres hispanos les dieron a sus niños cuando eran pequeños, es correspondido cuando son adultos. En muchas familias hispanas, se puede encontrar a un abuelo o a una abuela que vive con una o más generaciones de parientes. En general, no es una práctica común meter a nuestros padres ancianos a un hogar de ancianos.

Los cuentos tradicionales populares sirven para reforzar las conductas que valoramos y queremos que se repitan. El cuento "La nuera" en el libro *Cuentos from My Childhood* de Paulette Atencio, ilustra como el ciclo recíproco de amor continúa de una generación a la otra. En el cuento, un niño pequeño les enseña a sus padres la importancia de mantener su promesa de cuidar a sus padres en su vejez. Cuando la madre quiere que su suegro se vaya de la casa, el niño les construye una imagen de cómo planea él, a su vez, tratarlos a ellos cuando envejecen, al arreglarles un catre viejo con cobijas hechas jirones para cama. Luego coloca dos platos rajados de madera encima de una mesa vieja. Con esto, los padres recuerdan el dicho, *Joven eres y viejo serás, según lo hiciste, así lo verás.* Esto les hace llorar y pedirle perdón al abuelito del niño por haber querido rechazarlo. Juran nunca volver a faltarle el respeto, porque descubrieron que hay cierta verdad en el dicho, *Si respetas a tus mayores, te respetan tus menores.*

Mi madre y mi tío se turnaron para cuidar a mi abuelo Papayo en sus hogares cuando envejeció y hasta su fallecimiento. Yo admiro a los latinos que con ternura y cariño sostienen a sus mamitas envejecidas del brazo al llevarlas a diferentes lugares o cuando hacen una gran fiesta para ellas en sus cumpleaños o en el día de la Madre. Yo solía llevar a mi madre para acompañarme en algunos de mis viajes de negocio fuera de la ciudad. Nunca se me olvidará un viaje en particular, a Nueva York. Mi madre y yo nos reímos tanto al sostenernos una de la otra, al tratar de mantenernos en pie y no caer al ir patinando por las aceras cubiertas de hielo, hechizadas por los bellos adornos navideños y por los ligeros copos de nieve que se nos caían suavemente encima. Ahora que mi mamá se está acercando a los ochenta años de edad, todas su hijas se turnan para llevarla a comer, de compras, o en busca de gangas en las ventas de garaje, lo cual es su pasatiempo favorito. Una vez al año tomo el tiempo de hacer una venta de garaje en mi casa, donde ella puede vender, a tres veces el precio que ella pagó, todos los objetos que ella ha comprado en otras ventas de garaje. Su continua presencia en la vida de nuestros niños ha enriquecido a nuestras familias ya que ella constantemente imparte palabras de sabiduría acerca de su conducta, o sobre el respeto a Dios. Nuestro fuerte vínculo afectivo proviene de interacciones tempranas y las acciones amorosas que mi madre impartió a través de mi juventud.

La tercera etapa—"Háblame": El desarrollo de la comunicación—de los tres hasta los diez meses de edad

Ésta es la etapa durante la cual la interacción con el mundo humano se hace con más sentido, más intención o decisión. Después de que un niño establece su primer amor verdadero, ahora puede interesarse por establecer relaciones con otros. Durante esta etapa, usted sigue jugando un papel importante en la enseñanza del proceso de comunicación, donde el padre y el niño se turnan para hablar y escuchar. Éste es el período de interacción recíproca, cuando usted y él repetirán los sonidos que el otro produce, descifrarán sus señales respectivas, y aprenderán que cierta acción o expresión produce alguna reacción. Trate de ser responsivo a sus señales al seguir sus intereses.

Como seres humanos, los niños también poseen una amplia gama de emociones, desde la felicidad y el orgullo, hasta la tristeza, los celos, y la ira. Los niños sentirán éstas y muchas otras emociones a través de sus vidas. Ya para los tres meses de edad, los niños comienzan a experimentar con una variedad de emociones y son más o menos capaces de calmarse solos. Durante esta etapa, un niño comienza a darse cuenta que su madre y su padre no podrán responder a sus necesidades todo el tiempo. Cuando usted no lee correctamente las señales de su niño, o no le da lo que él quiere, él le informará a través de sus armas emocionales como los gritos, o al estallar en una rabieta.

El hogar es el lugar de entrenamiento para enseñarles a los niños cómo lidiar efectivamente con sentimientos negativos y aprender cómo comportarse para que no lo cataloguen como "el malcriado". Dentro del hogar es donde él comenzará a controlar sus emociones. Los niños deben experimentar con sus emociones en un medio ambiente seguro y amoroso si es que van a aprender cómo responder a ellas en futuras situaciones sociales. No les niegue a sus niños su amor y atención cuando están explorando sus sentimientos. No lo proteja excesivamente ni lo controle demasiado ni tampoco sea pasivo durante estos momentos. Cuando su niño se mete en las posesiones de sus hermanos, distraiga su atención con algo más interesante o con una actividad que producirá alegría a través de movimiento.

Los hispanos llaman a alguien grosero, malcriado, o mal educado si le faltan las habilidades sociales apropiadas para interactuar adecuadamente con otras personas. Se puede encontrar el origen de esta deficiencia al mirar los primeros meses de vida, cuando sus señales emocionales y sus deseos de comunicación se quedaron sin respuestas. Esto tiene fuertes implicaciones para los padres que tienen bebés, pero tienen que trabajar, ya que deben no sólo encontrar el tiempo para realizar una interacción íntima con sus niños, sino también asegurarse de que sus niños asistan a una guardería de buena calidad, y que las personas que los cuidan sean cálidas y afectuosas, personas que comunicarán afectuosamente con sus niños. Alguien debe tomar el tiempo para interactuar efectivamente con sus niños, ayudarles a sentir la alegría de la comunicación y aprender que ellos pueden provocar un impacto en el mundo.

Tal como declaré anteriormente, los niños cuyas sonrisas, peticiones, y exigencias consistentemente no se toman en cuenta, eventualmente se darán por vencidos y dejarán de interactuar con otros. Aun si usted y las otras personas que cuidan a su niño no siempre interpreten correctamente las señales de su niño, ni respondan siempre a las mismas, siempre y cuando lo hagan la mayoría de las veces, él aprenderá que puede tener una influencia sobre las personas. No todos los bebés tienen las mismas necesidades emocionales. Para un bebé que es muy activo y emocional, es importante que un padre se pase el tiempo necesario para calmarlo y atraer su atención antes de comenzar la interacción. Con el tiempo, el niño podrá regular sus propias emociones. Para el bebé que es tímido y reservado, se requerirá más creatividad para lograr que se muestre un poco más comunicativo. Un niño necesita "enamorarse" de alguien que le provocará alegría, satisfacción, y entusiasmo. Esta persona debe responder a sus sentimientos de tristeza, desilusión, y dolor. En el capítulo V, incluí unos juegos, rimas, y estrategias que le ayudarán a pasar momentos preciosos con su niño durante este muy importante período. Recuerde que las reglas generales son muy sencillas: háblele a su niño, juegue con él, y ámelo.

LA CUARTA ETAPA: EL SURGIMIENTO DE UNA ORGANIZADA CONCIENCIA DE SÍ MISMO—DE LOS NUEVE HASTA LOS DIECIOCHO MESES DE EDAD

Ésta es la etapa cuando la conducta se vuelve organizada. Durante esta etapa, la conducta del niño se vuelve más compleja y organizada, más deliberada y "fuera de control". Éste es un período que pone a prueba la paciencia y puede ser desquiciante, ya que es cuando los niños se dan cuenta que son personas individuales, separadas, y únicas, distintas de las demás personas y de los objetos. Al cumplir los ocho meses de edad, el niño entra a la etapa de "ansiedad de separación", cuando se da cuenta que la madre es una persona separada y se vuelve ansioso cuando no está allí. Quizá llore al instante de darse cuenta que su mami está fuera de su vista. Antes de esta etapa, se aplicaba el principio de "fuera de vista, fuera de mente".

A través de este período, el niño tendrá una gran necesidad de explorar y experimentar. Éste es un período cuando es muy expresivo. Si su niño está enojado, no solamente llorará, sino también golpeará, aventará, lloriqueará, y pataleará. Su amor no sólo se expresa con radiantes sonrisas, sino también con abrazos, besos, y suaves pellizcos. Comienza a comprender que las personas que lo cuidan tienen diferentes papeles y funciones y que tienen autoridad. Éste es un período importante durante el cual los padres deben dividir las responsabilidades y su tiempo con el niño, para que él no identifique solamente a su mami como enfermera, cocinera, compañera de juego, y chofer. Ambos padres pueden aliviar los dolores con un beso o con la rima amorosa *sana, sana, colita de rana, si no sana ahora, sanarás mañana.* Por medio de la observación, su niño también aprende que los objetos también tienen diferentes funciones. El ruido de las llaves quiere decir, "vámonos", y el repiqueteo del teléfono quiere decir que alguien está hablando por el otro lado. Si el niño le trae un pañal, quiere decir que necesita ser cambiado, o si trae un biberón, le está diciendo que tiene hambre. Todas estas observaciones pueden ser utilizadas más tarde como parte de sus juegos imaginarios y para asegurarse de que sean satisfechas sus necesidades.

Durante esta etapa, un niño aprende a conectar pequeñas unidades de sentimientos y de conducta social para formar unos patrones más grandes, complejos, y orquestados. A través de esta conducta más organizada, iniciará actividades por su propia cuenta, creará cosas, y se expresará de manera singular. Comienza a separarse de sus padres para explorar sus alrededores, siempre y cuando pueda mantener una sensación de seguridad con relación a sus padres, al poder verlos y escucharlos cerca.

Durante esta época, un niño puede descubrir cómo conseguir lo que quiere de sus padres al combinar sus habilidades motrices con otros sentidos, como cuando apunta hacia un objeto que lo entusiasma. Su falta de dominio provocará frustración e ira. Por otro lado, su capacidad de dominar tales habilidades como caminar, apilar, o hacerse entender, producirá sentimientos de orgullo, satisfacción, y una sensación de firmeza y confianza.

Los niños de esta edad pueden sacar de quicio a sus padres al explorar un repertorio completo de emociones. Por momentos son dulces, bondadosos, y juguetones, y a ratos están enojados y necios. Es importante hacerles felices a los niños, pero no a expensas de su seguridad, su bienestar, y su desarrollo. Se necesita controlar la conducta fuera de control de los niños. Los padres necesitan establecer los límites de lo que ellos consideran una conducta apropiada. Deben inmediata y consistentemente expresar su disgusto ante cualquier cosa que no consideran aceptable. ¿Recuerde lo que le acarreó la curiosidad al gato? Esté siempre vigilante con relación a dónde está el niño cuando anda en sus exploraciones cotidianas dentro y fuera de la casa.

Si usted quiere prevenir la conducta negativa de su niño, utilice la técnica de Greenspan de "ojo a ojo". Mire a su niño directamente a los ojos con una mirada de disgusto. Dígale "no" con firmeza y menee la cabeza. Baje un poco la cabeza, apriete los labios, y levante una ceja. Cuando una madre o un padre levanta la ceja y mira a su niño directamente a los ojos, llama su atención. Sea firme y consistente. Eventualmente su niño comprenderá que usted está serio y que está decidido a controlar su conducta, si él no lo puede hacer por cuenta propia.

Cada etapa de Greenspan construye sobre las anteriores. Para que los límites se puedan establecer más fácilmente al regular las emociones de su niño, cálmelo, consiga su atención, y ayúdele a enfocarse en sus señales mientras mantenga una conexión emocional con él. Su niño aceptará más fácilmente sus reglas y valores si son presentados en un ambiente de amor y seguridad. Aun si se disgusta cuando usted le pone límites con relación a la televisión o lo manda a dormir a cierta hora, puede mantener esa conexión emocional, ese vínculo afectivo, con usted, si usted se sigue esforzando por mantener una relación sólida. Después de que se haya calmado, trate de reconciliarse con él y luego esfuércese por mantener abiertas las puertas de la comunicación para mantener sólida y fuerte la relación.

Utilice el lenguaje especial y suave de los padres (*parentese*), para comunicarle que se identifica con sus sentimientos lastimados. Sea comprensivo y empático con relación a sus sentimientos. Refleje sus sentimientos al expresar lo que usted piensa que él está sintiendo: "Ah, estás muy disgustado porque no te quieres bañar. Yo sé que preferirías jugar, pero todos tenemos que bañarnos todos los días. Vamos por tu patito". "No debemos romper los libros. Los libros son para leer, y debemos cuidarlos. No podremos leerlos si están rotos. Vamos a pegar esto con cinta".

En las familias donde no se cultivan las emociones, los niños y los padres pueden ponerse de mal humor, un estado de ánimo silencioso donde uno comunica que está lastimado por las acciones de otro al hacer mohines. Este resentimiento se puede ir acumulando hasta estallar en otras formas inaceptables. Es la responsabilidad del padre maduro ayudar al niño a calmarse, volver a captar su atención, y convertir una situación negativa en una positiva al acariciarlo, acurrucarlo, o distraerlo. Su niño será más receptivo a lo que usted quiere que haga o se volverá más curioso e independiente si su relación con él se mantiene sólida y él siente amor y seguridad.

De acuerdo a Greenspan, se deben comenzar a establecer los límites a los ocho meses de edad. Al cumplir los doce o trece meses de edad, su niño debe reconocer su autoridad y comenzar a aceptar los límites que usted impone. Los niños necesitan vivir en un mundo organizado. Necesitan que usted les diga cómo funcionan las cosas y las razones por las cuales usted quiere que se porten de cierta manera. Aun si no entienden todas sus palabras, percibirán su disgusto a través del tono de su voz y sus expresiones. No debe simplemente dar órdenes como "¡no!" "¡quieto!" "¡no seas malo!" "pórtate bien" "¡calma!" "¡tranquilo!" y "¡silencio!" También debe proveer el porqué de las cosas, por ejemplo: "Duele cuando le pegas a alguien", "Papi está tratando de dormir", y "Las camas son para dormir, no para brincar". Sin embargo, el establecimiento de límites no significa usar la fuerza física o pegar.

Algunos padres comienzan a establecer los límites demasiado tarde. Ellos quizá piensen que un niño menor de un año no es capaz de comprender lo que dice un adulto cuando habla. Muchos padres hispanos que asistían a AVANCE solían decir: "Los niños no entienden". No se daban cuenta de que estaban perdiendo una maravillosa oportunidad. Es más fácil moldear la conducta de los niños cuando son pequeños porque le aceptan y respetan como una figura de autoridad y porque lo quieren mucho por ser la persona que satisface sus necesidades. Aceptarán cualquier cosa que usted les diga sin ninguna pregunta. Algunos padres comienzan a establecer los límites años después, cuando es mucho más difícil, y en algunos casos, demasiado tarde.

Los padres deben determinar qué consideran conducta apropiada e inapropiada. Necesitan estar preparados para enseñarles a sus niños cuándo y dónde son apropiadas ciertas emociones y los momentos y los lugares donde no lo son. Por ejemplo, quizá usted le diga a su hijo: "El expresar tu entusiasmo con gritos y corriendo está bien fuera de la casa, en tu recámara o en el cuarto de juegos, pero no está bien en ningún otro cuarto de la casa". "El jugar con figuras de acción o un saco de arena para soltar tu ira esta bien, pero no está bien pegarle a tu hermano o a tu hermana". Proporciónele una alternativa: "En lugar de golpear y gritar, ¿por qué mejor no me dices lo que te molesta?" El tiempo y el esfuerzo que se utiliza para enseñar, orientar, y establecer límites mostrará su provecho más adelante en el desarrollo de una persona que es socialmente competente, un niño bien educado. Usted está construyendo los cimientos para futuras interacciones sociales y para que sepan sus niños cómo comportarse en una situación social. Muestre empatía y apoyo, al ayudarle a su niño a organizar su mundo para que sea seguro, pacífico, cariñoso, y ordenado.

La quinta etapa: Produciendo imágenes mentales–creando ideas emocionales–de los dieciocho hasta los treinta y seis meses de edad

Durante esta etapa, el niño crece y avanza en su desarrollo—va de jugar con sensaciones físicas y acciones concretas a expresar sus sentimientos y explorar las interacciones por medio del juego imaginario, el cual incluye lenguaje, gestos, y relaciones espaciales. Podrá comunicar mejor sus emociones porque ahora posee nombres para ellas: "Estoy enojado" o "Yo quiero un helado". Él podrá recordar los sentimientos cálidos que tiene para su mamá, y esperar con entusiasmo el momento cuando ella pasa por la puerta. Quiere la pelota, aun cuando no la puede ver, porque recuerda la alegría que le provoca jugar con ella. Vacilará al querer agarrar la empanadita que su mami le dijo que no comiera hasta después de la cena, porque tiene una imagen mental de cómo se mira su madre cuando está enojada.

Ésta es la etapa cuando un niño descubre el juego imaginario. El niño de dos años primero jugará solo o al lado de otro niño, cada uno en su propio mundo de fantasía. Al cumplir los tres años de edad, los niños son menos egocéntricos y son capaces de jugar con otros niños. El juego imaginativo de un niño lo prepara para diferentes papeles y relaciones. Por medio del juego, él explora su mundo, prueba sus límites, y descubre sus talentos e intereses. Él hace una representación de cómo funcionan los objetos, y practica emociones que él observa y los combina para formar patrones. Los niños hispanos pueden aprender los papeles de hombres y mujeres de esta manera. Al jugar a la casita, el niño aprende a ayudarle a su esposa a cocinar y a mecer al bebé. Él le da suavemente el biberón al bebé al mecerlo para que se duerma. Otra escena también puede ser representada durante el juego imaginario. Si un niño agarra a un muñeco y le grita o le pega, bien puede estar actuando lo que mira en su hogar o cómo se siente. Si el padre es distante de la familia, y no participa en la crianza de los niños, su niño quizá represente esas acciones en su juego y en su vida real. Las acciones que ha visto y las palabras que ha escuchado de su madre y su padre, en la televisión, o en la casa de un vecino, pueden ser repetidas y representadas en su juego imaginario.

Puede expandir el juego de su niño para que contenga escenas más complejas y ayudarle a describir las emociones que está expresando y las características y las funciones de los objetos. Puede unirse a su juego para mostrarle cómo mecer, alimentar, e interactuar con el bebé, y enseñarle lenguaje y otras conductas que quiere que aprenda. Los niños hispanos pueden beneficiarse al tener como modelo a un hombre noble que permite una expresión abierta de sentimientos y de dominio de sí mismo. Usted puede reconocer y responder a gestos transmitidos al mecer, tararear, o acariciar, así demostrándole al niño una comprensión de las emociones que le ha comunicado. Puede ayudarle a expresar sus temores y preocupaciones por medio de las palabras en lugar de golpear, patalear, o aventar las cosas. Su niño también puede aprender a lidiar con sus temores y ansiedades por medio del juego, al representar el papel del médico que trata de calmar y reconfortar a su paciente, cuando necesita lidiar con sus sentimientos sobre el hecho de que mami volvió al trabajo. Puede ayudarle a resolver algunas de las preocupaciones que surgen de su juego al "convertirse en" uno de los personajes de su juego. A través del juego, también puede ayudarle a establecer límites, por ejemplo, puede usar un muñeco de peluche para "decirle" a otro muñeco de peluche qué tipos de conducta deben usarse en diferentes situaciones. Pero esté consciente del hecho de que algunos niños por naturaleza son más agresivos que otros, y necesitan oportunidades para mostrar su ira a través del juego. Si nos les permite mostrarlo de esta manera, surgirá en una conducta más indeseable más adelante.

Por medio del juego, un niño comienza a utilizar los juguetes u otros objetos para crear patrones e imágenes con relación a las personas, y las cosas, y sus características y funciones. Los bloquecitos pueden representar personas, casas, calles, o animales que ha visto en el pasado. Por medio del juego, él aprende cómo funciona su cuerpo en el espacio, cómo identificar y comprender diferentes emociones. Él describe características sensoriales de cómo la persona o el objeto se siente, huele, suena, y se mira. Su juego, lenguaje, y desarrollo conceptual crecen de ser de una forma fragmentada y sencilla a ser una historia más compleja, con patrones y temas organizados. Él puede hacer que un solo personaje represente muchos papeles o que muchos personajes desempeñen una sola actividad, como jugar a las comadritas, o a la escuelita. Mi hijo Steven separaba sus monitos en dos equipos y jugaba fútbol; Vanessa jugaba a la escuelita con sus muñecos; Sal era el director de todos los muñecos de peluche, los cuales él colocaba en filas.

Éste también puede ser un período muy difícil para usted y para su niño. Después de darse cuenta que es una persona aparte, él comienza a imponer su autonomía. "¡Yo hacerlo!" y "¡Mío!" son algunas palabras que se escuchan con frecuencia entre los niños de dos años. Tal como no tiene ningún control sobre su vejiga o sus evacuaciones, el niño tampoco ejerce control sobre sus emociones. Es muy impulsivo y dice "¡No!" a todo lo que usted le pide hacer. No sabe compartir, y quizá trate de cargar todas sus posesiones con él para que nadie las mire siquiera. Debido a su incapacidad de comunicar sus sentimientos, es muy impulsivo, a punto de gritar, rasguñar, y morder si se siente amenazado. Ésta es una conducta normal para los niños pequeños. Durante este período del desarrollo de un niño, él no es muy sociable con otros niños. Sobre todo, quizá no se lleve bien con sus hermanos, quienes están compitiendo para los juguetes, la comida, y aun el tiempo y la atención de sus padres.

Es un período muy difícil para los padres de un niño de dos años de edad, pero, *con paciencia se gana el cielo*. Uno debe ser paciente y tranquilizador, al aumentar extraordinariamente el lenguaje del niño, y sus habilidades motrices se desarrollan al mismo tiempo. Durante este período, un niño quizá sienta mucha ansiedad, frustración, y temor a aprender nuevas habilidades. Los padres deben ayudar a sus niños a crecer y desarrollarse intelectualmente, lingüísticamente, y físicamente, al apoyarlos durante este período de desequilibrio. Deben pasar mucho tiempo con sus niños para ayudarlos a volver a un estado de seguridad que les permitirá avanzar en su desarrollo. Entre más se desarrollen las habilidades lingüísticas y las habilidades motrices de un niño, mejor podrá comunicar sus necesidades, y más feliz será. Todos los niños tienen la necesidad de alcanzar logros y el éxito. Con cada pequeño logro y cada gran éxito, él gana una confianza que se muestra con una cara orgullosa y radiante de felicidad. Reconozca que está orgulloso de su niño al besarlo, abrazarlo, y aplaudirlo cuando logra una meta. Dígale: "Mi hijito, debes sentirte tan orgulloso de que pudiste hacerlo tú solito".

Un niño seguirá necesitando que usted le asegure entender lo que él siente. Algunos niños sufren un retroceso en su desarrollo cuando están tratando de dominar algo nuevo. Quizá tenga que volver varios pasos atrás para ayudarle a su niño a recuperar esa sensación de seguridad. A veces puede lograr cambiar a su niño de ser llorón o "cabezudo", al mostrarle que comprende sus sentimientos. Siga reflejando sus sentimientos con comentarios como: "Yo sé que te sientes mal porque tu perrito se fue. Pobre perrito, yo te llevaré en el carro a buscarlo". "Yo sé que te sientes enojado porque Juanito rompió tu juguete". Los niños que se vuelven inseguros y se aferran a uno, pueden ser alentados a jugar cerca de uno al principio, pero poco a poco debe animarlos a alejarse más para jugar, asegurándoles que usted está cerca. Por ejemplo: "Mami no se va a ir a ningún lado. Mami está aquí cocinando. Puedes jugar en el otro cuarto y me puedes oír cantando". Si su niño tiene rabietas, puede imponer los límites y aplicar el castigo, pero luego volver a captar su atención y decir: "¿Te sientes mejor ahora? ¿Estás listo para venir a jugar conmigo?" Cuando viene hacia usted, abrácelo y acurrúquelo.

Usted juega un papel importante en ayudar a su niño a progresar por el continuo del juego hacia las actividades más largas y más complejas, las cuales le conducirán a la siguiente etapa de desarrollo. Recuerde, del capítulo sobre el desarrollo cognoscitivo, que un juego de tortillitas puede avanzar a un juego de "Víbora de la mar", al volverse más complejas las habilidades intelectuales, lingüísticas, y motrices de un niño. Por medio de experimentar con el uso de muchas emociones en su juego imaginario, él podrá transferir lo que ha aprendido en su mundo imaginario a su mundo verdadero, donde la capacidad de expresar las ideas emocionales de uno forma una parte crítica del proceso de llegar a ser socialmente competente.

La sexta etapa: El pensamiento emocional—La base para la fantasía, la realidad, y el amor propio—de los treinta hasta los cuarenta y cinco meses de edad

Ésta es la época cuando su niño comienza a desarrollar un sentido de individualidad y cuando su amor propio verdaderamente comienza a formarse. Quizá vea a su niño mirándose al espejo con mucha frecuencia, fijándose en las facciones que lo distinguen de los demás niños. Ayúdele a hacer dibujos de sí mismo, utilizando colores y poniendo detalles que reflejan su singularidad. Recuérdele lo guapo que es él, o lo linda que es ella. El amor propio de los niños proviene de las primeras interacciones y opiniones de los familiares. Asegúrese de decir cosas positivas a su niño porque los comentarios negativos, como "estás feo", "no seas estúpido" o "no seas un bobo", hacen que el niño se sienta despreciable y quizá comience a representar estas conductas si se llega a identificar con ellas. Elogie a su niño cuando realiza algo bueno.

Ayúdele a sentirse bien acerca de quién es. Esto lo preparará para soportar las crueldades que los niños a veces ocasionan. Su niño tal vez venga a casa y le diga con lágrimas: "Mami (o Papi), Juan me dijo que tengo las orejas grandes". "Los niños me dicen gordo". Es importante que usted le ayude a su niño a aceptarse tal como es, con sus talentos y habilidades. Aun si su niño percibe que tiene defectos, o si tiene algún impedimento físico, si las personas significativas en su vida le dicen que es especial, guapo, e importante, es más fácil para él creerlos a ellos y hacer caso omiso de los comentarios negativos de los otros niños. En la película *Forrest Gump*, el papel que hizo la madre del personaje principal, quien lo alentó constantemente a pesar de la percepción que tenían otros de él por ser minusválido, ilustra la importancia de este apoyo en el desarrollo del amor propio positivo de un niño. Los niños son influenciados por lo que dicen sus padres, así que es muy importante que usted tenga conversaciones repletas de comentarios positivos que levanten su ánimo, no que lo desanimen.

Ésta es la etapa del pensamiento lógico emocional. El niño comienza a pensar de una manera más compleja al combinar muchas ideas, sentimientos, y experiencias para formar temas y patrones que ofrezcan una representación más real de la vida. Ahora puede organizar y manipular sus ideas para lograr una comprensión de causa y efecto con relación a sus emociones. Tal como el desarrollo intelectual, el desarrollo emocional y social se fomentan a través de las relaciones, además de a través de los patrones y las conexiones que se forman en el cerebro. Durante esta etapa, su niño puede comenzar a distinguir entre las cosas que son reales y las que no son.

Al completar los tres años de edad, su niño es capaz de jugar con otros niños. Durante esta etapa, se les vuela la imaginación. Por ejemplo, el médico, el maestro, el policía, el bombero, y el astronauta todos son personajes cuyos papeles son representados en el mundo de fantasía de un niño. Ésta es la época cuando los padres deben observar qué intereses tienen sus niños, y luego proporcionar los accesorios necesarios para ellos, además de conseguirles libros sobre los temas que más les fascinan.

Durante los siguientes tres años, los niños harán un millón de preguntas. Tratan de encontrarle sentido a su mundo, a comprenderlo, y ponen a prueba los límites de su ambiente social, emocional, y físico. Son muy observadores y siempre están tratando de descubrir cómo conseguir lo que quieren. Están comenzando a saber y a comprender "causa y efecto". Un niño pequeño que toca suavemente la mejilla de su padre, le da un beso, y le expresa su amor, probablemente conseguirá lo que quiere. Un niño que grita y patalea pronto se dará cuenta que este tipo de conducta no produce resultados deseables.

Éste es el principio de la consciencia moral. Es una época cuando un niño se puede imaginar lo que ocurrirá si hace algo indebido. Ahora puede distinguir entre sus sentimientos y aquéllos de los demás. Durante este período, un niño les pondrá atención a sus padres y obedecerá las reglas, porque no quiere ser castigado o porque quiere ser premiado. Entenderá que ciertas acciones producen premios de corta duración o cierto castigo. Sin embargo, sí hará cosas indebidas, pero tendrá mayor cuidado de que nadie se dé cuenta. Mirará por todos lados para ver si está cerca el padre o esconderá detrás de la espalda la galleta que sabe bien que no debe comer hasta después de la cena. Pero cuando lo agarre justo en el acto de agarrar la galleta, le mira con ese aire de culpable. Si fuera un poco mayor, el padre o la madre probablemente le diría: "No lo niegues, *porque cuando digo que la mula es parda es porque traigo los pelos en la mano*". Es importante mantener una relación sólida y positiva con sus niños. Al mismo tiempo, enséñeles qué es la conducta correcta y qué es inaceptable, y qué son los valores que usted quiere que tengan. Al hacer esto, los niños desarrollaran un sentido del bien y el mal. Es crítico que los padres impongan reglas, valores, y normas de conducta entre los tres y ocho años de edad, y que lo hagan en una manera amorosa, consistente, y racional.

Durante esta etapa, un niño puede reconocer otros puntos de vista y se vuelve más empático. Comienza a desarrollar el sentido de vergüenza y culpabilidad, al darse cuenta del impacto que su conducta tiene en otras personas. Comienza a controlar sus impulsos, porque sabe que sus acciones pueden causar dolor, y que las consecuencias son reales. Esto lo fuerza a planear para el futuro, porque está motivado a lograr un resultado final que le pueda ayudar a portarse de otra manera. Se vuelve más enfocado, más tolerante, más determinado a lograr sus metas deseadas.

Durante esta etapa, un niño comienza a organizar su mundo por tiempo (hoy, mañana, o la próxima semana). Está comenzando a aprender a esperar algo. Puede anticipar lo que va a pasar en el futuro cuando su madre dice: "Espera a que vuelva a casa tu papi", o "Puedes comer un dulce más tarde". Aprenderá que las acciones actuales pueden estar relacionadas con alguna conducta previa cuando escucha a su madre o padre decir: "Vas a jugar con tu hermano por treinta minutos porque lo pegaste, y no se debe pegar ni lastimar a nadie".

Cuando se enoja su niño, ayúdele a aprender cómo controlar y regular su ira. Utilice una voz firme y un equilibrio entre la empatía y la compasión al establecer los límites. Mantenga el control y muéstrele que usted puede controlar sus emociones la mayor parte del tiempo. Levante una ceja y utilice el método ya mencionado que Stanley Greenspan llama la técnica de "ojo a ojo", cuando uno le mira al niño directamente a los ojos, hasta que se calme y se controle. Utilice una voz firme, o quizá pueda distraerlo de lo que le hizo enojar. Ponga en claro que el castigo será por la infracción, un castigo como negarle el privilegio de mirar las caricaturas a la mañana siguiente, o mandarle a su cuarto por un "descanso", hasta que se calme. Dígale que todavía lo quiere, y comuníquele las razones de su disgusto. Permita que se exprese. Si usted no trata de volver a entablar una conversación con él, su resentimiento y rebeldía pueden acumularse. Éstos luego surgirán de nuevo, más tarde, a través de la agresión pasiva, en la forma de juegos de poder o ira sublimada.

Los niños siempre intentarán que sus padres se enfrenten. Los padres tienen que estar unidos en la manera de socializar a sus niños. Es crucial que la madre y el padre estén de acuerdo con relación a los valores y las reglas que quieren para sus niños, además de imponerlos y hacerlos cumplir. Cuando los padres no están de acuerdo, no existe un apoyo mutuo ni una consistencia en la crianza de sus niños. Un padre quizá utilice al niño para desquitarse de su pareja al formar una alianza con el niño. Este tipo de acción puede eventualmente llevar a la separación de la familia. Esto luego implica un enorme peso de culpabilidad para el niño que está metido en medio de ellos. A veces aun cuando los esposos están unidos y ambos desaprueban la conducta del niño, uno de ellos puede identificarse con las emociones del niño por medio de la empatía y la compasión, tratando de replantear, en una manera racional, las razones por su acción. La pareja que está fuera de la disputa puede servir de mediador y ser la fuente de seguridad para el niño además de ser el que ayuda a mantener la harmonía en la familia.

EL ÁRBOL QUE CRECE TORCIDO, NUNCA SU RAMA ENDEREZA

El papel de los padres en el desarrollo emocional y social es de suma importancia durante estos primeros años de vida. Igual a un árbol que requiere un tronco recto y fuerte con raíces profundas, su niño necesita mucha orientación cuando es pequeño, para proporcionar una dirección apropiada en el futuro. Durante los primeros cuatro años de vida, los padres necesitan construir los cimientos esenciales para el desarrollo de una personalidad sana que ayudará a su niño a funcionar como parte de la sociedad más adelante. A través de incontables interacciones con sus padres, los niños pueden desarrollar un sentido de confianza, amor, amor propio, autocontrol, y compasión que les ayudará más adelante en su vida. Al recibir una combinación sana de disciplina y amor, los niños pondrán a prueba sus límites pero aprenderán a controlar sus emociones y conducta.

LA IMPORTANCIA DEL EQUILIBRIO PARA EL DESARROLLO SOCIAL Y EMOCIONAL

Nuestra meta, como padres, es ayudar a nuestros niños a llegar a ser personas emocionalmente competentes. En un mundo de dos culturas, esto incluye lograr y mantener un delicado equilibrio entre dos fuerzas que frecuentemente compiten una contra la otra. Todos los niños necesitan establecer un equilibrio entre ser independientes, responsables, autodisciplinados y competitivos y ser adaptables, interdependientes, compasivos, y empáticos. Los niños hispanos que crecen en un medio ambiente tradicional tal vez tengan que enfrentar la presión adicional de mensajes sociales que refuerzan sólo algunas de estas cualidades. Debe existir un equilibrio entre el colmar a nuestros niños de demasiada atención y no darles ninguna, entre forzarlos a aprender todo por sí mismos y hacer todo por ellos. Debemos encontrar un punto medio entre imponer límites rígidos y severos, y no imponer ninguno, y entre no alentarlos a tener éxito y exigir demasiado.

A veces los padres tratan de evitar las rabietas al cumplir todos los deseos de sus niños, sin enseñarles a tener dominio de sí mismos. Ellos quizá descubran más adelante que sus niños toman decisiones con consecuencias devastadoras, tal como escoger asociarse con la gente equivocada, o tomar drogas, porque no supieron regular sus deseos al considerar las consecuencias de sus actos. Quizá no se den cuenta del efecto que las acciones de otros tengan sobre ellos o viceversa, hasta que sea demasiado tarde. Algunos niños, que tuvieron la oportunidad de tener una vida productiva, están en la prisión hoy porque estaban en el lugar equivocado, en el momento equivocado, y con personas que los manipulaban. Son parecidos a Juan Bobo, incapaces de tomar decisiones sabias y hacer evaluaciones apropiadas porque no pueden hacer la conexión entre las acciones y las consecuencias. Su falta de prudencia y valor los convierte en blancos perfectos para ser víctimas del abuso. El dicho *El camarón que se duerme, se lo lleva la corriente* describe lo que les pasa a los niños a quienes les falta la fortaleza de carácter para navegar por la vida porque sus padres fueron muy permisivos. El dicho *Detrás de la desconfianza está la seguridad* aconseja a los niños sobre la seguridad como resultado de ser precavidos y de saber que existen los límites y las consecuencias a nuestras acciones.

Aquellos niños que están acostumbrados a conseguir todo lo que quieren cuando son pequeños, crecen pensando que el mundo les debe todo lo que desean. Quizá roben o intimiden a otros para conseguir lo que quieren, sin pensar nunca que están haciendo algo indebido. Tal vez no les importe lastimar a quien sea, porque solamente se preocupan por sí mismos. Yo he visto a niños buenos meterse en problemas porque nunca se detuvieron a pensar en cómo sus acciones no solamente les lastimarían a ellos mismos, sino que también les ocasionarían un gran dolor a sus padres, agotarían los recursos de sus padres, y destruirían la estabilidad y la felicidad de su familia. Los niños necesitan ver y comprender la relación entre las acciones y las consecuencias.

Mientras que los niños necesitan amor y atención, los padres necesitan saber que el dar demasiado amor y demasiada atención puede ser igual de dañino que no dar suficiente. Cuando estamos constantemente encima de nuestros niños o tratamos de hacer todo por ellos, no podrán pensar, descubrir, y aprender por sí mismos. Los niños no son perfectos. Ellos cometerán errores, pero requerirán espacio para aprender de esos errores. Recuerde el dicho *El error sólo es fracaso cuando no se convierte en experiencia*. Ayúdeles a descubrir sus talentos y su potencial. Los padres que son demasiado exigentes y controladores pueden provocar una sensación de ansiedad, culpabilidad, e inseguridad en sus niños. Quizá sientan que es imposible lograr a alcanzar las expectativas y las normas tan altas de sus padres. Los padres que protegen excesivamente y consienten pueden producir unos niños arrogantes, egoístas, y malos, quienes serán rechazados por sus compañeros y tal vez no puedan funcionar independientemente ni sostener relaciones íntimas.

Del otro lado del espectro, si los padres no son suficientemente responsivos a las necesidades de sus niños durante estos años formativos críticos, las repercusiones en el desarrollo también pueden ser serias. Los niños a veces se sentirán impulsados a portarse mal, a causa de la ira o la rebeldía. Los niños necesitan tener reglas y límites, tanto como necesitan recibir amor y atención. Necesitan disciplina firme, justa, y consistente de parte de padres amorosos.

Mientras que sea crucial siempre proveerles a los niños un amor incondicional y atención, después de los ocho meses de edad ellos también deben aprender a lidiar con la frustración, el rechazo, y la desilusión, como resultado de no siempre conseguir todo lo que desean. A veces cuando los padres quieren que todo sea ideal, de ensueño, todos los días, sus niños quizá no puedan encarar el mundo verdadero, que no es siempre perfecta, y donde ocurren cosas que están fuera de su control. Yo he conocido a niños provenientes de familias muy estables que intentan suicidarse porque no supieron aceptar el rechazo de su primera novia, la admonición de un maestro firme, o un fracaso personal.

Después de los tres años de edad, los niños deben tener contacto con otros niños para aprender habilidades sociales efectivas. No los podemos resguardar de las emociones negativas. Algunos de los padres de AVANCE, igual a muchas otras familias hispanas, tenían la tendencia de mantener encerrados a sus niños, lejos y protegidos de la influencia negativa de otros. Por medio del arreglo de un tiempo de juego supervisado para sus niños, para que puedan tener interacción con otros niños, los padres pueden aprender los beneficios de estas interacciones. Si los niños aprenden cómo lidiar con las emociones intensas cuando son pequeños, dentro del contexto del ambiente seguro y de apoyo de su hogar, del hogar de unos amigos de confianza, o de una guardería, ellos aprenderán que estas emociones forman una parte de la vida normal. Si sienten las emociones como el rechazo, el fracaso, y la frustración cuando son pequeños, serán mejor capacitados para lidiar con ellas en el futuro.

Tal como noté antes, los niños que nunca han sentido el amor no pueden dar a su vez algo que no poseen. Si son víctimas del abuso y la negligencia, tal vez estén programados para más adelante abusar a sus propios niños y para transferir una enorme cantidad de ira, resentimiento, y dolor a otros. Éstas son las personas que lastimarán y manipularán a los más débiles sin sentir ningún remordimiento. Los niños requieren un equilibrio de amor, atención, comprensión, éxitos, límites, y reglas.

ATENCIÓN: ¡MÍRAME!

Cuando los padres no responden a las señales de sus bebés, sus niños son afectados de una manera adversa por este rechazo. Si no reciben la atención social y emocional que buscan y necesitan, al principio tal vez se sientan desilusionados y frustrados, y luego, con el tiempo se retraen a un estado de protección de sí mismos donde juegan con sus manos o se maman el dedo. Se vuelven introvertidos, retraídos y con una barrera de inseguridad que los mantiene aislados de la gente. Igual a los niños estudiados en la investigación sobre los orfelinatos, cuyas necesidades físicas se satisfacían pero no así sus necesidades emocionales de ser tocados y estimulados, estos niños quizá no se desarrollen bien bajo tales condiciones.

Los padres necesitan estar conscientes de que a veces el tipo de atención que ellos les proporcionan a sus niños se ve afectado por su propio estado emocional. En algunas familias, un niño puede convertirse en la víctima de una madre que sufre de depresión, ansiedad, o de mucha tensión como resultado de abuso de parte de su esposo, o a causa de violencia en la comunidad, o de problemas económicos. La madre no tiene la energía necesaria para interactuar con su niño, demostrar su cariño, o darle a su niño la atención que él necesita. Si ella fue víctima de abuso cuando era niña, quizá maltrate a sus propios niños, o bien tal vez trate de sobrecompensar por esto al darles demasiada atención al crecer. A veces una madre no quiere formar vínculos afectivos muy estrechos con su niño, porque él le recuerda a una persona que provoca emociones fuertes, como un esposo que la abandonó, un padre que la maltrató, o un niño que falleció. A veces el resentimiento que las hermanas sienten hacia los hermanos varones porque no tenían que hacer mucho en la casa, puede dirigirse hacia sus hijos varones más adelante. Puede ser necesario que las madres o los padres reciban terapia de un servicio profesional de la salud mental para poder enfrentarse a estos sentimientos negativos y resolver sus conflictos internos que pueden producir ansiedad e ira, antes de que afecte adversamente a sus niños. Los padres deben tratar de ser fuertes, física y mentalmente, porque cómo se sienten puede afectar su comportamiento.

Los padres tienen tres opciones con relación a cómo tratar a sus niños: pueden proveerles una atención positiva, una atención negativa, o ninguna atención. Los niños poseen una necesidad tan grande de ser reconocidos y de que los tomen en cuenta que tratarán de conseguir atención a como dé lugar, aun una atención negativa. Aunque lo mejor es darles a sus niños atención positiva la mayor parte del tiempo, los niños se sentirán impulsados a portarse de una manera que provocará un castigo, si ellos sienten que ésa es la única forma de conseguir atención. Desdichadamente, muchos padres caen en la trampa de reforzar y premiar la mala conducta, al sólo responder a los niños que rompen las reglas. Un padre debe hacer caso omiso de la mala conducta con la que quiere acabar, pero sólo si no le causa ningún daño a su niño ni a nadie más, como en el caso de una rabieta. En vez de eso, debe ser como un detective y buscar la buena conducta para premiarla, como cuando guarda sus juguetes o ayuda a sacar los trastes del lavaplatos. A través del elogio y la atención positiva, los padres refuerzan la conducta deseada, la que quieren que se repita. Si un niño recibe atención positiva, no tiene necesidad de portarse mal para conseguir la atención de su mami y su papi.

Los premios pueden ser tan sencillos como una sonrisa, una palmadita, o unas cuantas palabras bondadosas: "Tú y tu hermano están jugando tan bien"; "Gracias por ayudarme a poner la mesa"; "Eso es, *todo tiene su lugar y todo en su lugar*"; "Hiciste un buen trabajo de guardar todos tus juguetes donde pertenecen"; "Mira qué guapo te ves con tu cabello todo peinadito"; "Me gusta cómo hueles después de bañarte"; "Ah, mi hijito, qué bonita casa construiste"; "Gracias por estar tan calladito mientras yo dormía al bebé".

Un importante consejo para recordar es que debe compartir actividades con sus niños de vez en cuando—como leer un libro o dibujar algo juntos—para poder darles la atención que necesitan. Pase tiempo de calidad y de uno a uno, de este tipo, con cada uno de sus niños. Con demasiada frecuencia, los padres dejan a sus niños sentados enfrente de la televisión por horas, sin tomarlos en cuenta para nada, mientras hagan sus quehaceres. Los padres pueden estar tan ocupados que se pasan todo el día sin pasar cuando menos treinta minutos de tiempo de calidad con sus niños. Apague la televisión. Guarde el periódico. Mire a su niño y tenga una interacción con él. De otra manera, la próxima vez que tenga una interacción con él, puede que sea para darle un castigo.

En muchas familias hispanas, la expresión de ciertos tipos de emociones no es algo fácil, es más, en algunos hogares, está muy mal visto. Los padres quizá no muestren fácilmente el gusto ni le dan un elogio a su niño, por temor a convertirlo en un niño mimado, o un niño orgulloso que se cree mucho. Muchos padres hispanos sí crean un equilibrio sano entre elogiar y hacer lo que necesitan para mantener humildes a sus niños. En mi familia, mi madre siempre solía decir: "Ay, qué bonitas están mis hijas", pero el momento en que ella pensaba que las palabras se nos subían a la cabeza, inmediatamente decía, "No se chiflen" (no se pongan mimadas), o "no se descompongan" (no pierdan los estribos). Ella decía que aunque estaba muy orgullosa de nuestros logros, no se miraba bien alardear de eso todo el tiempo. Ella se suscribe al dicho *Alabanza en boca propia es vituperio*. Por un lado, ella quería que fuéramos competitivos, que ganáramos, y que probáramos que somos tan buenos como cualquier otra persona; sin embargo, por otro lado, ella no quería que diéramos la impresión de que pensábamos que éramos mejores que los demás.

Ella creía y nos enseñaba, de igual manera que los aztecas enseñaron a sus niños, que tenía que haber un equilibrio. *Todo con moderación.* Tal como se dice de la veladora, *ni tanto que queme al santo, ni tanto que no lo alumbre.* Unos padres que colman a sus niños de elogios y les dan todo lo que quieren, corren el riesgo de que sus niños crezcan mimados, malos, y egoístas, o bien, les quebrantan el espíritu. *Todo el que a su hijo consiente, va engordando una serpiente.* Mientras que lo ideal es lograr un equilibrio, es mejor pecar *ligeramente* por el lado de dar demasiado, que el de no dar suficiente. Así que proporcióneles a sus niños atención y reconozcan su existencia, sus talentos, y sus éxitos, pero recuerde la importancia del equilibrio.

LA NECESIDAD DE LOGRAR EL ÉXITO: EL DESEO DE APRENDER

Todos los niños tienen la necesidad de lograr el éxito, desarrollarse, aprender, y descubrir, tal como se discutió en el capítulo anterior. Tienen un impulso innato de crear, inventar, y experimentar, además de sentir una sensación de competencia. Tienen el anhelo de dominar las cosas, y de controlar su medio ambiente. También tienen la necesidad de descubrir quiénes son, qué son sus puntos fuertes, sus limitaciones, y su potencial. Los niños exploran algo nuevo a cada oportunidad por la euforia y la satisfacción que derivan al tener un impacto en su medio ambiente. Mientras que a su niño quizá le gusten sus palabras de elogio, él es persistente y determinado a lograr sus metas porque sus logros le provocan un sentido de confianza y competencia. Sus cariños son importantes para reconocer sus esfuerzos, pero su papel es también proveer un medio ambiente estimulante en el cual él tendrá desafíos y motivaciones. Los niños necesitan sentir que usted está allí para apoyarlos a intentar algo nuevo. Necesitan que usted esté allí cuando fracasan, no sólo como un cojín emocional, sino para ayudarles a sobreponerse a sus fracasos y a aprender de ellos.

Cuando sus niños logran algo, elógielos inmediatamente. Ponga énfasis en sus logros y reconozca sus nuevos talentos. Cuando ellos crean, construyen, e inventan cosas, exponga sus obras en el refrigerador u otro lugar prominente donde todos las puedan mirar. Cuando uno de sus niños alcance un logro mayor, como caminar o comer solo, reúna a la familia para aplaudirle y darle un abrazo. Pregúntele cómo se siente. Cuando mis niños alimentaban o bañaban a los perros, yo les decía: "¡Buen trabajo! Son tan responsables. Buffy tiene mucha suerte al tener a personas que lo quieren y lo cuidan". A todos les encantaba el reconocimiento. Cuando no lograban éxito en algo, yo les animaba a intentar de nuevo, y los apoyaba sin ser entrometida o metiche. Los padres necesitan tener cuidado de no empujar a sus niños más allá de sus límites, ni de impulsar a sus niños a lograr el éxito sólo para lograr sus propias aspiraciones. Uno tiene que respetar la individualidad de cada uno de sus niños y ayudarles a descubrir sus propios intereses, y ayudarles a lograr su potencial individual.

Los padres deben tener expectativas realistas de cuánto pueden hacer sus niños, basadas en su etapa de desarrollo y sus intereses. De vez en cuando, yo les daba a mis niños una pista sobre cómo resolver una adivinanza o crucigrama o algún misterio, un gesto que no siempre me agradecían. A veces los padres tienen que esperar mucho para que completen alguna tarea sus niños, un proceso que puede parecer insoportable al principio. En algunas ocasiones, una sugerencia en el momento apropiado es bien recibida.

Algunas cosas eran muy difíciles para mis niños, y necesitaban ayuda para evitar sentirse frustrados, así que yo dividía la tarea que yo quería que hicieran, en partes. Por ejemplo, cuando ellos estaban intentando ponerse los calcetines, comer solos, ir al excusado, o llevarse bien con sus hermanos, yo los elogiaba o premiaba a cada paso que los acercaba a su meta. Si usted quiere que su niño se ponga solo los calcetines, necesita premiarlo por simplemente lograr meter los deditos del pie dentro del calcetín. Dígale: "Yo sabía que podías hacer eso. Ya eres un niño grande, casi te pusiste los calcetines tú solito". Más adelante, lo alienta a ponérselo un poco más, tal vez logrando hacerlo hasta el tobillo, y luego dice, "Casi lo hiciste, mi hijito. Pudiste poner el calcetín hasta el tobillo. Eso está muy bien. La próxima vez podrás hacerlo todo tú solo". Cuando por fin logra completar la tarea sin ayuda, prémielo otra vez con una sonrisa y un abrazo. Pregúntele cómo se siente ahora que lo puede hacer solito. Él tiene que interiorizar esa sensación agradable que le provoca alcanzar su meta.

Después del calcetín, trate de enseñarle la diferencia entre el zapato derecho y el izquierdo. Luego desafíele a aprender a amarrarse las agujetas. Cuando logre dominar esta tarea, le puede decir que se ponga sus calcetines y sus zapatos, y todos los pasos encajarán automáticamente. Mi esposo y yo estábamos allí para apoyar y animar a nuestros niños lo más que podíamos, cuando dieron sus primeros pasos, construyeron una torre de bloquecitos, o cuando anduvieron solos en bicicleta.

Poco a poco los animamos a ser valientes y a atreverse a salir solos, comenzado por las veces aterrorizadoras e inseguras, cuando nuestros niños nos envolvían las piernas con sus brazos, o se aferraban de mi falda y no la querían soltar. Necesitamos ayudarles a arriesgarse, apoyarles cuando fracasan, y ayudarles a aprender de sus errores. Los niños necesitan tener éxito para sentir que son competentes. Con cada conquista, se dan cuenta de que pueden dominar su medio ambiente. No es saludable negarles a los niños la libertad de expresar sus verdaderos sentimientos. Usted debe alentarlos a pensar en diferentes maneras de resolver un problema. Permítales tomar decisiones con relación a las cosas que los afectan a ellos. Asígneles tareas y responsabilidades; manténgase firme en sus expectativas y no haga usted lo que es la responsabilidad de ellos hacer. Los padres dañan a sus hijos cuando no les enseñan acerca de las consecuencias de no ser responsable. La mejor manera de ayudar a nuestros niños es permitirles tomar decisiones y hacerlos responsables de ellas. Los padres tienen el derecho de estar en desacuerdo y ejercer su derecho de "veto" cuando se trata de decisiones "mayores" que pueden provocarles daño a sus niños. Pero es importante que les animen a sus niños a tomar decisiones y a alcanzar un sentido de responsabilidad. Hágales preguntas como: "¿Cuál camisa quieres que te compre?" o "Aquí está el dinero, ¿vas y pagas la película, por favor?"

COMPRENDA A SU NIÑO

Los niños necesitan sentirse comprendidos. Antes de que un niño tenga la capacidad de hablar, sus padres sólo pueden adivinar qué problemas tiene por las señales que él les da. Puede patalear y gritar para avisarle qué es lo que desea. La persona con quien ha establecido vínculos afectivos y que ha satisfecho sus necesidades, también le ayudará a ser comprendido y a comprender.

Al crecer un niño y tener interacción con el mundo fuera de la familia, sus sentimientos se verán afectados de gran manera por las palabras y las acciones de otros. Necesitará tener a padres que mostrarán que comprenden por lo que está pasando. Los padres necesitarán proveer el apoyo para ayudarle a sobreponerse a contratiempos, fracasos, y rechazos. No es fácil para los niños expresar sus emociones con palabras, ya sean expresivos por naturaleza, o no. Ellos tal vez decidan no compartir sus sentimientos. De nuevo, los padres tienen que ser como detectives. Tienen que descifrar qué es lo que le está molestando al niño que vuelve a casa de mal humor, con los hombros caídos, o con un genio tal que se nota que va a estallar con la más pequeña provocación. Usted sabe que está disgustado cuando avienta la puerta, o empuja los muebles hacia un lado. Hágale saber que comprende su ira al reflejar sus sentimientos. Dígale: "Estás realmente enojado. ¿Te gustaría platicar?" o "Parece que alguien hizo o dijo algo que te molestó mucho, ¿te gustaría hablar de ello?"

Cosas como perder un juego, no ser aceptado al equipo, no ser aceptado o no caerle bien a alguien o ser intimidado por alguien, todos estos son temas que los padres tendrán que ayudarles a sus niños a enfrentar. Sin embargo, no les puede resolver directamente sus problemas. Al crecer, tendrán que encontrar o descubrir sus propias soluciones. Si no le están invitando a una fiesta, quizá el motivo sea su propia actitud y conducta ofensiva, las cuales sólo él puede cambiar. La actitud de un padre es igual de importante que el consejo que ofrece. El tomar el tiempo para escuchar, poner atención, preguntar, y contestar preguntas, les hace saber a sus niños que ellos son importantes, que usted se preocupa por ellos, y que los comprende. Una vez que se establezca esta relación de comunicación, usted puede sugerir amorosamente una conducta alternativa o correctiva.

También lo contrario es cierto. Los padres que poseen una actitud negativa, pueden afectar adversamente a sus niños. Las palabras duras provocan sentimientos de incompetencia, falta de valía, impotencia, y baja autoestima. Provocan que los niños sean más tímidos, defensivos, o malos que lo normal. Una imagen propia negativa será muy difícil de cambiar cuando el niño crece, y quizá él escoja asociarse con otros que dan validez a su imagen propia negativa. Las palabras duras y las acciones severas también provocarán a los niños ira, agresión pasiva, una falta de motivación, y la postergación. El burlarse de nuestros niños, o reaccionar de manera excesiva, cuando algo sale mal les hará darse por vencidos y negarse a intentarlo de nuevo, pero la crítica constructiva en realidad es beneficiosa, si se hace en una manera sensible y amorosa.

EL SENTIDO DE PERTENECER: LA FAMILIA, LOS AMIGOS, Y LA RELIGIÓN

Hay un refrán que dice, *lo que viene del mar, al mar vuelve*. Esta pequeña sabiduría me recuerda el consuelo que acompaña al sentido de pertenecer, el cual todo el mundo ansia. Todos los niños necesitan sentirse seguros al pertenecer a algo más grande que ellos mismos para poder sentir su valía, su dignidad.

Primero, necesitan sentirse parte de una familia que les da validez, los acepta, los valora, y muestra preocupación por su bienestar. Necesitan tener una familia que les ayudará a sentir alegría por medio de experiencias memorables. Desde que el mundo es mundo, las personas han tenido la necesidad de pertenecer a un clan o a una familia extensa que les protegerá, cuidará, y apoyará. Como hispanos, nuestra sólida conexión a la familia y la comunidad nos puede servir para proporcionarles a nuestros niños el sentido de seguridad que todos los seres humanos anhelan.

La familia se convierte en un remanso de paz, donde los niños pueden "soltarse la melena" y donde pueden crecer y desarrollarse. (Véase la sección sobre "la familia".) Cuando los niños sufren rechazos o dolores, siempre pueden contar con la familia para proporcionarles afirmación y asistencia, y para reabastecerlos. Dentro de la familia, los niños deben ser amados, aceptados incondicionalmente, y tratados con igualdad y justicia. Cuando no lo son, los niños le harán saberlo a través de sus acciones o sus palabras: *"O todos hijos, o todos entenados"*.

Nuestras tradiciones y creencias establecen una conexión entre nuestros niños y sus antepasados, y les hace sentir que forman parte de un continuo de la vida. Al crecer los niños, también es importante ayudarles a sentir una conexión con el mundo fuera de la familia. Se puede lograr esto al permitirles participar en grupos como los niños exploradores, "Boy Scouts" o "Girl Scouts", "Boys' Club" o "Girls' Club", o las organizaciones para jóvenes de las iglesias, o en equipos deportivos. Es necesario que desarrollen relaciones y que adquieran un sentido de pertenecer y validez que extiende más allá de la familia inmediata. Se ha encontrado que la espiritualidad protege en contra de la tensión y la depresión.

Desdichadamente, algunos niños no tienen una asociación con familia, amigos, ni religión; quizá sientan que nadie los toma en cuenta para nada, aun pueden sentirse totalmente aislados. Aun cuando los padres estén juntos, tal vez no siempre están allí, disponibles para sus niños. A los niños se les dan cosas materiales, pero no el tiempo, la atención, y la energía que son necesarios para tener un sentido de familia. El dinero no puede comprar el amor y el respeto de nuestros niños. Si ellos no logran un sentido de pertenecer, aceptación, y amor de la familia y otras instituciones importantes, lo buscarán fuera de la familia, quizá en una pandilla.

Los padres hispanos a veces tienen dificultad para soltar a sus niños cuando ya son adultos. Con frecuencia quieren tenerlos cerca para ejercer más control sobre ellos, un sentimiento que existe tanto en el caso de los hijos varones como el de las hijas. Quizá teman que "algo terrible" les pueda pasar al estar solos en una ciudad extraña sin la familia no para ayudarles. Mi madre creiá que todos su hijos eran diferentes y requerían una orientación distinta. Algunos niños requieren más orientación que otros, pero, comenzando por los primeros años, los padres deben darles a todos sus niños suficiente libertad dentro de límites seguros, para permitirles explorar, experimentar, tomar decisiones, y arriesgarse, para que puedan crecer y desarrollarse bien. Aun si nuestros niños están fuera de la casa, en la escuela, en un campamento, o en la universidad, nuestras interacciones tempranas con ellos deben establecer la seguridad que necesitan para sentirse cómodos en su trato con otros y al estar lejos de la familia.

LA RIVALIDAD ENTRE HERMANOS: DE LA RIVALIDAD A LA HERMANDAD

Dos gatos en un costal, juntos no pueden estar. Si usted tiene a más de un niño, puede anticipar que habrá rivalidad entre ellos. Desde la época de Caín y Abel, y José y sus muchos hermanos envidiosos, los hermanos han caído fuera de feliz harmonía. Nuestros niños van a pelear, atormentarse, discutir, molestarse, y hacerse burla unos a otros. En algún momento, un niño quizá desee que otro nunca hubiera nacido. Se persiguen alrededor de la casa, gritándose y riéndose a la vez.

Yo he escuchado a mis angelitos decir: "Mamá, mira lo que hizo ella. ¡Haz algo!" Han gritado: "¡Él fue el que comenzó!" "¡Yo lo tenía primero!" "¡Él tiene todos los privilegios!" "¡Nunca haces que ella haga nada!" "¡Mami me quiere más a mí que a ti!" "¡Él me tocó!" "¡No toques a mi papi!" Algunos padres a veces tienen ganas de simplemente levantar los brazos y llorar de frustración, y del temor que algún día sus niños se van a matar. ¡La rivalidad entre hermanos puede enloquecer a los padres! Yo he escuchado a algunas madres decir: "Mis niños están bárbaros, son terribles y caranchos. ¿Qué voy a hacer con ellos?" Bueno, no puede regalar a sus niños. Están aquí para quedarse. Y, probablemente ni usted tendrá un ataque de nervios ni sus niños se matarán. Sin embargo, sí debe mantener la calma y tratar de comprender por qué se portan sus niños de esta manera.

Hay muchas razones por las cuales los niños aparentan ser egoístas y malos y por lo cual parecen estar siempre en un estado de guerra con sus hermanos. Quizá se sientan enojados o irritables porque tienen hambre o sueno, o están cansados. La causa puede radicar en algo que comieron, como un alimento con mucho azúcar o con colorante artificial, ambos de los cuales los pueden hacer muy activos. Tal vez sientan celos o envidia de algo que hizo otro o algo que posee. Quizá estén lo que algunas madres hispanas llaman "chipilones", como resultado de los celos provocados por la llegada de un hermanito recién nacido. Quizá exijan toda la atención de los padres, o tal vez teman perder su atención o amor a causa del recién llegado. A veces la agresión o el resentimiento acumulado en contra de alguien más grande, es desviado y dirigido al hermano más débil o indefenso. Puede parecer que los niños de vez en cuando simplemente quieren pelear para crear un poco de excitación o porque sienten curiosidad sobre qué pasará si pellizcan a uno de sus hermanos o arruinan uno de sus dibujos.

A veces sin darnos cuenta, nosotros los padres podemos ser la causa de la rivalidad entre los hermanos cuando inadvertidamente le asignamos a uno como "el hijo favorito, el consentido". El niño recibe más atención, mientras que a los otros no se les toma en cuenta, o se les rechaza. Los padres hispanos a veces realzan las imperfecciones de sus niños al llamarles cosas como *llorona* o *tonto*, o cuando se refieren al niño que consideran el más lindo o el más inteligente como *el chulo*, o *el más vivo*. Los sutiles comentarios despectivos pueden producir profundas cicatrices emocionales que pueden afectar las relaciones entre los hermanos por muchos años. Este resentimiento se puede transferir subconscientemente a otras personas más adelante.

Cuando las jóvenes, por ser las mujercitas, son obligadas a cuidar a sus hermanos varones, a cocinar para ellos, planchar sus camisas, o limpiar tras de ellos, ellas quizá más adelante dirijan este resentimiento no sólo hacia sus hermanos varones, sino hacia sus hijos varones también. Lo contrario también puede ocurrir con los niños a quienes no se les permite expresar sus emociones. Si lo hacen, son llamados chillón, o vieja, así que esconden sus sentimientos a como dé lugar. Ellos también quizá guarden resentimientos en contra de las hermanas que eran permitidas mostrar libremente sus emociones. Quizá también se les haya dicho que se portaran como "el hombre de la casa", lo cual es una expectativa no realista y más de lo que pueden lograr. Si no cumplen con las expectativas de la gente, comienzan a poner en cuestión su sexualidad. Todos los niños necesitan sentir amor y atención. Necesitan sentirse especiales y competentes, y que los quieran y los necesiten. Los padres deben tener expectativas altas pero realistas de todos sus niños basadas en sus intereses y talentos.

Hay otros factores que provocan coraje o tensión entre los hermanos. La personalidad de un niño, el orden de nacimiento de los hermanos, la edad, el sexo, y el medio ambiente, todos estos factores tienen una influencia sobre la conducta y pueden provocar competencia y rencor. Con mucha frecuencia, el primogénito tiene la tendencia de ser el más firme y el que tiene más confianza en sí mismo. Algunas investigaciones sugieren que es probable que el niño mayor sea el más exitoso de los hermanos. Muchos líderes y ejecutivos son primogénitos. Esto puede ser el resultado de la atención, el tiempo, la energía, y las altas expectativas que recibieron de sus padres.

Si los otros niños recibieran el mismo tipo de atención, también ellos podrían alcanzar su plenitud. Desdichadamente, algunos padres tienen que repartir su tiempo y energía limitados entre varios niños. Mi madre, quien tuvo ocho hijos, solía decir que después del tercer niño, se vuelve imposible mantener esa atención especial de uno a uno con solamente dos padres para proporcionarla. Ella creía que era importante enseñarles a los niños mayores a encargarse de algunas de las responsabilidades de cultivar y dar cariño. Mi suegra solía poner en parejas y tomados de la mano a sus niños cuando salían de excursión. Mi madre esperaba que los niños mayores ayudaran a los más pequeños con su tarea de la escuela. A veces, en los hogares hispanos de familia grande, quizá sean los más pequeños que estén mejor preparados para alcanzar su plenitud debido a toda la ayuda que recibieron de los mayores.

En la cultura latina, el mayor de los niños varones y de las mujeres generalmente tienen más privilegios, lo cual puede provocar celos. Esto es particularmente cierto cuando los padres les dicen a los más pequeños que no pongan en cuestión la autoridad de sus hermanos mayores. En muchas familias, los niños de en medio siempre tienen que luchar para conseguir atención. Esto puede provocar que sean más agresivos y manipuladores. La rivalidad tiene la tendencia de ser más intensa cuando es entre niños con un año y medio a tres años de diferencia y entre niños del mismo sexo. Los niños más pequeños generalmente son más protegidos por los padres y los hermanos los miran como mimados. Puede que una niña tenga una relación especial con su madre o tenga a su papi encantado con ella y deseoso de cumplir sus caprichos. Quizá la llamen la consentida.

La rivalidad entre hermanos forma parte del curso normal del desarrollo. Es un efecto secundario necesario en la lucha por autonomía de un niño, y de su necesidad de mirar profundamente dentro de sí mismo para descubrir quién es y qué tanto puede salirse con la suya. A los niños se les debe alentar a descubrir la amplia gama de emociones que poseen, desde el amor, la bondad, y el entusiasmo, hasta la agresión, el resentimiento, y los celos o la envidia. Usted debe orientarlos en la expresión de sus sentimientos y la resolución de sus propios problemas dentro de los confines seguros del hogar. Es dentro del hogar donde primero podrán controlar su ira y sus deseos impulsivos. La rivalidad entre hermanos, si se orienta por medio de límites, reglas, y amor incondicional, hasta puede ayudar a los niños a aprender a controlarse, a defenderse, y a ser firmes y fuertes en un mundo donde acechan los obstáculos. La rivalidad entre hermanos, dentro de un contexto seguro y amoroso, puede servir de vehículo para preparar a los niños a vivir en la sociedad.

Al establecer un hogar donde reina el cariño, el amor, y el orden, donde todos procuran el bienestar de los demás, los padres pueden alentar a sus niños a amarse unos a otros, a compartir, y a ser empáticos. Los hermanos mayores pueden servir de modelos de conducta a los más pequeños; pueden alentar, desafiar, enseñar, e inspirar. Con el tiempo, aprenderán la lección duradera de todos los hogares latinos: los hermanos se deben cuidar, amar, y apoyar uno al otro.

Los niños que no tienen hermanos pueden tener una ventaja emocional e intelectual, ya que tienen la atención total de los padres. Por otro lado, quizá tengan menos desafíos sociales, a menos que sus padres hagan arreglos periódicamente para que puedan estar en la compañía de otros niños. Los padres de un solo niño todavía pueden impartir los mismos valores de compasión, consideración, cooperación, y empatía cuando él está en compañía de otros. Esto puede ser en casa de parientes o vecinos, en una guardería, en un evento deportivo, en un campamento, o en un club para niños. Los padres también pueden "adoptar" a una familia o ayudar en un comedor de beneficencia y así enseñarle al niño la alegría de dar a otros.

El papel de los padres consiste en ayudar a su niño a controlar sus emociones e impulsos, a proporcionar amor, a comprender, y a ayudarle a descubrir su identidad y sus puntos fuertes. Así podrá tener mejor probabilidad de crecer y de llegar a ser un miembro competente y contribuyente de la sociedad. Una vez que logre esto, habrá alcanzado lo que Abraham Maslow llama la "realización propia" cuando una persona ha satisfecho la mayoría de sus necesidades, y le gusta su propia forma de ser, y acepta a otros. La realización propia significa tener relaciones que satisfacen y cambian, desarrollar la competencia, aprender a encauzar su propio camino, y tener un sentido de valores. Una persona que ha logrado la realización propia es una que se acerca a alcanzar su potencial y se siente satisfecha de sus logros y da de sí para crear un mundo mejor.

LA EXPERIENCIA PERSONAL: EQUILIBRANDO "EL SUBIBAJA" DE LA RIVALIDAD ENTRE HERMANOS

Usted ya sabe que las personalidades afectan la conducta de un niño. La personalidad fuerte de Steven lo inducía a volverse necio y a estallar en ira cuando algo lo molestaba. Tenía un genio vivo y era agresivo, y esas características le ayudaron en su papel de luchador por la justicia y la igualdad. La personalidad tranquila de Sal y su deseo de dicha eterna mantenía sus emociones refrenadas. Con frecuencia chocaba su personalidad tranquila con la personalidad extrovertida de Steven. Sin embargo, a través de la agresión pasiva trataba de desquitarse de Steven cuando menos lo esperaba él. Vanessa y Steven, con tres años de diferencia, han sido inseparables. Vanessa era la seguidora de Steven, sin embargo se le caía encima cuando se fastidiaba. Estas personalidades fuertes me mostraron que la rivalidad entre hermanos puede ser semejante al vaivén del subibaja.

Primero, un niño se sube por encima de sus hermanos para captar la atención de sus padres o conseguir lo que quiere, hasta que otro niño logre forzarse a la cima, a expensas del otro hermano. Vanessa aprendió rápidamente cómo mantener su posición en contra de sus hermanos. Ella utilizaba su posición como "la única niña" y como "bebé" para subir a la parte alta del subibaja y conseguir que Mamá y Papá intervinieran hasta que nos dimos cuenta que nos estaba manipulando. Sin embargo, Vanessa, por medio de sus habilidades para negociar, servía como mediadora en la competencia entre sus hermanos varones. Ella resultó ser la que lograba volver a establecer la harmonía en la casa cuando sus hermanos peleaban. Ella poseía un sentido más claro del bien y del mal a una edad más joven, a diferencia de Steven, que siempre estaba buscando cómo salirse con la suya. Al paso de los años, Steven se volvió más calmado, Sal se volvió más agresivo, y Vanessa se volvió más impredecible cuando cumplió los doce años de edad. La rivalidad entre hermanos se transfirió a Vanessa y Sal, probablemente porque se volvieron muy parecidos, y Steven se las arreglaba, cuando podía, para subirse a lo alto del subibaja como el "niño bueno". Mi familia es típica de otras familias cuyos niños luchan constantemente por estar en lo alto, lo cual ocasiona muchos desafíos para todos los padres que quieren llevar a sus niños de donde se encuentran, a donde deben estar.

El papel de los padres consiste en asegurarse de que cada niño está en lo alto del subibaja. También tiene que tratar de conseguir que sus hijos encuentren un término medio en el vaivén de la rivalidad entre hermanos, que logrará volver a unos más comunicativos y refrenar a otros de su conducta fuera de control. El equilibrio ayudará a nuestros niños a lograr su autonomía, a descubrir su identidad, y a tener confianza en sí mismos. Les ayudará a apreciar el valor de la interdependencia. Aunque pueda parecer muy frustrante, sí se puede lograr. Los niños pueden cambiar su conducta. Hay muchas estrategias que les pueden ayudar a manejar la rivalidad entre hermanos y que tienen el propósito de moldear la conducta de sus niños.

A veces los padres caen en la trampa de dejarse meter en los conflictos o discusiones de sus niños. Es tan fácil para los padres suponer quién es el culpable en un conflicto y a corregir una situación que parece estar escalando fuera de control. El método autoritario que utilizaba su padre con usted puede, bajo ciertas circunstancias, producir resentimientos que pueden provocar resultados indeseables, contrarios a lo deseado, más adelante, especialmente si el inocente es nombrado como culpable. Usted tendrá que guardar su energía para los asuntos mayores, más importantes. Cuando yo trataba de intervenir en las disputas entre mis niños, ambos lados invariablemente decidían que yo les había arruinado su juego. Luego me decían que si yo simplemente les hubiera dado más tiempo, ellos habrían solucionado sus propios problemas. El niño de cuyo lado yo me puse, defendía al otro y se quejaba que "todo estaba bien" hasta que yo llegué. Después de varias de estas experiencias donde miraba a mis niños terminar por reírse y abrazarse después de un pleito, yo decidí que comenzaría a implementar ciertas reglas nuevas: quedarme fuera y dejarlos resolver sus propios problemas. Porque tal como dice el dicho, *el mejor torero es el de la barrera.*

Por ejemplo, mi esposo y yo ya no íbamos a permitir más chismes ni acusaciones a menos que la situación fuera peligrosa o algo donde peligraba la vida de alguien. No íbamos a intervenir, ni ponernos de parte de nadie, ni convertirnos en árbitros ni jueces. Íbamos a dejar que ellos arreglaran las cosas para que aprendieran a resolver solos sus problemas. Lo más que haríamos como mediadores sería reconocer lo enojados que parecían estar y ayudarles a identificar el problema que necesitaba resolverse. Luego los alentaríamos a encontrar una solución satisfactoria para ambos. Es importante recordarles a sus niños que usted tiene la esperanza y la fe de que puedan encontrar ellos una solución. En mis experiencias, si ellos no podían hallar una solución, yo presentaba algunas sugerencias y les preguntaba cuál les parecía lo más justo. Juntos, logramos ponernos de acuerdo y establecer algunas reglas y límites, que se convirtieron en "la ley de la casa". Por ejemplo, había una regla que decía: "No se vale lastimar. Todos deben ganar, transigir, negociar, escuchar, y tratar de comprender". Otra regla mandaba que "Se vale estar en desacuerdo y disgustarse, pero es necesario respetar uno al otro y amarse incondicionalmente".

Cuando los niños son muy pequeños, usted los puede ayudar a resolver conflictos al separarlos y ponerlos en "descanso" en diferentes cuartos hasta que se calmen. Quizá tenga que distraerlos con otra actividad. Al crecer, tendrán que aprender a comunicarse y resolver sus propios problemas. Cuando los niños no son capaces de resolver sus propios problemas y si sus discusiones llegan a estar realmente fuera de control, tal vez tengan que enfrentarse a ciertas consecuencias, como la pérdida de privilegios. Quizá no sea permitido que miren la televisión, que usen la computadora, que jueguen con sus videojuegos, o que hablen por teléfono. Tenga precaución, que demasiado castigo puede debilitar una relación en la familia.

Con cada episodio de rivalidad entre hermanos, traté de repetir las admoniciones de mi abuelo y mi mamá. Ellos solían decirnos que no peleáramos y que intentáramos resolver nuestros problemas por medio de la comprensión y el perdón. Ellos decían: "Ustedes son hermanas, deben amarse y cuidarse. Somos familia y eso quiere decir que estamos unidos para ayudarnos mutuamente. No pueden quedarse enojadas. Deben perdonarse porque nosotros valoramos a la familia y valoramos a cada persona dentro de la familia". Eventualmente, estas palabras, en combinación con muchas otras lecciones, orientaron nuestra conducta.

Entre los hermanos, se desarrolla un vínculo afectivo especial que proviene de refrenar las necesidades de uno y los deseos de las posesiones ajenas, además de un dar y recibir que los permite escuchar, comprender, y empatizar. A los niños se les debe alentar a defenderse y a expresar sus opiniones, pero con el entendimiento que todos tienen un punto de vista legítimo y que no existen ni ganadores ni perdedores. A veces nos salimos con la nuestra, a veces cedimos, transigimos, y negociamos. Tuvimos que desarrollar las habilidades necesarias para comunicar nuestras necesidades. Cuando nuestros niños se dan cuenta que no siempre ganarán y que no siempre tienen la razón, comenzarán a comprender qué es lo que se necesita para formar vínculos afectivos y relaciones exitosas y duraderas.

Esas relaciones requieren un enfoque de dar y recibir que incorpora la paciencia y el perdón. Un hogar no debe ser un campo de batallas, un campo de fútbol, o una competencia de las Olimpiadas, con claros ganadores y perdedores. Es un lugar donde los niños pueden sentir la confianza de que todos ganan y donde el bien de todos es más importante que lo que uno solo puede ganar. El resultado de este tipo de interacción es una familia que está fuerte y sólidamente unida a través de su amor incondicional, su confianza, y su dependencia mutua.

El hogar prepara a los niños a vivir en la sociedad. Un hogar requiere a unos padres que les proporcionarán a sus niños las habilidades necesarias para vivir en harmonía con otras personas que poseen diferentes puntos de vista y necesidades. Los padres son responsables de establecer las reglas y los valores que orientarán la conducta de sus niños. A veces a mis niños no les han gustado las reglas, pero eventualmente han aprendido, tal como lo hice yo en mi casa, que las reglas se establecieron por su propio bien y por el mejoramiento de la familia. Es difícil para un padre ser fuerte y mantenerse firme en lo que instintivamente cree que es lo mejor. Esto es particularmente doloroso cuando significa tener que hacer caso omiso de las lágrimas tristes de un niño, o del estallido de ira de otro que dice: "Ya no te quiero". Los padres deben ser maduros y firmes al guiar a sus niños por el camino apropiado. Eventualmente nuestros niños se darán cuenta del beneficio, cuando a la larga, nuestra orientación logra cosechar lo que intentó sembrar. Todos los padres esperan que algún día sus niños podrán, con plena confianza, tomar decisiones sabias y prudentes.

Usted debe considerar todos los factores que puede ocasionar la rivalidad entre hermanos. ¿Usted recuerda algunas de sus propias batallas con sus hermanos cuando era joven? ¿Qué las provocó? ¿Estos episodios unieron más a los hermanos? ¿Era saludable de alguna manera la rivalidad?

Mi relación con mis hermanos es muy fuerte y sólida en la actualidad, porque lo bueno tuvo más peso que lo malo, sin embargo, lo malo era parte del crecimiento. Pueden haber algunos beneficios en una sana competencia y rivalidad, como se ilustra en los dichos *No hay rosa sin espinas* y *Más enseña la adversidad, que diez años de universidad.* Había ocho niños en mi familia, pero cinco nacimos con un año de diferencia. Yo soy la cuarta del primer grupo, todas mujeres. Dentro de ese grupo, yo era de las más pequeñas. Yo tenía a tres hermanas mayores que me cuidaban, me enseñaban, me inspiraban, y me protegían. Cuando mis dos hermanas mayores se casaron, yo era la segunda, en medio de las otras dos, y, por cierto, tenía las características típicas. Yo era más agresiva, aventurera, y extrovertida. Yo siempre estaba en el escenario, luchando por conseguir mi parte de la atención.

Como todas éramos mujeres, discutíamos sobre tener que compartir los juguetes, el tiempo y atención de mi madre, además de nuestra ropa, joyas, y medias mientras crecíamos. También teníamos mucho en común, como un interés por la ropa, el maquillaje, y salir con muchachos. Desarrollamos una relación muy estrecha, un sentido de sana competencia, y una fuente de inspiración. Cualquier cosa que hacían las hermanas mayores, las menores también tenían que hacer, ya fuera presentarse a una prueba para ser porrista, postularse como candidata a "Sweetheart Queen", o asistir a la universidad. Julia, mi hermana mayor, fue porrista, y tres de sus cuatro hermanas menores también fueron porristas. Julia se postuló como candidata para reina de la preparatoria, y Susie y yo le seguimos los pasos y fuimos reinas de la preparatoria, y yo, de nuevo en la universidad. Yo fui la primera para graduarme de la universidad, y en este caso, las mayores me siguieron a mí. Al escribir este libro, yo he inspirado a una de mis hermanas a escribir su propio libro. La rivalidad entre hermanos no siempre se trata de soltar agresión reprimida. También puede ofrecer una sana competencia y motivación. Sus niños pueden aprender valores importantes como la imparcialidad, la cooperación, la bondad, la paciencia, la justicia, y cómo compartir.

Mis hermanas y yo nos pasamos los días festivos riéndonos al recordar los episodios de rivalidad que compartimos. Yo tengo que admitir que en la mayoría de las ocasiones, yo fui la que comenzó los pleitos. Yo sabía muy bien que le molestaría a mi hermana si le agarraba sus cosas, pero lo hacía de todos modos. Una vez aun le vendí a mi hermana una caja de lindos pañuelos con encaje que pertenecían a mi otra hermana. Yo era agresiva y generalmente fuera de los límites. Me metí en problemas muchas veces y mi madre sabía que yo probablemente había instigado el pleito. Hacía mucho esfuerzo por mantenerme bajo control y hacer que fuera más bondadosa y considerada. Era dura conmigo y no me dejaba pasar mucho. Un día, mi hermana menor, Yolanda, se jactó de como ella podía lograr que mi madre me pegara. "¿Quieres ver cómo se enoja Mamá contigo?" me decía. Antes de poder contestarle, comenzaba a gritar a más no poder: "¡Mamá! ¡Mamá!" como si alguien la estuviera matando. Tal como ella lo predijo, entró como torbellino mi mamá y me dio una buenas. Al alejarse mi mama, mi hermana tenía una gran sonrisa burlona que realmente me provocaba ganas de matarla.

Lo que yo aprendí de ese episodio fue que los niños que son catalogados como peleoneros o buscapleitos pueden ganarse una reputación que se les queda y puede ser una fuente de tormento aun cuando no son culpables. Otro incidente involucraba a mi hermana Rosa Linda, quien solía enojarse si no cumplíamos con sus normas de limpieza. A Susie le hacían burla y se mofaban de ella porque siempre perdía las cosas, aunque eventualmente las encontraba. A pesar de las palabras duras y las batallas, cuando todo volvía a la calma, siempre quedábamos como mejores amigas. Por más que nos gustaba hacernos burla entre nosotras mismas, no tolerábamos que nadie fuera de la familia dijera nada sobre una de nuestras hermanas. Un día yo escuché a alguien en mi escuela decir que mi hermana (que era una "cheerleader") tenía "piernas de gallina". Yo me enojé mucho. El vínculo afectivo que existe entre mis hermanos y yo es tan bello y algo que siempre atesoraré.

Yo también fui testigo de muchos episodios de rivalidad entre mis propios niños, pero uno que recuerdo vívidamente ocurrió cuando Sal tenía cinco años de edad. Se volvió chipilón, o celoso, y se sentía amenazado ante la idea de perder su trono como hijo único. Yo leí libros con Sal para prepararlo para la llegada de nuestro chiquitín, por meses antes de que Steven naciera. Yo le compré regalos especiales cuando trajimos a Steven del hospital a la casa, y le dimos atención especial cuando los tíos y abuelitos venían a saludar al nuevo bebé. A pesar de todo lo que hicimos, Sal resintió mucho la llegada de su hermanito. El lenguaje de su cuerpo me informaba que no había aceptado fácilmente el cambio. Él me quería para él solito. Él se metía físicamente entre el bebé y yo cuandoquiera que me escuchaba haciendo cariños a Steven. Después de algún tiempo, cuando comencé a pedirle que fuera mi pequeño asistente, las cosas mejoraron. Pero todo el tiempo, yo sabía que él pensaba: "¿Por qué tuvo que venir él y arruinarlo todo para mí? La pasaba tan bien siendo el único niño. ¿Me dejará de querer mi mamá?"

Un día, en mi presencia, yo le vi agarrar uno de los dedos del bebé y doblarlo hacia atrás, provocando un fuerte grito. "¡NO vas a lastimar a tu hermano!" le dije. Sal se asustó con lo que había provocado y nunca lo volvió a hacer. Pero al crecer él, y al comenzar Steven a meterse en sus cosas, comenzaron los pleitos. Sal tenía una gran necesidad de privacidad, y yo sabía lo que iba a pasar cuando yo me di cuenta al mirar los ojos de Steven que él ansiaba meterse en las cosas de su hermano. Los primeros cinco años fueron muy difíciles para Sal, pero con el tiempo aceptó a su hermano y lo encontró útil de cierta manera. Cuando venían a la casa sus amigos, a Sal le gustaba que Steven los entretuviera. Desdichadamente, en ese momento Sal aprendió que podía meter a su hermano en problemas al desafiarlo a hacer cosas que no debía.

Una cosa importante que debe recordar cuando está preparándose para la rivalidad entre hermanos y cuando está lidiando con ella, es darles a sus niños claras y definidas reglas y guías, especialmente cuando los niños son demasiado pequeños para hacer evaluaciones apropiadas. Yo les había enseñado a mis niños que en caso de peligro o si alguien trataba de hacerles daño, que llamaran a 911. A veces los mensajes que mandamos pueden ser interpretados erróneamente.

Un día después de la escuela, mis tres niños estaban juntos, mirando la televisión en mi recámara, cuando un desacuerdo se volvió discusión, y Sal, quien en ese entonces contaba con doce años de edad, empujó a Steven, quien tenía siete años, al piso. Mi esposo me llamó y me dijo que tenía que salir para ir a su práctica para el coro, y yo estaba por llegar dentro de quince minutos. Yo siempre les había dicho a mis niños que se cuidaran uno al otro, que se respetaran, y que fueran considerados con respecto a los sentimientos de otros, tal como siempre me habían enseñado a mí. Desdichadamente, Steven recordó la pregunta que le hacíamos una y otra vez: "¿Qué debes hacer cuando alguien te está lastimando? Debes llamar a 911". Esto es exactamente lo que hizo nuestro hijo. Nunca olvidaré la experiencia de mirar a dos carros de policía acercarse a mi casa, con todo y las sirenas atronadoras, al poco rato de haberme metido a la entrada para coches. Los niños habían estado solos por menos de quince minutos. Allí en el porche estaban mis tres angelitos, con aires muy culpables y los ojos bien abiertos. Sal dijo: "Mamá, nunca vas a creer lo que hizo Steven ahora". Después de que me contaron lo que pasó, llegaron dos policías y con mucha vergüenza, traté de explicarles que todo el episodio era simplemente un caso de rivalidad entre hermanos y que él había marcado 911 porque su hermano lo lastimó. Él respondió: "Hágase a un lado, señora. Tengo que hablar con su hijo yo mismo". Huelga decir que cuando el oficial se enteró de lo que ocurrió, Steven recibió el sermón de su vida y de ahí en adelante pensaría dos veces cómo lidiar con la ira cuando las cosas no salían como él quería.

Yo estoy segura que usted tiene sus propias aventuras relacionadas con la rivalidad entre hermanos que le han provocado vergüenza, alegría, angustia, e ira. Tal como mis hermanos y los suyos, mis niños han establecido lazos más estrechos a causa del vaivén de la rivalidad entre hermanos.

LA DISCIPLINA: DE MALCRIADO A BIEN EDUCADO

Las culturas a través del mundo poseen diferentes creencias acerca de lo que es conducta aceptable o inaceptable dependiendo de sus propios valores singulares. Desde la época precolombina, los padres aztecas jugaron un papel importante en la crianza de sus niños, enseñándoles a ser obedientes, tener buenos modales, ser autodisciplinados, y sobre todo, a ser honorables. Jerry Tello, quien dirige un programa en Los Angeles, llamado "Cara y Corazón", describe las enseñanzas típicas de los padres aztecas a los padres hispanos. Todos los días, después del desayuno, los niños aztecas recibían instrucciones sobre cómo debían vivir. Esto incluía cómo respetar a otros, dedicarse a lo bueno y justo, evitar la maldad, y abstenerse de la perversión y la avaricia. Estos principios más tarde fueron reforzados por valores cristianos semejantes cuando llegaron los españoles.

Para las familias hispanas a través de los tiempos, la disciplina ha sido una herramienta principal en la socialización de los niños. Richard Griswold del Castillo observó que para las familias chicanas del siglo diecinueve en el sudoeste de los Estados Unidos, la disciplina era un aspecto distintivo de la vida, ya sea en el mundo público o privado. En ese mundo, el *respeto* era uno de los aspectos más valorados de la identidad de uno y no debía disminuirse. Para demostrar la validez de sus enseñanzas, los padres de esa época solían llevar a sus niños a que fueran testigos de las ejecuciones para mostrarles lo que podía ocurrir si cometían alguna fechoría. Mi suegro llevó a sus niños a las pizcas de algodón para mostrarles lo duro que tendrían que trabajar si no conseguían una educación universitaria.

En muchas familias, la disciplina todavía es considerada la manera más efectiva de cambiar a un niño de malcriado a bien educado. Sin embargo, mientras la disciplina sigue formando una parte importante de la crianza de los niños, debe ir de la mano con una comprensión acerca de las etapas de crecimiento de los niños y de sus necesidades básicas.

Durante los primeros años, un niño pequeño cree que las reglas impuestas por los padres son sagradas y no pueden ser cambiadas. Los niños eventualmente probarán los límites, y lucharán mientras adquieren la autonomía y la identidad. Si nosotros queremos que nuestros niños lleguen a ser miembros de la sociedad que desempeñan alguna función, necesitamos, como padres, proveer el tipo apropiado de medio ambiente para ayudarles a poder tomar las decisiones correctas y saber resolver problemas. Los niños necesitan aprender valores y desarrollar y fortalecer su carácter.

Usted puede aprender maneras más positivas de lograr que un niño sea bien educado sin las nalgadas, los rezongos persistentes, y los menosprecios. Puede prevenir las luchas por el poder, el resentimiento, y los arrebatos. Los siguientes son unos principios que le ayudarán a comprender el porqué del comportamiento de los niños. También les ofrezco una lista de estrategias que ayudarán a desarrollar la confianza y un autoestima positivo y a construir una relación positiva con otros. Como siempre, los niños cometerán algunos errores, pero permítales aprender de esos errores. Usted también cometerá errores y quizá vuelva a las estrategias inapropiadas que no funcionan. A través de suficiente práctica, mejorará.

1. Un niño necesita el amor incondicional, el poder confiar, y el ser aceptado.

    Todos los niños necesitan recibir amor incondicional para tener un sentido de seguridad, confianza en sí mismo, y aceptación. Ese amor se desarrollará al aprender los padres a ser más responsivos a las necesidades de sus niños, y por medio de muchas otras acciones, tal como darles un abrazo, un beso, un guiño, o mirarles a los ojos y sonreír. El vínculo afectivo entre los padres y el niño se convertirá en la base para futuras relaciones sociales. El amor necesita ser demostrado a los niños incondicionalmente al crecer ellos, sin tomar en cuenta lo que digan o hagan. *Odia el pecado, y compadece al pecador.*

2. Un niño se portará como se siente.

    La conducta de un niño es un reflejo de cómo se siente. La irritabilidad, semejante a los adultos, puede surgir si tiene hambre, sueño, temor, o se siente cansado, enfermo, aburrido, o triste. Además, puede estar letárgico por falta de ejercicio. La tensión, el trauma, una crisis o un cambio significativo en su vida como el comienzo de la escuela, la llegada de un nuevo hermanito, el lidiar con el divorcio, la mudanza a una nueva casa, el enfrentarse al racismo o a la violencia o al fallecimiento de un ser querido—todas estas cosas pueden afectar la conducta de un niño. La tensión puede provocar síntomas físicas como dolores de estómago, diarrea, vómito, sudor excesivo, o falta de energía. Algunos médicos creen que tales síntomas pueden ser psicosomáticos, provocados por tensión emocional. Otros piensan que el dolor, asociado con una disminución de autoestima, se manifiesta por medio de señales de depresión y desesperanza que pueden conducir a demasiada actividad, el retraerse o recluirse de los amigos y las actividades, el fracaso escolar, el uso de las drogas, y el suicidio. Si usted nota estos síntomas en su niño, busque ayuda psicológica en una clínica de orientación o terapia para niños. Proporcione un medio ambiente que satisface las necesidades de su niño. Asegúrese de que no tenga alergia a nada, como el colorante vegetal o la cafeína. Ayude a prepararlo para los cambios de la vida que pueden ser muy emocionales para los niños.

3. Tenga expectativas realistas.

Antes de decidir si su niño es un niño malcriado que le está causando disgustos intencionalmente, pregúntese si está a un punto en su desarrollo que le capacita hacer lo que usted espera que haga. Es importante que tenga expectativas realistas de sus niños. Por ejemplo, no debe esperar que un niño de nueve meses ya no use pañales cuando la edad promedia para ese logro es de alrededor de los tres años de edad. Su niño no podrá compartir sus cosas con otros antes de los tres años de edad. Antes de los ocho a doce meses de edad, no puede aceptar límites. Durante la difícil y "terrible" edad de los dos años, habrá una lucha de voluntades entre usted y su pequeño niño, al intentar él volverse autónomo. Comprenda que no se puede esperar que los niños se mantengan sentados por un período largo de tiempo. Recuerde que tienen una necesidad incontrolable de jugar, aprender, explorar, y experimentar. No es realista que su niño piense que él puede conseguir todo lo que desea. Es importante que usted tenga expectativas realistas y que no empuje a su niño a ser la persona que usted quiere que sea. Su niño necesita que usted reconozca y elogie sus intereses, sus talentos, y sus habilidades, al apoyar su desarrollo.

4. Proporcione los apropiados modelos de conducta.

Su niño aprenderá lo que mira y escucha. Él aprenderá lo que usted valora y aprecia a través de sus palabras y acciones. Si usted le dice que no está bien robar, pero luego lo mira comiendo las uvas antes de pagarlas en el supermercado, o no devuelve las cosas que no le pertenecen, su niño estará confundido por la contradicción entre lo que dice y lo que hace. Si usted quiere que su niño sea paciente y considerado pero usted empuja para adelantarse en la fila, entonces usted puede estarle mandando un mensaje por medio de sus palabras, y otro totalmente opuesto por medio de sus acciones. Si usted grita, hace mohines, y avienta las cosas cuando se enoja, usted le está enseñando a seguir ese ejemplo. Si usted trata a su niño duramente, a través del abuso verbal o físico, su niño aprenderá a hacer lo mismo con otros. La manera en que usted se comunica con su pareja, la relación que tienen, también le enseñará a su niño cómo relacionarse con otros. Usted debe modelar tolerancia, bondad, paciencia, y amor. Todo lo que un niño mira, dentro y fuera de la casa, le causará una impresión, y afectará su conducta. Esté consciente de la violencia, el sexo, y el materialismo al que puede estar expuesto a través de la televisión, la música que escucha, los videojuegos que juega, y en la Internet. Los medios de comunicación pueden ser tan peligrosos como educativos. Además, póngalo en contacto con buenos modelos de conducta y personas con buen carácter e integridad.

5. Sea un detective y elogie y premie la buena conducta.
    Cuando su niño hace cosas positivas sin habérselo pedido, reconozca sus buenas obras, elogie sus acciones, y prémielo con algo especial o con palabras bondadosas. Siempre debe darle a su niño atención positiva, para que no tenga que portarse mal para que lo tomen en cuenta. Esto quizá signifique tener que estar atento y buscar la buena conducta, o dividir una conducta particular en partes y reconocer cada paso con un elogio.

    Se portará de manera aceptable si aprende que es la única manera de conseguir atención. Los comentarios negativos que avergüenzan, critican, y ridiculizan a su niño afectarán adversamente su autoestima y su relación con él. Dele espacio. No esté encima de él, ni constantemente fastidiándole, ni lo provoque. No debe haber ninguna manipulación, luchas por el poder, ni humillaciones. Un niño tiene una gran necesidad de amor y atención de cuando menos una persona que está loca por él. Por lo mismo, usted sea esa persona al escucharle, reconocer sus sentimientos, y elogiar su buena conducta.

6. Sea un buen entrenador para alentar una conducta deseable.
    Aliente a su niño a tomar buenas decisiones, a escoger lo correcto. Si vuelve a casa enojado porque algo ocurrió en la escuela, pregúntele qué piensa que pudo haber hecho diferente. Dígale que usted confía en que él podrá resolver sus problemas.

7. Conozca a los amigos de su niño.
    Al crecer su niño, es importante que usted conozca a los amigos con quienes se asocia. Invite a sus amigos a su casa. Procure conocer a sus familias. Cuando los hispanohablantes dicen: *"Dime con quién andas y te diré quién eres"*, están dando una advertencia sobre la influencia que puede tener una mala compañía.

8. Establezca reglas claras y consistentes.
    Los niños necesitan reglas y límites en su vida para proveer la estructura necesaria para su firmeza y agresión. Usted debe ayudarle a su niño a comprender las reglas. Al llegar a los doce meses de edad, un

niño acepta el papel de usted en el establecimiento de límites y reglas. Asegúrese de que sean claras. Sea consistente. No ceda. No asuma sus responsabilidades. Él necesita aprender cómo cumplir una tarea. Usted quizá necesite proporcionarle asistencia y entrenamiento. Enséñele las metas deseables de su hogar y de una sociedad civilizada, como la justicia, la igualdad, y la equidad. Enséñele que hay consecuencias a pagar por la conducta inapropiada, con un énfasis más fuerte durante los años críticos entre uno y ocho años de edad.

9. Proporcione una educación espiritual, morales, y valores.
   Desde el primer año de vida, su niño necesita tener contacto con las normas de conducta, la moralidad, y los valores que usted considera importantes. Su meta es que él llegue a ser autodisciplinado. Ayúdele a establecer un sentido del bien y del mal y a desarrollar una imagen mental de una persona que es bien educada.

10. Comprenda que cada niño es único y responde a la disciplina de diferente manera, dependiendo de su personalidad.

DIFERENTES TIPOS DE TÉCNICAS DE DISCIPLINA

1. La distracción
   Cuando su niño muy pequeño se va a meter en algún problema, distraiga su atención. Por ejemplo, si grita por que quiere algo, llévelo afuera a jugar en el columpio, léale un libro, o saque la botella de las burbujas.

2. Remover
   Remueva o quítele el objeto que está causando el problema, y explique por qué lo hace.

3. La separación
   Separe físicamente a un niño que se está portando mal, de la persona o de la actividad que ha provocado su frustración.

4. El descanso
   Mande al niño a su recámara hasta que pueda calmarse y portarse bien, o hasta que acepte las condiciones que usted le ha especificado.

5.   El método de "ojo a ojo" o "levante la ceja"
Mire a su niño directamente a los ojos de una manera que muestra
su disgusto, y dígale firmemente "¡no!" y dígale "no" también con la
cabeza. Baje ligeramente la cabeza, apriete los labios, o levante una
ceja, cualquier cosa que mandará un mensaje de disgusto. Sea firme
y consistente, directo, honesto, y serio. No juegue ni haga bromas
sobre las cosas que no le gustan y que quiere cambiar. A veces sólo
tiene que decir una o dos palabras: "¡No!" "¡Deja eso!" "Platos"
"Basura". Captará su atención y le hará entender que está serio, y no
jugando. Describa lo más sucintamente posible lo que necesita hacerse ("Pon la ropa sucia en el cesto", "¡Ponte los zapatos!") en lugar
de darle todo un sermón.

6.   Habilidades efectivas de comunicación
El primer paso hacia la comunicación efectiva es que los padres y los
niños se calmen antes de decir y hacer cosas de los cuales luego quizá
se arrepientan. Si los padres quieren poder enseñar, deben tener
paciencia mientras el niño está tratando de aprender nuevos valores,
costumbres, reglas, y modales. Evite criticar al niño utilizando palabras como tonto, llorona, bobo, estúpido, o idiota. Dé mensajes
con "me"—"No *me* gustó lo que hiciste. Le disgustó mucho a tu hermano que le quebraste su juguete". Evite iniciar las frases con palabras como "tú" y "¿por qué?" porque muchas veces estas palabras
serán seguidas por un ataque al carácter de su niño. Estas palabras
pondrán a su niño a la defensiva. Lea los mensajes que manda su
niño con el cuerpo y refleje sus sentimientos, para demostrar que
usted comprende y valora sus sentimientos: "Parece que eso te hace
enojar mucho". Esto le dará a su niño la oportunidad de expresarse
y de que usted escuche lo que quiere decir. Pregúntele si tiene una
solución. Haga sugerencias sobre maneras diferentes de hacer las
cosas. Enséñele la importancia de resolver el conflicto de manera
que no hay perdedores y de que sea justo para todos.
   Claro que hay veces cuando hay que decir basta y ser autoritario. Algunas soluciones pueden ser tan sencillas como el establecimiento de las leyes de la casa. Dígale que recoja ya sus juguetes en
vez de preguntarle si quiere hacerlo. Quizá tenga que ayudarle hasta
que adquiera la costumbre de recoger sus cosas. Otras soluciones
involucran temas más importantes y serios que pueden provocar
una confrontación. En estos casos, las decisiones y los acuerdos no
siempre son una situación donde todos ganan, cuando menos al
principio, pero a la larga será mejor para el niño también. Asegúrese

de que cuando tenga una confrontación con su niño, ha escogido asuntos que valen la pena discutir. Cuando se trata de asuntos menos importantes, usted puede ser flexible y negociar o ceder. Cuando se trata de algo más serio, como cuando un niño no quiere ir a recibir sus inmunizaciones, o vacunas, o cuando un preadolescente quiere quedarse despierto más allá de su toque de queda, los padres deben mantenerse firmes sobre lo que ellos saben que sus niños necesitan para lograr un desarrollo y crecimiento sanos en oposición a lo que ellos desean. Cuando necesita ser inflexible, reconozca los sentimientos de su niño y explique la razón de sus acciones y las reglas. Dígale que lo que está haciendo es por su propio bienestar y que está tomando esta acción porque lo quiere. Quizá no lo comprenda ahora, pero lo comprenderá más adelante. Sería beneficioso que las reglas se establecieran de común acuerdo entre toda la familia durante una junta familiar. De esta manera todos entienden y aceptan la importancia de las reglas y acceden a cumplirlas.

Cuando se porta mal su niño, dígale que lo quiere, pero que no le gusta su comportamiento. Describa la acción que no le gusta, pero no ataque al niño ni juzgue su carácter. Diga cosas como: "No puedo permitir que te portes así. Ya te he dicho que no debes pegar a nadie". Dígale la razón: "porque duele". "Lo que dijiste hirió sus sentimientos y fue de muy mala educación". Describa lo que quiere que haga. Ayúdele a tratar de resolver su problema o de portarse de cierta manera. Los niños necesitan aprender algo cada vez que se portan mal. La disciplina debe ser una enseñanza. Es mejor alentar que forzar, y ayudarles a aprender de sus errores, especialmente si lo que hay en juego es muy importante.

7. Las consecuencias naturales y lógicas: Los contratos
Un niño necesita recibir ayuda para entender que hay consecuencias a sus acciones. Si no pone la ropa sucia en el cesto, no habrán calcetines o ropa interior limpios. Si no cuida a su perro, no podrá tenerlo. Si no viene a comer con la familia, su comida será metida dentro del refrigerador para que él la caliente más tarde. Si no se porta bien, tendrán que irse de la fiesta. Si no hace su tarea o no la entrega, sacará una mala calificación. A veces los niños tienen que aprender por medio del fracaso. Como padres, quizá no nos guste esto o tener que ser "duros", pero para que nuestros niños puedan aprender responsabilidad e independencia, necesitamos ayudarles a aprender de sus errores y siempre alentarlos a ser perseverantes e intentar de nuevo.

Necesita ayudarles a sus niños a establecer sus propios objetivos y metas y ayudarles a averiguar qué necesitan hacer para lograrlos. Podrían firmar un contrato con usted, con su maestro, o con sus hermanos para lograr cierta conducta. Necesitamos darles libertad y hacerles saber que tenemos fe en su juicio y en su capacidad de tomar las decisiones correctas. Esto llevará a la disciplina interna, una consciencia de lo que está bien y lo que está mal, la responsabilidad, y una satisfacción intrínseca por haber alcanzado sus propias metas y por haber cumplido con sus propias exigencias.

8. Dé a los niños la oportunidad de elegir y de encontrar alternativas
A los niños hay que darles opciones entre las cuales pueden elegir en lugar de un ultimátum. Puede decir: "¿Quieres bañarte ahorita o en diez minutos? ¿Quieres ayudarme con aspirar la alfombra o con sacudir los muebles? ¿Quieres ponerte este vestido o aquél?" Ésta es otra manera de ayudarle a su niño a aprender a resolver sus propios problemas, a volverse decisivo, y a aprender a prevenir confrontaciones. Por ejemplo, quizá usted diga: "Tu maestra me dijo que te portaste muy mal en el patio de recreo. Me disgustó mucho que lastimaste a alguien. Tienes un problema y quiero que me digas cómo lo vas a resolver". Si no tiene una solución, ofrezca algunas opciones. "O tienes que darte cuenta que no puedes volver a pegarle a alguien o no vas a poder jugar". "Yo entiendo que agarraste algo que no te pertenecía. Tú sabes las reglas sobre el respeto a la propiedad ajena. ¿Qué vamos a hacer tocante a esta situación?" "Dime todas las soluciones posibles en las que puedas pensar para resolver el problema que tienes de llegar tarde a la escuela".

9. Los premios
Otra técnica para conseguir que un niño haga lo que usted quiere es premiarlo por su buena conducta. Cuando él hace algo bueno por su hermanita, como traerle su biberón o pañal, puede decirle que fue muy considerado. Está reforzando la buena conducta al hacer esto. Mantenga una hoja donde cada vez que hace algo bueno, lo registra al poner una carita feliz, una calcomanía, o una estrella junto a su nombre. Cuando se hace acreedor de cierto número de estrellas y calcomanías, recibe un premio, por ejemplo un helado o una película. Cuando un niño alcanza el cuadro de honor en la escuela, él puede seleccionar el restaurante donde la familia celebrará el acontecimiento. Los niños se sentirán bien al saber que la excursión a jugar bolos o para acampar, se realizó como resultado de su buena

conducta. Algunos padres premian las buenas calificacio[...]
dinero, al pagar cierta cantidad por una "A" y tanto por un[...]
usted tiene los recursos, un niño puede ganar cierta cantidad por
realizar ciertos quehaceres de la casa. Esta técnica para modificar la
conducta funciona hasta cierto punto. Usted tiene que seleccionar
los premios que pueden motivar a sus niños a comportarse de cierta
manera. Desdichadamente, los niños quizá sientan satisfacción por
haberse ganado el premio y no la satisfacción interna por haber
aprendido algo, por haber ayudado, o por haber sido bondadosos.

10. El castigo: La privación de los privilegios
El privar a los niños de algo que usted sabe que les gusta, como mirar
la televisión, o hablar por teléfono, o jugar los videojuegos, por portarse mal, es otra técnica para corregir la mala conducta. Es muy
importante que los niños comprendan las reglas y que las consecuencias están directamente relacionadas con el rompimiento de las reglas.

Hay veces cuando no puede cumplir con consecuencias lógicas,
como cuando un niño hace una rabieta en el supermercado y usted
no puede llevarlo a la casa inmediatamente si tiene un carrito lleno
de mandado. Y no puede dejarlo quedarse en casa si sigue perdiendo
el camión. Usted quizá tenga más suerte si lo priva de algo que tendría o haría más tarde. Por ejemplo, si grita en el supermercado, no se
le permitirá escoger su cereal favorito. No se le permitirá ir al cine si
pierde otra vez el camión. Su niño necesita darse cuenta de que hay
consecuencias negativas de la conducta inapropiada. Debe hacer
cumplir la consecuencia inmediatamente después de la infracción y
ser siempre consistente. Otra forma de castigo es dar nalgadas, lo cual
puede provocar resentimiento, ira, una necesidad de represalias, una
mala relación entre padres y niño, y falta de harmonía en la familia.

DAR NALGADAS O NO DAR NALGADAS: EL DILEMA DE LA DISCIPLINA

Muchos hispanos que crecieron en familias dentro de las cuales una nal-
gada o un golpe era la respuesta infalible a la mala conducta, se
enfrentan al difícil dilema hoy en día acerca de qué es la mejor manera
de disciplinar a sus niños. Lo que quizá no se les haya dicho es que
muchos expertas creen que cuando le da nalgadas a su niño, le está
enseñando que la violencia física es la única manera de resolver los problemas. Usted puede amonestarlo acerca de no pegarle a su hermano o
hermana cuando están peleando y de comunicar su ira por medio de pa-

labras corteses, pero se puede perder la efectividad de la lección en el instante de sacar el cinturón.

Las nalgadas no constituyen una forma positiva de disciplina. Les enseña a los niños a ser violentos y agresivos. Produce conductas antisociales que provocarán que otros eviten asociarse con su niño. El castigo físico les enseña a nuestros niños que está bien perder el control. Las nalgadas no provocan una sensación de culpabilidad ni una motivación a portarse bien o hacer algo bueno. No forman un sentido del bien y el mal. Las nalgadas pueden producir ira y resentimiento. Provocan actos de desafío, una agresión pasiva, deseos de venganza, y sentimientos lastimados. Si su niño se arremete contra usted después de las nalgadas, esto puede enfurecerle a usted aun más y se intensificará el conflicto. Siempre y cuando usted esté más grande, probablemente gane, ¿pero a expensas de qué? Las nalgadas no ayudan a mejorar la relación entre usted y su niño ni tampoco ayudan a su niño a aprender a tener dominio de sí mismo. Darle nalgadas a su niño también puede hacer que usted se sienta sumamente culpable por haberse pasado de la raya cuando ésa no era su intención. No quiera Dios que su niño termine en un hospital o muerto porque usted no pudo controlar sus propias emociones. De nuevo, es mejor mandarlo a su cuarto o privarlo de algún privilegio que darle nalgadas.

Si usted recurre a castigos corporales, está enseñándole a su niño a utilizar la parte más primitiva del cerebro, los centros límbicos que están localizados en la base del cerebro, los cuales son utilizados durante momentos de temor, pasión, trauma, o crisis. En lugar de eso, ayúdele a utilizar los lóbulos prefrontales, dentro de la neocorteza, localizados detrás de la frente, los cuales son utilizados para pensar, planear, y analizar. Cuando un niño se encuentra en un estado emocional intenso, sus hormonas le fuerzan a "pelear o huir". Se acelera el latido de su corazón, se le sube la presión, y sus músculos grandes se preparan a reaccionar y a atacar. Los centros límbicos nos provocan a reaccionar sin pensar mientras que los lóbulos prefrontales analizan y evalúan la situación y nos permiten pensar, organizar, y planear una respuesta apropiada. Muchos animales utilizan los centros límbicos para protegerse de los predadores. Pero los humanos están bendecidos con una mayor capacidad para enfrentar conflictos.

Lo que es más importante, haga todo en su poder para establecer y mantener una sólida y fuerte relación de amor y confianza, para que si de vez en cuando llega a perder la calma y hace y dice algo de lo cual más tarde se arrepiente, su niño sabrá que sus obras buenas pesan más que las malas. Cuando sienten mucha tensión, los padres pueden fácilmente volver a seguir las técnicas de disciplina de sus padres. Si usted le administra un castigo duro a su niño que le hace sentirse incómodo más tarde, encare a su niño después y dígale: "Quizá debí haber manejado la situación de diferente manera. Lo siento. Solamente quiero que sepas que lo que hiciste me disgustó porque te quiero y deseo lo mejor para ti". Si hizo o dijo algo de lo cual se arrepiente, está bien pedir perdón para mantener fuerte y sólida la relación.

Lo que no quiere hacer como padre es lastimar a sus niños o quebrantarles el espíritu y hacerles sentir que no son dignos de respeto. Nuestro idioma pone mucho énfasis en palabras de respeto, como *mándeme, a sus órdenes, si Dios quiere,* y *para servirle.* Esto puede ser percibido como respeto y bondad, un resultado de nuestra fuerte crianza religiosa. Aquéllos que las utilizan pueden ser percibidos como sumisos y pasivos por las personas de afuera que no conocen la cultura. Algunas personas afirman que esta conducta es negativa y se atribuye al hecho de que nuestra gente ha sido oprimida como un pueblo conquistado, o bien, por ser los inmigrantes más recientes a este país. Sin importar su punto de vista, la mayoría de nosotros no quiere que sus niños sean demasiado agresivos. Además, exigimos que respeten a los adultos. Sin embargo, necesitamos respetar los puntos de vista y las opiniones de nuestros niños. Necesitamos mantenerlos fuertes y llenos de confianza para que puedan defenderse contra quienes quizá interpreten mal sus modales y su bondad como debilidad. Necesitan sentirse bien acerca de sí mismos para poder enfrentarse a la discriminación y al racismo que todavía existen en este país. Como padres, necesitamos alentarles a nuestros niños a expresar sus sentimientos y a experimentar y a explorar con persistencia y determinación. No lastime a sus niños ni emocionalmente ni físicamente al punto de que no se valoren ellos mismos. Los niños a quienes se les dan nalgadas o les hacen burla no pueden crecer bien y llegar a ser los niños llenos de confianza que nosotros queremos que sean. El desafío para los padres es mantener un equilibrio entre nuestros valores culturales sólidos y al mismo tiempo capacitarlos a saber defenderse y ser firmes en un mundo competitivo.

Mi experiencia personal con las nalgadas y el mantenimiento de ese equilibrio

La disciplina puede ser efectiva si está arraigada en una relación sólida con la persona que administra la orientación. Mi abuelo Papayo asumió el papel de quien impone y mantiene la disciplina después del fallecimiento de mi padre. Él tuvo una gran influencia sobre mi vida al desarrollar una relación estrecha él y yo por medio de hacer muchas cosas juntos. Igual como él ocupó el lugar de mi padre, yo le serví de intérprete y de traductora cuando él tenía citas médicas o cuando pagaba sus cuentas. Por mis conocimientos de inglés, él solía premiarme al comprarme algo que necesitaba, como un par de zapatos, o al invitarme a comer a un buen restaurante. Él se convirtió en nuestro líder espiritual, formando en nosotros un sentido de lo correcto y lo incorrecto al asegurarse de que fuéramos a la iglesia todos los domingos. Participó personalmente en nuestro crecimiento espiritual al hacernos arrodillarnos y rezar, leer la Biblia, y cantar coros con él. Yo recuerdo como se arrodillaba todas las noches sin falta y rezaba por cada miembro de la familia. Yo esperaba ansiosamente junto a la puerta en espera de que llamara mi nombre. Nos contaba historias de la revolución y de la época en México cuando era un guardia de seguridad. Un hombre estoico y orgulloso con un bigote bien recortado, siempre vestía un abrigo café de lana y un sombrero café obscuro. Nos dio "a todos y a cada uno" mucho amor y nos recalcó que en este país teníamos la oportunidad de llegar a ser el tipo de persona que queríamos. Pero, igual como mi madre, él no quería que perdiéramos los valores que nos harían ser mejores personas.

Cuando se trataba de la disciplina, Papayo nos hacía saber exactamente cómo debíamos comportarnos. Se mantenía muy firme en sus creencias sobre el valor del respeto, especialmente con relación a mi madre, de saber cómo portarse en público y cómo planear para el futuro. Un día, cuando apenas estaba entrando a la adolescencia, le respondí mal a mi madre, y él inmediatamente entró al cuarto con el cinturón en la mano. Nunca antes me había pegado. Al mirarme con sus ojos grises llorosos y vidriosos, mi abuelo me dijo: "Gloria, esto me va a doler más a mí que a ti, pero te he dicho varias veces que debes respetar a tu madre". *Quien bien te quiere te hará llorar.* Lloré aun antes de que el cinturón tocara mi cuerpo, no por el dolor que iba a sentir, sino porque sabía que había decepcionado al hombre que adoraba. Aun mi madre, quien sabía que no quise decir lo que había dicho, estaba sorprendida de como este hombre, tan fuerte como una roca, podía sin embargo ser tan emocional. A causa del amor tan grande que yo le tenía, y el concepto tan dramático que logró establecer ese día, sí aprendí el significado de respeto. Me causó un impacto tan fuerte, que hoy en día cuando oigo a los adolescentes hablándoles groseramente a sus padres o abuelos, me siento horrorizada por lo mucho que esas palabras van en contra de los valores que están arraigados en mí. Cuando escucho esta falta de respeto es como el sonido que hacen las uñas al arañar el pizarrón. Yo no hubiera aprendido esos valores y otros, si no me los hubieran enseñado unas personas significativas en un ambiente de amor y respeto. En la actualidad, mi madre todavía recibe mi mayor respeto, y yo, a mi vez, trato de inculcarle ese principio a mis niños.

Yo sé que cuando era niña, dado mi carácter curioso y con tendencia a tomar riesgos, pude haber sido tentada a experimentar con cosas que me hubieran llevado hacia un camino de destrucción si mi madre y mi abuelo no hubieran estado allí para imponer los límites y darme la dirección apropiada. Me enteré del desafío tan enorme que es para los padres que viven en el barrio, proteger a sus niños del daño. Sin embargo, como dice el dicho, *por la vereda no hay quien se pierda.* Mi madre, al igual que mi abuelo, me dejó muy claro lo que esperaba de mí. Porque era consistente y mantenía una relación cálida y amorosa con nosotros, confiábamos en sus consejos y los seguimos a través del camino largo y estrecho que nos fijó. Claro que de vez en cuando, como la mayoría de los niños a esa edad, me hice como que no escuchaba sus sermones y admoniciones. Me quejaba cuandoquiera que se me mandaba a hacer algo que yo no quería hacer. Sin embargo, tal como la mayoría de los jóvenes, yo quería y necesitaba tener a alguien que estableciera los límites.

Muchos padres se sienten perdidos en el debate sinfín sobre la disciplina. Quizá se preocupen de que las nalgadas tendrán un efecto adverso en el desarrollo de sus niños. Muchos padres sienten que a ellos mismos les dieron nalgadas, sin que eso ocasionara ninguna consecuencia negativa, y que tal vez uno o dos golpes hasta hayan sido provechosos y les ayudaron cuando andaban por mal camino. Pero mientras que algunos fuimos afortunados en que los castigos corporales no nos afectaron adversamente, lo mismo no es cierto para muchos niños. En mi caso, rara vez me dieron nalgadas; y cuando me las llegaron a dar, no me causó un dolor severo. Se me hizo comprender lo que yo había hecho y a creer entonces que se hizo por mi propio bien. También se hizo dentro de un contexto de amor incondicional y aceptación. Aunque pude agradecer la disciplina que mi abuelo me dio, no todos los niños son iguales, y no todas las nalgadas son iguales. Pueden haber ocasiones cuando los padres, sin embargo, se pasan no intencionalmente de la raya.

Por ejemplo, una de mis hermanas, a quien le llamamos la abogada de la familia, a causa de su personalidad obstinada y atrevida, nunca olvidó la ira que sintió cuando mi abuelo una vez le hizo sangrar profusamente la nariz. Hasta este día, ella dice que lleva cicatrices emocionales causadas por la disciplina severa de mi abuelo aquel día. Cuando mis otros hermanos y yo hablamos amorosamente de mi abuelo, mi hermana dice que ella sólo recuerda que fue abusador. Lo que no siempre recuerda es que mi abuelo se preocupaba mucho acerca de los traficantes de drogas y de los muchos hombres que se congregaban en el complejo de viviendas subvencionadas donde vivíamos. A pesar de las advertencias de no salir de la casa, ella lo hacía de todos modos. Después de que esto ocurrió varias veces, mi abuelo, impulsado por su propio temor de que algo le podría pasar, no encontró otra manera de impactar sobre ella para que no saliera. En cuanto a mi hermana se concierne, mi abuelo se pasó de la raya, la lastimó física y emocionalmente y dañó irrevocablemente su relación con ella.

A pesar de los volúmenes de consejos en contra del uso de los castigos corporales, es muy fácil recurrir a las nalgadas cuando todo lo demás falla, especialmente para aquéllos que crecieron con el castigo físico. Los hispanos tienen dichos que reflejan el pasaje bíblico "spare the rod and spoil the child" (si no utiliza la vara, consentirá al niño). Los hispanohablantes también dicen, *"los padres que quieren a sus hijos, con más Vera los corrige"* (la Vera es un árbol de madera muy dura). También, *"si a tu hijo no le das castigo, serás su peor enemigo"*. Mi madre creía que estaba bien darles nalgadas a los niños de vez en cuando, como mi abuelo, y cuando la ponía de nervios o le sacaba de quicio, me aventaba su chancla, o trataba de usar el cinturón. Este método no funcionó muy bien al crecer yo, porque aprendí a correr y esquivarla, y mi madre no tenía muy buena puntería. La chancla era su forma de decir: "¡Ya basta!"

Mientras que las nalgadas pueden tener un efecto muy negativo sobre el niño, generalmente no funciona como forma de disciplina. Ciertamente no funcionó con mi hermana, ni con mi hijo Steven. Yo tengo que admitir que mi esposo y yo le dimos nalgadas en las cuantas ocasiones cuando no supimos qué hacer acerca de su conducta incontrolable. Cuando lo hicimos, no le perturbó en lo más mínimo, y ni siquiera dejó salir una sola lágrima. Solamente nos fulminaba con esa mirada iracunda suya. Mi esposo y yo nos dimos cuenta de que tendríamos más éxito en llegarle a Steven si lo hacíamos a través de su corazón y su mente. Le poníamos énfasis a los morales y los principios y lo pusimos en contacto con la espiritualidad y con modelos de conducta apropiados, quizá a mayor grado que a nuestros otros niños.

Yo recuerdo como mi madre, mi abuelo, y mi hermana mayor, Julia, solían utilizar las mismas estrategias conmigo en sus intentos de enseñarme un sentido de lo correcto e incorrecto. Ellos me decían: "Gloria, tú sabes mejor que eso. Se te ha enseñado lo que está bien y lo que no, y tú sabes que lo que hiciste está mal". Siempre y cuando las personas no me gritaban y me explicaban cómo mis acciones afectaban a otros, y lo hacían de manera calmada y racional, yo escuchaba. Los adultos me podían alcanzar más efectivamente cuando apelaban a mi mente y mi corazón tal como lo había hecho mi abuelo cuando fue directo y abierto sobre cómo mi conducta les afectaba a él y a otros. Más adelante, cuando me encontraba frente a una situación tentadora, yo todavía podía escuchar su voz, aun cuando ya no estaba.

En tiempo de remolinos se ve subir la basura. Este refrán les advierte a los padres que deben estar conscientes de los momentos cuando la intensidad de sus emociones parece estar aumentando, fuera de control, y que deben tomar un poco de tiempo para calmarse para poder manejar la situación de una manera más racional. Deben entender que cuando uno está cansado o enfermo, o bajo mucha presión, tiene la tendencia a irritarse más fácilmente. A veces utilizaba el idioma como barómetro para determinar qué tan disgustada estaba en determinada situación. Cuando yo cambiaba de inglés a español y se me subía la ceja, mis niños sabían que estaba muy disgustada. "¡Salvador!" gritaba. "¿Qué estás haciendo? ¡Pórtate bien!" A veces el idioma inglés simplemente no me permitía expresar mis verdaderas emociones cuando estaba disgustada. Como yo hablé principalmente español durante los primeros seis años de mi vida, mi lengua materna es mi lengua emocional, la cual utilizo para expresar mis más profundos sentimientos, como el amor, el temor, y la ira. Algunos de mis amigos bilingües me han dicho: "¡Vaya! Cuando mi madre me hablaba en español, yo sabía que hablaba en serio, y cuando decía maldiciones en español, ¡mucho cuidado!"

Igual como muchos padres, mi abuelo amaba a mi hermana y creyó que sus intenciones eran buenas el día que la abofeteó. Él estaba pensando en su bienestar. Pero los padres pueden fácilmente pasarse de la raya, ponerse violentos, y cometer un abuso en un momento de ira, del cual luego se arrepentirán. En este país, donde por ley se tiene que reportar el maltrato a los niños, se reportan 2.8 millones de casos cada año, y 2,000 niños fallecen a causa del maltrato y la negligencia. Para asegurarse de que los padres participantes de AVANCE no se lleguen a encontrar en estas situaciones, aconsejamos a los padres que es mejor nunca darles nalgadas y les enseñamos métodos más efectivos de disciplina. Muchos padres a quienes les dieron nalgadas cuando eran niños, tenían la creencia inquebrantable que las nalgadas eran la mejor forma de evitar que sus niños se volvieran malcriados. Tuvimos que encontrar técnicas alternativas de disciplina que resultaran ser más efectivas. Aunque sea mejor encontrar una manera más apropiada que los castigos corporales para modificar la conducta, si usted se encuentra en una situación que siente que requiere *algo más*, yo sugiero que aplique los siguientes pasos para disminuir los efectos negativos que las nalgadas pueden tener sobre su niño y sobre su relación con él:

1. Cuente hasta diez o veinte.

2. Haga cualquier cosa necesaria para calmarse: salga del cuarto y vaya a caminar, pruebe algunas técnicas de relajamiento como la respiración profunda y la meditación, para soltar la tensión y la ira, o llame a alguien en quien usted confía para hablar del asunto.

3. Después de calmarse, explíquele a su niño que usted lo quiere *a él*, pero no le gusta su conducta.

4. Explíquele qué conducta quiere que aprenda y por qué.

5. Nunca le pegue a un niño en la cara o en la cabeza. Nunca lo patee. Nunca le aviente objetos. No use un cinturón para pegarle.

6. Si siente que tiene que darle nalgadas, hágalo con la mano abierta en las nalgas.

7. Trate de reparar y renovar la relación, al abrazarlo y decirle que lo perdona y lo quiere. Para cada acción negativa, tiene que haber muchas más que sean positivas.

LOS ESTILOS DE CRIANZA Y EL DESARROLLO DEL CARÁCTER

De acuerdo a R. R. Sears y E. E. Macoby en su libro *Patterns of Child Rearing*, es más probable que los niños desarrollen una consciencia y sufran de sentimientos de culpabilidad, si los padres utilizan el razonamiento y la culpabilidad, o si les dejan de dar afecto y aprobación. Sin embargo, si utilizan las nalgadas, las amenazas, o la privación de privilegios para disciplinar a sus niños, los niños tienen la tendencia de ser más agresivos. Diana Baumrind identificó tres estilos de crianza que incluyen el autoritario y el permisivo.

Padres autoritarios utilizan el castigo o la culpabilidad para seguir reglas absolutas; quieren controlar estrechamente a sus niños para que se adhieran a unas normas estrictas de conducta. Los padres son distantes, más controladores, y menos cariñosos que otros padres. Sus niños tienen la tendencia de ser más conformistas, más infelices, retraídos, y desconfiados.

Padres permisivos se les permite hacer todo lo que quieren. Con pocas reglas y casi nada de castigos, quizá lleguen a ser más ansiosos, inseguros, manipuladores, e inmaduros porque no han tenido un compás o mapa para orientarse. Su conducta es motivada por premios exteriores y por evitar el castigo, más que por gratificación interna.

Muchos investigadores están de acuerdo en que un niño que crece con rechazos, sin ningún entrenamiento, ni contacto con las reglas, ni consistencia con respecto a las reglas, los valores, y las expectativas, puede crecer con una falta de principios o llegar a ser impulsivo, egocéntrico, y vulnerable a la delincuencia. Los niños delincuentes son descritos como personas que no sienten culpabilidad, insensibles o crueles, y agresivos, que no han logrado interiorizar ninguna norma de conducta moral. En lugar de eso, quizá estén atrapados dentro de la etapa donde sólo tienen un sentido de culpabilidad o de incompetencia. La delincuencia juvenil está asociada con ciertas técnicas de crianza y patrones de relaciones familiares. Sin importar el nivel socioeconómico, la delincuencia juvenil puede surgir en cualquier hogar donde los padres disciplinan dura y esporádicamente, donde no participan en la vida de su niño, y no siguen de cerca ni supervisan las actividades de su niño.

Pero un carácter positivo nace en un hogar que es consistentemente democrático y que tiene relaciones familiares amorosas. Tal modelo está relacionado con el último estilo de crianza que Baumrind identifica: el de *autoridad*. Este modelo quizá sea diferente al modelo de autoridad con el cual muchos hispanos han crecido, pero no rechaza los valores que lo motivan. Los padres que tienen autoridad son amorosos, firmes, exigentes, consistentes, y respetuosos en su disciplina. Utilizan una disciplina indulgente y racional, explicándole al niño las razones por sus normas y sus posturas. Los padres que tienen autoridad le permiten a su niño expresarse y respetan sus opiniones, sus intereses, y su personalidad singular. Los padres de autoridad producen niños que son socialmente responsables, porque (1) ellos confrontan explícitamente a sus niños acerca de las cosas que les pueden resultar dañinos, (2) son consistentes al hacer cumplir los mandatos y las reglas, (3) son directos y honestos y no son manipuladores ni indirectos, (4) requieren obediencia a la autoridad, (5) su uso consistente de su autoridad de padres los convierten en modelos de conducta atrayentes para sus niños.

LA RELIGIÓN Y EL DESARROLLO DE LA CONSCIENCIA Y LA CONDUCTA DESEABLE

Las prácticas y las creencias religiosas, sin importar la religión específica, pueden servir como herramientas fuertes para el desarrollo moral. Cada religión tiene su valor, y cada una apoya normas y verdades universales con relación a la conducta moral. En el caso de mi familia, los diez mandamientos y la Biblia sirven como guías a la conducta apropiada y son unas fuentes de sabiduría. Las oraciones son fuentes de la fortaleza interna. Los niños que reciben una educación espiritual, incluyendo una asistencia habitual a la iglesia, adquieren y refuerzan algunos de los valores y los principios que son enseñados en el hogar. La "regla de oro" existe en todas las religiones.

Satisfacer la necesidad espiritual de los niños les ayudará a desarrollar un fuerte sentido de compasión y bondad además de una consciencia y un sentido de culpabilidad. La religión les provoca a los niños una consciencia de las fuerzas del bien y del mal que tiran del niño y luchan por ganarse la voluntad, el intelecto, y las emociones del niño, para que él haga cosas buenas o malas.

El personaje bueno en esta lucha se conoce por muchos nombres y se encuentra en muchos dichos hispanos que sirven de guía al comportamiento moral y a la conducta apropiada. Los padres utilizan esta fuerza poderosa para formar una consciencia en sus niños cuando dicen, *Bien sabe Dios tus mañas aunque pienses que lo engañas*. Este dicho les indica a los niños que no pueden nunca hacer cosas que queden desapercibidas porque Dios siempre está mirando. *Déjaselo a Dios* y *Cosas a Dios dejadas, son bien vengadas*, son dichos que ayudan a los niños a disminuir o disolver su ira.

El personaje malo que también tira de la consciencia por el temor, también es conocido por muchos nombres: Satanás, el Diablo, Lucifer, o Belcebú. Hay también dichos sobre él, como *el diablo no duerme*. La cultura hispana también tiene una riqueza de cuentos populares acerca de la facilidad con que las personas pueden ser tentadas por la maldad, una fuerza que a veces representa el papel de este personaje en un cuento para estimular a nuestros niños a portarse bien.

"Not Only One But Two Devils", *"The Devil Takes a Bride"*, y "El guapo extranjero" forman parte de una colección de cuentos populares por Juan Sauvageau en *Stories That Must Not Die*. Son cuentos populares tradicionales hispanos sobre el diablo, que provocan risa y temor a los niños, al mismo tiempo de transmitir lecciones sobre la moralidad. El cuento popular llamado *"Not Only One But Two Devils"* ("No solamente uno, sino dos diablos") se trata de un hombre que trataba muy cruelmente a su esposa e hijos cuando se emborrachaba. Motivada por la desesperación, la esposa les dice a los dos hermanos de ella que divorciará a su esposo si vuelve otra vez a la casa borracho. Para darle una lección, los dos hermanos se visten como diablos y lo asustan, atándolo y jalándolo hacia una pequeña hoguera que habían construido cerca del camino. Lo están calen-

tando antes de llevarlo a su destino eterno en el infierno por la vida de borracho que ha llevado. Pudo convencerlos de permitirle despedirse de su esposa y sus niños y pedirles perdón por su conducta tan terrible. La esposa acepta las disculpas sinceras del esposo y le ruega a los diablos que le den otra oportunidad. Los diablos ceden pero juran llevarlo derechito al infierno la próxima vez que toma. El hombre nunca más volvió a tomar.

"El guapo extranjero" es un cuento sobre una joven hermosa pero vanidosa, que deriva placer de hacerles daño a los hombres. Su madre le advierte que no debe jugar con los sentimientos de los hombres, pero ella sólo se ríe del consejo. Una noche la madre, quien presiente que algo malo le va a pasar a su hija, le ruega que no vaya al baile. Por fin decide acompañar a su hija, quien se mantenía firme acerca de hacer acto de presencia. Cerca de la medianoche, un hombre muy guapo entra al salón y va directamente hacia la hija, quien se sonroja de orgullo, porque él la ha escogido por encima de todas las demás muchachas. El hombre guapo baila con la hija aun después de terminar la música, dándole vueltas y vueltas, cada vez más velozmente, hasta que una nube de humo envuelve a la pareja. Cuando la nube desaparece, el extranjero se ha desaparecido y la hija está tirada en el piso, muerta. Todos hablan todavía acerca de que el "guapo extranjero" con quien bailó la hija era el mismo Satanás. Este cuento popular es similar al que contaban los niños de mi barrio, excepto que el hombre guapo tenía patas de gallo. Este cuento y otros como "La Llorona" y "La lechuza" eran algunos de los que provocaban más temor y que se contaban cada noche de Todos los Santos (*Halloween*) en el barrio.

BIEN EDUCADOS

Al ser el primer factor que ayuda a socializar, usted tiene la responsabilidad de enseñarles a sus niños a la edad más pequeña posible, lo que usted considera una conducta apropiada, enseñándoles la manera de vivir con relación al bien y al mal. Yo pienso en el pasado para recordar cómo mi madre trató de socializarnos a mis hermanos y a mí para que llegáramos a ser bien educados, a comportarnos según las buenas costumbres en la casa y en público. En la opinión de mi madre, el ser bien educado significaba tener un buen carácter, integridad, y honestidad. Iba más allá de conseguir una educación formal y adquirir una licenciatura, una maestría, o un doctorado. Ella estableció una norma de conducta, una manera de vivir que ella esperaba que nosotros cumpliéramos y siguiéramos. "La regla más importante de esta familia", ella decía, "es el respeto". Tener una falta de educación significaba una falta de respeto. Aprendimos muy temprano en la vida que se esperaba que respetáramos a nuestros abuelos, a nuestros padres, y a otras personas de autoridad. Ella también ponía énfasis en la importancia de respetar a aquéllos menos afortunados, emocionalmente, socialmente, y físicamente. Ella citaba las palabras de Benito Juárez, "el respeto al derecho ajeno es la paz", para enseñarnos que no debíamos agarrar ni dañar las cosas que no nos pertenecían. Ella nos enseñó la importancia de la dignidad y de sentirnos dignos de respeto.

Aparte del respeto, un niño hispano que es bien educado, necesita tener buenos modales. Él debe decir "por favor" y "gracias", no interrumpe, sí comparte, y es empático y generoso. Comprende cómo portarse con diferentes personas y bajo distintas circunstancias. Sabe cuándo hablar y cuándo no, como se ilustra por medio de refranes como *Al hablar como al guisar, su granito de sal*. Otro refrán relacionado a la acción de hablar es *Antes de hablar, es bueno pensar*. Unos dichos aconsejan que a veces es mejor estar callado al decir, *en boca cerrada, no entran moscas*, y también, *el poco hablar es oro, el mucho hablar es lodo*.

Estar bien socializado significa estar bien equilibrado. Mi madre quería que tuviéramos orgullo y confianza en nosotros mismos, que lográramos éxitos y que fuéramos competitivos. Pero al mismo tiempo, recalcaba la importancia de la humildad, de nunca pensar que éramos mejores que otras personas. Siempre nos decía que podíamos ser cualquier cosa que deseáramos si tan sólo nos esforzábamos mucho y nos educábamos, pero no debíamos jactarnos de nuestros logros, *ninguno diga quién es, que sus obras lo dirán*. *En árbol caído todos se suben a sus ramas* o *del árbol caído todos hacen leña*, son dichos que les enseñan a los niños hispanos que el orgullo derrocado sólo inspira desprecio y desdén, por eso deben ser modestos. Steven una vez puso en cuestión el valor de la modestia que tiene mi madre, al decirle: "Pero, Abuelita, mi entrenador de fútbol americano nos dice que debemos pensar que somos mejores que todos para mentalizarnos para ganar el juego". Ella respondió, como lo hacía frecuentemente, al decir: "Sea valiente como un león, sabio como un águila, y bondadoso como la paloma. Como jugadores de fútbol, la gente sabrá que son mejores si se esfuerzan mucho, si desarrollan y utilizan sus buenos talentos, y más importante, si *anotan más puntos* que el otro equipo". Como dice el dicho, *en el modo de montar se conoce al que es jinete*. Muestre su valor a través de sus acciones, no sus palabras.

En el mundo materialista de hoy, podemos dañar a nuestros niños cuando les damos todo lo que quieren. Nuestros niños podrían "volverse como serpientes" y mordernos si les damos todo, tal como dice el dicho, *todo el que a su hijo consiente, va engordando una serpiente*. Yo también soy culpable de darles más a mis niños de lo que necesitan y no he sido consistente con relación a hacerles trabajar para lo que quieren. Los niños necesitan desear algo. Deben aprender a luchar para ganar lo que quieren, para realmente apreciarlo. Quizá por nuestra condición económica humilde, mis hermanos y yo aprendimos muy temprano en la vida que teníamos que trabajar para lo que queríamos y que teníamos que contribuir a la familia. De las sabias palabras de nuestros mayores, aprendimos que debíamos apreciar lo que teníamos y lo que se nos daba, porque si no lo apreciábamos, no éramos bien criados, tal como se escucha frecuentemente en el dicho *No es bien nacido, el que no es agradecido.* También aprendimos que *la felicidad es querer todo lo que tienes y no tener todo lo que quieres.* Por supuesto, si queríamos más, sabíamos que teníamos que trabajar para conseguirlo.

En mi familia, se recalcaba mucho el valor del trabajo. Nunca olvidaré el verano antes de que cumpliera los dieciséis años de edad. Era el primer día de vacaciones de la escuela, y yo anticipaba con entusiasmo la idea de relajarme y tirarme en el sofá enfrente del aire acondicionado que funcionaba con agua, al estilo de antes, cuando mi madre entró al cuarto y me dijo: "Levántate y busca trabajo". Estaba desconcertada porque todavía faltaba un mes antes de que yo tuviera la edad para trabajar legalmente, sin embargo, ella no quería desperdiciar el tiempo, quería prepararme. Ya nos había inculcado el valor de trabajar fuera de la casa. De niña, había trabajado haciendo la limpieza en la casa de una vecina anciana y también vendiendo los aretes de lentejuelas que hacía mi madre, en adición a los mucho productos que vendíamos, como los de Stanley y Avon, y los vestidos de los catálogos.

En mi primer trabajo ese verano, de mesera, yo gané más dinero en propinas de lo que jamás podría haberme imaginado. Mi madre me aseguró que habría aun mejores trabajos para mí más adelante, que ése era tan sólo el principio. Después fui una vendedora en una tienda. Este trabajo pagaba mejor, pero requería que trabajara los jueves por la noche, y volviera a la casa en el camión. Era difícil para mi madre dejar que sus niños salieran al mundo lleno de crimen y violencia, especialmente por las noches. Ella respiraba hondo, nos dejaba en las manos de Dios, y le pedía a Dios que nos protegiera contra los peligros y las tentaciones que podríamos enfrentar. Tal como un gorrión en su nido, me dejó volar, pero a veces la miraba esperándome junto a la cerca en nuestra casa, donde me saludaba con un "bendito sea Dios" o "gracias a Dios".

Se nos enseñó que cada uno tenía que contribuir un porcentaje de cualquier dinero que ganaba, para el beneficio de la familia. Con frecuencia le oímos a mi madre decir: "Cuando yo trabajaba, le entregaba todo a mi mama. Cuando yo era joven", ella decía, "yo le daba todo mi cheque a mi madre, porque ella conocía mejor las necesidades de la casa. Ella manejaba el presupuesto familiar y se aseguraba que todos tuviéramos lo que necesitábamos y queríamos, incluyendo los vestidos que ella permitía que apartara y que pagábamos en abonos". Como resultado de su educación, mi madre alentaba, pero no exigía, que cada uno de nosotros le diera la mitad de sus ganancias. Todas mis hermanas obedecieron sin chistar, pero yo no.

Yo ponía en duda que yo debía darle dinero a ella, cuando algunas de mis amigas recibían una mensualidad de sus padres. Yo pensaba que porque ella creció durante la "depresión", la familia de mi madre tuvo que hacer un fondo común con todos sus recursos para sobrevivir, pero de ninguna manera sentía yo que nosotros fuéramos pobres. No era que yo no quería contribuir económicamente al bienestar de la familia, simplemente quería tener yo el control sobre el dinero que yo ganaba y quería determinar para qué se usaba. Yo quería comprarle a mi madre las cosas especiales que yo sabía que ella no se compraría a sí misma o para la casa. Nunca se quejó y siempre agradeció todo lo que le daba. Durante todo el año pagaba los abonos de los regalos que había apartado para su cumpleaños o para la Navidad. En retrospectiva, yo ahora me doy cuenta que mi madre sabía mejor qué eran nuestras necesidades, pero *cada cabeza es un mundo*, y yo siempre he querido ser la jefe y estar al mando. Mi madre enseñó, a través de su ejemplo, la importancia de economizar, ahorrar, y manejar el dinero, y muchas otras madres han enseñado a través de dichos tales como *¡Ahorra! No hay poco que no llegue, ni mucho que no se acabe; Guarda los centavos, que los pesos llegarán; Muchos pocos, hacen un mucho.*

Mi hermana Rosa Linda fue la única de la familia que siguió con la práctica de pedir un cierto porcentaje de las ganancias de sus hijos cuando trabajaban. En lugar del cincuenta por ciento, que había pedido mi madre, ella pedía un tercio. Ella realmente no necesitaba el dinero para cumplir su presupuesto y llegar a fin del mes; lo hizo porque quería enseñarles a sus niños la lección de dar de sí mismos, y de ayudar a sus hermanos que se quedaban en la casa haciendo los quehaceres. Su esposo llevaba a sus hijos varones al trabajo con él cuando eran pequeños para que aprendieran el oficio de la construcción de las aceras. Al final del día, le daba a cada uno veinte dólares. En cuanto sus niños le daban a ella la parte que le correspondía, ella a su vez les daba el dinero a los más pequeños. Mi hermana tenía un hijo obstinado que, al igual que yo, ponía en duda la práctica de darle su dinero. Ella le respondió al decir: "Tú tienes una responsabilidad de cuidar a tus hermanos menores".

Los padres deben enseñarles a sus niños los principios importantes, como por ejemplo, tener una sólida ética de trabajo, ahorrar el dinero, y ser el cuidador de sus hermanos. Un niño no puede aprender, de la noche al día, el valor del trabajo, cuando cumple los dieciséis años o cuando se gradúa de la universidad. La ética de trabajo comienza temprano en la vida. Los niños no pueden simplemente hacerse responsables del cuidado de sus hermanos si se lo pide su padre en su lecho de muerte. Al contrario, estos valores deben estar firmemente establecidos en la mente de los niños cuando son muy jóvenes. Encuentre maneras de enseñarles estos valores importantes, lo cual requiere de tiempo, consistencia, e ingenio.

El valor de la educación también debe ser recalcado en el hogar. Por ser hermanas, se esperaba que mis hermanas y yo nos ayudáramos con relación a nuestra educación. La forma que tenía mi madre de inculcarnos la importancia de la educación era de motivarnos a tratar de conseguir mejores trabajos. "Claro", ella decía, "cualquier trabajo es bueno. Pero", añadía siempre, "yo quiero que mis hijos trabajen en un lugar respetable con aire acondicionado y alfombra". Antes de darnos cuenta, estábamos luchando por algo mejor, y pronto nos enteramos de que el tipo de trabajos a los cuales ella refería, requerían una educación. Ella influía de una manera increíble sobre nuestras aspiraciones para algo mejor. Nos empujaba suavemente a soñar y a lograr metas más altas, pero nunca nos presionaba a hacerlo. Cuando yo gané un concurso de belleza, para ser "Miss Fiesta" para el desfile de Flambeau en San Antonio, mi madre sugirió con toda tranquilidad que no parara allí, que compitiera para el título de "Miss America". Cómo me reí. Ya para entonces, yo estaba determinada a forjar mis propias metas y a formar mis propias expectativas. Aunque no competí para ser "Miss America", sí me gradué de la universidad y me convertí en maestra en un cuarto con aire acondicionado y alfombra.

LAS ETAPAS DEL DESARROLLO DE LA MORALIDAD

Usted, como padre, tiene la responsabilidad principal de enseñar las buenas costumbres y la moralidad. Usted es la persona que enseñará primero a sus niños cómo vivir con relación al bien y al mal. Pero, ¿por dónde comienza uno? Quizá por saber y comprender que sus niños pasan por diferentes etapas de desarrollo moral. Los padres deben saber y comprender cómo aprenden, crecen, y se desarrollan los niños, y los muchos factores que afectan su conducta. Deben estar conscientes de las diferentes etapas del desarrollo moral, intelectual, social, lingüístico, y físico.

Toda esta información formará el marco que orienta las actitudes y las prácticas de los padres en la crianza de sus niños.

De acuerdo al psicólogo Jean Piaget, el niño primero es impulsivo y no tiene ningún concepto de obligaciones ni de reglas cuando es muy pequeño. ¿Recuerda cuando yo mencioné lo importante que es que alrededor de los ocho meses de edad, comience a enseñarle a su niño a tener dominio de sí mismo? Necesitamos ayudarle a ser menos impulsivo y no hacer todo lo que quiere. Necesitamos enseñarle a hacer lo que debe hacer, y qué es la conducta apropiada, y los deberes de la vida. Primero acepta estas reglas como sagradas e inalterables cuando son impuestas por los adultos. A la edad de nueve años, las reglas pueden ser más flexibles y se basan en el respeto mutuo. Por último, un niño desarrolla un interés en las reglas.

De acuerdo a Lawrence Kohlberg, un niño no se da cuenta en un principio, que es un ser separado, aparte, de los objetos y de sus padres. A la edad de dos años, comienza a afirmar su identidad separada. ¿Recuerde la etapa de "mío"? Esto les ocurre a los niños, como ilustré antes cuando puse a Vanessa como ejemplo. Durante esta etapa, su niño quizá sea más impulsivo e incontrolable. A esta etapa le sigue la etapa de "protegerse a sí mismo", durante la cual anticipa premios y castigos de corta duración. Probará los límites y hará cosas que sabe que no debe hacer. El dicho *Carita de santo, los hechos no tanto*, se aplica a los niños de esta edad. Vulnerable y cauteloso, trata de evitar que lo pillen. Mirará a su alrededor para ver si sus padres están allí antes de hacer algo malo. Pero *el mal y el bien en la cara se ven*. A esta etapa le sigue la etapa "conformista", durante la cual él puede ver la conexión entre su propio bienestar y el de la familia o el grupo. Él sabe que para formar parte de la familia, él tiene que hacer su parte. Luego, él desarrollará sus propias normas y verá los puntos de vista de otras personas. La etapa de "autonomía" marca el período cuando un niño desarrolla un respeto por la autonomía y la independencia. Por último, la etapa de "integración" es el período de realización propia, una época cuando un niño se siente seguro y feliz consigo mismo e intenta llegar a otros para ayudarles.

Los hispanos de ambos sexos alcanzan esta etapa mucho más temprano por su singularidad. Tal como he mencionado antes, Carol Gilligan, la profesora de Harvard, explora la diferencia entre los niños y las niñas. Los niños varones tienen la tendencia de ser más competitivos, más preocupados por las reglas, luchando para alcanzar logros e independencia. Las niñas, por otro lado, tienen una fuerte sensibilidad hacia otros, por naturaleza son más cariñosas, y les gusta cooperar más que competir o lograr a expensas de otra persona.

Al leer el libro de Gilligan *In a Different Voice*, yo concluí que las características que describe para las niñas quizá, hasta cierto punto, tengan que ver con la definición que tiene la madre hispana de lo que es un niño bien educado. Los hispanos tradicionalmente han reforzado estas características como parte de su cultura. Gilligan dice que los varones, desde el comienzo del complejo de Edipo, quieren separarse de su madre, y por eso no son tan cariñosos, desde ese momento luchando por la independencia y la autonomía. No es así en el caso de las niñas, ella dice. Ellas, como los hispanos, se preocupan mucho por las relaciones y desarrollan su personalidad dentro del contexto de los vínculos afectivos y la afiliación con otros.

No hay duda que noté una diferencia entre mi hija y mis hijos varones desde su nacimiento, sin embargo yo deseaba lo mismo para todos. A la vez quería que Vanessa fuera más competidora y firme y que mis niños varones fueran más cariñosos y comprensivos. Como padres nuestra meta para ellos debe ser que tengan un equilibrio entre los papeles tradicionales del varón y las calidades femeninas así como indican investigadores como Gilligan.

Por ejemplo, en mi familia mi madre me permitió ser una niña poca femenina. Yo solía jugar con canicas, subirme a los árboles, jugar deportes competitivos como el béisbol a mitad de la calle con los niños en el barrio. Yo luchaba por mis derechos y ponía en duda las reglas de todos los juegos que jugaba, desde la línea que teníamos que cruzar en el juego de tira y afloja con una cuerda en "La víbora de la mar" hasta los parámetros de "La roña". Mi hija es igual de competitidora con los niños varones y puede mantener el paso de ellos en todos los deportes. Sin embargo, yo, igual a mi madre, he recalcado la importancia de ser bondadoso, considerado, y empático. En muchos respectos este mundo sería mejor si nuestros niños fueran menos agresivos y competitidores, y más cooperativos.

LA ENSEÑANZA DE LOS VALORES, LA MORALIDAD, Y LAS COSTUMBRES

Los padres deben determinar qué significa para ellos ser bien educado. Los padres son los primeros maestros de la moralidad, los que imparten sus valores, sus principios, y sus costumbres. Son los primeros para transmitir los valores culturales y de conducta, los cuales influyen sobre la manera en que sus niños se deben portar y el tipo de vida que sus niños deben llevar. Por eso, es crucial que los padres tengan una imagen de cómo quieren que sus niños se porten. Deben formular y verbalizar las expectativas que tienen con relación a sus niños. Deben tener una idea acerca de los conocimientos que quieren que tengan. Por ser los primeros factores que ayudan a socializar, los padres moldean la conducta de sus niños para que se conforme con lo que ellos y la sociedad consideran importantes. Ellos establecen los cimientos para el desarrollo de carácter, la moralidad, y los valores. Los padres deben presentar una comprensión clara de lo que es correcto e incorrecto y enseñar por medio del ejemplo además de las palabras.

Un padre forma la conducta de un niño cuandoquiera que enseña modales y conducta apropiada como: "Di por favor y gracias; no te piques la nariz; tápate la nariz cuando estornudas; no interrumpas, espera tu turno; no le pegues a tu hermano; comparte; y sé bueno". La enseñanza de una conducta apropiada es una manera de socializar a un niño. Nuestros niños aprenden también a través de los mensajes negativos que les transmitimos. Cuando usted a sabiendas deja que el cajero le devuelva más cambio que lo debido en la presencia de su niño, o trata de hacerlo pasar por tener cierta edad para evitar tener que pagar el precio para un adulto en el cine, le está enseñando pequeñas mentiras. Tal como dice el dicho *Verdades a medias, mentiras enteras*, las mentiras pequeñas y los robos o delitos menores pueden fácilmente aumentar y convertirse en mentiras o delitos mayores. No debemos decir "No harás" con la boca y "Sí harás" con nuestras acciones. Nuestras acciones tienen que corresponder a nuestras palabras, tal como se nos dice en el dicho *Predicar con el ejemplo es el mejor argumento*.

La mayoría de los padres crían a sus niños de acuerdo a la manera en que sus padres los criaron a ellos. Aquellas lecciones tempranas no se olvidan fácilmente. Otros padres querrán leer y aprender lo más posible sobre la crianza de los niños. Las enseñanzas espirituales que se aprenden en el hogar, la iglesia, o la sinagoga, tales como la bondad, la honestidad, y la compasión, en realidad sirven como una orientación para la conducta. La regla de oro, "Haz a otros como tú querrías que te hicieran a ti", es un principio común entre muchas religiones. Se considera una necesidad para tener harmonía y paz. Los valores tales como la justicia, la bondad, la responsabilidad, y el respeto deben ser enseñados lo más temprano posible. Para que una sociedad civil y democrática prospere, debe ser compuesto de personas que abrazan estos principios y virtudes. Es importante que los padres comprendan el significado de cada una de estas virtudes. Dígales a sus niños claramente lo que espera de ellos. Ayúdelos a comprender y a adquirir estas características. Es la responsabilidad principal de los padres enseñarles a sus niños estas virtudes y fomentar el desarrollo moral y espiritual de sus niños.

Haga una lista de aquellas cualidades y virtudes que usted quiere que sus niños aprendan. Invite a su pareja a hacer lo mismo. Asegúrese de que usted y su pareja los pongan en orden de importancia para decidir cuáles consideran más importantes. Comprenda que tiene que ser flexible y darse cuenta que algunos valores estarán en conflicto debido a prioridades y falta de tiempo. Por ejemplo, la limpieza, el orden, y la organización a veces tendrán que hacerse a un lado para que su familia pueda sentir alegría, unidad, y apoyo al crecimiento y desarrollo de cada uno. Si se enfoca tanto en alcanzar una cierta virtud, quizá no le quede ni tiempo ni energía para los otros valores que usted considera importantes.

Lo más temprano posible, invite a sus niños a participar en establecer una lista de valores familiares que cada miembro de la familia accede a seguir. Discuta la razón para cada uno de estos valores y las consecuencias naturales que pueden ocurrir si no los siguen: "Si no tienes una recámara ordenada, no podrás encontrar tus cosas", "Dormirás más cómodamente si cambias tus sabanas una vez por semana". Quizá pueda intentar hacer un teatro improvisado para que sus niños puedan aprender cómo se siente cuando no son tratados con bondad o cuando alguien no respeta su propiedad. Ponga énfasis en el significado opuesto de cada valor para que sus niños puedan reconocer qué no deben hacer en ciertas situaciones, y por qué.

Los niños, dependiendo de su edad, quizá no tengan las mismas normas que usted. Únase a ellos para limpiar su cuarto cuando son pequeños. Haga el esfuerzo de modelar para ellos la paciencia, la bondad, y el respeto. Siempre trate de demostrar el valor de lo que les está tratando de enseñar. Por ejemplo, puede escribir los nombres de todos los miembros de la familia en una hoja grande. Cada vez que ocurre una acción que usted quiere reforzar, ponga una estrella dorada junto al nombre de la persona que lo demuestra.

Aliente, premie, y refuerce la buena conducta cuando ésta ocurre. Utilice comentarios como "Se siente bonito dar, ¿verdad?" "Ayudar a cortar el césped de los vecinos mientras están fuera de la ciudad es un acto de bondad. Estoy seguro que te lo agradecerán mucho". También: "Gracias por ayudarme a poner la mesa, te lo agradezco mucho". "Hiciste muy buen trabajo al guardar los juguetes donde pertenecen".

LA ENSEÑANZA A TRAVÉS DE LOS DICHOS

Mi madre y mi abuelo tenían muy claros los valores que nos querían transmitir. Como muchos hispanos a través de los siglos, nos enseñaron normas de conducta, virtudes, y valores al utilizar los dichos, los cuales se usaban para imprimir carácter. La autoridad y el respeto afuera de la institución familiar, se ganan a través de las virtudes y la bondad, como se declara en el dicho *Con virtud y bondad se adquiere autoridad*. El tipo de persona que llega a ser uno, es evidente a través de su carácter, porque *el árbol se conoce por su fruta*. Cuando los padres les enseñan virtudes a sus niños, están plantando las semillas que sus niños cosecharán más adelante al tener una vida sana y productiva. Los siguientes son unos valores que mi esposo y yo hemos tratado de inculcarles a nuestros niños, junto con algunos dichos que los ilustran:

Compasivos, bondadosos, y sensibles

El regalo más grande que le puede obsequiar a su niño es el amor incondicional, para que él, a su vez, lo pueda dar a otros. Queremos que cuiden a aquéllos con necesidad, y que sean generosos y agradecidos. Queremos que den de su tiempo, sus talentos, y sus recursos, para el beneficio de otros, y que aprendan el significado del perdón. Como dijo Madre Teresa, queremos que amen "hasta que duela".

- Ama a tu vecino y te amará.
- Ama a tu prójimo como a ti mismo.
- Amor con amor se paga.
- Amor de padre y madre, que lo demás es aire.
- Cortesía de boca mucho consigue y nada cuesta.
- Costumbres y dinero hacen a los hijos caballeros.
- Cuando hay corazón hay lugar en tu casa.
- El que da primero da dos veces.
- El que parte y comparte se queda con la mejor parte.
- Haz bien sin mirar a quién.
- La caridad para dar comienza en el hogar.

Trabajadores

Queremos que nuestros niños tengan motivación, determinación, y perseverancia, que usen la iniciativa y el entusiasmo para mejorarse y lograr el éxito. Deben resistir los impulsos y las tentaciones, y sobreponerse a los obstáculos y a las dificultades, para alcanzar sus metas deseadas. Queremos que sean dignos de confianza, formales, y responsables con relación a completar sus tareas (tarea escolar, quehaceres, pasatiempos) de comienzo a final, y hacerlo de una manera aceptable y apropiada sin la necesidad de recordatorios, y sin excusas. Los niños necesitan tener compromisos claros para establecer metas realistas, planear, y tomar los pasos necesarios para lograrlos. Una persona que es responsable se da cuenta de sus acciones y acepta las consecuencias. Se da cuenta que tiene la responsabilidad de saber quién es y qué son sus talentos, de respetar su nombre y mantener su palabra, y reconocer sus obligaciones a sí mismo, a la familia, a los amigos, a sus empleadores, a su patria, y a los necesitados. Debe utilizar su tiempo, su energía, y sus talentos sabiamente para lograr todas las metas que se fijen y que les harán sentirse realizados. Debe darse cuenta de que su vida es importante y que tiene un propósito.

- Al que madruga, Dios lo ayuda.
- Cada cual es hijo de sus obras.
- Como siembras, segarás.
- De lo dicho al hecho hay mucho trecho.
- El caballo corredor no necesita espuelas.
- El trabajo es virtud.
- Hombre precavido, jamás vencido.
- No dejes para mañana lo que puedas hacer hoy.
- Más vale pájaro en mano que ciento volando.
- Temprano se moja, tiene tiempo para secarse.
- Trabajar para más valer, estudiar para más saber.
- Ninguno diga quién es, que sus obras lo dirán.

Valientes y responsables

Los niños necesitan tener fortaleza para mantener inquebrantables sus valores e ideales y para tomar responsabilidad de sus acciones. Con esta virtud, podrán rechazar las drogas, el alcohol, el sexo, la violencia, y las pandillas. Queremos que tengan el valor y la confianza para tomar los riesgos necesarios para poder aprender, mejorarse, y crecer.

- Cuando una puerta se cierra, dos mil se abren.
- Cuando todas las puertas se cierran, una ventana se abre.
- Cumple con tu deber, aunque tengas que perder.
- Los cobardes mueren cien veces antes de morir.
- Más vale morir parado que vivir de rodillas.
- No dé un paso adelante sin ver para atrás.
- No hay mal que por bien no salga.
- No hay peor lucha que la que no se hace.

Educados

Los conocimientos se adquieren por medio de los consejos, la experiencia, y una educación formal. Con una buena educación, los niños podrán pensar de manera crítica, analizar, tomar buenas decisiones, planear, y establecer metas futuras. Tendrán confianza. Una buena educación da la llave para salir de la pobreza y lograr una mejor calidad de vida. Sirve como vehículo para una sociedad civil. En última instancia, la educación nos da la llave a la libertad. Se dice que en la vida las personas pueden quitarle a uno todas sus posesiones, despojarle de sus títulos y negarle su próximo aumento de sueldo, *pero nadie le puede quitar su educación.*

- Dichos de los viejitos, son evangelios chiquitos.
- El alfabetismo es enemigo de la esclavitud.
- El error sólo es fracaso cuando no se convierte en experiencia.
- El hombre que sabe hacia dónde va, el camino se abre para dejarlo pasar.
- El hombre que sabe dos idiomas vale por dos.
- El niño aprende cada día cosas que no sabía.
- El que adelante no mira, atrás se queda.
- El que bien tiene, y mal escoge, por mal que le vaya, que no se enoje.
- Lo que se aprende en la cuna, siempre dura.
- Los libros nos dan la ciencia y la vida la experiencia.
- Más sabe el diablo por viejo que por diablo.
- Mientras puedo, ¿quién dijo miedo?
- No hay que andarse por las ramas estando tan grueso el tronco.
- No vengo a ver si puedo, sino porque puedo vengo.
- Quien no oye consejos, no llega a viejo.
- Saber es poder.

Frugales y concienzudos con relación al dinero

Los niños necesitan aprender cómo manejar sus bienes, gastar juiciosamente, y ahorrar el dinero para cuando lleguen las vacas flacas.

- ¡Ahorra! No hay poco que no llegue, ni mucho que no se acabe.
- Compra con tu dinero, no con el del banquero.
- Cuentas arregladas, amistades largas.
- El que nada debe, nada teme.

- El que paga lo que debe, sabe lo que tiene.
- Guarda los centavos, que los pesos (dólares) llegarán.
- La ambición del dinero hace al hombre pecador.
- Poseer es ser poseído.
- Presta dinero a un enemigo y lo ganarás; préstaselo a un amigo y lo perderás.

Sanos

Llevar una vida sana significa comer bien, hacer ejercicio, y evitar los hábitos dañinos como fumar, tomar, o consumir otras sustancias que hacen daño. Significa hacer todo con moderación. Si uno es sano quiere decir que es feliz y tiene buen estado de ánimo. La apariencia exterior de uno muestra lo que uno siente por dentro. Mi esposo y yo queremos que nuestros niños disfruten de la vida porque la vida es muy corta. Queremos que nuestros niños puedan reírse, tener tiempo libre para pararse a oler el perfume de las rosas, a apreciar la belleza y las maravillas del mundo. Queremos que viajen y que conozcan a personas para aprender acerca de las diferentes culturas a través del mundo. Queremos que piensen, hablen, aprendan, y crezcan en un mundo pacífico, justo, y democrático.

- Cada cosa se parece a su dueño.
- Como te ven, así te tratan.
- Desayuna bien, come más, cena poco y vivirás.
- El que mucho abarca, poco aprieta.
- La que come manzana, se cría sana.
- Salud y alegría crían belleza.
- No te apures, para que dures.
- Si quieres vivir sano, acuéstate y levántate temprano.
- Se come para vivir, no se vive para comer.
- Tanto baja el cántaro al agua hasta que se quiebra.
- Una onza de alegría vale más que una libra de oro.

Exitosos con relación a la amistad y otras relaciones humanas

Queremos que nuestros niños sean exitosos socialmente y que tengan muchos buenos amigos. Queremos que sientan que pertenecen y que tienen la capacidad de contribuir a la sociedad como personas, como padres, como trabajadores, como vecinos, y como ciudadanos. Queremos que tengan muchas relaciones exitosas y que sean leales a su familia, sus amigos, sus vecinos, la comunidad latina, la comunidad en general, y al país. Las relaciones pueden servir como fuentes de apoyo y compañía que sean mutuamente beneficiosas, porque dependemos unos de otros y ningún hombre puede vivir solo y aislado, como se ilustra a través de estos dichos:

- Acompáñate con los buenos y serás uno de ellos.
- Amigo en la adversidad, amigo de verdad.
- Aquéllos son ricos que tienen amigos.
- El pueblo unido jamás será vencido.
- Entre más amistad, más claridad.
- El caballo y el amigo no hay que cansarlos.
- El que a buen árbol se arrima, buena sombra le cobija.
- La amistad sincera es un alma repartida en dos cuerpos.
- ¿Quién es tu hermano? Tu vecino más cercano.
- Vida sin amigos, muerte sin testigos.

Ordenados y organizados

Cada cosa tiene su lugar, y todo en su lugar. Los niños necesitan aprender a organizar sus posesiones, su tiempo, y sus pensamientos de una manera estructurada. Necesitan establecer prioridades, fijar horarios, trazar planes, y desarrollar sistemas, procedimientos, y rutinas en la vida. Necesitan ser considerados y respetuosos con otros al ser silenciosos y ordenados.

Respetuosos, honestos, y justos

Como padres, queremos que nuestros hijos traten a las personas con dignidad y respeto, al ser imparcial y justo. Igualmente importante, queremos que sepan que ellos también son merecedores de recibir dignidad y respeto, y que bajo la Constitución de los Estados Unidos, tienen ciertos derechos a la vida, la libertad, y la búsqueda de la felicidad. Queremos que estén familiarizados con la Constitución y sus diez primeras enmiendas para que puedan proteger a otros y a sí mismos en contra de la injusticia y la desigualdad.

Queremos que sean cautelosos, alertos, y agresivos, al tener trato con aquéllos que se quieren aprovechar de ellos o causarles daño. Los niños necesitan aprender a respetarse a sí mismos junto con sus talentos únicos además de respetar a sus padres, sus vecinos, las personas de autoridad, y las leyes.

- El respeto al derecho ajeno es la paz.
- Bienes mal adquiridos a nadie han enriquecido.
- De juez de poca conciencia no esperes justa sentencia.
- Detrás la desconfianza está la seguridad.
- Más vale mancha en la frente que mancilla en el corazón.
- Para ser justo, hasta con el diablo.
- Tu conciencia es testigo, juez, y jurado.

Religiosos, con fe y fortaleza espiritual

Mi esposo y yo queremos inculcarles a nuestros hijos un fuerte sentido de fe, esperanza, y confianza que proviene de su religión y crecimiento espiritual. Queremos que sepan que Dios los ama, que siempre estará a su lado, y que siempre pueden mirar hacia Él cuando necesitan ayuda. Además, que Dios ha creado a todos como personas únicas y con un propósito. Cuando las cosas salen mal, queremos que puedan voltearse a Dios porque Él puede hacer que cualquier situación negativa se convierta en una positiva. Cuando uno tiene que enfrentarse a una terrible pérdida o mala fortuna, puede derivar fortaleza de su fe. Un día al estar escribiendo esta sección del libro, recibí la noticia de que mi mejor amiga de treinta años, mi comadre, mi vecina, Carmen Prieto Cortez, había fa–llecido en un terrible accidente automovilístico. Yo acababa de leerles esta sección a mis hijos, incluyendo la parte de pedirle a Dios su ayuda para aceptar aquello que no podemos cambiar, cuando recibimos la desafortunada llamada. A través de la tragedia, pude mostrarles a mis hijos cómo la fe puede ayudarle a uno a soportar el sufrimiento y el dolor que forman una parte inevitable de la vida, la cual a veces no queremos aceptar.

- Ayúdate que Dios te ayudará.
- Cada quien es como Dios lo hizo.
- Como el arcoiris, siempre sale después de la tempestad (la esperanza).
- Cosas a Dios dejadas son bien vengadas.
- Cuando Dios no quiere, santo no puede.
- Dejárselo en las manos de Dios.

- Dios habla por el que calla.
- El que no habla, Dios no lo oye.
- El hombre propone y Dios dispone.
- No se mueve la hoja sin la voluntad de Dios.
- Tiene más Dios que darnos, que nosotros que pedirle.

LA ENSEÑANZA A TRAVÉS DE LOS CUENTOS POPULARES

Los cuentos no sólo son reconocidos como unos de los mejores conservadores de nuestro idioma y nuestros recuerdos culturales, sino también son maravillosos asistentes en el proceso de socialización, enseñando a nuestros niños las a veces difíciles lecciones sobre cómo relacionarse con la gente y qué ocurre cuando las virtudes son puestas a prueba o son enfrentadas una contra otra. Muchos hispanos han crecido escuchando las historias de Juan Bobo y aprendiendo de sus contratiempos. Estas historias son sólo unos ejemplos de los innumerables cuentos populares de Latinoamérica (además de todos aquéllos que han sido modificados a través de las generaciones y adaptados en los Estados Unidos) que contienen importantes mensajes sociales que usted puede compartir con sus niños.

Algunos cuentos populares tratan de contestar de manera fantasiosa o juguetona los porqués de la vida, como por ejemplo, por qué el cielo es azul, o cómo consiguió sus manchas el sapo. En el caso de este último, captado en una colección de Genevieve Barlow en *Legends from Latin America/Leyendas de Latinoamérica*, un sapo aventurero se mete a hurtadillas dentro del estuche de la guitarra de un cuervo musical que iba a una reunión de sus amigos emplumados en el cielo. Al ser descubierto en la fiesta, el sapo es aventado inmediatamente fuera del cielo y se cae al suelo encima de un montón de piedras puntiagudas que dejaron marcada con cicatrices para siempre su piel antes tersa. Sin embargo, hasta la fecha, el pequeño sapo inquisitivo y valiente es admirado por todos los animales por su vuelo atrevido, y sus manchas son consideradas como una marca de valentía.

A veces los cuentos antiguos proveen lecciones básicas en la supervivencia y en el aprecio a las bendiciones que le han sido otorgadas a uno. En el cuento *"Count Your Blessings"* ("Cuenta tus bendiciones"), versión y adaptación de Teresa Pijoan, en *La cuentista*, un padre muy pobre sale en un día frío, con un hacha, en busca de leña para su familia y cae accidentalmente dentro de un pozo. Recibe un golpe en la cabeza y cuando se despierta, se encuentra cara a cara con una víbora. Mirándose intensamente a los ojos, ambos hombre y víbora piensan ser matados por el otro. El hombre le dice a la víbora que no hay ninguna necesidad de que ambos se mueran congelados, y la avienta fuera del pozo. La víbora vuelve, trayendo a sus hijos, y amarrándose juntos todos, jalan al padre fuera del pozo. Todos regresan a la casa del hombre, y a pesar de la poca leña para calentar la casa, la víbora y el padre tienen muchas bendiciones que agradecer: la vida, la familia, y los amigos.

En *"How the Brazilian Beetles Got Their Coats"* ("Cómo consiguieron los escarabajos brasileños sus caparazones [abrigos]"), del libro *The Moral Compass* de William J. Bennet, Elsie enseña acerca de utilizar los dones que Dios nos ha dado y de tener la confianza para atreverse a salir por el mundo a pesar de las probabilidades. El escarabajo consiguió sus bellos colores como premio al ganar una carrera contra la gran rata. En lugar de hacer la carrera corriendo, el escarabajo utiliza sus alas para volar a la línea de la victoria. "Nadie dijo que teníamos que correr", le dijo tan gallito a la rata, al revelar sus atributos ocultos. Porque este insecto decidió usar sus dones, los escarabajos ahora tienen un caparazón (abrigo) de bellos colores mientras las ratas aún tienen su pelaje gris y sin brillo.

Las madres y las abuelas por siglos han utilizado el cuento popular maya *"The Story of Mariano the Buzzard"* ("El cuento de Mariano el zopilote"), en el libro de James D. Sexton, *The Mayan Folktales: Folklore from Lake Atzlán*, para enseñarles a los niños a trabajar y a no ser flojos. El cuento se trata de una pareja de casados que son muy flojos y casi no tienen nada que comer. Mariano, el marido, se acostaba entre las hierbas, mirando el cielo y añorando ser como un zopilote para no tener que trabajar para conseguir su comida y simplemente cernerse en busca de animales muertos. Un día el zopilote oye al hombre y se ponen de acuerdo para cambiar lugares al cambiarse las chaquetas. El verdadero zopilote se da cuenta que no quiere ser un ser humano, se quita la chaqueta humana enfrente de la esposa del hombre y se aleja volando. La esposa cree que su verdadero esposo se ha convertido en zopilote por ser tan flojo. Cuando su esposo vuelve a casa como un zopilote, intenta hablar con su esposa pero no puede. La esposa estaba tan disgusta e irritada con los sonidos que hacía el zopilote, que agarró un trozo de leña y lo mató.

"The Late Bloomer" ("La planta de flor tardía"), otro cuento encontrado en el libro *The Moral Compass* de William J. Bennett, es un cuento popular mexicano sobre un cactus que está consternado por su apariencia fea y su falta de utilidad y propósito en el desierto caluroso. La luna

se une a un coro de animales que se burlan del cactus, y se jactan de su utilidad. Luego, de repente, en la punta del cactus, una bella y gloriosa flor se abre como una brillante corona y libera una maravillosa fragancia. Todos se paran a admirar al bello cactus porque nunca han visto tanta belleza. Entonces se oye la voz del Señor que reconoce la paciencia del cactus, y le dice: "El corazón que busca hacer el bien refleja mi gloria, y siempre traerá al mundo algo que vale la pena, algo de lo cual todos se pueden alegrar—aun si por un sólo momento".

Éstos son sólo unos cuantos cuentos de los que se han pasado de generación en generación y han ayudado a moldear la manera a través de la cual los niños hispanos aprenden los valores, la moralidad, y las creencias de sus antepasados, al mismo tiempo de utilizar su imaginación. Un viaje a casi cualquier biblioteca pública puede dejar al descubierto una riqueza de cuentos populares hispanos, ya sea en libros o en cassettes. Muchos narradores con frecuencia trabajan en las bibliotecas, los museos, y los centros comunitarios.

La enseñanza a través de los poemas y las cartas

Otra manera de enseñar o reforzar la moralidad y los valores es al escribir cartas o poemas a sus niños que les llegarán al alma y ayudarán a renovar su relación con ellos durante los momentos de sus mayores logros. De manera similar, los niños pueden utilizar las cartas para expresar sus sentimientos. Siguen dos cartas, una que yo le di a mi hijo Steven cuando él participó en un campamento religioso, y la segunda carta es para mi esposo, de nuestro hijo Sal, cuando él tenía veintidós años de edad.

Querido Steven,

Este fin de semana sirve para que estés lejos de la familia y los amigos y para que hagas una reflexión y renovación de tus juramentos cristianos. También es el momento propicio para que comuniques con Dios acerca de la dirección y el propósito de tu vida y para que le pidas su bendición.

Este retiro me proporciona una oportunidad para decirte cuánto te quiero, Steven, y para decirte lo mucho que significas para mí, y lo contenta que me siento al ser tú mi hijo. Siempre te he dicho que eres muy especial y que Dios tiene un propósito y un plan muy especial para ti y para tu vida. Él te hizo tan compasivo, brillante, ingenioso, aventurero, y guapo. Tienes una personalidad que te hace resaltar dondequiera que estés. Siempre has estado rodeado de amigos que parecen seguirte y respetarte como un líder. Nunca te has preocupado por las cosas materiales y has estado satisfecho con lo que te hemos podido proveer. Lo que admiro más de ti es tu dinamismo y tu determinación. Cuando quieres algo, luchas duro para conseguirlo, a veces aun trabajando toda la noche, o estando afuera en el sol caliente. Ya sea en el salón de clase o en el campo de fútbol, tu desempeño refleja tu búsqueda de la excelencia. Has tenido suficiente fortaleza para resistir las tentaciones que hay en este mundo: los cigarros, las drogas, el alcohol, el sexo, y las pandillas. Tu padre y yo estamos tan orgullosos de que no te hayas hecho ningún daño a ti mismo, ni hayas ocasionado ni dolor ni sufrimiento a la familia. Estamos muy orgullosos de lo bien que estás aprendiendo a hablar español, y de lo bien que sabes bailar al compás latino. Nos encanta el respeto tan grande que tienes por la vida, las personas, los animales, y el medio ambiente. Eres gracioso y divertido por naturaleza, y les has provocado mucha risa y alegría a otros. Cuando yo estoy tensa y cansada, tú me haces reír.

Steven, todas estas cualidades y atributos maravillosos, Dios te los ha dado por alguna razón. Posees todos los ingredientes apropiados para llegar a ser alguien muy especial en el futuro. Eras un potro salvaje cuando eras pequeño. Yo rezaba que algún día pudieras refrenar esos impulsos incontrolables y llegar a ser el joven fino, maduro, respetable, y responsable en el que te estás convirtiendo. Necesitarás siempre poseer integridad y carácter, si es que vas a lograr el éxito y cumplir con el propósito de tu vida.

Pídele Dios que te llene con Su Gracia y Espíritu para comenzar el resto de tu vida, caminando por el camino cristiano con buenos principios y valores. Jesucristo vino a la tierra para mostrarnos a todos cómo vivir. Él fue paciente, bondadoso, y lleno de paz, alegría, y amor. Él utilizó los dones que Dios le dio para curar y ayudar a otros. Él ayudó a los pobres, los débiles, los ciegos, y los niños pequeños. Steven, debes luchar por ser lo más semejante a Jesucristo que puedas. La única manera de lograr esto es al pedirle a Dios que te llene de Su Espíritu y Gracia. Te quiero y estaremos pensando en ti mientras crezcas espiritualmente, con Cristo.

Con amor,
Mamá

Querido Papá,

Bueno, ¿cómo va el retiro hasta ahora? Ojalá y bien. Me alegro que me dijeron que te escribiera una carta, ya que rara vez tengo la oportunidad de realmente hablar contigo de una manera así de directa y abierta. Creo que no soy de las personas que realmente muestran mucha emoción, pero yo sé que tú sabes cuanto te quiero.

La verdad es que hoy por la noche estuve hablando con una amiga y le estaba diciendo que no sé como podría seguir mi vida sin ti, Mamá, Steven, o Vanessa. Me he dado cuenta que tengo la familia perfecta. Quiero decir, yo sé que a veces discutimos y peleamos, pero cuando todo sea dicho, yo sé que honestamente nos queremos y nos preocupamos unos por los otros mucho más que la mayoría de las familias soñaran siquiera. También sé que quizá yo no sea siempre perfecto, pero me alegro tanto de que tú y Mamá me hayan inculcado los valores y los principios necesarios para ser una persona exitosa y próspera, tanto en este mundo como a los ojos de Dios. Cuando mis amigos ven lo mucho que nosotros nos queremos y la relación estrecha que tenemos como familia, sólo les queda decir: "Híjole, Sal, qué suerte tienes". Yo quiero que sepas que no doy eso por descontado para nada. Le doy las gracias a Dios todos los días por haber sido tan afortunado de haber nacido en este mundo como parte de una familia tan amorosa y cariñosa, y que apenas ahora me estoy dando cuenta de lo mucho que ustedes realmente sí nos quieren.

Un día de estos, espero ser tan buen padre para mis hijos y tan buen esposo para mi esposa, como lo eres tú. Ha de haber sido difícil soportarnos de adolescentes. Me duele de verdad saber que les causé tanta angustia y por eso quisiera pedir disculpas. Para terminar, sólo quiero que sepas que verdaderamente te quiero muchísimo y estoy extremadamente agradecido por todo lo que has hecho y harás por mí.

Tu hijo que te quiere,
Salvador Rodríguez

Mi esposo escribió este poema, el cual después convirtió en una canción, para Vanessa cuando ella tenía un año de edad.

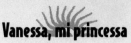

Vanessa, mi princessa

Tengo una niña muy linda
    Que nos mandó el Señor,
Para completar la familia,
    Y darle mucho amor.

Se llama Gloria Vanessa,
    La que me inspira a cantar.
Le gusta oír mi guitarra,
    Para ponerse a bailar.

Nació ya con dos hermanos,
    Que siempre la van a cuidar.
Con Salvador y Estéban,
    El amor nunca le faltará.

(Coro)
Y cuando está dormidita,
    No hay otra princesa igual.
Le cantan los angelitos,
    Con música celestial.

Mi muñequita tan linda,
    Eres un gran placer.
Vanessa, mi princesa,
    Que siempre tengas tu querer.

Ya que se está desarrollando,
    Sus gustos se proclamarán.
Expresa con una voz fuerte,
    "Denme leche con un pan."

Se divierte con sus libros.
    También trata de escribir.
Pero cuando llega su padre,
    Sus brazos le va a pedir.

Vanessa es muy cariñosa,
    Abrazos y besos ya da.
No le quites su juguete,
    Porque su modo cambiará.

Le gusta ver pajaritos,
    Cuando cantan su canción.
Camina con sus pasitos,
    Con gracia y precaución.

Sus labios son muy pequeños,
    Los ojos relumbran de amor.
Y con sus dientitos de perla,
    Come con mucho sabor.

Su pelo es muy fino y chino,
    Se ve bien con un prendedor.
Y cuando usa sus gorritas,
    Ya se ve como una flor.
(Coro)

Es linda como su madre,
    Le gusta la atención.
Y el pobre con quien se enamore—
    Cuidado con su corazón.

Y cuando se encuentre un hombre
    Que quiera hacerla felíz,
Le damos consejos de padres,
    Que ese amor no deje cicatriz.

Las aspiraciones de un padre
    Para su linda mujer,
Serán que goce de la vida,
    Su mejor trate de hacer.
(Coro)

Anuncian ya las trompetas,
    Las puertas se van a abrir;
Para que entre mi princesa,
    La Reina del porvenir.

LA DISCRIMINACIÓN Y EL PREJUICIO

Ayudar a su niño a funcionar en el mundo significa prepararlo para enfrentar a las personas en este mundo que quizá se nieguen a aceptarlo, quizá aun lo odien, simplemente por el color de su piel, el sonido de su apellido, el idioma que habla, su acento, sus creencias, y sus costumbres culturales. El racismo puede manifestarse de numerosas maneras, y sus semillas pueden ser plantadas a una edad muy temprana. Aunque algunos actos de racismo tal vez se desvanezcan de la memoria de su niño, hay cicatrices menos visibles que pueden perdurar toda la vida. Un niño expuesto al prejuicio, ya sea dirigido a él o a otra persona, puede recibir un golpe catastrófico a su amor propio, su sentido de pertenecer, y su sentido de confiar en el mundo a su alrededor. Su capacidad de lograr el éxito puede sufrir en muchas áreas de la vida bajo estas circunstancias. En el área social, la discriminación puede afectar la buena disposición del niño para asociar con otras personas más adelante en su vida por el temor de ser rechazado o alienado. Puede provocar que él catalogue a las personas con estereotipos, por pensar que todos los miembros de un grupo piensen de igual manera. Su hijo necesita saber que hay bueno y malo en todos los grupos y que el racismo y el prejuicio no son un reflejo de sus propios defectos sino que nacen de la ignorancia de otros.

Desde las tierras que fueron arrancados de nuestros antepasados a través de maneras ilegales y racistas, hasta las escuelas segregadas o con fondos desiguales, instalaciones públicas separadas y la explotación crónica en muchos campos de trabajo, los hispanos han sufrido bastante de discriminación y racismo a través de la historia. En la actualidad, el racismo y la discriminación quizá sean un poco más sutiles y menos fáciles de definir. Quizá surjan como ataques a los inmigrantes, continua falta de igualdad en las oportunidades educativas y el llamado "English Only Movement" (un movimiento para conseguir que se hable solo el inglés), el cual intenta negarnos el derecho de hablar nuestro propio idioma. Generalmente, durante tiempos económicos difíciles que ocasionan incertidumbres e inseguridad, hay la tendencia de haber un chivo expiatorio para ser el culpable de las condiciones. Los hispanos, especialmente porque somos los inmigrantes más recientes, somos los primeros de ser culpados por los males que achacan la sociedad, un hecho que es importante recalcar al hablar con sus hijos acerca de temas relacionados al prejuicio y la discriminación.

Mi experiencia personal con la discriminación

Cuando yo estaba creciendo, me vi confrontada a una situación donde una persona, a quien yo llamo un "guardián", pudo haber cambiado el curso de mi vida a causa de sus acciones. A pesar de que yo sacaba calificaciones de "A" y "B" y era una líder en mi escuela, el director de mi escuela de preparatoria les dijo a los representantes de un programa universitario que estaba luchando contra la pobreza, llamado "Project Teacher Excellence", que él no me recomendaba para el programa porque "yo no tenía madera de estudiante universitario". A pesar de su recomendación adversa, fui aceptada y me gradué con éxito en tres años y medio fui incluída en la lista *Who's Who in Colleges and Universities*, y más tarde participé en un curso de posgrado, donde ambos estábamos estudiando para conseguir el certificado para director.

Como madre, de nuevo tuve que enfrentarme con muchos "guardianes" en la educación de mis hijos, maestros o consejeros que pensaban que mis niños no pertenecían en ciertas clases, programas, o escuelas. Cuando Sal estaba cursando el tercer año de primaria en una escuela privada muy prestigiosa, se hizo muy evidente a los ojos de varios de nosotros, que una maestra en particular sentía que los hispanos y los negros no debían estar en esa escuela. Un año, las calificaciones de mi hijo bajaron, de casi todas "A" por tres años seguidos, hasta tener dos "D". Me enteré que la maestra había estado tratando injustamente a mi hijo y a una niña afroamericana, ninguno de los cuales, quizá ella haya pensado, pertenecía en esa escuela. Un día llegué a la escuela sin haber avisado de antemano y me enteré que Sal había sido mandado afuera al pasillo, y se le había ordenado quedarse allí todos los días por las primeras dos semanas del año escolar. Después de quejarme con el director y pedirle a un consejero que le hiciera a la maestra que fuera consciente de sus acciones y de los efectos que estos tenían sobre sus estudiantes, la conducta de la maestra cambió y el desempeño académico de mi hijo mejoró. Pasé por algo similar con mis otros dos niños, cuando no se les permitió tomar clases avanzadas o participar en los programas para niños superdotados. En estas ocasiones, yo les hice saber a los "guardianes" que yo quería la llave para abrirles la puerta a mis niños. Tuve éxito, pero sólo después de convencerlos de que mis niños merecían la oportunidad de participar en clases de enriquecimiento.

Como hispanos, necesitamos enfrentarnos al hecho de que nuestros niños probablemente sufrirán discriminación. Necesitamos ayudarles a lidiar con eso, porque puede ocurrir cuando y donde menos se espera, como en un campamento, por ejemplo. Mi hijo Steven estaba en un campamento con jóvenes anglosajones e hispanos y oyó a uno de los anglosajones decir en voz alta, "Más vale que cuidemos nuestras cosas, porque a los mexicanos les gusta robar". Otros comentarios que me han contado que les han dicho son "Frito Bandido", "Beanie", "Wetback", "¿Está mojada tu espalda por cruzar el Río Grande?" Un año alguien puso un cartel en la pared en la escuela de mi hijo que decía, "Hispanos y negros, vuelvan a México y África de donde vinieron". En un intento de meter a Steven en problemas para que no lo dejaran jugar en un juego importante de fútbol americano, un estudiante anglosajón le quebró un huevo en la cabeza. Fueron sus amigos anglosajones y negros que salieron en su defensa. Cuando mi hijo Sal asistía a la universidad de Texas A&M, dos estudiantes anglosajones estaban peleando afuera del recinto universitario y su amigo hispano trató de separarlos. Los policías vinieron y arrestaron al hispano. Todos estos hechos han sido temas de conversación en nuestro hogar, con relación a la discriminación.

Cuando existen tantos estereotipos en los medios de comunicación que representan a los hispanos como matones, miembros de la mafia mexicana, prostitutas, hombres estilo Don Juan, narcotraficantes, y "low-riders", no es de sorprenderse que existan actitudes tan negativas entre los jóvenes. En la televisión y en las películas, demasiados de los papeles que juegan los hispanos son limitados a los criados, niñeras, jardineros, o amantes voluptuosas, lo cual puede provocarles a nuestros niños a sentir que no son merecedores de trabajos profesionales. Los hispanos son representados como unos haraganes flojos que usan sombreros y se montan en burros. A muchos hispanos les perturban los personajes como Speedy Gonzalez, la Chiquita Banana, y Juan Valdez. En los años sesenta los hispanos se organizaron para formular una queja en contra del "Frito Bandido", y recientemente algunos hispanos se han ofendido con los comerciales de Taco Bell que muestran un chihuahueño con orejas puntiagudas que habla español y se llama Dink y dice, "Yo quiero Taco Bell". Quizá sea gracioso y a muchas personas les encantan los chihuahueños, pero es lo que dice, cómo lo dice, y lo que se viste, como un traje al estilo de los revolucionarios, lo cual provoca imágenes sutiles de lo que algunas personas quieren proyectar sobre los México-americanos o las personas de México. El reciente comercial de Jack-in-the-Box acerca de los frijoles y lo que les pasa a las personas que los comen de ninguna manera no me causa gracia y lo encuentro ofensivo.

Lo que los hispanos, como yo, queremos es que represente a nuestra cultura de una manera más fiel y respetuoso. No quieren la creación de nuevo estereotipos asociados con animales graciosos con voces chillantes o jalapeños verdes que hablan. Esto es una burla sutil de nuestra cultura. Necesitamos más modelos de conducta positivos e imágenes en la televisión y en los medios de comunicación que inspirarán y motivarán a nuestros niños y les harán enorgullecerse de quienes son. Nosotros como un grupo debemos hacer nuestra parte para educar al público en general sobre lo que verdaderamente significa ser hispano.

Afortunadamente, hoy en día, hay más películas que son escritas, dirigidas, y representadas por hispanos, las cuales destacan a nuestra gente en papeles más positivos y describen historias que reflejan de manera más fiel la belleza y fortaleza de nuestra cultura. En un intento por capturar el mercado hispano de 350 billones de dólares, las corporaciones ahora se están utilizando a empresas hispanas de mercadotecnia para crear comerciales como los que yo he visto que efectivamente captan los aspectos positivos de nuestra cultura, como nuestra devoción a la familia, y el alto valor que le asignamos al respeto.

Aun como adultos profesionales de la clase media, muchos de nosotros hemos sentido los efectos de los ataques a los inmigrantes. Una vez estaba yo tratando de bajar mi equipaje del depósito de almacenamiento de un avión que acababa de aterrizar en San Antonio proveniente de Nueva York, cuando un hombre muy grosero me empujó hacia un lado y dijo, "Propuesta 187, aquí estamos, en Texas. *Todos ustedes* deberían volver a México, de donde vinieron". No importó que yo venía en primera clase ni que traía un traje de apariencia profesional, aún formaba parte de una categoría de personas que este hombre detestaba porque soy hispana. Yo eché una mirada de desaprobación y decidí hacerle caso omiso.

Una conocida profesional de Colombia compartió conmigo su experiencia de vivir en un barrio de clase media alta en Michigan donde ella era la única hispana. Ella provenía de una familia grande cuyos miembros de su familia extensa la visitaban a menudo. Los vecinos no podían creer que algo que no involucraba el narcotráfico era la razón de tanta gente que iba a su casa, y la reportaron a las autoridades correspondientes, quienes mandaron un agente a su casa. Yo he escuchado historias donde a hispanos prominentes y de clase media se les han dicho que pasen a la cocina cuando llegan a una fiesta o se les han pedido ver sus papeles de legal estadía cuando en realidad son ciudadanos legales. Muchos han sido discriminados o les han rechazado sus aplicaciones cuando han tratado de comprar una casa en alguna área predominantemente anglosajona. A pesar de orden de la Corte Suprema en 1954, y el Título VI y VII (Title VI and VII) de la Ley de los Derechos Civiles (*Civil Rights Act*) aprobado por el Congreso en 1964, el cual prohibió la

práctica de métodos injustos y discriminatorios en alojamientos públicos, tales como escuelas, lugares de empleo, crédito, viviendas, o
cualquier institución que recibe fondos federales, basados en la raza, el
origen nacional, el credo, y el color, todavía vemos propuestas en las
urnas que intentan negar a nuestra gente sus derechos.

Ya sea que vivimos en un barrio pobre o en los suburbios, seamos
ricos o pobres, muchos de nosotros nos veremos afectados por las actitudes negativas que persisten con respecto a los hispanos. Estamos
pasando por muchos cambios, causados por fuerzas internas y externas,
los cuales pueden ser una amenaza para nuestra gente en el futuro, y
debemos preparar a nuestros niños para que estén preparados para
enfrentarse a ellos. Uno es el cambio demográfico en los Estados Unidos
que ofrece muchas oportunidades al mismo tiempo de plantear muchos
desafíos a la cantidad cada vez más grande de hispanos. El otro es que
Latinoamérica está ganando más importancia económica a escala
mundial, debido a los tratados como el North American Free Trade
Agreement, o NAFTA. O podemos quedarnos a un lado y permitir que
estos cambios nos arrollen, o podemos participar y formar parte de ellos
al asegurarnos que las políticas y normas que se están aprobando sean
sensibles a los hispanos.

Como padres, debemos de escuchar los mensajes verbales y no verbales de nuestros niños, discutir estos asuntos abiertamente con ellos
y enseñarles cómo hacerles frente de una manera que no sea violenta.
Nosotros, como padres, tenemos la responsabilidad de enseñarles a
nuestros niños a ser bondadosos y respetuosos. Podemos ayudarles a
tener fortaleza a través de la espiritualidad y la unidad de la gente. Sin
embargo, tenemos que hacerlos conscientes de que la hostilidad racial
y la discriminación sí existen en nuestro país y alrededor del mundo,
por una variedad de razones. A veces la mejor manera de hacerle
frente al racismo y la discriminación es mirar hacia el pasado para ver
cómo ha afectado a diferentes personas. Hábleles a sus niños acerca de
como otros grupos también han sido víctimas de la discriminación,
por ejemplo, la gente en Chiapas, Bosnia, Rwanda, Somalia, y
Alemania.

No sólo les hablamos a nuestros niños acerca de las atrocidades que
el hombre ha cometido en contra de otros hombres, sino que queríamos
que ellos miraran con sus propios ojos. Un año mi familia fue de vacaciones a Alemania, con la intención de llevar a nuestros niños al campo
de concentración de Dachau, para que pudieran ver por sí mismos las
atrocidades de las cuales fueron víctimas los judíos durante el holocausto. Mis niños recorrieron las mismas duchas de gas y los hornos donde

innumerables judíos perecieron. Yo les expliqué a mis niños que se había preservado el campo de concentración para que las personas de todo el mundo pudieran ver lo que ocurrió y se aseguraran que la historia nunca se repitiera. Yo quería ser sensible al trato de todas personas, incluyendo al de los hispanos. Este viaje, realizado cuando él era muy joven, tuvo un impacto en Steven cuando ya era un poco más grande. Un año, varios años después, Steven volvió a casa disgustado por la discusión que tuvieron en su clase de historia acerca de la Propuesta 187. Hubo discusión acerca de como se iban a expedir unas tarjetas de identificación para identificar a aquellos hispanos que no fueran ciudadanos americanos. "Primero, nos harán identificarnos con estas tarjetas de identificación, igual a como los judíos tuvieron que identificarse con la Estrella de David. Luego nos pondrán en campos de concentración. Tenemos que hablar en contra de esto antes de que sea demasiado tarde", dijo él.

Al mudarnos a comunidades de diversos grupos étnicos y nuestros niños asistan a escuelas con jóvenes de más diversos antecedentes, cada uno tendrá que ayudar a sus niños a aprender que siempre habrá personas que quizá digan o hagan cosas que les provoquen dolor. Su niño puede volver a casa un día, llorando porque alguien le dijo "greaser", "spic", o "wetback", o porque alguien le dijo que volviera a México, Cuba, África, o Puerto Rico, o "dondequiera que veniste". Las palabras llenas de odio pueden causarles a nuestros niños un gran dolor y afectar su autoestima. Esté preparado para ayudarle a su niño a comprender que hay diferentes tipos de personas en el mundo, tal como mi madre me enseñó a mí.

Las personas que digan esas cosas muchas veces tuvieron a padres que no les enseñaron a ser bondadosos y considerados, ni a respetar a sus semejantes. Quizá ellos tampoco recibieron ni amor ni bondad. A veces un niño que usa epítetos raciales ni siquiera sabe lo que dice, sino que simplemente está repitiendo lo que ha escuchado decir a sus padres, *no dice la criatura sino lo que oye tras el fuego*. Las personas que tienen mucho odio por dentro y que agarran como blancos a los que ellos consideran débiles o vulnerables, son personas inseguras, a quienes les falta confianza en sí mismos y quienes no han aprendido a preocuparse por otros o sentir empatía. Debido a su inseguridad, tratan de conseguir un sentido de superioridad y poder, al aprovecharse de otros y manipularlos. Quizá insistan que son superiores a otros, pero en la realidad, ellos mismos son los que se sienten inferiores y sin amor. Siguen unas maneras en que usted puede ayudarle a su niño a hacerle frente a la discriminación y al racismo. (También véase la "Lista de recursos" al final de este libro.)

1. La tolerancia y el pacifismo comienzan en el hogar

El buen juez por su casa empieza. La eliminación de la discriminación comienza en el hogar, al enseñarles a nuestros niños principios y valores, incluyendo la fraternidad, el respeto mutuo, y la responsabilidad social. Debemos ayudar a nuestros niños a canalizar su agresión de una manera constructiva. Cuando los niños tienen su primer conflicto con sus hermanos, están comenzando a aprender a resolver sus disputas y a vivir en harmonía bajo un mismo techo. Ese concepto debe extenderse afuera de la familia, para que puedan aprender a vivir juntos con diferentes personas de diversos grupos en el campo de béisbol, en la escuela, en la comunidad, y en el mundo.

Debemos enseñarles a nuestros niños a enorgullecerse de quienes son, de donde vinieron, y hacia donde van. La mejor herramienta que les podemos dar a los niños en contra de la conducta y las actitudes destructivas y llenas de odio, es darles una fortaleza sólida que proviene de nuestro amor, aceptación, y apoyo, y de una sólida educación espiritual. Como dice el dicho, *cuando el viento sopla, el árbol se limpia,* y después de asentarse el polvo, lo que queda, son aquellas características que le mantienen a uno erguido, fuerte, y con cimientos sólidos. Necesitamos ayudarles a nuestros niños a llegar a ser fuertes, tenaces, y audaces, y ayudarles a lograr poseer una fortaleza interna para poder hacerles caso omiso a las personas que intentan lastimarlos. A pesar de lo que otras personas le digan a ellos o digan sobre ellos, asegúreles que usted está allí para apoyarles. Ayúdeles a expresar sus sentimientos al hablar, al escribir, o al darle golpes a un saco de arena, o al patear una pelota diseñada específicamente para ayudar a soltar las emociones. Los niños necesitan saber que quizá los rechacen, su burlen de ellos, o los lastimen en algún momento de su vida, por su origen étnico, y que a veces la mejor defensa es presentar una demanda, desde el más bajo nivel de autoridad hasta la Corte Suprema.

Necesitamos enseñarles a nuestros niños que en algún momento de sus vidas tendrán que adoptar una postura en contra del odio expresado por algunas personas. Discuta la manera en que se ha discriminado a diferentes grupos de personas a través de la historia. Asegúrese de que sepan sobre líderes hispanos como el doctor Hector Pérez García, el fundador del G.I. Forum, y César Chávez, un activista de derechos civiles para los trabajadores agrícolas, quien luchó en contra de la discriminación y la injusticia social. Además, discuta acerca de cómo los grandes líderes como Martin Luther King, Jr., y Mohandas Gandhi lograron cambios sociales a través de medios pacíficos.

2. Hay que saber y conocer sus derechos

Saber es poder. Usted necesita saber que puede defender y apoyar los derechos que tienen sus niños a la dignidad y al respeto, y a igualdad de protección bajo la ley. Yo presentaba demandas a las autoridades cuando mis niños eran pequeños y recibieron un trato injusto. Les alenté a resolver sus propios problemas y a hablar por sí mismos cuando eran más grandes. Sepa que tiene derechos y recursos de ayudar si se discrimina a su niño. Sus niños no pueden aprender en la escuela si sienten temor. Acuda a algún representante de la directiva de la escuela o aun a la Oficina de Derechos Civiles (Office of Civil Rights—OCR), en Washington, D.C. (véase la "Lista de recursos" para conseguir la dirección). De acuerdo a la Oficina de Derechos Civiles, uno tiene 180 días después de un incidente para presentar una demanda, lo cual se hace al dar la siguiente información: (1) su nombre y dirección, (2) una descripción general de la persona lastimada por la(s) acción(es) o la clase de persona lastimada por el presunto acto, o actos, discriminatorio(s), (3) el nombre y la ubicación de la institución que cometió el acto, o actos, discriminatorio(s), (4) una descripción del acto, o actos, discriminatorio(s) con suficientes detalles para saber qué ocurrió, cuándo ocurrió, y qué piensa usted que fue la base del acto, o actos (raza, color, origen nacional, sexo, impedimento físico o retraso mental, o edad). Si usted se enfrenta a unos problemas muy graves, y están ocurriendo a más de una persona, recuerde que hay más fuerza cuando hay más personas involucradas. Puede organizar un grupo para poner una demanda o juntos pueden ejercitar una acción civil.

Usted y su familia tienen derechos en este país para protegerlos contra la hostilidad racial y la discriminación. Si usted o un miembro de su familia es tratado con hostilidad racial o discriminación de parte de los oficiales de inmigración, acuda al Servicio de Inmigración y Naturalización (Immigration and Naturalization Service—INS), al área de "Processing, Holding and Public Access" para conseguir una forma donde puede exponer sus quejas, o bien, llame el número gratuito que se encuentra dentro de la "Lista de recursos" al final de este libro. Es ilegal tomar represalias en contra de una persona que ha presentado una demanda en contra de la discriminación, que participa en una investigación sobre actos discriminatorios, o se opone a una práctica ilegal de empleo. Entérese de sus derechos civiles.

3. Los padres son los primeros modelos de conducta y maestros del pacifismo

El buen padre en la casa comienza. Los padres enseñan por medio de sus palabras y sus acciones. Los padres deben ser buenos modelos de la tolerancia, la paciencia, la bondad, y la compasión. Al refrenarse de utilizar el castigo corporal, al discutir las razones por las cuales tomó cierta postura, y al luchar para encontrar una solución, los padres les están enseñando a los niños a hacer lo mismo cuando quiere señalar algo. Algunos dichos que los padres pueden utilizar para enseñarles a sus niños empatía y compasión, incluyen los siguientes: *Sea grande o chica, la espina pica.* Esto enseña que quizá no sea evidente lo que una persona siente por dentro. *Sólo el que carga el costal sabe lo que la carga lleva adentro.* No diga ni se ría de chistes raciales o étnicos, ni permita a sus niños hacerlo tampoco. Hable en contra de cualquier persona que lo haga. No apruebe los comentarios racistas por medio de su silencio.

4. Discuta abiertamente el tema de la discriminación

Hombre prevenido nunca fue vencido. Debe sensibilizar a sus niños desde una edad pequeña, al hecho de que la discriminación y el racismo todavía existen y de que ellos pueden ser sus víctimas. Aliente a sus niños a discutir los temas relacionados con la discriminación, ya sean incidentes que a ellos les han ocurrido o problemas del mundo que necesitan ser tratados con mayor respeto mutuo, compasión, y cooperación. Enséñeles a sus niños a hablar en contra del odio y la discriminación, a decir lo que piensan. Aun si ellos no sean el blanco de la discriminación y el odio, deben ser enseñados a no tenerle temor a tomar una postura en contra de ello. Dígales las palabras del pastor Martin Niemoller, el presidente del Consejo Mundial de Iglesias, quien pasó varios años en un campo de concentración, a causa de su oposición a Hitler.

En Alemania vinieron primero por los comunistas, y no hablé porque yo no era comunista. Luego vinieron por los judíos, y no hablé porque yo no era judío. Luego vinieron por los sindicalistas, y no hablé porque yo no era sindicalista. Luego vinieron por los católicos, y no hablé porque yo era protestante. Luego vinieron por mí, y ya para entonces, no quedaba nadie más para hablar.

5. Aliente a sus niños a servir y a proveer servicios para la comunidad

Quien no sirve para servir, no sirve para vivir. La vida de uno debe ser dedicada al servicio, porque una persona que no sirve, no está viviendo bien. Los niños deben ser alentados a vivir. Deben ser sensibilizados a las dificultades y las penurias que sufren algunas personas en su comunidad y en el mundo, comenzando por los pobres, los que no tienen hogar, los ancianos, y los que tienen algún impedimento—los que viven en su propia ciudad y los que sufren en tierras lejanas. Los niños aprenden a convivir y a cuidar a su prójimo cuando han dado de su tiempo, sus talentos, y su energía, para ayudar a alguien menos afortunado. Aliénteles a ayudar a darles clases particulares a los niños, a organizar juegos recreativos para los niños minusválidos o los niños del barrio, o a darles clases de piano a los necesitados. Invítelos a unirse a usted para servir a los que no tienen hogar en el comedor de beneficencia, o a entregar los regalos a los pobres. Adopte a una familia necesitada para que sus niños comprendan cómo unos actos benévolos pueden influir sobre las vidas de las personas y cuánto agradecimiento puede resultar de tales actos de bondad. Ayúdeles a sentir la satisfacción proveniente de hacer algo bueno sin esperar nada a cambio. Dígales "Haz bien y no mires a quién".

6. Enseñe habilidades para resolver los conflictos

Más vale perro vivo que león muerto. Ayúdeles a sus niños a aprender a resolver sus problemas de una manera constructiva. Aliéntelos a hacer un teatro improvisado con situaciones dentro de los cuales deben pensar muy bien lo que harían si fueran enfrentados con una situación similar. No es fácil evitar algunas situaciones cuando están burlándose o mofándose de uno. *Más vale un cobarde en casa que un valiente en la cárcel o en el cementerio,* es un dicho que se utiliza para enseñarles a los niños a alejarse de una situación antes de convertirse en un valiente arrepentido o muerto. Es mejor mantenerse alejado del peligro, porque "jugar con fuego es peligroso".

7. Analice y sea crítico acerca de lo que sus niños miran en la televisión

El diablo no duerme. El que evita la tentación, evita el pecado. Estos son sólo un par de dichos que las madres hispanas utilizamos para ayudar a nuestros niños a darse cuenta y ser conscientes de los vicios que existen en el mundo.z Los niños necesitan supervisión y orientación. No les permita a sus niños mirar la televisión sin ningún tipo de sistema de monitorización. Siéntese con ellos a mirar la televisión y discuta las diferentes imágenes estereotípicas, el odio, y la violencia que salen en la televisión. Controle cuáles programas pueden mirar. Se han dado casos en los cuales los niños que miran la violencia en la televisión se vuelven violentos y atacan después de mirar tal programa. Proteste y escríbales a los productores de programas, comerciales, y música que son ofensivos y violentos. Lleve a cabo estas actividades con sus niños.

8. Aliente y fomente el respeto a la diversidad

Haz bien sin mirar a quién. Aliente a sus niños a asociarse con niños de otros grupos étnicos, raciales, y religiosos, para que puedan sobreponerse a los estereotipos ellos mismos y tener mayor comprensión y respeto por las diferencias. Aliéntelos a ir a campamentos, escuelas, o programas donde hay niños con diferentes antecedentes y líderes sensibles, para que sus niños puedan aprender a vivir juntos en harmonía y respeto. Viaje cuando sea posible, para que sus niños puedan tener contacto con diferentes personas y diversas culturas. La mejor manera para atacar los estereotipos que provocan los prejuicios y la discriminación es a través de los conocimientos y la información.

LO MEJOR DE AMBOS MUNDOS

No todos los hispanos crían a sus niños de la misma manera, ni tampoco estamos todos de acuerdo con relación a los valores principales que deseamos inculcarles. Pero tal vez casi todos los padres hispanos estén de acuerdo de que nuestra cultura compartida es rica en tradiciones y valores, los cuales incluyen la lealtad hacia la familia, los niños, y la comunidad, además de la obediencia, la interdependencia, el respeto, la compasión, la cooperación, la espiritualidad, y, para muchos, la preservación del idioma español. Los padres hispanos en los Estados Unidos también están socializando a sus niños en la cultura occidental dominante, la cual pone énfasis en la competencia, la agresividad, la firmeza, la individualidad, la independencia, y, claro, el idioma inglés. Aunque estos valores quizá a veces estén en conflicto, hay un mérito al poseer ambos sistemas de valores para lograr un equilibrio cultural.

Mi madre hablaba de la necesidad de tener un equilibrio cuando nos daba dos mensajes opuestos para crear ese equilibrio: "No te creas mucho" y "ten orgullo". "Ten respeto y espera respeto". Mientras la determinación, la agresividad, y la firmeza son características que deben ser mantenidas, tal y como son alentadas en el mundo anglosajón, debemos preguntarnos a nosotros mismos y a nuestros niños, ¿con qué fin van a ser utilizados? ¿Serán utilizados sólo para el bien individual, o pueden ser utilizados para el bien común de la familia y de la comunidad? ¿Serán utilizados para mantener nuestra libertad, democracia, igualdad, y justicia? Como padres tenemos que ayudar a los niños a desarrollar un sentido de competencia, autonomía, e independencia, y ayudarles a sentir que pueden participar y contribuir a la sociedad. Pero qué tal si todos se criaran para ser egocéntricos, con la creencia que deben ser completamente autónomos e independientes, siempre pensando en sí mismo, ¿cómo podrían sentir que formaban parte de algo? ¿Qué tipo de ciudadanos serían? ¿En qué tipo de sociedad viviríamos? Nuestros niños necesitan aprender que viven en un mundo social donde las personas deben depender unos de los otros si es que van a vivir y prosperar en una sociedad civil con harmonía.

Mientras que ambos mundos abogan por una ética laboral, yo creo que los hispanos tradicionalmente trabajan para vivir y no viven para trabajar, un principio que es importante recordar. El éxito y los logros han sido inculcados en la psique de los hispanos por generaciones, pero no a expensas de la destrucción de relaciones personales, las cuales valoramos mucho. Esta nación necesita a más personas que poseen los valores y los principios que están tan arraigados en la cultura latina. Necesitamos las habilidades de negociación, compromiso, y sensibilidad para evitar una aniquilación. Necesitamos tener líderes morales que se preocupan y que buscan el bien de todos, y que saben la importancia de la cooperación y la interdependencia.

Al mismo tiempo, debemos tratar de mantener nuestros derechos, dignidad, y lugar en la sociedad. Uno de nuestros derechos es el de hablar español en adición al inglés. Si vamos a lograr éxito en las próximas décadas, necesitamos poder comunicarnos en ambos idiomas. También se va a esperar que los líderes empresariales y de la política sean bilingües si es que quieren comunicarse con la porción de la población de este país que está creciendo con más rapidez, y con los ciudadanos de los países latinoamericanos que ahora están conectados a nuestro país más que nunca antes.

Necesitamos enseñarles a nuestros niños a ser socialmente competentes, a poder moverse dentro y afuera de ambos mundos, el hispano y el anglosajón, y a tratar con diferentes personas en diferentes situaciones. Mi esposo es un buen ejemplo de esta habilidad. Cuando él hablaba con sus padres o con las viejitas en el barrio, les hablaba en español, de manera respetuosa. Cuando me hablaba a mí, me hablaba de una manera coloquial, en ambos idiomas, inglés y español, mezclando los idiomas porque él sabía que ambos podíamos comunicar en ambos idiomas con soltura. Cuando hablaba con sus amigos ingenieros, hablaba de una manera muy profesional y técnica que sólo ellos podían entender. Cuando iba al barrio, saludaba a sus amigos con: "¡Órale, bato! ¿Qué tal?" Debido a sus habilidades sociales y lingüísticas, él podía comunicarse con mucha más gente, y bajo circunstancias muy diversas. No quería rechazar o negar sus raíces, su cultura, o su familia y amigos. Era una persona mejor porque tenía la habilidad de cambiar si era necesario, dependiendo de la situación.

Uno no tiene que asimilarse completamente, ni renunciar a la cultura o al idioma de uno para tener éxito en un mundo donde existen las "mayorías" y las "minorías". Si uno rechaza su cultura o su idioma, se rechaza a sí mismo. Como padres, queremos que nuestros niños sean bilingües y que tengan dos culturas, para obtener lo mejor de ambos mundos. Queremos que sean bondadosos y compasivos, pero también sí queremos que sean firmes y que exijan sus derechos y su lugar merecido en la sociedad. Mientras que queremos que valoren la humildad, no pueden ser tan humildes que no sean suficientemente firmes para conservar sus derechos constitucionales a la vida, la libertad, y la búsqueda de felicidad. Puede ser bilingüe y poseer dos culturas y tener la habilidad de moverse dentro y fuera de ambos mundos, seleccionando y haciendo suyo lo mejor de ambos, con confianza y orgullo.

Tercera parte

Los tres pilares de una crianza efectiva:

El matrimonio, la familia,

y la comunidad

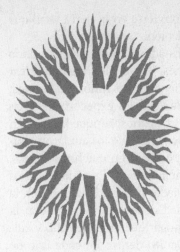

Capítulo VII

El matrimonio

El contrato, el compromiso, y la comunicación

LA BODA HISPANA

De un buen matrimonio, florecen las semillas. Este refrán, sencillo pero profundo, refleja la idea que es central en la manera hispana de ver a la familia. Igual a una planta que crece y se vuelve fuerte con los nutrientes en un suelo fértil, la fortaleza de un niño proviene del vínculo afectivo entre el esposo y la esposa. El amor y el respeto que se expresan uno al otro posibilitarán al niño a salir al mundo y tener una vida próspera. Es por eso que es tan crítico mantener un matrimonio sólido y sano. El vínculo afectivo entre los esposos, en el matrimonio, es un componente básico en la crianza efectiva de los niños. La estabilidad en el matrimonio es uno de los pilares para una crianza exitosa.

En una parábola bíblica acerca del cosechador y la semilla, se nos dice que la semilla que cae sobre terreno rocoso no se desarrollará bien por falta de humedad. La semilla que cae entre las espinas crecerá pero eventualmente será ahogada con las espinas y morirá. Sin embargo, la semilla que cae sobre tierra fértil desarrollará raíces fuertes y se multiplicará por cien. Si los jardineros se comprometen a producir una buena cosecha, deben plantar la semilla en una tierra rica y fértil y nutrirla para que la planta crezca sanamente. Un matrimonio que tiene sus orígenes en el amor, la confianza, y el respeto, se convierte en la tierra fértil que ayudará a los niños a crecer y desarrollarse bien.

Hoy en día, las familias latinas en los Estados Unidos están pasando por enormes transformaciones y presiones, las cuales pueden crear mucha tensión en el matrimonio y en la crianza de los niños, y a la larga, en el medio ambiente de los niños. Los papeles, las expectativas, y las responsabilidades de las madres y los padres hispanos, aunque basados en las experiencias con sus propios padres y personas que los cuidaron, exigen una nueva gama de habilidades y perspectivas. En muchos sentidos, estos métodos de crianza difieren enormemente de los que nuestros padres utilizaron con nosotros. Para demasiadas parejas, la educación, la carrera, y la participación en la comunidad deben equilibrarse con la responsabilidad de los padres de crear un hogar que ofrece cariño y cultiva a los niños para asegurar su éxito. Oculto dentro de cada uno de estos temas se encuentra el factor atenuante de la cultura. Mientras que todos queremos que nuestros niños sobresalgan en un mundo cuyo idioma principal es el inglés, muchos de nosotros queremos que mantengan un sentido de su cultura y su lengua materna, lo cual sirve de conexión para unirlos a ambos el pasado y el futuro. Esperamos que nuestros niños logren tener éxito en una sociedad donde se valora la competencia, la autonomía, y el éxito individual. Al mismo tiempo, queremos inculcar en ellos las virtudes tradicionales de la cooperación, el respeto, y la lealtad a la familia. Si uno no cuenta con alguna orientación, el camino que se recorre para criar a los niños en un mundo de dos culturas puede producir ansiedad e incertidumbre, y puede perturbar la tierra delicada necesaria para el desarrollo y crecimiento sanos.

Este libro se trata de ayudar a los padres latinos a comprender que es posible criar a sus hijos exitosamente en los Estados Unidos, sin abandonar sus valores culturales tradicionales. Con respecto al matrimonio, esto significa entablar un compromiso de toda una vida, el cual apoya las ideas tradicionales de la permanencia, la obligación, y la lealtad a la familia, de tal manera que no niega las necesidades y las metas personales. Dentro de este nuevo esquema para las familias latinas, las asociaciones iguales pueden estar basadas en tres elementos esenciales: el contrato, el compromiso, y la comunicación.

Mientras yo sí aliento a los lectores a hacer todo en su poder para conservar su matrimonio "por el bien de los niños", tal como lo hicieron nuestros padres, al mismo tiempo reconozco que los problemas a los cuales nos enfrentamos en la actualidad no son los mismos a los cuales se enfrentaban nuestros padres. Los sistemas tradicionales de apoyo no existen para muchas familias hispanas móviles, como existieron hace treinta años. Además, algunas madres y algunos padres que están criando a sus niños sin pareja han logrado criar bien a sus niños, a pesar de las probabilidades en su contra. Sin embargo, lo importante para el propósito de este libro es explorar la idea de que los matrimonios sólidos producen mejores resultados para los niños que uno deshecho o en condiciones poco sanas. A través de los veinticinco años que tengo trabajando con familias, yo he observado que si los matrimonios son sólidos, generalmente se verán resultados positivos en los niños.

Como mencioné antes, Urie Bronfenbrenner, de la Universidad de Cornell, una vez dijo que todos los niños necesitan tener a cuando menos una persona en su vida que está loca por él. Pero como se ha demostrado a través de innumerables investigaciones, es mucho mejor tener a dos padres unidos que a uno solo, económicamente, educativamente, emocionalmente, y físicamente, para ambos padres e hijos. Por ejemplo, el Reporte de Coleman, el cual fue una investigación pionera al nivel nacional, de 570,000 niños en 1965, encontró que la familia nuclear tuvo una mayor influencia sobre los logros académicos que cualquier otro factor, incluyendo la cualidad del programa de estudios, los libros, los edificios, y los programas de entrenamiento para los maestros. Esto significa que sin tomar en cuenta la posible superioridad de los maestros y el programa de estudios de una escuela, el éxito de su niño será más influenciado por las experiencias que recibe en su familia.

Pero los efectos de un matrimonio y una familia sólidos y sanos van mucho más allá del ruedo académico. También les proporciona a nuestros niños las habilidades personales para comunicar y formar relaciones con otros. Los padres que se respetan y se apoyan uno al otro están enseñándoles a sus niños valores básicos como lo son la lealtad, la honestidad, y la responsabilidad, todos los cuales son esenciales en una sociedad civilizada. Ocurren los conflictos en todos los matrimonios, pero cuando estos se resuelven de manera considerada y racional, los padres están mostrando las virtudes de tolerancia, compromiso, cooperación, y bondad. También apoyan las virtudes de la compasión y la generosidad cuando se escuchan mutuamente y trabajan juntos para encontrar la manera de satisfacer las necesidades y las metas de cada uno. Esta conducta a favor de la sociedad, determina cuanto éxito tendrán los niños con respecto a relacionarse con otros en la sociedad, particularmente con los miembros del sexo opuesto, más adelante en su vida. Uno quizá diría que el estado del matrimonio es un reflejo del estado de la sociedad en general, ya que la familia es la unidad básica de la sociedad. Una de las mejores cualidades que una persona puede tener en su trato con otros es la confianza, un sano sentido de confianza que ocurre al crecer dentro de una familia que se mantiene unida tanto en tiempos buenos como en los malos.

Todos los matrimonios tendrán sus momentos buenos y malos. Si las parejas no reconocen esto desde un principio, pueden fácilmente darse por vencidos y su matrimonio fallará, tal como sí ocurre en el 65 por ciento de los matrimonios nuevos en los Estados Unidos. Establezcan estrategias para lidiar con los muchos desafíos que surgen con la crianza de los niños en un mundo de dos sociedades, donde las presiones de ambos lados pueden ser abrumadoras. Como mencionamos antes, de acuerdo a los datos demográficos recopilados por el Departamento de Salud y Servicios Humanos de los Estados Unidos, un 74 por ciento de los hogares hispanos con niños están encabezados por dos padres. Sin embargo, el hecho de que se haya convertido en algo tan fácil abandonar y dejar a un lado el matrimonio representa un desafío para nuestros valores sobre tener y mantener una familia sólida. Esta política para el divorcio llamada "ninguna culpa", permite que uno rompa el contrato matrimonial más fácilmente que rompería un acuerdo de renta, o un contrato para comprar un refrigerador o un carro.

Los padres deben preguntarse en momentos de inseguridad y dudas: "¿Vale la pena salvar este matrimonio? Dado que esta persona es la madre o el padre de mis hijos, ¿es eso tan importante como para hacer el esfuerzo de arreglar las cosas? ¿Encontraré quizá a alguien peor que mi pareja? Como dice el dicho, *no te vayas de Guatemala a Guatepeor*. Si siente la tentación de dejar a su pareja y niños por otra persona que le parece más tentadora o atractiva, no dejes el camino por la vereda, no abandone un matrimonio de muchos años por algo que ni sabe si va a funcionar. Vale más malo por conocido que bueno por conocer. ¿Cómo sentiré con respecto a mis acciones en diez o veinte años, si me divorcio? ¿Qué efectos tendrá el divorcio sobre mis niños, mi salud, mi condición económica, y mi estabilidad emocional? ¿Y qué de las relaciones que hemos construido juntos a través de los años? ¿Perderé el contacto con nuestros amigos mutuos o la familia extensa? ¿Vale la pena?"

Mientras que muchas de estas preguntas son difíciles de contestar, algunas investigaciones han intentado examinar los efectos que tiene el divorcio sobre los niños. En el libro de J. Thomas Fitch, *Second Chances Men, Women* y el de Judith Wallerstein y Sandra Blakeslee, *Children a Decade After Divorce*, los autores encontraron que las probabilidades que tienen los hombres divorciados de morir de una enfermedad del corazón, un derrame cerebral, o cáncer, son dos veces mayores, son cuatro veces mayores sus probabilidades de morir en un accidente automovilístico o del suicidio, siete veces mayores sus probabilidades de morir de cirrosis hepática o pulmonía, ocho veces mayores sus probabilidades de morir asesinados, y diez veces mayores sus probabilidades de sufrir de una enfermedad psiquiátrica. Aunque las mujeres divorciadas eran menos propensas a las enfermedades físicas que las mujeres solteras, sí sufrieron más de condiciones crónicas y pasaron más días en cama debido a enfermedad. Son dos o tres veces mayores sus probabilidades de morir de cáncer de la boca, de los órganos digestivos, de los pulmones, y de los senos.

LOS EFECTOS QUE TIENE EL DIVORCIO SOBRE LOS NIÑOS

Después de un divorcio, los niños ven disminuir el presupuesto familiar en un 37 por ciento. Diez años después del divorcio de sus padres, uno de cada tres niños varones y una de cada diez niñas muestran una conducta delincuente. Los niños de padres divorciados tienen casi dos veces más probabilidad de tener un mal desempeño escolar que los niños que vienen de hogares con los dos padres. Las mujeres criadas en familias de un solo padre tienen sesenta y cuatro veces más probabilidad de tener a niños fuera del matrimonio ellas mismas. Aquellas mujeres que sí se casan tienen noventa y dos veces más probabilidad de divorciarse que las mujeres con familias de dos padres. Los presos de las prisiones estatales tienen dos veces más probabilidad de haber crecido en hogares con un solo padre o madre. Las hijas entre las edades de doce y dieciséis años que viven con madres que no están casadas tienen cuando menos dos veces la probabilidad de llegar a ser madres solteras también. Las investigaciones han relacionado la enfermedad mental, el suicidio, la enfermedad física, el consumo de drogas, el fumar cigarros, la falta de vivienda, el crimen juvenil, y el fracaso escolar, con matrimonios deshechos.

A veces los padres piensan que al divorciarse tendrán la oportunidad de encontrar una mejor pareja y que las condiciones mejorarán. Pero más de la mitad de los niños de padres divorciados son testigos de la violencia física entre sus padres; mientras que antes del divorcio la mayoría nunca había presenciado violencia en el hogar.

Quiero que quede claro que no estoy diciendo que todos los matrimonios deben mantenerse juntos sin tomar en cuenta las circunstancias, porque verdaderamente hay excepciones importantes que considerar. Simplemente quiero señalar que el conocimiento de las consecuencias negativas del divorcio, debe provocar que las parejas estudien más detenidamente la situación antes de dar un paso tan importante. Lo que a veces parece una cláusula de salida, o una "salida fácil", puede frecuentemente traer como resultado más problemas y sufrimientos. Muchas generaciones jóvenes de latinos hoy en día, al no estar totalmente comprometidos a la manera cultural de ver el matrimonio, la cual refuerza su permanencia, deciden probar otras alternativas. Quizá prueben vivir con sus parejas antes de casarse o simplemente no casarse. Cada vez más jóvenes se meten a este tipo de situaciones pensando que van a aprender algo acerca de su futura pareja que les preparará para un compromiso más adelante. Sin embargo, esta creencia no ha sido apoyada por ninguna de las recientes investigaciones.

De acuerdo a la Encuesta Nacional de Familias y Hogares (*National Survey of Families and Households*) realizada por la Universidad de Wisconsin, entre las 14,000 personas que fueron entrevistadas que vivían con sus parejas, el índice de divorcio o separación era 50 por ciento más alto que los matrimonios que no vivieron juntos antes de casarse. Casi el 40 por ciento de las parejas se separaron antes de siquiera llegar al altar. La duración promedia de la relación era de 1.3 años. Así que, ¿en qué radican las claves de un buen matrimonio? Simplemente, en el contrato, el compromiso, y la comunicación. Todo comienza con el examen y la revelación personal de sus propios valores, expectativas, y esperanzas antes de casarse uno.

INVENTARIO PERSONAL Y PREMATRIMONIAL: ANTES QUE TE CASES, MIRA LO QUE HACES

Mientras que el enfoque principal de este libro consiste en los padres que tienen niños menores de doce años, también está diseñado para aquellas personas que están pensando seriamente en el matrimonio (o casarse de nuevo), con la intención de algún día tener niños. A aquel grupo de personas les digo lo mismo que mi madre nos dijo a mí y a mis hermanos, "*Antes que te cases, mira lo que haces*". Cuando yo era una mujer joven y soltera, quería ser muy cuidadosa con respecto a escoger a la persona con quien compartiría el resto de mi vida. Quería que el matrimonio perdurara. Tenía una lista de características que buscaba en una pareja, y revisaba esa lista con todos los hombres con quienes salía.

No pude creer lo cerca que llegó mi esposo a mi hombre ideal. Éramos *como agua para chocolate*, parecía que estábamos destinados uno para el otro. Un día le anuncié a mi familia que estaba locamente enamorada y que había encontrado al hombre perfecto. Luego la voz se me bajó, y dije abruptamente: "Bue-e-eno, excepto por una sola característica". No era tan alto como yo esperaba que fuera mi príncipe azul. Yo recuerdo que fui a ver al padre Albert Kippes, el sacerdote católico que eventualmente nos casó, para que me diera un poco de orientación. Yo le dije: "Padre, creo que encontré al hombre perfecto, con la excepción de un detalle menor". Él contestó: "En un lado de una hoja de papel, escriba todas las cosas de él que te gustan; en el otro lado escribe lo que no te gusta. Luego platicaremos".

Yo seguí sus instrucciones, llenando el lado izquierdo de mi lista con todas las cosas que me gustaban de Sal. En el lado derecho, escribí una sola cosa: que era chaparro. El padre Kippes se rió cuando vio mi lista. "Las cosas que son importantes, como su carácter, no cambiarán", él dijo. "Los atributos físicos sí cambian. Todos nos ponemos chaparros, gordos, y pelones al envejecer. Quizá perdamos una pierna o un brazo en un accidente. Pero el corazón se mantendrá constante". Me miró y enérgicamente me dijo que me casara con él. Dicho y hecho, tal como recomendó el padre Kippes, me casé, y el 17 de junio de 1997, celebramos veinticinco años de casados. "¡Qué aguante!"

Uno de los mejores consejos que se le puede dar a alguien que está contemplando el matrimonio y que quiere que dure cuando menos veinticinco años, es hacer un inventario prematrimonial, el cual es ofrecido por los pastores y consejeros de muchas iglesias, para determinar qué tan compatibles son. *Si no escoges el mejor, por lo menos no el peor.* Querrá encontrar a alguien que le ayudará a usted a proveer el mejor ambiente para sus niños. Habrá tensión y problemas en cualquier relación, pero entre mejor se conozcan, mejor será su relación más adelante. Aun por su propia cuenta, puede hacer un recuento de esperanzas, actitudes, y expectativas personales. Haga una lista mental (o en una hoja de papel) de las cosas que usted valora más en la vida y las cosas que por las cuales quiere luchar: una educación, una carrera y/o una familia. Discuta las cosas que son importantes para cada uno y las cosas que no tolerarán, por ejemplo el adulterio. Todas las cosas que plantean se utilizarán más adelante para crear un plan para su matrimonio, para establecer metas, y para negociar el beneficio de ambos, un terreno común. Las parejas que están pensando en el matrimonio deben discutir sus puntos de vista sobre los papeles y las responsabilidades que cada persona asumirá, antes de firmar el contrato matrimonial. Entre más temprano comprenda cada uno de las posturas del otro con respecto a asuntos como las finanzas, la educación, su carrera, y el número de niños que quieren tener, mejor podrán resolver los conflictos más adelante. Si no se le presta la debida atención y consideración, las preguntas y las dudas bien pueden convertirse en resentimientos y hostilidad y pueden fácilmente brotar una gran cantidad de problemas.

Algunas de las preguntas que se deben preguntar son las siguientes:

- ¿Utilizaré el apellido de mi esposo o mantendré el mío?
- ¿Ambos tendrán igual oportunidad de luchar por alcanzar sus metas educativas y de su carrera?
- ¿Está dispuesta cada persona a mudarse a una ciudad o aun a un país distinto si al otro le ofrecen un trabajo o una oportunidad educativa?
- ¿Cómo se dividirán las finanzas? ¿Se compartirán equitativa- mente, o se esperará que cada uno contribuya una "parte justa"? ¿Está dispuesto uno a mantener al otro por años si es necesario? ¿Cuánto ahorraremos o invertiremos? ¿Tendremos tarjetas de crédito? ¿Cuántas? ¿Con un límite de cuánto?
- De los muchos quehaceres necesarios para mantener un hogar ordenado, ¿quién hará qué? ¿Debemos buscar ayuda de afuera?
- ¿Tendremos niños? Si vamos a tenerlos, ¿cuándo y cuántos? ¿Cómo los vamos a disciplinar? ¿Serán bilingües? ¿Cuáles costum- bres y creencias tradicionales queremos pasarles a nuestros niños?
- ¿Qué será el papel de los miembros de la familia extensa?
- ¿Dónde vamos a vivir? ¿Vamos a vivir cerca de nuestro sistema de apoyo, incluyendo las casas de nuestros padres, o un poco alejado?
- ¿Vamos a mantener ciertas costumbres y creencias tradicionales?
- ¿Qué religión vamos a practicar? Si decidimos mantener dife- rentes religiónes, ¿cuál de ellas practicarán nuestros niños cuando son pequeños?
- ¿Qué haré si mi pareja comete adulterio, me maltrata, o llega a ser alcohólica?
- ¿Dónde y cómo celebraremos los días festivos importantes (Navidad, día de las Madres, Pascua)?
- ¿Y qué tal los suegros? ¿Cómo aseguraremos mantener fuerte nues- tra relación con ellos?

Otros asuntos esenciales incluyen las relaciones sexuales, las amis- tades, y el uso del tiempo libre. Los papeles y las responsabilidades abar- carán desde temas tan complejos como la disciplina hasta algo que parece muy trivial, como lavar los platos. Tan difícil como quizá sea hablar sobre algunos de estos temas, platicar acerca de ellos puede ser muy útil para ayudar a explorar su terreno común. Aun las cosas que parecen insignificantes pueden convertirse más adelante en problemas significativos que pueden causar un rompimiento en su relación.

Para aquéllos que ya están casados, como dice el popular dicho, *te casaste, te fregaste*. Ahora lo importante es hacer que funcione. Siguen unos consejos, algunas observaciones que le pueden ayudar a mantener sólido su matrimonio.

LATINAS: LA SACRIFICADA Y LA "SUPERMAMÁ"

Las mujeres hispanas de la actualidad están definiendo de nuevo y haciendo más firme su posición en la sociedad. A través de la historia, las madres latinas han sido veneradas como el corazón de la familia, las que proporcionan cariño y cuidado, las que estabilizan, y las que se encargan de la gran tarea de mantener unida la familia. Pero su autoridad nunca competía con la de su marido, quien siempre tenía la última palabra en la casa. El modelo de ser sacrificada y sumisa, continúa afectando la posición de las mujeres hispanas en los Estados Unidos. Era ése el modelo con el cual yo crecí en mi barrio, el que todas, desde mi abuela hasta mi madre, hasta el momento en que se convirtió en testigo de Jehová, aceptaba y representaba sin chistar. Su nueva religión le dio la fortaleza necesaria para volverse firme, en el nombre de hacer "el trabajo de Jehová".

Más adelante, al ser madre y una mujer profesional que trabajaba, yo supe que la igualdad, la cooperación, y la comunicación iban a ser esenciales en mi familia y que la negociación de una relación de igualdad no iba a ser fácil. Las mujeres latinas de hoy en día exigen y esperan ser tratadas con igualdad, con dignidad y respeto. Tienen el impulso, como cualquier americano, de aprovechar al máximo las libertades y las oportunidades que la vida en este país les brinda. Sin embargo, una gran cantidad de barreras, ambos dentro y fuera de la familia, han hecho que éste sea un camino difícil. Como resultado, muchas mujeres hispanas se enfrentan a enormes dificultades al asumir nuevos papeles para complacer a un mundo de dos culturas distintas, cada una con sus propias expectativas. Es muy fácil sentirse abrumada.

Mi cuñado, quien está casado con mi hermana Yolanda, me dijo desde el principio de su matrimonio que sólo le permitiría a ella trabajar si la casa estaba limpia y había un plato de comida caliente en la mesa cuando él volvía del trabajo. Mi cuñada, Hope, una mujer muy tradicional, está siempre a la entera disposición de su esposo. Ella es considerada "pura mujer" a los ojos de algunos. Su marido le truena los dedos y no sólo *ella* brinca, sino también sus hijas. Ella ha aceptado el papel tradicional casi sin queja ni necesidad de adaptación, con una sola e importante diferencia: ella trabaja tiempo completo, no porque quiere, sino porque las exigencias económicas de la familia lo hacen necesario. Para algunos, este arreglo puede ser satisfactorio. Pero a un número cada vez más grande de hispanos, representa un escenario que causa preocupación.

En el terreno social de tan rápidos cambios, de los Estados Unidos, las mujeres hispanas están aprovechando la oportunidad de estrenar nuevos papeles y tener nuevas experiencias. Cada vez más, están descubriendo su potencial fuera del hogar. De acuerdo al Ministerio de Trabajo de los Estados Unidos, las mujeres hispanas componen uno de los grupos de mujeres que está aumentando más rápidamente dentro de la fuerza laboral de los Estados Unidos. El número de mujeres hispanas empleadas aumentó en un 65 por ciento entre 1986 y 1996. Por cierto que estos cambios drásticos implican unas enormes repercusiones en la estructura de la familia. Desdichadamente, estos cambios no se discuten fácilmente, y con más mujeres esperando más tiempo para tener niños, los temas de trabajo y la familia no siempre son aclarados desde el principio del matrimonio.

No me molestó representar el papel maternal tradicional cuando tenía sólo un niño y cuatro empleados, porque como soy una persona que gusta de cuidar y proporcionar cariño, quería dar todo lo que podía de mí misma. Cuando ambas familias, la de AVANCE y mi familia más cercana, crecieron, ya no podía ser todo para todos y aún mantener la cordura. Llegué a aceptar el hecho de que yo no era una supermamá, y lo que era más, no quería serlo. Solamente cuando protesté, comenzó mi esposo a asumir más responsabilidades con relación al cuidado de los niños, como bañarlos y cocinar para ellos. Lo que él odiaba era hacer los quehaceres de la casa. A través del proceso de la comunicación, en lugar de estar callada, yo le dije todas las cosas que yo necesitaba que se hicieran, y como no tenía yo ni el tiempo ni la energía para hacerlo todo. Igual como he hablado en voz alta a favor de los niños y de las familias a través de los años y he luchado por la supervivencia y el crecimiento de AVANCE, yo me encontré utilizando esta firmeza en mi propio hogar, con la gente a quien más quería. Mi esposo asumió una carga más pesada en nuestro intento por mantener un hogar ordenado, sin embargo se negó rotundamente a lavar los platos hasta que compramos un lavaplatos automático, y aun entonces, él tenía algo en contra de lavar esos platos. Al crecer los niños, se repartieron los quehaceres entre todos los miembros de la familia, además de conseguir una trabajadora doméstica que viniera cuando menos una vez por semana a encargarse de hacer el trabajo más pesado que nosotros odiábamos hacer—¡como lavar los baños!

Yo he pasado a engrosar las filas de muchos otros hombres y mujeres latinos que están convencidos que los cambios verdaderos deben ocurrir en varios sectores de la sociedad para que las mujeres hispanas consigan la igualdad de condiciones económicas y sociales que merecen. Romper con las barreras discriminatorias en la educación y en los lugares de trabajo, y hacer que las políticas en los empleos tomen más en consideración a las madres que trabajan, son dos ejemplos de cambios que necesitan efectuarse. Dentro de la familia, también será necesario que nuestros hombres vuelvan a evaluar sus papeles para ayudar a las mujeres a encontrar un punto medio entre ser la mujer sacrificada y la supermamá. El foco central del proceso de ponernos firmes y volver a definir qué son "nuestros lugares", como madres, esposas, y trabajadoras productivas en el próximo siglo, es hacer más fuertes nuestras voces para que nos oigan en nuestras familias y más allá.

EL HOMBRE HISPANO: REPLANTEANDO EL MODELO "MACHO"

Por generaciones, el machismo se ha asociado con un hombre que es muy firme y dominante en el hogar. Él es alguien que vive por sus propias leyes, las cuales nadie pone en duda, mucho menos la esposa. Mientras que esta reseña es muy conocida, el modelo del machismo consiste en mucho más.

La palabra raíz de "macho" proviene de la palabra náhuatl precolombina *mati*—conocer, y *macho*—ser conocido. Entre los aztecas, la valentía y el valor eran virtudes que los hombres se esforzaban a alcanzar, para lograr prominencia y reconocimiento. Los hombres hispanos de la actualidad aún son reconocidos por su valentía al poseer muchos de ellos una *Congressional Medal of Honor* (Medalla de Honor otorgada por el Congreso) por su valor. Además, de acuerdo al autor Earl Shorris, los valores, o *virtus*, por los cuales querían ser reconocidos los hombres aztecas incluían "valentía, vigor, fortaleza en la adversidad, logros públicos, orden, disciplina, felicidad, fortaleza, justicia, y por encima de todo, la reclamación de los derechos propios y los conocimientos, y el poder necesario para asegurar su satisfacción".

Se dice que los aspectos negativos del machismo surgieron después de la conquista, durante la cual los hombres, como líderes de la sociedad, perdieron su nombre, religión, cultura, y familia. En muchos aspectos, perdieron su identidad y su dignidad. El hombre que siente la necesidad de mostrar sus virtudes positivas, pero no puede, se esconde detrás la máscara del alcoholismo. Inflige violencia y terror en su familia y sus amigos, quienes él percibe como más débiles que él. No puede expresar su ira a su "patrón", ni siquiera las injusticias, y no tomará una postura ante una discriminación obvia. Esto puede llevar al alcoholismo para insensibilizarse al dolor, o bien, a la violencia familiar para soltar la ira.

Hay una leyenda azteca que ilustra el fenómeno de esconderse detrás de una máscara de vergüenza y culpabilidad. Había un monje bueno de Tula, a quien el dios malvado, Tezcatlipoca, logra engañar para que se emborrachara. No estando en su sano juicio, Tula abusa sexualmente a su hermana. A la mañana siguiente, avergonzado, esconde la cara detrás de una máscara de jade, se va al mar, y le prende fuego a su barco. Luego se convierte en un pájaro emplumado llamado Quetzalcoatl. Esta leyenda es análoga a lo que les ocurre a muchos hombres hispanos quienes han sido despojados de su identidad, su dignidad, y su amor propio, por medio de la opresión, la discriminación, o la incapacidad de mantener a su familia. Todos queremos que nuestra vida tenga un significado y un propósito. Pero cuando un hombre no puede satisfacer ni las necesidades básicas de su familia, ni saber quién es realmente, se esconde detrás de una máscara de vergüenza y desvía su ira en contra de las personas que ama. Por eso es tan crítico que la sociedad les proporcione a todos sus ciudadanos las oportunidades educativas y los trabajos para satisfacer apropiadamente sus papeles de padre con relación a ser el sostén de la familia. También es importante que los hispanos sepan desde muy pequeños quiénes son y se sientan orgullosos de su cultura.

En este país, existe un mejor equilibrio entre la madre, quien generalmente ha sido percibida como la que cuida y da cariño y educa a los niños, y el padre, quien tradicionalmente ha tenido el papel de imponer y mantener la disciplina, y de sostener a la familia. Si ocurre este equilibrio, ambos deben ser venerados y honrados por sus niños por los papeles que jugaron para mantener el hogar. *De un buen matrimonio, florecen las semillas*. Los niños tendrán un sentido de seguridad cuando los padres demuestran amor y respeto, uno para el otro.

Sin embargo, cuando a una mujer hispana la hace sentirse débil un hombre inseguro que expresa sus sentimientos de ineptitud al maltratarla física y emocionalmente, la familia se mueve fuera de equilibrio y se vuelve disfuncional. A veces el hombre, quien no puede encontrar un trabajo que pague lo suficiente para mantener a la familia, se da cuenta que no puede solo con la carga y esconde sus inseguridades, causadas por su incapacidad de cuidar a su familia, con los aspectos negativos del machismo. Cada familia necesita tener a dos personas fuertes para poder aplicar la antigua costumbre náhuatl conocida como Etzli-Yollotl, o *cara y corazón*. Cada persona debe tener una cara (dignidad y respeto) y un corazón (confianza y amor) para poder funcionar bien. La gente azteca náhuatl creían que si una persona siente dolor, quizá por la mala fortuna o la guerra, tiene que recobrar sus fuerzas a través de *cara y corazón*. Tenía que curarse para volver a ser un macho otra vez.

Igual como nuestros antepasados pudieron considerar el aspecto positivo del machismo como una manifestación exterior de virtud, en la actualidad, hay personas como el terapeuta familiar Jerry Tello, de Los Angeles, California, que están reconsiderando qué significa ser un hombre latino. Tello desarrolló un sistema de conexiones para hombres hispanos y un programa para los padres en la crianza de los niños que se llama *Cara y Corazón*, cuyo propósito es ayudar a los hombres hispanos a curarse del dolor que proviene de la discriminación, la falta de educación o de habilidades comerciales de trabajo, o la falta de empleo. Está intentando ayudarles a recobrar su cara y corazón para que puedan ser mejores padres, esposos, trabajadores, y ciudadanos. Como creían los aztecas, "el hombre maduro es el que tiene un corazón tan sólido como una roca, y una cara sabia. Debe ser capaz y comprensivo". Cuando a una persona la describen con frases como "no tiene cara para hablar y no tiene corazón", se dice que no tiene cara o corazón, o que le falta carácter. Pero el tener cara y corazón significa ser sabio, capaz y compasivo, y tener dominio de sí mismo. Es ser el hombre ideal, "un hombre noble".

En su libro *La Morenita, Evangelizer of the Americas*, el padre Virgilio P. Elizondo señala que los niños aztecas fueron aceptados como parte del clan desde su nacimiento, y recibían una cara (conocimiento de las tradiciones y las costumbres del grupo, lo cual les confería dignidad y respeto) y un corazón (una voluntad que les predisponían a tomar la dirección de la autodisciplina y la bondad). Desde una edad muy pequeña, los niños aztecas fueron enseñados el concepto de *virtus*—a dedicarse a lo que era bueno y justo, a evitar la maldad y a refrenarse de la perversión y la codicia. También se enseñaban los principios de la moderación y el dominio de sí mismo. En un pasaje extraído del texto náhuatl del *Códice Florentino*, un padre azteca enseñó a su hijo a abstenerse del sexo al comparar a su niño a una planta de maguey. "Si se abre antes de crecerse y se le extrae el líquido, ya no tiene sustancia. No produce líquido, es inútil. Antes de que se abra para extraerle el agua, debe permitirse que crezca y alcance su tamaño completo. Luego se le extrae toda su agua dulce en buen momento". La lección azteca concluye con:

"Antes de que conozcas a una mujer, necesitas crecer y ser un hombre completo. Entonces, estarás preparado para el matrimonio; tendrás hijos de buena estatura, sanos, ágiles, y lindos". Nuestros antepasados nos enseñaron que el verdadero hombre macho se había socializado bien y enseñado a tener dominio de sí mismo antes y después del matrimonio, la antítesis del aspecto negativo de ser macho.

Mientras sí existen algunos aspectos negativos de la imagen del hombre latino, tal como ocurre en muchas culturas, debemos recordar que para los hispanos, un hombre noble, como primero les fue enseñado a nuestros ancestros, era alguien que era un líder y un protector. En la actualidad, los padres hispanos todavía pueden ser las personas que gobiernan a sus niños, pero también pueden ser las personas que los cuidan y les dan cariño y no temen mostrar su afecto a su familia. Éstas son características que, por el valor que tienen, deben mantenerse y no ser descartadas o menospreciadas como algo "para las viejas". Los esposos y los padres deben explorar la parte del macho que pone énfasis en el respeto, el orgullo, y la responsabilidad. Aunque la mujer hispana es venerada por ser la que tradicionalmente mantiene unida la familia, es importante que el hombre comparta un lugar de honor al participar más en el cuidado y la educación de sus niños.

En su libro *Fatherlessness in America*, David Blankenhorn, un especialista social y el presidente del *Council on Families in America*, del cual yo soy miembro, escribió que no hace mucho, al morir un padre, la sociedad subrayó el papel del padre al ir con la familia para ofrecer asistencia y apoyo emocional. Yo crecí en tal comunidad. Cuando falleció mi padre, no fue una sola persona, sino muchos hombres y mujeres en el barrio quienes sintieron la obligación de ocupar su lugar. Ellos, juntos con mi madre, asumieron el papel de mi padre como las personas que imponían y mantenían la disciplina, sostenes de la familia, consejeros espirituales, modelos de conducta, y mentores. Esto de describe claramente con el dicho *El muchacho malcriado dondequiera encuentra padre*. Desdichadamente, en la actualidad, dice Blankenhorn, cuando un padre se va, en muchas familias su ausencia se acepta con indiferencia. La ausencia de los padres, él observa, se ha convertido simplemente en otro problema social que está más allá de nuestro alcance. Se percibe con demasiada frecuencia como simplemente un hecho más de la vida.

Hoy en día, en muchos sentidos, las expectativas que se tienen del hombre hispano son mayores que nunca. Al prepararnos para ser el grupo de minoría más grande de los Estados Unidos, los hombres hispanos, como sus parejas femeninas, se enfrentan al enorme desafío de mantener fuerte a la familia durante una época cuando adversas fuerzas económicas y sociales parecen estar destrozando a las familias. Demasiados jóvenes hispanos se están convirtiendo en padres a una edad muy joven o en víctimas del señuelo de las pandillas y las pistolas en un intento vano de encontrar un significado y un propósito a sus vidas. El macho hispano debe volver a su valor y su fortaleza para luchar, aguantar, y sacrificar por el bienestar de la familia y de los niños. No habrá mayor batalla ganada, ni mayor reconocimiento alcanzado cuando ambos madre y padre hacen todo lo posible dentro de un matrimonio sólido para ayudar a sus niños a tener éxito en la vida. Un hombre noble es uno que es bastante fuerte para mantener a su familia unida, en harmonía, y funcionando bien.

Mi madre creía que un esposo traía respeto al hogar. Ella creía que muchas personas se aprovechan de las mujeres solas, especialmente en el barrio. Se volvió a casar varios años después del fallecimiento de mi padre, por la importancia que ella le daba al tener a un hombre en la casa para protección, seguridad, y compañía. Para ella, una pareja de casados era un símbolo de respeto y bienestar. Su filosofía es corroborada por investigaciones que relacionan las familias y los matrimonios sólidos con la buena salud física y mental. Funciona como una protección en contra de la pobreza, la falta de vivienda para jóvenes, el crimen juvenil, y el abuso sexual. Las investigaciones también demuestran que tener a un esposo que proporciona apoyo, puede servir para amortiguar los efectos de la tensión y la depresión.

Hablo por mí misma cuando digo que yo sé que no podría mantener los horarios que tengo, ni lograr tanto como he logrado, sin el amor y el apoyo de mi esposo. Él me ha alentado, ha tenido fe en mi, me ha mantenido los pies firmemente plantados sobre la tierra, y ha sido mi caja de resonancia. Siempre ha estado a mi lado, ha sido mi fortaleza, y me ha ayudado a realizar mis sueños y mis metas más grandes. Sal y mis niños han sido mi fuerza estabilizadora y mi refugio de las fuerzas externas y las tensiones de la vida. Me siento tan afortunada y bendecida por tener a un esposo que ha apoyado tanto mi desarrollo personal y que no se siente amenazado con mis logros. Simplemente, es un hombre muy seguro y con mucha confianza en sí mismo.

Con respecto a su papel de padre, mi esposo también lo ha tomado muy en serio. Cuando yo he estado trabajando tarde, de viaje, o trabajando en mi doctorado y en mi libro, él ha asumido el papel principal de la crianza de nuestros niños. Mi esposo ha preparado biberones, cambiado pañales, y llevado a nuestros niños al médico cuando estaban enfermos. Ha cocinado para ellos, ha asistido a conferencias con los maestros conmigo o sin mí, y ha sido el entrenador de los niños. Mis niños han establecido una sólida relación con su padre por el tiempo tan precioso que ha pasado con ellos.

Muchos esposos han permitido que los compromisos de trabajo les prevengan participar en actividades con sus niños, y han perdido una gran oportunidad de sentir la misma satisfacción, gratificación, y amor que sienten las madres al dar de sí mismos a sus niños. El dicho *Sin dolor, madre sin amor*, también se puede aplicar a un padre. Satisfacer las necesidades de sus niños, y ayudarles a crecer, en momentos buenos y malos, desarrollará una relación inestimable entre padres y niños. Los niños no quieren simplemente la satisfacción de sus necesidades físicas, ni tampoco que les colmen de cosas materiales. Ellos quieren y necesitan el tiempo, apoyo, y orientación y asistencia emocional de ambos padres. Debe haber amor incondicional de ambos padres, y ambos deben ser responsables de satisfacer las necesidades que tienen sus niños para tener un crecimiento y desarrollo sanos. Los padres necesitan saborear la alegría y la satisfacción que provienen de participar plenamente en la vida de sus niños. Al mismo tiempo, aunque están ocupando la posición de matriarcas hispanas, las esposas necesitan soltar algunas de sus responsabilidades y ayudarles a sus hombres a encontrar maneras para asumir su parte justa de la crianza de los niños. Cuando yo lo hice, mi esposo aprendió a tener una relación más estrecha con sus niños, comprendiéndolos como personas individuales y forjando vínculos de amor y confianza con ellos. Estas cosas, él me ha dicho, han enriquecido enormemente su vida, como padre y también como ser humano.

ACABAR CON LAS TRADICIONES "TÁCITAS"

Cuando son jóvenes, los niños varones hispanos en algunas familias frecuentemente son alentados a tener relaciones sexuales y por lo general no tienen que enfrentar las consecuencias de sus acciones. Mi suegra les decía a sus vecinos: "Cuiden a sus pollitas, porque ahí vienen mis gallos". Los hombres, al igual que las mujeres, deben ser responsables con respecto a asuntos sexuales, una lección que necesita enseñarse en el hogar cuando son jóvenes. Muchas veces, cuando mis niños y yo mirábamos las telenovelas, me encontraba ante la necesidad de señalar mi oposición fuerte a la infidelidad. Mirábamos las novelas como manera de aprender el español. Pero lo que también vieron eran una representaciones de maridos infieles que hacían un deporte de tener aventuras extramatrimoniales. Mi hija, Vanessa, y yo nos poníamos furiosas con los hombres al ver su tratamiento de las mujeres y también nos enfurecían las mujeres por no ser más firmes.

Antes hablé acerca de algunos de los aspectos positivos del machismo que con frecuencia son pasados por alto, además de aquellas cosas que necesitan ser añadidas a la definición que tiene nuestra cultura de la identidad masculina hispana. Sin embargo, otro factor muy real relacionado con el machismo que debe ser discutido es la tradición del adulterio y el abuso. Sus orígenes provienen de aquellos dichos antiguos que afirman que los hombres básicamente eran como los gallos, libres para hacer lo que quisieran, y que era la mujer que tenía la responsabilidad de protegerse. La infidelidad es tolerada en Latinoamérica y aún persiste en los Estados Unidos. Yo me enteré que en México es común para un hombre tener a una "querida", y tener a uno o más niños ilegítimos. Cuando mi abuelo era un hombre joven en México, era un mujeriego. Su esposa toleró sus actos de sinvergüenza por muchos años. En aquella época, tenía pocas opciones. No fue hasta que mi abuelo, que era un católico poco entusiasta, se convirtió en un devoto pentecostalista que mi madre y mi abuela vieron una profunda transformación en él. Pero éste no era siempre el resultado para otras familias. Mientras cumplían con sus deberes formales, a los hombres generalmente les perdonaban sus aventuras extramatrimoniales. A veces, las mujeres que se atrevían a oponerse recibían golpes de sus maridos como castigo.

A través de mi vida y especialmente de mi trabajo, yo he escuchado a mujeres hispanas hablándose en voz baja acerca de los problemas que tenían con sus maridos. Aunque las situaciones variaban, muchas veces las palabras eran las mismas. "Pues una tiene que aguantar", dirían. O bien: "Ya me tocaba sufrir". Hoy en día, tal idea es inaceptable. No existe una sola justificación para que una mujer se quede al lado de un hombre que la maltrata, ya sea física o emocionalmente. Yo he instado a algunas madres participantes de AVANCE, quienes eran víctimas del abuso físico, a no tolerar tales actos de brutalidad. "¡Tú no eres una pelota para que te pateen!" Yo les decía: "Tú eres un ser humano con sentimientos y derechos. Lo que te ha hecho tu esposo está mal, y él necesita ayuda. No cambiará su conducta hasta que consiga ayuda. Piensa en ti misma y ante todo, piensa en tus niños". En cuanto mencionaba a los niños, las mujeres miraban su situación con un ojo más crítico y tomaban la acción apropiada.

María era una madre con seis niños que venía a AVANCE llena de moretones, con anteojos obscuros y mangas largas para esconder sus ojos morados y los moretones. Cuando le preguntaba acerca de sus heridas, nunca admitía que su esposo las había causado. Pero al asistir a las clases y aprender acerca de sus opciones, comenzó a comprender y apreciar su valor y potencial. Eventualmente dejó a su esposo, completó su educación de preparatoria y siguió su educación hasta conseguir su licenciatura. Después admitió que el maltrato a las esposas había existido por generaciones en su familia y que nunca supo que las cosas podrían ser diferentes hasta que vino a AVANCE. Dijo que al participar en el programa de AVANCE, aprendió que no tenía que vivir en "esa rutina sofocante" o callejón sin salida.

Es importante que las mujeres que se encuentran en estas situaciones, tomen las medidas necesarias para salir inmediatamente. En los Estados Unidos, el maltrato es causal de divorcio. Punto final. Lo mismo para el adulterio. Esta conducta nunca debe ser aceptada como una manera de vivir. Cada persona merece ser tratada con dignidad y respeto. Por medio de la educación, la propugnación, y un legado de victorias legales, nuestra sociedad ha logrado, hasta cierto punto, darle final al silencio que rodeaba el abuso doméstico y ha luchado por darles a las mujeres la herramienta necesaria para tomar medidas en su contra. Pero estas salidas sólo tienen éxito en la medida en que las mujeres tienen las fuerzas necesarias para dar el primer paso. El surgimiento de las enfermedades de transmisión sexual y el SIDA también han reforzado, para las mujeres, la importancia de la fidelidad en el matrimonio, ahora más que nunca. Las mujeres no pueden darse el lujo de ser sumisas cuando se trata de su vida. Deben mantenerse erguidas y firmes en contra de todo tipo de maltrato, incluyendo el adulterio, porque es su bienestar y el bienestar de sus niños que están en juego. Una de las cosas más importantes que debe considerar al tomar una decisión sobre su relación es que se trata de enseñarles a sus niños cómo un hombre y una mujer deben tratarse. Si usted se queda en una relación abusiva, sus acciones—o bien, falta de ellas—servirán de modelo de conducta a su niño.

LOS TIEMPOS CAMBIAN

A través de los años, he observado a las mujeres hispanas volverse más firmes y los hombres hispanos participar más en las cosas del hogar—algo que no se veía hace dos o tres décadas. Si los hombres ayudaban a sus esposas, lo hacían sólo cuando nadie los miraba. El marido de mi hermana Rosa Linda bajaba las persianas cuando le ayudaba a hacer tamales para la Navidad porque no quería que los vecinos o la familia lo miraran "con las manos en la masa". Aunque le encantaban los tamales caseros, él se veía forzado a aceptar el hecho de que, con su parte de los deberes correspondientes a criar a cinco niños además de mantener un trabajo de tiempo completo, mi hermana no podía hacerlos sin su ayuda. A través del tiempo, él pudo hacer estas cosas sin pensar dos veces en lo que pensarían o dirían los demás.

COMUNICAR, COOPERAR, Y NEGOCIAR

Con cada vez más frecuencia, encontrará a parejas que están comunicando abiertamente, negociando, transigiendo, y dándose cuenta que algunas cosas tienen que ser diferentes. Al tomar este camino de negociación las parejas, habrán algunos desacuerdos. La construcción de un matrimonio sobre cimientos sólidos requiere unas tremendas habilidades de comunicación y resolución de conflictos. Durante nuestros veinticinco años de vida de casados, mi esposo y yo hemos tenido bastantes discusiones. En momentos de ira, desilusión, frustración, o tensión, muchas personas tienen la tendencia de decir cosas que realmente no quieren. Yo me di cuenta de esto cuando justo después de nuestra luna de miel, me encontré declarando, "Yo quiero el divorcio", al tener nuestra primera discusión. De hecho, hasta la fecha no puedo recordar por qué estaba tan disgustada. Por fortuna, igual a nuestros padres, mi esposo y yo compartíamos la creencia fundamental que nuestro matrimonio iba a ser para siempre, hasta la muerte. El día de esa discusión determinamos que la palabra "divorcio" no existía y que nunca más se volvería a mencionar como una opción. Estábamos determinados a hacer que nuestro matrimonio funcionara.

A veces estábamos en desacuerdo acerca de proyectos no terminados, el manejo de las finanzas, la disciplina de nuestros niños, y sí, una vez aun un momento pasajero de celos insignificantes. En otros momentos, los conflictos eran a causa del uso de tiempo libre y de los quehaceres de la casa. Es natural que las parejas tengan discusiones. Sin embargo, no es saludable que uno de ellos se quede con todo por dentro. Todas las parejas deben desarrollar una estrategia y su propio "idioma" para utilizar con el otro en momentos de conflicto. Algunos pasos que nosotros seguimos son:

- Cuando aumenta mucho la tensión, tome un momento para calmarse. Vaya a otro cuarto, salga a caminar, escuche música, cualquier cosa que sabe que le calmará los nervios. Encontrará que es más fácil comunicar sus sentimientos después de tomar un momento para calmarse.

- Utilice un poco de ese tiempo para reflejar sobre el punto de vista de la otra persona, sin condenar el propio.
- Aunque a veces cuesta trabajo, trate de encontrar las palabras y el tiempo para que cada persona declare su postura y unas posibles soluciones. Evalúe la situación para decidir si puede funcionar para ambos.
- Comunique sus necesidades y preocupaciones claramente, sin pena y con confianza. No tema decir que estaba equivocado o pedir disculpas.
- Nunca haga burla, ni eche la culpa, ni haga sentir culpable a la otra persona.
- Siempre trate de restablecer la relación antes de acostarse.

Sólo al seguir estas estrategias nos dimos cuenta de que lo que parecía en el momento algo insoportable, resultaba ser algo relativamente insignificante, o un simple malentendido. Aprendimos tomar en cuenta, cambiar malos hábitos, o ceder a los deseos del otro. Para encontrar un terreno común uno tiene que aprender a comunicar, a cooperar, y a negociar. Si hay algún mensaje central en esta lección, es que un buen matrimonio está basado en un dar y recibir.

LIDIAR CON EL CONFLICTO A TRAVÉS DE LA COOPERACIÓN: LA MATRIARCA HISPANA—LA DOÑA

> No es bueno que el hombre esté solo. Yo haré una pareja apropiada para él… Luego el Señor hizo la mujer… Un hombre dejará a su padre y a su madre y se unirá a su esposa, y serán una sola carne. (Génesis)

De decir y hacer, hay mucho que ver. Es más fácil decir que hacer que un esposo hispano deje a su familia después de casarse. Cuando una mujer hispana se casa con su esposo, se casa con la familia de su esposo, y con todos sus parientes a través de dos generaciones (véase el capítulo sobre "La familia"). Esto también es cierto para los hombres hispanos.

Por más que luchen juntas para quitar las barreras entre ellos y para resolver los conflictos, las parejas quizá aún tengan conflictos fuera de la familia nuclear, particularmente con los miembros mayores de la familia.

En mi caso personal, estos conflictos eran más fuertes con mi suegra, ya que tenemos personalidades muy similares. La matriarca de una familia hispana tiene una relación muy sólida con sus hijos, especialmente con los varones. Mientras que a los padres hispanos se les hace pensar que son los reyes del castillo, es muy obvio que en la mayoría de las familias hispanas las mujeres, en muchos sentidos, son las cabezas del clan. Ellas son las astutas que generalmente gobiernan y toman las decisiones principales.

Esta creencia es capturada a través de maneras juguetonas en los cuentos populares hispanos donde las mujeres son las que tienen el papel dominante. Por ejemplo, *"In the Days of King Adobe"*, una historia contada por Joe Hayes en su libro titulado *Watch Out for Clever Women, Cuidado con las mujeres astutas*, una mujer anciana se burla de dos hombres que tratan de robar su jamón, por el cual había tenido que ahorrar por mucho tiempo. La mujer, quien había oído por casualidad el complot, cambia el jamón que ya habían metido en su bolsa, por unos ladrillos. El día siguiente los hombres le dicen riéndose que habían soñado de un rey llamado Jamón Primero. Ella les dice que ella también soñó de un rey llamado Jamón Primero, pero que en el sueño de ella, la gente lo destronó y lo echaron del reino, reemplazándolo con Adobe Magno. Los dos hombres no supieron a qué se refería hasta que descubrieron los ladrillos en su bolsa. Se dieron cuenta de lo que había querido decir, y juraron nunca volver a portarse mal con las ancianitas—especialmente las mujeres hispanas astutas.

"The Day It Snowed Tortillas" es otro cuento popular relatado por Joe Hayes que ilustra la astucia de una mujer que siempre saca a su marido de líos. Después de decirle a su marido que no le diga a nadie sobre el oro que encontraron junto al camino, él lo hace, e inevitablemente, los ladrones quienes perdieron el dinero vienen a buscarlo. En anticipación a su visita, ella esconde el oro y hace una gran cantidad de tortillas. Le dice a su marido, no tan listo, que había nevado tortillas. Cuando los ladrones piden el oro, ella les dice que no sabe de qué están hablando. Cuando voltean a mirar al marido, él le pregunta a su mujer: "¿Dónde está el oro que encontramos el día antes de que nevó tortillas?" Los ladrones los tiran a locos y se van sin el oro.

Mientras que el ser fuerte y astuto es claramente una ventaja, puede a veces ser la causa de conflictos cuando una madre y su nuera están tratando, ambas, de señalar o hacer hincapié en algo. Todavía recuerdo cuando vino a la casa un día mi suegra con unas tortillas caseras y le dijo a mi esposo, en un tono que más bien parecía dirigida a mí: "Pobrecito, mi hijito. Aquí te traje unas tortillitas calientes". Yo pensé para mis adentros: "Cuando una tiene tiempo limitado y puede comprar tortillas casi tan deliciosas como las caseras, en el supermercado, ¿para qué hacerlas?" Pero hice como que ni oí el comentario y disfruté de las tortillas, con mi esposo.

Después de que tuve un accidente de carro que dejó destrozado mi carro, mi suegra me aventó otra piedrita, cuando me dijo que Dios estaba tratando de hacerme comprender que mi lugar apropiado era "en la casa", cuidando a su hijo y a sus nietos. No fue fácil abstenerme de contestarle algo a mi suegra, pero por respeto lo logré. Ni tampoco fue fácil "deshacer" algunos de los malos hábitos que mi esposo había adquirido en su casa. Cuando mi esposo dejó salir por primera vez aquellas palabras que ni quiero recordar, "los hombres *no lavan* los platos", yo supe que ambos íbamos a tener que hacer muchos compromisos y adaptaciones. Pero al pasar el tiempo, logramos encontrar un equilibrio que satisfacía las necesidades y expectativas de ambos. Uno de los pasos más difíciles en el camino a lograr ese equilibrio es saber cómo mantenerse firmes con los parientes que muestran desaprobación, particularmente aquéllos que tradicionalmente inspiran el mayor respeto.

Mi suegra era la doña. Cada domingo ella esperaba que nosotros fuéramos a su casa después de misa para almorzar con ella y sus otros siete hijos y sus respectivas familias. Tenía todo un banquete preparado. Si no aparecíamos, yo sabía que ella me miraría a mí, la nuera, como la culpable. En ocasiones ella hacía un llamado a una junta familiar, a la cual se esperaba que asistieran todos, sin falta, y que estuviéramos de acuerdo con ella en cualquier asunto que mencionaba. Después del anuncio de nuestra boda, mi suegra llamó a la familia para que se reunieran con el solo propósito de planear mi boda. Yo estaba asombrada e indignada, pero me abstuve de hablar durante la reunión, hasta que llegó el momento de seleccionar el color de los vestidos de mis damas. A pesar de que yo siempre había deseado el color rosa, me encontré diciéndome por amarillo sólo para contradecir a mi suegra, quien quería rosa. Esta reunión siguió por un par de horas, y yo no podía creer lo que estaba ocurriendo, ni que mi futuro esposo lo permitiera. Salvador, quien estaba acostumbrado a la manera dominante de su madre, no veía nada de malo en cómo se estaban manejando las cosas.

Cuando volvimos a mi casa, yo le dije a Salvador que aunque lo quería mucho y quería casarme con él, no iba a seguir con los planes para casarnos si su mamacita iba a controlar nuestras vidas. De acuerdo, el día de nuestra boda era sólo un día entre muchos que compartiríamos como marido y mujer, pero para mí, era un momento que definiría el resto de nuestra vida juntos. Yo apelé a su sentido de razón y justicia al dejarlo solo para meditar sobre la situación. Yo sabía que tenía que encontrar la manera de resolver un choque potencial que podría haber dañado a nuestra nueva familia, pero sin abandonar el respeto que yo sentía que le debía a mi suegra y la familia extensa. Cuando volví, Sal accedió a darle las gracias a su madre y pedirle respetuosamente que permitiera que nosotros planeáramos nuestra boda. Aunque se sintió al principio, su madre comprendió que se había pasado sus límites con esta "caprichosa", que era muy parecida a ella.

Mi propia madre resultó ser igual de metiche que la de Sal. Yo recuerdo lo inflexible que se mostró con respecto a no querer que usara el vestido de color marfil que yo escogí para hacerle juego a mi velo de encaje español color marfil que llegaba hasta el suelo. En la opinión de mi madre, no usar un vestido blanco o no ponerse flores de azahar en su velo implica que una no es virgen, y que sería escandaloso declararlo abiertamente a aquéllos que asisten a la boda. "¡Ay, qué vergüenza!" eran las palabras que yo miraba en la expresión de su cara, a pesar de que yo no tenía nada de que avergonzarme. Como yo me mantuve firme acerca de usar el vestido, ella se pasó toda la noche cosiendo azahares en mi velo. "Los azahares significan que la novia es honrada y decente", ella dijo. Para algunas personas, las costumbres son muy importantes. Juntos, Sal y yo logramos abrazar otras tradiciones típicas de una boda hispana. Tuvimos padrinos y madrinas, trece monedas, las arras, las cuales simbolizan la prosperidad, y un lazo que simboliza la unidad. La música incluyó una Ave María y la canción *"We've Only Just Begun"*. Había mole de gallina, mariachis, y el baile del dólar. Había tantos parientes y amigos, y claro, los niños a mitad de la pista de baile, bailando solos o con sus padres. Pero al final de cuentas, uno de los momentos más especiales fue cuando nos arrodillamos para recibir la bendición de los padres de ambos. En ese momento supimos que los compromisos valieron la pena.

Años después, al reflejar sobre el carácter tan fuerte y la firmeza de estas dos mujeres, pude mirar de cerca también mis propias palabras y acciones. Ahora yo he sido profesionalmente entrenada para darles a los jóvenes el espacio que necesitan para crecer. Sin embargo, yo me oigo imponiendo la ley acerca de cómo deben hacerse las cosas de la casa, a veces sin permitir que mis hijos pongan en duda mi autoridad y mi sabiduría. Cuando una persona sigue haciendo algo a pesar de saber que no está bien, se hacen patentes las influencias culturales. Como una futura suegra, yo tengo que recordar el dicho, *guarda tu ayuda para quien te la pida*. Tendré que ser sensible, y al mismo tiempo mantener mi papel como la doña, manteniendo unida la familia. Con mi personalidad tan fuerte, estoy segura que no será fácil.

Podemos mantener los valores tradicionales tan apreciados por nuestros padres sin renunciar a nuestras propias expectativas. Piense por un momento sobre las características de sus padres que más admiraba. Quizá era su capacidad de recuperación en los momentos difíciles, su ingenio, o el orgullo que les provocaba su identidad. Quizá valore usted su sentido de lealtad a la familia, su compasión, su sentido del respeto, su esperanza.

Ahora piense en las situaciones de su vida cuando estas características le pueden beneficiar más. Puede ser al tener trato con personas fuera de su familia, con su pareja, o con los niños que tiene, o espera tener. Encontrará que con la negociación y la voluntad de tomar decisiones juntos, como marido y mujer, los valores tradicionales no tienen que necesariamente estar en conflicto con sus nuevos papeles, sino que más bien, pueden realzarlos y hacerlos más fuertes. Sin embargo, si mira a sus padres como el máximo y absoluto ideal, quizá no pueda enfrentarse a las nuevas realidades en su mundo de dos culturas. Después de todo, al inspeccionarse más de cerca, el control del hogar no es siempre lo que parece ser.

Mi madre, por ejemplo, siempre permitió que mi padrastro creyera que él era el jefe de la familia. Enfrente de la familia y los amigos, y particularmente enfrente de los extraños, ella asumía un papel de mujer sumisa. Pero en privado, mi padrastro siempre defería a mi madre las decisiones principales como la mudanza a una casa nueva, o los problemas asociados con los niños. Mi hermana Yolanda, quien está casada con un mexicano tradicional, me fascina con su habilidad para hacerle a su marido pensar que todas las decisiones que se toman en la familia son ideas suyas, cuando de hecho, son de ella. Ella nunca quiso que él perdiera su papel aparentemente prominente ni su respeto por ser el "jefe" de la familia. Ella sentía que era importante, cuando menos para mantener la paz en la familia, mantener alguna semblanza de tradición, aunque de acuerdo a sus propias condiciones. Su experiencia, aunque muy diferente a la mía, me ha hecho consciente de cómo la cultura de uno forma el equilibrio del poder en un matrimonio. Yo aprendí que las parejas pueden hacer adaptaciones que funcionan al beneficio de todos.

Yo siempre creí que mi esposo y yo compartíamos papeles iguales en nuestro hogar, hasta que mis niños me recordaron que "Papá es el hombre de la casa. Él hace las reglas". Estoy convencida que hay ciertas sutilezas culturales que se mantendrán con nosotros.

En cada familia, ya sea que se les permite a los padres jugar un papel activo o no, se mantienen dentro de nosotros ciertas maneras de pensar y actuar que reflejan las actitudes de nuestros padres y su manera de enfocar los problemas de la vida. Lo importante es que nosotros estemos conscientes de estas influencias, y que aprendamos cómo adaptarlas a situaciones nuevas. Con una mejor comprensión sobre las maneras en que ha sido acondicionado, a enfocar su autoridad de padre, puede comenzar a desarrollar nuevas herramientas para formar y fortalecer la relación entre usted y su pareja de una manera que es beneficiosa para ustedes y para sus niños.

El proceso nunca es fácil, y muchas veces requiere la negociación y la cooperación de ambas partes o, en ocasiones, simplemente seguir la corriente. Durante la primera de las reuniones familiares de mi esposo, a la cual asistí antes de nuestra boda, yo recuerdo haberme sentido molesta por el hecho de que los hombres estaban sentados todos juntos en un cuarto, tocando sus guitarras y trompetas y cantando, o mirando un juego de fútbol americano. Todas las mujeres estaban en la cocina preparando la comida, charlando acerca de sus niños o planeando la próxima reunión familiar y simplemente comadreando y chismeando. Yo puse en duda este arreglo porque yo quería estar con mi futuro marido. Rompiendo con las normas culturales, yo me senté con Salvador y recibí sutiles pero profundas sanciones de parte de todos, menos de Sal. Después de un rato, me sentí tan incómoda que eventualmente volví a "mi lugar", con las mujeres en la cocina. La lección que aprendí ese día: *A la tierra que fueres, haz lo que vieres.* Tuve que acostumbrarme a la idea de que mientras estaba en la casa de mis suegros, los hombres eran los artistas y los que entretenían, y las mujeres éramos las espectadoras y animadoras. Debíamos, cuando menos aparentemente, servir a nuestros hombres y niños, antes de pensar en nosotras mismas. Yo seguí la corriente y le serví a mi futuro marido antes de servirme a mí misma. Éste era tan sólo *un* mundo, y en cuanto a mi propio hogar, yo sabía que ése sería distinto. Y sí lo ha sido, porque en ocasiones no sólo ha cocinado mi esposo, sino también me ha servido a mí. Aunque, generalmente servimos los alimentos todos juntos, incluyendo los niños.

En la serie continua de conflictos potenciales que han surgido a través de nuestro matrimonio, yo he ganado algunas batallas a honra de los principios que yo sentía eran importantes, y he perdido otras que sentía que eran más negociables. Si usted se siente seguro, dentro de una relación donde ambos tienen igualdad de derechos, y cada uno está dispuesto a hacer ciertos sacrificios por el otro, será más fácil hacer concesiones de vez en cuando. De nuevo, la lección es que el matrimonio es un dar y recibir. Para ambas partes, hay cierta verdad en el dicho *Más vale doblarse que quebrarse.* Y yo estoy aquí para decirle que aunque se doble un poco, si el vínculo afectivo es suficiente fuerte, no se quebrará. ¡Transigir no significa darse por vencido!

Al paso de los años, al adaptar, mi esposo y yo, los valores culturales a situaciones nuevas, aprendimos a negociar los papeles, las responsabilidades, y las expectativas, y resolvimos comunicar nuestros sentimientos y preocupaciones. Ha sido mucho más fácil para nuestros niños seguir el ejemplo. Aunque mis hijos varones a veces bromean conmigo, diciendo que preferirían casarse con una mujer como su tía Hope, la que salta cuando el marido le truena los dedos, se sienten más cómodos cocinando y aspirando la alfombra o realizando otros quehaceres del hogar si miran a su padre hacerlo. Mi hija, quien siempre ha exigido el mismo trato que sus hermanos, es alentada a alcanzar sus metas, a ser firme en sus necesidades, y a expresar su singularidad. Por encima de todo, nuestros niños han aprendido que está bien cometer errores, porque han sido testigos de los obstáculos por los cuales han pasado su madre y su padre, al pasar por nuevas experiencias, creando y probando nuevas reglas por el camino, y al final, triunfando. Ellos comprenden que se encuentran en el medio de dos mundos, con un pie en cada uno, y como resultado de sus experiencias, estarán mejor preparados para representar nuevos papeles en un matrimonio, cuando les llega su momento.

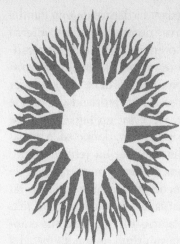

Capítulo VIII

La familia

Con la familia, hay
amor y sabiduría

Casi dos décadas antes de que la administración de Bush dirigió la atención nacional al desmoronamiento de la familia, yo viajaba por el país dando discursos, hablando de la importancia de la familia y cómo todas las familias necesitan apoyo para mantenerse sólidas. Yo me di cuenta en aquellos tiempos que los padres hispanos estaban siendo afectados de manera adversa por las fuerzas sociales, lo cual tenía un impacto negativo en los niños. Yo comencé AVANCE, Programa de Educación y Apoyo a las Familias, para fortalecer a las familias hispanas en algunas de las comunidades más pobres de este país, y para dirigir la atención nacional a los problemas que separan y destrozan a muchas familias. Cuando yo recibí un premio para "madres destacadas que trabajan", otorgados por *Working Mother* magazine, me preguntó el periódico local cómo me sentía acerca de este premio. Yo les dije que después de Dios, quiero a mi familia y que encuentro mucha gratificación a través de mi trabajo de madre porque yo siempre he considerado el papel de las madres como uno de los más importantes. Además, las esperanzas y los sueños que yo tengo para mis hijos, los tengo para todos los niños. Los resultados que busco y por los cuales abogo para los niños de AVANCE, son los mismos que quiero para mis propios hijos: verlos llegar a ser personas responsables, compasivas, y competentes.

La familia es la unidad básica de la sociedad. Es dentro de una familia que un bebé frágil y dependiente sobrevive, desarrolla, y descubre su identidad, sus talentos, y sus intereses. Su potencial sólo puede ser alcanzado, y su lugar bajo el sol sólo puede ser determinado, si la familia construye unos cimientos fuertes y sólidos. Una familia debe ser un lugar donde un niño aprende a confiar, donde se siente protegido, y donde tiene un sentido de valor y de pertenecer. Debe ser un lugar donde se aprenden valores importantes y se forma su carácter, donde se le transmite su cultura y su patrimonio. La familia debe ser un refugio seguro donde los miembros de la familia sienten una calidez, y una sensación de pertenecer. Es un lugar donde la gente puede encontrar refugio de las tensiones de la vida, y disfrutar de la compañía de los demás al crear maravillosos recuerdos juntos. Uno puede relajarse allí, expresar sus emociones, y probar sus límites, además de una multitud de emociones. La familia se convierte en la incubadora de la cual surgirán todas las futuras relaciones con otras personas. Será el terreno de pruebas para aprender a controlar las emociones y los impulsos de uno, y cómo enfrentarse a las frustraciones y a los fracasos. La familia, si es fuerte, preparará adecuadamente al niño para llegar a ser un miembro productivo que contribuye a la sociedad.

En la cultura latina, la familia es sagrada. Uno sólo tiene que entrar a un hogar latino y mirar las paredes para determinar qué valoran más. Encontrará allí docenas de fotos de hijos, nietos, padres, abuelitos, tíos, primos—la familia extensa completa. La sala de mi suegra estaba repleta de fotografías familiares que estaban divididas por categorías. En una pared estaban todos los nietos, en otra, todos los retratos de graduación, y aun otra mostraba a las mujeres vestidas de novia. Había una sección reservada para los tíos y los hijos valientes que habían ido a la guerra. Una fotografía de página completa, a todo color, de un artículo periodístico donde salí yo como "Miss Fiesta of San Antonio" cuelga en la sección de su casa que ella ha llamado "la pared de la fama", junto con otros premios otorgados a otros miembros de la familia. En el marco de madera de una puerta uno puede leer los nombres con sus respectivas estaturas de cada niño por un período que abarcaba varios años. Las huellas de las manos de miembros de la familia estaban marcadas en las aceras de cemento como aquéllas de las estrellas en Hollywood. Todas estas cosas transmiten el mensaje que el orgullo del hispano es la familia. Este sentido de orgullo de la familia no era nada diferente en la casa de mi madre. Cuando éramos niños, también nos sentimos orgullosos al vernos en la galería de fotos de la familia. Dentro de un barrio donde había influencias negativas en las calles, ninguno de nosotros sentíamos que necesitábamos formar parte de una pandilla para lograr una sensación de pertenecer, porque ya sabíamos que teníamos un lugar en la familia. Mi hermana Yolanda, quien llegó a ser una decoradora de interiores, autorizada, aprendió que no era "apropiado" colocar retratos familiares en la sala. Sin embargo, debido al valor que le asociamos a la familia, nuestros retratos generalmente son el eje de la decoración, sin tomar en cuenta quién diga que no es apropiado. Yo soy una persona hispana, profesional, de la clase media, y tengo los retratos familiares en mi sala al lado de otros cuadros y arreglos florales.

La familia consiste en hasta tres generaciones de parientes bajo el cuidado y la vigilancia de una fuerte y amorosa abuela y un venerado abuelo. En el libro de Lominitz y Perez titulado *A Mexican Elite Family, 1820–1980*, se le llamó la "grandfamily". Cuando alguien se casa con un hispano, se casa con dos generaciones de familia de ambos lados, el del padre y el de la madre. Parte de la cultura latina significa que la familia apoya a los padres en la preparación de nuestros niños para salir al mundo para convertirse en miembros competentes, responsables, y productivos de la sociedad. Los niños nunca son totalmente independientes de la familia por sus necesidades emocionales, económicas, y sociales, y por su sentido de identidad. Esto incluye los ritos compartidos, las interacciones sociales estrechas, la asistencia económica, el apoyo emocional, y las celebraciones compartidas. La familia hispana gira alrededor de cuando menos uno de los abuelos. Cuando ambos abuelos fallecen, el hijo o la hija mayor se convierte en el (la) cabeza de la nueva "grandfamily".

LA PROXIMIDAD A LOS PADRES

Después de casarnos, mi esposo y yo nos mudamos cerca de la casa de mis suegros. Como hispanos, estar cerca de la familia era muy importante. Mientras sea común ver a la gente no hispana salir de su casa y frecuentemente ir lejos, en cuanto llegan a la edad legal de hacerlo, uno generalmente observa lo contrario entre los hispanos. Esto fue cierto para nuestros padres—mi madre vivía en la casa al lado de la de su padre. Después de fallecer mi padre y mi abuela, mi madre se mudó al lado de mi tío y mi tío construyó un cuarto en su casa para mi abuelo para que ambos él y mi madre se turnaran para cuidarlo cuando envejecía. Los abuelos de mi esposo y todas sus hijas casadas vivían dentro de un área de tres manzanas. A pesar del hecho que mi esposo y yo éramos profesionales ambos, decidimos vivir a una cuadra de mis suegros en el barrio por un año. Rentamos una casa hasta que pudimos ahorrar suficiente para pagar la cuota inicial para nuestra primera casa, la cual estaba a menos de dos millas de la casa de mi madre. Muchos de mis amigos que no son hispanos se asombran al enterarse de que la mayoría de nuestros hermanos viven en la misma ciudad, y uno o dos de cada lado de la familia que no vive en el mismo estado.

Hoy en día, es más común cuando la gente logra la aculturación y alcanzan más seguridad económica, que se muden lejos de sus padres. Más hispanos se mudan fuera de la ciudad para aprovechar las oportunidades educativas y económicas. Otros quieren alejarse para descubrir su propia identidad e independencia, apartados de la familia. Sin embargo, lo que todavía es típico, es que muchos escogen no alejarse demasiado de la familia.

También he visto a muchos hispanos jóvenes y profesionales que se alejan del hogar, sólo para volver cerca después de conseguir su educación o experiencia de trabajo. Me cuentan que valoran su relación con su familia más que el dinero, la fama, y la gloria. Cuando ellos vuelven al hogar, no es para renunciar a algo, sino para tener una vida más completa, con una carrera y también la familia.

Los padres hispanos que están tratando de criar a sus niños de acuerdo a la norma tradicional de mantenerlos cerca de la casa hasta que se casen, se enfrentan con un conflicto al introducirse sus niños a una cultura mayoritaria que apoya la temprana independencia y separación. Yo viví con mi familia hasta que me casé. Mi esposo se alejó de la casa para asistir a la universidad, pero cuando se convirtió en ingeniero profesional, volvió a la casa con sus padres para poder ahorrar el dinero para comenzar su propia familia. Aunque espero que lo mismo pase con mi hijo, yo veo que esta generación de niños, de ambos lados de la familia, se está adhiriendo a la presión abrumadora de la aculturación. No están hablando sólo de querer tener sus propios departamentos sino también de vivir con novios o novias. "Cómo cambian las cosas" y "¡Qué vergüenza!" son los comentarios que se escuchan frecuentemente entre las viejitas en el barrio. Se vuelve más difícil para nosotros como padres criar a nuestros niños con ciertas normas y valores cuando sus compañeros y los padres de ellos no ven nada de malo en la cohabitación.

Durante unas vacaciones de primavera, mi hijo Salvador trajo a un grupo de amigos de la universidad a pasar el fin de semana en la casa. Esto no fue nada fuera de lo común, con la excepción de que en esta ocasión, el grupo incluía una pareja de jóvenes que no estaban casados, y esperaban dormir juntos en mi casa. Steven y Vanessa, quienes en ese tiempo contaban con trece y diez años de edad, respectivamente, querían saber cómo iba yo a manejar la situación. Ambos mi esposo y yo nos mantuvimos firmes en nuestras convicciones y le dijimos a nuestro hijo que sus amigos tendrían que dormir en habitaciones separadas. Yo me di cuenta, como padre, que los valores se extinguen lentamente si uno no es consistente y firme con respecto a sus creencias. Sus niños pequeños aprenderán lo que usted valora y aprecia a través de sus acciones, o bien su falta de acción.

LA "MUJER QUE CENTRALIZA"

En el libro *A Mexican Elite Family, 1820–1980*, la familia Gómez, igual a la mayoría de las familias hispanas, considera a su vida entera, incluyendo su prestigio social y de su empresa, como una bendición que fue otorgada sólo por el bien de sus niños. Tal como la familia Gómez, generaciones de hispanos han estado estructuradas alrededor de una persona, la "mujer que centraliza", la que organiza las actividades y reúne a la familia. Con frecuencia esa persona es la abuela. En la actualidad esas responsabilidades pueden ser divididas entre muchas. Por ejemplo, cada año, mi cuñada Lupe compraba veinte boletos para el desfile para que la familia pudiera sentarse juntos durante los desfiles anuales que tiene San Antonio durante la época de "fiesta". Ella ayudaba a mi suegra a organizar las reuniones familiares, y les decía a todos qué traer. Cuando falleció mi suegra, la hija mayor, Dolores, asumió su papel de mantener unida la familia. Cada noche de Fin de Año, la familia se reúne en su casa a comer los tradicionales buñuelos y menudo además de un festín de todo tipo de platillos.

En mi familia, ya que mi madre es testigo de Jehová y no cree en la celebración de actividades religiosas y cumpleaños, yo me convertí en la organizadora, y Lisa, mi sobrina, me ayudaba al ocupar mi lugar cuando yo estaba demasiado entretenida con mi trabajo. Cada año, para la celebración del día de la Acción de Gracias, Lisa prepara la lista de los miembros de la familia para el intercambio de regalos en Navidad. Ella aun ha mandado un boletín a la familia, con información sobre los acontecimientos especiales y recordatorios de cumpleaños.

La "mujer que centraliza" es considerada como la figura más respetada en la genealogía debido a su papel tradicional de reunir y transmitirle información sobre la familia y porque ella es a quien acuden para consultarla como la autoridad con respecto a la sabiduría y las tradiciones de la familia. Esta mujer circula la información, organiza, y promueve los acontecimientos sociales. Esa tradición aún continúa al reunirse las mujeres alrededor de la mesa en la cocina o en las reuniones familiares para planear el próximo acontecimiento social. Yo aprendí muy pronto del clan de los Rodríguez que, en su familia, los cumpleaños se celebran con una cena y un pastel, y el clan sin duda aparecerá cargado de regalos. Mi cuñada Dolores, igual a Lisa, mandaba a la familia unos boletines, informando a los parientes de lo que ocurría. Ahora, con la llegada de la Internet, la familia puede comunicar más a menudo. Con "chat rooms" (cuartos para charlar) y cámaras digitales que pueden transmitir fotografías a través de la computadora, la familia está más cerca que nunca.

Cuando un miembro de la familia que vive fuera de la ciudad viene de visita, la mujer que centraliza notificará a todos los miembros y organizará una celebración familiar. Si un miembro de la familia tiene una relación seria con una novia o novio, esa persona organizara una reunión para juntar a toda la familia para conocer a la "persona especial". Esto ocurrió con mi sobrina Mónica cuando se puso seria con un hombre que conoció a través de la Internet. ¡Vaya! ¡La familia tenía mucho interés por saber quién era este extraño de Canadá! Yo sentí lástima por él. Aquí estaba ese pelirrojo tan simpático que medía seis pies cuatro pulgadas, quien tuvo la oportunidad de ver todo lo que incluía el paquete si se casaba con una hispana. Después de pasar la interrogación con gran éxito y de sobrevivir la impresión, se planeó una fiesta para la boda, y toda la familia asistió a la ceremonia para celebrar.

EL APOYO ECONÓMICO

Otro aspecto de la familia hispana que todavía existe en los países latinoamericanos en la actualidad es el fuerte sistema económico entre los miembros de la familia. Muchas empresas que son propiedades de hispanos son manejadas por miembros de la familia. Una razón para esto, yo creo, es que los negocios así permiten la libertad de participar en los asuntos familiares y de la comunidad, además de utilizar el negocio como vehículo para ayudar a otros, especialmente a miembros de la familia.

En *A Mexican Elite Family, 1820–1980*, el tener a la familia como parte de la nómina era una manera para continuar cuidando a los miembros de la familia, especialmente a las mujeres. Si los miembros de la familia formaban parte de la empresa, entonces el jefe entendería cuando llegaban tarde o tenían que ausentarse para resolver asuntos de la familia. Esto es cierto para mi hermano, Tony, quien trabaja en una peluquería, propiedad de la familia. Él tiene la libertad de dejar de lugar de empleo para participar en la vida de sus niños. Un miembro de la mesa directiva de AVANCE, José Medellín, tiene a su esposa, varios de sus hermanos, y su hija, la futura presidenta de la compañía, manejando su imprenta, la cual tiene un valor de varios millones de dólares, mientras él participa activamente en la comunidad y disfruta de la vida. Desde que era un joven, su madre le dijo que como él era el mayor, él tenía la responsabilidad de cuidar a sus hermanos y hermanas. Cuando tenía poco más de veinte años, mudó a toda la familia de Laredo a San Antonio a vivir con él, y desde entonces ha estado cumpliendo la petición de su madre.

A veces los miembros de la familia hispana quieren trabajar juntos por el apoyo mutuo. Por veinticinco años, yo he trabajado al lado de mi hermana mayor, Julia, en AVANCE. Ella comenzó como voluntaria cuando una empleada dejó abruptamente su empleo el día antes de la apertura de AVANCE. Fueron apreciados los talentos, la creatividad, y la lealtad de Julia además de su compromiso a la gente, y mi supervisora le pidió que se quedara. Antes de trabajar en AVANCE, mi hermana Susie y yo enseñamos en la misma escuela por dos años.

EL APOYO EMOCIONAL DE LA FAMILIA

No existe mejor protección para los padres y los niños que la familia. Con frecuencia llamaba a miembros de mi familia extensa para apoyar a mi marido cuando estaba cumpliendo su papel de "Sr. Mamá", y a veces simplemente para que se enteraran cómo estaban él y los niños. Él cumplía perfectamente, pero yo quería tener un respaldo, en caso de urgencia. En otras ocasiones, la familia extensa hacía el papel de niñera. Mi madre y mi hermana cuidaban a Vanessa en mi casa durante su primer año de vida. A veces algún pariente pedía llevarse a uno de los niños a alguna excursión. Nosotros agradecíamos estas invitaciones cuando mi esposo y yo necesitábamos tener un poco de tiempo para los dos solos. Igual a como la familia extensa venía en nuestra ayuda, yo también devolvía el favor cuando me necesitaban. Yo solía recoger a los niños de mis hermanos después del divorcio, y los llevaba a los desfiles o a excursiones con nuestra familia, tal como lo hicieron mis tíos para mi madre cuando ella estaba sola con nosotros.

Hay veces cuando sus hermanos pueden servir de mediadores y ayudarles cuando usted o sus niños necesitan calmarse después de que ellos hayan probado los límites de su paciencia. Cómo lo agradecía cuando mis hermanos hablaban con mis hijos, les aconsejaban, y rezaban con ellos cuando se necesitaba controlar su conducta. Este tipo de apoyo puede ser una manera de reforzar los mensajes que usted está tratando de transmitirles a sus niños. Los miembros de su familia pueden ser personas imparciales que posibilitarán a la familia a resolver los conflictos y a permitir que queden abiertas las líneas de comunicación. Mi esposo y yo resolvemos nuestros propios problemas con nuestros hijos, pero aquellas pocas veces cuando intervinieron los parientes eran cuando *verdaderamente* los necesitábamos. Mi esposo y yo simplemente estábamos demasiado cerca de la situación. Generalmente, la persona mayor de la familia extensa asumiría el papel del mediador, en la ausencia de los abuelos. De manera más frecuente, los abuelos llamaban para ver cómo estaban los nietos, reforzando la conducta deseable, o reprendiendo aquéllas que eran indeseables. Cuando les digo a mis niños que su abuela quiere hablar con ellos, dicen, "Ahí viene el sermón", porque mi madre siempre cita de la Biblia. "Sí, Abuelita", dice Vanessa. "Está bien. Sí, yo también te quiero. Ten, Steven. Es tu turno". Una de mis sobrinas fue a vivir con mi madre por un período cuando estaba pasando por sus años rebeldes de la adolescencia, tal como mi hijo se fue a quedarse en casa de mi hermana por un día para calmarse. Los niños pueden hacer caso omiso o rechazar los consejos de los padres, pero generalmente no rechazan el consejo de la familia extensa. Escucharán a una abuelita o a una tía que muestra imparcialidad y un poco de comprensión.

Julia Álvarez, la autora del libro *How the Garcia Girls Lost Their Accents*, escribió sobre las ventajas de tener una familia latina grande. Su familia tenía tantos miembros, ella reveló, que cuando algún pariente estaba enojado con ella, siempre había alguien más a quien recurrir. Uno tan sólo tiene que mirar unas cuantas telenovelas para ver cómo la familia extensa está repleta de válvulas de escape para los niños.

Todos los padres se enfrentan a tribulaciones. La familia es importante para ayudarle a uno a lidiar, a soportar, y a sobreponerse a los desafíos de la vida cuando éstos ocurren. Yo fui recipiente de esta maravillosa asistencia cuando perdí a mi primera niña, quien falleció de un defecto congénito del corazón tres meses después de nacer. Parientes de ambos lados de la familia se reunieron en el hospital con nosotros por horas durante la delicada operación que habíamos esperado que le salvara la vida. Se fueron sólo después que nos avisaron que la cirugía fue exitosa y que lo peor ya había pasado. Desdichadamente, siete horas más tarde mi hija de tres meses de edad falleció; pero la familia nunca nos dejó solos hasta estar seguros que íbamos a poder sobreponernos a nuestra tragedia. Tenía tantos deseos de dormirme y de estar deprimida, pero nunca permitieron que eso ocurriera. Mi madre estuvo a mi lado por días enteros y les dijo a mis hermanas que hicieran lo mismo durante aquella primera semana tan difícil. Ella sabía por lo que yo estaba pasando porque ella también perdió un bebé poco después de su nacimiento. Las familias extensas de ambos lados, además de amigos, se estaban turnando para traer comida, tratar de hacernos hablar, o intentar alegrarnos un poco. Con el tiempo y el apoyo, el dolor se fue apagando y seguimos nuestras vidas.

Mi hermana Susie pasó por un verdadero suplico cuando unos miembros de una pandilla intentaron atraer a su hija de doce años y convencerla a unirse a ellos. Después de que Susie dejó a su hija con una amiga en la pista de patinaje, la amiga la llevó a una reunión de pandilleros. Por setenta y dos horas, los pandilleros trataron de lavarle el cerebro a mi sobrina, diciéndole que ellos eran su nueva familia y que iban a satisfacer todas sus necesidades. Todos de ambos lados de la familia llegaron a su rescate. Mi hermana Yolanda y su familia volaron de Dallas a San Antonio para brindar su apoyo. Mi madre de setenta y dos años se unió a mi hermana Rosa Linda, con todo y binoculares, para buscar a mi sobrina en los sitios donde dijeron sus amigos del barrio que los pandilleros solían congregarse. Los parientes se unieron a los agentes de la policía, y hasta oficiales del F.B.I., y los hermanos de mi cuñado, quienes eran policías, todos asistiéndonos para tratar de averiguar su paradero. Algunos parientes trajeron comida, otros hicieron volantes, y aun otros se pusieron en contacto con miembros de la iglesia, quienes hicieron una vigilia de veinticuatro horas para mi sobrina. Finalmente, fueron mi cuñado y mi valiente hermana Rosa Linda quienes se encontraron con los secuestradores, cara a cara, y los convencieron de soltarla. Afortunadamente, debido a la profunda unidad y voluntad de la familia, los pandilleros no pudieron devorar a mi sobrina como han podido hacerlo con tantos niños que no han tenido el beneficio de una familia sólida.

LAS CELEBRACIONES Y LOS RITOS

Nuestra familia extensa también ha sido fuente de maravillosos recuerdos y momentos alegres. Yo recuerdo las reuniones de fin de semana en casa de mi suegra donde los primos retozaban en el patio, mientras los adultos charlaban, comían, o participaban en juegos de equipo como básquetbol, béisbol, y voleibol. Los miembros de la familia también se sentaban juntos en los desfiles anuales para vitorear a sus hermanos y primos que marchaban en las bandas. Todo el clan asistía a las graduaciones y a las ceremonias de premios. Cuando otras familias tenían unas cuantas personas asistiendo, nosotros teníamos a las abuelitas, los tíos, las tías, los primos—cuando menos veinte personas—todos tomando fotos de la persona de honor. Fueron a ver a los hijos de los otros jugar deportes o bailar en los bailes folclóricos en las fiestas.

La familia viajaba en una caravana de carros en las vacaciones, de excursión, o a visitas a parientes fuera de la ciudad. Ir a acampar era especialmente divertido y agradable. La mesa estaba tan llena de comida que no quedaba ni una pulgada de espacio vacío. Mientras algunos de los hombres mayores se quedaban asando la carne, y algunas de las mujeres mayores preparaban el resto de la comida, los niños se iban con los demás adultos a jugar deportes, a nadar, a caminar, o en búsqueda de criaturas del bosque, como las ranas y las culebras. La mejor parte de la excursión era simplemente sentarse enfrente de la fogata escuchando el chisporroteo del fuego, mirando las estrellas en la noche y despertando al amanecer al aire fresco con aroma de pino y el olor del tocino cocinándose. Al día siguiente, quemados por el sol y exhaustos, los campistas se sentaban a jugar a las cartas o juegos de mesa.

Parecía que cualquier excusa era buena para celebrar o reunirnos como familia. Una vez fuimos a una "luau" en honor a mis suegros cuando iban a ir a Hawaii a visitar a su hijo que estaba allí de permiso de Viet Nam. Mi cuñada y su hijo recién nacido se unieron a mis suegros. También recuerdo una reunión de bienvenida a casa con mole y enchiladas servidos en una vajilla de porcelana fina, celebrada en honor a una sobrina que volvió de Alemania. En éstas y otras maneras, tratamos de reforzar la idea de que todos son especiales en la familia, y que a nadie lo dejan a un lado. A los niños hispanos se les enseña desde muy pequeños, por medio de acompañar a sus padres, que uno debe visitar a los miembros de la familia que son ancianos, viudos, o enfermos.

Escucho frecuentemente en las juntas profesionales que muchos de los problemas actuales se relacionan con el desmoronamiento de la familia y con frecuencia se proclama que hay una necesidad urgente de fortalecer la familia extensa. Yo me he parado en estas juntas y he descrito orgullosamente a los demás las maneras en las cuales mi familia y otros hispanos han mantenido una sólida y fuerte conexión con la familia. A menos que reconozcamos a la familia extensa como algo que nos da fortaleza, nosotros también la perderemos, junto con todos sus beneficios.

Los beneficios que usted y sus niños pueden derivar de una sólida familia extensa valen el tiempo y el esfuerzo que se necesita para conservar ciertas tradiciones, costumbres, y valores que sirven para formar vínculos entre los miembros de la familia extensa, y mantenerlos fuertes. Celebrar con nuestros seres queridos nos proporciona oportunidades para construir relaciones que proveen apoyo. Nos ayuda a establecer una conexión con nuestras raíces, nuestra familia, nuestros amigos, nuestros vecinos, y nuestro lado espiritual. Al reunirnos como familia, compartimos recuerdos alegres que enriquecen nuestras vidas, y nos ayudan a escapar, como dice mi hijo, "aunque sea por un momento", de los problemas y las aflicciones de la vida cotidiana. Puede ser tan poco emocionante como llamarle por teléfono a un pariente en su cumpleaños, lo cual le da a entender que a usted le importa, o bien puede ser una celebración de algún día festivo que toma una gran cantidad de planificación y preparación.

Cuando yo me doy cuenta de todo el tiempo y esfuerzo necesario para mantener fuertes la familia y las tradiciones, pienso en lo fácil que sería darnos por vencidos y mirar como todo desvanece lentamente, junto con todo lo que nos hace ser únicos y fuertes. Usted también quizá se haya dado cuenta temprano, como padre o madre, al igual que mi esposo y yo, que no quiere criar a sus niños sin el apoyo de la familia extensa y un sistema social fuerte de personas que los cuiden y amigos fuera de la familia. La crianza de los niños puede ser una responsabilidad formidable y abrumadora, si uno trata de hacerlo solo. La mayoría de las familias tienen muchas tribulaciones y un horario muy exigente. Podrá manejar mejor algunos de estos desafíos o tener unas experiencias educativas más enriquecedoras si obtiene la ayuda de sus parientes, quienes pueden influir sobre sus niños y mostrarles mucho amor.

LA FAMILIA NUCLEAR FRENTE AL CLAN

Tan lejano en el pasado como las primeras experiencias de la caza de animales y la junta de alimentos en las sociedades agrarias, ha sido la responsabilidad del clan mantener a las familias y cuidar a los niños. Bruce Perry del Colegio de Medicina de Baylor en Houston, ha hecho observaciones sobre el significado evolutivo del clan. Él dice que a través de la historia, los seres humanos han sido programados para trabajar y jugar en grupos.

Muchos hispanos se enfrentan a obstáculos cuando a veces se ven forzados a escoger entre mantener una proximidad cercana a la familia extensa en una ciudad, y aceptar un trabajo en otro estado o asistir a una universidad lejana. Si usted ha dejado a su familia extensa en otra ciudad, es importante mantenerse en contacto a través de cartas, visitas, y llamadas telefónicas. Hoy en día, los avances tecnológicos, como el correo electrónico y el fax, facilitan mantener el contacto con los miembros de la familia alrededor del mundo y al mismo tiempo resulta relativamente económico. Algunas familias organizan boletines informativos para mantener a todos informados sobre las actividades familiares. Visite a sus seres queridos cuando menos en ocasiones especiales para que sus niños puedan formar parte de algunas de las tradiciones de la familia. Invite a su familia a visitarlos, y juntos, hagan a sus niños participar en la preparación de tamales, buñuelos, pasteles, y otros platillos especiales, para mantener vivas ciertas tradiciones.

Desde la industrialización, más mujeres trabajan fuera de su casa y más familias han sido separadas debido a la movilización y la inmigración. Muchos padres ahora se enfrentan a la dificultad de tener que criar a sus niños dentro de la familia nuclear solamente. Igual como la mayoría de las familias donde ambos padres trabajan, a los hispanos que han perdido el contacto con la familia extensa, les está resultando formidable y abrumadora la tarea de criar y educar a sus niños. Hoy en día es aun más crucial que nunca que la familia nuclear funcione bien.

Un método que puede utilizar para ayudar que así sea, es crear un credo o una declaración de misión, usted y su familia. Steven R. Covey, un reconocido asesor de gestión empresarial y autor del libro *The 7 Habits of Highly Effective Families*, recomienda la declaración de misión como una manera de ayudar a las familias a delinear sus objetivos y valores compartidos. Para las familias hispanas, una declaración de misión es ideal para criar a sus niños en un mundo de dos culturas donde los valores y las expectativas tradicionales pueden a veces chocar, estar en conflicto con las otras normas. El documento podría servir como un contrato que está diseñado a ayudar a los miembros de la familia a navegar por ambos lados de la línea divisora cultural. Pueden decidir juntos lo que creen ser las metas de la familia y para qué debe luchar en su propia vida cada miembro de la familia. Los miembros de la familia aun pueden establecer guías con respecto a lo que ellos creen es una conducta aceptable y lo que no lo es. Al ayudar a establecer estos parámetros, sus niños estarán abriéndose paso para explorar sus intereses y talentos, desarrollar su carácter, y volverse seguros, sabios, compasivos, trabajadores, y respetuosos. La declaración de la misión alienta a los miembros de la familia a crear un medio ambiente amoroso, cómodo, ordenado, y de apoyo, un lugar donde pueden desarrollarse en todos los aspectos. Si todos en la familia tienen participación en la declaración de misión, harán mayor esfuerzo para lograr el ideal de la familia que todos han elaborado juntos. Los miembros de la familia deben tener una comprensión común de la importancia y el propósito de la unidad familiar y comprometerse a hacer lo posible por conservarla y hacerla funcionar apropiadamente. De acuerdo a Steven Covey, la declaración de la misión se convierte en una guía para pensar y para gobernar a la familia. "Cuando surgen los problemas y las crisis", él escribe, "está allí la constitución para recordarles a los miembros de la familia las cosas que son más importantes y para proveerles una orientación para resolver y tomar decisiones, basándose en principios firmes". Dos veces cada año, los miembros de la familia de Covey evalúan su declaración de la misión familiar para ver qué necesitan hacer para alcanzar sus metas y poner en práctica sus valores.

No es fácil lograr que muchos miembros de una familia vivan en harmonía bajo un solo techo. En nuestra familia de dos carreras, nos estaba resultando muy caótica la vida a veces, hasta que nos enfrentamos con los asuntos como los papeles tradicionales que están cambiando. Encontramos maneras de organizar nuestro tiempo limitado, dividiendo más equitativamente nuestras responsabilidades. Cada miembro de la familia posee una personalidad distinta, y diferentes necesidades e intereses, los cuales pueden fácilmente entrar en conflicto, unos con los otros. La comunicación es vital para planear acontecimientos que satisfacen las necesidades e intereses de todos. Es importante tener las herramientas para coordinar y organizar las actividades familiares.

Una de dichas herramientas que hemos encontrado ser muy útil es un calendario familiar, el cual mantiene un registro de los acontecimientos diarios. Es muy difícil recordar cuáles días voy a estar fuera de la ciudad, cuándo tiene práctica de coro Sal, cuándo tenían juegos de básquetbol y fútbol americano Vanessa y Steven, o cuándo Sal (hijo) iba a venir a la casa de la universidad, además de recordar todos los cumpleaños y nuestro aniversario. Un calendario también puede ser útil para ayudar en los detalles logísticos que necesitan ser considerados cuando se planea un acontecimiento. Muchas actividades requieren una división de responsabilidades entre los diferentes miembros de la familia y una buena lista de los miembros de la familia a quienes se les va a mandar invitaciones a los acontecimientos especiales.

Otra herramienta útil para mantener una familia fuerte y sólida son las reuniones familiares. Durante estas reuniones, podemos usar nuestro calendario para orientar muchas de nuestras decisiones sobre asuntos que varían entre las calificaciones y las visitas a la abuelita. Ése es el momento cuando se discuten todas las decisiones principales que afectan a todos los miembros de la familia: viajes familiares, compras grandes, fiestas, o cuando alguien hizo algo que tendrá un impacto sobre otros miembros de la familia.

Debido a que muchas familias tienen horarios agobiantes, es sumamente importante que se reúnan para compartir los alimentos cada vez que les sea posible. Las horas de comer—sin tener una televisión en el fondo—son momentos para dar las gracias por las bendiciones del día y son momentos para realizar una buena comunicación familiar. Éste es el momento cuando todos pueden ayudar en la preparación de los alimentos y en la limpieza después.

Las familias pueden hacer mucho por construir sus propias tradiciones, y enfrentarse a los problemas juntos. Pueden viajar juntos para aprender sobre nuevas culturas y explorar diferentes partes del mundo. Nosotros hemos tenido inolvidables vacaciones familiares a México, Europa y África, y a través de los Estados Unidos, y mi esposo y yo hemos ido juntos a Sudamérica y a Israel. Aun cuando no nos han acompañado, hemos compartido nuestras experiencias con nuestros hijos, después de los viajes.

Su viaje no tiene que ser una vacación a todos los rincones del mundo. Mientras que estos viajes han ampliado su percepción del mundo, mis niños dicen que sus mejores momentos los han pasado cuando hemos ido de excursión o cuando acampamos en los parques o en las playas. Era dentro de estos sitios naturales, las montañas coronadas por nieve, los cerros cubiertos de hierba, los manantiales vigorizantes, las cascadas de agua, y los arroyos, además de las bellas y extraordinarias flores, que sentimos lo más impresionados por el ambiente. La pesca, los paseos en barcos, y la natación—todas eran cosas que teníamos que hacer durante el verano. A los niños les encanta ir a acampar, para mirar las estrellas, escuchar el silencio de la noche, y oler el aire fresco y puro. Al crecer, se interesaron por el golf y el tenis. Muchas veces, trajeron a sus amigos para disfrutar de un buen juego de básquetbol.

A través de estas experiencias, aprendimos que las relaciones pueden alcanzar su plenitud solamente si las personas hacen el esfuerzo y dedican tiempo para estar juntos y cultivarlas. Estos lindos recuerdos con mi familia y mi familia extensa son las que atesoraré para siempre. Como Barbara Bush una vez dijo: "No será el número de casos que ha ganado, ni el número de juntas a las cuales asistió, lo que recordará y atesorará, sino el tiempo que pasó con aquellas personas que significan tanto para usted: su familia y sus amigos". En el caso de los latinos, es la lealtad a la familia que ha ayudado a muchos de nosotros a sobrevivir, a tener éxito, y a lograr una vida más completa, rica, y feliz. Debemos hacer lo necesario para mantener la solidez de la familia extensa. El valor de la familia es uno de nuestros puntos más valiosos y uno de los cimientos para una crianza efectiva.

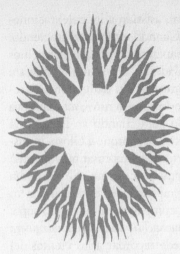

Capítulo IX

La comunidad

El muchacho malcriado dondequiera encuentra padre

Un conocido dicho mexicano, *el muchacho malcriado dondequiera encuentra padre*, recalca el papel importante que la gente del pueblo tiene en la crianza de los niños. Dentro de nuestra cultura, si un niño se porta mal, es la responsabilidad de todos corregirlo y enseñarle la manera apropiada de comportarse. Todos los niños pertenecen a la comunidad y, por lo mismo, todo el que pertenece a la comunidad comparte la responsabilidad de cuidarlos y procurar su bienestar. Hay mucha preocupación y atención puesta en los niños. Los vecinos se toman el tiempo para fijarse en lo que están haciendo y corregirlos si están haciendo algo indebido. Para que esto funcione bien, los vecinos deben conocerse como hermanos. *¿Quién es tu hermano? Tu vecino más cercano. Amigo en la adversidad es amigo de verdad.* Estos dichos recalcan el papel tan importante que los vecinos juegan en cuidarse unos a otros, y especialmente en el cuidado de nuestros niños. Los vecinos deben desarrollar la confianza, la unidad, y la comunicación. Deben llegar al acuerdo común que tienen una responsabilidad colectiva por el bienestar de todos los niños.

El barrio donde yo crecí estaba estructurado con estas ideas en mente. Todos se conocían de nombre. Había un gran sentido de comunidad donde los vecinos se ayudaban mutuamente. Los vecinos pedían prestados huevos, leche, y herramientas entre sí. Protegían las casas, los unos a otros, apoyaban los esfuerzos de cada cual, asistían a las celebraciones de todos, y cuidaban a los niños entre sí. Cuando estábamos creciendo, nunca podíamos hacer nada que pasara desapercibido porque los vecinos eventualmente platicarían nuestras maldades y travesuras a nuestra madre antes de llegar nosotros a la casa siquiera. Un día que me entretuve un rato después de la escuela, platicando con un niño, mi madre ya sabía exactamente lo que estuve haciendo para cuando yo llegué a la casa. Una vecina le dijo: "¡Ay, Luz! ¡Ten cuidado, porque a Gloria le gustan mucho los muchachos, y si no te cuidas, se te va a casar muy joven!" Debido a su preocupación, ¡yo fui la última de casarme! Si me ponía demasiado maquillaje o faldas muy cortas, mi madre se enteraba por las vecinas. El día que comencé a llevar mala compañía, mi madre lo supo. Hay una verdad en ese dicho de que *el muchacho malcriado dondequiera encuentra padre*. Cada uno de nosotros puede recordar a las viejitas del barrio y a las vecinas que se preocupaban por nosotros.

Desde la época de nuestros antepasados, la comunidad ha cuidado a sus niños. Los aztecas aceptaban a los niños del pueblo como miembros del clan y les daban cara y corazón. Los socializaban, enseñándoles tradiciones, el dominio de sí mismos, y que fueran buenos, y les ayudaban a desarrollar una identidad y personalidad singular. Era el grupo que le daba vida al niño y lo sostenía. El niño, a su vez, tenía que cumplir con su parte de asegurar que la comunidad sobrevivía y funcionaba bien. Virgilio Elizondo, en su libro *La Morenita*, escribió que la supervivencia y el bienestar del grupo era la responsabilidad de cada uno de los miembros del grupo. Cada uno sabía sus deberes y responsabilidades, los cuales tenía que cumplir para lograr que el grupo funcionara bien.

Al paso de los años, algo le pasó al espíritu fuerte del pueblo hispano. En demasiadas comunidades, los niños hispanos ya no son el foco central de la atención del pueblo. Muchos no son conocidos por sus vecinos, y prevalece la apatía y la indiferencia. Los niños son subvalorados y hechos caso omiso por la comunidad en general. Como resultado, muchos niños han caído víctimas del crimen y la violencia debido a la falta de atención y la negligencia de parte de los padres, los vecinos, y los líderes de la comunidad. De alguna manera, se está perdiendo el sentido de la comunidad en todos los barrios, ricos y pobres. Los padres desconfiados encierran a sus niños dentro de la casa y no conocen a sus vecinos ni se comunican con ellos. En muchas comunidades en la actualidad, los padres están aislados socialmente y sufren de depresión como resultado.

Una de mis metas cuando establecí AVANCE en 1973 era volver a crear, en los barrios pobres, ese sentido de comunidad del cual fui parte yo cuando era una niña, y del cual todavía formo una parte en mi barrio actual donde doctores, profesores, y empresarios viven unos al lado de otros y se ofrecen apoyo. Yo me di cuenta que la familia y la comunidad fueron factores importantes que le brindaron fortaleza a mi madre, lo cual a su vez le ayudó a ella a criarnos más efectivamente.

En el complejo de viviendas subvencionadas de Mirasol, donde se estableció el primer programa de AVANCE en San Antonio, las personas de la comunidad estaban tan aisladas, unas de otras, que a los adolescentes delincuentes y a los narcotraficantes les habían permitido un paso libre y reinaban sobre las calles. Mirasol se había convertido en un barrio donde los padres ni se conocían ni se hablaban. Los narcotraficantes vendían su mercancía en las esquinas de las calles, en los edificios vacíos, y alrededor de los patios de las escuelas. Cometían actos de vandalismo en las casas y en los carros y aterrorizaban a la gente que vivía a su alrededor. Después de muchos años de sentir que sus hogares estaban sitiados, la mayoría de la gente estaba demasiada atemorizada para hacer algo para cambiar las cosas, por temor a las represalias. Cuando una valiente madre de tres niños, una de las primeras madres para participar en el programa de AVANCE, tuvo el valor de quejarse a los directores de la asociación del complejo de viviendas subvencionadas, sobre todas las actividades atroces que veía a su alrededor, las consecuencias fueron devastadoras. Pocos días después de haberla conocido, me enteré que algunos pandilleros la sacaron a rastras de su casa y la mataron enfrente de sus niños, utilizando su muerte como una advertencia de lo que podía ocurrirles a los demás si se atrevían a quejarse de sus terribles maldades. Los padres habían renunciado lentamente a sus derechos y habían perdido su libertad. Ni siquiera las puertas cerradas con llave ni las protecciones de hierro forjado en las ventanas mantenían a los villanos fuera de sus hogares. Día con día, se empeoraba la situación en la comunidad.

Yo he visto este mismo escenario desarrollarse en las comunidades a través de los Estados Unidos. Cuando los vecinos dejan de hablarse y apoyarse, el barrio comienza a deteriorarse y a desintegrarse. Los elementos malos de la sociedad toman control. Los padres pierden el control de sus calles. Al paso del tiempo, los padres comienzan a sentirse indefensos, deprimidos, y sin poder. Están demasiado debilitados para mostrar su amor, para disciplinar, o para pasarles a sus niños las tradiciones que les ayudarán a desarrollarse y llegar a ser adultos fuertes. Igual a la parábola bíblica que compara a los niños a unas plantas de semillero, estas semillas caen sobre el suelo rocoso, y cuando crecen, se marchitan o se atrofian debido a la falta de un medio ambiente seguro, estimulante, que las cultive y las cuide.

Se me hizo cada vez más evidente, al implementar el programa de AVANCE, que iba a tener que mirar mucho más allá de simplemente educar a los padres, de uno a uno, sobre el crecimiento y desarrollo de los niños. Mejorar y ampliar sus conocimientos y habilidades de crianza no era suficiente. Sus barrios estaban en un estado de deterioro y habían caído víctimas de las drogas y la violencia. Sus escuelas se estaban desmoronando como instituciones de aprendizaje, debido a la falta de maestros y recursos. Los negocios se estaban alejando del área debido a la violencia, la cual había llegado a tal grado que aun los policías temían entrar a la comunidad, lo cual dejaba a los padres, especialmente aquéllos que estaban criando a sus niños sin pareja, a defenderse solos. Los niños nunca tendrían mucha probabilidad de lograr el éxito si vivían bajo estas condiciones.

Sin embargo, yo también sabía, por haber vivido en el mismo barrio, que al diseñar un programa para ayudar a los niños y a las familias, no iba a tener que comenzar de la nada. A diferencia de aquéllos que habían dado por perdido el barrio, porque sólo miraban las cicatrices de la pobreza y la apatía, yo sabía que en el barrio había mucha fortaleza sobre la cual construir. Detrás del temor y la frustración, yo sabía que aún permanecía un gran amor por los niños y una devoción inmensa a la familia y la comunidad que habían sido inculcados en sus almas a través de generaciones.

Con su libro en 1995, de gran éxito de ventas, la primera dama, Hillary Rodham Clinton, ayudó a volver a popularizar la idea de que "se necesita a todo el pueblo para criar a un niño". Pero para los hispanos, la idea de que el pueblo es estrechamente vinculado al bienestar de las familias y los niños siempre ha sido una parte integral de nuestra cultura. De hecho, el vecino ayudando al vecino, es una tradición que ha representado quizá el papel principal a través de nuestra historia ambos en nuestros lugares de origen y en los Estados Unidos. Por ejemplo, al final del siglo diecinueve, las comunidades mexicanas del sudoeste de los Estados Unidos formaron "mutualistas", unas sociedades donde se prestaban ayuda mutua. Consistían en unos grupos de familias que juntaban todos los recursos que podían para ayudarse en tiempos de crisis, ya sea una enfermedad, un fallecimiento, o la ruina económica. En la Ciudad de Nueva York, se organizaron una variedad de asociaciones, incluyendo algunas hermandades, para ayudar a nuevos inmigrantes, originarios de Puerto Rico. Aunque fueron diseñados como una protección social, estos grupos también eran una manera para que la gente se reuniera a realizar celebraciones familiares y de la comunidad. Eran los sistemas naturales de asistencia, antes de que fueran llamados *"social support networks"* (sistemas de apoyo social), que mantenían unidas a las familias y a las comunidades. Estos sistemas informales eran semejantes a los

"Settlement Homes" que eran patrocinados por el gobierno para apoyar a la gente que llegaba a la Isla Ellis. Estos arreglos les ayudaban a aprender el idioma y a encontrar un hogar y un trabajo, y les enseñaba el funcionamiento del "Sistema Americano". En algunas comunidades, los hispanos han tenido que hacer estas cosas principalmente por su propia cuenta, basado en el valor que le ponen a prestar ayuda a nuestra gente o a tener una comunidad fuerte. Sin embargo, en otras comunidades donde la gente y el gobierno sufren de apatía, se ven muchas comunidades en un estado de deterioro.

Después de varias generaciones, este sentido de la comunidad, desdichadamente, ha disminuido. Las iglesias también están cambiando. Antes solían prestar más apoyo directo a los oprimidos, a las viudas, y a los huérfanos. En muchas iglesias, la segunda colección que se realizaba tradicionalmente para los pobres, ya ni se hace. Con ambos padres trabajando, se ha vuelto cada vez más difícil para la gente dar de sí mismos a la comunidad. La tradición hispana del compadrazgo no es la misma que era para nuestros antepasados. Hoy en día, los compadres que son seleccionados como padrinos, no siempre tienen el tiempo para cumplir su papel como "segundos padres", después del bautismo.

A través de AVANCE, hemos podido reavivar el espíritu del compadrazgo y del pueblo en la comunidad de Mirasol y en muchas otras comunidades a través de los Estados Unidos. Presentamos a los padres con sus vecinos y proporcionamos un lugar y una razón por la cual reunirse y aprender cómo mantener a sus niños sanos, felices, y exitosos en la escuela y en la vida. Debido al amor, las esperanzas, y los sueños que los padres tienen para sus niños, las madres y los padres asisten a un programa sobre la crianza de los niños que tiene una duración de nueve meses. Comenzando por el sencillo hecho de reunirse, los padres pueden fortalecerse a sí mismos y a sus familias, en contra de las influencias de las pandillas, las drogas, y las pistolas, y en contra de la nube negra del aislamiento, la desesperanza, y la desesperación.

Por medio de asistir a las clases de AVANCE, los padres del primer programa comenzaron a hablar abiertamente de los problemas que estaban sufriendo en sus hogares y en la comunidad. Luego organizaron grupos de apoyo para buscar soluciones comunes. En el proceso, se dieron cuenta que no podían resolver todo por su propia cuenta. Las familias de AVANCE se aliaron y formaron un programa de "Community Watch" para proteger las casas unos a otros y reportar los robos cuando estos ocurrían. Cansados ya de mirar como los ladrones se metían a las casas de sus vecinos a robar, día tras día, un grupo de padres se organizó para llevar un registro del tiempo que tomaba la policía para responder a sus llamadas. Cuando los policías esperaron hasta las siete de la mañana para responder a una llamada de robo que se había hecho a las once de la noche anterior, los padres de AVANCE repartieron volantes, convocaron juntas, y establecieron unas estrategias para hacer más responsables a los oficiales y dirigentes de la comunidad y la ciudad, de lo que estaba ocurriendo. Convocaron una conferencia de prensa para aumentar la consciencia del público sobre el problema. A la mañana siguiente, había tantos policías en el barrio que casi fui atropellada por ellos. Finalmente, la mayoría de los narcotraficantes recibieron el mensaje de que su "negocio" no seguiría prosperando en este barrio y se fueron. Quizá se fueron a una comunidad más vulnerable donde los vecinos no se conocían, no se comunicaban, y no tenían un compromiso para apoyarse.

Poco a poco, más cambios comenzaron a ocurrir. En un barrio donde más de mil niños no tenían ni un columpio para jugar, los padres se organizaron y forzaron a los directores de la asociación del complejo de viviendas subvencionadas a apartar fondos para construir un área de juego para que sus niños tuvieran un lugar seguro donde jugar. Todavía había una continua amenaza de represalias, pero al pasar el tiempo, los padres se dieron cuenta que eran mayores en número a los pandilleros, y que juntos, eran más poderosos que cualquier narcotraficante. A través de sus esfuerzos, aprendieron el significado del dicho *un lápiz se puede quebrar muy fácil, pero muchos juntos no se pueden.* Por medio de la unidad, los padres se volvieron más fuertes. Hoy en día, los padres orgullosamente lucen camisetas y anillos especiales que señalan su membresía en la "familia AVANCE". Celebran los días festivos juntos, hacen desfiles en el barrio, se ayudan y se apoyan en momentos de crisis, cuidan a los niños entre sí, lamentan las pérdidas de los demás, y comparten las victorias de todos.

En el Programa Afiliado de AVANCE en el Valle del Río Grande, fuimos testigos de las deplorables condiciones de vida que tenían que soportar algunas de las familias en las colonias. Sin calles pavimentadas, ni agua potable, ni servicios de higiene, la mayoría de las familias viven en condiciones de "tercer mundo". Muchos niños nacen con daño cerebral y defectos físicos causados por los desechos tóxicos que a las maquiladoras les han permitido tirar en los ríos que corren por zona fronteriza. La falta de hacer cumplir algunas medidas ecologistas convierte la vida en una pesadilla para mucha gente. Los niños no pueden ni jugar en sus calles sin exponerse a la contaminación. Como resultado, los casos de hepatitis B que se han registrado, han llegado a un predominio que es tres veces mayor en esa área que en todo el resto de Texas. Tal como lo hicieron en San Antonio, los padres de AVANCE se organizaron y se presentaron ante los oficiales gubernamentales del condado para exigir la instalación de tuberías para agua potable en sus barrios. Su petición fue concedida. La falta de edificios para proveer los servicios a los padres, en esta área rural, no nos impidió ser una influencia. Una vez que los padres escucharon sobre los éxitos de la comunidad cercana, ellos también se organizaron, y un grupo de madres principalmente (con unos pocos padres hábiles) reconstruyeron un edificio viejo y deteriorado para albergar un proyecto de AVANCE.

Con cada acto mutuo de asistencia, las familias de AVANCE reavivan su espíritu de esperanza y comunidad. Adquieren conocimientos y habilidades. Fortalecen sus sistemas de apoyo social. Aprenden que los miembros de la comunidad necesitan hacer su parte para que se produzcan políticas, programas, y servicios adecuados que les ayudarán a ellos cumplir su papel de padre. El pueblo ha crecido y se extiende más allá de un área geográfica pequeña. Las comunidades en al actualidad incluyen a muchas personas, organizaciones, e instituciones. Pero tal como lo era con nuestros antepasados, los niños deben estar al centro de nuestro mundo donde todos los valoran y cuidan de su bienestar.

Actualmente, yo vivo en un suburbio, al lado de otros profesionales hispanos, anglosajones, y afroamericanos, y yo veo que muchos padres han traído consigo este sentido de la comunidad. Yo veo que nuestros niños se sienten libres para visitar los patios y las casas de los vecinos y jugar mientras los adultos observen. Los padres ocasionalmente piden prestados huevos, leche, herramientas, y escaleras, entre sí. Cuidamos a los niños, unos a otros, compartimos el deber de utilizar por turnos el coche de cada uno para trasladarnos a diferentes sitios, nos dejamos unos a otros al aeropuerto, y mantenemos un ojo vigilante cuando los vecinos están fuera, de vacaciones. Yo observo a mis vecinos que se ponen a la disposición de un vecino anciano para asegurar su salud y bienestar, cuidan a las mascotas y cortan el césped cuando los vecinos están ausentes. A veces, simplemente charlan afuera, tal como lo hacían nuestros padres en el barrio. También organizamos un "Neighborhood Watch", y una vez al año los vecinos se reúnen al final de la cuadra y tienen un picnic. Nuestros vecinos más cercanos tienen una llave en caso de alguna urgencia.

LAS IGLESIAS

Para los hispanos, el vínculo entre la iglesia y la familia siempre ha sido muy fuerte. Algunos de mis primeros recuerdos de la iglesia consisten en los hombres y las mujeres que cumplían su parte para mantener fuerte y sólida la congregación. Yo recuerdo al hermano García, quien, a petición de mi abuelo, venía a nuestra casa a llevarnos a mis hermanos y a mí a los oficios religiosos semanales en su pequeña iglesia protestante. Él hacía un esfuerzo adicional por cuidarnos a nosotros y a otros miembros de la comunidad. Un día cuando yo tenía once años, él me pidió que le ayudara a una madre soltera que estaba postrada en cama, quien acababa de tener un bebé, quizá mi primer acto de apoyo familiar.

Una de las metas principales de mi abuelo era asegurarse que cada uno de nosotros estuviera rebosado del mismo espíritu que él creía responsable de haber cambiado su vida cuando llegó a los Estados Unidos. A pesar de que fuimos bautizados como católicos, él nos llevaba a los renacimientos espirituales llevados a cabo en una carpas en la comunidad pentecostés. Yo recuerdo haberme sentido llena de asombro ante la intensa energía proveniente de la multitud de creyentes fieles que se meneaban al sonido rítmico de los tambores y los címbalos que resonaban en el aire. Algunos se caían al suelo, "dado muerte en el espíritu", otros simplemente elevaban las manos en oración, animados por su fe. Al final del oficio religioso, yo recuerdo lo aliviados y felices que parecían todos, como si una tremenda carga se acababa de levantarse de sus hombros. Allí en la iglesia, o en sus hogares, los hermanos colocaban las manos sobre los enfermos y oraban por ellos. De alguna manera, las personas parecían aliviarse, y ellos a su vez, más adelante se unían al grupo que curaban por medio de la intercesión. Esta congregación amorosa era una comunidad de personas sencillas que extendían las manos para ayudarse mutuamente, incluyendo a padres con niños pequeños.

Las iglesias pueden hacer mucho en sus esfuerzos por alcanzar a las familias, darles apoyo, y fortalecerlas, ya sea a través de encuentros matrimoniales, terapia, u oficios espirituales que todas las familias necesitan para enfrentarse más efectivamente a los obstáculos de la vida. En adición a ser un lugar para hacer oficios religiosos, la iglesia debe servir como un centro de hermandad donde se establecen relaciones, donde se enseñan y se refuerzan los valores y la moralidad. Algunas de las actividades ofrecidas por la iglesia incluyen grupos familiares para los padres divorciados o separados, actividades para los jóvenes, y diferentes tipos de ministerios como las visitas a los enfermos en los hospitales, o bien, como mi cuñado Jim, quien visita a los prisioneros en la cárcel. "Hay que lograr". Aproveche todas las organizaciones de apoyo en las iglesias cuya intención es fomentar los buenos valores.

Muchos padres están mandando a sus niños a escuelas religiosas con el mismo propósito de reunirse con familias con similares valores y creencias religiosas. Los miembros de la iglesia, y de organizaciones fraternales y cívicas, podrían trabajar juntos para ayudar a las familias.

LAS ESCUELAS

La estructura y la calidad de las escuelas también afecta enormemente el futuro de un niño. Por décadas, la estructura de la familia ha estado cambiando debido al aumento de movilidad y las mujeres que entran a la población activa. Sin embargo, demasiadas escuelas no han respondido a esos cambios. La escuelas todavía están diseñadas para apoyar a la familia agraria, cuyos niños necesitaban estar en casa por tres meses para cosechar las siembras. Muchos edificios escolares están vacíos en las noches y los niños dejados a defenderse y cuidarse solos mientras sus padres trabajen. Algunos abuelos y la familia extensa ya no están tan fácilmente disponibles para asistir en este importante papel del cuidado de los niños. Las políticas que les permiten a las escuelas quedarse abiertas todo el año y por períodos más largos durante el día para apoyar a las familias donde ambos padres trabajan, deben adoptarse a una escala más amplia. En la actualidad, algunos distritos escolares sí ofrecen calendarios diferentes que extienden los días que van a la escuela los niños a abarcar todo el año, con numerosos descansos más cortos.

Las decisiones que toman nuestros líderes con relación a los salarios de los maestros, los requisitos para los maestros, y la proporción de maestros con respecto a estudiantes, también tendrán una influencia sobre la capacidad de aprendizaje de los niños. Los maestros juegan un papel muy importante en la formación del carácter y el amor propio de un niño. Yo fui muy afortunada por haber tenido tres maestros excepcionales quienes me afectaron de manera positiva durante un período muy vulnerable de mi vida. Cuando me otorgaron el premio de "Woman of the Year" (Mujer del Año), de parte de nuestro periódico local, yo les agradecí a mis maestros de sexto y séptimo año, el señor Ben Mata y el señor y la señora Daniel Villarreal, cuyas palabras de aliento y apoyo tuvieron una gran diferencia sobre mí y sobre muchos niños en el barrio. Más adelante, durante mis años de preparatoria, las palabras bondadosas del señor Don Connell, en contra de un director que intentó disuadirnos a mí y a muchos otros hispanos de asistir a la universidad, también tuvieron un impacto positivo en mi vida.

Mientras la Investigación Coleman recalcó la importancia de la familia en la educación de los niños, muchos hispanos de comunidades pobres han sido afectados adversamente por la calidad de los edificios escolares, los salarios más bajos de los maestros y los cursos limitados sobre ciencia y matemáticas, debido a la incapacidad para atraer y poder pagar a los maestros titulados para estos cursos, además de recursos limitados, tales como computadoras y libros inadecuados en las bibliotecas. Como miembro de la Comisión Presidencial para la Excelencia Educativa para los Hispanoamericanos, yo escuché los numerosos testimonios de personas sobre las condiciones educativas deplorables a las cuales se han visto sometidos muchos hispanos sólo por vivir en áreas de pobreza. Existe tanta disparidad entre las escuelas de áreas prosperas en oposición a aquéllas de áreas pobres, que afectan el aprendizaje entre unas y otras. Por ejemplo, el Edgewood Independent School District, al cual asistí yo, llevó el caso de la desigualdad y la injusticia con relación a las finanzas escolares hasta la Corte Suprema, bajo *Edgewood v. Kirby* (*United States v. Texas, 1971; Edgewood ISD, et al. v. Kirby, et al., 1987*). De 1970 a 1971, por cada estudiante, los gastos por año por un estudiante en Edgewood sumaban $418.00, mientras que en Alamo Heights sumaban $913.00. Por años los hispanos han estado tratando de conseguir un reparto más justo de fondos para las escuelas. Las organizaciones como *Intercultural Development Research Association* y *Mexican American Legal Defense and Educational Fund* (MALDEF), por décadas han estado abogando por una igualdad educativa y mejores oportunidades para los hispanos.

Una oportunidad educativa que quizá quieran explorar e investigar los padres hispanos es la escuela "charter". Este tipo de instituciones, las cuales existen actualmente en comunidades a través del país, son escuelas públicas especiales, establecidas por maestros, padres, y grupos locales, que tratan de proveer alternativas a los sistemas educativos tradicionales. Muchas enfocan a las necesidades de los niños de diversos antecedentes al utilizar un programa de estudios que incorpora el idioma y la cultura de los niños. El *National Clearinghouse for Bilingual Education* (El Centro Nacional de Intercambio de Información Sobre la Educación Bilingüe) sigue la creación de estas escuelas y mantiene una lista de ellas en su *website*.

EL NEGOCIO DE AYUDAR A LOS JÓVENES

Cuando yo estaba creciendo en el barrio, los comerciantes y hombres de empresa en la comunidad apoyaban a los niños. Don Benito Romo nos obsequiaba pollitos pintados que se convertían en nuestras mascotas hasta que mi abuelo los mataba para una comida algún domingo, al retorcerles el pescuezo. Las empresas locales ayudaban a los niños en el barrio a ganar dinero adicional al apoyar su espíritu emprendedor y darles un trabajo.

Yo me di cuenta desde muy joven que tenía un talento para vender. Yo vendía bellos aretes de lentejuelas que mi madre hacía además de productos de catálogos de vestidos, Avon y Stanley, entre otros. No sólo los vecinos compraban lo que les vendía cuando tocaba a sus puertas, sino que los dueños del restaurante de la esquina que servía a los clientes en su propio automóvil, me permitían vender los aretes a sus clientes. Yo recuerdo al hombre anglosajón que entregaba el hielo y el supervisor de mantenimiento de la escuela, también anglosajón, de quienes yo me hice amiga. Ambos me decían: "Ahí viene la niña de la sonrisa de un millón de dólares". Cada vez que me miraban, compraban aretes. Sólo Dios sabe a quién le regalarían tantos aretes.

Yo vivía cerca de un cementerio donde había varias florerías, todas propiedades de la misma familia extensa. Varios de mis hermanos trabajaron para "Chelo" Alejandro, quien era muy buena y paciente, muy diferente a su madre. Me contrató su madre a la pequeña edad de nueve años para realizar diferentes quehaceres en una de sus florerías. Nunca olvidaré a la "Señora Elizondo". El primer día que trabajé para ella, se quejó enfrente de los clientes acerca de la calidad de trabajo que había hecho al barrer. La escoba probablemente estaba del doble de mi tamaño. Sin embargo, no me gustó la forma en que me habló, así que renuncié al trabajo a sólo unas horas de haber comenzado. Yo exigí mi pago prorrateado de $1.00. Tenía la creencia firme en ese entonces, como lo tengo hoy en día, que las personas deben ser tratadas con dignidad y respeto. Yo sentía en aquella época que sólo mi madre me podía llamar la atención. Pero ahora me doy cuenta que ella, como otros propietarios de negocios en la comunidad, sentía que tenía la responsabilidad de enseñar a los jóvenes a prepararse para el mundo del trabajo. Cuando un incidente similar me ocurrió varios años más tarde cuando estaba trabajando como vendedora con la señora Brown, cuando no doblaba los suéteres a su satisfacción, me sentí dolida, pero me quedé y aprendí a doblar aquellos suéteres de la manera que ella quería.

Hoy en día, los pequeños negocios familiares se están reemplazando por corporaciones grandes. Sin embargo, las empresas pueden y deben hacer más para apoyar a los jóvenes. Pueden patrocinar grupos comunitarios y eventos locales. Pueden alentar a sus empleados a participar en los programas de mentores para niños y jóvenes o establecer unos fondos para becas. Uno de los mejores ejemplos de la participación de una corporación en el bienestar de los jóvenes hispanos es el *National Hispanic Scholarship Fund* (El Fondo Nacional de Becas para los Hispanos). Iniciado por Ernest Robles, el fondo ahora recibe donativos de varias corporaciones. Esta ayuda económica les ha proporcionado a miles de jóvenes una ayuda para comenzar su educación y les ha brindado una esperanza a los padres jóvenes que quieren lo mejor para sus niños. Las asociaciones profesionales deben alentar y servir de mentores a los niños para que exploren y luchen para obtener sus carreras. A través de la *Texas Alliance of Mexican-American Engineers* (la Alianza de Ingenieros México-Americanos en Texas), mi esposo y otros ingenieros profesionales funcionan como mentores para los jóvenes en los campos de matemáticas y ciencia. Manuel Berriozábal de San Antonio inició el programa, ganador de premios, llamado Texas-Prep y Prep-Proyecto, un programa de ingeniería en el cual participan los estudiantes de secundario, el cual es apoyado por el gobierno, la fuerza militar, las universidades, y el sector empresarial que prepara a muchos estudiantes hispanos para seguir las carreras de matemáticas e ingeniería.

AVANCE recibe apoyo directo y en especie de los sectores privados y públicos. Las empresas nos han hecho contribuciones de dinero además de donativos de artículos como camionetas (vans) y equipos de juego para los niños. Han proporcionado fondos para la compra de juguetes para los niños, han patrocinado las celebraciones para Navidad y para el día de Acción de Gracias, y han reparado nuestros edificios. Sus empleados han trabajado como voluntarios y mentores, y han "adoptado" a niños, a familias, y a centros enteros. Han mandado a oradores y mentores para inspirar y motivar a los jóvenes.

Más allá de contribuir a esfuerzos que valen la pena y de alentar a sus empleados a realizar un servicio a la comunidad, los empleadores deben facilitarles a los hispanos encontrar maneras de crear un lugar de trabajo que beneficia a la familia, incluyendo horarios flexibles, permisos cuando es necesario para la familia, horarios partidos de trabajo, cuidado para los niños en el sitio del trabajo, y permiso de maternidad o para padres. Muchas corporaciones grandes les permiten tiempo a sus empleados para visitar las escuelas de sus niños.

Al apoyar a los empleados con políticas que benefician a la familia, los empleadores cosechan sus propios beneficios con una fuerza laboral más productiva, menos faltas al trabajo, y mayor retención de empleados. Al invertir en los niños, el sector empresarial, de manera global, contribuye a la construcción de comunidades más sanas y más fuertes.

EL GOBIERNO

Mientras que no creo que el gobierno debe jugar un papel dominante en la vida de los niños, sí creo que nuestras agencias públicas y nuestros funcionarios electos pueden y deben hacer más de lo que hacen en la actualidad para apoyar a las familias. En 1989, yo me uní a Hillary Clinton como parte de una delegación de doce miembros que fueron a Francia para aprender acerca del sistema de guarderías del país, el cual se considera uno de los programas de los sectores empresariales y gubernamentales más exitosos del mundo. En Francia, nos enteramos que un 95 por ciento de los niños entre los tres y cinco años de edad asisten a una guardería universal y gratis. Miramos a los niños usando equipos de juego asombrosos, adentro y afuera, equipos que promueven la creatividad, el desarrollo de las habilidades motrices mayores, el aprendizaje y juego social. Me impresioné de manera particular con el edificio tan bien diseñado y la calidad del programa y del personal, ya sea en una comunidad de nivel económico bajo o medio. Las educadoras en las guarderías francesas son consideradas profesionales, y son pagadas como tal. El campo es competitivo y requiere una educación formal extensa. Los empleados tienen la oportunidad de subir en su carrera, con más entrenamiento. A diferencia de los Estados Unidos, tienen un porcentaje muy bajo de empleados que renuncian a sus puestos.

Lo que más me impresionó fue la manera en que los franceses divisaron un sistema global que conectaba el cuidado de los niños con los sistemas nacionales de la salud y de servicios sociales. Todas las familias con dos o más niños, sin importar sus ingresos, recibían una prestación familiar si obtenían cuidado prenatal y demostraban que sus niños estaban recibiendo sus inmunizaciones fijadas y sus exámenes físicos apropiados. Las guarderías tenían médicos públicos asignados a cada centro. Francia también apoya a sus familias con beneficios como dieciséis semanas de permiso maternal.

Cuando la delegación americana se reunió con los líderes políticos y empresariales de Francia y preguntaron sobre su espectacular sistema de cuidado a los niños, parecían sorprendidos ante la curiosidad y explicaron que simplemente no podían darse el lujo de no invertir en el recurso más grande de su país—sus niños. "Estamos preparando a los futuros trabajadores, líderes, y ciudadanos", nos dijeron. Podemos aprender de éste y muchos otros países que apoyan más a las familias que nosotros. Con la nueva *Family Leave Policy, Americorp Programs*, aumentos en asistencia para las guarderías y los estudiantes universitarios, y un sueldo mínimo mayor, nuestro país está comenzando a tomar pasos positivos.

El gobierno tiene la responsabilidad social de encarar y tratar los problemas sociales y económicos de la sociedad. El trabajo que se realiza en AVANCE se trata de conferirles poderes a las personas para que puedan ayudar a sus niños, ayudarse a sí mismas, y ayudar a su comunidad, y es parcialmente apoyado por el gobierno. Los líderes políticos deben darse cuenta que apoyar a los padres por medio de conocimientos y asistencia con relación al crecimiento y desarrollo de los niños, alfabetismo, y entrenamiento de trabajo, es un buen uso para los dólares de los contribuyentes además de una inversión en el recurso más importante de la nación: su gente.

A nosotros nos afectan las políticas, las leyes, y las regulaciones que el gobierno aprueba. Algunas de estas leyes afectan los alimentos que comemos, el aire que respiramos, el agua que tomamos, la música que escuchamos, y las películas que miramos. Mientras que estamos logrando algunos progresos con respecto a algunas políticas muy buenas sobre la familia, como el *Family Leave Act*, el cual beneficia a todos los americanos, otras políticas no han sido tan buenas para los hispanos. Nos hemos convertido en los más recientes blancos de ataques contra los inmigrantes a causa de las más recientes leyes sobre inmigración que han sido aprobadas. A través de la historia, en momentos de dificultades económicas, los grupos de inmigrantes han sido los chivos expiatorios para los problemas económicos del país. La Propuesta 187, junto con el movimiento para "English Only" y una revocación de la Acción Afirmativa, afectan adversamente a los hispanos. La iniciativa Unz, o la Propuesta 227, fue un esfuerzo que se hizo en California para eliminar la educación bilingüe. Afortunadamente, estas acciones han unido a muchos hispanos para levantar su voz para exigir sus derechos. Las organizaciones como MALDEF y LULAC utilizan los tribunales para buscar la justicia y la igualdad de derechos para los hispanos.

Como padres, debemos participar activamente en el proceso político y enseñarles a nuestros niños por medio del ejemplo, la importancia de ejercer nuestro derecho como ciudadanos, de votar. Debemos emitir nuestro voto y conseguir que nuestros parientes y amigos hagan lo mismo. Hay tanto poder en el voto y cada voto sí ejerce una influencia sobre las políticas, las leyes, y los programas que son apoyados y que les afectan a usted y a sus hijos. Willie Velázquez nos enseñó que "su voto es su voz". El *Southwest Voter and Education Fund* está disponible para ayudarle a registrarse para votar y para enseñarle cómo usar las máquinas para votar. También puede asistir a los foros donde diferentes candidatos declararán sus posturas con relación a temas importantes. Debemos elegir a personas éticas, responsables, y sensibles, que tomarán decisiones prudentes que apoyarán a todos sus ciudadanos, conservar nuestra democracia, y apoyar los derechos humanos de la gente a través del mundo. También es crítico que comencemos a preparar ahora a un grupo de jóvenes hispanos que asumirán los futuros papeles políticos de liderazgo, para asegurar que las necesidades especiales y los intereses de los hispanos sean encarados adecuadamente en los gobiernos locales, estatales, y nacionales.

LOS MEDIOS DE LA COMUNICACIÓN: EL FIN DE "NINJA MANIA" Y SPEEDY GONZÁLEZ

Le incumbe al gobierno idear políticas que apoyan a la familia, tal como mantener a la radio y a la televisión más decente y apropiada para la familia. Las organizaciones de los medios de comunicación también tienen la responsabilidad social de regular el material ofensivo, incluyendo los discos compactos, las películas, y los programas de televisión que debilitan los esfuerzos de los padres de inculcarles a sus niños valores positivos, buena moralidad, y autoestima. Sin importar lo preparado que usted pueda ser como padre o lo mucho que se esfuerce, sus esfuerzos pueden ser regulados por otras fuerzas de la comunidad en general.

La violencia que se hace pasar por "entretenimiento para los jóvenes" es a veces difícil de evitar, por más esfuerzo que haga. Aun cuando yo le prohibí a mi hijo Steven que fuera a ver las películas de los *Ninja Turtles*, porque él tenía la tendencia de practicar las patadas de karate con su hermana, todavía no podía protegerlo del impacto de estas criaturas, cuyas imágenes estaban estampadas en las mochilas, los relojes, los juguetes, las piñatas, y los disfraces.

La cultura popular está tan afianzada en la violencia que pocas personas podían ver la influencia negativa que estaban creando los *Ninja Turtles* o los *Power Rangers*. Había mucha presión sobre mí, como madre, de no privar a mis niños de lo que ellos consideraban inofensivas figuras de acción. No podía creer lo que escuchaba cuando yo trataba de proteger a mi niño en contra de esas influencias. Otras personas los miraban como héroes, mientras yo los veía como demasiado violentos y agresivos. Me mantuve firme en mi postura, pero no fue fácil. Un día Steven, de seis años de edad, cayó víctima de la enorme cantidad de publicidad y trató de robar un reloj de los *Ninja Turtles* de una tienda, y convenció a su hermana de tres años de unirse a él. Le hicimos devolver ambos relojes al propietario de la tienda para pedir disculpas personalmente por su fechoría.

Años más tarde, yo estaba en una junta cuando Paul Simon, senador de los Estados Unidos, dijo que Japón no permitía que las películas de los *Ninja Turtles* entraran a su país con toda esa violencia y que los productores habían respondido con una versión de la película que no contenía las partes violentas. En nuestro país, parece que aceptamos generalmente la violencia sin ponerla en duda, y que ya nos hemos insensibilizado a la misma. Los niños son afectados por toda la violencia, tal como hemos visto en el reciente caso de los dos jóvenes de una secundaria en Arkansas que se pusieron a disparar violenta y frenéticamente y al final, había cuatro muertos y muchos heridos. Muchos creyeron que una escena violenta similar que los dos jóvenes habían visto en una película los había influenciado.

En adición a estos peligros, los medios de comunicación están llenos de imágenes negativas de los hispanos. Ya antes mencioné algunas de estas imágenes. Los hispanos se han representado como personas flojas que usan sombreros o andan en burros o se pasean en los carros *low-riders* como villanos, criadas, o pandilleros. *Speedy González, el Frito Bandido, Chiquita Banana* y *Juan Valdez* producen imágenes estereotípicas de los hispanos, igual como *Amos y Andy* representaban a los negros cuando yo crecía.

Los niños de hoy están expuestos a demasiado sexo, materialismo, y vulgaridad. Los niños de hoy, igual como los de mi época, imitarán lo que ven. La imagen del padre irresponsable, incompetente, y débil es representada en programas como los *Simpsons* y *Married with Children.* ¿Acaso produce asombro que los padres, ambos hispanos y otros, quizá tengan dificultad para llegarles a sus niños con el tipo de imagen de los padres que se representa en esos programas? Qué diferencia entre aquéllos y *Father Knows Best*, un programa donde se percibía al padre como un jefe de familia fuerte, responsable, decisivo, y compasivo. El programa de *Beavis and Butthead* es la antítesis de los *Waltons*, con el desafío y la falta de respeto como la base para la comedia.

Hay algunos programas educativos muy buenos en la televisión, como *Sesame Street* y programas en el Discovery Channel. Sin embargo, los padres necesitan controlar la cantidad de televisión que permiten a sus niños mirar. Los padres deben determinar sus creencias, e inculcarles estos valores a sus niños a través de los programas que miran. No pueden permitir que sean sometidos a la inmoralidad y la violencia en la televisión, la radio, los comerciales, los discos compactos, los cassettes, y la World Wide Web.

Yo asistí a una conferencia en Aspen con algunos de los ejecutivos principales de los medios de comunicación quienes intentaron decirles a los líderes hispanos presentes que los medios de comunicación sólo reflejan la cultura americana y que es a petición del público que se lleva a cabo la producción de películas, discos, y productos que muchos padres consideran ofensivos. Añadieron que la Primera Enmienda de la Constitución de los Estados Unidos no permite la censura de sus productos. Yo estoy en desacuerdo. Tal como uno no puede gritar "fuego" en un cine cuando no existe, la industria del espectáculo también tiene la responsabilidad corporativa de no proyectar el tipo de conducta que conduce a la violencia. Los ejecutivos de los medios de comunicación deben esforzarse para asegurar que sus productos reflejen el tipo de cultura y carácter que queremos para nuestro país y para nuestros niños.

Por supuesto que ellos forman una fuerza poderosa que puede luchar en contra de los valores que tratamos de inculcar, pero usted no es impotente para proteger a sus niños. Puede unirse a otros padres en una protesta en contra de la violencia, el sexo, y el lenguaje obsceno en los medios de comunicación. Si no nos quejamos, y si continuamos comprando los productos que no reflejan nuestros valores, la industria del espectáculo percibirá nuestra falta de acción como una señal de aprobación. Unidos, podemos ser la voz de nuestros niños y de nuestra sociedad.

LAS ORGANIZACIONES COMUNITARIAS: MANTENIENDO VIVO AL PUEBLO HISPANO

Este país en un lugar donde las personas y las organizaciones locales juegan un papel importante en el apoyo a los niños y a las familias. La sociedad necesita tener recursos comunitarios para apoyar a los padres que tiene preocupaciones e intereses especiales. Éstas incluyen organizaciones que apoyan a los padres que están criando a sus niños sin pareja, los que tienen niños minusválidos, los que tienen niños que fueron víctimas del abuso o matados, y los padres alcohólicos, entre otros. Debemos unirnos como comunidad, para ayudar a aquéllos que sienten dolor y necesitan apoyo. Si un niño en la comunidad sufre, todos sufriremos. Si un niño es vulnerable, todos nos volveremos vulnerables. A veces el problema tiene que estar enfrente de nosotros para provocar que hagamos algo, tal como lo descubrió uno de los hombres más prominentes de San Antonio al salir de un juego de básquetbol de los *Spurs* una noche. Un grupo de pandilleros le puso una pistola en la cara enfrente de sus cuatro nietos. Después, habló en contra de la violencia y comenzó a organizar a la comunidad para encarar este problema.

Alexis de Tocqueville, un gran pensador político francés, escribió en su libro *Democracy in America*, en 1835, que nuestra democracia y las virtudes de la libertad están asociadas no sólo con enseñarles a nuestros niños las lecciones que los prepararán para su libertad sino también con la participación cívica. Escribió sobre los miles de asociaciones voluntarias que existían en los Estados Unidos en esa época que proveían entretenimiento, enseñaban principios, distribuían libros, y fundaban hospitales, iglesias, prisiones, y escuelas—todas las cuales produjeron una mejor sociedad civil para ayudar en la conservación de nuestra democracia. Sin embargo, él nos advirtió que nuestra democracia iba a peligrar debido a una manera cultural individualista y si estas asociaciones dejaran de existir o si nuestros niños no fueran enseñados virtudes importantes.

Para los padres, esto significa que deben encontrar el tiempo para participar en su comunidad, desde pertenecer a la P.T.A., hasta los sindicatos, los clubes, y las asociaciones locales. Significa asistir a juntas en el ayuntamiento e informar a los funcionarios elegidos lo que usted siente que hace falta para lograr que su comunidad se mantenga fuerte y sólida, ya sea por medio de unas farolas, un parque, una biblioteca, mejores calles, un mejor sistema de alcantarillado, o más protección policíaca. Usted tiene el poder de organizar a un grupo de personas para asegurar que sus voces sean escuchadas por sus funcionarios elegidos. Si ellos no responden a las necesidades de la comunidad, ustedes tienen el poder de reemplazarlos. Juntos tienen una voz más fuerte y suficiente fuerza para provocar que sus funcionarios elegidos los representen con eficacia. Ésta es la verdadera democracia. El gobierno es para la gente y por la gente. Desdichadamente, por demasiado tiempo ha habido mucha apatía entre la gente. Cada vez menos personas votan o participan en actividades comunitarias. Si esto continúa, estamos permitiendo que el interés propio y una cultura individualista prosperen a expensas de nuestra democracia. Los padres deben unirse para asegurar que los niños y las familias estén al frente de cada decisión que hace el gobierno de los Estados Unidos, desde los problemas medioambientales, hasta los alimentos que comemos, los comerciales, las películas, y la música a los cuales están expuestos nuestros niños. Ya es hora de que los padres hagan sentir su presencia. Es hora de que tengan una voz activa con relación a la calidad de la vida en sus comunidades, la calidad de sus escuelas, y el tipo de gobierno que desean. Esto solamente se puede lograr si hacemos responsables a nuestros funcionarios elegidos, y si participamos en los asuntos comunitarios.

Como padres, debemos hacer todo lo que podemos para mantener a las instituciones sin fines de lucro que ofrecen apoyo. Estas organizaciones son dirigidas por voluntarios bondadosos que se preocupan por su comunidad. Desde las organizaciones nacionales como *Red Cross*, *March of Dimes*, y *Mothers Against Drunk Drivers*, hasta las organizaciones que prestan ayuda predominantemente a los hispanos, como AVANCE, SER, y Cara y Corazón, muchos grupos participan en el apoyo a las personas y a las familias. El *National Latino Children's Institute, Intercultural Development Research Association, The Thomas River Center*, HACU, y *el National Council of La Raza*, quienes apoyan y abogan diariamente por nuestros niños. Las actitudes, los conocimientos, la conducta, y vidas completas se están cambiando por medio del apoyo que proviene de las organizaciones sin fines de lucro, ubicadas en la comunidad.

Algunas organizaciones ubicadas en la comunidad que sirven a familias hispanas están citadas al final del libro. Éstas incluyen organizaciones que ayudan a los inmigrantes a aprender cómo funciona el sistema americano, algo semejante a los *Settlement Homes* de antaño. Éstas son organizaciones que ayudan a los hispanos que han sido víctimas de la discriminación y otros grupos que les ayudarán con sus derechos civiles y legales. Las organizaciones fraternales y cívicas como ASPIRA, *League of United Latin American Citizens*, G.I. *Forum, Mexican American Legal Defense and Educational Fund (MALDEF)*, y el *Puerto Rican Forum* se han organizado para encarar las necesidades especiales de los hispanos. Hay programas para los jóvenes y grupos culturales que les enseñan a sus niños arte, música de mariachi, y baile folclórico. Existen organizaciones sin fines de lucro que ayudan a los padres a aprender inglés, obtener la ciudadanía, adquirir su equivalencia a diploma de escuela preparatoria (high school), asistir a la universidad, participar en programas de entrenamiento, y encontrar empleo. Otras proveen talleres sobre la crianza de los niños, la salud mental, y servicios de orientación o terapia.

A veces la mejor ayuda que recibimos proviene no de grupos organizados ni de programas comunitarios, sino de los actos sencillos de generosidad, las palabras de sabiduría, y la orientación de parte de hombres y mujeres ordinarios que sirven como mentores, y sirven en las mesas directivas de estas organizaciones sin fines de lucro. Recuerde: la palabra "pueblo", además de significar una aldea o ciudad pequeña, también significa "la gente". Una comunidad consiste en cada persona que cumple con su parte para lograr que sea más que un lugar donde la gente duerme y come, para que sea un lugar donde pueden vivir y disfrutar su libertad.

Los cambios que han ocurrido en AVANCE han sido como las ondas de una laguna, cada una provocando otra reacción positiva, una tras otra. Todo comenzó con el amor que recibí de mi madre y mi abuelo, quienes a su vez lo habían recibido de otros. Ese amor generó compasión y preocupación por otros. Produjo una visión y una pasión de hacer todo lo que podía para mejorar las condiciones de los hispanos por medio de AVANCE. Desde los cocineros a los tenedores de libros hasta los directores, y los líderes voluntarios de la comunidad y los patrocinadores que compartieron mi visión, juntos reunimos un fondo común de energía y compasión, para brindar luz y esperanza a la gente de AVANCE. A pesar de los enormes obstáculos asociados con la pobreza y la discriminación, los hispanos pueden construir muchas defensas dentro de la comunidad si reciben el apoyo de una comunidad generosa.

A partir de esa comunidad generosa, provendrán más piedritas que producirán más ondas en la comunidad. Por ejemplo, debemos fortalecer el vínculo entre los esposos, quienes son los primeros maestros de sus niños. Hemos logrado realzar el amor entre los padres y sus niños. Por medio de interacciones cálidas entre los padres y los niños, que proveen cariño y cuidado y educación, sus niños llegarán a ser más compasivos y tendrán la capacidad de producir sus propias ondas al dar de sí mismos para lograr un mundo mejor. Hemos logrado tener un impacto sobre la relación y el trato entre vecinos. Cuando los vecinos se conocen por nombre y se sienten cómodos para hablarse en momentos de adversidad, se fortalecen y pueden alcanzar grandes logros juntos. Cuando los adultos pongan atención, muestren preocupación, y cuiden a todos los niños, en muchas comunidades, este país se convertirá en una nación aun más grande, una de la cual todos nos podremos enorgullecer.

Al mirar ahora el pasado y todos los cambios positivos que han ocurrido en los barrios a través de las últimas dos y media décadas, desde el comienzo de AVANCE, estoy convencida que si estas cosas pudieron ocurrir en algunas de las comunidades más pobres de los Estados Unidos, no hay duda de que pueden ocurrir en todas las comunidades, dondequiera que estén. Debemos recordar que, igual como Hillary Clinton dijo del "pueblo", el "pueblo" hispano no consiste tan sólo en un matrimonio sólido, la familia nuclear y extensa, o la tiendita de la esquina. Consiste en las escuelas, las iglesias, las empresas, el gobierno, los medios de comunicación, los voluntarios individuales, y las organizaciones comunitarias, todos luchando juntos para encontrar maneras de lograr un mejor futuro para nuestros niños.

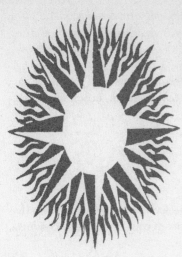

Lista de recursos para los padres

GRUPOS DE APOYO Y DEFENSA

ASPIRA
1444 I Street N.W., Suite 800
Washington, D.C. 20005-2210
(202) 835-3600
Un grupo de apoyo para los jóvenes hispanos, que provee apoyo educativo y promueve el liderazgo. Tiene oficinas en Bridgeport, Chicago, Miami, Newark, New York, Philadelphia, y Río Piedras, PR.

AVANCE
301 S. Frío, Suite 380
San Antonio, TX 78207
(210) 270-4630
Provee servicios globales de educación y apoyo familiar, ubicados en la comunidad, y a familias predominantemente hispanos. Esto incluye servicios de educación sobre la crianza de los niños y sobre la infancia, un programa para los padres y para parejas, alfabetismo, visitas a casa, y entrenamiento para el trabajo. Tiene programas afiliados a través del estado de Texas y en Kansas City. Además, provee entrenamiento y asistencia técnica, disemina información y un programa de estudios bilingüe a personas y organizaciones a través de los Estados Unidos y Latinoamérica.

Cara y Corazón
3270 Richview Drive
Hacienda Heights, CA 91745
(626) 333-5033
Provee entrenamiento a organizaciones y personas sobre el programa para padres, Cara y Corazón, además del *Hispanic Men's Network*, utilizando la práctica náhuatl conocida como "Etzli-Yollotl".

Catholic Big Brothers
45 E. 20th Street, 9th Fl.
New York, NY 10003
(212) 477-2250
Pone en contacto a jóvenes entre los siete y dieciocho años de edad, de familias de un solo padre, con adultos voluntarios que sirven como modelos de conducta.

Council of Latino Agencies
2309 18th Street N.W., Suite 2
Washington, D.C. 20009
(202) 328-9451
Este grupo reúne a 29 organizaciones comunitarias con tendencias latinas, desde escuelas de *high school* multiculturales a servicios de salud bilingües en el área de Washington, por medio de programas educativos y de apoyo, realizados en conjunto.

Educational Equity Concepts
114 East 32nd Street, Suite 306
New York, NY 10016
(212) 725-1803
Materiales educativos multiculturales, con un énfasis en la incapacitación.

Girls Incorporated
National Headquarters
30 East 33rd Street
New York, NY 10016-5397
(212) 689-3700
www.girlsinc.org
Una organización nacional que provee programas, educativos entre otros, para ayudar a las niñas a realizar su potencial. Tiene más de 1,000 afiliados a través del país.

Hispanic Association of Colleges and Universities
4204 Gardendale Street, Suite 216
San Antonio, TX 78229
(210) 692-3805
fax: (210) 692-0823

HACU@Hispanic.com
www.HACU2000.org
Provee oportunidades educativas a los hispanos.

Intercultural Development Research Association
5835 Callaghan Road, #350
San Antonio, TX 78228
(210) 684-8180
Provee investigaciones y servicios educativos para los hispanoamericanos. Participa en las políticas relacionadas con la educación bilingüe y el financiamiento de las escuelas.

La Leche League International
P.O. Box 4079
Schaumburg, IL 60168
(847) 519-7730 ó (800) LALECHE
www.lalecheleague.org
Provee información y apoyo a aquellas mujeres que desean amamantar a sus niños.

Multicultural Connections
y cosas hispánicas
Bilingual Books for Kids
P.O. Box 653
Ardsley, NY 10520
(800) 385-1020
www.bilingualbooks.com
Una selección de libros, cassettes, y juegos en español e inglés. Diseñados para ayudarles a los niños a aprender un segundo idioma además de aprender sobre la cultura hispana.

National Catholic Educational Association
1077 30th Street N.W., Suite 100
Washington, D.C. 20007-3852
(202) 337-6232
Una fuente de información y apoyo a grupos e individuos interesados en la educación católica desde el nivel de kinder hasta el posgrado.

National Clearinghouse for Bilingual Education
U.S. Department of Education Office of Bilingual Education and Minority Language Affairs
Información disponible a través del World Wide Web y por medio de un boletín informativo semanal llamado *Newsline*.
www.ncbe.gwu.edu

National Coalition of Hispanic Health and Human Services Organizations (COSSMHO)
1501 Sixteenth Street, N.W.
Washington, D.C. 20036
(202) 387-5000
www.cossmho.org
Su membresía consiste en numerosas organizaciones de salud y servicio social que sirven a las comunidades hispanas. Ofrece servicios que incluyen educación e investigación con relación a la salud maternal y de los niños, y las inmunizaciones. También tiene una línea directa para asuntos prenatales y sobre el radón.

National Council of La Raza
810 First Street N.E., Suite 300
Washington, D.C. 20002-4205
(202) 289-1380
fax: (202) 289-8173
Busca mejorar las oportunidades para los hispanoamericanos y conduce investigaciones sobre los temas que afectan a los hispanos, incluyendo la inmigración.

National Hispanic Scholarship Fund
One Sansome Street, Suite 100
San Francisco, CA 94104
(415) 445-9930
Otorga becas a los estudiantes universitarios y de posgrado hispanos.

National Information Center on Deafness
Gallaudet University
800 Florida Avenue N.E.
Washington, D.C. 20002-3695
(202) 651-5052
www.gallaudet.edu

National Latino Children's Initiative
1611 W. 6th Street
Austin, TX 78703-5059
(512) 472-9971

Parents Helping Parents
3041 Olcott Street
Santa Clara, CA 95054-3222
(408) 727-5775
Ayuda a las familias de los niños que tienen necesidades especiales, incluyendo a aquéllos que tengan alguna minusvalía o enfermedad grave.

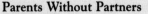

Parents Without Partners
401 N. Michigan Avenue
Chicago, IL 60611-4267
(312) 644-6610
Un grupo de apoyo para los padres que están criando a sus hijos sin pareja. Tiene programas afiliados a través del país. Las cuotas varían entre $17 y $45.

Puerto Rican Family Institute
145 W. 15th Street
New York, NY 10011
(212) 924-6320
Asiste a las familias con una variedad de servicios, incluyendo terapia psicológica.

Puerto Rican/Hispanic Genealogical Society
25 Ralph Avenue
Brentwood, NY 11717-2424
(516) 834-2511
Ayuda a aquéllos que quieren investigar la historia de su familia. La cuota anual es $20.

Service Employment and Redevelopment, SER Jobs for Progress
100 Decker Drive
Irving, TX 75062
(972) 541-0616
Un apoyo a las familias con un énfasis sobre el empleo de jóvenes y adultos.

Southwest Voter Registration and Education Project
403 E. Commerce, #220
San Antonio, TX 78205
(210) 222-0224
Educan a los hispanos sobre la importancia de registrarse para votar y ejercer su derecho de votar.

The Hispanic Mother-Daughter Program
Arizona State University
P.O. Box 870512
Tempe, AZ 85287-0512
(602) 965-6547
Está diseñado para las niñas de octavo año escolar y sus madres, en las comunidades locales. Lucha por construir sólidas relaciones entre las madres e hijas, al alentar a ambas a seguir una enseñanza superior.

EL MATRIMONIO

Marriage Enrichment and Family Life Conferences
Información: (800) 795-LOVE
Enriquecimiento de matrimonio: (800) 634-8325
Conferencia sobre la vida familial: (501) 223-8663

National Marriage Encounter
4704 Jamerson Place
Orlando, FL 32807
(407) 282-8120
(800) 828-3351
Ofrece retiros de fin de semana a parejas de casados y al clero para promover la comunicación y el crecimiento religioso/espiritual.

PREPARE/ENRICH
P.O. Box 190
Minneapolis, MN 55440
Ofrece retiros para parejas comprometidas.

Worldwide Marriage Encounter
2210 E. Highland, #106
San Bernadino, CA 92404
(909) 863-9963
Tiene 16 grupos regionales. Ofrece retiros de fin de semana para parejas católicas que desean explorar su relación y su fe.

DISCRIMINACIÓN Y DERECHOS CIVILES

American Civil Liberties Union
132 W. 43rd Street
New York, NY 10036
(212) 944-9800
fax: (202) 244-3196
Defiende los derechos de todos los ciudadanos como garantizados por la Constitución y la Declaración de Independencia.

American G.I. Forum
2711 W. Anderson Lane, #205
Austin, TX 78405
(512) 302-3025

Center for Democratic Renewal
P.O. Box 50469
Atlanta, GA 30302
(404) 221-0025 ó (404) 221-6614
Sigue de cerca las actividades de grupos de odio y ayuda a las comunidades a
luchar en contra de la violencia provocada por el odio.

Center for the Study of Biracial Children
2300 S. Krameria Street
Denver, CO 80222
(303) 692-9008
Conduce investigaciones y disemina información sobre niños de dos razas y
cómo les va dentro de una sociedad consciente de las razas.

LULAC (League of United Latin American Citizens)
701 Pennsylvania Avenue N.W., #1217
Washington, D.C. 20004
(301) 589-2222
www.lulac.org
Lucha para promover el bienestar de los hispanos en numerosos terrenos,
incluyendo el otorgamiento de poder, la educación, la salud, y los derechos
civiles. Ofrece un sistema de centros de orientación educativa para los jóvenes
a través de los Estados Unidos.

Mexican American Legal Defense and Educational Fund (MALDEF)
634 S. Spring Street, 11th Fl.
Los Angeles, CA 90014
(213) 629-2512
Defiende los derechos civiles de los hispanos en campos como la educación, el
empleo, la inmigración, y los derechos para votar. También conduce entrenamiento para el liderazgo. Tiene oficinas en Chicago, Los Angeles,
Sacramento, San Antonio, San Francisco, y Washington, D.C.

National Alliance Against Racist and Political Repression (NAAPR)
11 John Street, Suite 702
New York, NY 10038
(212) 406-3330
(212) 406-3542
Se opone a la represión de los derechos humanos y lucha por ponerle fin a la
hostilidad en contra de los trabajadores que son inmigrantes ilegales, y la
deportación de los mismos.

Northern California for Immigration Rights
995 Market Street, Suite 1108
San Francisco, CA 94103

(415) 543-6767 ó (415) 243-8215
fax: (415) 243-8628
Grupo de apoyo y defensa para los inmigrantes.

National Institute Against Prejudice and Violence
31 S. Greene Street
Baltimore, MD 21201
(410) 328-5170
fax: (410) 328-7551
Se opone a la violencia y la intimidación motivadas por prejuicios, por medio de la investigación, la educación, el entrenamiento, y la diseminación de información sobre programas y la legislación.

National Network for Immigrant and Refugee Rights (NNIRR)
310 8th Street, Suite 307
Oakland, CA 94607
(510) 465-1984
www.nnirr.org/news
Se compone de coaliciones de organizaciones interesadas en apoyar y defender a los inmigrantes y refugiados. Lucha por promover políticas justas para los inmigrantes y refugiados.

New York Association for New Americans (NYANA)
(212) 425-5051
(888) 2-HALT-DV
webmaster@nyana.org
Ofrece servicios de educación y entrenamiento de empleo a los inmigrantes y refugiados que vienen a este país, y sigue de cerca las políticas y difunde información sobre las políticas que afectan a los inmigrantes y refugiados.

EL Presidente de los Estados Unidos
The White House
1600 Pennsylvania Avenue N.W.
Washington, D.C. 20500
(202) 456-1414
(202) 456-1111 para informarles su postura sobre algún asunto

Puerto Rican Legal Defense and Education Fund
99 Hudson Street, 14th Fl.
New York, NY 10013
(212) 219-3360
Lucha por salvaguardar los derechos civiles de los puertorriqueños y otros latinos. Los campos que abarca incluyen la educación, el empleo, y la vivienda. También remite asuntos o preguntas legales a otras agencias.

U.S. Commission on Civil Rights
1121 Vermont Avenue N.W.
Washington, D.C. 20425
(202) 376-8177
Reúne datos con relación a la discriminación o denegaciones de igualdad de protección de las leyes debido a raza, color, origen nacional, u otros factores. Reporta al Congreso y al presidente sobre la eficacia de las leyes federales y los programas para igualdad de oportunidades.

U.S. Department of Education Office of Civil Rights
Customer Service Team
Mary E. Switzer Building
330 C Street S.W.
Washington, D.C. 20202
(202) 205-5413
fax: (202) 205-9862
Hace cumplir los estatutos que prohiben la discriminación en los programas y las actividades que reciben asistencia económica federal, lo cual incluye discriminación a causa de raza, color, origen nacional, minusvalía, o edad.

United States Immigration and Naturalization Services
1-800-755-0777
Responsables por hacer cumplir las leyes que regulan la entrada de personas nacidas en el extranjero a los Estados Unidos y administran los beneficios de naturalización y a refugiados. Acepta quejas de discriminación o acoso o hostilidad de parte de los dirigentes de inmigración.

ORGANIZACIONES CULTURALES

Association of Hispanic Arts
173 E. 116th Street, 2nd Fl.
New York, NY 10029
(212) 860-5445
Promueve las artes hispanas por medio de asistencia a las organizaciones y a artistas individuales y promueve representaciones y exposiciones comunitarias que reflejan la historia, la cultura, y los temas sociales de los hispanos.

Bilingual Foundation of the Arts
421 North Avenue, #19
Los Angeles, CA 90031
(213) 225-4044

Patrocina producciones de teatro en español e inglés, basadas en el trabajo de artistas hispanos, incluyendo a un grupo que hace giras para visitar a los jóvenes en las escuelas.

Campanas de América
1422 Buena Vista
San Antonio, TX 78207
(210) 224-0258
Promueve y enseña la instrumentación de la música de los mariachis a más de 3,000 escuelas a través del país.

Caribbean Cultural Center
408 W. 58th Street
New York, NY 10019
(213) 307-7420

Fine Arts Latin Association, Inc.
1123 Jocalyn
Houston, TX 77023

Florida Museum of Hispanic and Latin American Art
40006 Aurora Street
Coral Gables, FL 33146
(305) 444-7060
www.latinweb.com/museo
Pone un énfasis en el aprendizaje a través de las artes, con actividades como cursos, conferencias, y presentaciones de música y libros.

Grupo de Artistas Latino-Americanos
P.O. Box 43209
1625 Park Road N.W.
Washington, D.C. 20010
(202) 234-7174

Guadalupe Cultural Arts Center
1300 Guadalupe Street
San Antonio, TX 78207
(210) 271-3151
www.guadalupeculturalarts.org
Una institución comunitaria de las artes que incluye una variedad de programas diseñados para los jóvenes y las familias.

Hispanic Fashion Designers
1000 Thomas Jefferson Street N.W., #310
Washington, D.C. 20007
(202) 337-9963

Houston Society of Flamenco Arts
7016 Culmore
Houston, TX 77087
(718) 640-1089

Instituto Cultural Mexicano
600 Hemisfair Plaza
San Antonio, TX 78204
(210) 227-0123

Latino Resources at the Smithsonian
Si quiere recibir un folleto sobre artículos en las colecciones del Smithsonian
que fueron hechos por o sobre latinos, escriba a:
Smithsonian Institution
SI Building, Room 153, MRC 010
Washington, D.C. 20560
www.si.edu/resource/tours/latino/start.htm

Mexican Fine Arts Center Museum
1852 W. 19th Street
Chicago, IL 60614
(312) 738-1503
Contiene una colección de arte popular mexicano. Ofrece conferencias y representaciones.

LIBROS Y CASSETTES PARA NIÑOS PEQUEÑOS

Alacon, Francisco X. *From the Bellybutton of the Moon/Del Ombligo de la Luna*.
San Francisco: Children's Book Press, 1998. $15.95.

Alacon, Francisco X. *Laughing Tomatoes and Other Spring Poems/Jitomates Risueños y Otros Poemas de Primavera*. Illustrated by Maya Christina Gonzalez.
San Francisco: Children's Book Press, 1997. $15.95.

Castañeda, Omar S. *Abuela's Weave*. Illustrated by Enrique O. Sanchez. New York: Lee & Low Books, Inc., 1993. $15.95.

Cepellín, Ricardo Gonzalez. *Rondas Infantiles*. Cepellín DML-C9355. 1996 Orfeón Videovox, S.A.

Cisneros, Sandra. *Hairs/Pelitos*. Illustrated by Terry Ybañez. New York: Alfred A. Knopf, 1994. $15.00. Softcover $6.99.

Compañía Fonográfica. *Coro del Valle de México. Juegos y Rondas Infantiles.* Internacional, S.A..

Elizondo, Evangelina, Del Campo, Yolanda, y Conjunto de Carlos Oropeza. *Juegos Infantiles. 15 Éxitos. Coro Label.* Compañía Fonográfica. Internacional, S.A. de C.V. Sanctorum No. 86-B. Argentina, Mexico D.F.C.P.

Delacre, Lulu. *Arroz con Leche: Popular Songs and Rhymes From Latin America.* English Lyrics by Elena Paz. Musical arrangements by Ana-Maria Rosado. New York: Scholastic, 1989. $15.95. Softcover $4.95.

Delacre, Lulu. *Vejigante Masquerader.* New York: Scholastic, 1993. $15.95.

Delgado, María Isabel. *Chave's Memories/Los Recuerdos de Chave.* Illustrated by Yvonne Symank. Piñata Books, Arte Público Press. University of Houston, 1996. $14.95.

Dorros, Arthur. *Abuela.* New York: Dutton's Children's Books, 1991. $15.99. Softcover $4.99.

Dorros, Arthur. *Tonight Is Carnaval.* Illustrated by members of the Club de Madres Virgen del Carmen of Lima, Peru. New York: Dutton Children's Books, 1991. $4.99.

Garcia, Maria. *The Adventures of Connie and Diego/Las aventuras de Connie y Diego.* San Francisco: Children's Book Press, 1987. $14.95.

Garza, Carmen Lomas. *Family Pictures/Cuadros de familia.* San Francisco: Children's Book Press, 1990. $14.95. Softcover $6.95.

Garza, Carmen Lomas. *In My Family/En Mi Familia.* San Francisco: Children's Book Press, 1996. $15.95.

Gonzalez, Lucia. *The Bossy Gallito/El Gallo de Bodas.* Retold by Lucia M. Gonzalez. Illustrated by Lulu Delacre. New York: Scholastic, 1994. $14.95.

Gonzalez, Ralfka, and Ruiz, Ana. *Mi Primer Libro de Dichos/My First Book of Proverbs.* San Francisco: Children's Book Press, 1995. $15.95.

Harper, Jo. *The Legend of Mexicatl.* New York: Turtle Books, 1998. $15.95.

Hinojosa, Tish. *Cada Niño.* Niños catalog, NS 8032.

Jaramillo, Nelly Palacio. *Grandmother's Nursery Rhymes/Las Nanas de Abuela*. *Niños* Catalog NS 1115.

Lachtman, Ofelia Dumas *Pepita Thinks Pink/Pepita y el Color Rosado*. Houston: Arte Público Press, 1998. $14.95.

Martinez, Alejandro Cruz. *The Woman Who Outshone the Sun/La Mujer que Brillaba Aun Más Que el Sol*. San Francisco: Children's Book Press, 1991. $14.95. Softcover $6.95.

Mora, Pat. *A Birthday Basket for Tía*. Illustrated by Cecily Lang. New York: Macmillan Publishing Co., 1992. $13.95.

Mora, Pat. *Pablo's Tree*. Illustrated by Cecily Lang. New York: Macmillan Publishing Co., 1994. $14.95.

Mora, Pat. *Delicious Hullabaloo/Pachanga deliciosa*. Illustrations by Francisco X. Mora. Houston: Piñata Books, Arte Público Press, 1998. $14.95.

Mora, Pat, & Berg, Charles Ramírez. *The Gift of the Poinsettia/El Regalo de la Flor de Nochebuena*. Houston: Piñata Books, 1995. $14.95.

Orozco, José-Luis. *De Colores and Other Latin-American Folk Songs for Children*. Illustrated by Elisa Kleven. New York: Dutton Children's Books, 1994. $17.00. *De Colores* (cassette). *Niños* catalog NS 2131. $10.95.

Pfister, Marcus. *El Pez Arco Iris*. Switzerland: North-South Books Inc., 1994. $16.95.

Ramirez, Michael Rose. *The Little Ant/La Hormiga Chiquita*. Illustrated by Linda Dalai Sawaya. New York: Rizzoli, 1995. $12.95.

Sáenz, Benjamín Alire. *A Gift from Papá Diego/Un Regalo de Papá Diego*. El Paso: Cinco Puntos Press, 1998. $10.95.

Soto, Gary. *Chato's Kitchen*. Illustrated by Susan Guevara. New York: G.P. Putnam's Sons, 1995. $15.95.

Soto, Gary. *Too Many Tamales*. Illustrated by Ed Martinez. New York: G.P. Putnam's Sons, 1993. $14.95.

Tripp, Valerie. *Josefina Series of the American Girls Collection*. Middleton: Pleasant Co., 1997. $5.95.

Winter, Jeanette. *Diego*. New York: Dragon Fly Books, 1991. $5.95.

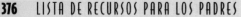
LIBROS A NIVEL INTERMEDIO

Barlow, Genevieve. "The Toad's Spots." En *Legends from Latin America/Leyendas de Latinoamérica*. Illustrated by Robert Borja and Julia Scarf. Lincolnwood (Chicago), Illinois: National Textbook Company, 1995.

Lankerford, Mary D. *Quinceañera: A Latina's Journey to Womanhood*. Photographs by Jesse Herrera. Brookfield, CT: Millbrook Press, 1994. $20.90.

Nye, Naomic Shihab, ed. *The Tree Is Older Than You Are: A Bilingual Gathering of Poems & Stories From Mexico*. With Paintings by Mexican Artists. Simon and Schuster, 1995. $19.95.

Phillis, Tashlik, ed. *Hispanic, Female, and Young: An Anthology*. Houston: Piñata Books, 1994. $14.00.

FUENTE PARA LOS LIBROS BILINGÜES

Éstas son sólo unas cuantas fuentes de libros bilingües. Ya que éste es un campo que está creciendo, hay más editoriales y librerías que venden libros bilingües:

American Girls Collection. Josefina Collection. Pleasant Company. 8400 Fairway. Middleton, WI 53562, 1-800-845-0005. www.americangirl.com.

Bilingual Books for Kids. P.O.Box 653. Ardsley, NY 10520, (800) 385-1020. www.bilingualbooks.com.

Cinco Puntos Press. 2709 Louisville, El Paso, TX 79930. (800) 566-9072.

Children's Book Press. 246 First Street, Suite 101, San Francisco, CA 94105, (415) 995-2200, 1-800-788-3123.

Lind, Beth Beutler. *Multicultural Children's Literature: An Annotated Bibliography*. *Grades K–8*. Jefferson, N.C.: McFarland & Company, Inc., 1996. $34.50.

Piñata Books, Arte Público Press. University of Houston, Houston, TX 77204-2090, (800) 633-2783.

Scholastic. 55 Broadway. New York, N.Y. 10012 (212) 343-6100.

Turtle Books. 866 United Nations Plaza, Suite 525, New York, NY 10017, (212) 644-2020, 1-800-788-3123.

LIBROS DE DICHOS

Aranda, Charles. *Dichos. Proverbs and Sayings From the Spanish*. Santa Fe: Sunstone Press, 1977. $4.95.

Aroroa, Shirley L. *Proverbial Comparisons and Related Expressions in Spanish*. Folklore Studies 29. Los Angeles: University of California Press, 1977.

Burciaga, José Antonio. *In Few Words/En Pocas Palabras. A Compendium of Latino Folk Wit and Wisdom*. San Francisco: Mercury House, 1997. $14.95.

Cobos, Rubén. *Southwestern Spanish Proverbs*. Sante Fe: Museum of New Mexico Press, 1985. $11.95.

Coca, Benjamí. *Book of Proverbs*. Montezuma: Montezuma Press, 1983.

Gómez Maganda, Alejandro. *¡Como Dice el Dicho! Refranes y dichos mexicanos*. Mexico City: Talleres Litográficos E.C.O., 1963.

Martinez Perez, José. *Dichos, Dicharros y Refranes Mexicanos*. Mexico City: Editores Mexicanos Unidos, 1981. 30 pesos.

Rivera, Maria Elisa Diaz. *Refranes Más Usados en Puerto Rico*. Puerto Rico: Editorial de la Universidad de Puerto Rico, 1984. $11.95.

Sellers, Jeff M. *Proverbios y dichos mexicanos/Folk Wisdom of Mexico*. San Francisco: Chronicle Books, 1994. $9.95.

Índice

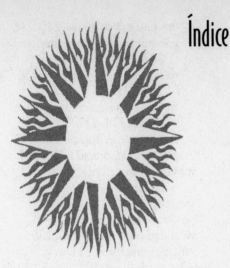

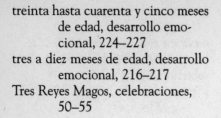